HANDBOOK OF
Neonatal Intensive Care

Fourth Edition HANDBOOK OF
Neonatal Intensive Care

Gerald B. Merenstein, MD, FAAP

Professor of Pediatrics,

Senior Associate Dean, Education,

Director, The Lula O. Lubchenco Center for Perinatal
  Research, Education, Followup, and Epidemiology,

University of Colorado School of Medicine,

Denver, Colorado

Sandra L. Gardner, RN, MS, CNS, PNP

Neonatal/Perinatal/Pediatric Consultant,

Director, Professional Outreach Consultation,

Aurora, Colorado

with 246 illustrations

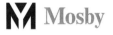 Mosby

St. Louis Baltimore Boston Carlsbad Chicago Minneapolis New York Philadelphia Portland
London Milan Sydney Tokyo Toronto

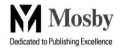

Mosby
Dedicated to Publishing Excellence

A Times Mirror
Company

Vice President and Publisher	**Nancy Coon**
Editor	**Barry Bowlus**
Developmental Editor	**Cynthia Anderson**
Project Manager	**Dana Peick**
Production Editor	**Jeffrey Patterson**
Design Coordinator	**Amy Buxton**
Manufacturing Supervisor	**Karen Boehme**

Fourth Edition

Copyright 1998 by Mosby–Year Book, Inc.
Previous editions copyrighted 1993, 1989, 1985

Printed in the United States of America
Composition by Graphic World
Printing/binding by R.R. Donnelley

Mosby-Year Book, Inc.
11830 Westline Industrial Drive
St. Louis, Missouri 63146

Library of Congress Cataloging-in-Publication Data
Handbook of neonatal intensive care / [edited by] Gerald B. Merenstein, Sandra L. Gardner.—4th ed.
   p.   cm.
  Includes bibliographical references and index.
  ISBN 0-8151-3696-X (pbk.)
  1. Neonatal intensive care.   I. Merenstein, Gerald B.   II. Gardner. Sandra L.
   [DNLM: 1. Infant, Newborn, Diseases. 2. Intensive Care, Neonatal. 3. Patient Care Team.
    WS 421 H236 1998]
  RJ253.5.H36 1998
  618.92'01—dc21
  DNLM/DLC
  for Library of Congress   97-20146
                                         CIP

98 99 00 01 02 / 9 8 7 6 5 4 3 2 1

Contributors

Steven H. Abman, MD
Professor of Pediatrics,
University of Colorado School of
  Medicine/The Children's Hospital,
Denver, Colorado

Karen Adams, RN, BSN
Research Study Coordinator,
Section of Neonatology,
Department of Pediatrics,
Baylor College of Medicine,
Houston, Texas

Eugene W. Adcock III, MD
Professor of Pediatrics,
Associate Dean for Professional Affairs,
Vice President, Planning and Program
  Development,
Bowman Gray School of Medicine of
  Wake Forest University;
North Carolina Baptist Hospital,
Winston-Salem, North Carolina

Rita Agarwal, MD
Assistant Professor, Anesthesiology,
University of Colorado School of
  Medicine/The Children's Hospital,
Denver, Colorado

Nancy Allen, MSRD, CNSD
Neonatal Nutritionist,
Children's Mercy Hospital,
Kansas City, Missouri

**Joanne Marino Bartram, RN,
MS**
Instructor, Parent-Child Nursing,
University of New Mexico College of
  Nursing,
Albuquerque, New Mexico

Kathy Bendorf, RN, BSN
Nutrition Support Nurse Coordinator,
Section of Gastroenterology,
The Children's Mercy Hospital,
Kansas City, Missouri

Denis D. Bensard, MD
Assistant Professor of Surgery,
University of Colorado School of
  Medicine and Affiliated Hospitals
Denver, Colorado

David D. Berry, MD
Associate Professor, Pediatrics,
Bowman Gray School of Medicine of
  Wake Forest University,
Winston-Salem, North Carolina

W. Woods Blake, MD
Associate Professor of Pediatrics
Chattanooga Unit, University of
  Tennessee College of Medicine,
Chattanooga, Tennessee

Melvin Bonilla-Felix, MD
Assistant Professor, Pediatrics,
University of Texas Health Science
  Center at Houston,
Houston, Texas

Patricia Brannan, RN, CNN
Clinical Coordinator, Pediatric
  Nephrology,
Hermann Hospital,
Houston, Texas

Brian Carter, MD
Associate Professor, Pediatrics,
Medical College of Georgia,
Augusta, Georgia

Susan Clarke, MS, RNC
Clinical Nurse Specialist for Children's
  Services,
The Children's Hospital,
Denver, Colorado

Shannon Collins, RN, BSN
Professional Research Assistant,
Neonatal Clinical Research Center,
University of Colorado Health Sciences
  Center,
Denver, Colorado

Carol Ann Consolvo, RN, MS
Nursing Practice and Education
  Coordinator,
The North Carolina Baptist Hospital,
Winston-Salem, North Carolina

**Sharla C. Cooper, RN,
MSN, NNP**
Assistant Professor,
Radford School of Nursing,
Community Hospital of Roanoke
  Valley,
Roanoke, Virginia

Audrey J. Costello, MSW, LCSW
University of Colorado Health Sciences
  Center,
Denver, Colorado

**Elaine Daberkow-Carson, RN,
MS**
Pediatric Cardiology Clinical Nurse
  Specialist,
Lucile Salter Packard Children's
  Hospital,
Stanford University,
Pale Alto, California

David J. Durand, MD
Division of Neonatology,
Children's Hospital of Oakland,
Oakland, California

Loretta P. Finnegan, MD
Senior Advisor on Women's Issues,
National Institute on Drug Abuse,
National Institutes of Health,
Bethesda, Maryland

C. Gilbert Frank, MD
Co-Director, Neonatology,
Community Hospital of Roanoke
  Valley;
Assistant Professor of Pediatrics,
University of Virginia School of
  Medicine,
Roanoke, Virginia

Sandra L. Gardner, RN, MS, CNS, PNP
Neonatal/Perinatal/Pediatric Consultant,
Director, Professional Outreach
  Consultation,
Denver, Colorado

Mary I. Enzman Hagedorn, RN, PhD, CNS, CPNP
Associate Professor,
Beth El College of Nursing at
  University of Colorado, Colorado
  Springs,
Colorado Springs, Colorado

William H. Hay, Jr., MD
Professor of Pediatrics,
University of Colorado School of
  Medicine/The Children's Hospital,
Denver, Colorado

Randall M. Holland, MD
Pediatric Surgeon,
Spokane, Washington

Gary M. Joffee, MD
Director, Perinatal Medicine,
Lovelace Medical Center,
Albuquerque, New Mexico

Cynthia B. Johnson, RN, NNP, MS
Neonatal Nurse Practitioner,
The Children's Hospital,
Denver, Colorado

Marilyn Manco-Johnson, MD
Professor of Pediatrics,
University of Colorado School of
  Medicine/The Children's Hospital,
Denver, Colorado

Howard W. Kilbride, MD
Professor of Pediatrics,
University of Missouri School of
  Medicine;
Chief, Section of Neonatal Medicine,
The Children's Mercy Hospital,
Kansas City, Missouri

Ruth A. Lawrence, MD
Professor of Pediatrics and Obstetrics/
  Gynecology,
University of Rochester School of
  Medicine,
Rochester, New York

Cyndi J. Lepley, RN, MSN, PhD
Texas Women's University,
Denton, Texas

Lula O. Lubchenco, MD
Professor Emerita,
Department of Pediatrics,
University of Colorado School of
  Medicine/The Children's Hospital,
Denver, Colorado

Carolyn Houska Lund, RN, MS, FAAN
Neonatal Clinical Nurse Specialist,
Intensive Care Nursery,
Children's Hospital, Oakland,
Oakland, California

Anne L. Matthews, RN, PhD
Director, Genetic Counseling and
  Family Studies Core Programs,
Case Western Reserve University,
Cleveland, Ohio

Jane E. McGowan, MD
Associate Professor of Pediatrics,
MCP-Hahnemann School of Medicine,
Allegheny University of the Health
  Sciences,
Philadelphia, Pennsylvania

Gerald B. Merenstein, MD
Professor of Pediatrics,
Senior Associate Dean, Education,
Director, Lubchenco Perinatal Centers,
University of Colorado School of
  Medicine,
Denver, Colorado

Paul Moe, MD
Professor of Pediatrics,
University of Colorado School of
  Medicine/The Children's Hospital,
Denver, Colorado

Claudia A. Moore, BA, BSN, RN
Consultant,
Denver, Colorado

Judith A. Murray, RNC, MSN
Neonatal Nurse Practitioner,
T.C. Thompson Children's Hospital,
Chattanooga, Tennessee

M. Gail Murphy, MD
Director, Clinical Pharmacology,
Merck Research Laboratories,
Philadelphia, Pennsylvania

Susan Niermeyer, MD
Associate Professor, Pediatrics,
University of Colorado School of
  Medicine/The Children's Hospital,
Denver, Colorado

Miriam Orleans, PhD
Professor Emerita,
University of Colorado School of
  Medicine,
Denver, Colorado

Patti L. Paige, RN, MSN
Neonatal Clinical Nurse Specialist,
Wolfson Children's Hospital
Jacksonville, Florida

William H. Parry, MD, PhD
Medical Director,
Children's Ambulatory Services,
Santa Rosa Health Care,
San Antonio, Texas

Leslie Perry, RNC, MS
Perinatal Clinical Nurse Specialist,
Lovelace Health System,
Albuquerque, New Mexico

Gary Pettett, MD
Professor of Pediatrics and
  Neonatology,
University of Missouri School of
  Medicine;
Medical Director, CareForce Neonatal
  Transport Service,
The Children's Mercy Hospital,
Kansas City, Missouri

John R. Pierce, MD, COL, MC, USA
Deputy Commander for Clinical
  Services,
Director, Medical Education,
Walter Reed Army Medical Center,
Washington, DC

Ronald J. Portman, MD
Director of Pediatric Nephrology and
  Hypertension,
Associate Professor of Pediatrics,
University of Texas Health Sciences
  Center at Houston,
Houston, Texas

Frances N. Price, RN, BSN
Pediatric Surgery Nurse Clinician,
The Children's Hospital,
Denver, Colorado

Donna J. Rodden, RN, BSN
Senior Professional Research Assistant,
Neonatal Clinical Research Center,
University of Colorado Health Sciences
  Center,
Denver, Colorado

Roberta Siegel, MSW
Perinatal Social Worker,
The Children's Hospital,
Denver, Colorado

Sally Sewell, RNC, BSN
Transport Nurse,
CareForce Neonatal Tranport Service,
The Children's Hospital,
Kansas City, Missouri

B.J. Snell, RN, PhD, CNM
Associate Professor, Department of
  Nursing,
Director of Nurse Midwifery,
University of Southern California,
Los Angeles, California

John W. Sparks, MD
Professor and Chairman,
Department of Pediatrics,
University of Texas Health Science
  Center at Houston,
Houston, Texas

Eva Sujansky, MD
Associate Professor of Pediatrics,
Co-Director of the Division of Pediatric
  Genetics,
University of Colorado School of
  Medicine/The Children's Hospital,
Denver, Colorado

Julie Sandling Swaney, M Div
Chaplain,
Clinical Instructor,
Departments of Medicine and
  Psychiatry,
University of Colorado School of
  Medicine,
Denver, Colorado

Ellen Tappero, RNC, MN, NNP
Lutheran Medical Center,
Wheatridge, Colorado

Susan F. Townsend, MD
Associate Professor of Pediatrics,
University of Colorado School of
  Medicine/The Children's Hospital,
Denver, Colorado

Barbara S. Turner, RN, DNSc, FAAN
Associate Dean, School of Nursing,
Director, Nursing Research Center,
Duke University,
Durham, North Carolina

Reginald L. Washington, MD
Associate Clinical Professor,
Pediatric Cardiology,
University of Colorado School of
  Medicine/The Children's Hospital;
Rocky Mountain Pediatric Cardiology,
Denver, Colorado

Susan M. Weiner, RNC, MSN, CS
Perinatal Clinical Nurse Specialist,
Instructor of Nursing,
Thomas Jefferson University,
College of Allied Health Sciences,
  Department of Nursing,
Philadelphia, Pennsylvania

Leonard E. Weisman, MD
Director, Neonatal-Perinatal Medicine
  Fellowship Program,
Head Section of Neonatology and
  Professor, Department of Pediatrics,
Baylor College of Medicine,
Houston, Texas

Jan Zimmer, RN, MSN
Director of Patient Care Services,
Santa Rosa Health Care,
San Antonio, Texas

Notice Since some of the drugs mentioned in this book have not been approved by the FDA for use in neonates, caution should be exercised in their use. We have tried to ensure that the dosage schedules provided are accurate and meet current conventional standards. Changes in treatment may occur with new information from research or clinical experience. The reader should consult the package insert for changes in dosage, indications, and contraindications.

Preface

The concept of the team approach is important in neonatal intensive care. Each health care professional must not only perform the duties of his or her own role but must also understand the roles of other involved professionals. Nurses, physicians, other health care professionals, and parents must work together in a coordinated and efficient manner to achieve optimal results for patients in the neonatal intensive care unit (NICU).

Because this team approach is so important in the field of neonatal intensive care, we believe it is necessary that this book contain input from both major fields of health care—medicine and nursing. Therefore it has been coedited by a physician and a registered nurse. In addition, the chapters have been contributed by both physicians and nurses and other health care professionals.

The book is divided into six parts, all of which have been reviewed, revised, and updated for the fourth edition. Part I presents evidence based practice and the need to scientifically evaluate neonatal therapies emphasizing randomized controlled trials as the ideal approach. Parts II through V are the clinical sections, and this edition contains several additions, including new chapters on pain and pain relief and on skin and skin care.

The combination of physiology and pathophysiology and separate emphasis on clinical application in this text is designed for neonatal intensive care nurses, nursing students, medical students, and pediatric, surgical, and family practice housestaff. This text is comprehensive enough for physicians and nurses yet basic enough to be useful to all ancillary personnel.

Part VI presents the psychosocial aspects of neonatal care. The medical, psychologic, and social aspects of providing care for the ill neonate and family are discussed. This section, in particular, will benefit social workers and clergy who frequently deal with family members of patients in the NICU. Of course, it will also be a valuable resource for all other involved health care professionals.

In this handbook we present physiologic principles and practical applications and point out areas as yet unresolved. Material that is clinically applicable is set in boldface type so that it can be easily identified.

Gerald B. Merenstein
Sandra L. Gardner

Contents

Introduction

The Goals of Neonatal Intensive Care

"What are the goals of neonatal intensive care for this patient?"

Most fundamental to the inquiry of what is best for an individual baby in the NICU, however the question may be phrased, is the ability to speak to the goals of care for the particular patient. These goals, although individualized for the patient's needs, must reach beyond the isolated clinical considerations of the health care professionals at work in the NICU environment. They must reflect a discernment and incorporation of those values and goals sought by the family on behalf of their newborn child, and they must be pursued within the context of more broadly held, but perhaps poorly expressed, societal goals for the provision of health care for women and infants.

Daily we may ask ourselves, or hear others around us asking, "Are we doing the right thing for this baby?" "What else can we do for this patient?" "Why are we doing this?" "Should we stop?" "What do the parents want?" "What are we trying to accomplish here?"

These questions raise issues that are central to our individual perception as valued health care professionals trying to serve patients, families, and a broader society. They call on us to address the values of our profession, ourselves, and those we serve. To ignore these issues is to fail to recognize their significance in shaping our professional lives and affecting our human interactions. But beyond that, failing to answer these questions will perpetrate our inability, or unwillingness, to responsibly address the value-laden charge we have to each other. **It is no small thing to profess the willingness to help a vulnerable and sick newborn; to devote our lives toward service; and to be educated and trained to practice our art with scientific rigor, technologic skill, and human caring, even in the face of medical uncertainty.** Ignoring these questions, however, will lead to moral uncertainty and quite possibly moral angst, causing us to do things against our own better judgement.

Despite well over a quarter of a century providing "modern" neonatal intensive care, it is difficult to answer the questions regarding the goals of neonatal intensive care. This lies at the root of many of our problems in working through challenging cases and situations, as well as addressing parental and societal concerns. I do not believe that we can simply state our goals as "to save all babies" or "to reduce infant mortality."

Throughout the interactions of every health care professional in dealing with issues in the NICU, consideration should be given at all times to the goals of specific monitoring, diagnostic tests, therapies, or even research protocols that are part of what we do. **The goals of care should be patient- and family-centered. It is the patient we treat, but it is the family, of whatever construct, with whom the baby will go home. Indeed, it is the family who must live with the long-term consequences of our daily decisions in caring for their baby.**

The goals of neonatal intensive care include more than simple application of critical care technology (such as ventilators, monitors, medications, invasive devices, a multiplicity of laboratory measurements, etc.) to sick and premature newborn infants. **These goals include the provision of skilled professional care. An effective neonatal intensive care team consists of trained professionals of many disciplines—no one of us can do it alone. This care is, however, to be extended over a necessarily limited, rather than endless, period of time.**

The ends to which this care is provided include the initial stabilization of the newborn and, ultimately, the facilitation of transition to normal, extrauterine, neonatal physiology. Obviously, this transition takes longer for some infants than others and may require significant intervention and support. Similarly, the reversal of acute disease processes such as infection and respiratory distress is a recognized end. Minimizing chronic or debilitating outcomes (including iatrogenic sequelae of applied neonatal intensive care), also falls within these goals. We need to recognize the potential impact of iatrogenic effects that include (1) the environment in which the baby is managed; (2) the mode of ventilation; (3) the types, doses, and effects of medications used; (4) the short- and long-term effects of certain procedures, foreign bodies, or devices used; and (5) ways to meet the baby's nutritional needs.

All of this care should be provided with a reasonable expectation of steady improvement. Care should proceed with the absence of excruciating pain and unnecessary suffering and develop toward a capacity for the newborn to enjoy and participate in the human experience over a life prolonged beyond infancy.

These goals seek to maintain a focus upon the best interests of the child. In determining the best interests of the child, the parents are generally considered to be the spokespersons. Hence, their opinions should be sought, values discerned, and goals considered.

Shared decision making should be the commonly employed process, requiring shared information among relevant health care professionals and a willingness and capability to effectively and regularly communicate with parents. This process also suggests the need for outcome data. Such data should be relevant to the population seeking care at a given institution. It is not always valid to rely on nationally reported data outside the local practice setting since both populations and practices may neither be constituted nor controlled in the same fashion that yours may be. Both the provision of care, decided upon by local clinical and population data, and determination of best interests—or what can be viewed as either effective, beneficial, and appropriate care versus ineffective, burdensome, or inappropriate care—demand the availability of data from which to make these determinations with parents. Until such data are available, we should be frank in recognizing and communicating some uncertainty in our decision-making process with parents.

From inquiries into "What are we doing?" let's move toward defining our goals for our patients. **Each patient's care should be based upon his or her best interests, consonant with professional goals, societal norms, and institutional mission, through a process of mutually derived goals with the parents and/or family.** This requires time, thoughtful reflection, communication with families, and advocation for our patients' benefit. In so doing, the good with which we all seek to provide for our patients hopefully will become apparent to all concerned.

Brian S. Carter, MD

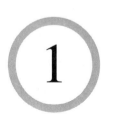

1

Evidence Based Clinical Practice Decisions

Miriam Orleans, Ellen Tappero, Gerald B. Merenstein

The rapid spread and high cost of new technologies have led practitioners to ask questions about the benefits of many new as well as old clinical practices. As neonatal advocates, many physicians, nurses, therapists, and parents often hope that new treatments will improve the health and future development of the newborn. It is often assumed that traditional clinical practices have been well-studied in appropriately selected populations of sufficient size to inform practitioners of their efficiency, benefits, safety, side effects, and costs.

When clinical practices are widely diffused and accepted, it is difficult to raise challenging questions. William Silverman has described how painfully slow the development of skepticism and use of the scientific method and experimentation were until we reached our present views of how to ask and answer clinical questions:[27]

> Spectacular therapeutic disasters have made it clear that informal let's-try-it-and-see methods of testing new proposals are more risky now than ever before in history. Since there are no certainties in medicine, it must be understood that every clinical test of a new treatment is, by definition, a step into the unknown.

Quality of Evidence

As we increase our knowledge regarding the health and health problems of newborn infants and as new therapies reach the marketplace and are quickly integrated into "state-of-the-art" practice, we must learn to overcome our impatience with uncertainty. We must ask questions about the quality of the evidence regarding the use and benefit of these new clinical practices. Questions will arise with careful reading of our own research literature. Questions can best be answered by the careful design and conduct of clinical studies.

It is not the purpose of this chapter to review the various research designs that allow strong scientific inference. Rather, it is the purpose of this chapter to (1) encourage careful assessment of the research that supports or argues against the use of both new and older clinical practices and (2) challenge our clinical observations and wisdom by subjecting them to systematic study.

Sinclair[29] has suggested four levels of clinical research to evaluate safety and efficacy based on their ability to provide an unbiased answer. In ascending order these include (1) single case or case series reports without controls, (2) nonrandomized studies with historic controls, (3) nonrandomized studies with concurrent controls, and (4) randomized controlled trials (RCTs). An RCT, the strongest design for evaluating the effect of therapy, tests a hypothesis utilizing randomly assigned treatment and control groups of adequate size to test the efficacy and safety of the new treatment. Tyson has suggested criteria for therapies as proven[31] (Box 1-1).

We know that clinical observations, although valuable in sharpening our questions, often suffer from our selective perception, our wish to see a strategy work (or fail to work). We also know that in some situations we can learn a great deal from carefully maintained databases when we have formed these databases with clear intentions and when they contain the needed data. For a variety of good reasons, case-controlled and prospective studies with historic controls are sometimes the only feasible way to answer clinical questions.[15,17] Although there is a rapidly growing point of view that RCTs provide the best scientific evidence on which to base clinical decisions, it is often difficult to overcome our impatience with delays in introducing innovative therapies.

Pressures to Intervene

The pressures to intervene before studies are conducted or completed have many sources. I. Chalmers,[8] in considering the struggle to gather scientific evidence in a climate of firmly held beliefs, has illustrated some of the pressures facing the scientific investigator (Fig. 1-1). Unfortunately, these pressures to intervene often become reasons not to do scientific studies.

Other authors have described various attitudes toward controlled trials that have inhibited their development. Bryce and Enkin discuss myths about RCTs, which become reasons not to do them.[7] Among such myths is the belief, often heard in clinical circles, that randomization is unethical. This may be true in some instances but not if there is poor evidence for adopting the commonly used strategy in the first place. To alternate a strategy whose benefit is not scientifically supported (but widely acclaimed) with one that is openly called "experimental" is not unethical. In fact both are "experimental." It is the use of an unstudied intervention that might more readily be labeled "unethical."

Believing that an infant is in trouble, we intervene; sometimes a cascade of interventions may follow,[21,24] one leading to the next, each carrying its own risk as well as benefit. One of the most frequently cited examples of this cascade is the epidemic of blindness associated with the use of oxygen in newborns. Silverman provides extensive details in two of his books.[26,27]

Oxygen had been used since the early 1900s for resuscitation and cyanotic episodes, but in the 1940s it was noted to "correct" periodic breathing in premature infants. After World War II when new gas-tight incubators were introduced, an epidemic of blindness occurred, resulting from retrolental fibroplasia (RLF). Silverman has pointed out that although many etiologies were suspected, it was not until 1954 that a multicentered controlled

---

Box 1-1

Proven Therapies

- Reported to be beneficial in a well-performed metaanalysis of all trials
  or
- Beneficial in at least one multicenter trial or two single-center trials

Modified from Tyson JE: Use of unproven therapies in clinical practice and research: how can we better serve our patients and their families? *Semin Perinatol* 19: 98, 1995.

Figure 1-1 Pressures to intervene. (From Chalmers I: *Birth* 10:151, 1983.)

trial confirmed the association between high oxygen concentration and RLF. Frequently forgotten, however, is that in subsequent years infants cared for in restricted oxygen environments had an increased mortality and that many of the survivors had spastic diplegia. The introduction of micro techniques for measuring arterial oxygen in the middle to late 1960s permitted more rational monitoring of oxygen therapy, with a reduction in RLF, now called retinopathy of prematurity (ROP), mortality, and spastic diplegia. ROP is now usually limited to extremely-low-birth-weight (ELBW) infants, and it may not be preventable,[26] although current research continues to explore other etiologies, preventive measures, and treatments (see Chapter 22).

The desire to see an intervention "work" permeates much of health care as well as research and encourages both practitioners and investigators to seek early signs of improvement of problems. Neonatology is not alone in focusing on the short-term effects of an intervention immediately after its introduction. Long-term effects of treatment are rarely sought for a number of reasons. The ultimate results in those studies may not have been foreseen. Consider the unfortunate effects of diethylstilbestrol (DES). **For many years hormones such as DES were given to pregnant women to prevent miscarriage, fetal death, preterm delivery, and other adverse outcomes of pregnancy. In the 1950s the use of DES in pregnant women was thought to be effective after a number of uncontrolled studies. Controlled trials occurring during that same time period were the subject of an overview (metaanalysis) by Goldstein et al[16] (Table 1-1). Clearly, DES was not effective, but it continued to be offered to pregnant women until the 1970s when the FDA finally disapproved of its use. Children of DES mothers have been found to have genital tract abnormalities, including vaginal adenosis, vaginal adenocarcinoma, decreased female fertility, and structural abnormalities of the cervix, vagina, uterus, and ovaries. Male children have epididymal cysts, hypotrophic testes, and relative infertility.**

T. Chalmers[12] has noted that this was not the only time that physicians have ignored the evidence and continued to use therapies that have been shown in RCTs to be of no benefit. The costs of

Table 1-1
Effects of DES on Pregnancy Outcomes

	Typical Odds Ratio*	95% Confidence Limits
Miscarriage	1.2	.89-1.62
Stillbirth	.95	.50-1.83
Neonatal death	1.31	.74-2.34
All three	1.38	.99-1.92
Prematurity	1.47	1.08-2.00

*An odds ratio is an estimate of the likelihood (or odds) of being affected by an exposure (e.g., a drug or treatment), compared with the odds of having that outcome without having been exposed. Women receiving diethylstilbestrol (DES) did not have fewer stillbirths or miscarriages than women who were untreated. The only statistically significant improvement that was seen was in the reduction of prematurity. Modified from Goldstein PA, Sacks HS, Chalmers TC: Hormone administration for the maintenance of pregnancy. In Chalmers I, Enkin M, Kerse M, editors: *Effective care in pregnancy and childbirth*, New York, 1989, Oxford University Press.

long-term studies or of follow-up surveillance are greater than those of short-term investigations. However, when delayed effects or effects that are measurable only later in the life of the child (psychologic problems, inability to function well in school, etc.) are likely, cost should not be the determining factor in selection of a study design.

Even when practitioners are assured that randomized trials show successful outcomes, often unanswered questions remain: Will a technology or treatment have the same effect in all settings? Has an "appropriate" target population been selected? Are there short-term side effects? Are there long-term foreseeable consequences?

Evaluation of Therapies

The evaluation of various therapies for respiratory distress syndrome (RDS) contrasts the value of controlled and uncontrolled trials. The major cause of death in premature infants is respiratory failure secondary to RDS (see Chapter 22). Previously called idiopathic respiratory distress syndrome (IRDS) or hyaline membrane disease (HMD), this syndrome was a mystery only 25 years ago. **The patient with IRDS was a premature infant in respiratory distress with expiratory grunting, nasal** flaring, chest wall retractions, and cyanosis that could or could not be ameliorated with high oxygen concentrations.[27]

Sinclair evaluated the popular methods of treatment of these patients in 1966.[28] He noted that these popular treatments were more frequently thought to be beneficial in uncontrolled studies than in controlled trials. In 19 *uncontrolled* studies, 17 showed "benefit." In 18 *controlled* studies only 9 showed "benefit." The untrained reviewer of the research would have reached faulty conclusions had he or she based clinical practice on the uncontrolled studies.

In contrast with many of the proposed treatments, surfactant therapy in premature infants has been well studied in randomized controlled trials. These studies have evaluated the efficacy of treatment of RDS with surfactant, the optimal source and composition, and prophylactic versus rescue treatment. Within these studies premature infant morbidity (including pneumothorax, periventricular and/or intraventricular hemorrhage, bronchopulmonary dysplasia [BPD], and patent ductus arteriosus) and mortality in the treatment and control groups have been compared. **In an overview of surfactant RCTs, Soll[30] noted increased survival, improvement in oxygenation and ventilation, and a decrease in the incidence of pneumothorax. Effects on BPD were unclear. There appeared to be no difference in outcomes when rescue and prophylactic treatments were compared (Table 1-2).**

RCTs involving thousands of newborns have clearly demonstrated the benefits of surfactant therapy in RDS. However, some unanswered questions remain, and further research is needed to define the optimal dose, optimal number of treatments, and most efficacious formulation.

Not only have treatment methods for RDS been examined, methods to prevent RDS have also come under close scrutiny. Antenatal administration of corticosteroids to pregnant women who threatened to deliver prematurely was first shown in 1972 to decrease the neonatal mortality rate and the incidence of RDS and intraventricular hemorrhage (IVH) in premature infants.[20] In 1990 Crowley et al used metaanalysis to evaluate 12 randomized controlled trials of maternal corticosteroid administration involving more than 3000 women. They showed that maternal corticosteroid treatment significantly reduced the risk of neonatal mortality, RDS, and IVH.[14] After two decades of published clinical trials[13,14,18] and the consensus development conference statement on "Effects of Corticosteroids for Fetal Maturation on Perinatal Outcomes" (1994), antenatal steroids have been shown to be effective and safe in enhancing fetal lung maturity and reducing neonatal mortality.[23]

To further reduce the incidence of RDS and chronic lung disease in very-low-birth-weight (VLBW) infants, investigations are under way to determine the efficacy and safety of thyrotropin-releasing hormone (TRH) as an additional prenatal treatment. Several studies have shown that antenatal TRH and corticosteroid administration reduce the risk of neonatal respiratory distress.[1,4,19,22] However, one of the largest randomized control trials conducted in Australia found that the TRH

Table 1-2
Mortality After Prophylactic Surfactant vs Surfactant Treatments

Author	Prophylactic	Treatment	Relative Risk*	95% Confidence Interval
Dunn	9/62	8/60	1.09	0.45,2.65
Kendig	29/235	49/244	.62	0.62,0.94
Merritt	29/102	23/101	1.25	0.78,2.00
Typical Effect			0.85	0.63,1.14

*In this table it can be seen that mortality was not different when the results of the two treatments were compared. None of the relative risk estimates were statistically significant.
Modified from Soll RF, McQueen MC: Respiratory distress syndrome. In Sinclair JC, Bracken MB, editors: *Effective care of the newborn infant,* Oxford, England, 1992, Oxford University Press.

treated group had an increased risk of RDS and need for ventilation. TRH administration was also associated with maternal nausea, vomiting, and rise in maternal blood pressure.[3] Why the sharp contrast in findings between these clinical trials? When examining the treatment procedures used in these studies, one notes that the Australian investigators administered a lower dose of TRH (200 μg vs. 400 μg) and gave it less frequently (every 12 versus 8 hours) than in other trials. Did this account for the discrepancies in efficacy and safety of the drug? This and many other questions remain to be answered. Currently, there is a large collaborative trial of antenatal TRH being undertaken in the United States. The results of this study together with those of a planned European trial should highlight the efficacy and safety of antenatal TRH for routine clinical use to reduce the severity of RDS and the risk of neonatal mortality.

Although extracorporeal membrane oxygenation (ECMO) was first reported for use in infants in 1976, it was not until 1984 that a randomized trial was reported.[56] Another "controlled" trial was reported in 1989.[25] Some care providers questioned the results of these trials based on sample size and study design. In 1990 the Committee on Fetus and Newborn of the American Academy of Pediatrics noted the expansion of ECMO centers and cautioned that its use should be limited to research centers.[2] Neither those who believed in the benefits nor those who argued against its use could turn to clear sufficient evidence to support their views. In 1993 a multicentered trial was organized in 83 collaborating British hospitals with the help of the Clinical Trial Service Unit at Oxford.[32] Mature infants with severe respiratory failure were randomly assigned to either one of five treatment centers or to continuing conventional care in the hospitals in which they were born. Each treatment center was experienced in the provision of long-term ventilatory support and capable of conducting cardiologic assessment, echocardiography, cranial ultrasound, ECMO and the care required for infants with severe respiratory failure. The benefit of ECMO was so clear that the external committee monitoring the data recommended that the trial be halted. Of the 93 infants assigned to ECMO 30 died, as compared with 52 of the 92 neonates receiving conventional care. This difference in

outcome meant that there was one extra survivor for every three to four infants assigned to ECMO care. This well-conducted single study was able to diminish the uncertainty regarding the use of ECMO. Granting that many practitioners will wish to see a repetition of the study in other settings, the example illustrates the way in which good studies resolve knotty problems.

Overviews

Chalmers and Sinclair conducted a rather disconcerting analysis of the perinatal literature several years ago.[9] When they considered perinatal trials as a proportion of all publications in selected obstetric, pediatric, anesthetic, and general journals published between 1966 and 1980, they found that reports of randomized trials were remarkably infrequent when compared with the attention given to other forms of study and commentary (Table 1-3).

Believing that the results of perinatal controlled trials had to be summarized in a manner useful to practitioners, Chalmers et al and other perinatal professionals from various countries developed a registry of randomized controlled trials. They reviewed a vast literature for published trials, sought out unpublished trials, and encouraged those who had begun, but not completed, studies to make them known to the registry. Once gathered, the studies' findings were summarized in "overviews."

Overviews (or metaanalyses) pool the results of independently conducted RCTs whose study meth-

Table 1-3 Controlled Trials in Perinatal Medicine as a Percentage of all Publications in Selected Journals, 1966-1980			
Journals	**1966-70**	**1971-75**	**1976-80**
5 Obstetric	1.7	1.6	3.0
5 Pediatric	0.9	1.0	1.6
5 Anesthetic	0.5	0.8	0.8
6 General	0.2	0.1	0.2

Modified from Chalmers I, Sinclair JC: Promoting perinatal health: is it time for a change of emphasis in research? *Early Hum Dev* 10:171, 1985.

ods are reasonably similar, both in the selection and characteristics of participants and in the treatments that are offered. Tables 1-2 and 1-3 were developed after pooling the results of different studies.

From these overviews, practitioners can learn of the strength or weakness of support for a claim of benefit or ill effect of a strategy. The result of Chalmers', Enkin's, and Keirse's efforts was a remarkably useful book entitled *Effective Care in Pregnancy and Childbirth.*[11]

It has become clear not only that trials are needed but also that their results must be organized and communicated. The National Perinatal Epidemiology Unit at Oxford (NPEU) and the National Institute of Child Health and Human Development (NICHD) have encouraged RCTs. In addition to providing support to individual investigators for RCTs, the NICHD has formed both neonatal and maternal-fetal medicine multicenter networks to conduct perinatal RCTs. This is particularly useful, providing an opportunity to see whether treatments have similar effects in different practice settings. It is also useful in that practitioners in individual settings may not always see enough cases to reach robust conclusions. Rare conditions and rare outcomes are better understood when trials are replicated and/or their findings are pooled.

At the end of the previously mentioned volume on pregnancy and childbirth, Chalmers, Enkin, and Keirse reported their own views based on conclusions formed in the preceding articles. They found that some strategies and forms of care were shown to be very useful but others were of questionable value. It is also evident that some interventions believed to be useful are in fact not useful—sometimes of little benefit—or, in fact, are even harmful. A companion publication, *Effective Care of the Newborn Infant,*[29] provides a compilation and review of neonatal RCTs.

> Since ours is the only species on the planet which has achieved rates of newborn survival which exceed 90 percent, it seems to me we must demand the highest order of evidence possible before undertaking widespread actions that may affect the full lifetimes of individuals in the present as well as in future generations. Here a strong case can be made for a *slow* and *measured* pace of medical innovations.[27]

References

1. Althabe F et al: Controlled trial of prenatal betamethosone plus TRH vs betamethasone plus placebo for prevention of RDS in preterm infants, *Pediatr Res* 29:200, 1992.
2. American Academy of Pediatrics, Committee on Fetus and Newborn: Recommendations on extracorporeal membrane oxygenation, *Pediatrics* 85:618, 1990.
3. Australian collaborative trial of antenatal thyrotropin-releasing hormone (ACTOBAT) for prevention of neonatal respiratory disease, *Lancet* 345:877, 1995.
4. Ballard RA et al: Respiratory disease in very-low-birthweight infants after prenatal thyrotopin-releasing hormone and glucocorticoid, *Lancet* 339:510, 1992.
5. Bartlett RH et al: Extracorporeal membrane oxygenation (ECMO) cardiopulmonary support in infancy, *Transactions of the American Society of Artificial Organs* 22:80, 1976.
6. Bartlett RH et al. Extracorporeal circulation in neonatal respiratory failure: a prospective randomized study, *Pediatrics* 76:479, 1985.
7. Bryce RL, Enkin MW: Six months about controlled trials in perinatal medicine, *Am J Obstet Gynecol* 151:6, 707, 1985.
8. Chalmers I: Scientific inquiry and authoritarianism in perinatal care and education, *Birth* 10:3, 151, 1983.
9. Chalmers I, Sinclair JC: Promoting perinatal health: is it time for a change of emphasis in research? *Early Hm Dev* 10:171, 1985.
10. Chalmers I et al, editors: *Oxford database of perinatal trials,* Oxford Electronic Publishing, Oxford, England, 1988, Oxford University Press.
11. Chalmers I, Enkin M, Keirse M: *Effective care in pregnancy and childbirth,* New York, 1989, Oxford University Press.
12. Chalmers T: The impact of controlled trials on the practice of medicine, *Mt Sinai J Med* 41:753, 1974.
13. Collaborative Group on Antenatal Steroid Therapy: Effect of antenatal dexamethasone administration on the prevention of respiratory distress syndrome, *Am J Obstet Gynecol* 141:276, 1981.
14. Crowley P, Chambers I, Keirse MJNC: The effects of corticosteroid administration before preterm delivery: an overview of the evidence from controlled trials, *Br J Obstet Gynaecol* 97:11, 1990.
15. Fletcher RH, Fletcher SW, Wagner EH: *Clinical epidemiology,* ed 2, Baltimore, 1988, Williams & Wilkins.
16. Goldstein PA, Sacks HS, Chalmers TC: Hormone administration for the maintenance of pregnancy. In Chalmers I, Enkin M, Keirse M, editors: *Effective care in pregnancy and childbirth,* New York, 1989, Oxford University Press.
17. Hulley SB, Cummings SB: *Designing clinical research,* Baltimore, 1988, Williams & Wilkins.
18. Jobe AH, Mitchell BR, Gunkel, JH: Beneficial effects of the combined use of prenatal corticosteroids and postnatal surfactant on preterm infants, *Am J Obstet Gynecol* 168:508, 1993.
19. Knight DB, Liggins GC, Wealthall SR: A randomized controlled trial of antepartum thyrotropin-releasing hormone and betamethasone in the prevention of respiratory disease in preterm infants, *Am J Obstet Gynecol* 171:11, 1994.

20. Liggins GC, Howie RN: A controlled trial of antepartum glucocorticoid treatment for prevention of the respiratory distress syndrome in premature infants, *Pediatrics* 50:515, 1972.
21. Mold JW, Stein HF: The cascade effect in the clinical care of patients, *N Engl J Med* 314:512, 1986.
22. Morales WI et al: Fetal lung maturation: the combined use of corticorsteroids and thyrotropin-releasing hormone, *Obstet Gynecol* 73:111, 1989.
23. National Institutes of Health Consensus Development Conference Statement: Effects of corticorsteroids for fetal maturation on perinatal outcomes, *JAMA* 273:413, 1995.
24. Orleans M, Haverkamp AD: Are there health risks in using risking systems? the case of perinatal risk assessment, *Health Policy* 7:297, 1987.
25. O'Rourke PP et al.: Extracorporeal membrane oxygenation and conventional medical therapy in neonates with persistent pulmonary hypertension of the newborn: a prospective randomized study, *Pediatrics* 84:957, 1989
26. Silverman WA: *RLF, a modern parable,* New York, 1980, Grune & Stratton.
27. Silverman WA: *Human experimentation: a guided step into the unknown,* New York, 1985, Oxford University Press.
28. Sinclair JC: Preventions and treatment of respiratory distress syndrome, *Pediatric Clin North Am* 13:711, 1966.
29. Sinclair JC Bracken MB: *Effective care of the newborn infant,* New York, 1992, Oxford University Press.
30. Soll RF: Overviews of surfactant treatment. In Chalmers I et al, editors: *Oxford database of perinatal trials,* version 1.2, records 5206, 5207, 5252, 5253, 5664, 5675. Oxford Electronic Publishing, Oxford, England, 1991, Oxford University Press.
31. Tyson JE: Use of unproven therapies in clinical practice and research: how can we better serve our patients and their families? *Semin Perinatol* 19:98, 1995.
32. UK Collaborative ECMO Trial Group: UK Collaborative trial of neonatal extracorporeal membrane oxygenation, *Lancet* 348:75, 1996.

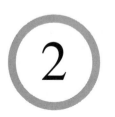

Part II *Support of the Neonate*

2 Prenatal Environment: Effect on Neonatal Outcome

Joanne Bartram, Gary M. Joffe, Leslie Perry

The human fetus develops within a complex setting. Structurally defined by the intrauterine/intraamniotic compartment, the character of the prenatal environment is largely determined by maternal variables. The fetus is absolutely dependent on the maternal host for respiratory and nutritive support and is significantly influenced by maternal metabolic, cardiovascular, and environmental factors. In addition, the fetus is limited in its ability to adapt to stress or modify its surroundings. This creates a situation in which the prenatal environment exerts a tremendous influence on fetal development and well-being. This influence lasts well beyond the period of gestation, often affecting the newborn in ways that have profound significance for both immediate and long-term outcome. There is great utility in the identification of maternal factors that adversely affect the condition of the fetus. Providers of obstetric care have long used this information to identify the "at-risk" population and design interventions that prevent or reduce the occurrence of fetal and neonatal complications. It is equally important that neonatal care providers obtain a clear picture of the prenatal environment and use this information before delivery to anticipate the newborn's immediate needs and make appropriate preparations for resuscitation and initial nursery care. After delivery, an awareness of the likely sequelae of environmental compromise helps to focus ongoing assessment and aids in clinical problem solving.

The purpose of this chapter is to help the neonatal care provider to evaluate maternal influences on the prenatal environment, identify significant environmental compromise, and anticipate the associated neonatal problems. Information on the assessment and treatment of specific neonatal problems is provided throughout this text and is not repeated here. For a more extensive discussion of perinatal physiology and the complicated pregnancy, refer to the references cited within this chapter.

Physiology

Two variables have a critical influence on fetal well-being throughout gestation: placental function and the inherent maternal resources. The interplay of these factors is a major determinant of fetal oxygenation, metabolism, and growth.

The placenta has a dual role in providing nutrients and metabolic "fuels" to the fetus. First, placental secretion of endocrine hormones, chiefly human chorionic somatomammotropin (HCS), increases throughout pregnancy, causing progressive changes in maternal metabolism. The net effect of these changes is an increase in maternal glucose and amino acids available to the fetus, especially in the second half of pregnancy. Second, the placenta is instrumental in the transfer of these (and other) essential nutrients from the maternal to the fetal

9

circulation and, conversely, of metabolic wastes from the fetal to the maternal system.

Fetal "respiration" also depends on adequate placental function. Respiratory gases (oxygen and carbon dioxide) readily cross the placental membrane by simple diffusion, with the rate of diffusion determined by the P_{O_2} (or P_{CO_2}) differential between maternal and fetal blood.

Although the placenta mediates the transport of respiratory gases, carbohydrates, lipids, vitamins, minerals, and amino acids, it is the maternal "reservoir" that is their source. Maternal-fetal transfer depends on the characteristics and absolute content of substances within the maternal circulation, the relative efficiency of the maternal cardiovascular system in perfusing the placenta, and the function of the placenta itself.[134] The fetal environment can be disrupted by inappropriate types or amounts of substances in the maternal circulation, decreases or interruptions in placental blood flow, or abnormalities in placental function.

Compromised Fetal Environment

Maternal Disease

Diabetes

The prevalence of diabetes mellitus and gestational diabetes mellitus (GDM) is increasing worldwide. Approximately 3% to 5% of pregnant women in the United States are diagnosed with GDM annually.[6] Despite major reductions in mortality over the past several decades, the infant of a diabetic mother (IDM) continues to have a considerable perinatal disadvantage. The physiologic changes in maternal glucose utilization that accompany pregnancy, coupled with either a preexisting hyperglycemia (as found in type I and II diabetes) or an inability to mount an appropriate insulin response (as seen in the gestational diabetic), result in a fetal environment that is markedly abnormal as a result of the increased level of maternal glucose, often in concert with episodic hypoglycemia and ketone exposure. Early in pregnancy this environment may have a teratogenic effect on the embryo, accounting for the dramatic increase in congenital malformations in the offspring of diabetic women with poor metabolic control.[45,58,123] During the second and third trimesters the mechanics of placental transport

dictate that fetal glucose levels depend on, but are slightly less than, maternal levels.[6,105] Assuming adequate placental function and perfusion, elevations in maternal glucose lead to fetal hyperglycemia and increased fetal insulin production. Repeated or continued elevations in blood glucose result in fetal hyperinsulinism, alterations in the utilization of glucose and other nutrients, and altered patterns of growth and development.[6,58,105]

In addition to the basic metabolic disturbances, diabetes predisposes the woman to a number of other complications, including hypertension, renal disease, and vascular compromise. **The various complications of diabetes are also associated with fetal and neonatal problems including prematurity, growth restriction, chronic hypoxia, cardiovascular problems, RDS, and intrauterine demise. In terms of predicting perinatal morbidity and mortality, the "Prognostically Bad Signs of Pregnancy," first identified by Pedersen in the 1960s, are especially significant. The occurrence of any of these signs, which include diabetic ketoacidosis, pregnancy-induced hypertension, pyelonephritis, and maternal noncompliance, continue to be useful predictors of increased fetal and neonatal risk.[31,105]**

In preparing for the delivery of an IDM, the neonatal team should consider the classification of maternal diabetes (type I, II, or gestational diabetic mother), the quality of metabolic control throughout the pregnancy and labor, maternal complications, and the duration of the pregnancy, along with indicators of fetal growth and well-being. Table 2-1 summarizes key maternal factors, their environmental implications, and the fetal and neonatal outcomes associated with diabetes in pregnancy.

Thyroid Disease

The thyroid hormones triiodothyronine (T_3) and thyroxine (T_4) cross the placenta in only small amounts. The significance of this transfer is unclear. Iodine is readily transferred from mother to fetus. The fetal thyroid concentrates iodine and synthesizes its own hormones as early as 10-12 weeks' gestation; this is independent of maternal thyroid function. Severe maternal hypothyroidism often results in infertility. Mild maternal hypothyroidism does not inhibit fetal thyroid function and generally poses little threat to the fetus. More severe

Table 2-1
Maternal Diabetes, the Prenatal Environment, and Perinatal Outcome

Maternal Factors	Environmental Implications	Fetal and Neonatal Consequences
Hyperglycemia		
Early	Exposure to elevated glucose levels during organogenesis	Increased incidence of congenital anomalies
Late	Availability of excess glucose, which leads to fetal hyperinsulinism, abnormal growth, and delayed surfactant production	Macrosomia, organomegaly, trauma during delivery, neonatal hypoglycemia, increased incidence of respiratory distress syndrome (RDS), polycythemia secondary to hypoxemia
Ketoacidosis	Fetal exposure to excess glucose and ketones, which can result in fetal diabetic ketoacidosis[58]	Fetal hypoxemia, intrauterine fetal demise
Hypertension, cardiovascular, and renal disease	Placental insufficiency secondary to vascular compromise, which results in diminished fetal oxygenation and nutrition	Growth restriction, fetal asphyxia, intrauterine fetal demise, prematurity
	Increased incidence of maternal urinary tract infections	Prematurity, RDS, sepsis

hypothyroidism has been linked to gestational hypertension, prematurity, and low birthweight.[72] Treatment with replacement hormone is well tolerated by the fetus and reduces these risks.[89,93,106]

Maternal hyperthyroidism presents a different situation. Thyroid-stimulating antibodies, commonly found in patients with Graves' disease, as well as many of the drugs used to treat hyperthyroidism, cross the placenta and can have a significant effect on the fetus. Antibodies, including long-acting thyroid stimulant (LATS) and thyroid-stimulating immunoglobulin (TSI), can cause an increase in fetal thyroid hormone production. High levels are associated with fetal and neonatal hyperthyroidism.[89,142] Untreated maternal thyrotoxicosis has been linked to preterm delivery, low birthweight, and stillbirths.[28] In rare cases the offspring of women with Graves' disease may themselves be afflicted with this condition. In the fetus and newborn, this is evidenced by elevations in heart rate, growth restriction, goiter, and congestive heart failure. Perinatal mortality is high.[106] Administration of antithyroid medication to the mother can decrease thyroid hormone production in both the mother and the fetus but may result in fetal hypothyroidism and goiter.[28]

Another maternal antibody, thyroid-stimulating hormone (TSH)-binding inhibitor immunoglobulin, also crosses the placenta and can prevent the expected fetal thyroid response to TSH. The result is a transient fetal and neonatal hypothyroidism.[84,89,142] Iodine deficiency in the mother is another cause of fetal and neonatal hypothyroidism and, in its severe form, cretinism because of the fetus's dependence on maternal iodine reserves.[55]

Phenylketonuria

Phenylketonuria (PKU) is a genetic disorder in which an enzymatic defect precludes the conversion of the essential amino acid phenylalanine to tyrosine. This metabolic derangement is evidenced by the accumulation of excessive amounts of phenylalanine in the blood and its subsequent excretion in the urine of affected persons. Historically, PKU resulted in virtually certain mental retardation; affected individuals were often institutionalized and rarely reproduced. With the advent of widespread neonatal screening and effective dietary treatment to prevent hyperphenylalaninemia during infancy and early childhood, genetically affected persons may now avoid the devastating effects of this disease, have relatively normal development, and become pregnant. However, even in women who were treated in childhood and are developmentally normal, maternal PKU poses a significant environmental risk for the fetus. The care of these women and their infants presents a unique perinatal challenge.

The offspring of women with PKU are frequently microcephalic and mentally retarded. They also have an increased incidence of growth restriction and congenital cardiac defects regardless of whether they are themselves affected with PKU.[69,70] The problem arises because although current recommendations are to maintain a low phenylalanine diet for life to avoid progressive deterioration and an increased risk of blindness, many phenylketonurics remain on this diet only through early childhood. However, during pregnancy elevated levels of phenylalanine in the mother are associated with fetal hyperphenylalaninemia. This prenatal exposure to excessive phenylalanine appears to be the primary mechanism of fetal injury. Maternal diet therapy offers the best hope for an unimpaired infant. **Phenylalanine levels drop quickly once dietary restrictions are instituted, and there is a strong correlation between maternal blood levels and neonatal outcome.[74,119] As with diabetes, control is ideally achieved before conception. Several studies have identified improved long-term outcomes when desirable phenylalanine levels (less than 2 to 8 mg/dl) are achieved before or early in pregnancy and maintained throughout.[26,70,110,119]**

Renal Disease

Maternal adaptation to pregnancy involves significant changes in renal function and structure. Plasma volume increases 40% to 50% with an associated increase in renal blood flow and a 50% increase in glomerular filtration rate (GFR).[85] There is increased retention of sodium and water. These changes place unique demands on the urinary tract; women with preexisting renal disease are often unable to tolerate this stress and may experience a deterioration in function. Furthermore, renal dysfunction complicates pregnancy and increases fetal risk.

Renal disease in pregnancy may occur as a result of urinary tract infections, glomerular disease, or as a complication of systemic diseases including diabetes and systemic lupus erythematosus (SLE). **Regardless of the underlying etiology, pregnancy outcome relates most closely to two factors: the presence of hypertension and the degree of renal insufficiency that existed before the pregnancy.[65,102,130,131]** Many women with renal disorders are hypertensive before pregnancy, and they often develop a superimposed pregnancy-induced hypertension leading to preeclampsia. Even those with previously normal blood pressures run an increased risk of developing hypertension during pregnancy.[54,59,102] The presence of hypertension in these pregnancies represents a significant risk to the fetus and is strongly associated with intrauterine growth restriction (IUGR), preterm delivery, and perinatal loss. Drug therapy to control chronic hypertension has been shown to have a beneficial effect on fetal outcome and is generally continued throughout pregnancy. Renal insufficiency, as measured by creatinine clearance or serum creatinine level, also has implications for fetal outcome. Mild to moderate renal insufficiency (serum creatinine <1.5 mg/dl) is associated with a generally favorable outcome, whereas severe insufficiency (serum creatinine >1.6 mg/dl) often carries an increased risk for perinatal death.[59,65,102] As a rule, the number of preterm deliveries and growth restricted infants increases with increasing blood pressure and decreasing renal function.[30,60,102]

Two special circumstances are dialysis during pregnancy and pregnancy after renal transplantation. Women undergoing dialysis rarely become pregnant. When pregnancy does occur, it is associated with significant perinatal morbidity and mortality with spontaneous abortions reaching 50%. Hemodialysis is also associated with numerous complications including placental abruption, polyhydramnios, IUGR, preterm labor, and pregnancy loss.[35,46,54,60,85] The risk may be lower with ambulatory peritoneal dialysis.[35,114] Pregnancy after transplantation is more common and has a better prognosis than pregnancy managed by dialysis.[27,102] Infants born after maternal transplantation are commonly preterm. Other complications may include growth restriction, RDS, congenital anomalies, adrenocortical insufficiency, hyperviscosity, seizures, and neonatal sepsis.[27,107,131] The criteria used to predict fetal outcome with other renal patients (i.e., hypertension and renal insufficiency) also have predictive value in posttransplantation pregnancies.

Neurologic Disorders

Neurologic disorders such as epilepsy, multiple sclerosis (MS), and myasthenia gravis generally have little effect on fertility; pregnancy can, and does, occur. The risks that accompany such pregnancies vary according to the individual disease entity and pertain to both the course of the mother's disease and the pregnancy outcome.

Maternal seizure disorders have been associated with increased fetal and neonatal risks, including prematurity, congenital defects, intrauterine demise, neonatal depression, and hemorrhage. These risks are in part attributable to the alterations in the fetal environment that occur as a result of either the seizure disorder itself or the administration of anticonvulsant drugs to the mother. An epilepsy-related genetic predisposition to certain major congenital defects may also be a factor.[63,101] A significant number of women experience an increase in seizure activity during pregnancy. This is most likely due to decreased compliance with medication regimens, physiologic changes associated with pregnancy, and gestational changes in plasma levels of anticonvulsant drugs.[11,63] There is evidence that maternal seizures compromise fetal oxygenation, possibly because of diminished placental blood flow or maternal hypoxemia secondary to postseizure apnea.[133] There are also data linking seizure activity during pregnancy to an increased incidence of poor pregnancy outcome.[98] For these reasons, control of maternal seizure activity with anticonvulsants is one of the primary goals of prenatal care.

Placental transport of anticonvulsants does occur, resulting in fetal levels that approximate or in some cases exceed maternal levels.[11,97] Many studies have demonstrated an increased incidence of congenital defects in the offspring of epileptic women treated with anticonvulsants.[11,63,98,101] These anomalies are most likely attributable in part to drug teratogenicity, but the influence of the seizure disorder itself, as well as genetic makeup, may also be a factor. Trimethadione is considered to be a potent teratogen, and its use is contraindicated in pregnancy. It is associated with spontane-

ous abortion, craniofacial anomalies, intrauterine growth restriction, hypoplasia of the fingers and nails, congenital heart defects, and mental retardation.[11,96,141] Valproic acid is associated with neural tube defects, craniofacial abnormalities, and several minor malformations.[97,132] Carbamazepine has also been linked to neural tube defects.[120] Other anticonvulsants, including hydantoins, primidone, and barbiturates, have been implicated in minor birth defects; specific syndromes have been associated with their use.

Infants born to mothers treated with anticonvulsants, especially barbiturates, may exhibit signs of generalized depression, including decreased respiratory effort, poor muscle tone, and feeding difficulties. They may also have symptoms indicative of drug withdrawal (see Chapter 8). These symptoms usually present in the first week of life and include tremors, restlessness, hypertonia, and hyperventilation.[7] In addition, there have been reports of abnormal clotting and hemorrhage in the offspring of women treated with phenytoin, phenobarbital, and primidone. This appears to be due to a decrease in vitamin K-dependent clotting factors. Hemorrhage usually starts within the first 24 hours, is often severe, and may result in death. Infants born to these mothers should have cord blood clotting studies done, vitamin K prophylaxis on admission to the nursery, and close observation.[11,101]

MS frequently strikes women during their reproductive years. The onset of MS is usually insidious; the course is marked by a seemingly capricious cycle of exacerbation and remission. A wide range of sensory, motor, and functional changes is associated with this disease; the type and severity of symptoms vary dramatically from one individual to another and in any one patient over time. The etiology of the disease is not well understood. Genetic, environmental, and immunologic mechanisms have been implicated; viral factors have also been suggested.[122] Pregnancy is usually well tolerated; however, a higher than expected number of relapses has been identified in the first six months after delivery.[112,122]

In women with MS, the disease process itself is not a threat to fetal or neonatal well-being. No increases in perinatal morbidity, mortality, or in the incidence of congenital defects have been demonstrated.[112,122] **The priority for neonatal care providers is to determine the extent of the mother's disability, including her level of fatigue and her ability to care for her infant. The availability of appropriate support systems, both personal and professional, should be assessed, and needed follow-up and referrals should be made.**

Even though the prognosis for these infants is excellent, there are some factors associated with MS that are potentially problematic. Bladder dysfunction, common in women with MS, often results in urinary tract infections during pregnancy. Associated fetal and neonatal problems include preterm delivery and sepsis. Early identification and prompt treatment with appropriate antibiotics should minimize these risks. An additional area of concern is the variety of drugs administered to MS patients. Immunosuppressants are frequently used during severe exacerbations. The placental transport and fetal risk vary with the individual agent used. Prednisone is generally considered safe for use in pregnancy; the safety of azathioprine is still in question.[10] Although there have been reports of healthy infants born after maternal azathioprine therapy, there have also been reports of fetal complications, including hypoplasia of the thymus, immunoglobulin deficiency, decreases in cortisol levels, and transient chromosomal abnormalities. Cyclophosphamide has been associated with skeletal defects, growth retardation, and preterm labor.[10,37] Both azathioprine and cyclophosphamide are best avoided during pregnancy. A final consideration is a long-term one: the incidence of MS in the offspring of a parent with the disease is somewhat higher than the incidence in the general population.

Myasthenia gravis is an autoimmune disorder in which a dearth of acetylcholine receptor (AChR) results in neuromuscular dysfunction.[115] Antibodies to AChRs have been found in most affected persons.[75] Distinguishing features include generalized weakness and muscle fatigue with activity. Persons with myasthenia gravis may also experience respiratory compromise and difficulty swallowing. In some cases pregnancy leads to deterioration; maternal deaths related to postdelivery myasthenic crisis have occurred.[111] **Infants born to myasthenic mothers may be affected by maternal drug therapy; an increased rate of preterm delivery**

has also been reported.[111] **An additional risk stems from transplacentally acquired antiacetylcholine receptor antibodies, which cause approximately 12% of these newborns to experience a transient, self-limited course of myasthenia gravis.[32,115] It is difficult to predict which pregnancies will result in an affected infant, although infants born to women with very high AChR antibody titers may be at highest risk. Affected infants usually present at birth or within the first 24 hours of life with generalized weakness, diminished suck and swallow, and a decreased respiratory effort that may require mechanical support.**

Systemic Lupus Erythematosus

SLE is an autoimmune disease that primarily presents in women of childbearing age. The clinical effects of lupus range from mild or subclinical disease to serious illness affecting multiple organ systems. In pregnancy, SLE is associated with increased rates of spontaneous abortion, preterm delivery, and stillbirths.[108] Outcome is best when pregnancy is not complicated by renal disease or hypertension.[29,108]

The neonatal manifestations of SLE are attributed to the placental transfer of maternal antibodies to the fetus. Findings in the newborn include a transient lupus-like rash, thrombocytopenia, and cardiac abnormalities.[138] A strong association has been established between maternal antiRo (SS-A) antibodies and congenital heart block in the offspring of women with SLE.[138] The heart block is often identified prenatally; infants are treated with cardiac pacemakers after delivery.

Heart Disease

Marked changes in cardiovascular function accompany normal pregnancy. Plasma and red blood cell volumes rise, heart rate and cardiac output increase, and peripheral vascular resistance falls. These changes facilitate increased uterine blood flow, placental perfusion, and fetal oxygenation and growth; they also increase maternal oxygen consumption and cardiovascular work load and can further compromise the cardiovascular status of women with preexisting serious heart disease.[90] Pregnancy also creates a risk for maternal cardiovascular complications, including an increased incidence of thromboembolism and sudden death.[87]

In some cases, such as Eisenmenger's syndrome and primary pulmonary hypertension, the risk to maternal survival is so great that pregnancy is contraindicated.[86] In general, how well the woman with heart disease tolerates pregnancy depends on the specific disease process and the degree to which her cardiac status is compromised.[15,66,90,139]

Maternal heart disease also affects the fetus. Fetal risks are the result of genetic factors, alterations in placental perfusion and exchange, and the effect of maternally administered drugs. **The genetic risk is demonstrated by the increased incidence of congenital heart defects that occur in the offspring of parents who have such a defect.** The exact risk depends on the specific parental lesion, mode of inheritance, and exposure to environmental triggers.[13]

Alterations in placental perfusion and gas exchange occur when the mother's condition involves chronic hypoxemia or a significant decrease in cardiac output. These factors increase the threat to the fetus, with fetal risk increasing as maternal cardiac status declines.[90] Chronic maternal hypoxemia results in a decrease in oxygen available to the fetus and is associated with fetal loss, prematurity, and IUGR.[139] Significant reductions in maternal cardiac output create decreased uterine blood flow and diminished placental perfusion with a resulting impairment in the exchange of nutrients, oxygen, and metabolic wastes.[4,90] **Possible fetal and neonatal consequences include spontaneous abortion, IUGR, neonatal asphyxia, central nervous system (CNS) damage, and intrauterine demise.**

A wide variety of drugs are used in the management of maternal cardiovascular disease. Although it is sometimes difficult to differentiate drug effects from the effects of the underlying disease, some associations between drug administration and fetal outcomes can be made. Anticoagulants are used to decrease the risk of thromboembolism, especially in women with artificial valves, a history of thrombophlebitis, or rheumatic heart disease. **Oral anticoagulants, specifically warfarin (coumarin), have been associated with fetal malformations, including nasal hypoplasia and epiphyseal stippling, when administered during the first trimester. They have also been associated with eye and CNS abnormalities when adminis-**

tered later in pregnancy.[52] The incidence of warfarin embryopathy is estimated at 15% to 25%. Warfarin is also associated with maternal and fetal hemorrhage. Heparin is generally considered the preferable agent for anticoagulation during pregnancy. Heparin does not cross the placenta and so does not result in fetal anticoagulation or neonatal hemorrhage (although maternal hemorrhage may still occur), nor has it been associated with congenital defects.[135]

Antiarrhythmic medications and cardiac glycosides used during pregnancy cross the placenta to varying degrees. They have not been implicated in fetal malformations and, although several have been associated with minor complications, are generally considered safe for use in pregnancy.[121,135] Reported complications include uterine contractions (quinidine, disopyramide), decreased birth weights (digoxin, disopyramide), and maternal hypotension with a sudden decrease in placental perfusion (verapamil).

Antihypertensives and diuretics have also been used in the treatment of cardiovascular disease during pregnancy. Propranolol, a beta-blocker commonly used to treat both hypertension and arrhythmias, acts as a uterine stimulant and is a possible cause of preterm labor.[90] It is also associated with neonatal depression, including decreased respiratory effort and bradycardia at the time of delivery, as well as with hypoglycemia, polycythemia, and hyperbilirubinemia in the newborn period.[90,121,140] Atenolol and metoprolol, selective beta-blockers that can also be used to treat chronic hypertension, appear to have fewer adverse consequences for the neonate and are preferable agents.[121,135] Diuretic use in pregnancy remains an area of some controversy. Fetal and neonatal compromise can result from diuretic-induced electrolyte and glucose imbalance and decreased placental perfusion secondary to maternal hypovolemia. The use of thiazide diuretics has been linked to neonatal liver damage and thrombocytopenia. In general, diuretic use is restricted to women with pulmonary edema or acute cardiac or renal failure.[90,135] Although a great number of possible complications have been listed here, it is important to remember that with few exceptions most of the drugs used in the treatment of maternal heart disease can be used in pregnancy if the maternal condition warrants it.

Respiratory Disease

Respiratory function is altered even in normal pregnancy. Changes include a decrease in lung volume and increases in both oxygen consumption and minute ventilation. Significant decreases in maternal respiratory function and oxygenation could have a negative effect on the fetus, but careful management of respiratory disease during pregnancy generally results in a favorable outcome.

Asthma is the most commonly occurring respiratory disease in pregnancy. Infants born to well-controlled asthmatics usually do well; unstable or worsening disease, especially status asthmaticus, increases fetal risk. Commonly used asthma medications, including corticosteroids, adrenergic bronchodilators (terbutaline, albuterol, epinephrine) and aminophylline are considered safe for use in pregnancy.[25] No teratogenic effects have been clearly demonstrated. Although avoidance of any drug, especially in the first weeks of pregnancy, is a good rule, the first priority in asthma is to maintain control of the disease throughout pregnancy. Asthma medications are used as needed to maintain control and avoid (or treat) acute episodes.[25] **Fetal risks related to maternal asthma include low birth weight and/or prematurity. However, with good control the occurrence rate of these problems is essentially the same as in nonasthmatic pregnancies.[129]**

Cystic fibrosis (CF) was once considered a lethal childhood disease, but the life expectancy of those with CF has increased, with more women surviving to conceive pregnancies. Pregnancy is not recommended for women with severe disease, since they often experience a marked deterioration during gestation. Patients with less severe disease and careful prenatal care may tolerate pregnancy well and achieve good neonatal outcomes. **Fetal risks include prematurity, IUGR, and perinatal death, caused primarily by maternal hypoxemia and infection. Women with CF frequently require treatment with antibiotics during pregnancy. Several antibiotics have been associated with fetal abnormalities and neonatal complications.[68] These include tetracycline (tooth discoloration and abnormal bone development), aminoglycosides (ototoxicity), and sulfonamides (hyperbilirubinemia). Trimethoprim is a folic acid antagonist and**
should be avoided because of the association between folic acid deficiency and neural tube defects. Penicillins and cephalosporins are generally considered safer for use in pregnancy. All infants born to mothers with cystic fibrosis will be heterozygous carriers for CF.

Maternal Behavior

Smoking

It is well established that maternal smoking is associated with reductions in both birth weight and length, as well as with an increase in the incidence of birth weights below 2500 g. The exact mechanism by which fetal growth is retarded is not entirely clear, but reductions in placental blood flow secondary to vasoconstriction, elevated carbon monoxide levels, and chronic fetal hypoxia may all play a role.[12,57,92] Maternal smoking is also associated with placental dysfunction, an increased incidence of placental abruptions and previas, premature rupture of the membranes, preterm labor, and intrauterine fetal demise. Fetal risk increases with the number of cigarettes smoked, maternal anemia, and poor nutrition.[91] **Eliminating or reducing smoking can improve fetal growth; women should be counseled to do so even relatively late in pregnancy.[125]**

Substance Abuse

Maternal drug and alcohol abuse place the fetus and newborn at risk for a plethora of structural, functional, and developmental problems. Perinatal morbidity is related to the direct effects of the abused substance on the developing fetus, its sudden "withdrawal," the interactions of multiple abused substances, the nutritional effects of addiction on the mother, and/or the social and health care implications of substance abuse. Alcohol is one of the most commonly abused substances during pregnancy. Alcohol in the maternal circulation crosses the placenta resulting in direct fetal exposure to alcohol and its metabolites.[1] **The exposed fetus may suffer a wide range of effects, including craniofacial malformations, growth restriction, CNS dysfunction, and organ or joint abnormalities.[1,61]** The mechanism of fetal injury is not entirely clear but is likely related to three main factors: a teratogenic effect, hypoxia as a result of increased oxygen consumption, and a diminished ability to use amino acids in protein synthesis.[1] The expression of fetal alcohol effects ranges from subtle to extreme and depends on the timing of exposure, the dose, and the genetic response of the mother and fetus to the effects of alcohol. Secondary factors, such as maternal age, nutritional status, general health, and the effects of other abused substances may also influence outcome. **When the more severe effects are exhibited the condition is known as fetal alcohol syndrome (FAS). FAS occurs in the offspring of chronic alcoholics and is defined by a triad of defects consisting of IUGR with microcephaly, facial anomalies (small palpebral fissures, low nasal bridge, indistinct philtrum, thin upper lip, shortened lower jaw), and CNS dysfunction, including mental restriction.[61] These infants may also exhibit tremors, irritability, and hypertonus related to alcohol withdrawal. The effects of prenatal alcohol exposure may be seen in postnatal life as continued abnormalities in motor, behavioral, and intellectual development.**

Drug use and addiction in pregnancy is a complex problem. Maternal reporting of drug use is often unreliable; frequently more than one substance is involved, and there may be a cycle of drug use and periodic abstinence during pregnancy. In addition, a host of medical and social problems are associated with maternal drug abuse. Substance abusers have generally poor health; infectious diseases, including pneumonia, sexually transmitted disease, urinary tract infections, and hepatitis are common. Anemia is frequently seen, and nutrition and prenatal care are often inadequate. These factors contribute to a poor pregnancy outcome and make it difficult to isolate the effects of any individual drug on the fetus. However, several generalizations are made. The majority of drugs used by the mother, including narcotics, stimulants, and depressants, cross the placenta and have an effect on the fetus. **Fetal risks include IUGR, malformations, intrauterine demise, prematurity, asphyxia, and CNS dysfunction; fetal addiction does occur and is associated with neonatal abstinence syndrome.[38,61,88,143]**

Maternal cocaine use merits special attention.

Cocaine is a CNS stimulant that produces vasoconstriction, tachycardia, and hypertension in both the mother and fetus. Its use during pregnancy has been linked to IUGR, genitourinary (GU) tract anomalies, placental abruption, stillbirths, and cerebral infarcts, as well as impaired performance on the Brazelton Behavioral Assessment tool.[18,19] See Chapter 8 for a more complete discussion of complications in the drug exposed neonate.

Maternal Malnutrition

Fetal nutrition is linked to maternal intake during pregnancy and to the existent maternal stores of various nutrients, as well as to placental function. In general, poorly nourished mothers have more perinatal losses and give birth to smaller babies; this is especially true of the markedly underweight woman who fails to gain adequate weight during pregnancy.[71,79,137] However, it is difficult to draw direct correlations between poor maternal diet and fetal growth unless the nutritional disturbances are severe. Many fetuses grow well despite suboptimal maternal nutrition, in part because of the complexities of placental transport and the ability of the fetus to be preferentially supplied with some nutrients.

Although reduced birth weight is associated with inadequate carbohydrate, protein, and total caloric intake, inappropriate amounts of other nutrients may also affect the fetus. Vitamin and mineral deficiencies have been linked to spontaneous abortion (vitamin C), congestive heart failure (thiamine), megaloblastic anemia (folic acid, B_{12}), congenital anomalies including neural tube defects (folic acid, zinc, copper), and skeletal abnormalities (vitamin D, calcium).[137] Vitamin overdosage, especially of the fat-soluble vitamins, has also been implicated in fetal abnormalities; vitamin A overdose has been associated with kidney malformations, neural tube defects, and hydrocephalus, and vitamin D overdose with cardiac, neurologic, and renal defects.[78,80,137]

Nutritional deficiencies (or excesses) should be identified before or early in pregnancy, and both weight gain and fetal growth should be monitored throughout gestation. When problems are identified, individualized intervention strategies should be implemented in an attempt to increase birth weights and improve perinatal outcome.

Obstetric Complications

Antepartum Bleeding

Maternal cardiovascular support is crucial to fetal well-being. Chronic blood loss can lead to maternal anemia and a related decrease in oxygen-carrying capacity. Uncompensated acute bleeding results in diminished blood volume, decreased systolic pressure, decreased cardiac output, and ultimately decreased placental perfusion. The net effect on the fetus is decreased oxygenation and impaired nutrient delivery.

The most common causes of hemorrhage late in pregnancy include placental abruption and placenta previa. In an abruption, a normally implanted placenta separates from the uterine wall before the time of delivery, resulting in maternal bleeding and a functional decrease in uteroplacental size. A relationship between cocaine use and an increase incidence of abruptions has been reported.[39] The separation may be partial or complete, involving peripheral and/or central portions of the placenta. Fetal compromise relates to the extent of the separation and to the frequent need for preterm delivery. When the abruption is small and bleeding is minimal, the pregnancy may continue without marked fetal compromise; however, it is important to remember that the decrease in uteroplacental surface area is irreversible and reduces the absolute placental capability. As the fetus grows or experiences additional stressors, its ability to tolerate the abruption may change. Extensive abruptions are poorly tolerated by both fetus and mother; the resulting maternal hemorrhage and decreased placental function lead to fetal asphyxia and, without immediate intervention, to intrauterine demise.[50]

A placenta previa exists when the placenta lies abnormally low in the uterus and to some extent covers or encroaches on the internal cervical os. In the latter part of pregnancy, the normal elongation of the lower uterine segment and changes in the cervix disrupt the attachment of the overlying placenta. This generally presents as episodic painless maternal bleeding, often accompanied by preterm labor. To avoid active labor with resulting maternal hemorrhage, fetal lung maturity is assessed at 35 to 36 weeks. If mature, a cesarean section is scheduled before the onset of labor.[116] Fetal compromise relates to the extent of the previa, severity of maternal hemorrhage, degree of the resulting fetal hypoxia, and gestational age at delivery.

Preeclampsia

Preeclampsia, a type of pregnancy-induced hypertension, is a condition in which hypertension, accompanied by proteinuria and edema, develops during the second half of pregnancy in women with or without preexisting hypertensive disease. It is most common in primigravidas, in women younger than 16 or older than 35, in multiple gestations and molar pregnancies, and in women with a family history of this disorder.[20] As a perinatal complication, preeclampsia is significant because of its high toll in terms of both maternal and fetal well-being.

Pregnancy is normally associated with vasodilation and decreased peripheral vascular resistance. The net effect is that even though there is a significant increase in blood volume, maternal blood pressure does not increase during pregnancy. In contrast, pregnancy-induced hypertension is associated with vasoconstriction and an increase in vascular resistance and arterial pressure. The result is a reduction in blood flow to the vital organs, including the kidney, liver, brain, and uterus; reduced maternal blood volume; and a host of maternal hepatic, CNS, and coagulation abnormalities. The major effect on the intrauterine environment is placental insufficiency caused by significant reductions in uteroplacental blood flow and the development of placental vascular abnormalities.[83,118] **Associated fetal and neonatal risks include IUGR, prematurity with all of its attendant problems, perinatal asphyxia, and perinatal death.[8,36,83,117,126] The risk to the infant increases with earlier onset and increasingly severe maternal disease, such as chronic hypertension with superimposed preeclampsia.[81] Maternal seizures (eclampsia) further compromise the fetus by promoting hypoxemia and acidosis, which can result in intrauterine demise.[118]**

HELLP syndrome, a severe form of pregnancy-induced hypertension manifested by *h*emolysis, *e*levated *l*iver enzymes, *l*ow *p*latelets, and renal function abnormalities, carries a high risk of fetal and maternal death. In milder cases of HELLP syndrome, conservative management may facilitate improvements in condition before delivery, but the risk of IUGR remains. However, in most cases of

HELLP syndrome, delivery is indicated regardless of the gestational age of the fetus.[127]

Drugs commonly used to treat pregnancy-induced hypertension include magnesium sulfate, hydralazine (Apresoline), labetalol, nifedipine, and other antihypertensives. Magnesium sulfate is the most commonly used agent in the United States for the prevention of maternal seizures. **Hypotonia and CNS depression have been reported as neonatal side effects, yet no correlation has been found between neonatal magnesium level and APGAR score.[118] These effects are more likely due to coexisting complications such as prematurity and asphyxia.[52,124]** Hydralazine and other antihypertensives are used in the treatment of severe maternal hypertension; actions include relaxation of the arterial bed, decreased vascular resistance, and decreased blood pressure. Maternal response to antihypertensives must be carefully monitored because precipitous decreases in blood pressure reduce placental perfusion and further compromise the fetus.[103]

Preterm Labor

Preterm birth, defined as any birth before 37 weeks' gestation, poses an unparalleled threat to neonatal survival and well-being. Its cost, both human and economic, is staggering, and its prevention is a primary focus of modern obstetric care. Prevention is best accomplished through an aggressive effort to identify women at risk and close follow-up to achieve early recognition and appropriate intervention should preterm labor occur.[56,77] Unfortunately, many women continue to receive inadequate prenatal care or no care at all. Even women who obtain early and ongoing care often fail to recognize the signs of preterm labor and delay reporting symptoms until intervention is difficult if not impossible.

Although in many specific instances a definitive cause cannot be identified, it is possible to identify several factors that are generally associated with preterm labor and delivery.[49,56,64] These factors are summarized in Box 2-1. When preterm labor cannot be halted, it culminates in the delivery of a physiologically immature infant. The result is a host of neonatal problems that relate largely to the degree of immaturity, but also to compounding problems such as infant anomalies or maternal disease, as well as to the events that led to the preterm delivery

---

Box 2-1
Factors Associated with Preterm Labor and Delivery

Maternal History
Chronic disease
Diabetes
Renal disease
Cardiovascular disease
Respiratory disease
In utero exposure to diethylstilbestrol
Reproductive tract anomalies
Underweight (before pregnancy)
Smoking
Age extremes (below 18, above 40)
Previous preterm labor
African-American race
Low socioeconomic status

This Pregnancy
Inadequate weight gain
Acute maternal illness
    Pregnancy-induced hypertension
    Urinary tract infection
    Chorioamnionitis, vaginal infection
Antepartum hemorrhage
Isoimmunization
Premature rupture of membranes
Multiple gestation
Polyhydramnios
Retained inatrauterine device

Fetal Factors
Fetal anomalies
Intrauterine fetal demise
Infection

(e.g., asphyxia secondary to a bleeding placenta previa). Problems commonly encountered in preterm infants include respiratory distress, asphyxia, hyperbilirubinemia, metabolic disturbances, fluid and electrolyte imbalance, neurologic and behavioral problems, infection, nutritional deficits and feeding problems, ineffective thermoregulation, cardiovascular disturbances, chronic respiratory disease, and hematologic disturbances.

Beta-sympathomimetic agents, such as ritodrine hydrochloride and terbutaline sulfate, are commonly used as a means of interrupting preterm labor. They achieve their tocolytic action by maximizing the beta$_2$-adrenergic effects on the uterus, with a resulting decrease in uterine smooth muscle contractility.[23,77] Although these drugs are effective in prolonging gestation, they are also associated with maternal, fetal, and neonatal complications.[9,14,23,76,77,113] Mothers may experience tachycardia and dysrhythmias, hyperglycemia, hypokalemia, anxiety, nausea, and vomiting. Myocardial ischemia and pulmonary edema are rare but serious maternal side effects. The fetus may also develop tachycardia and hyperglycemia. **Neonates born after beta-sympathomimetic therapy may develop a rebound hypoglycemia in response to in utero hyperglycemia and overproduction of insulin. No long-term problems have been identified.**

Magnesium sulfate has also been employed as a tocolytic. Magnesium sulfate decreases muscle contractility, thereby inhibiting uterine activity and effectively interrupting preterm labor.[23,109,124] **Neonatal consequences of maternal magnesium administration include decreased muscle tone and drowsiness, as well as decreases in serum calcium levels.**[51,104,109]

Prostaglandins play an important role in the onset of labor. Prostaglandin synthetase inhibitors, such as indomethacin, are a class of pharmacologic agents that interfere with the body's synthesis of prostaglandin, thereby inhibiting prostaglandin-mediated uterine contractions. These drugs have been used to treat preterm labor. They can cause in utero constriction, or closure, of the ductus arteriosus with resulting development of fetal pulmonary hypertension and congestive heart failure.[5,73,99,100] They may also lead to oligohydramnios and must be used with caution, especially late in the third trimester.[5,16,67] Other neonatal risks include decreased platelet activity and gastrointestinal irritation.[99]

Calcium antagonists, such as nifedipine, also have a demonstrated ability to interfere with the labor process. Uterine contractility is directly related to the presence of free calcium; increased calcium concentration enhances muscle contractility, whereas decreased calcium levels inhibit contractility.[23,40] Calcium antagonists block the entry of calcium into cells and inhibit uterine muscle

contraction. In animal studies, these drugs have been associated with fetal acidosis.[34,53]

Environmental Effects of Labor on the Fetus

Effects of Contractions

During labor, the dynamics of uterine contractions alter the intrauterine environment and influence the fetus. The "healthy" fetus is equipped to withstand the challenge of labor, but when the fetus is compromised or the labor, is dysfunctional, the fetus can be taxed beyond its capacity, placing it at risk for further compromise, asphyxia, or intrauterine death.

Strong uterine contractions are characterized by decreased blood flow through the intervillous spaces in the placenta.[21,43,95] As blood flow decreases, there is a corresponding decline in placental gas exchange, and the fetus must depend on its existing reserves to maintain oxygenation until placental blood flow is reestablished. The net effect is that fetal Pao$_2$ decreases as the consequence of uterine contraction. In the fetus with adequate reserves, the fall in Pao$_2$ is not drastic; the fetus remains adequately oxygenated and so is able to tolerate the stress of labor.

Fetal Reserve

The factors that influence fetal reserve fall into two general categories: those that diminish reserves and those that exhaust reserves. When fetal oxygen reserves are diminished, the fetus has less than optimal oxygenation at the onset of a contraction. This may occur as a consequence of any condition that decreases placental exchange, including reduced placental surface area caused by abruption, previa, or an abnormally small placenta[3,11,95]; decreased placental perfusion caused by maternal hypotension or hypertension; or maternal hypoxemia. Oxygen reserves can also be diminished as a result of a reduction in fetal oxygen-carrying capacity, as in severe anemia or acute fetal hemorrhage.

A fetal reserve that is adequate at the onset of labor can be exhausted by factors that place unusual demands on the fetus. Exhaustion of reserves occurs with contractions that last for a prolonged period of time, that are of extremely high intensity, or that occur with increased frequency and without an adequate recovery period between individual contractions.[3,11,95] This is often a consequence of the use of oxytocics to induce or augment labor.

Fetal Response to Contraction-Induced Hypoxia

When the fetal oxygen reserve is diminished or exhausted, uterine contractions can precipitate a marked fall in Pao_2. The fetus is quite limited in its ability to compensate for this hypoxemia. The adult mechanism, which involves increasing total cardiac output by increasing heart rate, does not play a major role in the fetal response.[48] Instead, the fetus responds with a redistribution of cardiac output as a means of maintaining critical function; blood flow to the brain and heart increases, whereas perfusion of less critical organs is reduced.[3,4,48,95] This mechanism enables the fetus to survive brief episodes of hypoxia, but severe and prolonged hypoxic episodes are poorly tolerated.

Acute hypoxemia leads to the development of acidosis and also produces a reflex bradycardia secondary to vagal stimulation, both of which further compromise fetal oxygenation. In addition, myocardial hypoxia has a direct bradycardic effect.[4,43] These mechanisms give rise to one of the classic signs of fetal distress, the late deceleration, in which the peak of uterine pressure, which also represents the nadir of intervillous blood flow and the onset of fetal hypoxemia, is followed by a decline in fetal heart rate.[3,21,43,48] Late decelerations are significant in that they help to identify the fetus unable to tolerate labor because of inadequate oxygen reserves, and they allow for the implementation of measures to enhance fetal reserve, improve placental perfusion, or interrupt labor.

Late decelerations are particularly ominous when accompanied by loss of fetal heart rate variability and/or fetal baseline tachycardia, since these findings are indicative of fetal acidosis. In the preterm infant, the findings of decreased variability and tachycardia, with or without late decelerations,

correlate highly with acidosis, depression, and low Apgar scores.[3,43,95]

Other Factors that Evoke a Fetal Response During Labor

Head Compression

Pressure on the fetal head during labor, especially with pushing efforts in the second stage, also produce a vagal response and a reflex slowing of the fetal heart rate.[3,21,43,95] In general, this does not indicate hypoxia or fetal compromise and is often seen in the healthy fetus. The deceleration that accompanies head compression, also referred to as an early deceleration, is differentiated from the late deceleration of fetal asphyxia by its timing in relation to a contraction. In early deceleration the heart rate begins to fall as a contraction builds, reaching its lowest point as the contraction peaks. As the contraction subsides, the heart rate returns to baseline. The result is a uniformly shaped dip that mirrors the shape of the contraction. In comparison, a late deceleration also has a uniform shape but lags behind the contraction, with the fall in heart rate beginning at or slightly after the contraction peak and continuing to fall as the contraction subsides. With a late deceleration the heart rate does not return to baseline until well after the contraction has ended.

Cord Compression

Compression of the umbilical cord occurs when the cord is looped around fetal body parts or is knotted, as a result of cord prolapse, or when there is scant amniotic fluid. During labor, cord compression may be exacerbated by contractions and by descent of the fetus, resulting in varying degrees of occlusion of the umbilical vessels and diminutions of blood flow. Partial venous occlusion may be manifested by fetal heart rate acceleration, whereas significant occlusion precipitates a rapid fall in heart rate, caused at least in part by vagal reflex.[3,21,43,62,95] Variable decelerations can be spontaneous, occurring anytime, or periodic, occurring with contractions. They typically have an abrupt descent in heart rate and may be either "V," "U," or "W" shaped, hence the term variable deceleration. Periodic variable decelerations are identified by a decline in heart rate that generally begins before the contraction peaks but, unlike early decelerations, falls rapidly and does not mirror the shape of the contraction. Typically, recovery of the heart rate is also rapid. However, when the occlusion is severe or of long duration, or the fetus has diminished oxygen reserves, recovery may be slow, indicating fetal hypoxia and in essence incorporating a component of late deceleration within the variable deceleration.[21]

Maternal Pain Medication

Maternal anesthesia and/or analgesia has the potential to affect the infant, either during labor and delivery or in the newborn period. The risk is increased if the fetus is preterm or otherwise compromised. This is not to say that there is no place for these drugs in obstetric care, only that they must be used judiciously and with a clear understanding of the risks and benefits involved. Table 2-2 summarizes the effects of commonly used analgesic and anesthetic agents on the fetus and the newborn.[44]

Assessment of Fetal Well-Being

Over the past 20 years the ability to assess fetal well-being has advanced from simple auscultation of the fetal heart to direct physiologic and biochemical measurement of fetal status. With these advances, an appreciation of the similarities between the fetus and the newborn, as well as a more complete understanding of the unique features of fetal life, has been gained. This knowledge reinforces the importance of viewing fetal physiology as a precursor of neonatal function, and especially as a significant influence on the success with which the fetus will complete the adaptations required by the birth process.

The goal of antepartum fetal surveillance is to answer the following questions: What is the safest environment for the fetus at the gestational age at which the testing is taking place? Is the fetus more likely to survive in utero for the week after testing, or does the fetus have a significant risk of in utero death based on the degree of environmental or intrinsic intolerance demonstrated through testing? In the case of preterm infants, this may mean delivery at a gestational age at which there is a high

---

Table 2-2
Fetal and Neonatal Effects of Maternal Analgesia and Anesthesia During Labor

Drug	Possible Fetal and Neonatal Side Effects
Narcotics	Fetal and neonatal effects are related to the dose, route, and timing of maternal administration and may be reversed by the administration of a narcotic antagonist (naloxone); they include the following: CNS depression Fetal bradycardia Depressed respiratory effort Decreased muscle tone and reflexes Decreased responsiveness
Paracervical block	Fetal bradycardia and asphyxia related to decreased uterine blood flow and direct fetal myocardial depression
Epidural and spinal block	Fetal bradycardia and asphyxia related to maternal hypotension Fetal neonatal toxicity
General (inhalation) anesthesia	Fetal and newborn effects related to the duration and depth of maternal anesthesia include the following: CNS depression Respiratory depression Decreased responsiveness

CNS, Central nervous system.

likelihood for respiratory, neurologic, cardiac, gastrointestinal, and immunologic immaturity requiring neonatal intensive care.

The obstetric practitioner has several tools available to help answer the above questions. First and foremost is the identification of maternal conditions that may predispose the fetus to in utero compromise. Examples of such conditions include Type I diabetes mellitus, chronic hypertension, collagen vascular disease, antiphospholipid antibody disease, maternal cardiac or pulmonary disease, preeclampsia, blood group isoimmunization, in utero infection, preterm rupture of membranes, and maternal substance abuse. This list is not all inclusive but demonstrates several commonly encountered conditions for which antepartum fetal surveillance is warranted.

Once the decision is made to assess fetal well-being, there are four different modalities available in general practice to help the practitioner and client answer the questions regarding the optimal environment for the fetus at any given time. These include fetal movement counts, the contraction stress test, the nonstress test, and the fetal biophysical profile. Two additional tools often used by maternal fetal medicine specialists in certain clinical situations are Doppler flow studies and percutaneous umbilical cord sampling. None of these tools are used as the sole determinant for delivery but rather are used in conjunction with the entire clinical picture. The choice of testing method is also clinically driven; each method is useful in certain clinical settings, but no one method is the correct choice in all situations.

Although most of the procedures used to monitor fetal well-being are decidedly high tech, the simple "kick count," or fetal movement survey, is a low-tech, low-cost screening tool. Many women with an intrauterine fetal demise have no identifiable risk factors that would place them in a fetal testing protocol. This is one reason why many institutions ask their clients to begin a fetal movement counting protocol at 26 to 32 weeks' gestation. Although there are continuing study results, some centers have demonstrated a significant decrease in the incidence of fetal mortality after the institution of a fetal movement counting protocol.

There are several different approaches to fetal movement counting. None has been shown to be superior.[2] One approach is to have the client choose a certain time every day to rest in the lateral position and count fetal movements. The perception of ten distinct fetal movements within two hours constitutes a reassuring session. The most important aspect of this type of testing is to emphasize to the client the importance of notifying her practitioner immediately if the fetal movement counting has not met the established criteria. A system must be in place where clients have immediate access to health care personnel 24 hours per day.

The contraction stress test (CST) is used in an attempt to evaluate fetal response to uterine contractions. The principle behind CST is that uterine contractions cause a transient interruption in utero placental perfusion. With normal placental reserve, this intermittent interruption is well tolerated. With inadequate or exhausted reserve, late fetal heart rate decelerations appear.[42] Because late decelerations during labor had been associated with fetal hypoxia and acidosis, it was reasoned that similar interpretations could be applied to contractions induced in the antepartum client. Thus the CST is considered a test of utero placento reserve.

During a CST, uterine contraction activity is evoked with either the use of maternal nipple stimulation or an intravenous infusion of oxytocin. The fetal heart rate is charted using graph paper attached to a monitor that uses a continuous wave ultrasound transducer placed on the maternal abdomen over the uterus. The minimum number of spontaneous or evoked contractions is necessary for adequate testing is three contractions of 40 seconds duration in a ten minute period. The results are interpreted as follows: a negative CST is one in which no late fetal heart rate decelerations occur during the exam. In a positive CST, late decelerations occur after 50% or more of the contractions, even if contraction frequency is less than three in 10 minutes.

A suspicious or equivocal finding is one in which intermittent late or significant variable decelerations occur. A CST result is considered unsatisfactory if fewer than three contractions occur per 10 minutes or a poor quality tracing is obtained. In many clinical situations a positive CST warrants delivery of the fetus because of suspected in utero hypoxemia during periods of uterine contraction. However, there are numerous exceptions to this rule. For example, if a positive CST is noted in the presence of maternal diabetic ketoacidosis, a correction of the underlying metabolic process may reverse the fetal acidosis and a negative CST may be subsequently obtained. Thus the delivery of a neonate who has metabolic acidosis and is preterm can be avoided.

The nonstress test (NST) is a tool used to indirectly assess the integrity of the fetal autonomic nervous system. The fetal heart is under the dual influences of the sympathetic and parasympathetic nervous systems. By approximately 28 weeks' gestation, 85% of fetuses will demonstrate fetal heart rate accelerations in response to fetal movement. Lack of these intermittent fetal heart rate accelerations usually indicates a fetal sleep cycle. However, there are many other intrinsic and extrinsic factors, including fetal acidosis, that may lead to an absence of these intermittent accelerations in heart rate. Examples include, but are not limited to, medication exposure, maternal smoking, uteroplacental insufficiency, and fetal structure or chromosomal anomaly. Factors leading to maternal acidosis (severe anemia, congenital heart disease, sepsis) can also result in fetal acidosis and a nonreactive NST.

The NST is performed with the client in a semi-Fowler or lateral tilt position. Like the CST, the fetal heart rate is monitored with an external transducer. NSTs are interpreted as either reactive or nonreactive. An accepted definition of a reactive NST is an increase in fetal heart rate of 15 beats per minute above the baseline heart rate occurring twice in a 20 minute period.[2] Some centers require that the fetal heart rate accelerations be associated with fetal movements as well as perceived by the maternal client.[33] A nonreactive test is defined as lacking the required fetal heart rate accelerations during a 40 minute period. Examples of clients who may be candidates for nonstress testing include those with insulin-requiring diabetes, pregnancy-induced hypertension, intrinsic renal disease, fetal IUGR, post dates pregnancy, or a maternal perception of decreased fetal movement.

The NST has certain advantages over the CST. It does not entail the production of uterine contractions, and so there are fewer potential problems or contraindications to the NST. Because the NST is quicker and easier to conduct, it is often the first-line screening test of fetal well-being. Its disadvantages are that it does not evaluate uteroplacental reserve and that it has a higher false positive rate than the CST.

When the NST is nonreactive, an option that is often used in lieu of the CST or delivery of the fetus is the biophysical profile (BPP) (Table 2-3). This test combines the NST with real-time ultrasound evaluation of the fetus. Although there are several different BPP scoring systems, the one most generally accepted assigns a numerical score of 0 or 2 for the absence or presence of five different

Table 2-3
Biophysical Profile Scoring

Biophysical Variable	Normal (2)	Abnormal (0)
Fetal breathing—At least one episode of at least 30 seconds during 30-minute observation	Present	Absent
Gross body movement—At least three body or limb movements during 30-minute observation	≥3	≤2
Fetal tone—One episode of extension or flexion of limbs or trunk during 30-minute observation	Present	Absent or sluggish movements
Reactive nonstress test—At least two episodes of 15 beats/min fetal heart rate accelerations during 30-minute observation	Yes	No
Amniotic fluid volume—At least one pocket of at least 1 cm by 1 cm in two directions	Present	Absent

Normal score: 8-10

parameters. These include fetal movement, tone, "breathing" movements, amniotic fluid volume, and the NST. One advantage to evaluation of several different fetal biophysical variables is enhanced specificity of testing with a diminished incidence of delivery for false positive results. The presence or absence of acute markers (movement, tone, breathing, NST) help reflect fetal status at the time of testing. Evaluation of amniotic fluid volume as a marker is indirect evidence that the portions of the fetal CNS that control that activity are intact and functioning and therefore not acidotic. However, the absence of a given marker may be difficult to interpret since it may simply reflect normal periodicity.

The biophysical activities that mature first in fetal development disappear last as acidosis worsens. Fetal tone (flexion and extension) is present at 7.5 to 8.5 weeks after the last menstrual period. This activity, as well as gross body movement, is mediated in the cortex and nuclei of the CNS. Fetal movement is present by 9 weeks. Fetal breathing movements (rhythmic breathing movements of 30 seconds or more) are generally seen by 20 weeks' gestation. The CNS center responsible for control of this activity is the ventral surface of the fourth ventricle. The final acute marker to mature is fetal heart rate acceleration in response to movement (reactive NST) seen in the later second trimester. The posterior hypothalamus and medulla control this activity. Given that the first marker to appear in development is the last to disappear with worsening fetal acidosis, the absence of fetal tone has been found to be associated with high perinatal morbidity and mortality.[136] Chronic sustained fetal hypoxia or acidosis may produce a protective redistribution of cardiac output away from less vital fetal organs (e.g., kidney and lung) toward the essential organs (e.g., brain, heart, and adrenal glands). Redistribution of fetal blood flow may be so profound that renal perfusion decreases to the point that oligohydramnios is established. When the largest vertical amniotic fluid pocket within the uterus is less than 1 cm, the perinatal mortality rate is as high as 110/1000.[17]

A BPP score of 8 or 10 is normal; 6 is equivocal and should be repeated in 12 to 24 hours. A score of 4 or less is abnormal. Management in the presence of an abnormal BPP is dependent upon the gestational age and the maternal and/or fetal factors contributing to the altered state.

The BPP takes advantages of real-time ultrasound to observe fetal behavior.[82] One of its major advantages is as an intermediate step in the evaluation of a fetus with a nonreactive NST before performance of the time-consuming CST. It is also a useful tool for those clients with contraindications to the CST, such as premature labor, premature rupture of membranes, unexplained vaginal bleeding, or multiple gestation. The modified BPP, which combines an acute marker (NST) with the chronic marker of fetal well-being (amniotic fluid index [AFI]), has been shown by some centers to be as equally predictive of fetal well-being as the full BPP. Since evaluation of the AFI is less time consuming and requires less technical skill, this may be an acceptable alternative for many centers.

No matter which of these testing modalities is used, the client should be counseled as to the predictive value of a "normal" test. The incidence of stillbirth within one week of a reactive NST is 1.4/1000; for a negative CST it is 0.4/1000; and for a normal BPP 0.6/1000.[2] Although some investigators have reported a decreased incidence of fetal mortality after initiation of a fetal movement counting program for "low risk" clients, there is not yet enough data available to apply these numbers to the general population.[94]

The role of Doppler flow assessment of the fetal arterial and venous systems in the prediction of in utero well-being remains controversial. At the present time, Doppler velocimetry is not required.[2] However, if used to assess umbilical arterial waveform, the absence of end-diastolic velocity may appear days before conventional antenatal tests become abnormal. In cases such as these, at a minimum, intensive fetal surveillance is advised.[41]

The dramatic improvement in ultrasound image quality over the past 10 years has also made it possible to directly sample fetal blood and tissue. The technique of percutaneous umbilical blood sampling (PUBS) has given the obstetrician access to the fetal circulation with relative safety for both the fetus and the mother. In this procedure, real-time ultrasound is used to guide the insertion of a needle into the umbilical vein or artery. Samples of fetal blood can be obtained or, as in the case of red cell isoimmunization, transfusions can be carried out. The fetal loss rate is generally quoted as 1% to 2%.[128] PUBS is now frequently used in specialized perinatal centers for assessment of fetal well-being.

References

1. Abel EL: Consumption of alcohol during pregnancy: a review of effects on growth and development of offspring, *Hum Biol* 54:421, 1282.
2. ACOG: Technical bulletin #188, Chicago, 1994.
3. Adelsperger D et al: Fetal heart monitoring principles and practice, Washington DC, 1993, AWHONN.
4. Battaglia FC, Meschia G: *An introduction to fetal physiology,* Orlando, Fla, 1986, Academic Press.
5. Besinger R et al: Randomized comparative trial of indomethacin and ritodrine for the long term treatment of preterm labor, *Am J Obstet Gynecol* 164:981, 1991.
6. Blank A et al: Effects of gestational diabetes on perinatal morbidity reassessed, *Diabetes Care* 18:127, 1995.
7. Bossi L et al: Plasma levels and clinical effects of antiepileptic drugs in pregnant epileptic patients and their newborns. In Johannessen SI et al, editors: *Antiepileptic therapy; advances in drug monitoring,* New York, 1980, Raven Press.
8. Brazy JE, Grimm JK, Little VA: Neonatal manifestations of severe maternal hypertension occurring before the thirty-sixth week of pregnancy, *J Pediatr* 100:256, 1982.
9. Brazy JE, Little VA, Grimm JK: Isoxsuprine in the perinatal period. II. Relationships between neonatal symptoms, drug exposure, and drug concentration at the time of birth, *J Pediatr* 98:146, 1981.
10. Briggs G: *Drugs in pregnancy and lactation: a reference guide to fetal and neonatal risk,* Baltimore, 1983, Williams & Wilkins.
11. Buehler BA, Stempel LE: Anticonvulsant therapy during pregnancy. In Rayburn WF, Zuspan FP, editors: *Drug therapy in obstetrics and gynecology,* ed 3, St Louis, 1992, Mosby.
12. Bureau MA et al: Maternal cigarette smoking and fetal oxygen transport: a study of P50,2,3-diphosphoglycerate, total hemoglobin, hematocrit, and type F hemoglobin in fetal blood, *Pediatrics* 72:22, 1983.
13. Burns J: Congenital heart disease; risk to offspring, *Arch Dis Child* 58:947, 1983.
14. Caritis SN et al: Pharmacodynamics of ritodrine in pregnant women during preterm labor, *Am J Obstet Gynecol* 147:752, 1983.
15. Cannobbio MM: Reproductive issues for the woman with congenital heart disease, *Nurs Clin N Am* 29:285, 1994.
16. Cantor B et al: Oligohydramnios and transient neonatal anuria, a possible association with the maternal use of prostaglandin synthetase inhibitors, *J Reprod Med* 24:220, 1980.
17. Chamberlin PFC et al: Ultrasound evaluation of amniotic fluid volumes. I. The relationship of marginal and decreased amniotic fluid volumes to perinatal outcome, *AM J Obstet Gynecol* 118:327, 1979.
18. Chasnoff IJ et al: Perinatal cerebral infarct and maternal cocaine use, *J Pediatr* 108:456, 1986.
19. Chasnoff IJ et al: Temporal patterns of cocaine use in pregnancy: perinatal outcome, *JAMA* 261:1741, 1989.
20. Chesley LC: Hypertensive disorders in pregnancy, *J Nurse Midwifery* 30:99, 1985.
21. Cibils LA: *Electronic fetal-maternal monitoring,* Littleton, Mass, 1981, PSG Publishing.
22. Cohen LF, di Sant'Agnese PA, Friedlander J: Cystic fibrosis and pregnancy, *Lancet* 2:842 1980.
23. Creasy RK: Preterm labor and delivery. In Creasy RK, Resnick R: *Maternal fetal medicine principles and practices,* ed 3, Philadelphia, 1994, WB Saunders.
24. Cunny GJ et al: Pregnancy and cystic fibrosis, *Obstet Gynecol* 77:850, 1991.
25. D'Alonzo GE: The pregnant asthmatic patient, *Semin Perinatol* 14:119,1990.
26. Davidson DC et al: Outcome of pregnancy in a phenylketonuric mother after low phenylalanine diet introduced from the ninth week of pregnancy, *Eur J Pediatr* 137:45, 1982.
27. Davidson JM: Renal transplantation in pregnancy, *Am J Kidney Dis* 9:374, 1987.
28. Davis LE et al: Thyrotoxicosis complicating pregnancy, *Am J Obstet Gynecol* 160:63, 1989.
29. De Swiet M: Systemic lupus erythamatosus and other connective tissue disorders. In De Swiet, editor: *Medical disorders in obstetric practice,* ed 3, Oxford, England, 1995, Blackwell Science Ltd.
30. Davison JM, Katz AL, Lindheimer MD: Kidney disease and pregnancy: obstetric outcome and long-term renal prognosis, *Clin Perinatol* 12:497, 1985.
31. Diamond MP et al: Reassessment of White's classification and Pedersen's prognostically bad signs of diabetic pregnancies in insulin-dependent diabetic pregnancies, *Am J Obstet Gynecol* 156:599, 1987.
32. Donaldson JO et al: Antiacetylcholine receptor anti-body in neonatal myasthenia gravis, *Am J Dis Child* 135:222, 1981.
33. Druzin ML: Antepartum fetal heart rate monitoring, state of the art, *Clin Perinatol* 16:627, 1989.
34. Ducasy CA et al: Effects of calcium entry blocker (nicardipine) tocolysis in rhesus macaques: fetal plasma concentrations and cardiorespiratory changes, *Am J Obstet Gynecol* 157:1482, 1987.
35. Elliott JP et al: Dialysis in pregnancy: a critical review, *Obstet Gynecol Surv* 46:319, 1991.
36. Eskenazi B et al: Fetal growth retardation in infants or multiparous and nulliparous women with preeclampsia, *Am J Obstet Gynecol* 169:1112, 1993.
37. Evans OB et al: Neurologic diseases. In Sweet AY, Brown EG, editors: *Fetal and neonatal effects of maternal disease,* St Louis, 1991, Mosby.
38. Finnegan LP: Drugs and other substance abuse in pregnancy. In Stern L, editor: *Drug use in pregnancy,* Balgowlah, NSW, Australia, 1984, Adis Health Science Press.
39. Fleming AD: Abruptio placentae, *Crit Care Clin* 7:865, 1991.

40. Forman A, Anderson KE, Ulmsten U: Inhibition of myometrical activity by calcium antagonists, *Semin Perinatol* 5:288, 1981.

41. Forouzan I: Absence of end-diastolic flow velocity in the umbilical artery: a review, *Obstet Gynecol Survey* 50:219, 1995.

42. Freeman R: Contraction stress testing for primary fetal surveillance in patients at high risk for uteroplacental insufficiency, *Clin Perinatol* 9:265, 1982.

43. Freeman RK, Garite TJ, Nageotte MP: *Fetal heart rate monitoring,* ed 2, Baltimore, 1991, Williams & Wilkins.

44. Frigoletto FD, Little GA: *Guidelines for perinatal care,* ed 2, Chicago, 1988, AAP and ACOG.

45. Fuhrmann K et al: Prevention of congenital malformations in infants of insulin-dependent diabetic mothers, *Diabetes Care* 6:219, 1983.

46. Gabert HA, Miller JM; Renal disease in pregnancy, *Obstet Gynecol Sur* 40:449, 1985.

47. Gandhi FA et al: Fetal cardiac hypertrophy and cardiac function in diabetic pregnancies, *Am J Ostet Gynecol* 173:1132, 1995.

48. Gimovsky ML, Caritis SN: Diagnosis and management of hypoxic fetal heart rate patterns, *Clin Perinatol* 9:313, 1982.

49. Gravett MG: Causes of preterm delivery, *Semin Perinatol* 8:246, 1984.

50. Green J: Placenta previa and abrupto placentae. In Creasy RK, Resnick R: *Maternal fetal medicine principles and practices,* ed 3, Philadelphia, 1994, WB Saunders.

51. Green KW et al: The effects of maternally administered magnesium sulfate in the neonate, *Am J Obstet Gynecol* 142:29, 1983.

52. Hall JG, Pauli RM, Wilson KM: Maternal and fetal sequelae of anticoagulation during pregnancy, *Am J Med* 68:122, 1980.

53. Harake B et al: Nifedipine: effects on fetal and maternal hemodynamics in pregnant sheep, *Am J Obstet Gynecol* 157:1003, 1987.

54. Hayslett JP: Interaction of renal disease and pregnancy, *Kidney Int* 25:579, 1984.

55. Hetzel BS: Iodine deficiency disorders (IDD) and their eradication, *Lancet* 2:1126, 1983.

56. Hiller SL et al: Association between bacterial vaginosis and preterm delivery of a low birth weight infant, *N England J Med* 333:1737, 1995.

57. Hoff C et al: Trend associations of smoking with maternal, fetal, and neonatal morbidity, *Obstet Gynecol* 68:317, 1986.

58. Hollingsworth DR: *Pregnancy, diabetes and birth: a management guide,* ed 2, Baltimore, 1992, Williams & Wilkins.

59. Hou SH, Grosman SD, Madias NE: Pregnancy in women with renal disease and moderate renal insufficiency, *Am J Med* 78:185, 1985.

60. Hsieh TT et al: Pregnancy outcome in patients undergoing longterm hemodialysis, *Acta Obstet Gynecol Scand* 70 (4–5):299, 1991.

61. Hutchings DE: Drug abuse during pregnancy: embropathic and neurobehavioral effects. In Braude MC, Zimmerman AM: *Genetic and perinatal effects of abused substances,* Orlando, Fla, 1987, Academic Press.

62. James LS, Yeh MN, Morishima HO: Umbilical vein occlusion and transient acceleration of the fetal heart rate, *Am J Obstet Gynecol* 126:276, 1976.

63. Janz D: Antiepileptic drugs and pregnancy: altered utilization patterns and teratogenesis, *Epilepsia* 23(suppl):S53, 1982.

64. Kaltreider DF, Kohl S: Epidemiology of preterm delivery, *Clin Obstet Gynecol* 23:17, 1980.

65. Katz AI et al: Pregnancy in women with kidney disease, *Kidney Int* 18:192, 1980.

66. Katz M et al: Outcome of pregnancy in 110 patients with organic heart disease, *J Reprod Med* 31:343, 1986.

67. Kirshon B et al: Long-term indomethacin therapy decreases fetal urine output and results in oligohydramnios, *Am J Perinatol* 8:86, 1991.

68. Kotloff RM, Fitzsimmons SC, Fiel SB: Fertility and pregnancy with cystic fibrosis, *Clin Chest Med* 13:623, 1992.

69. Lenke RR, Levy HL: Maternal phenylketonuria and hyperphenylalaninemia: an international survey of the outcome of untreated and treated pregnancies, *N Engl J Med* 303:1202, 1980.

70. Lenke RR, Levy HL: Maternal phenylketonuria—results of dietary therapy, *Am J Obstet Gynecol* 142:548, 1982.

71. Leonard LG: Pregnancy and the underweight woman, *MCN* 9:331, 1984.

72. Leung AS et al: Perinatal outcome in hypothyroid pregnancies, *Obstet Gynecol* 81:349, 1993.

73. Levin DL: Effects of inhibition of prostaglandin synthesis in fetal development, oxygenation and the fetal circulation, *Semin Perinatol* 4:35, 1980.

74. Levy HL, Waisbren SE: Effects of untreated maternal phenylketonuria and hyperphenylalaninemia on the fetus, *N Engl J Med* 309:1269, 1983.

75. Lindstrom JM et al: Antibody to acetylcholine receptor in myasthenia gravis, *Neurology* 26:1054, 1976.

76. Lipshitz J: Beta-adrenergic agonists, *Semin Perinatol* 5:252, 1981.

77. Lirette M, Holbrook RH, Creasy RK: Management of the woman in preterm labor, *Perinatol Neonatol* 10:30, 1986.

78. Luke B: Megavitamins and pregnancy: a dangerous combination, *MCN* 10:18, 1985.

79. Luke B: Nutritional influences on fetal growth, *Clinical Obstet Gynecol* 37:538, 1994.

80. Luke B: Maternal fetal nutrition, *Clinical Obstet and Gynecol* 37:93, 1994.

81. Mandeville LK, Trojano NH: *High risk intrapartum nursing,* Philadelphia, 1992, Lippincott.

82. Manning FA et al: Fetal assessment based on fetal biophysical profile scoring: experience in 12,620 referred high risk pregnancies. I. Perinatal mortality by frequency and etiology, *Am J Obstet Gynecol* 151:343, 1985.

83. Martin JN Jr, Perry KG Jr: Hypertension and preeclampsia. In Sweet AY, Brown EG, editors: *Fetal and neonatal effects of maternal disease,* St Louis, 1991, Mosby.

84. Matsuura N et al: Familial neonatal transient hypothyroidism due to maternal TSH-binding inhibitor immunoglobulins, *N Engl J Med* 303:738, 1980.

85. Maurer G, Ambriola D: Pregnancy following renal transplant, *J Perinat Neonat Nurs* 8:28, 1994.

86. McAnulty JH, Morton MH, Ueland, K: The heart and pregnancy, *Curr Prob Cardiol* 13:589, 1988.

87. McAnulty JH, Metcalfe J, Ueland K: General guidelines in the management of cardiac disease, *Clin Obstet Gynecol* 24:773, 1981.

88. Merker L, Higgins P, Kinnard E: Assessing narcotic addiction in neonates, *Pediatr Nurs* 11:177, 1985.

89. Mestman JH: Thyroid disease in pregnancy, *Clin Perinatol* 12:651, 1985.

90. Metcalfe J, McAnulty JH, Ueland K: *Heart disease and pregnancy: physiology and management,* ed 2, Boston, 1986, Little, Brown.

91. Meyer MB, Jonas BS, Tonascia JA: Perinatal events associated with maternal smoking during pregnancy, *Am J Epidemiol* 103:464, 1976.

92. Mochizuki M et al: Effects of smoking on fetoplacental-maternal system during pregnancy, *Am J Obstet Gynecol* 149:413, 1984.

93. Montoro M et al: Successful outcome of pregnancy in women with hypothyroidism, *Ann Intern Med* 94:31, 1981.

94. Moore TR, Piacquadio K: A prospective evaluation of fetal movement screening to reduce the incidences of antepartum fetal death, *Am J Obstet Gynecol* 160:1075, 1989.

95. Murray M: *Antepartal and intrapartal fetal monitoring,* Albuquerque, 1997, Learning Resources International.

96. Nakane Y et al: Multi-institutional study in the teratogenicity and fetal toxicity of antiepileptic drugs: a report of a collaborative study group in Japan, *Epilepsia* 21:663, 1980.

97. Nau H et al: Valproic acid and its metabolites: placental transfer, neonatal pharmacokinetics, transfer via mother's milk and clinical status in neonates of epileptic mothers, *J Pharmacol Exp Ther* 219:768, 1981.

98. Nelson KB, Ellenberg JH: Maternal seizure disorder, outcome of pregnancy and neurologic abnormalities in the children, *Neurology* 32:1247, 1982.

99. Niebyl JR: Prostaglandin synthetase inhibitors, *Semin Perinatol* 5:274, 1981.

100. Niebyl JR, Johnson JWC: Inhibition of preterm labor, *Clin Obstet Gynecol* 23:115, 1980.

101. Noronha A: Neurological disorders during pregnancy and the puerperium, *Clin Perinatol* 12:695, 1985.

102. Paller MS: Renal diseases. In Burrows GN, Ferris TF, editors: *Medical complications during pregnancy,* ed 2, Philadelphia, 1995, WB Saunders.

103. Patterson-Brown S et al: Hydralazine boluses for the treatment of severe hypertension in preeclampsia, *Br J Obstet Gynecol* 101:409, 1994.

104. Peaceman AM et al: The effect of magnesium sulfate tocolysis on the fetal biophysical profile, *Am J Obstet Gynecol* 161:771, 1989.

105. Pedersen J: *The pregnant diabetic and her newborn,* ed 2, Baltimore, 1977, Williams & Wilkins.

106. Pekonen F et al: Women on thyroid hormone therapy, pregnancy course, fetal outcome, and amniotic fluid thyroid hormone level, *Obstet Gynecol* 63:635, 1984.

107. Penn I, Makowski EL, Harris P: Parenthood following renal transplantation, *Kidney Int* 18:221, 1980.

108. Petri M and Allbritton J: Fetal outcomes of lupus pregnancy: a retrospective case-control study of the Hopkin's lupus cohort, *Rheumatol* 20:650, 1993.

109. Petrie RH: Tocolysis using magnesium sulfate, *Semin Perinatol* 5:266, 1981.

110. Platt LD et al: Maternal phenylketonuria collaborative study, obstetric aspects and outcome: the first 6 years, *Am J Obstet Gynecol* 166:1150, 1992.

111. Plauche WC: Myasthenia gravis, *Clin Obstet Gynecol* 26:592, 1983.

112. Poser S, Poser W: Multiple sclerosis and gestation, *Neurology* 33:1422, 1983.

113. Procianoy RS, Pinheiro CEA: Neonatal hyperinsulinism after short term maternal beta sympathomimetic therapy, *J Pediatr* 101:612, 1982.

114. Redrow M et al: Dialysis in the management of pregnant patients with renal insufficiency, *Medicine* 67:199, 1988.

115. Repke JT: Myasthenia gravis in pregnancy. In Goldstein PJ, Stern BJ, editors: *Neurological disorders of pregnancy,* ed 2, Mt Kisco, NY, 1992, Futura Publishing.

116. Resnick R, Morre TR: Obstetric management of the high risk patient. In Burrows GN, Ferris TF, editors: *Medical complications during pregnancy,* ed 4, Philadelphia, 1995, WB Saunders.

117. Rey E, Couturier A: The prognosis of pregnancy in women with chronic hypertension, *Am J Obstet Gynecol* 171:410, 1994.

118. Roberts J: Pregnancy-related hypertension. In Creasy RK, Resnick R, editors: *Maternal fetal medicine principles and practices,* ed 3, Philadelphia, 1994, WB Saunders.

119. Rohr FJ et al: New England maternal PKU project: prospective study of untreated and treated pregnancies and their outcomes, *J Pediatr* 110:391, 1987.

120. Rosa FW: Spina bifida in infants of women treated with carbamazepine during pregnancy, *N England J Med* 324:674, 1991.

121. Rotmensch HH, Elkayam U, Frishman W: Anti-arrhythmic drug therapy during pregnancy, *Ann Intern Med* 98:487, 1983.

122. Rudnick RA, Birk KA: Multiple sclerosis and pregnancy. In Goldstein PJ, Stern BJ, editors: *Neurological disorders of pregnancy,* ed 2, Mt Kisco, NY, 1992, Futura Publishing.

123. Sadler TW et al: Evidence for multifactorial origin of diabetes induced embryopathies, *Diabetes* 38:70, 1989.

124. Scardo JA et al: Favorable hemodynamic effects of magnesium sulfate in preeclampsia, *Am J Obstet Gynecol* 174:1249, 1995.

125. Sexton M, Hebel JR: Clinical trial of change in maternal smoking and its effect on birth weight, *JAMA* 251:911, 1984.

126. Sibai BM et al: Maternal-fetal correlations in patients with severe preeclampsia/eclampsia, *Obstet Gynecol* 62:745, 1983.

127. Sibai BM: The HELLP syndrome (hemolysis, elevated liver enzymes, and low platelets): much ado about nothing? *Am J Obstet Gynecol* 162:311, 1990.

128. Skupski DW, Wolf CFW, Bussel JB: Fetal transfusion therapy, *Obstet Gynecol Surv* 51:181, 1996.

129. Stenius-Aarniala B, Piirilä P, Teramo K: Asthma and pregnancy: a prospective study of 198 pregnancies, *Thorax* 43:12, 1988.

130. Surian M et al: Glomerular disease and pregnancy, *Nephron* 36:101, 1984.

131. Sweet AY: Diseases of the kidneys and urinary tract. In Sweet AY, Brown EG, editors: *Fetal and neonatal effects of maternal disease,* St Louis, 1991, Mosby.
132. Tein I, MacGregory DL: Possible valproate teratogenicity, *Arch Neurol* 42:291, 1985.
133. Teramo K et al: Fetal heart rate during a maternal grand mal epileptic seizure, *J Perinat Med* 7:3, 1979.
134. Tropper PJ, Petrie RH: Placental exchange. In Lavery JP, editor: *The human placenta, clinical perspectives,* Rockville, Md, 1987, Aspen.
135. Ueland K et al: Special considerations in the use of cardiovascular drugs, *Clin Obstet Gynecol* 24:809, 1981.
136. Vintzileos AM, Campbell WA, Rodes JF: Fetal biophysical profile scoring: current status, *Clinics in Perinatology* 16:661, 1989.
137. Wall RE: Nutritional problems during pregnancy. In Abrams RS, Wexler P, editors: *Medical care of the pregnant patient,* Boston, 1983, Little, Brown.
138. Watson RM, Lane AT, Barnett NK: Neonatal lupus erythematosus, *Medicine* 63:362, 1984.
139. Whittemore R: Congenital heart disease: its impact on pregnancy, *Hosp Pract* 18:65, 1983.
140. Witter FR, King TM, Blake DA: Adverse effects of cardiovascular drug therapy on the fetus and neonate, *Obstet Gynecol* 58(suppl):100S, 1981.
141. Zackai EJ et al: The fetal trimethadione syndrome, *J Pediatr* 87:280, 1975.
142. Zakarija M, McKenzie M: Pregnancy-associated changes in the thyroid-stimulating antibody of Graves' disease and the relationship to neonatal hyperthyroidism, *J Clin Endocrinol Metab* 57:1036, 1983.
143. Zuspan FP, Rayburn WF: Drug abuse during pregnancy. In Rayburn FP, Zuspan FP, editors: *Drug therapy in obstetrics and gynecology,* ed 3, St Louis, 1992, Mosby.

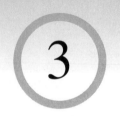

Regionalization and Transport in Perinatal Care

Gary Pettett, Sally Sewell, Gerald B. Merenstein

Regionalization

Regionalization can be defined as a process of resource allocation or service delivery based on geographic boundaries.[11,19] Frequently employed in the business and industrial sectors, regionalization improves service delivery and efficiency by reducing costly duplication of operations. Advocates have urged its implementation in a variety of health care settings for more than 60 years.[32] As the result of a series of legislative, professional, and local community efforts, regionalization emerged in the 1960s as the organizational model for efforts to improve the reproductive outcome of pregnant women.

In 1966 the American Medical Association (AMA) Committee on Maternal and Child Care focused attention on the relatively stagnant trend in infant mortality in the United States.[13] Despite its role as a leader in the industrialized world, infant mortality in the United States lagged significantly behind that of other westernized countries. The committee emphasized the need for the identification of risk factors and problems associated with prematurity; more efficient use of human resources; development of research in perinatal biology; and the education of obstetricians, pediatricians, and expectant parents on appropriate health care. Two major pieces of federal legislation related to regionalized health care were passed by the Eighty-ninth Congress. Public Law 89-239, Regional Medical Programs (RMPs), concentrated on delivery of service by disease category, and Public Law 89-749, Comprehensive Health Planning (CHP), dealt with plans for using resources. Unfortunately, neither act carried any significant administrative or fiscal authority.

In 1971 the AMA[2] policy statement, "Centralized Community or Regionalized Perinatal Inten-

sive Care," pressed for the development of centrally operated special care facilities. It encouraged the training of personnel, formulation of guidelines and evaluations, and development of adequate facilities. The AMA Maternal and Child Care Committee was directed to establish the necessary guidelines for regional perinatal programs.[3] In 1972, in conjunction with the National Foundation-March of Dimes, representatives of the American Academy of Pediatrics, the American College of Obstetricians and Gynecologists, the American Academy of Family Physicians, and the AMA met to draft these guidelines. Operating as the Committee on Perinatal Health, their recommendations were published in 1975.[52] In 1990, at the request of the American Academy of Pediatrics and the American College of Obstetricians and Gynecologists, the March of Dimes convened a new committee on perinatal health. Their recommendations were published in 1993.[33] In addition to continued support for regionalization, the committee emphasized the need for (1) health promotion and health awareness, (2) reproductive awareness, (3) perinatal regional structure and accountability, and (4) preconception and interconception care. Additional recommendations were also included. Federal expansion of Title V (Social Security Act of 1935) by Public Law 92-345 required each state to develop programs in intensive infant care that addressed the location of perinatal centers, type of care offered, type of transport systems used, and plans for regionalization.

Administrative and financial authority for regionalization was given new strength with the passage of Public Law 93-641, the National Health Planning and Resource Development Act. The intent of this legislation was to standardize effective methods of delivering health care, redistribute health care facilities, and offset the increasing costs of health care. Planning was facilitated by establishing Health Systems Agencies (HSA) or State Health Planning Agencies. Regional goals were to be developed by joint efforts of health care professionals and local citizenry working within a health department or HSA subunit. By 1979 there were approximately 200 regional neonatal centers in the United States.[51] Only four states had not developed a regional plan for perinatal care.[13] The success of regional programs in reducing neonatal mortality is well documented.*

The American Academy of Pediatrics and the American College of Obstetricians and Gynecologists have developed guidelines for the regional

organization of perinatal services.[22] A conceptual model based on these recommendations is shown in Figure 3-1. Level I facilities (basic care) provide continuing care for neonates with relatively minor problems not requiring advanced diagnostic or therapeutic support. Most level I units can also provide convalescent care for infants from level II and level III facilities. Level II facilities (specialty care) primarily provide neonatal expertise for moderately low-birth-weight babies (1500 to 2500 g, 32 to 36 weeks' gestation) from relatively healthy participants. Level III units (subspecialty care) provide a combination of neonatal and maternal fetal services to those at the highest risk (<1500 g birth weight or <32 weeks' gestation). Included in this latter category are women who

*References 9, 37, 40, 45, 50, 53, 57–59.

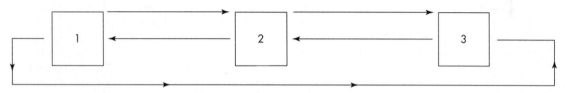

Level 1 to level 2

Complicated cases not requiring intensive care

Level 1 to level 3

Complicated cases requiring intensive care

Level 1 (responsibilities)

1. Uncomplicated maternity and neonatal care for areas not served by other units
2. Emergency management of unexpected complications

Special services

1. Early identification of high-risk patients
2. Preventive and social services

Level 2 to level 3

Complicated cases requiring intensive care
1. Labor less than 34 weeks' gestation
2. Severe isoimmune disease
3. Severe medical complications
4. Anticipated need for neonatal surgery

Level 2 (responsibilities)

1. Complete maternity and neonatal care for uncomplicated and most high-risk patients

Special services

1. 15-minute start-up time for cesarean section
2. 24-hour in-house anesthesia for obstetrics
3. Short-term assisted ventilation of newborn
4. 24-hour clinical laboratory services
5. 24-hour radiology services
6. 24-hour blood bank services
7. Fetal monitoring
8. Special care nursery

Level 3 or level 2 to hospital of origin

For growth and development of infants no longer requiring intensive care

Level 3 (responsibilities)

1. Complete maternity and neonatal care plus intensive care of intrapartum and neonatal high-risk patients

Special services

1. 24-hour consultation service for region
2. Coordination of transport system
3. Development and coordination of educational program for region
4. Data analysis for region

Figure 3-1   Consultation and possible transfer patterns in regional system. (From Ryan GM: *Am J Obstet Gynecol* 46:375, 1975.

require specialized medical care and/or fetuses with identified serious malformations. Unfortunately, regionalization has not fared well in the current economic environment. Traditional concepts of regionalization have frequently given way to the economic forces of a more competitive health-care market. The increasing availability of trained neonatal-perinatal specialists, wider dissemination of new technologies, and the growth of managed health care have encouraged many hospitals to expand their perinatal services, primarily in response to patient care activities. Integration of services within many of these new health-care plans and rapidly merging hospital systems has fostered the duplication of perinatal services in the guise of providing a "more competitive" market. Ironically, the result has often been a greater fragmentation of perinatal services. As the complexity of health care needs increases, access to specialized services within many plans and/or delivery systems actually becomes more restrictive and difficult to obtain. Within the same hospital there is often a wide disparity in the level of care for obstetric, neonatal, surgical, and other critical support services.[15] Whether managed care programs can provide critical care services as efficiently as they provide preventive services remains a serious and unanswered question.

Although this growing "deregionalization" of perinatal services may provide immediate benefits to local hospitals and perinatal professionals, the long-term advantage to the patient and community is less clear. Cost control and universal access are two of the most important issues affecting perinatal health care today. Despite the recent advances in perinatal care, neonatal mortality in the United States remains higher than in many European and Asian countries. In part this disparity reflects the uneven effect of improved perinatal care on the population. Racial and ethnic minorities continue to have neonatal mortality rates 1.5 to 2.0 times that of whites. Excess mortality is related to the persistent high rates of premature and low-birth-weight infants in the United States, particularly among disadvantaged minorities. Evidence suggests that this gap may be widening, with the burden of poor pregnancy outcome falling more acutely on those women or families least likely to have adequate financial resources or access to comprehensive care.

Rapidly increasing costs are an important problem for those who underwrite perinatal care. Newborn intensive care units are currently among the most expensive hospital services.[26,36,48,49] The development of specialized high-risk obstetric and neonatal units requires a substantial capital investment in both personnel and high-technology equipment. Continuing improvements in diagnostic and therapeutic techniques, such as high-resolution ultrasonography, magnetic resonance imaging, high-frequency ventilation, ECMO, and surfactant replacement therapy, add to the rising costs of neonatal-perinatal care. The central role of specialized perinatal facilities in lowering the infant and neonatal mortality rate has, to some extent, exempted them from cost containment efforts. However, as the bill for these services continues to increase, many federal, state, and commercial insurers may feel more compelled to consider methods for controlling perinatal costs.

How successfully we address these issues may largely determine the nature of neonatal and maternal-fetal medicine in the not-too-distant future. The need for more cost-effective utilization of resources and improved access to perinatal care is a strong argument for the continued support of regional organization. Perhaps as Merkatz suggested in 1976, it is time to more forcefully explore the incorporation of regional perinatal programs into our pluralistic system of health care.[38]

Despite current economic pressures, regionalization of perinatal care continues to provide a framework for ensuring that the relatively small number of perinatal patients at the highest risk for a poor outcome have timely access to the appropriate medical facilities, equipment, and personnel. The ultimate objective is to improve reproductive outcome by reducing perinatal morbidity and mortality in the most cost-effective and care-efficient manner.

Transport

Because of the increasing complexity of perinatal care and the emphasis on early access, triage of perinatal patients has assumed growing importance. High-risk perinatal patients need to be identified during the early prenatal period, intrapartum period, and neonatal period. Participating hospitals must establish criteria for the transfer of patients within the region and develop support systems for consultation, laboratory services, education, and patient transport.

An interhospital transport service is an essential component of a regional perinatal program. Based on established referral criteria, the transport service gives high-risk patients timely access to the appropriate services without interrupting their care. Return or "back" transports move recovering patients from tertiary centers to local community hospitals for completion of convalescent care in preparation for discharge from the hospital. The transport service is an important factor in the efficient management of regional bed space.

Maternal (Obstetric) Referrals

The identification of high-risk perinatal patients begins with antepartum surveillance. During the first prenatal visits the physician or nurse obtains medical, social, and demographic information pertinent to the mother's health and fetal well-being.[21,25,27] Early identification of factors that can affect pregnancy outcome is important in developing appropriate diagnostic and treatment plans to minimize potential maternal and neonatal morbidity.[23,38,41,43,46] A list of factors derived from the history and physical examination that may increase pregnancy and neonatal risk is included in Box 3-1.

Although there is a strong correlation between antenatal risk factors and subsequent outcome in large population studies, risk assessment does not reliably predict the outcome of an individual pregnancy.[24,56] Women who are found to be at high risk during the antepartum period should be considered candidates for further evaluation and closer surveillance. Where a risk of uteroplacental insufficiency exists, evaluation of fetal well-being (e.g., BPP, CST, NST) may be indicated (see Chapter 2.) Consultation and referral decisions will have to be made based on the results of a thorough evaluation of each individual patient.[10]

On the other hand, certain maternal conditions more predictably require specialized care in a perinatal center (Box 3-2).[8] Evidence of these disorders should prompt a more timely consultation and consideration for referral. Transfer to a combined obstetric-neonatal intensive care facility may be especially necessary when these conditions are accompanied by the potential for delivery of an infant before 34 weeks of gestation and/or at an estimated weight of less than 2000 g.

Neonatal Referrals

Despite efforts to identify high-risk perinatal patients during the antepartum period, as many as 30% to 50% of infants who ultimately require additional neonatal care will not be recognized until the late intrapartum or early neonatal periods.[31] The critically ill neonate must have immediate care and stabilization at the time of delivery. Supportive care needs to be maintained until either the infant is out of danger or the transport team has arrived and assumed care.

For high-risk infants who do not require immediate resuscitation, potential problems can be identified from a systematic assessment of birth weight and gestational age.[4,5,7,16,42] Additional problems may be identified through systematic observation of the newborn infant. Stabilization and intervention procedures should be directed toward the prevention or treatment of the most likely complications.[34,35]

The decision to transfer a high-risk neonate should be based on predetermined criteria. Premature infants less than 32 weeks' gestation will generally need specialized physiologic support and should be cared for in a well-equipped intensive care unit. Between 33 and 37 weeks' gestation, premature infants can frequently be managed in a less complicated environment. Attention to thermal support, glucose levels, fluid therapy, hematocrit, bilirubin, ventilation, and perfusion is important but may frequently be of a lower order of magnitude than in the very small infant.

Communication and Consultation

The communication system is an important factor in any regional perinatal program. The rapidly advancing field of telecommunications offers a wide variety of opportunities for transmitting medical information.

A central dedicated telephone line can provide direct and immediate access to the regional center and should be staffed 24 hours a day, 7 days a week. The line must be unencumbered by other requirements of the center. Access should be made as easy as possible. Utilizing a single telephone number to

---

Box 3-1

Maternal Risk Factors Frequently Elicited from High-Risk Pregnancies

I. Prenatal
A. History
  1. Sociodemographic
    a. Low socioeconomic status
    b. Ethnic minority
    c. Low educational level
    d. Emotional instability
    e. Substance abuse
      (1) Alcohol
      (2) Drugs
      (3) Cigarettes
    f. Age <15, >35
  2. Medical-obstetric
    a. Moderate to severe renal disease
    b. Chronic hypertension
    c. Moderate to severe toxemia
    d. Organic heart disease, class 2-4
    e. Prior Rh sensitization, prior erythro-blastosis fetalis
    f. Previous stillbirth
    g. Previous premature infant
    h. Previous neonatal death
    i. Previous cesarean section
    j. Habitual abortion
    k. Prior birth >10 lb
    l. Sickle cell disease
    m. History of tuberculosis (TB) or purified protein derivative (PPD) +
    n. History of genital herpes
B. Physical examination/prenatal follow-up
  1. Severe toxemia, hypertension
  2. Severe renal disease
  3. Severe heart disease, class 2-4
  4. Acute pyelonephritis
  5. Diabetes mellitus
  6. Uterine malformation
  7. Incompetent cervix
  8. Abnormal fetal position
  9. Polyhydramnios, oligohydramnios
  10. Abnormal cervical cytology
    a. Dysplasia
    b. Herpes
  11. Multiple pregnancy
  12. Rh sensitization
  13. Positive serology
  14. Vaginal bleeding
II. Intrapartum
A. Maternal
  1. Moderate to severe toxemia
  2. Polyhydramnios, oligohydramnios
  3. Amnionitis
  4. Uterine rupture
  5. Premature rupture of membranes
  6. Premature labor
  7. Labor lasting >20 hr
  8. Second stage of labor >2½ hr
  9. Precipitous labor (<3 hr)
  10. Prolonged latent phase of labor
  11. Uterine tetany
B. Placenta
  1. Placenta previa
  2. Abruptio placentae
  3. Postdates (>42 weeks' gestation)
  4. Meconium-stained amniotic fluid
C. Fetal
  1. Abnormal presentation
  2. Multiple pregnancy
  3. Fetal bradycardia
  4. Prolapsed cord
  5. Fetal weight <2500 g
  6. Fetal acidosis, pH <7.25
  7. Fetal tachycardia
  8. Operative/vacuum delivery
  9. Difficult forceps delivery

---

contact the center with subsequent distribution of calls simplifies the process for the referring community. Toll-free or "800" numbers can be employed. Appropriate consultants must be available at all times. The use of mobile phones, the ability to transfer calls or setup conference calls, and the ready availability of fax technology enhance access to consultants.

The success of the initial call may be crucial to the infant's intact survival. Ongoing stabilization of the infant before the arrival of the transport team is critical, particularly in those regions where service

---

Box 3-2

Maternal Conditions Requiring Specialized Perinatal Care

I. Obstetric complications
   A. Premature rupture of the fetal membranes
   B. Premature onset of labor
   C. Severe preeclampsia or hypertension
   D. Multiple gestation
   E. Intrauterine growth retardation with evidence of fetal distress
   F. Third-trimester bleeding
   G. Rh isoimmunization
   H. Premature cervical dilation
II. Medical complications
   A. Maternal infection that may affect the fetus or lead to premature birth
   B. Severe organic heart disease, class 3-4
   C. Thyrotoxicosis
   D. Renal disease with deteriorating function or hypertension
   E. Drug overdose
III. Surgical complications
   A. Trauma requiring intensive care
   B. Acute abdominal emergency
   C. Thoracic emergency requiring intensive care

---

immediate care plans. Ideally, staff at the receiving center would make frequent calls to the parents and referring staff, keeping them informed on both progress and problems. At all times a line of immediate contact must be available in case the patient's condition suddenly changes.

Preparation for Transport

The goal of every transport is to bring the high-risk or critically-ill patient to the tertiary center in stable condition. Federal guidelines enacted through COBRA (Congressional Budget Reconciliation Act) legislation now specify certain activities that must occur as part of the transport of any patient from one facility to another. Included in these guidelines are definitions of stable patients and a description of the types of communication that must occur to ensure the proper availability of services at the receiving hospital. Stabilization of patients for transport should actually begin before the transport team arrives. Specific areas of attention may be determined in initial communications between the referring physician and hospital and the transport team or its medical control officer.

The most common reasons for antenatal maternal referral include premature rupture of the membranes, premature onset of labor, and pregnancy-associated hypertension. Factors that require a thorough assessment before transport include fetal well-being, stage or likelihood of labor, and the probability of delivery en route. A good physical and obstetric examination, prenatal record review, and evaluation of fetal heart rate and activity would constitute a minimum evaluation. After consultation with the receiving hospital, further measures may be indicated before transport, depending on the referring hospital's capabilities. These may include an ultrasound examination, NST, fetal scalp pH, or amniocentesis. If indicated, magnesium sulfate, tocolytic agents, antibiotic agents, or antihypertensive agents may be administered. Although the reasons for neonatal referral may be quite diverse, the most common indications include respiratory distress, prematurity, congenital anomalies (surgical and nonsurgical), and suspected congenital heart disease. Stabilization and support of these infants may require frequent interhospital communication (referring

areas are large and transport times are long. The ability to assess the infant's condition accurately and to provide management can be facilitated by the use of a standard list of questions and information that should be obtained.

Whether the calls are received by a physician, transport team member, or professionally (medically) trained dispatcher will vary with different regional programs. Junior personnel (trainees) and staff members who are not active in newborn or maternal transport should not perform this function.

A final and frequently overlooked priority in communication occurs at the conclusion of a transport. Once the patient has arrived at the receiving center, a call should be placed to the referring physician, parents, and/or spouse. The purpose of the call is to relay information regarding the patient's condition and to indicate the scope of physician and transport medical officer) to identify specific interventions. Upon arrival of the transport team, the receiving hospital will generally assume control of the infant's care, although a certain degree of flexibility and cooperation with the referring staff will be maintained. A complete copy of the patient's records (hospital and prenatal), results of any laboratory tests, heart rate monitor strips, x-ray examination, and notation of all medications (with the times and doses given) should be ready to accompany the patient.

A properly fixed placenta should be sent to the receiving hospital for pathologic examination. The mother or infant should always remain at the hospital until the transport team arrives. It is never wise to send the patient ahead with plans to meet the transport team at an alternate location however expedient it may seem.

Whenever possible, the transport team should make contact with the parents (in a neonatal transport) or spouse (in a maternal transport) before departing for the center. This offers the parents or spouse the opportunity to meet the interim care team, ask questions, and receive information about where and how the patient will be cared for. The transport team leader can explain how the transport will occur, approximately how long it will take, and what will be done en route.

Information regarding the tertiary center should be left with the parents. This should include the following:

- Exact location of the unit—address, map
- Visiting hours and hospital rules
- Telephone numbers
- Names of individuals likely to be involved with the patient's care
- Information on the special care unit—what it is, what it does
- Location of parking facilities, nearby lodging, and rules regarding young children (siblings)
- Any particular rules or regulations regarding the special care unit

Transport Team

Transport teams may be composed of a variety of medical personnel, including neonatologists, neonatal nurse practitioners, registered nurses, respiratory therapists, paramedics, and emergency medical technicians.[41,55] There are two general categories of transport teams: dedicated and nondedicated. The decision of which type of team to use largely depends on institutional factors. These factors often include the unit's acuity of care, annual volume of transports, financial support, and state or local laws regarding the expanded role of nurses in health care. Regardless of the team composition, the team must have the cumulative expertise to resuscitate, stabilize, and provide critical care throughout the transport.[5]

Nondedicated teams are usually made up of staff nurses within the neonatal intensive care unit (NICU).[7,11] The advantage to having a unit based, nondedicated transport team is the large pool of trained personnel available around the clock. Qualifications of team members can be based on their daily bedside critical care experience and supplemental education such as certification as a neonatal resuscitation provider. When the neonate is critically ill and more advanced procedures may be anticipated, a physician or nurse practitioner may be added to the team.[20] The primary disadvantage to this team design is that the transport nurse's patient assignments must be absorbed by the unit until he or she returns. However, unit based teams are usually very cost effective because critical care skills are maintained during regular patient care, advanced skill training may be more focused, and the administrative oversight duties are diminished.

Dedicated transport teams originated in the 1980s when large metropolitan hospitals began to experience an increase in the demand for neonatal transports. These teams are often composed of a nurse designated as team leader and a second nurse or a respiratory therapist as a partner. Nurse-led teams have been shown to provide better continuity of care, improved documentation, better maintenance of transport equipment, improved team availability, stronger liaisons with referring hospitals, and reduced overall operating costs.[15] The principal advantage to dedicated teams includes their immediate around-the-clock availability and their advanced training in neonatal resuscitation and stabilization procedures. However, the additional personnel required for dedicated teams may make these teams expensive to maintain.

Participation on a transport team requires leadership qualities, an ability to prioritize and organize care, and skill in handling stressful situations. A minimum of 2 years of neonatal experience with 1 year of NICU experience is a basic requirement of most transport services. Nurses who specialize in neonatal transport should have a basic understanding of neonatal pathophysiology, stabilization and resuscitation techniques, ventilatory management, and x-ray interpretation. Nurses who function as team leaders should have advanced training in endotracheal intubation, umbilical vessel catheterization, and thoracentesis. When transport by aircraft is a service component, an understanding of flight physiology and flight safety is often required. Specific standards of care for neonatal transport have been developed by the National Association of Neonatal Nurses Practice Committee.[44] Written treatment protocols should be developed by each transport service. These protocols should be directed and authorized by the team's medical director and should be updated or expanded on a regular basis.

Because of the large volume of transports involving respiratory distress, respiratory therapists have been involved in a growing number of neonatal transports. Our service utilizes a nurse and a respiratory therapist as the basic dedicated transport team. The respiratory therapist has proven to be a valuable asset in pulmonary stabilization and airway or ventilatory management. Respiratory therapists possess a more detailed knowledge of the transport respiratory equipment, ventilators, and oxygen delivery systems, obviating the need for additional technical training of nurses. The respiratory therapist must acquire the same knowledge base as the nurse counterpart. Joint training and review sessions have allowed us to standardize our instructional programs and have provided the opportunity to engender a cohesive team attitude.

Continuing education is essential for all team members. Procedural skills training should be performed on a regular (annual, semiannual, quarterly, etc.) basis to maintain competency. Educational opportunities are also provided through periodic case reviews, topic-specific lectures, outreach teaching activities, and operational (clinical) research projects.

Equipment

The equipment and medications required for neonatal transport are similar to those used in the NICU. Box 3-3 provides a list of common transport equipment and medications. Essential items are those for physiologic (heart rate, respiratory rate, blood pressure, pulse oximetry) monitoring, temperature support, infusion therapy, and ventilatory support.

Because much of the major equipment is electronic, these units must be easily adaptable to the types of power supply used in transport. All electronic equipment used in transport should be supplied with battery-operated capability. The batteries should be able to support the equipment for the entire transport if no other power source is available. Conversion devices are often needed to adapt equipment to various ambulance and aircraft power supplies. Adequate grounding of electrical equipment is as important during transport as it is in the special care unit. Equipment used in air transport must also meet Federal Aviation Agency (FAA) requirements. Some of the monitoring devices on the market today may interfere with aircraft navigational equipment. Equipment of this type should not be taken on air transport, particularly where instrument flying may be necessary.

The transport incubator is the central piece of neonatal equipment. It must be capable of controlling the infant's immediate environmental condition and allowing sufficient access to manage a critically ill patient. If extremes in environmental temperature may be encountered, the transport team should understand the incubator's capabilities and limits. Transport incubators should be of double-wall design to assist with thermal wall support. Where extremely low temperatures might be encountered, additional equipment or insulation devices (thermal incubator hood, warming blanket and plexiglass, cellophane, and plastic "bubble heat shields) may be necessary. The incubator should be mounted on or built into an easily movable stand that can be locked into position during transport. Some transport modules are designed with incubator and ancillary monitoring equipment in a single configuration. Because the incubator and monitoring equipment will need to be lifted on and off the transport vehicle, total weight becomes an important factor in selecting these units. The unit must be light enough to be easily lifted by the crew or transport team.

Because many neonates are transported for reasons of respiratory distress, oxygen and air-

Box 3-3

Neonatal Transport Equipment

Equipment

Transport incubator*
Cardiorespiratory monitor*
Blood pressure monitor*
Suction apparatus*
Thermometer with skin probe*
Oxygen analyzer*
IV infusion pump*
Laryngoscope (various sizes)*
Transcutaneous oxygen monitor*
Pulse oximeter*
Oxygen hood
Nebulizer
Light source*
Oxygen/air cylinders
Stethoscope
Blood pressure transducers

Supplies

Suction catheters (6, 8, 10 Fr.)
Bulb/ear syringe
Feeding tubes (5, 8 Fr.)
Umbilical artery catheters (3.5, 5, 8 Fr.)
Thoracostomy tubes
DeLee suction catheter
Three-way stopcocks
Blunt needle catheter adapter (18–20 gauge)
Scalp vein needles (21, 23, 25 gauge)
Intracaths (22–24 gauge)
IV pump tubing
Alcohol swabs
Skin prep swabs
Povidine-iodine (swabs and solution)
Umbilical ligature
4-0 silk suture with needle
Tape (½, 1-inch)
Glucose screening strips
Lancets
Capillary tubes
Culture bottles (aerobic/anaerobic)
Syringes (various sizes)
Needles (various sizes)
Gauze pad (2 × 2, 4 × 4)
Monitor leads
IV filters
Sterile water vials
Bacteriostatic saline
Endotracheal tubes (2.5, 3, 3.5, 4 mm)

Endotracheal tube stylets
Heimlich valves
Flashlight batteries
Laryngoscope bulbs
Y-connectors
Oxygen tubing
Diapers
Blanket
Umbilical catheter tray
Plastic bag
Oxygen face mask (0, 1, 2 sizes)
Resuscitation bag
Chemical warming blanket

Drugs

Albumin 5%
Atropine multidose vial
10% Calcium gluconate solution
$D_{10}W$, 250 ml IV bags
D_5W, 250 ml IV bags
Digoxin, 0.5 mg ampule
Heparin, 1000 u/ml
Isuprel, 0.5 mg ampule
Tolazoline, 25 mg/ml
Lasix, 20 mg ampule
Lidocaine multidose vial
Narcan, 0.4 mg ampule
Sodium bicarbonate, 0.5 mEq/ml
Valium, 10 mg vial
Phenobarbital, 120 mg vial
Fentanyl
Ampicillin
Gentamicin
Aquamephyton, 10 mg ampule
Dopamine
Dobutamine
Pavulon
Epinepherine 1:10,000
Ringer's lactate, 250 ml
Prostaglandin, 500 µg/ml
Heparinized flush solution
Surfactant
Adenosine, 2 mg
Cefotaxime
Decadron, 4 mg/ml
Morphine, 2 mg/ml
Vecuronium, 10 mg

* Battery operated/back-up system.

blended mixtures are essential. The most convenient gas container for transport is the compressed gas cylinder. The FAA has strict regulations about compressed gas cylinders in aircraft. The transport team should be familiar with these regulations and use appropriately designed cylinders.[18,54] The capacity of standard gas cylinders and expected life of the cylinder at various flow rates are listed in Table 3-1. Table 3-2 gives the flow rates of oxygen and air required to produce various oxygen concentrations (FIo_2).

Regardless of the type of equipment purchased, maintenance and servicing are important considerations:

- Replacement parts should be readily available.
- Hospital biomedical engineers should be familiar with the equipment and provide routine preventive and reparative maintenance.
- Local equipment representatives should be available to service the equipment and provide technical updates to the transport team.

- Warranty and maintenance contracts should be easily obtained.
- Loan equipment should be available when major equipment is being repaired.

Maternal transports may require additional equipment to monitor and support both the mother and fetus. A list of additional items is provided in Box 3-4. At the completion of each transport, the equipment should be checked, batteries charged, and supplies restocked. A checklist of these functions kept with the transport equipment can help ensure timely completion and preparation for the next call. As the equipment used in the NICU has become more sophisticated, so has that in the transport environment. Portable, hand-held analysis instruments are now being used by a number of transport systems. Depending on the device used, these instruments provide the capability of measuring blood gases, glucose, hemoglobin, hematocrit, and electrolytes on small samples of blood obtained during transport. However, the opportunity to measure blood chemistries en-route also raises the problems of standardization and quality control. We

Table 3-1
Volume and Flow Duration of Oxygen in Two Sizes of Cylinders

	Full		¾ Full		½ Full		¼ Full	
Reading on cylinder pressure gauge								
Pressure (lb/in²)	244		183		122		61	
Cylinder type	E	H	E	H	E	H	E	H
Contents ((ft³)	22	244	16.5	183	11	122	5.5	61
(liters)	622	6900	466	5175	311	3450	155	1725
Approximate number of hours of flow								
Cylinder type	E	H	E	H	E	H	E	H
Flow rate (liters/min)								
2	5.1	56	3.8	42	2.5	28	1.3	14
4	2.5	28	1.8	21	1.2	14	0.6	7
6	1.7	18.5	1.3	13.7	0.9	9.2	0.4	4.5
8	1.2	14	0.9	10.5	0.6	7	0.3	3.5
10	1.0	11	0.7	8.2	0.5	5.5	0.2	2.7
12	0.8	9.2	0.6	6.7	0.4	4.5	0.2	2.2
15	0.6	7.2	0.4	5.5	0.3	3.5	0.1	1.7

From Segal S: *Transport of high risk newborn infants,* 1972, Canadian Pediatric Society.

Table 3-2
Effective Flo$_2$ Delivery from Various Combinations of Air and Oxygen Flow*

		VIo$_2$ V (oxygen flow in liters/min)								
		1	**2**	**3**	**4**	**5**	**6**	**7**	**8**	**9**
V$_{air}$ (air flow in liters/min)	10	0.93	0.87	0.82	0.77	0.74	0.70	0.67	0.65	0.63
	9	0.92	0.86	0.80	0.76	0.72	0.68	0.65	0.63	0.61
	8	0.91	0.84	0.76	0.74	0.70	0.66	0.63	0.61	0.58
	7	0.90	0.82	0.76	0.71	0.67	0.64	0.61	0.58	0.56
	6	0.89	0.80	0.74	0.68	0.64	0.61	0.57	0.55	0.53
	5	0.87	0.77	0.70	0.65	0.61	0.57	0.54	0.51	0.49
	4	0.84	0.74	0.66	0.61	0.56	0.53	0.50	0.47	0.45
	3	0.80	0.68	0.61	0.55	0.51	0.47	0.45	0.43	0.41
	2	0.74	0.61	0.53	0.47	0.44	0.41	0.39	0.37	0.35
	1	0.61	0.47	0.41	0.37	0.34	0.32	0.30	0.30	0.29

$$*Flo_2 = \frac{0.21\ VIo_2 + V_{air}}{V_{air} + VIo_2}$$

From Ferrara A, Harin A: *Emergency transfer of the high-risk neonate,* St Louis, 1980, Mosby.

have enlisted the assistance of our hospital to provide analytic standards and quality control monitoring to fulfill current Clinical Laboratory Improvement Act (CLIA) requirements. In addition, results obtained during transport can be downloaded directly to our laboratory computer and printed to the patient's medical record upon arrival.

Over the last 10 years, advances in respiratory support have included the development of patient-triggered ventilators, high-frequency ventilation, and ECMO. Although none have been specifically adapted to the transport setting, anecdotal reports of the use of high-frequency ventilation[1] and ECMO[14,17] during transport have appeared. As the need for these services becomes more apparent and interest in their use during transport increases, it is possible that specific transport equipment may be made available.

Specific Therapeutic Modalities

Surfactant

The endotracheal administration of exogenous surfactant, either prophylactically or as a rescue therapy, has been shown to significantly reduce morbidity and mortality from RDS (see Chapter 22). Its use in other neonatal respiratory disorders such as meconium aspiration and prolonged mechanical ventilation, though as yet unproven, is receiving increasing attention. Since respiratory disorders continue to account for the majority of neonatal transports, the use of surfactant in the transport setting deserves careful evaluation. Techniques for the administration of surfactant must be closely observed. Whether given by transport personnel or the referring hospital staff, experience with the method of administration is important. The endotracheal tube must be in proper location to ensure a uniform distribution of the surface active material as possible. Confirmation of proper tube placement via chest x-ray examination is an important safety check. In VLBW infants (<1500 g), surfactant may need to be administered in small aliquots to prevent airway occlusion and further respiratory compromise. After treatment, it is important to reestablish ventilatory stabilization. Effective therapy may produce fairly rapid changes in lung compliance. Failure to recognize clinical improvement with appropriate ventilatory adjustments increases the risk of alveolar overdistention and pulmonary airleaks (e.g., pneumothorax, pneumomediastinum). As a result, surfactant therapy may increase stabilization time at the referring hospital. If, however, respiratory control is improved, it may be time well spent.

Box 3-4

Maternal Transport Equipment

Equipment

IV infusion pump*
IV stand/poles
Blood pressure monitor*
Fetal heart rate monitor*
Portable light source*
Stainless steel buckets and basins
Speculum
Scissors

Supplies

Kelly clamps (4)
Cord clamps
Sponges (4 × 4)
Tape
Surgeon's gloves
Suture set
Assorted suture material
Pudendal block set
Tourniquet
Suction bulb
Adult oxygen masks and nasal cannula
Red-topped blood collection tubes
Povidinde-iodine sticks
0.5 Normal saline, 1000 ml
D₅W, 1000 ml
Ringer's lactate, 1000 ml

Blood administration set
Assorted syringes
Assorted needles
Assorted angiocaths
Adult arm boards

Drugs

Demerol, 50 and 75 mg ampules
Apresoline, 20 mg ampule
Narcan, adult, 0.4 mg ampule
Magnesium sulfate, 10% IV solution, 50% IM solution
Phenobarbital, 120 mg vial
Phenergan, 25 mg/ml
Diazoxide, 300 mg ampule
Lasix, 20 or 40 mg
Vistaril, 50 mg/ml
Pitocin, 10 u/ml
Calcium gluconate, 1 g/10 ml
Methergine, 0.2 mg/ml
Lidocaine, 1%, without epinephrine
Isoxsuprine, 10 mg/ml
Terbutaline, 80 mg in 500 ml D₅ ¼NS
Ritodrine, 150 mg/500 ml
Betamethasone

* Battery operated/back-up system.

Pulmonary hemorrhage as a result of improved lung compliance, reduced pulmonary vascular resistance, and increased left-to-right blood flow (patent ductus arteriosus [PDA], persistent foramen ovale [PFO]) is a significant, though infrequent, complication. Pretreatment with indomethacin to promote constriction of the ductus arteriosus has been suggested, but evidence of a true beneficial effect is as yet lacking.

In deciding to use or withhold surfactant, the transport team must carefully weigh the risks and benefits. At present we make decisions on a case-by-case basis. Surfactant is an expensive therapeutic agent. Once constituted, the manufacturer currently recommends only a single course per vial even though most small infants require much less than the full vial. Keeping a sufficient stock of surfactant for transport use or preparing surfactant in anticipation of its use do not seem to be practical alternatives. Our transport service restricts surfactant use to those infants in whom the medical control officer feels its use would be essential. Before leaving the receiving hospital, the transport team obtains surfactant from the hospital pharmacy but does not reconstitute the drug until the infant has been properly evaluated or an order to do so is obtained from the transport physician. At the completion of the transport, unused surfactant is returned to the hospital pharmacy where its utilization is closely monitored.

Prostaglandin E1

After respiratory distress, suspected congenital heart disease represents one of the next most common reasons for neonatal transport. Prostaglandin E1 is an effective drug for maintaining patency of the ductus arteriosus and in important palliative therapy for infants with ductal dependent heart lesions. Indications include cyanotic lesions, such as pulmonary artresia, transposition with intact septum, tricuspid artresia, and Tetralogy of Fallot, as well as acyanotic lesions including interrupted aortic arch, coarctation of the aorta, and hypoplastic left ventricle.

Unfortunately, confirmation of a defect or a description of the anatomy is often not available in the pretransport setting. Clinical indicators of congenital heart disease include persistent cyanosis (particularly that unresponsive to oxygen enrichment or ventilatory support), diminished peripheral pulses (weak or thready quality), poor perfusion and delayed capillary refill time, persistent metabolic acidosis, and hypotension. The absence of a heart murmur is not particularly reassuring, although its presence may be further suggestive of a heart defect. We have not found that the administration of prostaglandin on clinical grounds has significantly compromised the clinical course of infants even when no heart lesion is found on subsequent evaluation.

Prostaglandin must be given intravenously to be effective. Although this may include either a peripheral or central IV, we prefer the central (umbilical vein) route to ensure proper distribution and to provide central venous access for further therapy and support. The most common side effects of prostaglandin are bradycardia, cutaneous flushing, splotchy cutaneous rash, hyperthermia, hypotension, and apnea. Apnea tends to be most frequent in those infants who also have an elevated Pco_2. The transport team should be prepared to intubate or to provide additional inotropic support should serious complications occur.

Sedation and Paralysis

The use of sedative and paralyzing agents may be required to achieve adequate oxygenation and ventilation. Most frequently, this occurs in larger infants with meconium aspiration syndrome and/or persistant pulmonary hypertension. Many of these infants have only marginal respiratory gas exchange that is further compromised by agitation and asynchronous ventilation.

Among the most commonly used agents are fentanyl and morphine for sedation and pancuronium or vecuronium for paralysis. Fentanyl is a rapidly-acting drug that may be administered by either intravenous bolus or continuous infusion. It is a short-acting agent that can be reversed by discontinuing administration of narcan. It does not increase intracranial pressure but can produce bradycardia, hypotension, apnea, and muscle rigidity as side effects. Morphine, though similar to fentanyl, has a longer duration of action. Side effects include increasing intracranial pressure, decreased intestinal motility, respiratory depression, and peripheral vasodilation.

Pancuronium and vencuronium are neuromuscular blocking agents that act as cholinergic antagonists at the neuromuscular end-plate. Both have a near immediate onset of action. Several clinical states not uncommon to the transported infant may either potentiate or antagonize the effects of these medications. Although preterm infants may be particularly sensitive to neuromuscular blockade, acidosis, hypothermia, hypokalemia, and renal insufficiency may potentiate their effect even further. Antagonists include alkalosis, hyperkalemia, and the use of epinephrine. Paralyzing agents should not be used in the absence of sedation and/or analgesia since neither of these agents materially alters pain or pain perception. With the loss of spontaneous respiratory effort and chest wall stability, ventilatory support may need to be significantly increased after paralyzation. As with surfactant, restabilization of ventilatory support is often necessary before transporting paralyzed infants.

Nitric Oxide

The addition of small amounts (5 to 20 ppm) of nitric oxide (NO) to inspired gases of infants with pulmonary hypertension has been found to lower pulmonary vascular resistance and improve gas exchange (oxygenation).[28][29] Although it is still an experimental therapy, controlled clinical trials are currently underway to asses its efficacy and indication for administration. Inhaled NO is a particularly attractive therapy because of its selective action on the pulmonary vasculature. Prior therapeutic agents (e.g., tolazoline, priscoline) were of limited efficacy because of their generalized systemic and pulmonary vasodilatory actions.

The use of inhaled NO in the transport setting has received very little attention. A single anecdotal report involving six patients would indicate that this therapy may be adaptable to transport systems.[30] Pending the outcome of clinical trials and approval by the Food and Drug Administration, current usage of NO during transport should only be under properly approved protocol. Furthermore, since NO is a recognized noxious pollutant, its ultimate use during transport also requires adherence to safety considerations. The primary side effect of NO administration is the development of methemoglobinemia. However, the small quantities used and the relatively short duration of most neonatal transports would suggest that this will not be a major deterrent.

Mode of Transport

Selecting the proper mode of transport (ambulance, helicopter, or fixed-wing aircraft) may not always be a straightforward decision. Factors to consider include distance (round-trip), the severity of the illness, immediacy of specialty intervention (e.g., surgery, cardiac evaluation) and costs to the patient. As a general rule we have used ambulances for distances of up to 100 miles (one way), a helicopter for those from 100 to 200 miles, and fixed-wing aircraft for distances <200 miles. Weather becomes an important determinant for air transport. These decisions rest primarily with the pilot, as well they should. In some settings, different modes may be indicated for each leg of the transport. Nonavailability of aircraft or rapidly changing weather patterns may require a change in plans before the transport is completed.

Regardless of the mode of transport, there must be ample room to care for the patient. Smaller aircraft and low-topped ambulances frequently do not afford this capability. Helicopters have a major disadvantage. Once aboard a helicopter, the team and patient are exposed to an unusual amount of noise, vibration, and rotational forces. Many of these factors may have a direct effect on the critically-ill infant. Evaluation and monitoring of a patient may be almost impossible. On flights after dusk, lighting in the patient area may interfere with the pilot's night vision. If the mother or infant is not adequately stabilized before lift-off, they will not likely become so in flight. For patients whose condition is tenuous or who require constant attention, another mode of transport may be advisable.

Finally, there are a few miscellaneous cautions about selecting the transport vehicle. Never initiate a transfer with a crew that is unfamiliar with the craft. The FAA and many state or county health agencies have certifying procedures for ambulance or aircraft personnel. The regional center should always be sure that the patient and transport team are in the best possible hands for travel.

For each transport, alternative referral sites or temporary stops should be identified. Regardless of the amount of preparation, the possibility of vehicle malfunction or patient deterioration always exists. It may be necessary to stop temporarily for equipment or vehicle repair or for stabilization of the patient.

By whatever means the team is traveling, they should always have access to communication with the center. The center should be kept informed of their progress, the estimated time of arrival, any changes in the patient's condition, and the patient's anticipated needs on arrival.

Care of the Parents

The birth of a critically ill infant can be a devastating event for both the mother and the family. Transferring the infant to a distant hospital adds an element of physical separation that disrupts the normal process of maternal and family bonding. Parents often feel as though they have lost control of the situation and continually fear their infant will die. Parental attachment and family interactions may become dysfunctional. There are a number of things that the transport team can do to help parents cope with their infant's illness.

Before leaving the referring hospital, the parents should be encouraged to see and touch their infant. As soon as conditions persist, the parents need to be informed of their infant's condition in an honest and forthright manner. As soon as possible, the parents should be allowed to visit their child. Physical contact between parents and infant should be encouraged. Seeing, touching, and talking to their baby can be very therapeutic for the parents.

If the parents cannot visit, snapshots and/or a videotape of their baby can provide alternative contact for the parents.

When both mother and infant have been transported, the normal family support mechanisms for dealing with crisis are disrupted. The center should provide alternate mechanisms by involving the hospital's chaplains, social workers, and parent support groups.

Depending on the distance from the parents' home to the center, lodging and financial assistance may be needed. The referral hospital should maintain a listing and provide information about local support groups. Every attempt should be made to keep the parents informed, available, and involved in their child's care.

References

1. Allen PD, Turner DT, Brinck MJ: Ground transport of an infant on high-frequency ventilation: a case presentation, *Neonatal Network* 14:39, 1995.
2. American Medical Association: *Centralized community or regionalized perinatal intensive care (Report J).* Adopted by the AMA House of Delegates, June 1971.
3. American Medical Association Committee on Maternal and Child Care: *Action guide for maternal and child care committees,* Chicago, 1974, American Medical Association.
4. Amil-Tison C: Neurologic evaluation of the maturity of newborn infants, *Arch Dis Child* 43:89, 1969.
5. Ballard JL: A simplified assessment of gestational age, *Pediatr Res* 11:374, 1977.
6. Barth J: Staff preparation and training for high-risk neonatal transport. In Graven S, editor: *Newborn air transport,* Evansville, Ind, 1978, Mead Johnson.
7. Battaglia FC, Lubchenco LO: A practical classification of newborn infants by birth weight and gestational age, *J Pediatr* 71:159, 1967.
8. Bowes WA, Merenstein GB: *Recommendations and guidelines for the transport of high risk obstetrical patients,* Colorado Perinatal Care Council Transport Committee, March 1978.
9. Brann AW: Perinatal health care in Mississippi 1973. In sunshine P, editor: *Regionalization of perinatal care: report of the Sixty-Sixth Ross Conference on Pediatric Research,* Columbus, Ohio, 1974, Ross Laboratories.
10. Brown FB: The management of high-risk obstetric transfer patients, *Obstet Gynecol* 51:674, 1978.
11. Butterfield LJ: The impact of regionalization on neonatal outcome. In Smith JF, Vidyasagar D, editors: *Neonatal and perinatal medicine,* New Delhi, 1985, Inberprint.
12. Butterfield LJ: Newborn country U.S.A., *Clin Perinatol* 3:281, 1976
13. Butterfield LJ: Organization of regional perinatal programs, *Semin Perinatol* 1:217, 1977.
14. Clarke TA et al: Transcutaneous oxygen monitoring during neonatal transport, *Pediatrics* 65:884, 1980.
15. Cornish JD et al: Extracorporeal membrane oxygenation as a means of stabilizing and transporting high risk neonates, *ASAIO Transactions* 37:564, 1991.
16. Danzig D: Neonatal transport teams: a survey of functions and roles, *Neonatal Network* Oct. 1984, p. 41.
17. Dubowitz LMS, Dubowitz V, Goldberg C: Clinical assessment of gestational age in the newborn infant, *J Pediatr* 77:1, 1970.
18. Faulkner SC et al: Mobile extracorporeal membrane oxygenation, *Am Thorac Surg* 55:1244, 1993.
19. Ferrara A, Harin A: *Emergency transfer of the high-risk neonate,* St Louis, 1980, Mosby.
20. Ginsberg E: *The meaning of regionalization in health,* Regionalization and Health Policy, Department of Health, Education, and Welfare, Pub No (HRA) 77-263, 1977.
21. Gomez M: Hiring, staffing, and team composition. In McClosky K, Orr R, editors: *Pediatric transport medicine,* St Louis, 1995, Mosby.
22. Goodwin JW, Dunne JT, Thomas BW: Antepartum identification of the fetus at risk, *Can Med Assoc J* 101:458, 1969.
23. *Guidelines for perinatal care,* ed 3, Elk Grove Village, Ill, 1992, American Academy of Pediatrics and American College of Obstetricians and Gynecologists.
24. Harris TR, Isaman J, Giles HR. Improved survival in very low birth weight premature and postmature neonates through maternal transport, *Clin Perinatol* 26:180, 1976.
25. Hobel CJ: Perinatal health care in Mississippi 1973. In Sunshine P, editor: *Regionalization of perinatal care: report of Sixty-Sixth Ross Conference on Pediatric Research,* Columbus, Ohio, 1974, Ross Laboratories.
26. Hobel CJ et al: Perinatal and intrapartum high risk screening: prediction of the high risk neonate, *Am J Obstet Gynecol* 117:1, 1973.
27. Imershein AW et al: Covering the costs of care in neonatal intensive care units, *Pediatrics* 89:56, 1992.
28. *Infant death: an analysis by maternal risk and health care,* Washington, DC, 1973, Institute of Medicine, National Academy of Sciences.
29. Kinsella JP, Abman S: Inhalational nitric oxide therapy for persistant pulmonary hypertension of the newborn, *Pediatrics* 91:997, 1993.
30. Kinsella JP et al: Clinical responses to prolonged treatment of persistant pulmonary hypertension of the newborn with low doses of inhaled nitric oxide, *J Pediatr* 123:103, 1993.
31. Kinsella JP, Schmidt JM, Abman SH: Inhaled nitric oxide treatment for stabilization and emergency medical transport of critically ill newborns and infants, *Pediatrics* 92:773, 1995.
32. Ledger WJ: Identification of the high risk mother and fetus: does it work? *Clin Perinatol* 7:125, 1980.
33. Lewis CE: *Improved access through regionalization,* Regionalization and Health Care Policy 71-84, Department of Health, Education, and Welfare, Pub No (HRA) 77-263, 1977.
34. Little GA et al: *Toward improving the outcome of pregnancy, the 90s and beyond,* White Plains, 1993, March of Dimes.

35. Lubchenco LO, Hansman C, Boyd E: Intrauterine growth in length and head circumference as estimated from live births from 26-42 weeks, *Pediatrics* 47:831, 1971.
36. Lubchenco LO, Searls DT, Brazie JV: Neonatal mortality rate: relationship to birth weight and gestational age, *J Pediatr* 81:814, 1972.
37. McCarthy JT et al: Who pays the bill for neonatal intensive care? *J Pediatr* 95:755, 1979.
38. McCormick MC, Shapiro S, Starfield BH: The regionalization of perinatal services, *JAMA* 253:799, 1985.
39. Merenstein GB et al: An analysis of air transport results in the sick newborn. II. Antenatal and neonatal referrals, *Am J Obstet Gynecol* 128:520, 1977.
40. Merkatz IR, Johnson KG: Regionalization of perinatal care for the United States, *Clin Perinatol* 3:271, 1976.
41. Meyer HBP: Transportation of high risk infants in Arizona. In Sunshine P, editor: *Regionalization of perinatal care: report of the Sixty-Sixth Ross Conference on Pediatric Research,* Columbus, Ohio, 1974, Ross Laboratories.
42. Meyer HBP: Regional care for mothers and their infants, *Clin Perinatol* 7:205, 1980.
43. Mitchell RG, Farr V: The meaning of maturity and the assessment of maturity at birth. In Dawkins M, MacGregor WG, editors: *Gestational age, size, and maturity,* London, 1965, William Heineman.
44. Modenlow HD: Antenatal versus neonatal transport to a regional perinatal center: a comparison between matched pairs, *Obstet Gynecol* 53:725, 1979.
45. *Neonatal transport standards and guidelines,* 1992, National Association of Neonatal Nurses.
46. Paneth N et al: Newborn intensive care and neonatal mortality in low-birth-weight infants, *N Engl J Med* 307:149, 1982.
47. Pettett G: Outcome of maternal air transport. In Graven S, editor: *Maternal air transport,* Evansville, Ind, 1979, Mead Johnson.
48. Pettett G et al: An analysis of air transport results in the sick newborn infant. I. The transport team, *Pediatrics* 55:774, 1975.
49. Phibbs CS, Williams RL, Phibbs RH: Newborn risk factors and costs of neonatal intensive care, *Pediatrics* 68:313, 1981.
50. Pomerance JJ et al: Cost of living for infants weighing 1000 grams or less at birth, *Pediatrics* 61:908, 1978.
51. Reynolds EOR, Taghizadeh A: Improved prognoses of infants mechanically ventilated for hyaline membrane disease, *Arch Dis Child* 49 505, 1974.
52. Ross Planning Associates: *Referral centers providing perinatal and neonatal care,* Columbus, Ohio, 1979, Ross Laboratories.
53. Ryan GM Jr: Toward improving the outcome of pregnancy, *Am J Obstet Gynecol* 46:375, 1975.
54. Ryan GM Jr: Regional planning for maternal and perinatal health services, *Semin Perinatol* 1:255, 1977.
55. Segal S: *Transport of high risk newborn infants,* 1972, Canadian Pediatric Society.
56. Shenai J: Neonatal transport outreach educational program, *Pediatr Clin North Am* 40:275, 1993.
57. Sobol RJ et al: Clinical application of high risk scoring on an obstetric service, *Am J Obstet Gynecol* 134:904, 1979.
58. Stahlman MT et al: A six year followup of clinical hyaline membrane disease, *Pediatr Clin North Am* 20:433, 1973.
59. Stewart AL, Reynolds EOR: Improved prognosis for infants of very low birth weight, *Pediatrics* 54:724, 1974.
60. Usher RH: Clinical implications of perinatal mortality statistics, *Clin Obstet Gynecol* 14:885, 1976.

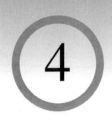

4 Delivery Room Care

Susan Niermeyer, Susan Clarke

The purpose of immediate delivery room care is to support the newborn's respiratory and circulatory systems during the transition from fetal to neonatal life. Normal physiologic changes at birth include lung expansion with initiation of gas exchange and closure of circulatory shunts that were necessary during intrauterine life. When delivery is complicated by perinatal conditions leading to asphyxia, resuscitation aims to reverse hypoxia, hypercarbia, and acidosis. The survival and outcome of distressed newborns depends on timely and effective intervention in the first few minutes after birth. Information in this chapter will provide the reader with a clearer understanding of the physiologic and pathophysiologic events that take place in the distressed neonate and the techniques and equipment used in delivery room resuscitation. The basic techniques of thermal control and airway management constitute the initial steps in all resuscitations.[1] Indications are discussed for supplemental oxygen administration, bag and mask ventilation, intubation, chest compressions, and use of medications and volume expansion. A discussion of delivery room emergencies integrates the basic elements of resuscitation as well as more advanced procedures sometimes called for during stabilization in the delivery room and transitional nursery. Finally, guidelines for care of the family and perinatal decision making are presented.

Physiology

Rapid physiologic transition from intrauterine to extrauterine environments must be made at birth. Effective, regular respirations should be initiated within 30 to 45 seconds of delivery. Environmental factors such as a relatively cool ambient temperature and tactile stimulation assist in initiating respiration. The changes in Pa_{O_2} and Pa_{CO_2} result-

ing from clamping the umbilical cord affect chemoreceptors and aid in the reflexive initiation of respiration. The initial breath may generate from 20 to 70 cm H_2O of negative intrathoracic pressure to expand the collapsed alveoli.[2] A rapid decrease in pulmonary vascular resistance and increase in pulmonary blood flow occur after lung expansion, resulting in increased pulmonary perfusion and oxygenation.[3] Removal and absorption of intrauterine lung fluid is also necessary. Resorption of fetal lung liquid across the respiratory epithelium accelerates during labor to result in net clearance of liquid from the potential airspaces.[4] Colloid osmotic pressure and the relatively lower postnatal hydrostatic pressure of blood within the pulmonary circuit assist in absorbing alveolar fluid after delivery. Fetal right-to-left shunts through the ductus arteriosis and forama ovale gradually close during this process (Fig. 4-1 and Table 4-1).

Asphyxia and Apnea

Asphyxia is defined as inadequate tissue perfusion, which fails to meet the metabolic demands of the tissues for oxygen and waste removal. Asphyxia is characterized by progressive hypoxia ($\downarrow Po_2$), hypercarbia ($\uparrow Pco_2$), and acidosis ($\downarrow pH$). Hypoxic tissues begin anaerobic metabolism, producing metabolic acids that are initially buffered by bicarbonate. When the bicarbonate supply fails, acidosis occurs. Initially, acidosis and hypoxia result in reflexive, compensatory changes. After an initial tachycardia, cardiac output decreases and a generalized peripheral vasoconstriction occurs to maintain a blood pressure adequate for perfusion of vital organs. Conversion from aerobic to anaerobic glycolysis takes place with the accumulation of lactate and the development of metabolic acidosis.[5]

Asphyxia may occur *in utero* or postnatally. In

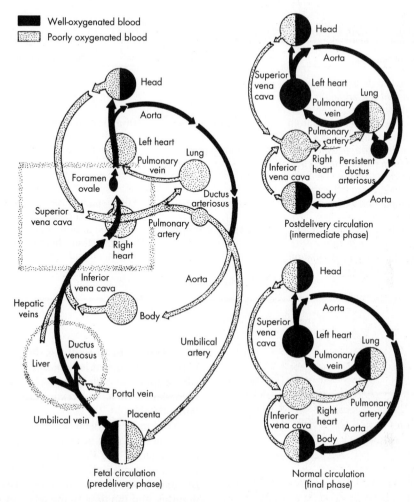

Well-oxygenated blood
Poorly oxygenated blood

Head
Aorta
Left heart
Pulmonary vein
Lung
Foramen ovale
Superior vena cava
Pulmonary artery
Right heart
Ductus arteriosus
Inferior vena cava
Aorta
Hepatic veins
Body
Ductus venosus
Liver
Umbilical artery
Portal vein
Umbilical vein
Placenta

Fetal circulation
(predelivery phase)

Head
Aorta
Superior vena cava
Left heart
Pulmonary vein
Lung
Pulmonary artery
Inferior vena cava
Right heart
Persistent ductus arteriosus
Body
Aorta

Postdelivery circulation
(intermediate phase)

Head
Aorta
Superior vena cava
Left heart
Pulmonary vein
Lung
Inferior vena cava
Right heart
Pulmonary artery
Aorta
Body

Normal circulation
(final phase)

Figure 4-1   Blood circulation before and after birth. (From Babson SG, Pernoll ML, Benda GL: *Diagnosis and management of the fetus and neonate at risk: a guide for team care,* ed 4, St Louis, 1980, Mosby.)

either circumstance, there follows a well-defined series of events (Fig. 4-2). After a brief period of rapid breathing, respiratory movements cease and a period of apnea designated as primary apnea follows. At the same time, heart rate falls and neuromotor tone diminishes. Intrauterine asphyxia may result in the passage of meconium. If the asphyxic insult continues, the heart rate falls further, blood pressure falls, hypotonia worsens, and a series of spontaneous deep gasps occurs. Gasping continues but becomes weaker, more irregular, and finally ceases.

After the last gasp occurs, there begins a period of apnea known as secondary apnea.[1]

Delivery may occur at any point in the progression of an asphyxial insult. If an infant is born in primary apnea, exposure to oxygen and stimulation will usually induce respirations. If delivery occurs during secondary apnea, the infant will not respond to stimulation. Spontaneous respirations will not resume until resuscitation is initiated with assisted ventilation and oxygen.[2] In the clinical setting, primary and secondary apnea are essentially indistinguishable from one another. In both,

Table 4-1
Comparison of Vascular and Pulmonary Functions Before and After Birth

Fetal Function	Body Structure	Extrauterine Function
Carries oxygenated and deoxygenated blood from left ventricle and pulmonary arteries to fetal organs and placenta	Aorta	Carries oxygenated blood from left ventricle into systemic circulation
Shunts most of the oxygenated blood from placenta to inferior vena cava	Ductus venosus	Disappears within 2 weeks after birth; becomes ligamentum venosum
Connects right and left atria; permits oxygenated blood from right atrium to bypass right ventricle and pulmonary circuit and go directly into left atrium	Foramen ovale	Functionally closes soon after birth; anatomically seals during childhood
Shunts blood from pulmonary artery directly into aorta	Ductus arteriosus	Functionally closes soon after birth; eventually becomes ligamentum arteriosum
Carry blood to and from placenta, the organ of respiration before birth	Umbilical arteries and vein	Clamped at birth, obliterating placenta connections; become ligaments
Collapsed; minimal pulmonary circulation; fetal respiratory movements	Lungs	Expanded and aerated; pulmonary circulation allows CO_2 and O_2 exchange; organ of respiration

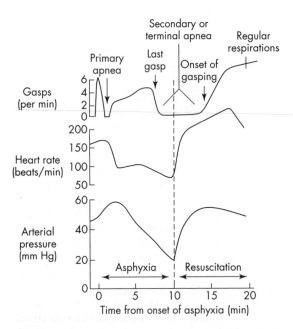

Figure 4-2   Changes in physiologic parameters during asphyxiation and resuscitation of Rhesus monkey fetus at birth. (From Klaus MH, Fanaroff AA: *Care of the high-risk neonate*, ed 4, Philadelphia, 1993, WB Saunders.)

the infant is not breathing, heart rate may be <100, and the infant is hypotonic. Thus any infant who is apneic at delivery must be assumed to be in secondary apnea, and resuscitation should begin immediately.

The longer artificial ventilation is delayed after an infant's last gasp in secondary apnea, the longer time required for the infant's first spontaneous gasp after resuscitation. For every 1-minute delay, the time to the first gasp is increased by about 2 minutes, and the time to the onset of spontaneous breathing is delayed by more than 4 minutes.[6] In the absence of effective resuscitation after delivery, apnea and decreased cardiac output will result in progressive biochemical deterioration:

- A plasma P_{O_2} of 0 in less than 5 minutes
- An increase in P_{CO_2} of 8 mm Hg/min
- A decrease in pH of 0.04 units/min
- A decrease in bicarbonate of 2 mEq/min

Severe fetal and neonate asphyxia impair the physiologic transitions to extrauterine life. The normally high fetal pulmonary vascular resistance may not decrease in the presence of persistent acidosis and hypoxemia and consequently the pulmo-

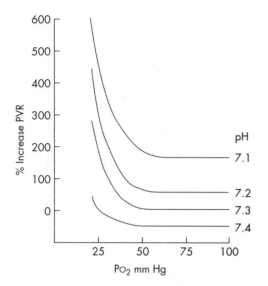

Figure 4-3   Pulmonary vascular resistance in calf. *PVR,* Pulmonary vascular resistance. (From Rudolph AM, Yuan S: *J Clin Invest* 45:399, 1966.)

Table 4-2
Conditions That May Require Availability of Skilled Resuscitation at Delivery

Intrapartum Problems
- Fetal distress
   Persistent late decelerations
   Severe variable decelerations without baseline variability
   Scalp pH <7.25
   Meconium-stained amniotic fluid
   Cord prolapse
- Prolonged, unusual, or difficult labor
- Emergency operative delivery
- Breech presentation with vaginal delivery

Medical/Obstetric/Genetic Problems
- Diabetes mellitus
- Suspected or confirmed maternal infection
- Substance abuse
- Third trimester bleeding
- Pregnancy-induced hypertension
- Abnormal amniotic fluid volume
- Prolonged rupture of membranes
- Multiple gestation
- Low-birth-weight infant
- Prematurity
- Isoimmunization
- Fetal congenital anomalies

nary circuit continues to carry low volumes of blood and remains hypoperfused (Fig 4-3).[4] **As part of persistent pulmonary hypertension of the newborn, normal closure of fetal shunts is delayed by low systemic vascular resistance, pulmonary hypoperfusion, hypoexpansion, and hypoxia, thus resulting in persistent right-to-left shunting through the ductus arteriosus and foramen ovale.** Lung fluid clearance may also be delayed because of poor lung inflation and/or pulmonary hypoperfusion. Additionally, intraalveolar fluid may accumulate as a result of leakage from damaged pulmonary capillaries resulting in pulmonary edema. **With worsening hypoxemia and acidosis, myocardial function begins to fail, cardiac output falls, and perfusion to vital body organs (brain, kidney, intestine) decreases, setting the stage for postasphyxial injury of these organs.**[7]

Preparation for Resuscitation

Immediate, effective resuscitation of the newborn infant can reduce or prevent morbidity and mortality. Much of neonatal resuscitation focuses on ventilation, oxygenation, and reversal of perinatal asphyxia. Application of basic procedures is often all that is necessary to successfully resuscitate a depressed infant. However, effective resuscitation requires anticipation and adequate preparation of equipment and personnel.[8,9,10]

Elements of the antepartum and intrapartum histories may identify the infant at risk for neonatal asphyxia (Table 4-2). Any normal pregnancy, however, may become high risk with the onset of previously unexpected or undetected complications during the intrapartum phase (e.g., maternal hemorrhage, prolapsed cord, meconium staining).

Prevention, detection, and treatment of fetal asphyxia is the responsibility of the obstetric team. Once fetal asphyxia is diagnosed, therapeutic intervention should be coordinated between obstetric and neonatal services to allow for a timely delivery and effective, coordinated resuscitation.

Box 4-1

Equipment Used During Neonatal Resuscitation

Thermal management
Radiant warmer
Warmed blankets or towels
Infant stocking caps

Airway
Bulb syringe
Mechanical suction
Suction catheters 5F or 6F, 8F, 10F
8F feeding tube and 20 ml syringe
Meconium aspirator/suction device

Breathing
Bag and mask ventilation
    Oxygen source with flowmeter and tubing
    Neonatal resuscitation bag with 100% oxygen
        capability and manometer or pressure re-
        lease valve
    Face masks, newborn and premature sizes
    Oral airways, newborn and premature sizes
    (Pulse oximeter)
Intubation
    Laryngoscope with extra batteries
    Straight blades No. 0 and No. 1 with ex-
        tra bulbs
    Endotracheal tubes 2.5, 3.0, 3.5, 4.0 mm ID
    Stylet
    Tape, skin preparation
    Scissors

Circulation
Stethoscope
Wall clock or stopwatch
Cord clamp
Medications (see Table 4-3)
Sterile gloves
Alcohol sponges
Umbilical vessel catheterization tray
Umbilical catheters 3.5F and 5F
Three-way stopcocks
Umbilical tape
Suture material
Intravenous catheters, tubing, fluid
Needles 25g, 23g, 22g, 20g, 18g
Syringes 1ml, 3ml, 5ml, 10ml, 20ml, 50ml
(Cardiorespiratory monitor)
(Procedure light)

In the mid-1980s the need for a national training program for neonatal resuscitation in the United States was addressed by the American Heart Association (AHA) and the American Academy of Pediatrics (AAP) through development of the Neonatal Resuscitation Program (NRP). The goal of the NRP is to provide the materials and training necessary for health care professionals to follow guidelines established and updated periodically at the National Conference on Cardiopulmonary Resuscitation and Emergency Cardiac Care.[11] The widespread acceptance of the NRP assures consistent use of current guidelines, awareness of proper equipment, and preparation of personnel to work as a team using shared cognitive knowledge and performance skills.

The NRP recommends that, "At every delivery there should be at least one person who has the skills required to perform a complete resuscitation." A second person should be present to assist with resuscitation, even in cases of an anticipated normal delivery. When asphyxia is anticipated, two persons whose sole responsibility is resuscitation of the infant should be present, and roles should be designated in advance. Multiple gestation deliveries require a full set of personnel (and equipment) for each infant.[1]

The pediatric staff should be familiar with the prenatal and intrapartum history of the mother and fetus (see Table 4-2), because these data will affect the initial level of resuscitation preparation.

Resuscitation equipment (Box 4-1) and drugs (Table 4-3) should always be readily available, functional, and assembled for immediate use in a designated location, ideally in a specific area of the delivery/birthing room. Consumable supplies and small equipment can be stored on specially constructed wall shelves or on a radiant warmer intensive-care bed equipped with easily accessible storage (Figs. 4-4 and 4-5, pp. 54 and 55).

Prepare for resuscitation by performing the following:

- **Preheat the radiant warmer.**
- **Assemble warm linens, bulb syringe, stethoscope, cord clamp.**
- **Check suction equipment for function, and set the wall vacuum regulator control not to exceed 100 mm.**

- Turn on the oxygen flow to the ventilation bag and check all connections, pop-off control valves, manometer function, and face masks.
- Check the laryngoscope for a bright light source and appropriate blades (size no. 0 for premature infants and size 1 for term infants); tighten the bulb.
- Check the availability of appropriately sized endotracheal tubes.
- Check the ancillary equipment (i.e., sterile trays, intravenous [IV] solutions, drugs).
- If the clinical situation warrants, draw up and label emergency medications for ready administration and obtain O negative packed red blood cells for emergency transfusion.
- Equip all members of the resuscitation team with appropriate personal protection (gloves, gown, goggles, and mask or face shield).

The steps of neonatal resuscitation follow the standard ABCs of resuscitation:

- A—Airway
- B—Breathing
- C—Circulation

With the ABCs as an overall framework for neonatal resuscitation, the components of the procedure can be examined sequentially.

- A—Establish an airway
  Positioning
  Suctioning of mouth, nose, and trachea (in some cases)
  Endotracheal intubation if necessary
- B—Initiate breathing
  Tactile stimulation
  Positive pressure ventilation
- C—Maintain circulation
  Chest compressions
  Medications

At each step of the resuscitation procedure, whether uncomplicated or extended, the cycle of evaluation/decision/action is repeated. Evaluation is based on the infant's respirations, heart rate, and color (Fig. 4-6, p. 56).

Apgar Score

The Apgar score, developed by Dr. Virginia Apgar in 1952, provides a comprehensive, objective, measure of the infant's condition in the first minutes after birth (Fig. 4-7, p. 56). The Apgar score is not used as an indicator of the need for resuscitation, but it may be used to assess an infant's response to resuscitative measures. Although asphyxia may be associated with low Apgar scores, it is possible for an infant to have a low Apgar score without having asphyxia.[13] For example, an infant born to a mother who received general anesthesia may be flaccid and have depressed reflexes and poor respiratory efforts. These infants usually respond rapidly to bag-and-mask ventilation, and no further intervention is necessary. Conversely, an infant may have an equally low Apgar score as a result of intrauterine asphyxia and require prolonged resuscitative efforts. An infant with a midrange Apgar score between 6 and 7 may be using all of his or her homeostatic mechanisms to maintain an adequate central blood pressure and cardiac output. Apgar scores should be assigned at 1 and 5 minutes and every 5 minutes thereafter until the score is 7. A complete description of resuscitative steps is vital to interpret a low Apgar score.

Initial Steps of Resuscitation

The initial steps of resuscitation should be performed at every delivery. They include (1) prevention of heat loss, (2) clearing the airway (positioning and suctioning), (3) initiation of breathing by tactile stimulation or bag and mask ventilation, and (4) evaluation of the infant.
  Prevent heat loss

- Place the infant under a radiant heat source.
- Dry the infant thoroughly and remove the wet linen.

Clear the airway

- Position the infant supine and flat with the neck slightly extended. A rolled blanket or towel may be used under the shoulders.
- Suction the mouth then the nose to clear the airway. The mouth is suctioned first to clear

Table 4-3
Medications for Neonatal Resuscitation

Medication	Concentration to Administer	Preparation	Dosage/Route*	Total Dose/Infant			Rate/Precautions	Indications for Use
Epinephrine	1:10,000	1 ml	0.1-0.3 ml/kg IV or ET	**Weight (kg)** 1 2 3 4	**Total ml** 0.1-0.3 0.2-0.6 0.3-0.9 0.4-1.2		Give *rapidly* May dilute with normal saline to 1-2 ml if giving ET	Heart rate <80 after 30 seconds adequate ventilation and chest compressions or heart rate zero
Volume expanders	Whole blood 5% Albumin-saline Normal saline Ringer's lactate	40 ml	10 ml/kg IV	**Weight (kg)** 1 2 3 4	**Total ml** 10 20 30 40		Give over 5-10 min	Evidence of acute bleeding with signs of hypovolemia
Sodium bicarbonate	0.5 mEq/ml (4.2% solution)	20 ml or two 10-ml prefilled syringes	2 mEq/kg IV	**Weight (kg)** 1 2 3 4	**Total dose (mEq)** 2 4 6 8	**Total ml** 4 8 12 16	Give *slowly* over at least 2 min Give only if infant is being effectively ventilated	Documented metabolic acidosis

Drug	Concentration		Dose/Route	Weight (kg)	Total dose (mg)	Total ml	Comments	Indications
Naloxone hydrochloride	0.4 mg/ml	1 ml	0.1 mg/kg (0.25 ml/kg) IV, ET IM, SC	1	0.1	0.25	Give rapidly IV, ET preferred IM, SC acceptable	Severe respiratory depression and history of maternal narcotic administration within past 4 hours
				2	0.2	0.50		
				3	0.3	0.75		
				4	0.4	1.00		
	1.0 mg/ml	1 ml	0.1 mg/kg (0.1 ml/kg) IV, ET IM, SC	1	0.1	0.1		
				2	0.2	0.2		
				3	0.3	0.3		
				4	0.4	0.4		

Drug	Dose/Route		Weight (kg)	Total µg/min	Comments	Indications
Dopamine	Begin at 5 µg/kg/min (may increase to 20 µg/kg/min if necessary) IV	$\dfrac{6 \times (\text{kg}) \times (\mu g/kg/min)}{\text{Desired fluid (ml/h)}} = $ mg of dopamine per 100 ml of solution	1	5-20	Give as a continuous infusion using an infusion pump Monitor heart rate and blood pressure closely Seek consultation	After initial resuscitation continued poor perfusion, thready pulses, evidence of shock
			2	10-40		
			3	15-60		
			4	20-80		

IM, Intramuscular; *ET*, endotracheal; *IV*, intravenous; *SC*, subcutaneous.
(From *Textbook of neonatal resuscitation* 1987, 1990, 1994 American Heart Association)

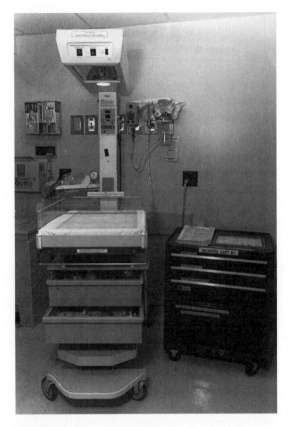

Figure 4-4 Labor/Delivery/Recovery (LDR) room resuscitation area consisting of radiant warmer with anesthesia bag and manometer and wall oxygen and suction outlets. Other supplies for airway suctioning and intubation are stored in the drawers of the radiant warmer. Resuscitation drugs and umbilical catheterization trays are kept in a separate resuscitation cart accessible from all LDR rooms.

the largest volume of secretions; when the nasopharynx is suctioned, a reflex cough, sneeze, or cry often results.
• Turn the head to the side to allow secretions to pool in the cheek, then remove with a bulb syringe or suction catheter. Deep pharyngeal suction (in a child not requiring positive-pressure ventilation or intubation) should not be performed during the first few minutes after birth to avoid vagal depression and resultant bradycardia.

Initiate breathing

• Provide tactile stimulation by rubbing the back or gently slapping the feet.
• If the infant remains apneic after stimulation once or twice, immediately begin bag-mask ventilation.
• Continue gentle rubbing of trunk, extremities, or head to support early respiratory efforts in a depressed infant.
• If adequate chest wall movement is observed, proceed to heart rate evaluation.
• If the infant remains apneic or has gasping respirations, continue positive-pressure ventilation.

Maintain circulation

• Count the heart rate in 6 seconds and multiply by 10 for the beats per minute. The heart rate may be monitored by auscultation with a stethoscope or by palpating the umbilical cord pulse. The individual assessing the heart rate should indicate each pulse by tapping the thumb and index finger together.
• If the heart rate is >100 beats/min, proceed to evaluation of color.
• If the heart rate is <100 beats/min, begin positive-pressure ventilation, even though the infant may have spontaneous respirations.
• If after 15 to 30 seconds of positive-pressure ventilation with 100% oxygen the heart rate is <60 or 60 to 80 beats/min and not rising, begin chest compressions, consider intubation, and prepare emergency drugs (see Table 4-3).

Evaluate the infant

• If the infant is centrally pink, continue to observe under guidelines for transition.
• If the infant has peripheral cyanosis (acrocyanosis), continue to observe; supplemental oxygen is not indicated.
• If the infant has central cyanosis (with spontaneous respirations and adequate heart rate), give free-flow oxygen.
• Assign an Apgar score at 1 and 5 minutes (see

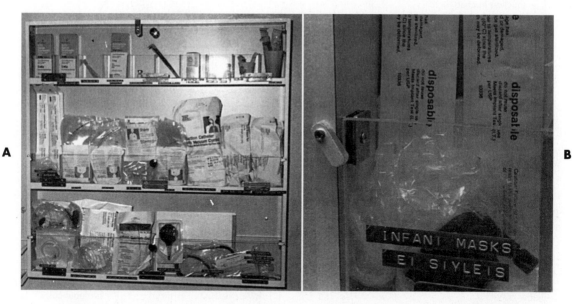

Figure 4-5   A, Wall-mounted storage bin. Unit consists of three plexiglas shelves; each shelf is divided by plexiglas into smaller compartments. Each compartment is labeled. Shelves can be opened for cleaning. Each shelf is held in place by hinge and magnet. **B,** Hinge and magnet device used to ensure closure of plexiglass shelves.

Fig. 4-7). Continue to assign an Apgar score every 5 minutes until it is ≥ 7.

Supplemental oxygen should be administered in a concentration of 100% at a flow rate of 5 L/min. Oxygen may be administered by mask or by holding the oxygen tubing in a cupped hand over the face. 100% oxygen at 5 L/min provides 80% to 100% oxygen to the infant when delivered via a mask or via tubing held 1/2″ from the nares and surrounded by a cupped hand. 100% oxygen delivered at 5 L/minute provides approximately 60% oxygen when the tubing is held 1″ from the nares or a mask is held loosely on the face and 40% oxygen if the tubing is held 2 inches from the nares or a mask is held away from the face. Once the infant becomes pink, gradually decrease the concentration of oxygen by withdrawing the tubing or the mask from the infant's face. If cyanosis persists, re-evaluate the quality of respirations and the heart rate; perform a brief physical exam; and consider bag-mask ventilation or intubation if there is evidence of respiratory distress.

Initial Steps of Resuscitation with Meconium-Stained Amniotic Fluid

Meconium-stained amniotic fluid most often occurs in infants >34 weeks' gestational age, especially in term and postterm neonates. Passage of meconium may be associated with asphyxia. Severe fetal acidosis can result in fetal gasping, leading to in utero meconium aspiration.[14] If meconium has not been aspirated in utero, meconium aspiration often can be avoided with thorough suctioning of the mouth and hypopharynx at delivery of the head[15,16] and again after delivery is complete. Tracheal intubation is indicated based on the character of the meconium (thick, particulate rather than uniformly dispersed through the amniotic fluid) and the vigorousness of the infant (depressed rather than crying).

Perform the following steps:

- Suction the nose, mouth, and posterior pharynx when the head is delivered and again on the radiant warmer.

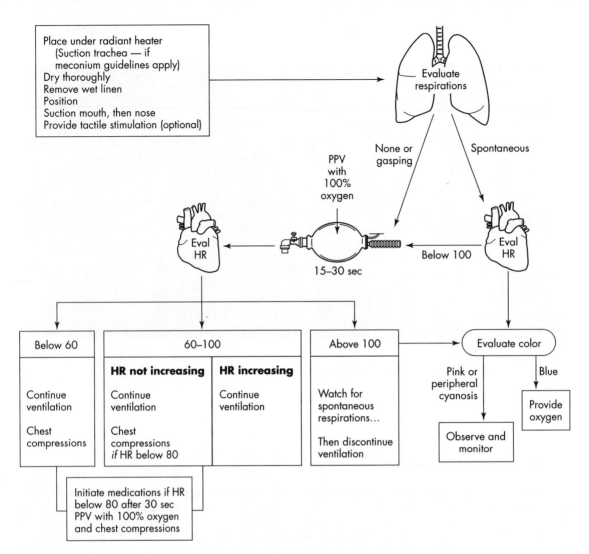

Figure 4-6 (From Bloom RS, Croplcy C, AHA/AAP Neonatal Resuscitation Program Steering Committee: *Textbook of neonatal resuscitation,* Dallas, 1994, American Heart Association.)

Sign		Score		
		0	1	2
A	Appearance (color)	Blue, pale	Body pink Extremities blue	Completely pink
P	Pulse (heart rate)	Absent	Below 100	Above 100
G	Grimace (reflex, irritability to suctioning)	No response	Grimace	Cough or sneeze
A	Activity (muscle tone)	Limp	Some flexion	Well flexed
R	Respiration (breathing efforts)	Absent	Weak, irregular	Strong cry

Figure 4-7 Practical epigram of Apgar score. (From Butterfield J, Covey M: *JAMA* 181:353, 1962.)

- If the infant is vigorous, thorough suctioning during and after delivery may be adequate.
- If the infant is depressed or the meconium is thick and particulate, suction the trachea under direct visualization using an endotracheal tube, adapter, and mechanical suction or meconium suction device (Fig. 4-8).
- Dry, stimulate, and remove the wet linen after airway suctioning is complete or positive-pressure ventilation is initiated.
- Suction the stomach when airway management is complete and vital signs are stable (usually after 5 minutes). Clearing residual meconium from the stomach decreases the risk of postnatal regurgitation and aspiration.

Controversy exists over the correct resuscitation of the vigorous infant with thick meconium.[13,14] Research continues actively in this area to attempt to answer the question whether vigorous babies born in the setting of thick meconium can be managed more safely without intubation. Any infant born in the setting of meconium-stained amniotic fluid who needs positive-pressure ventilation should first have the trachea suctioned and cleared of any meconium present.

Bag and Mask Ventilation

The indications for bag and mask ventilation include (1) apnea unresponsive to brief stimulation, (2) gasping respirations, and (3) heart rate <100 beats/min. The equipment for bag and mask ventilation can be either a self-inflating bag (240 to 750 ml) with an oxygen reservoir and pressure-relief valve or pressure gauge or an anesthesia bag (500 to 750 ml) with pressure gauge and flow-control valve. Self-inflating bags more reliably deliver tidal volume in the hands of providers who resuscitate babies infrequently[17]; however, self-inflating bags cannot be used reliably to deliver free-flow oxygen, and they require a special adapter to deliver continuous positive airway pressure (CPAP) (Fig. 4-9). Anesthesia bags require a complete seal between mask and face to deliver a tidal volume. They offer the advantages of ability to achieve high peak pressures, CPAP capability, and delivery of free-flow oxygen. The face mask should be selected to assure that it is appropriately sized to cover the chin, mouth, and nose, but not the eyes. Masks are commonly available in term and premature sizes and may be obtained to fit even VLBW infants. Flexible, translucent masks with a cushioned rim generally provide the best seal with minimal trauma and allow monitoring of mouth position and secretions.

Perform the following steps:

- Set the flowmeter to deliver 5 to 8 L/min with the capability of increasing to 10 to 12 L/min.

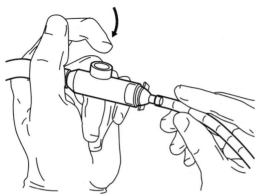

Meconium aspirator attached to wall suction

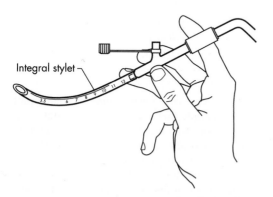

Integral stylet

Figure 4-8 Equipment for suctioning meconium from the airway—aspirator and meconium suction device. (From Bloom RS, Cropley C, AHA/AAP Neonatal Resuscitation Program Steering Committee: *Textbook of neonatal resuscitation*, Dallas, 1994, American Heart Association.)

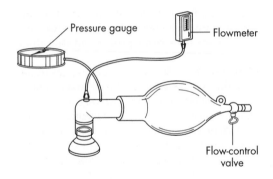

Pressure gauge

Flowmeter

Flow-control valve

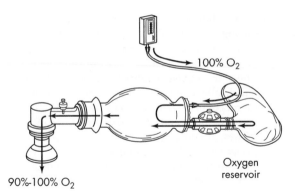

100% O₂

Oxygen reservoir

90%-100% O₂

Anesthesia bags. Anesthesia bags contain an inflatable gas reservoir that is refilled between breaths.
Advantages:
- The ability to deliver 100% oxygen and any desired inspiratory pressure
- The ability to maintain a positive end expiratory pressure
- In-line manometer

Disadvantages:
- Dependence on an external oxygen supply
- Practice and experience required for efficient and safe use
- Risk of pneumothorax with very high inspiratory pressures

Self-inflating bags. Self-inflating bags fill with ambient air and are independent of an external oxygen or compressed air source.
Advantages:
- Simplicity of use
- Self-inflation (useful backup system in case compressed oxygen source fails)

Disadvantages:
- The maximum pressure-limiting pop-off valve, usually set by the manufacturer at 30 to 35 cm H_2O, will preclude adequate ventilation in a noncompliant lung. (Some models have a manual override device that will allow increased inspiratory pressures.)
- A reservoir must be attached to deliver 100% oxygen.
- Free-flow oxygen cannot be delivered reliably through the patient outlet.
- The bags do not routinely deliver end expiratory pressure, and it is difficult to retrofit them with an in-line manometer.
- Higher pressures than the pop-off valve pressure are given with rapid ventilation.

Figure 4-9   Anesthesia bag and self-inflating bag. (From Bloom RS, Cropley C, AHA/AAP Neonatal Resuscitation Program Steering Committee: *Textbook of neonatal resuscitation,* Dallas, 1994, American Heart Association.)

- Test equipment before use. Equipment failure can cause resuscitation failure!
- Position the infant with the neck slightly extended and avoid compression of soft tissues of the neck by holding the mask to the face with the third, fourth, and fifth fingers resting along the mandible.
- If the infant has not initiated respirations, give an opening breath with pressures 30 to 40 cm H_2O and an inspiratory time of 1 to 3 seconds.
- Ventilate with pressures 15 to 40 cm H_2O and rate 40 to 60 breaths per minute.

- Observe chest expansion. If inadequate, (1) reapply face mask for better seal, (2) reposition the head, (3) suction secretions, (4) open the infant's mouth slightly, and (5) increase pressure.
- Reevaluate heart rate, respirations, and color.
- Insert an orogastric catheter (8 Fr feeding tube) after 2 minutes of bag and mask ventilation.
1. Measure the insertion depth of the catheter by holding the tip at the bridge of the nose and measuring to the earlobe, then to the xiphoid.

2. Insert the catheter through the mouth, not the nose.
3. Aspirate gastric contents with a 20 ml syringe and leave the catheter open.
4. Tape the catheter to the infant's cheek.

The adequacy of bag and mask ventilation must be continuously assessed by auscultation of breath sounds, visualization of chest wall movement, monitoring of heart rate, and observation of skin color. Peak inspiratory pressure should be limited to that necessary to visualize chest wall movement and auscultate breath sounds. Infants with collapsed or fluid-filled alveoli may occasionally require inspiratory pressures of 40 to 60 cm H_2O or higher.[18] Inspiratory pressures cannot be judged clinically; bags fitted with in-line pressure manometers are recommended in the delivery room. Data suggest that the neonatal respiratory system responds slowly to mechanical inspiratory pressure[19]; prolonged inspiratory times may be necessary to achieve an adequate inspiratory volume and establish functional residual capacity.

Potential complications of bag and mask ventilation include trauma to the eyes or face from improper size or position of mask, air leak (pneumothorax, subcutaneous air), intestinal distention elevating a normal diaphragm, or compressing the lung directly in the case of a diaphragmatic hernia (Table 4-4). Complications can be minimized by use of gentle technique and equipment of correct size, careful monitoring of pressures, and insertion of an orogastric tube when indicated.

Endotracheal Intubation

Endotracheal intubation is indicated when (1) there is a need for tracheal suctioning as with meconium-stained amniotic fluid, (2) bag and mask ventilation is ineffective, (3) there is a need for prolonged positive-pressure ventilation, and (4) diaphragmatic hernia is suspected.

Equipment for intubation is listed under Airway and Breathing in Box 4-1.

Select a noncuffed, uniform-diameter endotracheal tube of the correct size (Table 4-5). A variety of sizes (2.5 to 4.0) should be available, since estimated weights may be inaccurate or airway anomalies may exist. Orotracheal intubation is preferable to nasotracheal intubation dur-

ing acute resuscitation because it can be performed rapidly and without additional equipment. Perform the following steps:

- Shorten the selected endotracheal tubes to 13 cm and prepare the laryngoscope, tape, suction, oxygen, bag, and mask.
- Position the infant with the neck slightly extended.
- Provide free-flow oxygen.
- Holding the laryngoscope with the left hand, open the mouth with the right index finger and insert the blade.
- Lift the laryngoscope upward and outward so that the blade is nearly parallel to the surface beneath the infant.
- Visualize landmarks; identify the epiglottis, vocal cords, and glottis (Fig. 4-10). If the esophagus is seen, withdraw the blade until the epiglottis drops down. If only the tongue is visible, advance the blade further until it enters the vallecula or passes under the epiglottis.
- Gentle external pressure over the trachea may help visualize the vocal cords. This may be applied with the little finger of the intubator's left hand or by an assistant.
- Insert the endotracheal tube from the right corner of the mouth to the level of the vocal cord guideline at the tip of the tube.
- Limit each intubation attempt to 20 seconds to avoid hypoxia.
- Confirm endotracheal tube position by auscultation for bilaterally equal breath sounds in the axillae and absence of breath sounds over the stomach. Observe chest wall movement. Note the centimeter marking at the lip (Table 4-6).
- Secure the endotracheal tube with tape and obtain a chest x-ray examination.
- If necessary, shorten the endotracheal tube to 4 cm beyond the lips.

Complications of intubation include hypoxia caused by prolonged intubation attempts; lack of supplemental oxygen; tube malposition; apnea or bradycardia caused by hypoxia or vagal stimulation; and trauma to the oropharynx, trachea, vocal cords, or esophagus (see Table 4-4). Subglottic stenosis may result from prolonged, traumatic, or

Table 4-4
Complications During Resuscitation and Stabilization

Problem	Cause	Diagnosis	Remedies
Persistent cyanosis	Inadequate FiO$_2$	Check flowmeter (and blender)	Always administer 100% O$_2$
	Disconnected O$_2$ line	Check all connections	Reconnect line
	Empty O$_2$ cylinder	Check O$_2$ source	Replace O$_2$ cylinder
	Improper bag-and-mask ventilation		
	Insufficient insufflation pressure	Diminished breath sounds; little chest wall movement	Increase insufflation pressure until breath sounds are audible and chest movement seen
	Compression of airway	Diminished breath sounds; little chest wall movement	Apply upward force to mandible to counteract downward force holding face mask in place; tilt head backward
			Compression of lungs by distended stomach
			Place orogastric tube
	Inadequate face mask seal	Diminished breath sounds; little chest wall movement; air leak around mask	Readjust face mask; seal tightly against skin
	Inadequate ventilation Malpositioned ET tube	Check tube position with laryngoscope	Reinsert into trachea
		Check breath sounds	Adjust so breath sounds are bilaterally equal
			Tape ET tube in place
	Pneumothorax	Check breath sounds	Decompress tension pneumothorax
		Check for chest asymmetry	
		Transillumination	
		Chest x-ray examination	
Bradycardia	Same as cyanosis	Auscultation; electronic monitor or palpation	See above for cyanosis
			External cardiac compression if heart rate <80 beats/min with effective ventilation
	Perinatal myocardial ischemia	Lack of response to oxygenation and ventilation	Emergency medication administration
Hypothermia	Evaporative heat loss; conductive heat loss	Specific symptoms overlap those of asphyxia and shock	Dry infant
			Cover wet hair
		Low core temperature	Keep under radiant warmer
Hypoglycemia	Using glucose stores before birth or during resuscitation	Specific symptoms overlap those of asphyxia and shock	Infusion of D$_{10}$W at 100 ml/kg/24 hr
		Low blood glucose	
Hemorrhage	Inadequately secured umbilical arterial or venous line	Pallor	Keep all intravascular tubing connection sites in plain view
		Poor capillary filling	
		Leakage of blood	Tape UAC/UVC in place in addition to suturing lines
	Liver laceration		Perform chest compressions with correct position/depth

Table 4-5
Endotracheal Tube Size

Tube Size (mm) (Inside Diameter)	Weight (g)	Gestational Age (wk)
2.5	Below 1000	Below 28
3.0	1000-2000	28-34
3.5	2000-3000	34-38
3.5-4.0	Above 3000	Above 38

From Bloom RS, Cropley C, AHA/AAP Neonatal Resuscitation Program Steering Committee: *Textbook of neonatal resuscitation,* Dallas, 1994, American Heart Association.

repeated intubation. In order to prevent complications, provide free-flow oxygen during intubation, use gentle technique, and limit intubation attempts to 20 seconds.

Chest Compressions

Indications for chest compressions include (1) a heart rate <60 beats/min, and (2) a heart rate between 60 and 80 beats/min and not increasing despite ventilation for 15 to 30 seconds with 100% oxygen. It is important to follow the steps of (A) Airway, (B) Breathing, and (C) Circulation; before the heart rate is even checked, an airway should be established and ventilation begun if the infant is apneic. Often, adequate ventilation alone will result in a rapid increase in heart rate.[20]

Perform the following steps:

- **Position the infant with the neck slightly extended.**
- **Provide firm support for the back.**
- **Perform compressions by two-finger or thumb method (Fig. 4-11):**
    Position: lower third of sternum[21]
    Rate: 90 times/min
    Depth: 1/2 to 3/4 in
    Support: encircling fingers or hand under back
- **Provide 90 compressions/min and interpose 30 breaths/min with a 3:1 ratio of compressions to breaths (120 events/min).[11,22]**
- **Evaluate the heart rate after 30 seconds.**
- **Continue compressions until the heart rate is >80 beats/min.**
- **Administer medications if heart rate remains <80 beats/min despite at least 30 seconds of**

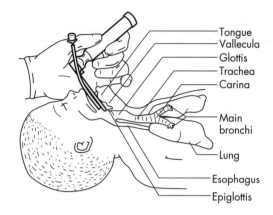

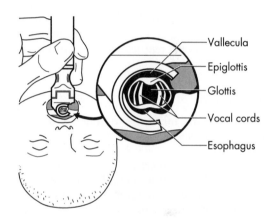

Figure 4-10 Anatomic landmarks that relate to intubation. (From Bloom RS, Cropley C, AHA/AAP Neonatal Resuscitation Program Steering Committee: *Textbook of neonatal resuscitation,* Dallas, 1994, American Heart Association.)

adequate ventilation with 100% oxygen and chest compressions.

When there is poor response to positive-pressure ventilation and chest compression, re-evaluate for technical problems and conditions interfering with ventilation. Confirm that 100% oxygen is connected properly (see Table 4-4). Assure that the airway is patent, the endotracheal tube is in proper position, and the ventilation pressures and rate are optimal. Evaluate the infant for pneumothorax, diaphragmatic hernia, or hypovolemia (see Delivery Room Emergencies, p. 63).

Complications of chest compressions include liver laceration, rib fractures, and pneumo-

Table 4-6
Depth of Endotracheal Tube Insertion

Weight (kg)	Depth of Insertion (cm from upper lip)
1	7
2	8
3	9
4	10

From Bloom RS, Cropley C, AHA/AAP Neonatal Resuscitation Program Steering Committee: *Textbook of neonatal resuscitation,* Dallas, 1994, American Heart Association.

thorax. In order to prevent complications, check the position of compressions, maintain contact with the chest during the release portion of the compression cycle, and avoid excessive force of compressions.

Medications

The indications for drugs during resuscitation include the following:

- Epinephrine: heart rate <80 beats/min despite at least 30 seconds of adequate ventilation with 100% oxygen and chest compressions; heart rate zero
- Volume expanders: evidence of acute bleeding and signs of hypovolemia; poor response to other resuscitative measures
- Sodium bicarbonate: documented or suspected metabolic acidosis in the presence of adequate ventilation
- Naloxone hydrochloride: severe respiratory depression and narcotic administration to the mother in the last 4 hours

Perform the following steps (see Table 4-3):

- Prepare each drug for administration, draw up the appropriate concentration and volume, and label.
- Calculate the correct dosage of each drug.
- Administer each drug by the correct route and at the proper rate.[23]
- Reevaluate for desired effect and take follow-up action.

Two-finger method: Use the tips of two fingers of one hand to compress the sternum, and use your other hand or a very firm surface to support the infant's back.

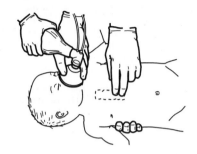

Thumb placement

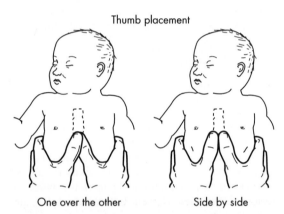

One over the other   Side by side

Figure 4-11   Two-finger method and thumb method of chest compressions. (From Bloom RS, Cropley C, AHA/AAP Neonatal Resuscitation Program Steering Committee: *Textbook of neonatal resuscitation,* Dallas, 1994, American Heart Association.)

Epinephrine increases the rate and strength of cardiac contractions; its principal action during resuscitation is that of a peripheral vasoconstrictor; thus it directs cardiac output to the central circulation and increases coronary perfusion pressure.[24,25] Expansion of the plasma and blood volumes may also be required to maintain cardiac output, blood pressure, and peripheral perfusion. Volume expansion should be considered when there is evidence of acute blood loss (e.g., abruptio placentae, fetal-maternal hemorrhage, umbilical cord tear, acute neonatal hemorrhage) or poor response to resuscitation (e.g., pallor, poor capillary filling, or hypotension unresponsive to oxygen and assisted ventilation). Although acidosis frequently persists after a prolonged resuscitation, many infants will correct an acidosis spontaneously once the asphyxiating circumstances are relieved and adequate ventilation is established. Metabolic correction of pH is a slow process that takes several hours, and treatment with $NaHCO_3$ is not mandatory.

Complications of drug administration include extravasation with intravascular administration, hepatic injury with low umbilical venous catheters, and unpredictable absorption with endotracheal and intramuscular administration. One must also be aware of the adverse pharmacologic effects of resuscitation drugs. Epinephrine, administered in high doses, increases the risk of significant hypertension and germinal matrix hemorrhage.[26] Epinephrine absorption after endotracheal administration is erratic.[27] Sodium bicarbonate results in worsened acidosis in the setting of impaired ventilation; bicarbonate may also worsen intracellular acidosis. Bicarbonate adds a high sodium load, which may directly depress myocardial performance.[28,29] Volume overload may result from administration of repeated doses of sodium bicarbonate or volume expanders. Naloxone hydrochloride is contraindicated in infants of narcotic-addicted mothers; administration can result in severe abstinence syndrome, including seizures.

Intraventricular hemorrhage has been associated with rapid volume expansion, producing acute elevation of systolic blood pressure[30] and high-dose epinephrine leading to prolonged hypertension.[26]

Distressed newborns have impaired autoregulation of cerebral blood flow, with the blood flow directly related to the systolic blood pressure. Increased cerebral blood flow and elevated systolic pressures may be responsible for intraventricular hemorrhage in the presence of a capillary bed insulted by acidosis and hypoxia.[31] Autopsy studies also suggest that increased cerebral venous capillary pressure can initiate intraventricular hemorrhage (Fig. 4-12). Volume expansion should be performed cautiously in preterm or asphyxiated infants, infusing 10 ml/kg aliquots of fluid over a 5- to 10-minute period and evaluating the response before administering repeated aliquots of fluid.

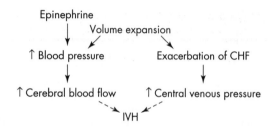

Figure 4-12 Potential adverse effects of rapid volume expansion.

The exception to this rule is the infant who has experienced acute perinatal hemorrhage with hypovolemia. These infants should have the circulatory fluid volume restored as rapidly as possible. Complications of medication administration can be prevented by choosing the correct dose, rate, and route of administration and positioning umbilical lines carefully. The infant should be evaluated for adverse effects after each medication dose. Calcium and atropine have little role in delivery room settings. Calcium is indicated for hypocalcemia or hyperkalemia, which are infrequent problems in the delivery room. Atropine may mask hypoxia-related bradycardia.[32,33]

Delivery Room Emergencies

Certain conditions can present as emergencies in the delivery room (Table 4-7).[34,35] These conditions may require extensive resuscitation or result in a poor response to resuscitation. Some situations require special intervention immediately; most merit pediatric or neonatology involvement for management. Surgical intervention is necessary to complete stabilization of diaphragmatic hernia, abdominal wall defects, and neural tube defects. See Box 4-2 for an outline of emergency procedures in the delivery room.

Care in Transition from Delivery Room to Nursery

After the infant is stabilized and vigorous, perform elective procedures, such as clamping and shortening the umbilical cord, footprinting and identifi-

Table 4-7
Delivery Room Emergencies

Conditions	Signs and Symptoms	Ongoing Problems	Initial Responses
Pneumothorax	Cyanosis, respiratory distress, unequal breath sounds	Continuing asphyxia, shock ($\downarrow$ venous return)	Perform needle thoracentesis, evaluate for chest tube placement
Choanal atresia and airway anomalies	Noisy respirations, pink when crying but cyanotic when quiet, inability to pass suction catheter per nares	Respiratory distress, intermittent cyanosis and bradycardia	Supplemental oxygen, oral airway, and prone positioning or intubation (lower airway anomalies may require emergency tracheostomy)
Extreme prematurity	Respiratory distress	Continuing hypoxia, hypothermia, possible sepsis, hypovolemia	Intubate, place umbilical lines, evaluate for use of artificial surfactant, begin antibiotics, consider transport to neonatal center
Sepsis	Respiratory distress, hypotonia, poor perfusion, foul odor	Continuing hypoxemia, shock	Intubate, place umbilical lines, administer antibiotics
Severe asphyxia	Prolonged apnea, poor perfusion, pallor, hypotonia, seizures	Hypoxemia, shock, multiorgan system injury	Intubate, place umbilical lines, give volume support and pressors for shock, consider transport to neonatal center
Hydrops fetalis	Body wall edema, ascites, pallor, poor perfusion, respiratory distress, possibly unequal breath sounds (pneumothorax), distant heart sounds (pericardial effusion)	Hypoxemia, anemia, shock, potential for multi-organ system injury	Intubate, perform posterolateral needle thoracentesis bilaterally if unable to ventilate, consider paracentesis; if ascites compromises ventilation, place chest tube for pneumothorax, place umbilical lines, evaluate need for partial exchange transfusion, consider transport to neonatal center
Pulmonary hypoplasia and oligohydramnios	Respiratory distress; flattened, deviated nose; infraorbital creases; low-set, crumpled ears; small chin; deformities of the extremities	Hypoxemia, pneumothorax, pulmonary hypertension	Intubate, place umbilical lines, monitor closely for pulmonary air leak, consider transport to neonatal center

cation, applying ophthalmic prophylaxis, or weighing. A vigorous, stable infant may be safely held by the parents and nursed at the breast. The infant may be placed next to mother's skin or wrapped in double blankets. A stocking cap prevents heat loss from the large surface area of the head and wet hair. Transport of the stable infant to the nursery can be done in the bassinet.

In the case of the infant who has required more extensive resuscitation in the delivery room, trans-

Table 4-7
Delivery Room Emergencies—cont'd

Conditions	Signs and Symptoms	Ongoing Problems	Initial Responses
Congenital diaphragmatic hernia	Respiratory distress with asymetrical breath sounds, barrel chest and scaphoid abdomen, point of maximal intensity (PMI) shifted to side opposite hernia	Hypoxemia, pulmonary hypertension, contralateral pneumothorax	Intubate, place umbilical lines, decompress bowel with orogastric suction to low intermittent suction, arrange transport to neonatal center
Abdominal wall defect	Midline abdominal wall defect at base of umbilical cord (omphalocele) or lateral to cord insertion (gastroschisis) with externalization of abdominal contents	Shock, respiratory distress, hypothermia, ischemic injury to externalized abdominal contents, infection	Protect exposed tissue with gauze soaked in warmed saline and covered with evaporative barrier; begin parenteral fluids at 1.5 X maintenance; place an orogastric tube to low intermittent suction, position infant side-lying with support of exposed organs, monitor temperature and urine output, arrange transport to a neonatal center with pediatric surgery
Neural tube defect	Open spinal defect (myelomeningocele), cranial defect with outpouching brain tissue (occipital or frontal encephalocele), failure of formation of skull and brain (anencephaly)	Prolonged apnea, infection, hypothermia	Provide supportive care unless prenatal diagnosis of lethal anomaly has allowed formulation of a plan for limited support; protect exposed tissue with gauze soaked in warmed saline and evaporative barrier; arrange transport to a neonatal center with specialists in spinal defects

fer the infant to the nursery when adequate spontaneous or controlled ventilation has been established, the heart rate is >100 beats/min, and the infant has been dried and protected from excessive heat loss. Note the time of the infant's first respiratory effort and sustained, regular respirations. Transfer the infant in a warmed transport incubator with continuation of required support measures (heart rate monitoring by stethoscope or pulse oximeter, supplemental oxygen or positive

---

Box 4-2

Emergency Procedures in the Delivery Room

A. Umbilical vessel catheterization (see Chapter 7)
B. Thoracentesis and chest tube placement (see Chapter 22)
C. Partial exchange transfusion for anemia (see Chapter 19)
  1. Indications[52]
    Profound chronic anemia (hct <25%), as in the setting of hydrops. Distinct from situations of acute loss of blood volume, chronic anemia results in normal blood volume per kilogram, necessitating partial exchange transfusion to rapidly raise the hematocrit.
  2. Procedure
    a. Obtain O-negative packed red blood cells (PRBCs) (emergency release). PRBCs should be as fresh as possible to minimize risk of hyperkalemia.
    b. Insert a low umbilical venous catheter, and attach a 4-way stopcock (exchange set).
    c. Perform an isovolumetric exchange by alternating withdrawal and infusion of 5 to 10 ml aliquots of patient blood and PRBCs to a total exchange volume of approximately 20 ml/kg The formula

    exchange volume = est. dry wt. × blood volume/kg (desired hct − current hct)/hct of PRBCs

    can be used to estimate the rise in hematocrit for a given exchange volume and a given hematocrit of exchange blood.
    d. Alternatively, place both low UVC and umbilical artery catheter (UAC). Withdraw from the UAC while infusing PRBCs per UVC at the same rate to the total exchange volume.
  3. Risks
    a. Thrombotic, embolic events
    b. Infection

c. Bleeding (secondary to mechanical complications or depletion of clotting factors)
d. Hyperkalemia (consider use of washed PRBCs for nonemergent partial volume exchanges)

D. Prophylactic administration of exogenous surfactant (see Chapter 22)
  1. Indications[55-57]
    a. Prematurity
    b. Respiratory distress
    c. Presumed surfactant deficiency
  2. Procedure
    a. Calculate the appropriate dose of surfactant based on birthweight
    b. Confirm correct endotracheal tube position by cm markings at the lip (see Table 4-6) and careful auscultation. Chest x-ray confirmation is ideal if surfactant is administered during stabilization in the nursery.
    c. Suction the endotracheal tube to clear secretions.
    d. Monitor heart rate and oxygen saturation with pulse oximetry.
    e. Administer surfactant according to manufacturer's directions or experimental protocol. Administration options include rapid bolus or gradual infusion combined with positioning of the infant and hand or mechanical ventilation.
    f. Refrain from suctioning for at least 4 hours after surfactant administration.
    g. Monitor chest wall rise, saturations, and arterial blood gases and adjust ventilator support accordingly.
  3. Complications
    a. Hypoxemia
    b. Air leak
    c. Pulmonary hemorrhage

---

pressure ventilation). Delay elective procedures until the infant is physiologically stable.[36]

In the intensive care nursery, place the infant on a preheated open warmer with servo control. Continue monitoring of heart rate with complete cardiopulmonary monitoring. Continue monitoring of oxygen saturation with pulse oximetry. Obtain a serum glucose by heelstick and a blood pressure by Doppler and blood pressure cuff. Evaluate for placement of umbilical venous and/or arterial lines for fluid administration, blood sampling, and arterial pressure monitoring. Begin a peripheral intravenous infusion if blood glucose is low or volume expansion is indicated; alternatively, consider rapid placement of a low umbilical vein catheter (UVC) to administer glucose or volume if umbilical lines are to be placed.

Care of the Family and Perinatal Decision-Making

Encouraging the presence of the father or of a mature support person in the delivery room is common obstetric practice and should not interfere with delivery room care. Ideally, the members of the resuscitation team should introduce themselves to the parents before the delivery. Parents have a great deal of anxiety concerning procedures performed on their newborn; a few moments spent describing routine procedures will help allay their fears and avoid misinterpretation. When problems are anticipated, a calm, professional explanation of neonatal assessment and life support measures is necessary. Parental awareness that the medical staff has expected and is prepared to care for possible problems can partially relieve their anxieties. Care must be taken, however, to avoid instilling undue alarm. Nonverbal cues such as tone of voice, body language, and comments to other staff members often give the parents a message different from the spoken word.[37]

If an infant requires resuscitation or prolonged physiologic assessment, the attending staff's primary obligation is to immediately administer this care. The presence of the father or a support team must not be allowed to interfere with or delay the delivery of care; however, the pediatric staff should tell the parents what is happening at the earliest possible opportunity. Lack of communication prolongs anxiety for the parents. A few brief statements to explain the procedure can relieve the anguish of silence.

When severe perinatal problems are anticipated, such as extreme prematurity, anencephaly, or trisomy 13 or 18, discussions may be held in advance with obstetric care providers and the family regarding limitation of resuscitative measures.[38] When problems are unanticipated or there has been no time for decision-making, intervention in the delivery room is usually warranted.[39,40] This approach allows time for complete information to be gathered and discussed with the family. If appropriate, support can be withdrawn later in the nursery.[41,42]

When an infant fails to respond to intensive resuscitative measures in the delivery room, the decision must be made when to stop support. Survival is unlikely in premature infants <750g who require cardiac compressions[13] and in term infants if no heart rate has been obtained by 10 minutes.[44] The probability of survival diminishes, and the probability of cerebral palsy increases with the length of time Apgar scores remain <4. If the Apgar score remains <4 at 20 minutes, the probability of cerebral palsy in surviving infants is >50%. If after 20 minutes of maximal resuscitative efforts the infant does not have a heart rate >100, consider discontinuing supportive measures. Parents should have the opportunity to receive answers to their questions from individuals present at the resuscitation.

References

1. Bloom RS, Cropley C, AHA/AAP Neonatal Resuscitation Program Steering Committee: *Textbook of neonatal resuscitation,* Dallas, 1994, American Heart Association.
2. Scarpelli EM: Perinatal lung mechanics and the first breath, *Lung* 162:61, 1984.
3. Rudolph AM: High pulmonary vascular resistance after birth I. Pathophysiologic considerations and etiologic classification, *Clin Pediatr* 19:585, 1980.
4. Bland RD, Nielson DW: Developmental changes in lung epithelial ion transport and liquid movement, *Ann Rev Physiol* 54:373, 1992.
5. Fisher DE, Paton JB: Resuscitation of the newborn infant. In Klaus MH, Fanaroff AA: *Care of the high-risk neonate,* ed 4, Philadelphia, 1993, WB Saunders.
6. Adamson K et al: Resuscitation by positive pressure ventilation and tris-hydroxymethylaminomethane of rhesus monkeys asphyxiated at birth, *J Pediatr* 65:807, 1964.
7. Carter BS, Haverkamp AD, Merenstein GB: The definition of acute perinatal asphyxia, *Clin Perinatol* 20:287, 1993.
8. Bailey C, Kattwinkel J: Establishing a neonatal resuscitation team in community hospitals, *J Perinatol* 10:294, 1990.
9. Price WR et al: Implementing a neonatal resuscitation quality improvement committee, *J Perinat Neonat Nurs* 7:57, 1993.
10. Wheeler CA, Tudhope AE: Development of a neonatal intensive care nursery resuscitation and triage team: impact on nursing care and infant outcome, *Neonat Net* 13: 53, 1994.

11. Emergency Cardiac Care Committee and Subcommittees, American Heart Association: Guidelines for cardiopulmonary resuscitation and emergency cardiac care. VII. Neonatal resuscitation, *JAMA* 268:2276, 1992.
12. American Academy of Pediatrics, American College of Obstetricians and Gynecologists: Antepartum and intrapartum care. In Poland RL, Freeman RK, editors: *Guidelines for perinatal care,* ed 3, Elk Grove Village, Illinois, 1992, American Academy of Pediatrics.
13. Jain L, Vidyasagar D: Controversies in neonatal resuscitation, *Pediatr Ann* 24:540, 1995.
14. Wiswell RE, Bent RC: Meconium staining and the meconium aspiration syndrome, *Pediatr Clin North Am* 40:955, 1993.
15. Carson BS et al: Combined obstetric and pediatric approach to prevent meconium aspiration syndrome, *Am J Obstet Gynecol* 126:712, 1976.
16. Hageman JR et al: Delivery room management of meconium staining of the amniotic fluid and the development of meconium aspiration syndrome, *J Perinatol* 8:127, 1988.
17. Kanter RK: Evaluation of mask-bag ventilation in resuscitation of infants, *AJDC* 141:761, 1987.
18. Vyas H et al: Determinants of the first inspiratory volume and functional residual capacity at birth, *Pediatr Pulmonol* 2:189, 1986.
19. Boon AW, Milner AD, Hopkins IE: Lung expansion, tidal exchange and formation of the functional residual capacity during resuscitation of asphyxiated neonates, *J Pediatr* 95:1031, 1979.
20. Perlman JM, Risser R: Cardiopulmonary resuscitation in the delivery room, *Arch Pediatr Adolesc Med* 149:20, 1995.
21. Orlowski JP: Optimum position for external cardiac compression in infants and young children, *Ann Emerg Med* 15:667, 1986.
22. Burchfield D et al: Why change the compression and ventilation rates during CPR in neonates? Neonatal Resuscitation Steering Committee, American Heart Association and American Academy of Pediatrics [letter], *Pediatrics* 93:1026, 1994.
23. Hasagawa EA: The endotracheal use of emergency drugs, *Heart Lung* 15:60, 1986.
24. Otto CW, Yakaitis RW, Blitt CP: Mechanism of action of epinephrine in resuscitation from asphyxiated arrest, *Crit Care Med* 9:321, 1981.
25. Paradis NA et al: Coronary perfusion pressure and the return of spontaneous circulation in human cardiopulmonary resuscitation, *JAMA* 263:1106, 1990.
26. Burchfield DJ et al: Medications in neonatal resuscitation, *Ann Emerg Med* 22:435, 1993.
27. Lucas VW Jr, Preziosi MP, Burchfield DJ: Epinephrine absorption following endotracheal administration: effects of hypoxia-induced low pulmonary blood flow, *Resuscitation* 27:31, 1994.
28. Hein HA: The use of sodium bicarbonate in neonatal resuscitation: help or harm? *Pediatrics* 91:496, 1993.
29. Howell JH: Sodium bicarbonate in the perinatal setting—revisited, *Clin Perinatol* 14:807, 1987.
30. Goldberg RN et al: The association of rapid volume expansion and intraventricular hemorrhage in the preterm infant, *J Pediatr* 96:1060, 1980.
31. Loe HC, Lassen NA, Friis-Hansen B: Impaired autoregulation of cerebral flow in the distressed newborn infant, *J Pediatr* 94:118, 1979.
32. Leuthner SR, Jansen RD, Hageman JR: Cardiopulmonary resuscitation of the newborn: an update, *Pediatr Clin North Am* 41:893, 1994.
33. Sims DG, Heal CA, Bartle SM: Use of adrenaline and atropine in neonatal resuscitation, *Arch Dis Child* 70:F3, 1994.
34. Khan NS, Luten RC: Neonatal resuscitation, *Emerg Med Clin North Am* 12:239, 1994.
35. Ringer SA, Stark AR: Management of neonatal emergencies in the delivery room, *Clin Perinatol* 16:23, 1989.
36. Kattwinkel J et al: Resuscitating the newborn infant. Perinatal Continuing Education Program, *Book I. Fetal evaluation and immediate newborn care,* Charlottesville, Va, 1995, Division of Neonatal Medicine, Department of Pediatrics, University of Virginia Health Sciences Center.
37. Kimberlin LV et al: The role of the neonatal intensive care nurse in the delivery room, *Clin Perinatol* 16:1021, 1989.
38. Southgate M, Annibale DJ: Clinical ethics and neonatology: integrating emerging disciplines, *Neonatal Intensive Care* 8:42, 1995.
39. Byrne PJ, Tyebkhan JM, Laing LM: Ethical decision-making and neonatal resuscitation, *Semin Perinatol* 18:36, 1994.
40. Sachs BP, Ringer SA: Intrapartum and delivery room management of the very low birthweight infant, *Clin Perinatol* 16:809, 1989.
41. Kattwinkel J: Very difficult questions in neonatal resuscitation, *NRP Instructor Update* 5(3 Part 2-Supplement):1S-2S, 6S, 1996.
42. Rivers RP: Decision making in the neonatal intensive care environment, *Br Med Bull* 52:238, 1996.
43. Davis DJ: How aggressive should delivery room cardiopulmonary resuscitation be for extremely low birth weight neonates? *Pediatrics* 92:447, 1993.
44. Jain L et al: Cardiopulmonary resuscitation of apparently stillborn infants: survival and long-term outcome, *J Pediatr* 118:778, 1991.
45. Kattwinkel J et al: Perinatal Continuing Education Program, *Book II. Newborn care: concepts and procedures.* Charlottesville, Va; 1995, Division of Neonatal Medicine, Department of Pediatrics, University of Virginia Health Sciences Center.
46. Greenough A: Where should the umbilical catheter go? *Lancet* 341:1186, 1993.
47. Shukla H, Ferrara A: Rapid estimation of insertional length of umbilical catheters in newborns, *AJDC* 140:786, 1986.
48. Squire SJ, Hornung TL, Kirchhoff KT: Comparing two methods of umbilical artery catheter placement, *Am J Perinatol* 7:8, 1990.
49. Schneider K, Hartl M, Fendel H: Umbilical and portal vein calcification following umbilical vein catheterization, *Pediatr Radiol* 19:468, 1989.
50. Kempley ST et al: Randomized trial of umbilical arterial catheter position: clinical outcome, *Acta Pediatr* 82:173, 1993.

51. Seibert JJ et al: Aortic thrombosis after umbilical artery catheterization in neonates: prevalence of complications on long-term follow-up, *AJR Am J Roentgenol* 156:567, 1991.

52. Quak JM, Szatmari A, van den Anker JN: Cardiac tamponade in a preterm neonate secondary to a chest tube, *Acta Paediatr* 82:490, 1993.

53. Arya H et al: Neonatal diaphragmatic paralysis caused by chest drains, *Arch Dis Child* 66:441, 1991.

54. Stephenson R, Zuccollo J, Mohajer M: Diagnosis and management of non-immune hydrops in the newborn, *Arch Dis Child* 70:F151, 1994.

55. Corbet A: Clinical trials of synthetic surfactant in the respiratory distress syndrome of premature infants, *Clin Perinatol* 20:737, 1993.

56. Mercier CE, Soll RF: Clinical trials of natural surfactant extract in respiratory distress syndrome, *Clin Perinatol* 20:711, 1993.

57. Pramanik AK, Holtzman RB, Merritt TA: Surfactant replacement therapy for pulmonary diseases, *Pediatr Clin North Am* 40:913, 1993.

5 Initial Nursery Care

Cyndi J. Lepley, Sandra L. Gardner, Lula O. Lubchenco

The content of this chapter presents the basis of newborn care in the first hours of life. The neonate must demonstrate a condition of well-being before being considered a normal low-risk infant. It is essential for health professionals involved in neonatal intensive care to understand the normal neonate in order to care for the sick neonate. The authors discuss the initial assessment, transitional period, and gestational age characteristics to teach the nurse to apply these concepts in initial nursery care.

Physical changes occur so rapidly after birth that the newborn examination can be divided into four time periods. Apgar [8,9] defined the first period in terms of seconds as "exactly 60 *seconds* after birth" and the next period in minutes. The transition period is considered in hours, and the hospital stay in hours or days. If one continues this logarithmic time span for newborns, one uses weeks for the first few follow-up visits, then months, and eventually one speaks of the child's age in years.

Each of these four newborn examinations has a specific purpose. One should consider these examinations in relation to the *age* of the infant rather than to the *location* of the mother and infant in the hospital—or to arbitrary nursery routines (delivery room versus birthing room, transition nursery versus mother's recovery room, rooming-in versus low-risk nursery, etc.) The examination at delivery is aimed at detecting life-threatening emergencies. The examination during the next few hours (transition period) is used to evaluate the infant's adjustment to extrauterine life and to estimate and anticipate likely morbidities. The complete newborn examination, at about 12 to 24 hours, is an important examination, because many findings can be treated or complications can be avoided.

The discharge examination is not as detailed as the complete examination. During this examination the professional demonstrates the baby's unique abilities and answers the parents' questions. This is a good time to provide support and encouragement as the parents begin to incorporate the new member into their family.

Examination at Delivery

Before the delivery occurs, one should obtain pertinent facts regarding the pregnancy, such as parity, gravidity, fetal losses, estimated birth weight and gestational age of the fetus, and, of course, any problems present in the current pregnancy.[43]

During labor one can observe the frequency and duration of contractions and the mother's reaction to contractions. Passage of meconium, rupture of membranes, fetal distress, etc., will alert the attendants to impending problems. At birth, record the amount and distribution of vernix, because it is quickly wiped off. The initial cry and tone, part of the Apgar evaluation, are noted even before 60 seconds, because one does not wait for the 1-minute Apgar to begin resuscitative procedures if the infant is limp and not breathing.[40] If the baby is vigorous, the care provider may place the baby on the mother's abdomen or in her arms—the Apgar score can be done there or in a bassinet or warmer.

The score is repeated at 5 minutes. Under some conditions, such as prolonged resuscitation, it is helpful to have a score at 10 or 15 minutes. Between the 1- and 5-minute Apgars, one systematically evaluates the baby for potential or apparent medical emergencies. Cardiac and respiratory problems were identified before the 60-second Apgar. With practice and experience the professional will be able to identify the approximate gestational age from the physical appearance. One quick and effective way to estimate gestational age is by measuring foot length.[28] Foot length of appropriate-for-gestational-age preterm infants has been correlated with gestational age (Table 5-1 and Fig. 5-1). In short gestation (i.e., 25th to 34th week) there is a consistent, incremental increase in the mean foot length of 0.5 cm every 2 weeks. Measurement of foot length (i.e., from the posterior prominence of the heel to the tip of the first [big] toe with a millimeter ruler) is a rapid and simple method of assessing maturation of all newborns, even the very ill, VLBW infant. With this method, like other physical measurements of gestational age, one must consider the standard deviation in interpretation of the results.

After turning the infant to a prone position, further inspection will reveal congenital abnormalities such as spina bifida, imperforate anus, skeletal abnormalities, or genital defects. Internal abnormalities should be suspected if there is an "empty"

or scaphoid abdomen (diaphragmatic hernia) or profuse oral or nasopharyngeal mucus (transesophageal [TE] fistula). Choanal atresia may present as apnea after respirations have been established. Closing the infant's mouth, which results in cyanosis and/or apnea, is a test for choanal atresia. Examination of the umbilical cord and vessels may give a clue to other abnormalities. The size and amount of Wharton's jelly, especially if the cord is thin, suggests problems in intrauterine nutrition. Persistent pulsation of the umbilical cord, best felt in the skin-covered stump, suggests inadequate ventilation (fetal circulation). A single umbilical artery may be a clue to other anomalies.

Physiology

Transitional Phases and Significance

With the first breath of life and the cutting of the umbilical cord, all neonates begin the transition from intrauterine to extrauterine life. The neonate is a recovering patient, similar to a patient recovering from anesthesia. The transitional phase of the neonate is closely monitored to recognize any abnormalities, initiate appropriate measures for referral, and screen the neonate for common problems in early neonatal life.

In 1966 Desmond et al[19] described temporal changes occurring in the behavior and physiology of the infant during the first few hours after birth. Figure 5-2 gives a summary of the physical findings noted during the first 10 hours of extrauterine life in a representative high-Apgar-score infant delivered with the mother under spinal anesthesia without prior medication. Vital signs, including the heart rate, temperature, and blood pressure, are so closely related to age after birth that the examiner can almost estimate the age of the infant from them when there are no problems in the transition to extrauterine life. Vital signs thus alert one to problems if the heart rate, respirations, temperature, and blood pressure do not follow the usual time course.

A heart rate of 160 beats/min at any time other than the first hour after birth should alarm the observer. And, of course, if this rate persisted, it would indicate some serious problem. In the

Table 5-1
Foot Length By Gestational Age*

| Gestational Age (wk) | N | Foot Length (cm) | | | |
		Mean	Median	SD	Range
24	6	4.22	4.1	.17	3.8-4.4
25	12	4.5	4.5	.08	4.4-4.6
26	16	4.72	4.7	.07	4.65-4.9
27	19	4.99	5.0	.14	4.8-5.2
28	18	5.23	5.2	.13	5.0-5.5
29	22	5.47	5.4	.129	5.3-5.7
30	27	5.75	5.75	.23	5.6-6.2
31	24	5.95	6.0	.19	5.7-6.23
32	21	6.22	6.2	.13	6.0-6.4
33	25	6.5	6.5	.26	6.3-6.9
34	24	6.77	6.8	.20	6.5-7.1
35	20	7.1	7.0	.15	6.8-7.3
36	22	7.27	7.27	.21	7.0-7.6
37	24	7.51	7.5	.24	7.4-8.0
38	40	7.92	8.0	.23	7.6-8.3
39	42	8.22	8.3	.32	7.9-8.6
40	56	8.6	8.7	.37	8.2-8.9
41	22	8.75	8.9	.30	8.3-9.1
42	12	9.1	9.2	.33	8.7-9.3
43	8	9.27	9.3	.25	8.9-9.6

*Applies to both male and female infants.
SD, Standard deviation.
From Hernandez, J et al: Footlength and gestational age in the very-low-birth-weight infant, *The children's hospital pediatric update*, September 1987, p 4.

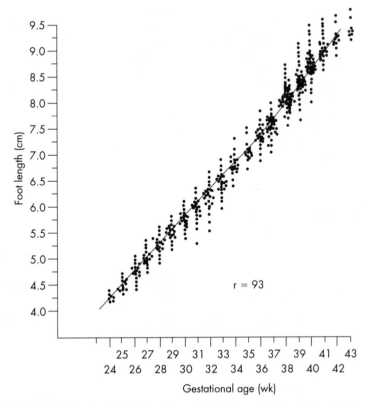

Figure 5-1   Foot length and gestational age: a positive linear correlation.(From Hernandez J et al: Foot length and gestational age in the very low birth weight infant, *The Children's Hospital Pediatric Update*, Sept. 1987, p. 5.

healthy infant shown on the graph in Figure 5-2, the rate falls to a more usual rate seen in newborns. Equally disturbing is the respiratory rate after birth. When one considers the pulmonary adjustments the infant must make immediately after birth, it is not surprising to see tachypnea, but it is disturbing to see barreling of the chest, which is usually indicative of extraalveolar air. The improvement, spontaneously, is just as surprising and gives us even greater respect for the ability of the newborn.

The temperature fall shown in Figure 5-2 may well be iatrogenic. The infant is already stressed by birth and all the adjustments he or she must make. Cold stress requires the infant to use sources of energy that are easily depleted, and if feeding is delayed, hypoglycemia may occur. Hypoglycemia is especially critical in the small-for-

gestational-age infant, whose stores of glycogen and fat are limited.

The newborn's activity during the awake and sleep states[33] can help the professional assess the neurologic development and the effect of stimuli on the newborn's ability to recover from the birth process. The infant is usually awake and alert for the first hours after birth and often indicates hunger by mouthing movements or hand-to-mouth contact. A term infant should be fed early in life before it enters its first sleep period. Bowel sounds are present within the first 30 minutes after birth, and the newborn can successfully feed during this time. After the first feeding the infant falls asleep for several hours and then begins its second stage of activity. The infant awakes from sleep and comes to an alert state if no problems exist. If there are

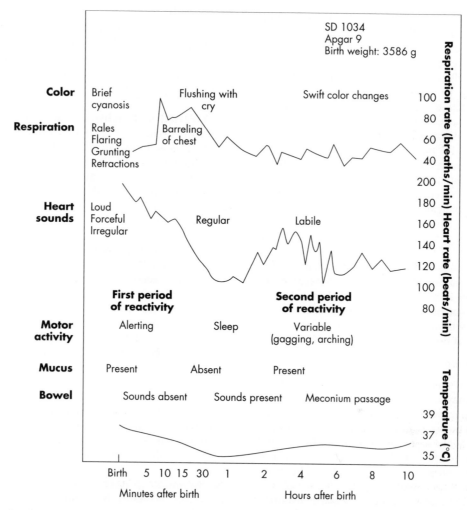

Figure 5-2   Neonatal transitional period. (From Desmond et al: *Pediatr Clin North Am* 13:656, 1966.)

medical problems, the infant will fluctuate between sleep and crying without an alert period in between. Feeding during a drowsy or fussing state will be unsatisfactory and gives us one of the earliest signs of illness—"poor feeding." More subtle signs of distress in the infant are closed eyes with hands tightly fisted and arms extended rather than kept toward the midline, peripheral or circumoral cyanosis, and regurgitation. The infant attempts to alleviate distress and quiet herself when she brings her hands to her face or mouth.

During these first hours, care providers begin to assess the risk of the infant for various morbidities. The assessment is aimed at anticipating or preventing problems that interfere with the infant's adjustment to extrauterine life. Warmth and comfort measures are, of course, indicated throughout this transition period.

The newborn infant responds to illness or stress by "turning off" reactions, and then the professional has a difficult time recognizing problems. Care providers must learn to suspect illness or problems from very few clues. For instance, illness is suspected when the infant is hypotonic, does not feed well, or is difficult to arouse or bring to an alert state. These signs are the same whether the infant has hypoglycemia,[31] polycythemia, or sepsis. Illness may be suspected but requires laboratory documentation to determine the cause. Hence many nurseries have adopted routines that include blood glucose determinations, hematocrit counts, x-ray films, etc. for the most common problems (blood pressure, heart rate, and respiratory rate are already routine). Blood and other cultures, blood typing, screening for congenital infections, and other tests may be indicated depending on the pregnancy history.

Bowel Activity

Bowel sounds are absent until about 1 hour of age. In some babies bowel sounds will occur earlier, especially if they were stressed during labor or delivery and passage of meconium occurred at this time. Auscultate the abdomen for the presence or absence of bowel sounds.

Temperature

The infant's temperature drops rapidly after delivery and may not begin to stabilize for several hours unless appropriate intervention occurs. A newborn needs to be dried off immediately after delivery to prevent heat loss caused by evaporation. Until the temperature has stabilized, maternal skin contact, a radiant warmer, or incubator should be used to maintain thermoneutrality (see Chapter 6). Bathing should be deferred until a normal transition has been achieved.

Pulse and Respirations

As the cardiopulmonary system changes from fetal to neonatal circulation, the transition from intrauterine to extrauterine life begins (see Chapter 4). Initially the neonate may exhibit grunting, flaring, retracting, and cyanosis that resolve in the first hour of life (see Figure 5-2). Also, rales may be heard in the normal newborn's chest. As lung fluid is absorbed, the chest sounds clear. Observe, evaluate, and record the infant's respiratory rate and effort. A normal respiratory rate is 30 to 60 breaths/min without grunting, flaring, or retracting. Auscultate and record the apical pulse. A normal pulse rate is 120 to 160 beats/min.

Motor Activity

A full-term infant who has not been subjected to medications or stress during labor and birth will be awake and alert immediately after delivery. Observe, evaluate, and record the baby's state and activity.

First Period of Reactivity. The first period of reactivity occurs during the first 1 to 2 hours after birth. This is an excellent time for parents to be with their baby and begin the bonding process. Although the neonate may be physiologically unstable, it is safe to allow the mother and baby to be together under the close observation of the professional staff.

Sleep Period. The baby becomes hungry, will nurse, then falls asleep after an initial awake period, and sleeps for several hours. Care providers should avoid disturbing the baby at this time with laboratory work, physical examinations, or feedings so that the infant can recover from the stress of labor and birth. Bathing should be postponed until the baby is awake and the temperature has stabilized.

Second Period of Reactivity. A second period of reactivity occurs between 4 and 6 hours of age. The infant frequently has significant mucoid secretions. The baby will awaken, begin to cry, and demand feeding. Suction secretions as needed.

Awake and Sleep States. Awake and sleep states affect the neonate's behavior and ability to respond to the environment. The newborn may go from one state to another quite frequently in the nursery and at home (see Table 12-3 for newborn states).

Etiology

Failure to make a normal transition to extrauterine life may be the result of obstetric anesthesia or analgesia, neonatal illness, or stress such as perinatal asphyxia and its sequelae. If the infant's pulse, respirations, color, and activity have not stabilized within the normal ranges after 1 hour of life, a problem should be suspected and investigated.

Prevention

Determination of the infant's gestational age provides a reference point for individualizing care. Whether the infant is term and admitted to the normal newborn nursery or preterm and admitted to the special care nursery, attention to care practices that support development and neurologic integrity is essential in preventing iatrogenic disruptions or injury.

In utero, the fetus depends on the mother's physiologic systems to automatically regulate its own. At birth, the neonate's basic physiologic needs (feeding, elimination, heat balance, communication) are met in new and different ways. Emerging from physiologic dependence into a physiologically independent neonate introduces new variables for both mother and baby in the development of their extrauterine relationship. For both term and preterm, the primary developmental task of the new born is to reestablish biorhythmic balance by (1) establishing homeostasis through self regulation of states (e.g., arousal and sleep and wake cycles); (2) processing, storing, and organizing internal and external stimuli; and (3) establishing a reciprocal relationship with primary care providers and the environment.

Although biorhythmic balance is internally determined, caretaking interaction between newborn and parent or caretaker either facilitates or disturbs this transition. After birth, balance is facilitated by contact with familiar surroundings (e.g., the mother's body). The mother's sensorimotor (e.g., auditory, tactile, visual), thermal, and nutrient stimuli provide regulatory effects on the infant's behavior (e.g., activity level, sucking, sleep and wake cycles, and circadian rhythms) and physiology (e.g., endocrine secretion, oxygen consumption, and cardiovascular status).[29] Full-term newborns placed on the mother's chest immediately after delivery display a stereotyped innate sequence of prefeeding behavior (e.g., no sucking activity in first 15 minutes, rooting and sucking activity begins and reaches maximum intensity at 45 minutes, first hand-to-mouth movement at 35 minutes, spontaneous and unassisted finding of nipple and initiation of breastfeeding).[65] Within the first 90 minutes after birth, neonates cared for in close body contact with the mother are quiet.[16,17] However, infants separated from their mothers during this period and cared for in a crib cry and exhibit a "separation distress call" (also seen in several other mammalian species) that ceases at reunion.[16,17]

Care practices (e.g., separation of mother and infant, gastric suction, supine positioning, noise levels in newborn nursery) that have become "routine" in maternal child care are (1) based on few scientific foundations,[36] (2) disrupt maternal and infant regulation and establishment of innate behaviors,[29,55,59,65,66] (3) may have hidden consequences that surpass human adaptability,[36] and (4) may contribute to behavioral deviations that result from violations of an innate agenda.[36,55,56,59] Gastric suction after birth evokes aversive reflexes (e.g., retching, combative movements, increased mean arterial blood pressure, varied heart rate including bradycardia), disrupts development of early feeding behaviors, is unpleasant, and has no advantages in the healthy, term infant after normal pregnancy, vaginal delivery, and clear amniotic fluid.[65]

During transition of the term neonate, prone position has been shown to improve oxygenation, decrease heart and respiratory rates, and encourage more favorable behavioral states.[57] In the newborn nursery the lack of diurnal rhythm in noise levels and care providing activities disrupts reestablishment of biorhythmic balance, sleep and wake cycles, and state liability.[24] Significant differences in nighttime sleep and wake patterns exist between newborns cared for in the nursery (exposed to more light, noise, crying, and noncontingent care) than for newborns rooming with mother (more quiet sleep and less crying).[32] In another study, 20 Caucasian term infants exposed to soothing music in the newborn nursery spent less time in high arousal states (i.e., nonalert waking and crying) and had fewer behavioral state changes.[30] Studies of outcomes of early discharge have not evaluated behavioral states, sleep and wake cycles, and state lability of infants at home versus infants hospitalized after birth.[11]

If adaptation to extrauterine life of the full term neonate is influenced either positively or negatively by nursery care practices, adaptation of the preterm or sick neonate may be even more influenced by early care and handling. Use of stress reduction techniques to prevent fluctuations in blood pressure, vital signs, and oxygenation are often not initiated till after the preterm has been admitted and stabilized in the NICU.[41,61] Individualized developmental care (e.g., dimmed lights, decreased noise, gentle handling, contingent stimuli) (see Chapter 12) may be delayed in the urgency of expeditious assessment, diagnosis, and life-supporting interventions by care providers in the delivery room and on admission to the nursery. However, the physiologic, anatomic, and psychologic transition to extrauterine life makes the neonate, especially the preterm or sick neonate, extremely vulnerable to the stress of resuscitation and initial nursery care.

Minimizing stress and conserving energy should accompany establishing and maintaining an airway, adequate oxygenation and ventilation, and circulatory support.[41,61] The immature preterm infant (<32 weeks' gestation) (see Chapter 12) who is physiologically unstable may deteriorate if not handled gently and protected from overstimulation. Rapid fluctuations in oxygenation and blood pressure, overwhelming stimuli, too rapid volume expansion, suction, unrelieved pain, and hypothermia contribute to the incidence of intraventricular hemorrhage that most commonly occurs in the first 24 hours after birth (see Chapters 4, 6, 7, 11, 22, and 25). In preterm infants, "routine" procedures such as bathing result in increased heart rate and blood pressure, motor stress behaviors, changes in stability and reorganizational behavior, hypoxia, and increased intracranial pressure.[18,50-52,58] Overwhelmed by external stimuli, the neonate's global response to stress may be apnea and bradycardia.

Based on the infant's ability to tolerate an intervention and the benefits of early assessment and intervention, the admission process should be prioritized to (1) provide life-supportive care (2) conserve energy, and (3) collect data and complete the health care record.[61] Table 5-2 outlines developmental interventions for neonatal admissions and initial nursery care that decrease stress, reduce energy consumption, improve oxygenation and respiratory and heart rates, and prevent iatrogenic stress and injury.

Knowledge of the normal vital processes of an infant's first 24 hours of life assists the care provider in early recognition of deviations from normal extrauterine life and in early initiation of corrective interventions.[25,42] Delay in recognizing

and initiating therapy increases morbidity and mortality.[63]

Data Collection

History

Good perinatal care requires the identification of social, demographic, and medical-obstetric risk factors that correlate with fetal outcome. This must be an ongoing process, because high-risk patients may be identified on the first prenatal visit, during follow-up prenatal visits, or not until the intrapartum and postpartum periods. Review of the perinatal history is important in determining significant factors for neonatal health management. Identification of an at-risk maternal situation is essential in order to plan and organize care for the at-risk neonate. Review of the perinatal history includes antepartum and intrapartum events (see Chapter 2) and events of the neonatal course such as normal or abnormal transition, timing and onset of symptoms, and the ability to feed.

Signs and Symptoms

Unlike the verbalizing adult patient, the nonverbal neonate communicates needs primarily by behavior. Through objective observations and evaluations the neonatal care provider interprets this behavior into information about the individual infant's condition. Assessment of the neonate includes the following:

- Estimation of gestational age
- Physical examination
- Neurologic examination
- Brazelton examination

All care providers must not only be familiar with these tools but also be proficient in performing and interpreting them.

Assessment of Gestational Age

An assessment of gestational age should be done on all newborns to assign a newborn classification, to determine neonatal mortality risk, to gen-

Table 5-2
Developmental Interventions During Admission and Initial Nursery Care

Oxygenation	Apply noninvasive monitor (see Ch 7)
	Titrate FiO$_2$ to maintain saturation at 92% to 94% (see Ch 7, 10)
	Handle gently, minimally (see Ch 12, 22)
	Position prone to maximize oxygenation (see Ch 12 and below)
	Delay or defer bathing[50,51,52] (see Ch 17)
Thermoregulation	Maintain temperature: axillary (36.5° C to 37.5° C in term infants); skin (36° C to 36.5° C in preterm infants) (see Ch 6)
	Prewarm linen, scales, radiant warmer, incubator (see Ch 6)
	Decrease heat loss with position (i.e., prone, flexion) (see Ch 6 & 12)
	Use warm water on skin before applying probe, electrodes (see Ch 17)
	Delay or defer bathing[50,51,52] (see Ch 17)
Nutrition	Screen at-risk and symptomatic infants for hypoglycemia (see Ch 14)
	Provide fluids and/or calories (orally or intravenously) (see Ch 13,14,15,16)
	Decrease energy expenditures by decreasing internal (i.e., hypothermia, hypoxia) and external (i.e., noise, light) stressors (see Ch 12 & 14)
Pain	Minimize painful stimuli (see Ch 11, 12)
	Relieve pain with pharmacologic management (see Ch 11)
	Provide comfort measures (e.g., pacifier, containment, grasping) (see Ch 11, 12)
Environmental stimuli	Tactile: (see Ch 12)
	Handle gently and minimally
	Support and contain in flexion
	Rest periods between procedures, handling
	Visual: (see Ch 12)
	Shield from bright, direct light
	Dim lights as soon as possible
	Cover oxygen hood, face with wash cloth
	Cover incubator with blanket or cover
	Auditory: (see Ch 12)
	Talk quietly
	Respond quickly to alarms
	Parents to softly talk to infant
	Keep ill neonates away from crying babies[32]
Position	Promote flexion in side-lying position with blankets, rolls (see Ch 12)
	Prone (oxygenation better; quiet; more restful sleep; decreased caloric expenditure; decreased reflux)[57] (see Ch 12)
	Swaddle (see Ch 12)
	Avoid supine (see Ch 12)
Assess and interpret infant cries	Assess avoidance and approach behaviors so that care is individualized (see Ch 12)
	Support infant strengths, adaptive and coping behaviors (see Ch 12)
	Modulate environmental and caregiver stimuli based on infant cues (contigent on cues rather than noncontingent stimuli and interaction) (see Ch 12)
	Teach parents infant cues (see Ch 12)

erate a problem list of potential morbidities, and to quickly initiate appropriate screening procedures and/or interventions for recognized morbidities.[10,20,44,62] Gestational age can be assessed by obstetric methods and by pediatric methods.

The obstetric methods for determining matu-

rity will have already been performed by the time the newborn reaches the nursery. However, the newborn's care providers should be familiar with dating a pregnancy. Dating the last menstrual period (LMP) could be the most accurate method if the mother is sure of the dates of her last menstrual period. Some women will have spotting or even a light period after becoming pregnant, making them unsure of the time of conception. The use of birth control pills may also make the time of ovulation and conception unknown; therefore pregnancy tests are useful in confirming the pregnancy and the time of conception. Although amniotic fluid analysis is used for gestational assessment, ultrasound examination is preferred because it confirms conception, assesses gestation, and evaluates fetal growth. Office ultrasound examination has improved the ability to assess the duration of gestation. The pregnancy can also be dated by auscultating fetal heart tones, measuring fundal height, and observing quickening.

Pediatric methods of determining gestational age are based on physical characteristics and neurologic examination. On admission to the nursery, every newborn should have an assessment of gestational age by physical characteristics. Numerous tables, charts, and graphs are available for determining gestation. Some tables are more subjective than others, but at least one form should be used by all nurseries caring for babies.

Three of the available charts for determining gestational age by physical characteristics are shown in Figures 5-3, 5-4 and 5-5. Figure 5-3 does not place much emphasis on the neurologic assessment, which may not be valid in the first 24 hours because of birth recovery.[3] To use this chart, an X or "" is placed in each appropriate slot. Then an age is assigned according to a line drawn through the point where most of the marks have been placed. The disadvantages of this system is the subjectivity of the chart; the advantage is that items relate to gestational age, not a score. The examiner must therefore be experienced to offset the possibility of error in the chart.

Figure 5-5 incorporates physical maturity and neuromuscular maturity on an equal basis. An X is placed in the appropriate box for each category. The score for the neuromuscular and physical maturity is added and noted under the maturity rating column. Weeks of gestation are assigned according to the maturity rating score.

To use these charts accurately the examiner must assess the following physical characteristics.[44,62]

Vernix

At 20 to 24 weeks, vernix is produced by sebaceous glands. Note the amount and distribution of vernix on the baby's skin (best done in the delivery room). Vernix is high in fat content and protects the skin from the aqueous amniotic fluid and bacteria. At 36 weeks, the white, cheeselike material begins to decrease and disappears by 41 weeks.

Skin

In early gestation the skin of the fetus is very transparent, and veins are easily seen. As gestation progresses, the skin becomes tougher, thicker, and less transparent. By 37 weeks, very few vessels are visible. From 36 weeks to delivery, fat deposits begin to form and grow. In the postterm infant, desquamation will be prominent at the ankles, wrists, and possibly palms and soles. As gestation progresses, the loss of vernix and subcutaneous tissue causes wrinkling. Note skin turgor, color, texture, and the prominence of vessels, especially on the abdomen.

Lanugo

At 20 weeks, fine downy hair (lanugo) appears over the entire body of the fetus. At 28 weeks, it begins to disappear around the face and anterior trunk. At term, a few patches of lanugo may still be present over the shoulders. Note the distribution of lanugo, first on the face and anterior trunk, then on the rest of the body.

Sole Creases

Sole creases develop from toe to heel, progressing with gestational age. An infant with IUGR and early loss of vernix may have more sole creases than expected. By 12 hours after birth, the skin has dried to a point that sole creases are no longer a valid indicator of gestational age. Note the development of sole creases as they progress from the superior to inferior aspects of the foot (Fig. 5-6, p. 82).

Hair on the Head

Hair appears on the head at 20 weeks. At 20 to 23 weeks the eyelashes and eyebrows develop. From 28 to 34 or 36 weeks the hair is fine and woolly and sticks together. It appears disheveled and sticks out in bunches from the head. At term the hair lies flat

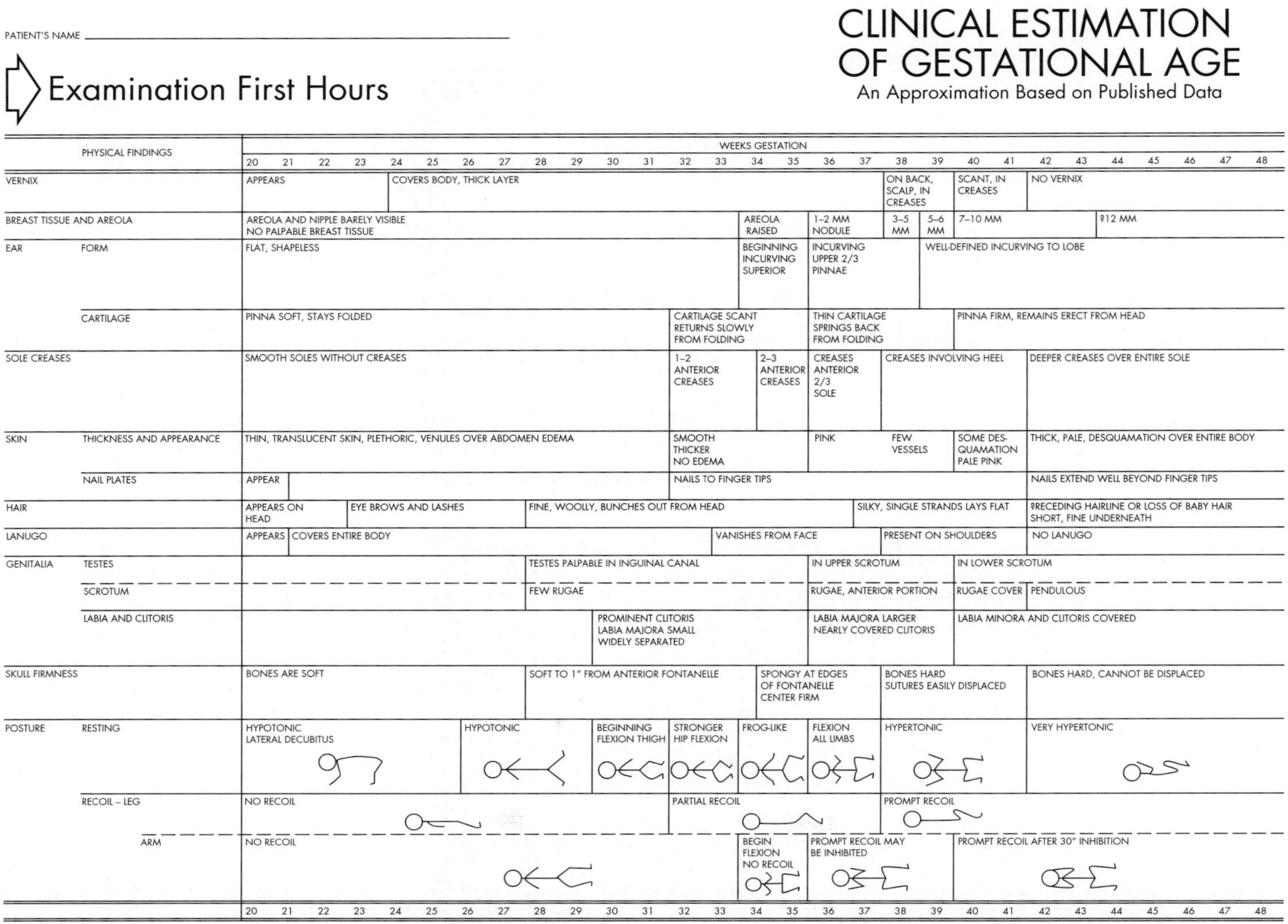

PATIENT'S NAME _____

⬆ Examination First Hours

CLINICAL ESTIMATION
OF GESTATIONAL AGE
An Approximation Based on Published Data

WEEKS GESTATION: 20 21 22 23 24 25 26 27 28 29 30 31 32 33 34 35 36 37 38 39 40 41 42 43 44 45 46 47 48

PHYSICAL FINDINGS	Findings across weeks gestation (20–48)
VERNIX	APPEARS (20) → COVERS BODY, THICK LAYER (24–37) → ON BACK, SCALP, IN CREASES (38) → SCANT, IN CREASES (41) → NO VERNIX (42)
BREAST TISSUE AND AREOLA	AREOLA AND NIPPLE BARELY VISIBLE, NO PALPABLE BREAST TISSUE (20) → AREOLA RAISED (34) → 1–2 MM NODULE (36) → 3–5 MM (38) → 5–6 MM (39) → 7–10 MM (40) → ≥12 MM (44)
EAR — FORM	FLAT, SHAPELESS (20) → BEGINNING INCURVING SUPERIOR (34) → INCURVING UPPER 2/3 PINNAE (36) → WELL-DEFINED INCURVING TO LOBE (38–40)
EAR — CARTILAGE	PINNA SOFT, STAYS FOLDED (20) → CARTILAGE SCANT RETURNS SLOWLY FROM FOLDING (32) → THIN CARTILAGE SPRINGS BACK FROM FOLDING (35) → PINNA FIRM, REMAINS ERECT FROM HEAD (39)
SOLE CREASES	SMOOTH SOLES WITHOUT CREASES (20) → 1–2 ANTERIOR CREASES (32) → 2–3 ANTERIOR CREASES (35) / ANTERIOR 2/3 SOLE (36) → CREASES INVOLVING HEEL (38) → DEEPER CREASES OVER ENTIRE SOLE (43)
SKIN — THICKNESS AND APPEARANCE	THIN, TRANSLUCENT SKIN, PLETHORIC, VENULES OVER ABDOMEN EDEMA (20) → SMOOTH THICKER NO EDEMA (32) → PINK (36) → FEW VESSELS (38) → SOME DESQUAMATION PALE PINK (40) → THICK, PALE, DESQUAMATION OVER ENTIRE BODY (43)
SKIN — NAIL PLATES	APPEAR (20) → NAILS TO FINGER TIPS (35) → NAILS EXTEND WELL BEYOND FINGER TIPS (43)
HAIR	APPEARS ON HEAD (20) → EYE BROWS AND LASHES (24) → FINE, WOOLLY, BUNCHES OUT FROM HEAD (28) → SILKY, SINGLE STRANDS LAYS FLAT (37) → RECEDING HAIRLINE OR LOSS OF BABY HAIR SHORT, FINE UNDERNEATH (42)
LANUGO	APPEARS (20) → COVERS ENTIRE BODY (22) → VANISHES FROM FACE (35) → PRESENT ON SHOULDERS (37) → NO LANUGO (42)
GENITALIA — TESTES	TESTES PALPABLE IN INGUINAL CANAL (28) → IN UPPER SCROTUM (36) → IN LOWER SCROTUM (40)
GENITALIA — SCROTUM	FEW RUGAE (28) → RUGAE, ANTERIOR PORTION (36) → RUGAE COVER (40) → PENDULOUS (41)
GENITALIA — LABIA AND CLITORIS	PROMINENT CLITORIS, LABIA MAJORA SMALL WIDELY SEPARATED (30) → LABIA MAJORA LARGER NEARLY COVERED CLITORIS (36) → LABIA MINORA AND CLITORIS COVERED (40)
SKULL FIRMNESS	BONES ARE SOFT (20) → SOFT TO 1″ FROM ANTERIOR FONTANELLE (28) → SPONGY AT EDGES OF FONTANELLE CENTER FIRM (34) → BONES HARD, SUTURES EASILY DISPLACED (38) → BONES HARD, CANNOT BE DISPLACED (42)
POSTURE — RESTING	HYPOTONIC LATERAL DECUBITUS (20) → HYPOTONIC (26) → BEGINNING FLEXION THIGH (29) → STRONGER HIP FLEXION (32) → FROG-LIKE (34) → FLEXION ALL LIMBS (36) → HYPERTONIC (38) → VERY HYPERTONIC (42)
POSTURE — RECOIL–LEG	NO RECOIL (20) → PARTIAL RECOIL (32) → BEGIN FLEXION NO RECOIL (34) → PROMPT RECOIL MAY BE INHIBITED (36) → PROMPT RECOIL (39)
POSTURE — ARM	NO RECOIL (20) → PROMPT RECOIL AFTER 30″ INHIBITION (40)

Figure 5-3 Clinical estimation of gestational age: examination in first hour.(From Kempe CH, Silver HK, O'Brien D: *Current pediatric diagnosis and treatment*, ed 3, Los Altos, Calif, 1974, Lange Medical.-

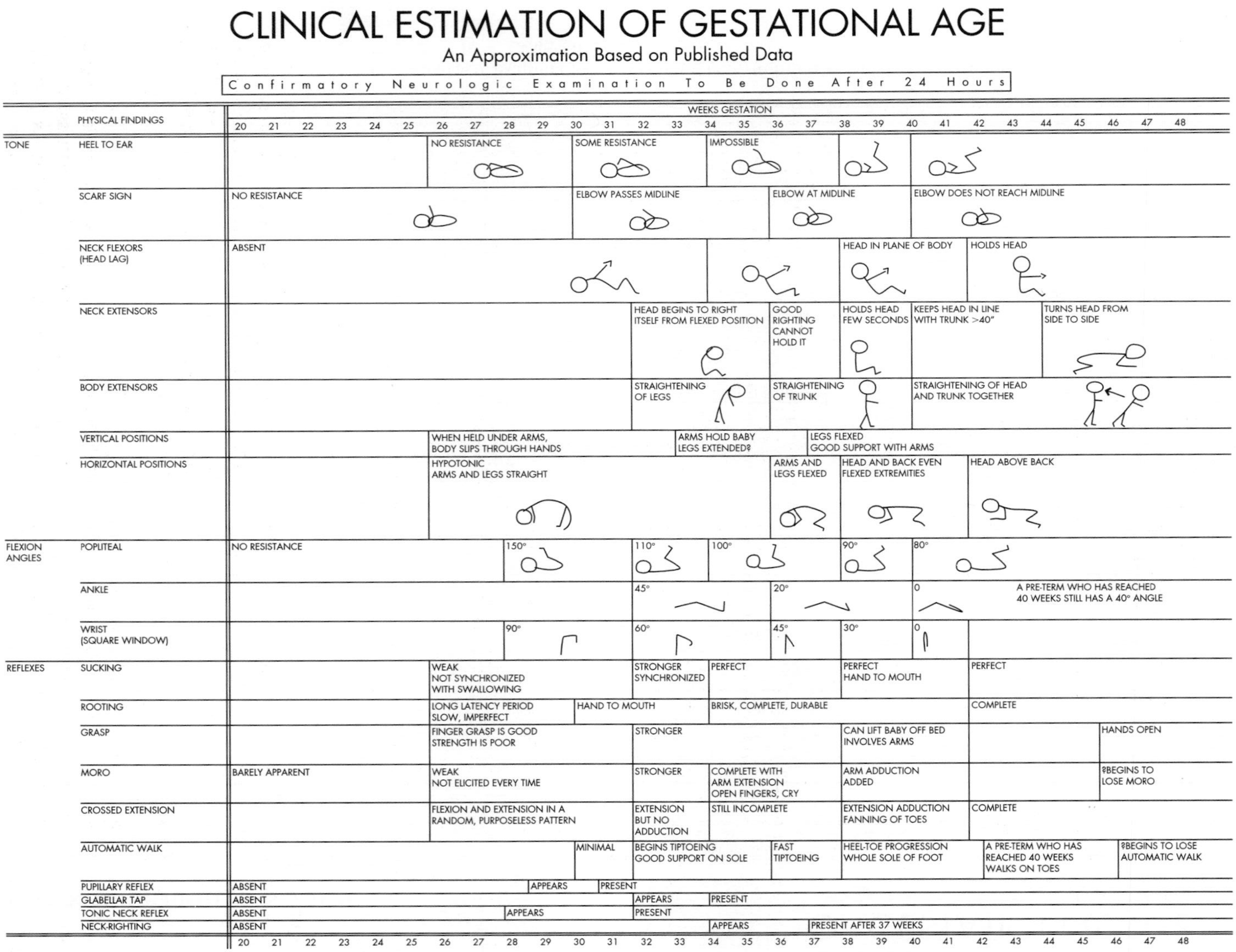
CLINICAL ESTIMATION OF GESTATIONAL AGE
An Approximation Based on Published Data
Confirmatory Neurologic Examination To Be Done After 24 Hours
PHYSICAL FINDINGS
WEEKS GESTATION
20 21 22 23 24 25 26 27 28 29 30 31 32 33 34 35 36 37 38 39 40 41 42 43 44 45 46 47 48
TONE
HEEL TO EAR
NO RESISTANCE
SOME RESISTANCE
IMPOSSIBLE
SCARF SIGN
NO RESISTANCE
ELBOW PASSES MIDLINE
ELBOW AT MIDLINE
ELBOW DOES NOT REACH MIDLINE
NECK FLEXORS (HEAD LAG)
ABSENT
HEAD IN PLANE OF BODY
HOLDS HEAD
NECK EXTENSORS
HEAD BEGINS TO RIGHT ITSELF FROM FLEXED POSITION
GOOD RIGHTING CANNOT HOLD IT
HOLDS HEAD FEW SECONDS
KEEPS HEAD IN LINE WITH TRUNK >40°
TURNS HEAD FROM SIDE TO SIDE
BODY EXTENSORS
STRAIGHTENING OF LEGS
STRAIGHTENING OF TRUNK
STRAIGHTENING OF HEAD AND TRUNK TOGETHER
VERTICAL POSITIONS
WHEN HELD UNDER ARMS, BODY SLIPS THROUGH HANDS
ARMS HOLD BABY LEGS EXTENDED?
LEGS FLEXED GOOD SUPPORT WITH ARMS
HORIZONTAL POSITIONS
HYPOTONIC ARMS AND LEGS STRAIGHT
ARMS AND LEGS FLEXED
HEAD AND BACK EVEN FLEXED EXTREMITIES
HEAD ABOVE BACK
FLEXION ANGLES
POPLITEAL
NO RESISTANCE
150°
110°
100°
90°
80°
ANKLE
45°
20°
0
A PRE-TERM WHO HAS REACHED 40 WEEKS STILL HAS A 40° ANGLE
WRIST (SQUARE WINDOW)
90°
60°
45°
30°
0
REFLEXES
SUCKING
WEAK NOT SYNCHRONIZED WITH SWALLOWING
STRONGER SYNCHRONIZED
PERFECT
PERFECT HAND TO MOUTH
PERFECT
ROOTING
LONG LATENCY PERIOD SLOW, IMPERFECT
HAND TO MOUTH
BRISK, COMPLETE, DURABLE
COMPLETE
GRASP
FINGER GRASP IS GOOD STRENGTH IS POOR
STRONGER
CAN LIFT BABY OFF BED INVOLVES ARMS
HANDS OPEN
MORO
BARELY APPARENT
WEAK NOT ELICITED EVERY TIME
STRONGER
COMPLETE WITH ARM EXTENSION OPEN FINGERS, CRY
ARM ADDUCTION ADDED
?BEGINS TO LOSE MORO
CROSSED EXTENSION
FLEXION AND EXTENSION IN A RANDOM, PURPOSELESS PATTERN
EXTENSION BUT NO ADDUCTION
STILL INCOMPLETE
EXTENSION ADDUCTION FANNING OF TOES
COMPLETE
AUTOMATIC WALK
MINIMAL
BEGINS TIPTOEING GOOD SUPPORT ON SOLE
FAST TIPTOEING
HEEL-TOE PROGRESSION WHOLE SOLE OF FOOT
A PRE-TERM WHO HAS REACHED 40 WEEKS WALKS ON TOES
?BEGINS TO LOSE AUTOMATIC WALK
PUPILLARY REFLEX
ABSENT
APPEARS
PRESENT
GLABELLAR TAP
ABSENT
APPEARS
PRESENT
TONIC NECK REFLEX
ABSENT
APPEARS
PRESENT
NECK-RIGHTING
ABSENT
APPEARS
PRESENT AFTER 37 WEEKS
20 21 22 23 24 25 26 27 28 29 30 31 32 33 34 35 36 37 38 39 40 41 42 43 44 45 46 47 48

Figure 5-4 Clinical estimation of gestational age: examination after first 24 hours.(From Kempe CH, Silver HK, O'Brien D: *Current pediatric diagnosis and treatment,* ed 3, Los Altos, Calif, 1974, Lange Medical.

Neuromuscular maturity

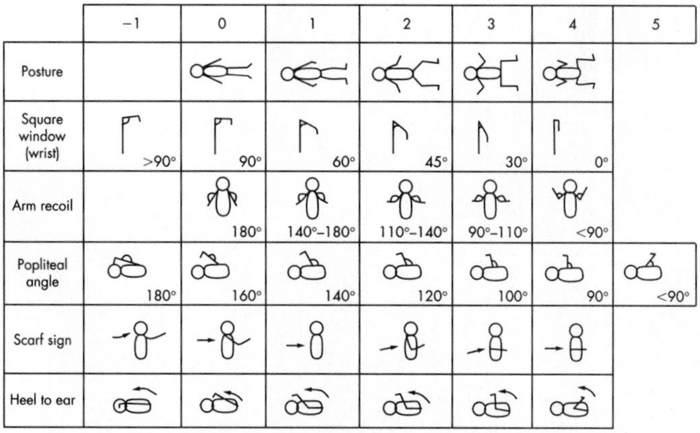

	−1	0	1	2	3	4	5
Posture							
Square window (wrist)	>90°	90°	60°	45°	30°	0°	
Arm recoil		180°	140°–180°	110°–140°	90°–110°	<90°	
Popliteal angle	180°	160°	140°	120°	100°	90°	<90°
Scarf sign							
Heel to ear							

Physical maturity

Skin	Sticky friable transparent	Gelatinous red, translucent	Smooth pink, visible veins	Superficial peeling and/or rash, few veins	Cracking pale areas rare veins	Parchment deep cracking no vessels	Leathery cracked wrinkled
Lanugo	None	Sparse	Abundant	Thinning	Bald areas	Mostly bald	
Plantar surface	Heel-toe 40–50 mm: −1 <40 mm: −2	>50 mm no crease	Faint red marks	Anterior transverse crease only	Creases ant. 2/3	Creases over entire sole	
Breast	Imperceptible	Barely perceptible	Flat areola no bud	Stippled areola 1–2 mm bud	Raised areola 3–4 mm bud	Full areola 5–10 mm bud	
Eye/ear	Lids fused loosely: −1 tightly: −2	Lids open pinna flat stays folded	Sl. curved pinna, soft, slow recoil	Well-curved pinna; soft but ready recoil	Formed and firm instant recoil	Thick cartilage ear stiff	
Genitals male	Scrotum flat, smooth	Scrotum empty faint rugae	Testes in upper canal rare rugae	Testes descending few rugae	Testes down good rugae	Testes pendulous deep rugae	
Genitals female	Clitoris prominent labia flat	Prominent clitoris small labia minora	Prominent clitoris enlarging minora	Majora and minora equally prominent	Majora large minora small	Majora cover clitoris and minora	

Maturity rating

Score	Weeks
−10	20
−5	22
0	24
5	26
10	28
15	30
20	32
25	34
30	36
35	38
40	40
45	42
50	44

Figure 5-5   Clinical estimation of gestational age (revised to include extremely premature infants). (From Ballard JL et al: *J Pediatr* 119:417, 1991.)

on the head, it feels silky, and single strands are identifiable. Note the quality and distribution of the hair and feel its texture.

Eyes

In the third month of fetal life the eyelids fuse and reopen between 26 and 30 weeks.

From 27 to 34 weeks of gestation, examination of the anterior vascular capsule of the lens is useful in assessing gestational age. Gestational age is determined by assessing the level of remaining embryonic vessels on the lens (Fig. 5-7). Before 27 weeks the hazy cornea prevents visualization of the vascular system. After 34 weeks, only remnants of the vascular system are visible. Because rapid atrophy occurs in the vascular system, an ophthalmoscopic examination should be performed during the first physical examination or within 24 to 48 hours after birth.

Ears

Before 34 weeks the pinna of the ear is a slightly formed, cartilage-free double thickness of skin. When it is folded, it remains folded. As gestation progresses, the pinnas develop more cartilage, resulting in better form so that they recoil when

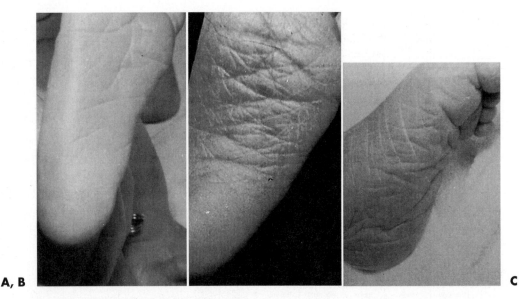

A, B   **C**

Figure 5-6   Sole creases at different gestational ages. **A,** Age 31 to 33 weeks' gestation. **B,** Age 34 to 38 weeks' gestation. **C,** Term.

folded (Fig. 5-8). Check ear recoil by folding the ear in half or into a three-corner-hat shape. Consistently folding it the same way helps the care provider develop a baseline for judging maturity. Note the form and cartilage development of the ear. Examine both ears to be sure they are the same and without defects.

Breast Development

Breast development is the result of the growth of glandular tissue related to high maternal estrogen levels and fat deposition. The areola is raised at 34 weeks. Note the size, shape, and placement of both breasts. Palpate the breast nodule and determine its size. If the infant is growth retarded, breast size may be less than expected at term.

Genitalia

Male Genitalia.   At 28 weeks the testes begin to descend from the abdomen. By 37 weeks they are high in the scrotum. By 40 weeks the testes are completely descended, and the scrotum is covered with rugae. As gestation progresses, the scrotum becomes more pendulous (Fig. 5-9). Note the pres-

ence of rugae on the scrotum and its size in relation to the position of the testes. When examining the baby for descended testes, put the fingers of one hand over the inguinal canal to prevent the testes from ascending into the abdominal cavity and palpate the scrotal sac with the other hand.

Female Genitalia.   Early in the female's gestation the clitoris is prominent with small and widely separated labia. By 40 weeks the fat deposits have increased in size so that the labia majora completely cover the labia minora (Fig. 5-10). Note the labial development in relation to the prominence of the clitoris.

Newborn Classifications

The clinical estimate of gestation is defined by weeks of gestation into the following categories (Figs. 5-11 and 5-12).

- Preterm (PR)—Through 37 completed weeks
- (Full) term (F)—38 through 41 completed weeks
- Postterm (PO)—42 weeks or more

Intrauterine growth curves for the 10th and 90th percentiles are represented in Figure 5-11. Small-for-gestational-age (SGA) infants are those below the 10th percentile. Appropriate-for-gestational-age (AGA) infants are those between the 10th and 90th percentiles. Large-for-gestational-age (LGA) infants are above the 90th percentile. Based on birth weight the infant's intrauterine growth will be SGA, AGA, or LGA.

Using the clinical estimate of gestational age (in weeks) and the birth weight (in grams), one determines the newborn's classification. Combining gestational age and weight criteria in Figure 5-11 forms nine possible newborn classifications: pre-term, full-term, and postterm large-for-gestational-age (PRLGA, FLGA, and POLGA); pre-term, full-term, and postterm appropriate-for-gestational-age (PRAGA, FAGA, and POAGA); and preterm, full-term, and postterm small-for-gestational-age (PRSGA, FSGA, and POSGA).

Using Figure 5-11 plot the newborn weight in grams against the clinical gestational age and mark an X on the chart. Determine to which of the nine categories the baby belongs. Then classify and note the newborn's classification on the record.

Neonatal Mortality Risk. Neonatal mortality risk (NMR), the chance of dying in the neonatal period, can be determined from graphs such as that shown in Figure 5-11 and is based on birth weight and gestational age. On the chart the area of least risk is the FAGA infant. Deviations from this area of least risk in relation to either weight or gestational age increase the newborn's mortality risk.

Over time there has been a change in mortality because of an increasingly physiologic basis of care coupled with sophisticated professional care, technology, transport systems, and aggressive management to handle increasingly at-risk populations. In Figure 5-13 on page 87, NMR graphs are useful in making decisions about potential viability and the appropriate level of care.[16] Babies with greater than 10% risk of neonatal mortality will usually require level II or III care. Note the infant's NMR on the chart (see Fig. 5-11) and record in the newborn record. NOTE: To determine the appropriate NMR, read to the right of the vertical lines and above the horizontal line.

Examination of NMR on Figure 5-11 also re-

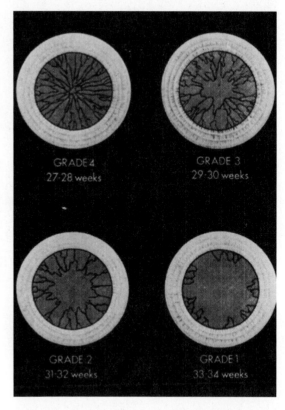

Figure 5-7 Anterior vascular capsule and gestational age. (From Hittner H et al: *J Pediatr* 91:455, 1977.)

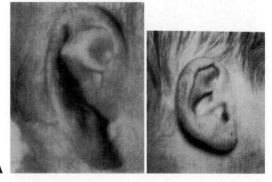

Figure 5-8 Ear form and gestational age. **A,** Age 34 to 38 weeks' gestation. **B,** Term.

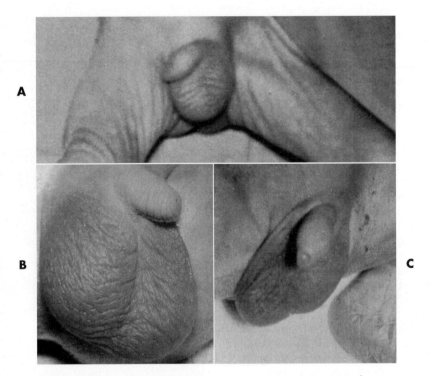

Figure 5-9   Male genitalia and gestational age. **A,** Age 28 to 35 weeks' gestation. **B,** Term. **C,** Age 42 or more weeks' gestation.

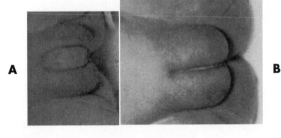

Figure 5-10   Female genitalia and gestational age. **A,** Age 30 to 36 weeks' gestation. **B,** Term.

veals that two infants with the same birth weight but with different gestational ages may have very different risks of death. For example, *infant A* may have a birth weight of 3000 g and a gestational age of 33 weeks. Plotting these values on Figure 5-11, one determines the NMR for this infant at 2%. *Infant B,* on the other hand, may also weigh 3000 g but have a gestational age of 40 weeks. The infant's risk is only 0.2%. *Infant A* thus has a mortality risk 10 times greater than *infant B,* even though they have the same birth weight.

Neonatal Morbidity Risk.   Neonatal morbidity risk (see Figure 5-12) is determined by deviations of intrauterine growth and newborn classification. Classification of the newborn assists in identification, observation, screening, and treatment of the most commonly occurring problems. For every newborn, formulate a problem list based on the morbidities common to the newborn classification. Observe, screen, intervene, and refer as necessary to prevent complications.

Physical Examination

The purpose of the physical examination is (1) to discover common variations of normal or obvious defects, (2) to quickly initiate intervention or referral for deviations from normal, and (3) to establish a database for serial observations and comparisons. The best data are obtained from the

Grams

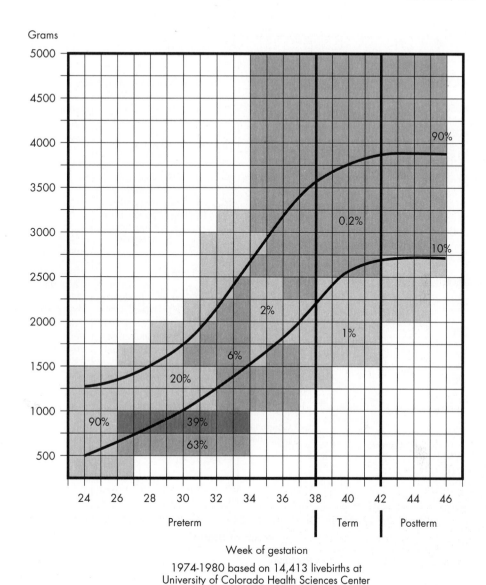

Week of gestation
1974-1980 based on 14,413 livebirths at
University of Colorado Health Sciences Center

Figure 5-11   Neonatal mortality risk by birth weight and gestational age.(From Koops BL et al: *J Pediatr* 101:969, 1982.)

neonate when the physical examination is organized to limit stress, maximize interaction with the examiner, and not overwhelm the newborn. To maximize data and minimize stress, the physical examination should entail observation, quiet examination, and head-to-toe examination.

The order of the first, thorough examination is

determined by using the least stressful items first to obtain optimal information on organ systems. However, the examination is usually recorded in an orderly manner from head to toe.

When one appreciates how stressful it is to the newborn to be undressed, it becomes obvious that as much as possible should be done without ex-

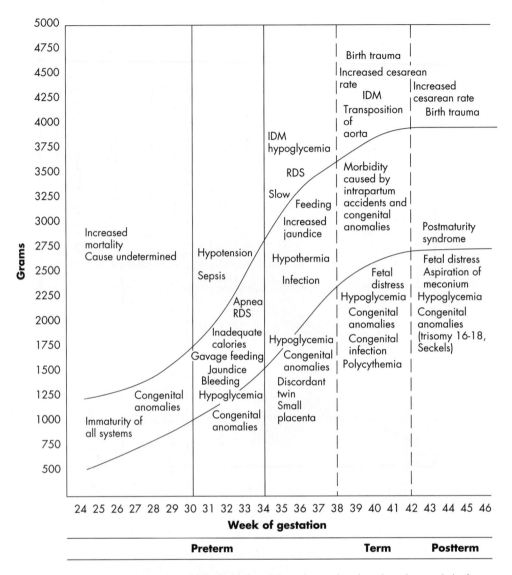

Figure 5-12   Specific neonatal morbidity by birth weight and gestational age based on statistics from Newborn and Premature Center at the University of Colorado Medical Center.(From Lubchenko LO: *The high-risk infant,* Philadelphia, 1976, WB Saunders.)

posing the infant. Warm hands and instruments are essential, and a warm environment helps. Before touching the infant or removing any covers, observe the face, head, and hands as they appear.

Observation

Observation of the neonate provides pertinent data without touching the newborn. General condition, anomalies, resting posture, and respirations of the infant should be observed.

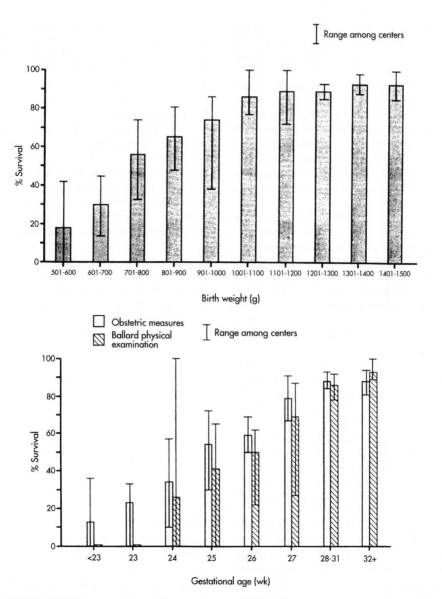

Figure 5-13   Survival of very-low-birth-weight (by gestational age) babies.(From Hack M et al: *Pediatrics* 87:587, 1991.)

General Condition.   The general condition of the infant should be assessed by noting the color, activity, and neonatal state.

Color.   The color of the newborn is normally pink. Acrocyanosis, peripheral cyanosis of the hands and feet, is commonly present in the first 24 hours of life and may be due to immature circula-

tion or cold stress. Ecchymotic areas, especially on the presenting part, are common; however, they may be confused with cyanosis. To differentiate the two, apply pressure to the area. An ecchymotic area remains blue with pressure, whereas a cyanotic area will blanch.

General cyanosis and central cyanosis of the

lips, mouth, and mucous membranes may indicate CNS, heart, or lung disease. Jaundice appearing at birth or within the first 12 hours of life is abnormal. Physiologic jaundice appears after 24 hours, but jaundice may indicate other abnormalities. Pallor at or directly after birth is a sign of circulatory failure, anoxia, edema, or shock. Pallor of anoxia is associated with bradycardia, and the pallor of anemia with tachycardia. Plethora, a beef-red color, may indicate polycythemia and is confirmed by hemoglobin and hematocrit determinations. However, lack of plethora does not rule out polycythemia or hyperviscosity.

Activity and Neonatal State.   Activity and the neonatal state at the beginning of the examination and appropriate changes throughout the examination should be observed. If the infant is asleep, is it quiet or rapid-eye-movement (REM) sleep? Spontaneous, symmetric movements are normal. Tremors and twitching movements of short duration are normal in relation to states of coldness or startling. Good muscle tone is established with adequate oxygenation soon after birth.

Flaccidity, floppiness, or poor muscle tone should be noted. Spasticity, hyperactivity, opisthotonos, twitching, hypertonicity, tremors, or convulsions may be indicative of CNS damage. Asymmetry may result from intrauterine pressure or birth trauma rather than a CNS insult. A lack of crying or evasive behavior in response to the manipulations of a physical examination is abnormal.[49]

Crying.   Attempts to calm and console the crying infant during this part of the examination assist in better data collection during the quiet examination. Acoustic qualities (e.g., melody, pitch, duration, latency, etc.)[52] reflect the newborn's neurophysiologic status and are general assessors of risk.[39,52] Crying is beneficial in (1) ductal closure and transition from fetal to neonatal cardiorespiratory status, (2) improving pulmonary capacity, (3) maintaining homeostasis, (4) facilitating vocal tract development, and (5) cueing and care-eliciting behavior.[52] Negative effects include (1) changes in cardiovascular (e.g., tachycardia, hypoxia, changes in cerebral blood flow) and endocrine systems, (2) stress production and energy drainage, (3) strong, sometimes negative feelings in care providers.[52]

Although uniquely individual, types of cries

that reflect the infant's state and contextual basis have been identified as birth, distress call, hunger, pain, spontaneous, and pleasure.[17,61,65,66] At birth, the term neonate has a loud, lusty cry, whereas the preterm's cry may be weak or absent. Observe the infant's ability to quiet himself or herself when crying.

A high-pitched cry suggests CNS irritation from increased intracranial pressure, injury, infection, or abnormality. Weak crying, no crying, or constant, irritable crying may indicate brain injury, infection, or abnormality. Hoarse cries or crowing inspirations result from laryngeal inflammation, injury or anomalies. A weak, groaning cry or expiratory grunt is indicative of respiratory disease.

Anomalies.   Obvious bodily malformations such as omphalocele, cleft lip and palate, imperforate anus, syndactyly, polydactyly, spina bifida, or myelomeningocele should be observed and recorded as anomalies. Odd facies or body appearances that are often associated with specific syndromes should also be noted.

Resting Posture.   Resting posture should be observed while the infant is quiet and not disturbed. The infant's posture systematically develops according to gestational age[3]: (1) from extension to flexion of the lower extremities, and (2) to flexion of the upper extremities. Asymmetry may result from intrauterine pressure or birth trauma. The infant may take a position of comfort assumed in utero.

Respirations.   Respirations should be evaluated while the infant is at rest and before any manipulation. The normal rate is 30 to 60 breaths/min. Count the respiratory rate and rhythm, noticing the infant's use of accessory muscles. Respiration is normally abdominal or diaphragmatic.

After the first hour of life a respiratory rate of more than 60 breaths/min indicates tachypnea. Tachypnea is the earliest sign of many neonatal respiratory, cardiac, metabolic, and infectious illnesses. Tachypnea, apnea, dyspnea, or cyanosis may indicate cardiorespiratory distress. Labored respirations include retractions, flaring nares, and expiratory grunt.[23]

If the infant is swaddled, the observation examination will not be as extensive as is possible when the infant is unclothed in an incubator or under a radiant warmer. If the infant is swaddled, unwrap gently so that observations of the thorax, abdomen, genitalia, and extremities may also be done during this phase of the examination.

Without touching the infant, one can rule out a multitude of conditions. In fact, over 80% of the newborn examination is made through observation.

Quiet Examination

Quiet examination is defined as any part of the examination in which data are best collected from the quiet, cooperative newborn. The heart, lungs, head and neck, scalp and skull, abdomen, eyes, and blood pressure are areas that should be checked during the quiet examination. Using pacifiers, warming hands and stethoscopes, and holding and gently manipulating the infant are ways to avoid overwhelming the baby and to prevent crying.

Auscultation

Heart. Auscultation of the heart, lungs, and abdomen is most effective when the infant is quiet. When the infant is quiet and at rest, auscultate the heart rate, rhythm, and regularity at the apex. The normal rate is 120 to 160 beats/min at a regular rhythm. Sinus dysrhythmia is normal and may be heard. The point of maximal intensity (PMI) of the neonatal heart is lateral to the mid-clavicular line at the third to fourth interspace. Note the PMI.

A rate of less than 120 beats/min is bradycardia that may be associated with anoxia, cerebral defects, or increased intracranial pressure. A rate greater than 160 beats/min is tachycardia that may be associated with respiratory problems, anemia, or congestive heart failure when accompanied by cardiomegaly, hepatomegaly, and generalized edema.

Murmurs are noted for loudness, quality, location, and timing. They are best auscultated at the base of the third or fourth interspace. Note dextrocardia—heart sounds audible on the right side of the chest. Pneumothorax, pneumomediastinum, dextrocardia, or diaphragmatic hernia result in muffled heart sounds or a shift in PMI.

Lungs. Normally the lungs and chest are resonant after birth, and fine rales may be present for the first few hours. Auscultation reveals bronchial breath sounds bilaterally. Air entry should be good, particularly in the midaxilla. A normal respiratory rate is 30 to 60 breaths/min.

Hyperresonance suggests pneumomediastinum, pneumothorax, or diaphragmatic hernia. Decreased resonance is a result of decreased aeration—atelectasis, pneumonia, or respiratory distress syndrome. Expiratory grunt suggests difficulty in aeration and oxygenation. Peristaltic sounds heard in the chest may be caused by a diaphragmatic hernia.

Abdomen. Peristalsis is normally heard shortly after birth.

Palpation. Palpation of the fontanels and abdomen is best accomplished before the infant begins crying, because guarded muscles and the normally tense fontanels of the crying infant give little useful data.

Head and Neck. The head and neck of the newborn make up 25% of the total body surface. The head is usually 2 cm larger than the newborn's chest. Normal head circumference ranges between 32 and 38 cm for an FAGA infant. Note the size, shape, symmetry, and general appearance.

Microcephaly is characterized by a small head size in proportion to body size. Craniosynostosis is a small head size caused by early closure of sutures. Hydrocephalus is a condition in which an increase in cerebrospinal fluid creates an abnormally large and growing head.

Scalp and Skull. Temporary deformation of the head is caused by pressures during labor and delivery. The head circumference measurements may be altered so that the occipitofrontal circumference (OFC) on the first day of life may be smaller than on the second or third. Caput succedaneum is an edematous area over the presenting part of the scalp that extends across suture lines and resolves in 24 to 48 hours. Cephalhematoma is a soft mass of blood in the subperiosteal space on the surface of the skull bone. The blood mass does not extend across suture lines and resolves in 6 to 8 weeks.

Deviating from the normal, skull fractures may be linear or depressed, palpable or nonpalpable.

The anterior fontanel, a diamond-shaped space normally measuring from 1 to 4 cm, may be gently palpated at the junction of the sagittal suture and coronal suture and between the two parietal bones. Normally the anterior fontanel softly pulsates with the infant's pulse, becomes slightly depressed when the infant sits upright and is quiet, and may bulge when the infant cries. Within 24 to 48 hours after birth, the initial molding of the head and overlap of the sutures resolve, resulting in a larger fontanel and in suture lines that should be palpated as depressions.

The posterior fontanel, formed at the juncture of the sagittal suture and the lambdoidal suture, is palpated between the occipital and parietal bones. Normally it is triangular shaped and barely admits a fingertip.

A bulging, tense, or full fontanel may be associated with increased intracranial pressure caused by birth injury, bleeding, infection, or hydrocephalus. A depressed fontanel, a very late sign in the newborn, may indicate dehydration. A third fontanel, located along the sagittal suture between the anterior and posterior fontanels, may be a sign of congenital infection, Down syndrome, or a normal variant.

Sutures are palpable ridges between skull bones. The coronal suture is located between the frontal and two parietal bones. The sagittal suture intersects the two parietal bones, and the lambdoidal suture lies between the occipital and the two parietal bones. With increasing gestational age, the suture edges become firmer and with gentle palpation are felt as hard ridges. Sutures may be open to a varying degree or may be overlapped because of molding. Lack of normal expansion may indicate microcephaly or craniosynostosis. Abnormally rapid expansion indicates hydrocephalus or increased intracranial pressure.

Abdomen.   The abdomen will appear slightly scaphoid at birth but will become distended as the bowel fills with air. Gentle palpation of the abdomen for organs or masses reveals that the spleen tip can be felt from the infant's left side and is sometimes 2 to 3 cm below the left costal margin. The liver is palpable 1 to 2 cm below the right costal margin. Superficial veins over the abdominal wall may be prominent.

A markedly scaphoid abdomen coupled with respiratory difficulty may indicate a diaphragmatic hernia. Abdominal distention and lack of bowel sounds may occur because of intestinal obstruc-tion, paralytic ileus, ascites, imperforate anus, meconium plug, peritonitis, omphalocele, Hirschsprung's disease, or necrotizing enterocolitis. The infant should be observed for abdominal wall defects such as umbilical hernia; omphalocele, a herniation into the base of the umbilical cord; and gastroschisis, a defect of the abdominal wall.

The umbilical cord may also be observed and inspected while the abdomen is being palpated. The diameter of the cord varies depending on the amount of Wharton's jelly present. Two arteries and one vein are normally present in the umbilical cord. The umbilical cord begins to dry soon after birth, becomes loose from the skin by 4 to 5 days, and falls off by 7 to 10 days. Redness, foul odor, or wetness of the cord may indicate omphalitis.

Inspection

Eyes.   Inspection of the infant's eyes is best accomplished when the infant is found in the quiet alert state or when the infant has been aroused to wakefulness during the examination. The eyes cannot be observed while the baby is crying. Tipping the baby backward and raising him or her slowly or shading the infant's eyes from bright light often causes the eyes to open.

The newborn's eyes open spontaneously, look toward a light source, fix, focus, and follow. Uncoordinated eye movements are common. Subconjunctival or scleral hemorrhages are a common result of the pressures of labor and birth. The size, shape, and structure of the eye should be noted.

The pupils of the normal newborn respond to light by constricting. Red reflex is normally present and indicates an intact lens. Tears are not normally produced until 2 months of age. The iris is usually dark blue until 3 to 6 months of age. Doll's eye maneuvers are normally associated with eyes that follow movement of the head, often with a lag and/or nystagmus.

Discharge from the eyes may represent irritation or infection. A lateral upward slope of the eyes with an epicanthal fold may indicate syndromes of mental, physical, or chromosomal aberrations. The absence of red reflex may indicate tumors or congenital cataracts accompanying rubella, galactosemia, or disorders of calcium metabolism.

Chorioretinitis is often found in congenital viral diseases such as cytomegalovirus and toxoplasmosis. White speckles on the iris known as Brushfield's spots are associated with Down syndrome and mental retardation or are a normal variant. Scleral blueness is associated with osteogenesis imperfecta and scleral yellowness with jaundice. Brain injury may be indicated by a constricted pupil, unilaterally dilated fixed pupil, nystagmus, or strabismus.

Blood Pressure.   Blood pressure with noninvasive Doppler devices is best determined before the infant is upset. The blood pressure should be checked in all four extremities of the infant's body to screen for coarctation of the aorta. Because the blood pressure proximal to the area of obstruction is higher than the blood pressure distal to the area of obstruction, blood pressure in the upper extremities is higher (>15 mm Hg) than in the lower extremities (Figs. 5-14 and 5-15).

Head-To-Toe Examination

The infant's crying will not affect the data to be gathered in the head-to-toe examination.

Skin.   As each body part is examined, the skin is also inspected. Vernix, a white, cheeselike material, normally covers the body of the fetus and decreases with increased gestational age. Discoloration of the vernix occurs with intrauterine distress, postmaturity, hemolytic disease, and breech presentations.

The color of the skin is normally pink. Mongolian spots caused by the presence of pigmented cells may cover the sacral-gluteal areas of infants of color (e.g., black, hispanic, Asian). The degree of generalized pigmentation varies and is less intense in the newborn period than later in life. Nevi may be present at the nape of the neck or on the eyelids.

Note the size, shape, color, and degree of ecchymosis, erythema, petechaie, or hemangiomas.

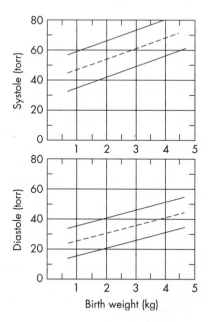

Figure 5-14 Aortic blood pressure during first 12 hours after birth. Linear regression *(broken lines)* and 95% confidence limits *(solid lines)* of systolic and diastolic blood pressures on birth weight in healthy newborn infants. (From Versmold H et al: *Pediatrics* 67(5):607, 1981.)

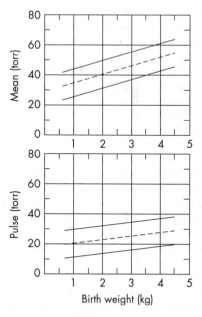

Figure 5-15 Mean aortic and pulse pressures during first 12 hours after birth. Linear regression *(broken lines)* and 95% confidence limits *(solid lines)* on birth weight n healthy newborn infants. (From Versmold H et al: *Pediatrics* 67(5):607, 1981.)

Meconium staining suggests prior fetal distress and anoxia. Erythema toxicum appears as a generalized red rash in the first 3 days of life. Milia caused by retained sebum are pinpoint white spots on the cheeks, chin, and bridge of the nose.

The normal texture of the neonate's skin is soft. A preterm infant's skin is more translucent than a term infant's skin. Slight desquamation may occur as skin becomes dry. Moderate to severe desquamation occurs in postterm infants with IUGR. Puffy, shiny skin is symptomatic of edema. Localized edema of a presenting part is caused by trauma and is only temporary. Edema should be distinguished from increased subcutaneous fat. Lanugo coverage decreases with increasing gestational age.

Tissue turgor is the sensation of fullness derived from the presence of hydrated subcutaneous tissue and intrauterine nutrition. Test the elasticity of the skin by grasping a fold of skin between the thumb and forefinger. When released, the skin should promptly spring back to the surface of the body. A loss of normal skin turgor resulting in peaking of the skin is a late sign of dehydration. A generalized hardness of the skin is a sign of sclerema that occurs in debilitated, stressed infants.

Ears.   Cartilage development and ear form progress according to gestational age. Observe the external ears for size, shape, and position. The angle of placement of the ears is almost vertical. If the angle of placement is greater than 10 degrees from vertical, it is abnormal. The level of placement is determined by drawing an imaginary line from the outer canthus of the eye to the occiput. If the ear intersects the line, it is placed normally. Slapping hands or other sharp noises will normally elicit a twitching in the eyelid or a complete Moro reflex.

Malformed or malpositioned (lowset or rotated) ears are often associated with renal and chromosomal abnormalities and other congenital anomalies. Abnormalities such as skin tags or sinuses may be associated with renal problems or hearing loss. Forceps or difficult deliveries may injure the outer ear. Congenital deafness is suspected if the infant does not respond to noise. It is confirmed by standardized hearing screening tests and follow-up.

Nose.   Note the shape and size of the nose. Deformities caused by intrauterine pressure may be temporary. Neonates are obligatory nasal breathers and must have patent nasal passages. Check the patency of the alae nasi by (1) obstructing one nostril, closing the mouth, and observing breathing from the open nostril; (2) placing a stethoscope under the nostrils that will "fog" the diaphragm and auscultate breathing; or (3) passing a soft catheter if necessary.

Abnormal configuration may be associated with congenital syndromes. Obstructions can be caused by drugs, infections, tumors, nasal discharge, and mucus. Choanal atresia, a membranous or bony obstruction in the nasal passage, may be unilateral or bilateral. Choanal atresia is characterized by the noisy breathing, cyanosis, and apnea of the quiet infant (mouth closed) as opposed to the pink color of the same crying infant (mouth open).

Mouth.   Examination of the mouth may be done here or at the end of the examination when the infant is crying loudly with a wide, open mouth. At birth the normal infant is able to suck and swallow (develops at 32 to 34 weeks' gestation) and root and gag (develops at 36 weeks' gestation). Elicit each.

Lips and mucous membranes are normally pink. Observe the lips and mucous membranes for pallor and cyanosis. If the infant is well hydrated, the membranes should be moist. Open the mouth to look for anomalies. Palpate the hard and soft palates for a membranous cleft or submucous cleft. Epithelial pearls are common along the gum margins and the palate.

Natal teeth may be present and may require removal to prevent aspiration.[35] A large tongue (macroglossia), cleft lip or palate (including submucous cleft), or high-arched palate may be associated with abnormal facies or be an isolated finding. Esophageal atresia and tracheoesophageal fistula are often present with drooling or distress in feeding.

Thorax.   Conformation of the newborn chest is cylindric with an anteroposterior ratio of 1:1. Note the shape, symmetry, position, and development of the thorax. Asymmetry of the chest may be caused by diaphragmatic hernia, paralysis of the diaphragm, pneumothorax, emphysema, pulmonary agenesis, or pneumonia. Fullness of the thorax caused by increased anteroposterior diameter occurs with an overexpansion of the lung. Retractions, an inward pull of the soft parts of the chest while inhaling, indicate air-entry interference or pulmonary disease.

Breasts. Breast tissue systematically develops according to gestational age. Enlargement of breasts because of maternal hormones occurs in either sex on the second or third day. Milky secretions may be present. Unilateral redness or firmness indicates infection.

Clavicles. Observe and palpate the area above each clavicle. A fracture of the clavicle is evidenced by a palpable mass, crepitation, tenderness at the fracture site, and limited arm movements on the affected side.

Genitalia. Male and female genitalia systematically develop according to gestational age.

Male. Inspect the genitalia for the presence and position of the urethral opening. Palpate the testes either in the inguinal canal or scrotum. The scrotum appears large and pendulous with the presence of descended testes. A tight prepuce may be found. In dark-skinned races, darker pigmentation of the genitalia is normal. Hypospadias exists if the urethral opening is on the ventral surface of the penis. Epispadias exists if the opening is on the dorsal surface.

Female. Inspect the genitalia for the presence and position of the urethral opening. The introitus is posterior to the clitoris. A vaginal skin tag is a visible hymenal ring.

Edema of the genitalia in both sexes is common in breech deliveries. Note the presence of a hydrocele or hernia. Fecal urethral discharge may indicate rectourethral fistulas. Note femoral pulses.

Rectum. Visualize and check the patency of the anal opening by gently inserting a soft rubber catheter (do not use rigid objects such as glass rectal thermometers). Observe the anatomy and feel the muscle tone. Meconium is normally present during the first days of life.

Imperforate anus, irritation, or fissures may be present. Meconium passage before birth suggests fetal intrauterine distress. Failure to pass meconium within 48 hours suggests obstruction. Meconium ileus is associated with cystic fibrosis.

Back. Place the infant in a prone position and observe for a flat and straight vertebral column. Separate the buttocks to observe the coccygeal area. To check incurving reflex, stroke one side of the vertebral column. The baby will turn the buttocks toward the side stroked. Deviations from normal include curvature of the vertebral column, pilonidal dimple, pilonidal sinus, spina bifida, or myelomeningocele.

Extremities

Upper Extremities. Note the size, shape, and symmetry of the arms and hands. Observe and feel for fractures, paralysis, and dislocations. Count and inspect the fingers. The hands are normally clenched into fists. The infant is capable of adduction, flexion, internal rotation, extension, and symmetry of movement. Note the tone of the muscles. Flexion develops with increasing gestational age.

Simian creases may indicate chromosomal abnormalities that are frequent causes of deformity. Polydactyly and syndactyly of the fingers may be found. Osteogenesis imperfecta is characterized by multiple fractures and deformities. Palsies caused by fractures, dislocations, or injury to the brachial plexus are recognized by limited movement of the extremity. Fractures may also be present with edema and palpable crepitus.

Lower extremities. Note the size, shape, and symmetry of the feet and legs. Note the normal position of flexion (develops according to gestational age) and abduction. Note symmetry of movement, thigh folds, and gluteal folds. A full range of motion is possible, including the "frog position," a rotation of the thighs with the knees flexed. Observe and feel for fractures, paralysis, and dislocations. Palpate femoral pulses.

Polydactyly and syndactyly of the toes may exist. Osteogenesis imperfecta results in multiple fractures and deformities. Paralysis of both legs is caused by severe trauma or congenital anomaly of the spinal cord. A unilaterally or bilaterally dislocated hip (more common in females) causes a hip click when the baby's legs are abducted into the "frog" position. Although soft clicks are common, a sharp click indicates dislocation. Fractures may be present and are characterized by limited movement and edematous, crepitant areas. Chromosomal abnormalities are frequent causes of deformity.

Recoil is a test of flexion development and muscle tone. Recoil systematically develops as flexion develops in the lower extremities first and then in the upper extremities. Extend the legs and then release. Both legs should return promptly to the flexed position in accordance with the gestational age of the infant. Extend the arms alongside the body. On release, prompt flexion should occur at the elbows.

Hypotonia causes the infant to become limp and "floppy" with little control. The extremities fall without resistance when the infant is raised off the bed. Recoil may be partial or absent. Hypertonia causes the infant to tremble and startle easily. The fists are tightly clenched, arms flexed, and legs stiffly extended.

Neurologic Examination

Clinical, electric, and anatomic studies of the nervous systems of premature and full-term neonates have confirmed the belief that the CNS of the human fetus matures at a fairly constant rate. Neurologic findings, clinical signs, and electroencephalogram (EEG) findings specifically correlating to gestational age have been established.[21,37,45] However, there are recognized limitations in clinical applications of the neurologic evaluation. The evaluation is of little value in the first 24 hours of life unless there is an obvious palsy or seizure. Because the newborn is recovering from the stress of birth, the neurologic examination is not valid until after the infant has successfully completed the transition to extrauterine life. Therefore the neurologic examination should be performed after the first 24 hours of life (see Fig. 5-4.) If the infant is ill or has obstetric anesthesia or analgesia, the neurologic examination may not be valid even after 24 hours.

Brazelton Examination

The Neonatal Behavioral Assessment Scale[12] assesses the interactive behavior of the newborn. This psychologic scale for the neonate enables as-

sessment of the infant's individual capabilities for social relationships. Clinical application of the Brazelton scale includes neonatal research and evaluation of infant capabilities after illness, prematurity, or maternal medications. A modified version of the Brazelton examination is useful in teaching parents about their individual infant's patterns of behavior, temperament, and states.[15,26,27,47]

By understanding the uniqueness of their infant, parents may more intelligently assess and interpret their baby's cues for interaction and distance. If the parents know their infant's individual strengths and weaknesses, they will be more capable of realistically reacting to their infant. It is important for the care provider to elicit the parents' assessment of their infant's behavior and responsiveness. Unrealistic expectations or incorrect parental perceptions may exist. The care provider therefore uses this opportunity for parent teaching, counseling, and possibly referral.[27,46]

The Brazelton examination is usually performed at 2 to 3 days of life, at discharge, or on the first follow-up visit at 1 to 2 weeks. This examination assesses the infant's best performance in response to stimulation and handling by the examiner. For research purposes, the scoring technique by a certified examiner is required. For clinical use, knowledge of the specific techniques and interpretation of results is all that is required. Because the state of consciousness influences the newborn's reactions, the most important variable in the examiner's observation is knowledge of the infant's state (see Table 12-3 for neonatal states). Performing the examination with the parents present provides the opportunity for parental participation and observation of their infant's response.

Interventions

After the newborn has been examined and assessed, certain admission procedures should be performed. Vital signs should include pulse, respirations, and skin or axillary temperature (never rectal). During the transitional period, vital signs should be recorded frequently enough to monitor the infant's condition and provide appropriate care:

• If the infant is distressed (elevated heart rate

or respiratory rate, retracting and/or nasal flaring), vital signs may be required every ½ to 1 hour.
- If the baby's vital signs are normal on admission (120 to 160 heart rate, 30 to 60 respiratory rate, and 36° C to 36.5° C [97.8° F to 98.6° F] temperature), they may be recorded once or twice during the transition.
- Vital signs should be recorded at least once every 8 hours.

- Rectal temperatures are contraindicated in the newborn infant because of the risk of rectal perforation (see Chapter 6).

Weight, length, and head circumference should be graphed on the appropriate intrauterine growth chart to show in which percentile the baby falls. The parameters should be set at less than 10%, between 10% and 90%, and greater than 90%. Determine the weight/length ratio (Fig. 5-16),

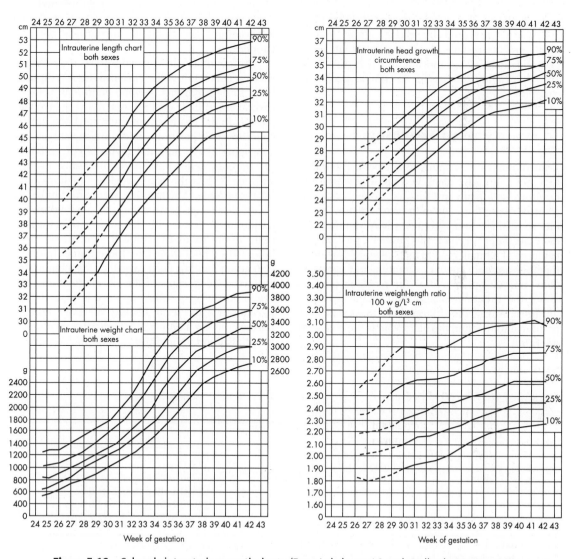

Figure 5-16 Colorado intrauterine growth charts. (From Lubchenco LO et al: *Pediatrics* 37:403, 1966. Original art published by Ross Laboratories, Columbus Ohio.)

which normally increases with fetal age because baby becomes heavier for length as term approaches. In intrauterine growth retardation the weight/length ratio decreases because the rate of growth in weight is affected more than length. Severe and prolonged intrauterine malnutrition may affect head, weight, and length ratios.

Complications

Complications of common morbidities (see Fig. 5-12) are prevented by classification, assessment, and screening of all newborns at birth. Complications of the morbidities in Figure 5-12 are thoroughly discussed in the appropriate chapters.

Parent Teaching

Transitional care, neonatal assessment, and initial care need not take place in a nursery where the newborn and family are isolated from each other. Alternative settings for initial care include birthing rooms, recovery rooms where family and baby are kept together, the mother's postpartum room, or at a home visit. In fact, keeping the family together not only facilitates bonding but also provides unique opportunities for teaching parents about the uniqueness and individuality of their newborn. At this time, parents are most receptive to information about the baby, who is the center of attention.

The assessments of gestational age and physical condition are best performed with the mother and father in attendance so that deviations from normal such as caput, cleft lip, cleft palate, or clubfoot can be explained. Eliciting parental cooperation is important. For example, when the major concern is whether the procedure "will hurt," a response such as "it is routine" will not comfort and reassure well-informed, noninterventionist consumers. Rather, a more physiologically oriented explanation about the condition being screened, why their particular infant is at increased risk, and what interventions are available encourages parental cooperation.

Professional care providers are only temporary caretakers. It is the care providers' responsibility to help parents become confident, primary caretakers of their own infants. Actively involving parents in the treatment of their newborn further solidifies their position as primary caretakers. Encouraging active parental involvement enhances the parents' self-esteem and confidence in their abilities,[26] thus the care providers' actions must tell the parents, "You are able to care for this baby."

At discharge, performing the physical examination in the room with the parents offers a final opportunity to teach, counsel, and advise them before they take their new baby home. Information about feeding, cord care, bathing, elimination patterns, safety, signs of illness, medications, and the importance of follow-up care is essential for parents of a full-term, healthy newborn and for parents taking home an infant after prolonged hospitalization. In addition, a modified version of

Table 5-3
Average Hospital Length of Stay

	1982*	1992†	1994-1995‡
Term	3.7 days	1.7 days	1.6 days
Preterm	>40 days	18 days	1750-2499 g = 1.6-2.4 days
			1500-1749 g = 13-24.3 days
			1000-1499 g = 40.6-42.8 days
			500-999 g = 70.9-72.2 days

*From Commission on Professional and Hospital Activities: *Length of stay by operation, United States, 1982,* Ann Arbor, Mich, Commission on Professional Hospital Activities, 1983.
†From HCIA Inc: *Length of Stay by Diagnosis and Operation, United States, 1994,* Baltimore, Md.
‡From HCIA Inc: *Length of Stay by Diagnosis and Operation, United States, 1996,* Baltimore, Md.

Brazelton's examination on all neonates enables parents to become familiar with a newborn's competencies for reacting to and shaping his or her environment and with strategies for parental intervention. Developing written materials for parents about normal newborn care and documenting teaching sessions and return demonstrations ensure that no important information is forgotten.[48,53,54]

Both term and preterm neonates are being discharged earlier (Table 5-3).

Although evidence of the safety, efficacy, and effectiveness of traditional hospital practices and procedures is lacking and has been questioned,[2,16,29,36,54,55,59,65] early discharge has been generalized from a birth alternative by a self-selected population to virtually all low-risk mothers and babies.[11] Concerns about the mother include (1) rest, (2) readiness to learn and assume self and newborn care (3) readiness to parent, and (4) availability of support systems. Concerns about the newborn include (1) transition from intrauterine to extrauterine life, (2) ability to feed and hydrate adequately, and (3) the early development and recognition of complications. Until scientific evidence is available, individualized discharge plans requiring strict predischarge screening and postdischarge follow-up are recommended[4,6,7,11,34,46,48] (Box 5-1). Because in the first 24 hours after delivery, women have transient deficits in cognitive function, particularly memory,[22] verbal instructions may be poorly remembered and should be augmented with written information.[4,5,7,22,48]

For preterm infants, the attainment of a weight of 5 pounds is no longer the criteria for discharge. Rather, the ability of the preterm or recovering neonate to maintain physiologic stability and the ability of the family to care for the infant's physiologic and developmental needs are the criteria for discharge[46] (Box 5-2). After meeting specific criteria, early discharge of preterm infants using advanced practice nurses who provide a comprehensive program of transitional home follow-up has been shown in a randomized clinical trial to (1) decrease hospital stay by 11 days (2) not increase rehospitalization or emergency room visits, and (3) reduce hospital charges by 27%.[13] In lieu of continued hospitalization, chronically ill VLBW infants were provided with 8 to 24 hours/day of home nursing care and were retro-

spectively found to have fewer rehospitalizations, emergency room and specialty clinic visits, and no doctor's office visits for illness in the first year of life.[13] As in other aspects of health care delivery, care of the high-risk infant from hospital to home is happening sooner with more technology and is more common. While reducing health care costs, earlier home care of these infants increases family burdens of care, expenses, and stressors and without collaborative follow-up, complications and problems may go undetected.[14]

Box 5-1

Criteria for Discharge Within 24 Hours of Delivery

Maternal

Uncomplicated vaginal delivery

Stable condition after delivery: normal vital signs, able to urinate and ambulate

Laboratory data obtained: Hgb/Hct; ABO blood group; Rh typing; RhIg administered

Support system available first few days after delivery

Demonstrates knowledge, ability, and skill in self and newborn care, recognizing complications and how to access care

Neonatal

Term (38 to 42 weeks, gestation), appropriate for gestational age newborn (2500 to 4500 g)

Examined by qualified health care provider and found to be normal

Newborn course: (1) normal and without complications, (2) normal thermoregulation, and (3) able to successfully feed

Follow-up for mother and newborn within 48 hours of discharge

Adapted from American Academy of Pediatrics & American College of Obstetricians and Gynecologists: *Guidelines for perinatal care*, ed 3, Washington, DC, 1992.

References

1. Abman S et al: Pulmonary vascular response to oxygen in infants with severe bronchopulmonary dysplasia, *Pediatrics* 75:80, 1985.
2. Alberts J: Learning as adaptation of the infant, *Acta Paediatr Suppl* 397:77, 1994.

Box 5-2

Criteria for Discharge of Preterm or Neonate With Special Needs

Infant

Maintain temperature between 36° C to 37° C axillary in an open crib

Maintain fluid and nutrition status—take in adequate calories to grow and maintain adequate weight gain (20 to 30 g/day)

Maintain oxygenation status
- in room air, without oxygen
- in nasal cannula oxygen to maintain saturation ≥92% to 95%
- pass room air challenge—able to maintain saturation ≥80% to 85% after 40 min in room air
- free of apnea and bradycardia for at least 5 days

Maintain oxygenation and ventilation status on home ventilator

Parents/Family

Demonstrates knowledge, ability, and skill to
- provide infant care: bathing, diapering, dressing, cord and circumcision care
- maintain infant's thermal state—able to take temperature and dress appropriately
- feed infant adequate calories to gain weight by breast, bottle, or alternative methods (e.g., nasogastric tube, gastrostomy)

- manage oxygen and oxygen equipment
- manage monitoring equipment (e.g., cardiorespiratory, apnea, or pulse oximetry)
- manage home ventilator equipment, suction and retrach procedure
- maintain safe environment
- administer medications in proper doses, at proper times, and know side effects
- recognize signs of illness, know when to call primary care provider
- administer CPR

Availability of support system to assist in infant's care (e.g., family, friends, or community resources)

Demonstrates emotional and relationship stability

Financial resources (e.g., insurance, Medicaid) available for equipment, medications, and ongoing care and services

Understands importance of follow-up care and knows when and who to call for problems or questions

Able to read and respond to infant cues for hunger, pain, more or less stimuli, increasing distress, sleep and wake cycles

3. Allen MC, Capute A: Tone and reflex development before term, *Pediatrics* 85(suppl):393, 1990.
4. American Academy of Pediatrics and American College of Obstetricians and Gynecologists: *Guidelines for perinatal care,* ed 3, Washington, DC, 1992.
5. American Academy of Pediatrics: Hospital stay for healthy term newborns, *Pediatrics* 96:788, 1995.
6. American College of Obstetricians and Gynecologists: *Statement on decreasing length of hospital stay following delivery,* Washington, DC, 1995.
7. American Nurses Association: *Home care for mother, infant, family following birth,* Washington, DC, 1996.
8. Apgar V: A proposal for a new method of evaluation of the newborn infant, *Anesth Analg* 32:260, 1953.
9. Apgar V: The newborn (Apgar) scoring system, reflections and advice, *Pediatr Clin North Am* 13:645, 1966.
10. Attico N et al: Gestational age assessment, *Am Fam Physician* 41:535, 1990.
11. Braverman P et al: Early discharge of newborns and mothers: a critical review of the literature, *Pediatrics* 96:716, 1995.
12. Brazelton TB: *Neonatal behavioral assessment scale,* ed 2, Philadelphia, 1984, JB Lippincott/Spastics International Medical Publishers.
13. Brooten D et al: A randomized clinical trial of early hospital discharge and home follow-up of very low-birth-weight infants, *N Engl J Med* 315:934, 1986.
14. Brooten D: Perinatal care across the continuum; early discharge and nursing home follow-up, *Journal of Perinatal Neonatal Nursing* 9:38, 1995.
15. Buckner E: Use of Brazelton neonatal behavioral assessment in planning care for parents newborns, *JOGN Nurs* 12:26, 1983.
16. Christensson K et al: Temperature, metabolic adaptation and crying in healthy full term newborns cared for skin-to-skin or in a cot, *Acta Paediatr* 81:488, 1992.
17. Christensson K et al: Separation distress call in the human neonate in the absence of maternal contact, *Acta Paediatr* 84:468, 1995.
18. Conway A: The effects of routine nursing procedures on the behavior of preterm infants in the NICU. In *Proceedings of the NAAN Clinical Update and Research Conference,* Washington, DC, 1992, NAAN.
19. Desmond M et al: The transitional care nursery, *Pediatr Clin North Am* 13:65, 1966.

20. Dodd V: Gestational age assessment, *Neonat Net* 15:27, 1996.
21. Dubowitz L, Dubowitz V, Goldberg C: Clinical assessment of gestational age in newborn infant, *J Pediatr* 77:1, 1970.
22. Eidelman A, Hoffman N, Kaitz M: Cognitive deficits in women after childbirth, *Obstet Gynecol* 81:764, 1993.
23. Estol P et al: Assessment of pulmonary dynamics in normal newborn: a pneumotachographic method, *J Perinat Med* 16:183, 1988.
24. Freudigman K, Thoman E: Ultra dian and diurnal cyclicity in the sleep states of newborn infants during the first two postnatal days, *Early Hum Dev* 38:67, 1994.
25. Galloway K: Early detection of congenital anomalies, *JOGN Nurs* 2:37, 1973.
26. Gardner SL: Mothering the unconscious conflict between nurses and new mothers, *Keep Abreast J* 3:192, 1978.
27. Gibes RM: Clinical uses of the Brazelton neonatal behavioral assessment scale in nursing practice, *Pediatr Nurs* 7:23, 1981.
28. Hernandez J et al: Foot length and gestational age in the very-low-birth-weight infant, *The Children's Hospital Pediatric Update,* Sept. 1987, pp. 3–7.
29. Hofer M: Early relationships as regulators of infant physiology and behavior, *Acta Paediatr Suppl* 397:9, 1994.
30. Kaminski J, Hall W: The effect of soothing music on neonatal behavioral states in the hospital newborn nursery, *Neonat Net* 15:45, 1996.
31. Karp T et al: Glucose metabolism in the neonate: the short and sweet of it, *Neonat Net* 14:17, 1995.
32. Keefe M: Comparison of neonatal nighttime sleep-wake patterns in nursery vs. rooming-in environments, *Nurs Res* 36:114, 1987.
33. Keefe M et al: Development of a system for monitoring infant state behavior, *Nurs Res* 38:344, 1989.
34. Kessel W et al: Early discharge: in the end, it is judgement, *Pediatrics* 96:739, 1995.
35. King MM: Prematurely erupted teeth in newborn infants, *J Pediatr* 114:807, 1989.
36. Kjellmer I, Winberg J: The neurobiology of infant-parent interaction in the newborn: an introduction, *Acta Paediatr Suppl* 397:1, 1994.
37. Koeingsberger R: Judgment of fetal age. I. Neurologic evaluation, *Pediatr Clin North Am* 13:823, 1966.
38. Koops B et al: Neonatal mortality risk in relation to birthweight and gestational age; update, *J Pediatr* 101:969, 1982.
39. Lester B et al: Early detection of infants at risk for later handicap through acoustic cry analgesis, *Birth Defects* 25:99, 1989.
40. Letko M et al: Understanding the apgar score, *JOGN Nurs* 25:299, 1996.
41. Little D, Riddle B, Saule C: The power in our hands: integrating developmental care into neonatal transport, *Neonat Net* 13:19, 1994.
42. Lubchenco L: Watching the newborn for disease, *Pediatr Clin North Am* 8:471, 1961.
43. Lubchenco L et al: Intrauterine growth in length and head circumference as estimated from live births at gestational ages from 26–43 weeks, *Pediatrics* 37:403, 1966.
44. Lubchenco L et al: Neonatal mortality risk: relationship to birthweight and gestational age, *J Pediatr* 81:84, 1972.

45. Lubchenco L: *The high risk infant,* Philadelphia, 1976, WB Saunders.
46. National Association of Neonatal Nurses: Draft: position statments in early neonatal discharge, *Neonat Net* 15:48, 1996.
47. Nugent J: The Brazelton neonatal behavior asessment scale: implications for interventions, *Pediatr Nurs* 7:18, 1981.
48. Nurses Association of the American College of Obstetricians and Gynecologists: *Standards for the nursing care of women and newborns,* ed 4, Washington, DC, 1991.
49. Parker S et al: Jitteriness in full-term neonates; prevalence and correlates, *Pediatrics* 85:17, 1990.
50. Peters K: Does routine nursing care complicate the physiologic status of the premature infant with RDS? *J Perinat Neonat Nurs* 6:67, 1992.
51. Peters K: Dinosaurs in the bath, *Neonat Net* 15:71, 1996.
52. Pineyard B: Infant cries: physiology and assessment, *Neonat Net* 13:15, 1994.
53. Pridham K et al: Early postpartum transition: progress in maternal identity and role attainment, *Res Nurs Health* 14:21, 1991.
54. Robinson T: Discharge teaching: sending babies home safely, *Neonat Net* 13:77, 1994.
55. Rosenblatt J: Psychobiology of maternal behavior: contribution to the clinical understanding of maternal behavior among humans, *Act Paediatr Suppl* 397:3, 1994.
56. Rosenblum L, Andrews M: Influences of environmental demand on maternal behavior and infant development, *Acta Paediatr Suppl* 397:57, 1994.
57. Schwartz R: Effect of position on oxygenation, heart rate, and behavioral state in the transitional newborn infant, *Neonat Net* 12:73, 1993.
58. Smail K: The effects of routine bathing on the behavior of preterm infant in an NICU, *NANN annual meeting procedure,* Sept. 1992, pp. 158–159.
59. Smotherman W, Robinson S: Milk as the proximal mechanism for behavioral changes in the newborn, *Acta Paediatr Suppl* 397:64, 1994.
60. Thoden C, Koivisto M: Acoustic analysis of the normal pain cry. In Murry M, Murry J, editors: *Infant communication: crying and early speech,* Houston, 1980, College Hill Press.
61. Tribotti S: Admission to the NICU; reducing the risk, *Neonat Net* 8:17, 1990.
62. Usher R et al: Judgement of fetal age. II. Clinical significance of gestational age and an objective method for its assessment, *Pediatr Clin North Am* 13:835, 1966.
63. Van Leewan G: The nurse in prevention and intervention in the neonatal period, *Nurs Clin North Am* 8:5089, 1973.
64. Wasz-Hockert O et al: The infant cry: a spectographic and auditory analysis. In *Clinics in developmental medicine 29,* Lavenham, Suffolk, 1968, Spastics International Medical Publications.
65. Widstrom A et al: Gastric suction in healthy newborn infants: effects on circulation and developing feeding behavior, *Acta Paediatr Scand* 76:566, 1987.
66. Wolff P: The natural history of crying and other vocalizations in early infancy. In Foss B, editor: *Determinants of infant behavior IV,* London, 1969, Metheum.
67. Zahr L, Montijo J: The benefits of home care for sick premature infants, *Neonat Net* 12:33, 1993.

6 Heat Balance

W. Woods Blake, Judith A. Murray

Optimal care of sick newborn and premature infants requires meticulous attention to detail. The consequences of overlooking some details may not as yet be clinically apparent, whereas other details may affect the very survival of the neonate. Such was the case early in the twentieth century when the beginning of the science of neonatology was marked by the discovery of the importance of maintaining adequate warmth in the newborn. The reports by Tarnier, an obstetrician in Paris and Lion in Nice during the late nineteenth century of improving the survival of premature infants using crude incubators to warm them were impressive first steps in attempting to control the fragile heat balance of weak preterm infants. Manual adjustment of the oil or gas flames that warmed these incubators (undoubtedly resulting in both hypothermia and hyperthermia) dramatically improved the survival rate of these infants.[30,48,11a] Building on these early findings, researchers have gained insight into the physiology of thermoregulation and developed the technology to maintain thermal neutrality in the tiniest and sickest neonates. Although the modern NICU has the expertise and equipment to avoid the consequences of inadequate thermoregulation, determining the most appropriate ways of attaining the best temperature balance is the subject of ongoing investigation.[5] This chapter discusses the current knowledge of the physiology and pathophysiology of neonatal thermoregulation and approaches to prevention and management of heat balance.

Physiology

Animals that maintain their body temperature within a narrow range through a wide range of environmental temperatures are known as homeotherms. Humans, as homeotherms, maintain a "normal" body temperature by balancing the amount of heat lost from the body with the amount of heat generated from within the body. Our ability to cope with changing thermal environments improves physically and physiologically with age. Eventually we are physically able to move to a different place with a more suitable environment or dress more appropriately when the temperature is uncomfortable. Babies, especially preterm or SGA babies, of course cannot physically respond as older children would, and even their physiologic responses are different and limited. Adults lose some thermoregulatory control during REM sleep. Since newborns spend a great deal of time in active sleep, loss of their ability to compensate for changes in environmental temperatures may be detrimental to their well being. Recent evidence suggests that thermoregulation is not impaired during active sleep, indicative of the developmental importance of both thermoregulation and active sleep in the maturation of newborn infants.[4] Physiologic responses to a cold environment involve metabolic reactions that consume substrate and oxygen and result in the production of heat. A *neutral thermal temperature* **is the body temperature at which an individual baby's oxygen consumption is minimized.** Thus a minimal amount of the baby's energy is expended for heat maintenance, and energy is conserved for other basic functions and growth. Minimal metabolic activity is possible within a narrow range of temperatures so that temperatures too high or too low add stress and increase metabolic rate. Extreme deviations from this range will overwhelm the thermoregulatory mechanisms, leading to body temperature changes and eventually death.

CAUTION: **All studies used to developed Figures 6-1 and 6-2 have been done under specific, controlled environments that may not exist in the clinical setting. The ideal temperature varies with**

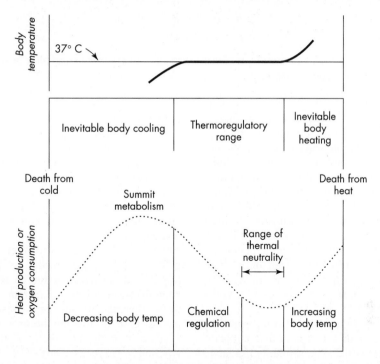

Figure 6-1 Temperature versus oxygen consumption. Effect of environmental oxygen consumption and body temperature. (From Klaus M, Fanaroff A: *Care of the high-risk neonate,* ed 2, Phildelphia, 1979, WB Saunders.)

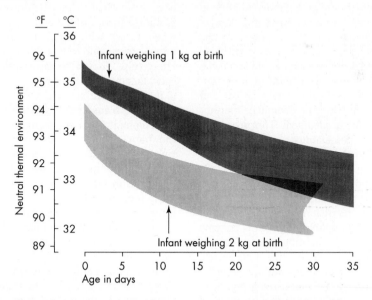

Figure 6-2 Thermal neutral environments. Range of temperature to provide neutral environmental conditions for infant lying naked on warm mattress in draft-free surroundings of moderate humidity (50% saturation) when mean radiant temperature is same as air temperature. Shaded area shows average neutral temperature range for healthy infant weighing 1 kg *(dark)* or 2 kg *(light)* at birth. Optimal temperature probably approximates to lower limit of neutral range as defined here. Approximately 1° C (34° F) should be added to these operative temperatures to derive appropriate neutral air temperature for single-walled incubator when room temperature is less than 27° C (80° F) and more if room temperature is much less. (From Katz G, Hey EN: *Arch Dis Child* 45:328, 1970).

the particular baby and environmental variables (e.g., relative humidity, type of incubator used, and clothing used).

The goal in controlling the neonate's environment is to minimize energy expended to maintain a "normal" temperature, thus eliminating thermal stress. This *neutral thermal environment* is the environmental air temperature at which a baby with a normal body temperature has a minimal metabolic rate and therefore minimal oxygen consumption. Both traditional indirect and the more accurate and sensitive direct calorimetry are used to study the production and expenditure of heat n newborns. Factors such as ambient air temperature, air flow velocity, relative humidity, and temperature of objects in direct contact with the infant or to which heat may be radiated compose the infant's thermal environment.

When exposed to a cold environment, the neonate senses the reduced skin surface temperature (using sensors in the skin, primarily the face), and reduces core body temperature (using sensors along the spinal cord and in the hypothalamus). Information from these various sensors is processed (probably in the posterior hypothalamus), including average temperature, rate of temperature change, and size of the stimulated area. Cold stress results in the initiation of a series of reactions to increase heat production and decrease heat loss. In adults the most significant involuntary method of heat production is shivering. Neonates rarely shiver and must rely on nonshivering, or chemical, thermogenesis to produce the needed heat. This process is initiated in the hypothalamus and transmitted through the sympathetic nervous system leading to the release of norepinephrine at the site of brown fat. Brown fat, found mostly in the nape of the neck, axilla, and between the scapulae of newborns, is a specialized type of fat that is unique in that it contains thermogenin, which is the key enzyme regulating nonshivering thermogenesis. Norepinephrine causes the release of free fatty acids, which with thermogenin undergo combustion in the mitochondria of brown fat cells, releasing heat. Lipoprotein lipase also provides further triglyceride substrate for heat production. When servocontrol is used, care must be taken not to place the thermistor over an area of brown fat, which may directly heat the overlying skin, causing a decrease in the amount of servocontroller heat output. Oxygen and glucose are also consumed during nonshivering thermogenesis. Thus an infant who already has low oxygen or glucose levels may become hypoxemic or hypoglycemic when faced with an added thermal stress. The tiniest premies may not have developed brown fat stores well enough to mount a significant heat production response to compensate for even minimal cold stress.[42]

Heat generated within the body is transferred by conduction through tissues along a gradient to cooler areas such as the skin surface. An initial response to a cold environment is to constrict superficial blood vessels to minimize the transfer of heat from the core to the surface of the body. Superficial vasoconstriction in response to cold stimulus gives a lower skin temperature reading to the thermocontroller and consequently causes an increase in the incubator temperature. The smaller the body size, the less effective vasoconstriction is in conserving heat. Compared with adults, newborns have a very large surface area/body mass ratio and therefore have a relatively large area exposed to the environment from which heat can be lost. More mature infants may try to minimize their surface area by changing positions when faced with cold stimulus, but immature infants are unable to flex the trunk and extremities effectively. They also have little insulation (i.e., subcutaneous fat tissue) preventing heat conduction to the body's surface where it is lost.[26]

Heat is transferred from the infant's body to the environment (i.e., everything in close proximity to the baby) along a temperature gradient from warmest to coolest. This transfer of heat occurs by four principal mechanisms: radiation, conduction, evaporation, and convection. Figure 6-3 illustrates these four mechanisms of heat loss and identifies interventions to minimize their effects.

The newborn calls on physiologic responses to an environment that is too warm much less frequently, and these responses are somewhat limited. As skin temperature rises, superficial blood vessels dilate, increasing the transfer of core body temperature to the surface. Increasing the temperature gradient between the skin and the environment increases heat loss from the body. When exposed to elevated environmental temperatures, babies less than 36 weeks' gestation are generally unable to

RADIATION   **EVAPORATION**

CONDUCTION   **CONVECTION**

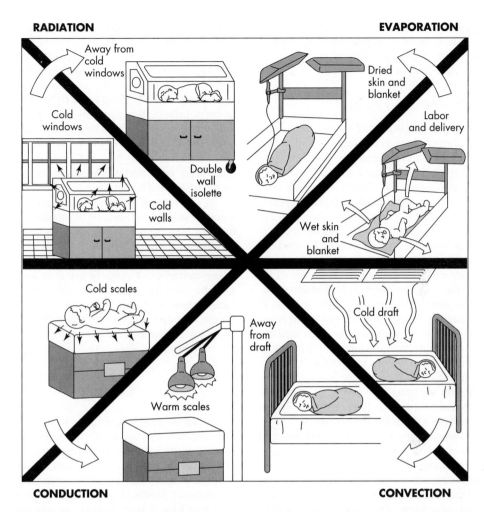

Away from
cold
windows

Cold
windows

Cold
walls

Double
wall
isolette

Dried
skin and
blanket

Labor
and delivery

Wet skin
and
blanket

Cold scales

Cold draft

Away
from
draft

Warm scales

Figure 6-3   *Radiation* or heat loss in the form of electromagnetic photons occurs from warm skin surfaces to a cooler object *not* in contact with the newborn (e.g., inside the incubator wall, nursery wall, or window). Radiant heat loss is independent of ambient air temperature and is the main source of heat loss because of the infant's large surface area. *Conduction* is the loss of heat to a cooler object in direct contact with the newborn (e.g., cold scale, unwarmed bed, stethoscope, or examiner's hand). *Convection* is the loss of heat to moving air at the skin surface and depends on the air's velocity and temperature. *Evaporation* of water from the skin and mucous membranes also causes heat loss, especially in the delivery room. The thinner stratum corneum layer of skin of VLBW infants makes evaporative heat and water loss and fluid management ongoing problems. (Original illustration courtesy Lynn Jones, RN.)

generate sweat to eliminate heat by evaporation. Maturing babies develop this eccrine gland function first on the forehead, followed by the chest, upper arms, and more caudal areas.[25]

Temperature Measurement

The neonate's temperature can be determined by various methods. Deep body (core) temperature may be measured in the rectum, in the esophagus, and on the tympanic membrane. Rectal thermisters are thin, flexible probes and must be inserted at least 5 cm to obtain an accurate reading. Insertion at this depth runs the risk of perforation because the sigmoid colon makes a right-angle turn approximately 3 cm from the anal opening.[39] Esophageal and tympanic readings are difficult to obtain and usually impractical. Noninvasive infrared thermometry, a rapid and painless method of determining tympanic membrane temperature in children, is not recommended for use in newborns at this time. Studies have failed to demonstrate an accurate correlation between infrared tympanic thermometer readings and axillary or rectal temperature readings in newborn infants.[55,56] Continuous monitoring of abdominal skin temperature when lying prone is a noninvasive method that has been reported to show good correlation with rectal temperatures.[15]

Rectal temperature can be obtained using a glass or electronic thermometer, but there are risks of vagal stimulation and rectal perforation.[19,39] Care must be taken that the thermometer is inserted less than 3 cm to avoid perforation at the site where the sigmoid colon turns. Rectal glass thermometers should be held in place at least 3 minutes to obtain an accurate reading. Electronic thermometers may provide a reading in less time. Because of the risks involved, rectal temperatures should not be taken on a routine basis in the neonate. Some nurseries routinely obtain rectal temperatures upon admission to check patency of the anus. However, a soft, flexible, red rubber catheter can easily maneuver the turns in the colon and would be a safer method of determining patency while reducing the risk of perforation.

Axillary temperatures are safe and easy to obtain and may be measured using glass, electronic, or disposable thermometers. The tip of the thermometer should be held firmly in the midaxillary area for at least 3 minutes in preterm infants and 5 minutes in term infants. When taken properly, axillary temperatures provide readings as accurate as rectal and core temperature methods. Axillary temperatures by consensus should be maintained at 36.5° C to 37.5° C (97.7° F to 99.5° F) in term infants. For preterm infants the normal axillary temperature ranges between 36.3° C and 36.9° C (97.3° F to 98.6° F).[2] Infants nursed under radiant warmers may have higher axillary readings compared with rectal measurements and compared with infants cared for in incubators.

In critically ill infants the skin temperature is usually routinely monitored in addition to regular axillary temperature readings. The skin probe is secured to the right upper quadrant of the abdomen. Because the infant responds to cold stress by vasoconstriction, a drop in the skin temperature may be the first sign of hypothermia. The core temperature may not fall until the infant is no longer able to compensate. The axillary temperature may remain normal because of close proximity to brown fat stores.

Etiology

The ambient temperature range in which a healthy full-term infant maintains a stable core temperature is narrower than the temperature range in which an adult maintains a normal temperature. When measures are taken to provide a *neutral thermal environment* for the neonate, thus avoiding excessive heat loss or gain, heat balance is maintained. Recognition of infants at risk for heat imbalance is essential in the prevention of thermal stress.

Premature infants have a limited ability to control body temperature and are extremely susceptible to hypothermia. Factors that contribute to temperature instability include very thin skin, large surface area relative to body mass, limited substrate for heat production, decreased subcutaneous tissue, and an immature nervous system. These infants often have multiple health problems that necessitate frequent interventions by health care providers with consequent disruption of the infant's neutral thermal environment.

The premature infant's very thin skin and larger surface area/body mass ratio allow for increased evaporative heat loss. Term infants can reduce surface area by flexing their extremities onto their trunk, a skill that increases with gestational age. Unable to maintain flexion, the preterm infant lies primarily with extremities extended. Care providers may reduce the infant's surface area by positioning infants in flexion and supporting them with blankets and rolls. Brown fat, lipid supplies, and subcutaneous tissue are limited because of shortened gestation. The immature nervous system delays or mutes the infant's response to thermal stress. The premature infant is likely to experience other complications (e.g., respiratory distress, sepsis, intraventricular hemorrhage, and hypoglycemia) that may increase basal metabolic rate and oxygen consumption, thus interfering with the ability to maintain thermal stability. Numerous procedures and interventions (e.g., medication administration, starting intravenous fluids, and obtaining vital signs) may impede efforts to maintain a neutral thermal environment. Care providers should routinely check the infant's temperature before initiating treatments. If the temperature is low, treatment should be delayed until a more normal temperature is obtained. If interventions are prolonged, temperature should be monitored frequently, an external heat source provided, and the intervention stopped if hypothermia occurs.

SGA infants, like the preterm infant, have a large surface area relative to body mass and decreased subcutaneous tissue, brown fat, and glycogen stores, all of which contribute to heat imbalance.[49] Decreased placental blood flow frequently contributes to the small size and possible intrauterine hypoxia.

The relatively large surface area of the SGA infant increases evaporative and radiant heat loss, whereas limited subcutaneous tissue and brown fat stores contribute to a decreased ability to produce heat. Some flexion of the extremities may be present because flexion depends on gestational age and not weight. SGAs have a higher metabolic rate compared with infants at similar weights but appropriate for gestational age. This is believed to be due to the larger brain size compared with body weight.[49] Hypoxia in utero may depress the infant's CNS and alter the ability to regulate temperature. Increased energy requirements coupled with limited glycogen stores may result in hypoglycemia

and limited ability to produce heat. SGAs may require numerous interventions that disrupt the neutral thermal environment. Care providers should ensure that the infant has a stable temperature before initiation of treatments. Should treatments be prolonged, temperature should be monitored frequently, an external heat source provided, and treatments stopped if hypothermia occurs.

Infants with neurologic damage or depression may experience difficulty maintaining a stable temperature. Hypoxia before, during, or after delivery, neurologic defects, and exposure to drugs such as analgesics and anesthetics may depress the infant's neurologic response to thermal stress.

Hypoxia decreases the effect of norepinephrine on nonshivering thermogenesis, the main route of thermal regulation in the newborn infant. Hypoxia may also reduce the oxidative capacity of the mitochondria in brown fat and skeletal muscles, which are involved in thermogenesis. Infants who have experienced hypoxia in utero may have increased norepinephrine concentrations, which result in peripheral vasoconstriction. This may cause a delayed metabolic response to cold stress and delayed vasodilation to heat stress.[11]

Neurologic defects that affect the hypothalamus also may interfere with heat balance. The hypothalamus coordinates temperature input from various sensors. Drugs (e.g., analgesics and anesthetics) cause CNS depression and reduce the infant's ability to respond to thermal stress. Neuromuscular blocking agents inhibit the infant's ability to maintain a flexed position, increasing exposed body surface and heat loss. **Care providers must be alert to the effect of drugs on the CNS and the infant's ability to regulate temperature.**

Septic infants may experience hypothermia or hyperthermia. In the newborn infant an elevated temperature may begin as a response to cold stress, with peripheral vasoconstriction and thermogenesis. Heat production continues as the infant attempts to achieve a higher body core temperature. Exogenous and endogenous pyrogens may enhance thermogenesis.[11]

Initially, the septic infant may feel cool to the touch and may have a low body temperature. As fever progresses, temperature may rise and the infant feels warm to touch. Infants nursed in servo-

controlled incubators may not have an elevated temperature. The lower heater output in response to increasing skin temperature (by manual or servocontrol adjustment) may mask a fever by keeping the incubator temperature within normal limits. The care provider should be alert to a sudden decreased need for incubator heat support in a previously stable infant.

Many times hyperthermia is iatrogenic, caused by inappropriate control of the neonate's environmental temperature. The most common cause is the use of external heat sources. Dehydration may also contribute to hyperthermia.

Infants nursed with the use of external heat sources should have their temperatures monitored frequently. Phototherapy, sunlight, and the use of excessive clothing and blankets contribute to overheating. Dehydration may be avoided by early recognition of infants at risk for increased fluid loss. Increased insensible water loss occurs in preterm infants because of increased skin permeability and use of phototherapy and radiant warmers. Vomiting, diarrhea, gastric suction, and ostomy drainage also increase fluid loss. These infants should receive additional fluids to replace the increased losses (see Chapter 13).

Prevention

Heat balance is determined by the amount of heat lost to the baby's environment offset by the amount of heat generated by the body plus the amount of heat supplied from outside sources. Because the smaller, more immature, and sicker baby is less able to regulate body temperature, it is crucial that care providers understand the physical and physiologic principles of heat balance and be able to maintain a *neutral thermal environment.* Two broad categories of interventions foster thermal neutrality: (1) blocking avenues of heat loss and (2) providing external heat and environmental support to maintain temperature within the normal range of 36.5° C to 37.5° C (97.7° F to 99.5° F). The theoretically neutral thermal environment required for neonates of 1 and 2 kg at a given age is listed in Figure 6-2. Newborns of less than 800 g are not adequately addressed in currently avail-

able tables but should have a starting environmental temperature setting of 36.5° C (97.7° F).

Attention to the details of these interventions begins in the delivery room, where the first step is to adjust the ambient delivery room temperature to 22° C (71° F) with a relative humidity of 60% to 65%. Warming the room and placing the resuscitation table away from doors or drafts minimizes convective heat loss. The newborn's skin temperature may drop by as much as 0.3°C/minute, with core temperature dropping more slowly after delivery.[2] At birth, the majority of heat lost is due to evaporation of amniotic fluid from the baby's skin surface. Drying the infant with prewarmed towels and immediately replacing them with dry warm towels minimizes evaporative heat loss. Dry towels conduct heat poorly when contacting the neonate's skin. However, cold examiner hands, stethoscopes, scales, and bare mattresses are good heat conductors and can add significant cold stress if not warmed before coming in contact with the newborn.

Skin-to-skin contact between mother and infant may reduce conductive and radiant heat loss. If the infant remains with the parents for an extended time, temperature should be monitored. In the case of a preterm infant in stable condition, the use of an additional heat source (e.g., a radiant warmer) enables parents to spend more time with their infant before transfer to the NICU.[51]

Resuscitation should take place on a preheated radiant warmer so that the adverse consequences of hypothermia are avoided. Because a significant amount of heat is lost through the surface area of the head with its abundant blood supply and the brain's high heat production, covering the infant's head with some insulating material conserves heat during transfer to the nursery or NICU and afterwards. Stockinette material is relatively ineffective for this purpose and provides poor insulation. The best material is thick, maintains its shape with use, and has a high percentage of air volume trapped in the fibers. Knitted wool caps or thinsulate® material may provide the best results.[14,20]

There are a variety of ways to maintain thermal neutrality. Accessability, insensible water loss, servocontrol versus manual control of temperature, and safety are major considerations when determining the method to use for an individual neonate.

Incubators

Incubators provide a controlled, enclosed environment, heated convectively with warm air. The temperature in an incubator may be servocontrolled to maintain a desired skin temperature or air temperature.[10] As the temperature varies from the desired "set point," proportional control units gradually increase or decrease heat output to maintain a constant temperature (without the wider temperature fluctuations seen with simple on-off controllers). **When servocontrolling the incubator to the desired skin temperature, the sensor should be attached to the right upper quadrant of the abdomen with temperature patches or tape. Do not place the sensor over areas of brown fat deposits because the higher-than-expected temperature information to the controlling unit results in a lower-than-desired heat output. Inadvertent cooling may take place if the sensor is covered with clothes or a blanket or if the baby lies on it. If the sensor becomes disconnected from the skin, unwanted heating may occur because an erroneously low temperature reading will cause an unwanted increase in heat output. One must also consider that when an insulated patch is used to cover the thermistor, skin temperature is sensed as being higher than if tape covers the thermistor, resulting in decreased heat output by the warming device.[16] The desired skin temperature used for skin servocontrol is generally 36.0° C to 36.5° C (96.8° F to 97.7° F).[34] Modern incubators can also be servocontrolled to a desired air temperature. This mode has been shown to provide a more stable thermal environment and less temperature variation when compared with skin servocontrol.[17,27] Air servocontrol maintains a constant ambient air temperature when other factors such as phototherapy, external radiant heat, unstable room temperature, or direct sunlight are not confounding variables. The question of air versus skin servocontrol or manual control is still debatable for any given situation, and probably neither is the perfect solution for all babies.[14]**
    Radiant heat loss to cooler incubator walls, especially in single-walled incubators, is a significant source of heat loss. Double-walled incubators (with the inner wall warmed to the ambient air temperature inside the incubator) result in less radiant heat loss from the baby.[6,37] With a skin-set servocontrol temperature, the decreased radiant heat loss (because of warmer incubator walls) is offset by increased convective heat loss (because the ambient air temperature required for the desired skin temperature is lower[9]). Consequently there is no net change in the mean environmental temperature. **Double-walled incubators provide less temperature fluctuation when doors are open, thus providing a more stable caretaking environment. Evaporative heat loss is not appreciably different with single- and double-walled incubators. One may increase the humidity in incubators to decrease the infant's metabolic rate only if a neutral thermal environment cannot be achieved by increasing the ambient temperature. The tiniest neonate has a large evaporative heat loss, and maximum air temperature is limited by the incubator controls (thus making it impossible to reach an air temperature high enough for thermal support). In such cases hypothermia can be avoided by increasing the ambient humidity within the incubator by (1) using the water reservoir or (2) supplying warmed humidified air into the incubator with respiratory humidifiers. Careful attention should be given to preventing bacterial growth in the humidification system[21] (see Chapter 21). Incubator temperatures may also be controlled manually by estimating the appropriate temperature for the baby's age and weight from the chart shown in Table 6-1 and setting the incubator to that temperature. Regardless of whether one is using skin or air servocontrol or manual temperature adjustments, the baby's temperature and the air temperature must be monitored and recorded regularly. The incubator should be kept away from air conditioning ducts, direct sunlight, and cool windows that may cool or warm the incubator. Room temperature should be kept between 22.2° C and 24.4° C (72° F and 76° F). Alarms for both high and low temperature levels should always be turned on.**
    The principal disadvantage of maintaining sick newborns in incubators is the limited access to the

Table 6-1
Neutral Thermal Environmental Temperatures

Age and Weight	Starting Temperature (°C)	Range of Temperature (°C)
0-6 hr		
Under 1200 g	35.0	34.0-35.4
1200-1500 g	34.1	33.9-34.4
1501-2500 g	33.4	32.8-33.8
Over 2500 g (and >36 wk)	33.9	32.0-33.8
6-12 hr		
Under 1200 g	35.0	34.0-35.4
1200-1500 g	34.0	33.5-34.4
1501-2500 g	33.1	32.2-33.8
Over 2500 g (and >36 wk)	32.8	31.4-33.8
12-24 hr		
Under 1200 g	34.0	34.0-35.4
1200-1500 g	33.8	33.3-34.3
1501-2500 g	32.8	31.8-33.8
Over 2500 g (and >36 wk)	32.4	31.0-33.7
24-36 hr		
Under 1200 g	34.0	34.0-35.0
1200-1500 g	33.6	33.1-34.2
1501-2500 g	32.6	31.6-33.6
Over 2500 g (and >36 wk)	32.1	30.7-33.5
36-48 hr		
Under 1200 g	34.0	34.0-35.0
1200-1500 g	33.5	33.0-34.1
1501-2500 g	32.5	31.4-33.5
Over 2500 g (and >36 wk)	31.9	30.5-33.3
48-72 hr		
Under 1200 g	34.0	34.0-35.0
1200-1500 g	33.5	33.0-34.0
1501-2500 g	32.3	31.2-33.4
Over 2500 g (and >36 wk)	31.7	30.1-33.2

infant when extensive procedures are required. Incubators may also be perceived by mothers as a barrier between them and their infants and prolong feelings of fear and insecurity compared with heating methods that provide easier access to the baby.[46] We also now have an increasing awareness and concern regarding the high noise levels within incubators. Such noise poses a potential deleterious effect on the hearing development of preterm infants (see Chapter 12). Improved alarm technology minimizes the risk of inappropriate heating, but malfunctions still occur occasionally. When care is provided by experienced nurses, infants can be appropriately managed in incubators using any of the three modes of temperature control.

Weaning an infant from an incubator to an open crib is an important step in preparing for discharge. Few studies have been conducted that demonstrate when it is safe to begin the weaning process. A recent study supported by AWHONN demonstrated that infants could be successfully weaned if they weighed at least 1500 g, had 5 days of consistent weight gain, were free of medical complications, tolerated enteral feedings, and did not require assisted ventilation. Infants were dressed in a hat, shirt, diaper, and two blankets for several days

Table 6-1
Neutral Thermal Environmental Temperatures—cont'd

Age and Weight	Starting Temperature (°C)	Range of Temperature (°C)
72-96 hr		
Under 1200 g	34.0	34.0-35.0
1200-1500 g	33.5	33.0-34.0
1501-2500 g	32.2	31.1-33.2
Over 2500 g (and >36 wk)	31.3	29.8-32.8
4-12 days		
Under 1500 g	33.5	33.0-34.0
1501-2500 g	32.1	31.0-33.2
Over 2500 g (and >36 wk)		
4-5 days	31.0	29.5-32.6
5-6 days	30.9	29.4-32.3
6-8 days	30.6	29.0-32.2
8-10 days	30.3	29.0-31.8
10-12 days	30.1	29.0-31.4
12-14 days		
Under 1500 g	33.5	32.6-34.0
1501-2500 g	32.1	31.0-33.2
2-3 wk		
Under 1500 g	33.1	32.2-34.0
1501-2500 g	31.7	30.5-33.0
3-4 wk		
Under 1500 g	32.6	31.6-33.6
1501-2500 g	31.4	30.0-32.7
4-5 wk		
Under 1500 g	32.0	31.2-33.0
1501-2500 g	30.9	29.5-32.2
5-6 wk		
Under 1500 g	31.4	30.6-32.3
1501-2500 g	30.4	29.0-31.8

From American Academy of Pediatrics and American College of Obstetricians and Gynecologists: *Guidelines for perinatal care,* ed 2, Evanston, Ill, 1988, American Academy of Pediatrics and American College of Obstetricians and Gynecologists. Data from Scopes JW, Ahmed I: Minimal rates of oxygen consumption in sick and premature infants, *Arch Dis Child* 41:407, 1966; Scopes JW, Ahmed I: Range of critical temperatures in sick and premature newborn babies, *Arch Dis Child*: 417, 1966. For their table, Scopes and Ahmed had the walls of the incubator 1° to 2° warmer than the ambient air temperatures. Generally speaking, the smaller the infants in each weight group require a temperature in the higher portion of the temperature range. Within each time range, the younger the infant, the higher the temperature required.

before the weaning process. The incubator was placed on manual control, and the temperature in the incubator was slowly lowered over several days. Optimal abdominal skin temperature was 36° C to 37° C (96.8° F to 98.6° F). The incubator temperature was lowered if the skin temperature was greater than 37° C (98.6° F). When the incubator temperature was as low as possible and the infant's skin temperature was stable at 36° C to 37° C (96.8° F to 98.6° F) for 8 to 24 hours, the infant was placed in a crib in a draft-free environment. Some infants required an extra blanket. After weaning to a crib, the infant's temperature was monitored every 15 minutes for the first hour and then every 3 to 4 hours when stable. Weight was recorded daily to detect signs of increased caloric consumption secondary to hypothermia. Infants were placed back in an incubator if their skin temperature fell below 36° C (96.8° F) while covered with four blankets.[38]

Radiant Warmers

Radiant warmers provide infrared energy to heat the baby's skin while he or she lies naked on an open bed. The radiant warmer must generate enough energy to offset the tremendous amount of radiant heat lost to the room by a naked baby lying in an open environment. **Heat output can be servo-controlled or manually controlled. Manual control utilizes no feedback from the infant and poses a greater risk of overheating or overcooling. Therefore manual control should not be used routinely except for short periods of time (e.g., initiating resuscitation). The servocontrol sensor measuring skin temperature must be protected from the infrared heat source or the probe will sense a temperature higher than the skin temperature and decrease radiant heat output, leading to cold stress. Conversely, insulating the sensor with an aluminum reflective patch protects the underlying skin from the radiant heat and keeps the protected skin cooler than the surrounding skin. When the skin under the patch is warmed to the desired temperature, the rest of the skin may be overheated. Vasodilation may then increase convective heat loss, resulting in an effective, though precarious, heat balance.**

Insensible water loss (IWL) under radiant warmers is increased by 40% to 50% compared with losses in incubators. Directly related to the amount of heat required from the warmer, this loss is also influenced by other factors (e.g., relative humidity and convective air currents) on an open bed. With very premature infants, severe dehydration may occur if water intake is not increased to replace the inordinate IWL (see Chapter 13). Plexiglass heat shields and polyethylene blankets (plastic wrap) have been used in an attempt to prevent the large IWLs; studies have shown them to be somewhat effective for this purpose.[7,8,18] However, the microenvironment created by these blankets undergoes drastic change every time the blanket is removed. Even without such blankets the baby will experience wide swings in heat balance when the infrared heat is blocked from reaching the newborn by hands, heads, or drapes during a procedure.

Incubators and radiant warmers both are effective in maintaining an appropriate thermal balance in sick and preterm infants. The method chosen should be individualized to the infant and to the situation. Experience, skill, and nurse preference often influence the choice of heating methods. These factors also influence the extent to which incubators are perceived to interfere with the performance of care providers' tasks. Basic principles of care (e.g., keeping bed linens dry to prevent evaporative heat loss) apply to use of both heating methods. Radiant warmers provide easy access for performing procedures, a definite advantage over incubators, in which procedures must be done through portholes. Fluid management is easier in infants in incubators because humidity is easily added to the enclosed environment. The large flux of heat exchange between radiant heat source, the baby, and the environment make wide fluctuations in heat balance more likely when compared with the more easily and controlled temperature within an incubator. Oxygen consumption using these two heating methods has many variables, but the metabolic rate and oxygen consumption of infants under radiant warmers is slightly higher than in incubators. However, the clinical significance of this finding is uncertain. Infection rates are comparable between the two methods.[29,36,52] Regardless of the type of heat supplied, care must be taken to minimize thermal instability during nursing interventions. Radiant warmers may be able to rewarm a baby faster than an incubator with convective heating after a procedure. Organizing interventions so their frequency and duration limit as much as possible the exposure to a thermally unstable environment can minimize this instability.[40,47]

Other Methods

In the tiniest preterm infants, a conductive heat source (e.g., a heating pad) may also be needed to raise and maintain body temperature. Heated water mattresses provide a neutral thermal environment for less critically ill babies lying in open cribs (making access easier than in closed incubators).[44] This may also provide a feasible and effective means of rewarming hypothermic infants. Heated, water-filled mattresses are most useful in the newborn units of developing countries.[45]

Swaddling materials include various types of infant wrappings (e.g., blanket, clothing, foil, or bubble wrap). Use of swaddling materials makes observation of the infant more difficult and blocks heat from overhead radiant warmers. Before one

wraps the infant in insulating materials, the infant must be warm, because these merely retain body warmth and do not generate heat.

Oxygen and air delivered to the neonate should be warmed and humidified to minimize convective and evaporative heat loss (see Chapter 22).

Skin-to-skin (kangaroo) care provides a safe and effective alternative method of caring for prematures.[3] The infant, dressed only in a diaper and hat, is held upright against the mother's or father's bare chest and covered with the parent's shirt or a blanket. Both AGA and SGA infants experience a beneficial warming effect and a stable skin and core temperature when held skin to skin.[1,32,33,53,54] Mothers exhibit thermal synchrony with the infants, so that their body temperature increases or decreases to maintain the infant's thermal neutrality.[3,32,33] In one study, each mother's skin temperature met the neutral thermal environmental zone of her particular infant.[32] Mothers also preferred this method for holding their infant compared with the traditional method of being wrapped in a blanket and cradled in the parent's arms.[31]

Transport

The same principles of heat balance that apply to infants in an NICU apply to infants during transport. Infants should have a stable temperature before transport. The infant should be transferred from nursery to transport incubator rapidly to prevent prolonged exposure to an uncontrolled thermal environment. Transport incubators that can provide thermal stability inside the transport vehicle must be used. Oxygen provided during transport should also be warmed and humidified. Monitor temperature continuously or at least every 30 minutes.[23] Thin plastic wrap may be useful in decreasing IWL or convective and radiant heat loss. Chemically heated mattresses can also be used to provide a short-term heat source.[28]

Data Collection

Anticipation and early recognition of the infant at risk for temperature instability is important in the management and prevention of complications associated with both hypothermia and hyperthermia.

The perinatal history and ongoing neonatal evaluation identify events and early clinical indicators of temperature instability.

History

Events during pregnancy and the early neonatal period may increase an infant's risk for thermal instability. Review of the maternal history should include estimated date of confinement because preterm infants at delivery are at increased risk for hypothermia. Exposure to viral agents (e.g., herpes) as well as vaginal and cervical colonization increases the risk of acquiring an infection before or during delivery (see Chapter 21). Intrapartum use of analgesics and anesthetics may depress the infant's CNS and mute the thermoregulatory ability.

Fetal stress manifested as fetal decelerations, meconium-stained fluid, or low Apgar scores may suggest an impaired thermoregulatory response.

Neonatal interventions that may depress the CNS and thermal response include resuscitation and administration of analgesics, anesthetics, or neuromuscular blocking agents. Invasive procedures (e.g., endotracheal intubation and umbilical catheterization) increase the infant's chance for infection and need for prolonged use of antibiotics. Poor hand washing by care providers may also contribute to infectious nursery outbreaks, such as outbreaks of necrotizing enterocolitis (see Chapter 21).

Physical Examination/Signs and Symptoms

Physical assessment of the infant should include not only gestational age but also appropriateness of size. Evaluation of the infant's neurologic status (tone, activity, alertness, etc.) may give the caretaker an indication of the extent of the neurologic impairment. Hypotonia results in decreased flexion, with an increased exposed surface area and resultant heat loss.

Temperature Determinations

Temperature determinations may need to be made as often as every 30 minutes until stable. After that, temperatures should be recorded every 1 to 3 hours in low-birth-weight and preterm infants and every 4 hours in the healthy term infant. Critically ill infants should have continuous monitoring of skin temperature, with axillary determinations every 1 to 2 hours.[2] Documentation should include environmental temperature (e.g., air temperature in the incubator or radiant warmer settings). Measuring the skin and core temperatures simultaneously may help to differentiate fever as a result of disease versus environmental overheating. Noting that the baby's servocontrolled skin temperature is relatively stable but that the environmental temperature has dropped may also be indicative of fever as the incubator responds to the high probe reading by cooling the infant's environment.

Hypothermia

As the infant attempts to conserve heat by vasoconstriction, he or she may be pale and feel cool to touch, particularly on the extremities. Acrocyanosis and respiratory distress may occur as the infant increases oxygen consumption in an attempt to increase heat production. If hypothermia continues, apnea, bradycardia, and central cyanosis may occur. The hypothermic infant may initially be irritable but may become lethargic as cold stress continues. Other behavioral changes that may occur include hypotonia, apnea, weak cry, weak suck, increased residuals, abdominal distention, or emesis. Infants generally do not shiver in response to cold stress, but shivering may occur in the presence of severe hypothermia. Chronic hypothermia may result in poor weight gain.

Hyperthermia

The hyperthermic infant may feel warm to touch, and skin color may be red as the infant attempts to increase heat loss by vasodilation. Sweating may occur in the term infant but generally is not present in infants less than 36 weeks' gestation. Sweating may first appear on the forehead followed by the chest, upper arms, and lower body.[25]

The hyperthermic infant may be irritable, lethargic, hypotonic, apneic, have a weak or absent cry, and be a poor feeder. Tachypnea may be seen as the infant attempts to increase heat loss.

Infants with thermal instability should be closely watched for changes in behavior, feeding patterns, and respiratory status. Temperatures should be monitored frequently in any infant exhibiting these symptoms or who feels cool or warm to touch. Early recognition of thermal instability may prevent further consequences and possibly permanent injury or death.

Laboratory Data

The following laboratory data should be used to evaluate metabolic derangements associated with thermal instability:

- Arterial blood gas (to assess for hypoxemia and metabolic acidosis)
- Complete blood count (to asses for sepsis)
- Blood glucose level (to assess for hypoglycemia)
- Electrolytes (to assess for hyperkalemia)
- Blood urea nitrogen (BUN) (elevated with dehydration)
- Serum and urine osmolality (to assess hydration)

Treatment and Intervention

Hypothermia

To avoid the complications of hypothermia, rewarming of cold infants should begin immediately by providing external heat. Rewarming too rapidly, however, may further compromise the already cold-stressed infant and result in apnea. Oxygen consumption is minimal when the difference between the skin and the ambient air temperature is less than 1.5° C (35° F).[24] Avenues of heat loss should be blocked, temperatures should be monitored, and investigations into iatrogenic or pathologic causes should be conducted.

If hypothermia is mild, slow rewarming is preferred. External heat sources should be slightly warmer than the skin temperature and gradually increased until the neutral thermal environmental temperature range is attained. Efforts to block heat loss by convection, radiation, evaporation, and conduction should be initiated. Skin, axillary, and environmental temperatures should be measured and recorded every 30 minutes during the rewarming period. For more extreme hypothermia (i.e., core temperatures less than 35° C) more rapid rewarming with radiant heaters (servocontrol = 37° C) prevents prolonged metabolic acidosis or asymptomatic hypoglycemia and decreases mortality.[23,41,50]

Hyperthermia

The usual approach to treating the hyperthermic infant is to cool by removing external heat sources and by removing anything that blocks heat loss. The most common causes of hyperthermia in intensive care nurseries are iatrogenic. Check the heating controls for proper function and thermistors for proper position. Consider sources of heat (e.g., direct sunlight, heaters, and lights) as possible causes of hyperthermia. Excessive bundling with blankets and a hat and elevated environmental temperature can cause a newborn's body temperature to rise into the febrile range. When evaluating the treatment options in the hyperthermic infant, one should consider removing extra blankets or swaddling materials.[12] Nonenvironmental causes of hyperthermia (e.g., infection, dehydration, or CNS disorders) should be considered. During the cooling process, skin, axillary, and environmental temperatures should be monitored and recorded every 30 minutes.

Complications

Hypothermia

Acute cold stress results in the release of norepinephrine, which causes vasoconstriction to reduce heat loss and initiate thermogenesis. As glycogen stores are depleted and oxygen consumption increases, the infant uses anaerobic metabolism to increase heat production, resulting in lactic acid production (metabolic acidosis). Pulmonary vasoconstriction, accentuated by metabolic acidosis, is associated with hypoxia, decreased surfactant production, and further acidosis (see Chapter 22). Blood flow to vital organs is diminished, and pulmonary hemorrhage and death may occur if hypothermia continues.[35]

Hyperbilirubinemia and kernicterus may occur as nonesterified free fatty acids from brown fat

metabolism compete with bilirubin for albumin binding sites. Acidosis not only decreases the affinity of albumin for bilirubin but also increases the permeability of the blood brain barrier, allowing bilirubin to enter brain tissue. If hypothermia continues, carbohydrate, protein, and fat supplies will be utilized for heat production instead of growth.[22]

Close monitoring of the hypothermic infant is essential for early identification and prevention of complications. Evaluation of vital signs, arterial blood gas, and oxygen saturation may give early indication of hypoxia and metabolic acidosis. The infant may be dusky or bright red as failure of dissociation of oxyhemoglobin occurs at low body temperature. Respirations may be rapid, shallow, and grunty accompanied by bradycardia. Oxygen and ventilation should be initiated as needed to reduce hypoxia. Sodium bicarbonate may be given to correct metabolic acidosis. Seizures may occur as a result of hypoxia, requiring the administration of anticonvulsants.

IV glucose may be necessary to prevent or correct hypoglycemia. Blood glucose levels should be monitored hourly until stable (see Chapter 14).

Blood pressure and urine output should be measured to evaluate hydration and kidney function. An elevated BUN and hyperkalemia may be indicators of decreased renal perfusion and impaired renal function. As fluid is retained, edema of the extremities and face may occur.

Bilirubin should be monitored on a regular basis, and phototherapy may be initiated at a lower-than-usual level to prevent kernicterus. Adequate nutrition to promote growth should be given either intravenously or enterally. While the infant is hypothermic, nipple feeds should be avoided to conserve calories and energy for heat production and growth and to avoid aspiration.

During the rewarming process the hypothermic infant should be observed for hypotension as vasolidation occurs. Volume expanders may be needed to maintain an adequate blood pressure. Apnea and seizures may occur as a result of hypoxia or decreased cerebral blood flow after vasodilation.

Hyperthermia

Vasodilation to increase heat loss may also cause hypotension and dehydration secondary to increased IWL. Seizures and apnea may also occur as a result of high core temperature.

Fluid status should be monitored by assessing intake, output, electrolytes, serum and urine osmolality, skin turgor, and mucous membranes. Fluids should be adjusted to include IWL. Blood pressure should be assessed for hypotension, and volume expanders should be administered as needed.

Cardiorespiratory monitoring to detect apnea should be used. Ventilation may be needed if apnea persists or is unresponsive to stimulation. Subtle signs of seizures may include facial grimacing, nystagmus, tremors, apnea, opisthotonic posturing, tongue thrusting, or staring (see Chapter 25).

Parent Teaching

Parents should be taught the importance of maintaining a normal temperature. Temperature should be taken before parents touch the infant through the portholes of the incubator or hold the infant. While the infant is outside the incubator, monitor the skin temperature continuously with a telethermometer. Unwrapping the infant to check the temperature exposes the baby to cold stress. Additional heat sources (e.g., a radiant warmer, a hat, and extra blankets) may be needed while parents hold the infant. Teach parents to monitor their infant's temperature and notify the nurse if it rises or falls.

Before discharge, teach parents to take an accurate axillary temperature and to notify their physician if it drops below 36° C (96.8° F) or rises above 37.8° C (100° F). A rectal temperature should not routinely be taken by a parent. The temperature should be taken whenever the infant feels cool or warm to touch. The nurse should observe the parents taking the infant's axillary temperature before discharge.

The home environment should be kept at a temperature that prevents heat and cold stress. A room temperature that is comfortable for the parent is usually suitable for the infant. The infant should be in clothing appropriate for the room temperature. For example, if the parent requires a sweater to be comfortable, then the infant probably also requires a sweater. Parents often overdress the infant or overheat the home and cause hyperthermia. Give parents written instructions before discharge on how and when to take an axillary temperature, when to call the physician, and how to maintain a comfortable environment for their infant.

References

1. Acolet D, Sleath K, Whitelaw A: Oxygenation, heart rate and temperature in very low birthweight infants during skin-to-skin contact with their mothers, *Acta Paediatr Scand* 78:189, 1989.
2. American Academy of Pediatrics and American College of Obstetricians and Gynecologists: *Guidelines for perinatal care,* ed 2, Evanston, Ill, 1988, The American Academy of Pediatrics.
3. Anderson GC: Current knowledge about skin-to-skin (kangaroo) care for preterm infants, *J Perinatol 21(3):216, 1991.*
4. Bach V et al: Regulation of sleep and body temperature in response to exposure to cool and warm environments in neonates, *Pediatrics* 93:789, 1994.
5. Baker JP: The incubator controversy: pediatricians and the origins of premature infant technology in the United States, 1890 to 1910, *Pediatrics* 87(5):654, 1991.
6. Baumgart S et al: Effect of heat shielding on convective and evaporative heat losses and on radiant heat transfer in the premature infant, *J Pediatr* 99(6):948, 1981.
7. Baumgart S: Reduction of oxygen consumption, insensible water loss, and radiant heat demand with use of a plastic blanket for low-birth-weight infants under radiant warmers, *Pediatrics* 74(6):1022, 1984.
8. Bell EF et al: Heat balance in premature infants: comparative effects of convectively heated incubator and radiant warmer, with and without plastic heat shield, *J Pediatr* 96(3):460, 1980.
9. Bell EF, Rios GR: A double-walled incubator alters the partition of body heat loss of premature infants, *Pediatr Res* 17:135, 1983.
10. Bell EF, Rios GR: Air versus skin temperature servocontrol of infant incubators, *J Pediatr* 103(6):954, 1983.
11. Bruck K: Neonatal thermal regulation. In Polin R, Fox W, editors: *Fetal and neonatal physiology,* Philadelphia, 1991, WB Saunders.
11a. Butterfield LS et al: Martin Covney's story revisited, *Pediatrics* 100:159, 1997.
12. Cheng T, Partridge J: Effect of bundling and high environmental temperature on neonatal body temperature, *Pediatrics* 92:238, 1993.
13. D'Apolito K: Hats used to maintain body temperature, *Neonat Net* 13:93, 1994.
14. D'Apolito K: Temperature control: servo versus nonservo: which is best? *Neonat Net* 15:75, 1996.
15. Dollberg S et al: A trancutaneous alternative to rectal thermometry for continuous measurement of core temperature in preterm infants, *Pediatr Res* 35:222A, 1994.
16. Dollberg S et al: Effect of insulated skin probes to increase skin-to-environment temperature gradients of preterm infants cared for in convective incubators, *J Pediatr* 124:799, 1994.

17. Ducker DA et al: Incubator temperature control: effects on the very low birthweight infant, *Arch Dis Child* 60:902, 1985.
18. Fitch CW et al: Heat shield reduces water loss, *Arch Dis Child* 59:886, 1984.
19. Frank J, Brown S: Thermometers and rectal perforation of the neonate, *Arch Dis Child* 53:824, 1978.
20. Greer P: Head coverings for newborns under radiant warmers, *J Obstet Gynecol Neonatal Nurs* 17(4):265, 1988.
21. Harpin VA, Rutter N: Humidification of incubators, *Arch Dis Child* 60:219, 1985.
22. Kanto WP, Calvert LJ: Thermoregulation of the newborn, *Am Fam Phys* 16(5):157, 1977.
23. Kaplan M, Eidelman AI: Improved prognosis in severely hypothermic newborn infants treated by rapid rewarming, *J Pediatr* 105(3):470, 1984.
24. Klaus MH, Fanarof AA: *Care of the high-risk neonate,* ed 3, Philadelphia, 1986, WB Saunders.
25. Lane A: Sweating in the neonate. In Polin R, Fox W, editors: *Fetal and neonatal physiology,* Philadelphia, 1991, WB Saunders.
26. LeBlanc MH: Neonatal heat transfer. In Polin R. Fox W, editors: *Fetal and neonatal physiology,* Philadelphia, 1991, WB Saunders.
27. LeBlanc MH: Skin, rectal, or air temperature control in the neonate: which is the preferred method? *J Perinatol* V(2):2, 1985.
28. LeBlanc MH: Evaluation of two devices for improving thermal control of premature infants in transport, *Crit Care Med* 12(7):593, 1984.
29. LeBlanc MH: Relative efficacy of radiant and convective heat in incubators in producing thermoneutrality for the premature, *Pediatr Res* 18(5):425, 1984.
30. LeBlanc MH: Thermoregulation: incubators, radiant warmers, artificial skins, and body hoods, *Clin Perinatol* 18(3):403, 1991.
31. Legault M, Goulet C: Comparison of kangaroo and traditional methods of removing preterm infants from incubators, *J Obstet Neonat Nurs* 24:501, 1995.
32. Ludington-Hoe SM, Anderson GC, Hadeed A: Synchrony in maternal and premature infant temperature during skin-to-skin contact. Poster presented at the American Nurses Association Council of Nurse Researchers Conference, Chicago, Ill, September, 1989.
33. Ludington-Hoe SM: Hadeed A, Anderson GC: Physiologic response to skin-to-skin contact in hospitalized premature infants, *J Perinatol* 11:19, 1991.
34. Malin SW et al: Optimal thermal management for low birth weight infants nursed under high-powered radiant warmers, *Pediatrics* 79(1):47, 1987.
35. Mann TP, Elliott RIK: Neonatal cold injury due to accidental exposure to cold, *Lancet* 1:299, 1957.
36. Marks KH et al: Energy metabolism and substrate utilization in low birth weight neonates under radiant warmers, *Pediatrics* 78(3):465, 1986.
37. Marks KH et el: Oxygen consumption and temperature control of premature infants in a double-wall incubator, *Pediatrics* 68(1):93, 1981.
38. Medoff-Cooper B: Transition of the preterm infant to an open crib, *J Obstet Neonat Nurs* 23:329, 1994.
39. Merenstein G: Rectal perforation by thermometer, *Lancet* 1:1007, 1970.
40. Mok Q et al: Temperature instability during nursing procedures in preterm neonates, *Ach Dis Child* 66:783, 1991.
41. Motil KJ et al: The effects of four different radiant warmer temperature set-points used for rewarming neonates, *J Pediatr* 84(4):546, 1974.
42. Nedergaard J, Cannon B: Brown adipose tissue: development and function. In Polin R, Fox W, editors: *Fetal and neonatal physiology,* Philadelphia, 1991, WB Saunders.
43. Rao M et al: Direct calorimetry for the measurement of heat release in preterm infants: methods and applications, *J Perinatol* 15:375, 1995.
44. Sarman I et al: Providing warmth for preterm babies by a heated, water filled mattress, *Arch Dis Child* 64:29, 1989.
45. Sarman I et al: Rewarming preterm infants on a heated, water filled mattress, *Arch Dis Child* 64:687, 1989.
46. Sarman I et al: Mothers' perception of their preterm infants treated in an incubator or on a heated water filled mattress: a pilot study, *Act Pediatr* 82:930, 1993.
47. Sequin J, Vieth R: Thermal stability of premature infants during routine care udner radiant warmers, *Arch Dis Child* 74:F137, 1996.
48. Silverman WA: Incubator-baby side shows, *Pediatrics* 64(2):127, 1979.
49. Sinclair J: Heat production and thermoregulation in the smaller-for-date infant, *Pediatr Clin North Am* 17(1):147, 1970
50. Sofer S et al: Improved outcome of hypothermic infants, *Pediatr Emerg Care* 2(4):211, 1986.
51. Vaughans B: Early maternal-infant contact and neonatal thermoregulation, *Neonat Net* 8(5):19, 1990.
52. Walther FJ et al: Cardiovascular changes in preterm infants nursed under radiant warmers, *Pediatrics* 80:235, 1987.
53. Whitelaw A: Skin-to-skin contact in the care of very low birthweight babies, *Matern Child Health* 7:242, 1986.
54. Whitelaw A et al: Skin-to-skin contact for very low birthweight infants and their mothers: a randomized trial of "kangaroo care," *Arch Dis Child* 63:1377, 1986.
55. Weiss ME et al: Infrared tympanic thermometry for neonatal temperature assessment, *J Obstet Gynecol Neonat Nurs* 23:978, 1993.
56. Yetman et al: Comparison of temperature measurements by an aural infrared thermometer with measurements by traditional rectal and axillary techniques, *J Pediatr* 122:769, 1993.

7 Physiologic Monitoring

John R. Pierce, Barbara S. Turner

Since the clinical usefulness of the umbilical vessels was first demonstrated by Diamond in 1947 when exchange transfusions were being performed to prevent kernicterus, many advances have taken place. In most nurseries it is a matter of routine to use the umbilical artery for monitoring blood gas status and arterial blood pressure. Because of the frequency and clinical significance of complications, alternatives to indwelling artery catheters have been vigorously sought. The development of noninvasive oxygen saturation monitoring has been a major step toward this goal.

The purpose of this chapter is to review the procedures for using indwelling umbilical catheters and to look at advances in physiologic monitoring.

Physiology

Pulmonary

Gas exchange takes place in the alveolus of the lung. Ventilation is the movement of air in and out of these air spaces. Diffusion is the movement of oxygen from the alveolar space into the pulmonary capillary and the movement of carbon dioxide from the pulmonary capillary into the alveolar space for eventual exhalation. Pulmonary perfusion is the flow of blood through the pulmonary capillaries that surround the alveolar spaces. Once oxygen diffuses through the alveolar lining cells and into the capillaries, it is bound to hemoglobin within the red blood cell.

Oxygen content in the arterial blood is the sum of the amount of oxygen dissolved in the plasma and the amount bound to hemoglobin. Approxi-

mately 3% of the oxygen content is dissolved in the plasma, with the remaining 97% bound to hemoglobin. Pao_2 is the partial pressure of the oxygen dissolved in the plasma. Fetal hemoglobin has a higher affinity for oxygen than does adult hemoglobin; therefore at any given Pao_2 more oxygen is bound to adult hemoglobin (Fig. 7-1). Oxygen saturation (Sao_2) is the percentage of oxygen bound to hemoglobin.

Noninvasive Blood Gas Monitoring

Oxygen

Noninvasive monitoring of oxygenation can be accomplished by using two monitoring technologies. Oxygen saturation monitoring is the most common and widely used method for assessing oxygenation status. This technology relies on a pulsating arterial vascular bed between a dual light source and a photoreceptor.[1] As blood passes between the light source and the photoreceptor, different amounts of red and infrared light are absorbed, depending on the percentage of oxygen saturation. This difference in light absorption is electronically processed and displayed by the monitor as arterial hemoglobin oxygen saturation.[13]

The second method of noninvasive monitoring of oxygenation is transcutaneuos oxygen tension, which relies on the principle of oxygen diffusing from the skin capillaries through the dermis to the surface of the skin. To measure the oxygen, it is necessary to heat the skin, which then dilates the local capillaries and arterializes the capillary bed as well as promotes faster diffusion of the oxygen from the skin.[13]

Carbon Dioxide

As with noninvasive monitoring of oxygen, carbon dioxide can also be assessed using two types of

The opinions and assertions in this chapter are those of the authors and do not necessarily represent those of the Department of the Army or the Department of Defense.

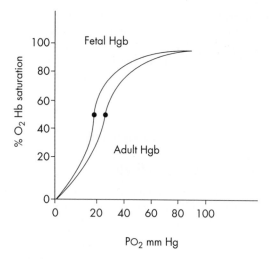

Figure 7-1 Oxygen dissociation curve for fetal hemoglobin (Hgb) *(left)* and adult hemoglobin *(right)*.

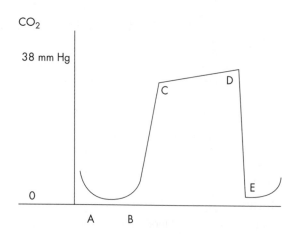

Figure 7-2 Variations in the content of carbon dioxide during phases of the respiratory cycle. *A*, End of inspiration. *B*, beginning of exhalation; *C*, end of mixed gases washout (deadspace and alveolar gases); *D*, end of expiration of alveolar gases; *E*, inspiration.

monitors. Transcutaneous carbon dioxide works under similar principles as transcutaneous oxygen monitoring. Although heating of the skin is not required for carbon dioxide, the values are more reliable and valid if a heated probe is used.[3] A second method used to measure the content of the carbon dioxide in the respiratory gases during the respiratory cycle is called end-tidal carbon dioxide (PetCO$_2$) monitoring. The carbon dioxide content varies widely with the phase of the respiratory cycle. During inspiration there are minimal amounts of carbon dioxide, whereas at the end of expiration the carbon dioxide values are at their maximum level (Fig. 7-2). Until recently the relatively fast respiratory rate of the newborn combined with the small tidal volumes resulted in inaccurate values when measured by end tidal carbon monoxide monitors. Recent advances in technology have improved the reliability of this monitoring technique for the newborn infant.

Cardiorespiratory Monitoring

The electrical activity of the infant's heart is picked up by chest leads (usually three) placed on the infant and is recorded by the cardiorespiratory monitor. The recording is displayed on a visual screen as the infant's electrocardiographic pattern.

The infant's respiratory pattern is also recorded, because the chest leads electronically detect movement of the infant's chest with each respiration.

Blood Pressure Monitoring

Systolic blood pressure (measured in millimeters of mercury) is the pressure at the height of the arterial pulse and coincides with left ventricular systole. Diastolic blood pressure (measured in millimeters of mercury) is the lowest point of the arterial pulse and coincides with left ventricular diastole. Mean arterial pressure is the diastolic pressure plus one third the pulse pressure. Central venous pressure is the blood pressure in the right atrium and may be approximated by the blood pressure in any of the large central veins.

Data Collection

The indications for using the various techniques for physiologic data collection depend on the infant's clinical situation.

Umbilical Artery Catheters

A UAC is placed in those infants requiring frequent blood gas determinations. Infants who are candidates for indwelling catheters are those suffering from congenital heart disease or disorders that cause respiratory insufficiency, such as surfactant deficiency, meconium aspiration syndrome, persistent pulmonary hypertension, and diaphragmatic hernia.[8] Although use of an indwelling umbilical artery catheter allows arterial pressure monitoring and accessibility for parenteral infusions, it is not acceptable to place a UAC for these indications alone.

Umbilical Vein Catheters

UVC use is reserved for exchange transfusions, central venous pressure monitoring, and administration of emergency fluids or chemicals in delivery room resuscitation. There are more complications associated with umbilical venous lines than with umbilical arterial lines, but the complications are less severe.[3,8,18] UVCs are being used with increasing frequency for initial management of extremely low-birth-weight infants. There is a need for research into their efficacy and safety.

Noninvasive Oxygen Monitoring

Oxygen monitoring is indicated in the infant receiving oxygen for any reason. Acute monitoring is used in management of acute respiratory disorders. Chronic monitoring is used to wean infants with chronic lung disease from oxygen. During transportation of infants, noninvasive oxygen monitoring is helpful. Carbon dioxide monitoring is useful in the infant with a respiratory disease in which retention of carbon dioxide may become clinically significant.

Cardiorespiratory Monitoring

Cardiorespiratory monitoring should be used in any infant who requires intensive or intermediate care and in any infant at risk for apnea.

Blood Pressure Monitoring

Blood pressure monitoring should be used in the infant requiring surgery and in the infant acutely ill with cardiorespiratory distress or with any other illness in which hypotension may be a significant contributor to the pathologic state. Central venous pressure should be monitored in infants who potentially may experience an excess or loss of blood volume.

Interventions

Umbilical Artery Catheters

Determine the size and length of the catheter to be inserted. For infants weighing more than 1250 g use a no. 5 Fr catheter, and for infants weighing less

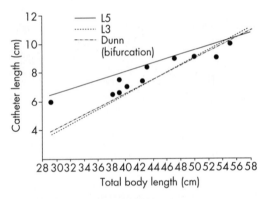

Figure 7-3 Graph for distance of catheter insertion from umbilical ring for low placement. (From Rosenfeld W et al: *J Pediatr* 96:735, 1980.)

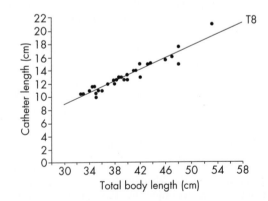

Figure 7-4 Graph for distance of catheter insertion from umbilical ring for high placement (T8). (From Rosenfeld W et al: *J Pediatr* 98:627, 1981.)

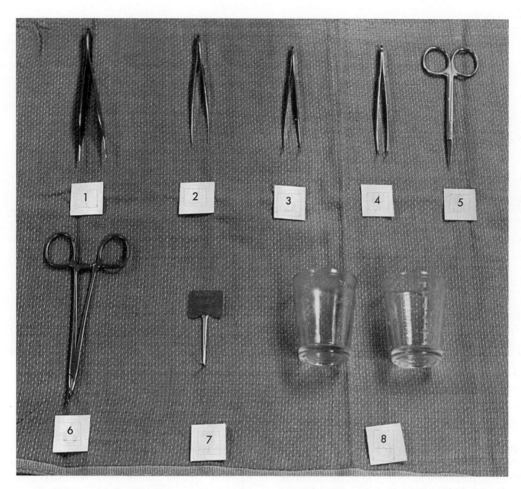

Figure 7-5   Mini-umbilical vessel catheterization tray. *1,* Adson's tissue forceps; *2,* straight iris forceps without teeth; *3,* half-curved forceps with teeth; *4,* full-curved forceps without teeth; *5,* iris scissors; *6,* curved mosquito clamp; *7,* vein flag; *8,* two containers for antiseptic.

than 1250 g use a no. 3.5 Fr catheter. (Refer to Figures 7-3 and 7-4, which correlate total body length to the length of the catheter to be inserted.) Place the infant in a supine position on a radiant heater or in an incubator. Skin temperature should remain between 36° C and 37° C (96.8° F to 98.6° F). Provide appropriate oxygenation and ventilation. Restrain the infant's hands and feet. This prevents the infant from contaminating the sterile field and interfering with the placement procedure. Wash hands before and after the procedure. Put on a gown and gloves. Open the catheterization tray. Catheterization tray contents are shown in Figures 7.5 and 7.6. Supplementary needs that are not shown are a tape measure, twelve 4- by 4-inch gauze pads, and two towel drapes. To minimize dead space in the catheter, the flared end of the catheter can be trimmed and a blunt end needle adapter can be inserted securely. The catheter and adapter are connected to the stopcock; the entire system is flushed and filled with flush solution. The stopcock is turned off to the catheter to prevent fluid from draining out of the catheter during insertion and securing of the catheter. Prepare the catheter by flushing it with a flush solution. Prepare the cord and base of the umbilicus with povidine-

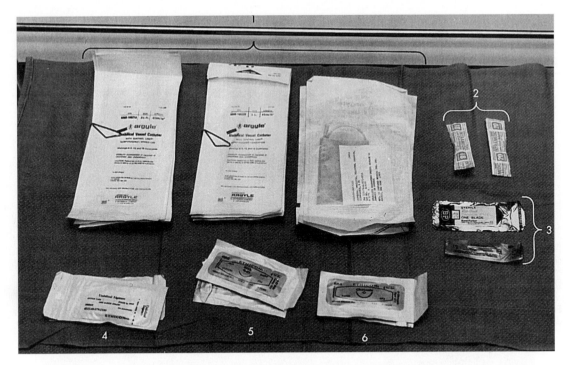

Figure 7-6 Supplemental sterile equipment for umbilical vessel catheterization. *1,* Umbilical vessel catheters sizes 3, 5, and 8 Fr; *2,* Luer stub adapters, 18- and 20-gauge; *3,* knife blades, sizes 15 and 20; *4,* umbilical ligature; *5,* silk suture on curved needle; *6,* chromic suture on curved needle.

iodine (Betadine) and then alcohol. Infants weighing less than 1000 g may experience iodophor skin burns; therefore an excess of povidine-iodine should be avoided so that the infant is not lying in the solution during the procedure. Any residual iodophor should be carefully washed off the infant after the procedure is completed. Drape the infant by placing an eye sheet over the umbilicus. Use additional sterile drapes as necessary. Ensure that the infant's head and feet remain visible during the procedure to assess the infant's color. A small eye drape with adhesive backing (Steri-Drape) has the advantage of being transparent so that the infant's color can be seen and temperature can be maintained. Towel drapes may interfere with a radiant heat source used for temperature regulation.

Because the tie will be left in place, umbilical tape should be tied around the base of the cord to ensure that the tape is not around skin. The tape is used to control bleeding. A single overhand knot that allows tightening as needed is preferred.

Using tissue forceps, pick up the cord and cut it with a scalpel about 1 to 1.5 cm above the base. Arterial spasm allows only minimal bleeding. Identify the vessels. There are usually two arteries and one vein. The arteries are small, thick-walled, and constricted. The vein is larger, thin-walled, and usually gaping open. If the vein is at the 12 o'clock position, the arteries are usually at the 4 and 8 o'clock positions (Fig. 7-7). Stabilize the umbilical stump by grasping the cord between the thumb and index finger or grasping the edge of the stump with a mosquito hemostat. Ensure that the hemostat does not crush the umbilical vessels. With iris forceps, dilate one of the arteries by placing the tips of the forceps in the artery and gently allowing them to spring open. This procedure may need to be repeated several times. While grasping one side of the wall of the dilated artery, gently insert the catheter or insert the catheter between the open prongs of the forceps, dilating the artery. Instructional aids

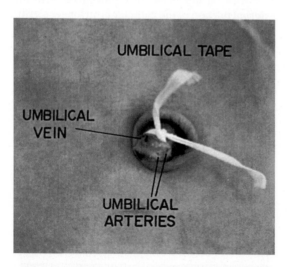

Figure 7-7 Umbilical tape and position of umbilical vessels.

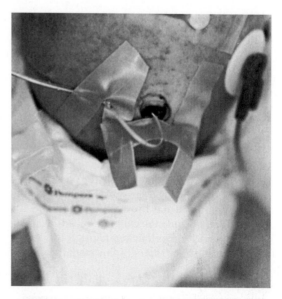

Figure 7-8 Umbilical artery catheter secured in "goal post" design.

such as Baby Umb* and the Umbilical Artery Catheterization Slide-Tape Neonatal Educational Program† are helpful. As the catheter passes into the artery, resistance may be met at several different points:

- At the umbilical tape—The tape may be tied too tightly. Loosen slightly.
- At the point where the umbilical artery turns downward (caudal) into the abdomen—Steady gentle pressure is important, because forceful pressure may cause the catheter to perforate the artery wall and create a false channel.
- At the point where the umbilical artery joins the external iliac artery—Once again, steady gentle pressure is important.

Insert the catheter to the predetermined length. Aspiration on the syringe should provide immediate blood return. Lack of blood return may indicate the following:

* Medical Plastics Laboratory, Inc., P.O. Box 38, Gatesville, TX 76528.
† Charles R. Drew Postgraduate Medical School, 1621 E. 120th St., Los Angeles, CA 90059.

- The catheter is not inserted far enough. Insert farther.
- The vessel wall has been perforated, or a false channel has been created. If the catheter has pierced the vessel wall, repeat the procedure using the other artery.
- The catheter is kinked. Pull back slightly and then advance.
- The stopcock is turned off. Correct the stopcock position. Return aspirated blood to the infant and flush until the catheter clears.

Observe the feet, legs, and buttocks of the infant for signs of vascular compromise. If any blanching or blueness occurs, follow the steps outlined under complications on p. 125. Secure the catheter by making a "goalpost," using skin-prep on the skin (Fig. 7-8). Properly secured by the "goalpost" taping method, the catheter is secure, and foreign bodies such as sutures are avoided. (Many centers, however, use sutures to secure the catheter.) Connect the stopcock to the intravenous (IV) solution and set an appropriate infusion rate. Ensure that no air is in the tubing, stopcock, or catheter. All connections must be secure. A tongue blade may be used to stabilize and secure this connection. Automatic infusion pumps must be used for UACs. Determine catheter placement by an abdominal x-ray examination. Figure 7-9 shows how the UAC will appear on lateral x-ray film. Note that the catheter enters the umbilicus and travels inferiorly before turning superiorly. This "leg loop" is characteristic of an arterial catheter. Optimal placement is L3-4 for a low catheter and T8 for a high catheter.[8,18] A large study found that over 56% of practitioners preferred high placement for UACs.[8] Figure 7-10 shows high catheter placement, and Figure 7-11 shows low catheter placement. If the catheter is too high, measure on the x-ray film the distance from the tip of the catheter to the desired level and pull the catheter back the appropriate distance. Some clinicians multiply this length by 0.8 to account for radiographic magnification. If

the catheter is placed too low, the catheter cannot be advanced but must be removed because the external portion of the catheter is no longer sterile.

Teaching Model

The umbilical cord can be used for teaching the procedure of both arterial and venous catheterization. Many of the steps can be effectively carried out using a fresh placenta.

Special UACs and monitors are available for continuous Pao_2 and/or oxygen saturation monitoring.

Nursing Care and Use of Umbilical Artery Catheters

Infants can be positioned on their sides or their backs. The abdominal position is avoided, because accidental slipping, kinking, and removal of the

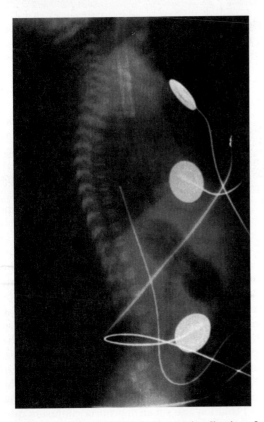

Figure 7-9   High catheter demonstrating "leg loop."

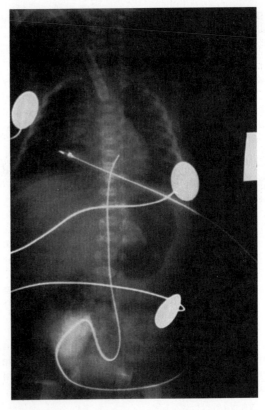

Figure 7-10   Umbilical artery catheter in high position (T8).

catheter may occur without being immediately apparent. Care needs to be taken that the infant is adequately restrained so that the catheter cannot be accidentally removed. Soft wrist restraints that restrict the range of movement will prevent the infants' fingers from grasping the catheter or connections. Diapers are an effective mechanism for preventing the feet and toes from becoming entangled in the catheter. The diaper is folded below the umbilicus. If the infant is receiving phototherapy and thus not diapered, leg restraints may be indicated. A dressing over the umbilicus is unnecessary. Dressings inhibit inspection of the umbilicus and evaluation of the catheter. The IV tubing, connecting tubing, and stopcock should be changed daily. Clots form in the stopcock, so changing it daily prevents the likelihood of emboli forming. Blood backing into the catheter can be caused by the following:

- Increased intraabdominal pressure commonly caused by the infant crying vigorously
- Disconnection of tubing
- Stopcock turned in wrong direction
- Infusion pump malfunction
- Leak in filter or tubing

The procedure for drawing blood gases from an umbilical catheter must be kept sterile. It requires one syringe flushed with heparin, and one filled with flush solution. Syringes are used for aspirating fluid and blood from the line, collecting blood gas samples, and flushing the line.

Procedure for Drawing Arterial Blood Gas

Turn the stopcock so that the IV solution stops flowing. Aspirate 1 to 2 ml from the catheter into the dry syringe (Fig. 7-12). The IV fluid is prevented from infusing, and aspiration clears the catheter of its IV fluid. Turn the stopcock to the neutral position (Fig. 7-13), remove the syringe, and replace it with the heparinized syringe. The neutral position of the stopcock prevents contaminating the sample with IV fluid and prevents blood loss from the infant. CAUTION: Never allow blood to drip from an open stopcock. Using steady, even pressure, aspi-

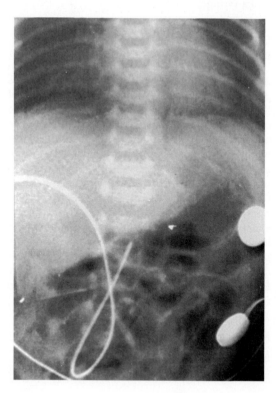

Figure 7-11 Umbilical artery catheter in low position (L3).

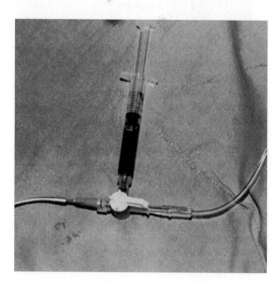

Figure 7-12 Stopcock off to IV solution; 1 to 2 ml aspirated into syringe.

rate blood into the heparinized syringe. Turn the stopcock to the neutral position and remove the syringe (Fig. 7-14). Remove the air from the syringe, cap the end, and chill it to preserve values. Usually 0.2 to 1 ml of blood is needed, depending on the

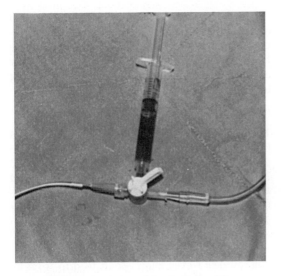

Figure 7-13 Stopcock in neutral position.

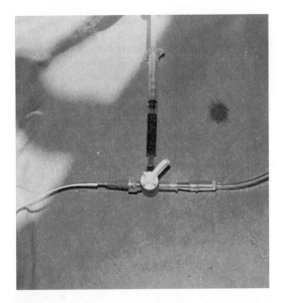

Figure 7-14 After blood is aspirated into heparinized 1-ml syringe, stopcock is placed in neutral position before syringe is removed.

laboratory requirements. Replace the syringe that has the aspirated blood in it with the syringe filled with flush solution. Turn off the stopcock to the IV. Slightly aspirate to remove any air in the stopcock and slowly insert it. After infusing the flush solution, return the stopcock to the neutral position. Record the amount of blood removed from the infant. Replace the syringe filled with flush solution with a clean, dry syringe. Turn the stopcock so that the IV can be infused.

To ensure the integrity of all connections, the stopcock and other connections must be visible at all times. Do not place the stopcock and other connections under linen, because this would hamper the immediate detection of an accidental disconnection that would cause severe blood loss in the infant. Immediately remove any air in the tubing or catheter, because air is a potential embolus. It is best removed through the stopcock. If the air has passed the stopcock, it can be easily aspirated back into a syringe.

Umbilical Vein Catheter Placement Procedure

A no. 5 Fr catheter is normally used in the UVC placement procedure. To determine the length of the catheter to be inserted, the distance from the umbilicus to the sternal notch should be measured and multiplied by 0.6. Complete steps for the placement procedure are found in this chapter's section on UACs. The only difference is that the vein is used instead of the artery up to the point of stabilizing the cord. The vein is usually gaping open and does not require dilation. The catheter can be easily advanced to the desired position. The catheter should lie in the inferior vena cava that UVCs is above the diaphragm but below the heart on x-ray film. UVCs do not have the "leg loop" found on the lateral x-ray film of the UACs. The catheter should be taped in the same manner as a UAC.

Nonivasive Oxygen/Carbon Dioxide Monitoring

End-Tidal Carbon Dioxide Monitoring[19,20]

End-tidal CO_2 monitors use either side stream or mainstream analysis.[10-12] For side stream analysis the endotracheal tube has a second narrow lumen, which opens at the end of the endotracheal tube. Gases are analyzed from samples taken from the end of the tube. The advantages of this system are that there is no increased dead space in the ventilator circuit and less chance of inspiratory gases contaminating the sample. The disadvantage to this method is the possibility that secretions that pool at the tip of the endotracheal tube may occlude the sampling port. The response time to changes in carbon dioxide content is slower than that used with mainstream analysis.

Mainstream analysis of carbon dioxide samples gases in the ventilator circuit. These gases are thought to be reflective of gases at the tip of the endotracheal tube. This method requires a separate chamber attached to the end of the endotracheal tube adapter, thus adding increased dead space and additional weight at the endotracheal tube adapter.

When side stream and mainstream analysis of end-tidal CO_2 were compared, it was found that distal values were higher than proximal values and that distal values correlated more closely with Pa_{CO_2} values. This discrepancy was thought to be due to the mixing of end-tidal gases with fresh gases in the ventilator circuit. In the infant with a large A-a gradient, $PetCO_2$ monitoring cannot be relied upon for accuracy. In premature infants, it may be useful if the lung disease is mild to moderate; in infants with normal lung function this method is reliable.

The waveform output of the end-tidal CO_2 monitor can be used clinically if the clinician understands how the waveform corresponds to the exchange of gases in the lung. The waveform has a sharp rise on expiration that reflects the carbon dioxide content of the alveolar gases. This expiration is followed by a plateau that reflects the cessation of dead space gases and the measurement of alveolar gas. At the end of the plateau is a sharp drop that reflects the inspiration of fresh gases with minimal carbon dioxide content.

When using the monitor, the clinician should recognize that a sharp rise indicates compromised exhalation. Partial plugged endotracheal tubes and dislodged tubes will change the angle of rise on the capnogram.[5] The plateau phase of the capnogram can be altered by severe hypotension or decreased cardiac output, whereas a leak around the endotracheal tube will alter the slope of the drop of the

waveform caused by entrainment of tracheal carbon dioxide.[5]

Transcutaneaous Oxygen/Carbon Dioxide Monitoring

Skin oxygen tension (TcP_{O_2}) and carbon dioxide tension (TcP_{CO_2}) are measured by using one or two electrodes, depending on the model and brand of the monitor. The electrodes, once positioned on the skin, heat the area under the probe and cause certain physiologic changes as previously discussed. Oxygen and carbon dioxide that diffuse through the heated skin are measured by the electrode, and the value is digitally displayed on the monitor. If intervals between calibration are longer than 4 hours, the readings are subject to drift. The calibration procedures vary with the instruments used. Inherent in the calibration process is the necessity to change the position of the skin electrode on the infant. In the clinical setting the correlation of the TcP_{O_2} and Pa_{O_2} has been reported to vary from $r = .84$ to as low as $r = .16$.[16] Better correlations are found when the instrument is calibrated every 4 hours, the temperature is set correctly, and the infant is well perfused and normothermic. If the temperature of the probe cannot be maintained at $43°$ C to $44°$ C, a lower temperature should be selected to avoid possible burns. At a lower temperature the TcP_{O_2} monitor can be used to monitor trends but should not be interpreted as actual arterial Pa_{O_2} values. The range of accuracy of TcP_{O_2} monitors is limited; hypoxia (less than 40 mm Hg) and hyperoxia (more than 120 mm Hg) may not be accurately reflected.[17]

In an infant with suspected significant right-to-left shunting through a patent ductus arteriosus such as in persistent pulmonary hypertension, two transcutaneous oxygen electrodes can be placed on the infant: one preductally (right shoulder) and the other postductally (lower abdomen or legs). Significant right-to-left shunting through the patent ductus arteriosus is present when the preductal oxygen tension is significantly higher than the postductal oxygen tension.

The disadvantages of the use of transcutaneous monitoring are that the instrument requires frequent calibration, requires the use of a heated electrode, requires a 15-minute period after calibration to heat the skin to the correct temperature, and has a 15- to 20-second delay in the readings as compared with the patient's real-time values. The advantages are that it is not invasive, does not require the removal of blood for analysis, and displays a continuous readout of skin oxygen/carbon dioxide tensions.

Nursing Care of Infants with Noninvasive Monitors

The electrode can be placed on any portion of the infant's body as long as good contact between the electrode and the skin is maintained. Uneven areas of skin such as skin over bones should be avoided because of poor contact between the membrane and the skin surface. The infant should not lie on the electrode. Placing the infant on top of the electrode increases the pressure on the underlying capillaries, thus affecting the flow of blood under the probe and resulting in a drop in $TcPo_2$ values. Because of the heat generated by the electrode (43° C to 44° C), small red areas are produced on the infant's skin. To minimize trauma to the infant's skin, the electrode should be repositioned every 2 to 4 hours depending on the infant's skin sensitivity. Grouping of nursing interventions has resulted in minimizing the time that the infant receives less than optimal oxygenation.

Oxygen Saturation Monitoring

Oxygen saturation is monitored by placing a small sensor on the infant in such a manner that the infant's finger, toe, foot, or wrist comes between the light source and the photoreceptor. The light source and receptor must be directly opposite each other to have a pulse detected.

The monitor does not require any heat source or warm-up period; nor does it require calibration or changing of the probe position. Oxygen saturation monitoring provides the care provider with continuous and instantaneous readout of the oxygen saturation in the infant. In comparison with a blood gas analyzer, which calculates the relative oxygen saturation based on established nomograms, the oxygen saturation monitor measures the actual saturation of the hemoglobin. Calculated values using standard nomograms do not reflect shifts in the affinity of oxygen for hemoglobin based on changes in the patient's temperature, pH, Pco_2, or 2.3-DPG.

The oxygen saturation monitor relies on ad-

equate perfusion to the site and the ability to detect arterial pulsations; thus if it is placed distal to a blood pressure cuff, there will be an inaccurate reading while the cuff is inflated. There may be incorrect readings when the probe is placed under or near infrared heat lamps and under phototherapy lamps.[2] The light from these external sources interferes with the light receptor on the infant's extremity. Newer neonatal probes have built-in external light source protectors that are not found on adult probes.

Oxygen saturation is more indicative of the total oxygen content of the blood than is Pao_2 and is the most sensitive to hypoxemia when it is on the steep part of the oxygen dissociation curve (see Fig. 7-1). Keeping the Sao_2 at 90% to 92% will keep the infant in a normoxemic state under most conditions.

There are no complications associated with the use of oxygen saturation monitoring other than the potential for skin trauma caused by adhesive on the probe. Newer probes held in position by gentle elastic pressure have no adhesive touching the infant's skin.

Oxygen saturation monitoring by pulse oximetry is reliable and practical for use in infants over a wide range of birth weights and postnatal ages.[1,2,7,14] There is one report in recent literature of an infant with meconium-stained skin in whom pulse oximetry produced a false low reading because the meconium staining absorbed more red, thereby filtering the infrared light.[9]

Cardiorespiratory Monitoring

The chest leads are applied in a triangular pattern on the infant's chest. Integrity of the leads must be ensured. Allowing the contact gel to dry or inadvertently dislodging the lead during procedures such as x-ray examination, echocardiography, and lumbar puncture may account for inaccurate tracings. Various components of the electrocardiogram (ECG) pattern may be diagnostically helpful. The QRS complex should be monitored for baseline height. A sudden decrease in QRS complex height that is not caused by artifact may be an indication of pneumothorax. The QT interval is helpful in diagnosing hypocalcemia in some infants. Other portions of the strip may be evaluated for electrolyte imbalance and possible cardiac ischemia. Changes registered on the visual display or strip recorder should be verified by a 12-lead ECG.

Blood Pressure Monitoring

Arterial pressure monitoring may be accomplished via the UAC attached to a transducer and monitor. Newer transducers require calibration only once daily. Central venous pressure monitoring may be carried out in the same manner. The same transducers may be used for either arterial or venous pressure recording.

Event Monitoring

The advancement of physiologic monitors with memory capability has enhanced the ability of the practitioner to review the physiologic status of the infant on multiple physiologic parameters for the past 24 to 48 hours. In many NICUs the monitor output is integrated into the electronic or computerized chart. This integration allows the care provider to "pull" the data from the monitors into the chart at preselected times either prospectively or retrospectively. When the monitors are programmed with critical value ranges, any deviation outside these ranges is noted as an "event," which can then be reviewed, tallied, or otherwise annotated. For care providers at the bedside, the challenge is to keep iatrogenic events (such as lead removal, excessive activity of the infant, a stopcock turned the wrong direction) minimized such that the infant's record is as valid a reflection of their actual physiologic status as possible. Any circumstances noted at the time of the event that may produce false readings should be recorded so that when the infant's record is reviewed, these events can be placed in context of the circumstances at the time.

Complications*

UACs act as foreign bodies, causing fibrin deposition and thrombus formation around the catheter.

---

* References 8, 18.

Although most catheters are associated with thrombus formation, it is of clinical significance in less than 10% of patients. The most common problem associated with major complications of UACs is ischemic disease resulting from emboli or spasms. In such cases the catheter should be removed immediately, and heparin therapy should be considered. Although vasospasm is quite common, usually it does not require immediate removal of the catheter. Blue discoloration is seen rather than blanching. Obviously a hemorrhage may occur when the catheter slips out or when any of the various connections loosen. For reasons such as these, UACs require constant attention.

If the extremities or buttocks blanch, the catheter should be removed immediately, and heparin therapy should be considered. To prevent bleeding once the catheter is removed, pressure should be applied immediately below the umbilicus. When the color has returned to the affected area and the infant is stable, replacement of the catheter can be considered. If vasospasm occurs in one leg or foot, apply warm wraps (diapers wet with warm water) to the opposite leg or apply wraps to the upper extremities, thereby producing a reflex vasodilation to the legs. Inherent in this action, however, is the hazard of obscuring recognition of compromise in that extremity. The wraps need to be reheated every 10 to 15 minutes until the spasm has resolved. The skin temperature of the infant must be greater than 36° C for wraps to be effective. Infants with UACs need blood available for immediate transfusion.

UVCs may cause thrombi. Clots may form in the portal vessels, resulting in portal hypertension. Hepatic necrosis, gut ischemia, and hemorrhage have been associated with UVCs.[15]

Transcutaneous blood gas monitoring may cause burns to the skin.

Controversies

Complications involving high catheter placement (T8) are fewer but more severe than the complications involving low catheter placement (L3-4).[18] Prophylactic antibiotic agents are not indicated. Use of the UAC for infusion of antibiotic agents, calcium, hyperalimentation solutions, or blood varies, and no definite studies are available. Blood cultures drawn from the UAC are accurate for 6 hours after insertion. The use of heparin in the infusate is controversial. Practices vary widely, and definite studies are lacking; however, it appears safe to feed infants enterally with an UAC in place.[6] Routine monitoring on all infants is the standard of care. Indwelling catheters for blood pressure monitoring have the advantage of continuous readout, but external cuffs are less invasive.

Parent Teaching

As for the many other invasive procedures in neonatology, permission is obtained from the parents for umbilical vessel catheterization. This may be the clinician's first contact with the family and thus sets the atmosphere for future contacts. Although parents are initially hesitant about umbilical catheter placement, they are generally comforted to learn that it will result in a painless way of drawing blood. Before visiting the infant, parents need to be told what the umbilical catheter, transcutaneous monitors, cardiorespiratory monitors, and blood pressure monitors look like in place and what they are registering. Often parents are confused as to where the catheter goes once it enters the umbilicus and what the purpose of other monitoring devices is. Some parents are uncomfortable with the arm and leg restraints on their infant. It may be unwise for parents to hold their infant while an umbilical catheter is in place because manipulating the infant may accidentally dislodge the catheter, and subsequently the infant may lose blood. Also, when the infant is being held out of the incubator and is wrapped in blankets, the integrity of the catheter and connections cannot be evaluated.

References

1. Anderson JV: The accuracy of pulse oximetry in neonates: effects of fetal hemoglobin and bilirubin, *J Perinatol* 7: 309, 1987.
2. Barrington JK, Finer NN, Ryan CA: Evaluation of pulse oximetry as a continuous monitoring technique in the critical care unit, *Crit Care Med* 16:1147, 1988.
3. Cassady G: Transcutaneous monitoring in the newborn infant, *J Pediatr* 103:837, 1987.
4. Comer DM: Pulse oximetry implications for practice, *Obstet Gynecol Neonat Nurs* 21(1):35, 1992.
5. Cote CJ, Ryan JF: *A practice of anesthesia for infants and children,* Philadelphia, 1993, WB Saunders.
6. Davey AM et al: Feeding premature infants while low umbilical catheters are in place: a prospective, randomized trial, *J Pediatr* 124:795, 1994.
7. Emery JR: Skin pigmentation as an influence on the accuracy of pulse oximetry, *J Perinatol* 7:329, 1987.
8. Fletcher MA et al: Umbilical arterial catheter use: report of an audit conducted by the Study Group For Complications of Perinatal Care, *Am J Perinatol* 11(2):94, 1994.
9. Johnson N et al: The effect of meconium on neonatal and fetal reflectance pulse oximetry, *J Perinat Med* 18(5):351, 1990.
10. McEvedy BA et al: End tidal CO_2 measurements in critically ill neonates: a comparison of sidestream and mainstream capnometers, *Can J Anaesth* 37:322, 1990.
11. Meredith KS, Monaco FJ: Evaluation of a mainstream capnometer and end-tidal carbon dioxide monitoring in mechanically ventilated infants, *Pediatr Pulmonol* 9:254, 1990.
12. Paige PL: Noninvasive monitoring of the neonatal respiratory system, *Clinical Issues in Critical Care Nursing* 1(2):416, 1990.
13. Poets CF, Southall DP: Noninvasive monitoring of oxygenation in infants and children: practical consideration and areas of concern, *Pediatrics* 93(5):737, 1994.
14. Ramanathan R, Durand M, Larrazabal C: Pulse oximetry in very low birth weight infants with acute and chronic lung disease, *Pediatrics* 79:612, 1987.
15. Rejjal AR et al: Complications of parenteral nutrition via umbilical vein catheter, *Eur J Pediatr* 152:624, 1993.
16. Rooth G, Huch A, Huch R: Transcutaneous oxygen monitors are reliable indicators of arterial oxygen tension (if used correctly), *Pediatrics* 79:283, 1987.
17. Turner BS: Nursing procedures. In Nugent J, editor: *Acute respiratory care of the neonate,* San Rafael, Calif, 1991, NIC.
18. Umbilical Artery Catheter Trial Study Group: Relationship of intraventricular hemorrhage or death with the level of umbilical artery catheter placement: a multicenter randomized clinical trial, *Pediatrics* 90(6): 881, 1992.
19. Watkins AMC, Weindling AM: Monitoring of end tidal CO_2 in neonatal intensive care, *Arch Dis Child* 62:837, 1987.
20. Weingarten M: Respiratory monitoring of carbon dioxide and oxygen: a ten year perspective, *J Clin Monit* 6(3):217, 1990.

8

Drug Withdrawal in the Neonate

Susan M. Weiner, Loretta P. Finnegan

The epidemic of maternal substance abuse over the last 30 years has continued to escalate at an alarming rate. The extent of drug use during pregnancy is often underestimated, as are the effects on the fetus and neonate. This lack of awareness is related, in part, to a tendency of human nature to minimize the existence of socially undesirable problems, especially among those of higher socioeconomic standing. Nevertheless, the sequelae of both licit and illicit substance abuse by the mother during pregnancy must be recognized and addressed in order to provide optimal medical care of the neonate. Stereotypic biases should not interfere with the diagnosis or treatment. Drug dependence in pregnancy crosses all socioeconomic and racial barriers. Therefore health care providers should not rule out drug exposure in any neonate who is exhibiting symptoms at birth related to withdrawal or exposure to drugs.

Opioid addiction of the mother during pregnancy has been studied in detail for the past three decades in terms of its effects on the woman, the fetus, and the developing child.* However, as time, circumstances, and knowledge change, other factors need to be considered when treating the neonate. Diagnostic data can no longer be gathered on the assumption that one drug or substance was used. Polydrug use and the combination of illicit substances with those that are legal are more the norm. The impact on the fetus and neonate is not necessarily minimized by the legality of the substance.[5] Patterns of abuse, purity of the illicit drug, and sometimes potent or poisonous additions to them may also cause catastrophic sequelae in the newborn.

A new phenomenon studied by Franck and Vilardi concerns iatrogenic neonatal abstinence syndrome (NAS), a condition caused by the abrupt withdrawal of analgesics and sedatives administered during the neonatal period.[30] Recent advances in neonatology have continued to broaden the period of viability as many more premature infants are being kept alive. However, due to the complexity and number of procedures that are performed on these infants, narcotic sedation is utilized, causing narcotic dependence (see Chapter 11).

This chapter presents current information about treatment issues surrounding the drug-exposed neonate with the main focus on opioid withdrawal. The effects of other substances such as stimulants, hallucinogens, nonopioid CNS depressants, tobacco, and alcohol will be addressed when symptoms deviate from those of NAS.

Physiology

Because of their low molecular weight and lipid solubility, all drugs of abuse reach the fetal circulation by crossing the placenta, causing direct toxic effects on the fetus.[1] Although certain drugs may produce specific effects, many abused drugs produce similar manifestations of fetal and neonatal disease. In addition, the effects of legal drugs such as tobacco, caffeine, and alcohol may confound simple drug-effect relationships.[41] A hostile intrauterine environment may also be caused by adverse effects of the mother's drug addiction and must be considered when diagnosing the neonate's problems. **Examples of factors that could impact on neonatal outcome include lifestyle, homelessness, physical and/or sexual abuse, prostitution, poverty, poor or no prenatal care, polydrug abuse, intravenous drug abuse, binge and withdrawal cycles, anorexia, poor maternal nutrition, pica, dehydration, alcoholism, sexually transmitted dis-**

---

* References 19, 24, 28, 38, 41, 44, 46, 48, 61, 69.

eases, dental abscesses, HIV positive or AIDS infection, and hepatitis B.[24,39,41,48,70,71]

Opioid Substances

When the major opioid drugs such as heroin, methadone, morphine, and meperidine cross the placenta, the fetus may become passively addicted. Morphine, the major metabolite of heroin, and methadone have been identified and measured in amniotic fluid, cord blood, breastmilk,[15] neonatal urine, and meconium.[7,20,46,72] Stimulants (amphetamines and cocaine) have been found in breastmilk in extremely high levels.[15] Nonopioid CNS depressants (benzodiazepines, barbiturates), and the minor opioids (codeine and propoxyphene) have all been identified in neonatal urine and meconium.* Ethanol and its primary metabolite, acetaldehyde, have been identified in placental tissue and amniotic fluid.[13,37,54,64,65]

Human and animal studies have shown that use of opioids during pregnancy directly affects fetal growth. Heroin is associated with IUGR with only a slight reduction in gestational length. However, the mechanism by which heroin inhibits growth is not known.[20,41] Studies comparing methadone-exposed infants with nonexposed infants have found that methadone-exposed infants had lower birth weights.[19] But infants born to methadone-maintained women have been reported to have higher birth weights than those born to women using heroin.[20,43] Decreased head circumference has been an inconsistent finding with theses babies. However, at the 18 month follow-up there was no catch-up growth, and they continued to exhibit a head circumference below the third percentile.[2,4,5,18,36,57] Kandall and colleagues reported a significant relationship between first trimester maternal methadone use and birth weight. This study indicated that methadone may promote fetal growth in a dose-related fashion even after maternal heroin use, whereas heroin itself has been found to induce fetal growth restriction that may persist beyond the period of addiction.[19,60]

Neither heroin nor methadone has been associated with congenital malformations or a specific dysmorphic syndrome in offspring.[5,41]

Fetuses who are heroin-exposed are born with meconium-staining more often than methadone-exposed infants.[41] Usually, antenatal passage of meconium reflects fetal withdrawal rather than fetal hypoxia and acidosis.[41] Heroin exposure during pregnancy has also been reported to accelerate fetal lung maturity.[31,41] However, it is not known whether this occurs from the direct heroin exposure or from the growth restriction and chronic stress.[31,41]

Neonatal withdrawal from all the substances that the fetus is exposed to occurs in varying degrees. Several studies have shown that symptoms of NAS in heroin-exposed infants occur earlier than in those infants of methadone-maintained mothers. This is a result of heroin's shorter half-life.† NAS, resulting from in utero exposure to opioids, may be severe and necessitate pharmacologic intervention.

Nonopioid Substances

Cocaine crosses the placenta by simple diffusion. This occurs because of its high lipid solubility, low molecular weight, and low ionization at physiologic pH.[70] Cocaine has a marked vasoconstrictive property, which decreases blood flow to the placenta and fetus, contributing to fetal growth retardation and hypoxia.[40,52,70] These infants have an increased risk of prematurity, perinatal cerebral infarctions, abnormal EEGs at birth, nonduodenal intestinal and anal atresias, necrotizing enterocolitis, terminal limb defects, cardiovascular effects, and genitourinary anomalies.‡ Maternal cocaine abuse has also been shown to produce neuromotor deficits, which include impaired muscle tone leading to abnormal movement patterns and tremors.[18,35,58]

Alcohol has been shown to cause diminished deoxyribonucleic acid (DNA) synthesis, disruption of protein synthesis, and impaired cellular growth, differentiation, and migration. These cellular effects can be seen with both ethanol and acetaldehyde and are instrumental in inducing fetal malformations. Alcohol interferes with the transport of amino acids across the placenta to the fetus. Thus

---

* References 3, 41, 47, 52, 53, 72, 74.

† References 5, 14, 21, 22, 24, 25, 26, 31, 60, 70.
‡ References 1, 2, 4, 5, 18, 34, 35, 36.

embryonic organization is altered with IUGR and chronic fetal hypoxia as the result.[54] Alcohol causes many of the same anomalies that are observed in cocaine-exposed neonates. When marijuana is added, the incidence of delivering an infant with the features of FAS are increased nearly fivefold.[2,71]

When cocaine and alcohol are used together, as often is the case, a unique metabolite, cocaethylene, is formed.[63] Cocaethylene is reported to be 10 times more potent than cocaine alone, which also suggests that it is more toxic in its effects on the growing fetus.[63] Snodgrass also reports that cocaethylene plasma concentrations may exceed those of cocaine alone and has a longer half-life in humans (i.e., 2 to 3 hours). In light of these data, the expression of fetal cocaine effects or nonspecific anomalies could be expected to increase when the parturient is combining cocaine with the teratogen ethanol.[63]

Amphetamines and methamphetamines known as "crystal," "ice," or "crank" are abused by pregnant women in many geographic areas in the United States with the same frequency as cocaine.[8] Like cocaine and "crack," the amphetamines are potent stimulants and effects on the fetus and neonate are similar.[5,8] Bell and Lau discuss in their 1995 article *Perinatal and Neonatal Issues of Substance Abuse* how in utero amphetamine exposure can lead to congenital brain lesions, which include hemorrhage, infarction, or cavitary lesions.[5] They also describe the sites of these lesions as frontal lobes, basal ganglia, posterior fossa, or general atrophy with the effects of the lesions not being exhibited until the child is older.[5]

A review of the most recent literature documents lack of prenatal care as the hallmark of maternal cocaine and amphetamine use with an increase in maternal morbidity and mortality as its consequence.* The use of these stimulants prove to be toxic to the fetal brain, and there is an increase in sudden infant death syndrome (SIDS) and neonatal seizure activity.† These infants also demonstrate poor state control, difficulty with habituation, and impairment in a number of neonatal reflexes.[1,2,5,35,67]

---

* References 1, 2, 3, 5, 6, 8, 9, 34, 36, 40, 48, 53, 63, 70, 71.
† References 2, 3, 5, 36, 47, 48, 53, 70, 73.

Etiology of Neonatal Abstinence Sydnrome

NAS is presently occurring in two ways: first, by the passive exposure to opioids in utero as a consequence of maternal addiction to heroin, methadone, and other narcotic analgesics and second, iatrogenically, by the administration of opiates such as fentanyl, morphine, and methadone to the neonate for analgesia and sedation.[30] Infants born to heroin- or methadone-dependent mothers have a high incidence of NAS. Less potent opioids or opioidlike agents also have been implicated in the development of NAS (see Box 8-1 for a complete list). **Neonatal abstinence is described as a generalized disorder characterized by CNS hyperirritability, gastrointestinal dysfunction, respiratory distress, and autonomic dysfunction man-**

Box 8-1
Drugs Associated with NAS

Opioids
Heroin
Fentanyl
Methadone
Morphine
Meperidine (Demerol)

Less Potent Opioids and Opioidlike Agents
Propoxyphene hydrochloride
Codeine
Pentazocine (Talwin)

Nonopioid Central Nervous System Depressants
Tranquilizers and sedatives
Bromides
Chlordiazepoxide (Librium)
Desipramine (Pertofrane; Norpramin)
Diazepam (Valium)
Ethchlorvynol (Placidyl)
Glutethimide (Doriden)
Hydroxyzine HCl (Atarax)
Oxazepam (Serax)
Alcohol

Box 8-2

Factors Influencing the Onset of Passively Acquired NAS

Drugs used by the mother
Both the timing and the dose of the drugs before delivery
Character of labor
Type of analgesia and/or anesthesia given during labor
Maturity, nutritional status, and the presence of intrinsic disease in the neonate

NAS, Neonatal abstinence syndrome.

Box 8-3

Factors Influencing the Onset of Iatrogenic Acquired NAS

Prolonged opiate sedation for mechanical ventilation
Duration of opioid analgesia use during extracorporeal membrane oxygenation
Type of opiate used
Maturity and presence of intrinsic disease in the neonate

NAS, Neonatal abstinence syndrome.

---

ifesting vague symptoms such as yawning, hiccups, sneezing, mottled color, and fever.[21,22,38,41]

When narcotics cross the placenta, an equilibrium is established between maternal and fetal circulations. Before birth, the drug is cleared from the infant's circulation primarily by the mother's excretory and metabolic mechanisms.[27]

The onset of withdrawal symptoms varies from minutes or hours after birth to 2 weeks of age, but the majority of symptoms appear within 72 hours. Many factors influence the onset of NAS and are mentioned in Boxes 8-2 and 8-3.

Once the umbilical cord has been cut, the neonate is no longer exposed to the drug and symptoms of withdrawal can be expected. Because heroin is not stored in appreciable amounts by the fetus, signs of heroin withdrawal usually are apparent shortly after delivery and generally within 48 hours. However, methadone is stored in the fetal lung, liver, and spleen, facilitating the slow decline of methadone levels, but the rate of metabolic disposition varies for each infant, making the age of onset of NAS unpredictable.[20,26,41,56] Withdrawal may be mild and transient and delayed in onset, or it may increase stepwise in severity. Symptoms may be intermittently present or follow a biphasic course characterized by acute NAS signs, followed by improvement and then the onset of a subacute withdrawal reaction.* Withdrawal seems to be more severe in infants whose mothers have taken

large amounts of drugs for an extended time period. **In general, the closer to delivery a mother takes the drug, the more severe the symptoms and the greater the delay in their onset.**[14]

The origin of NAS lies in the abnormal intrauterine environment. A series of steps appears to be necessary for the onset of NAS and thus the recovery of the infant. The growth and ongoing survival of the fetus is threatened by the continuing or episodic transfer of addictive substances from the maternal to fetal circulation. During this time, the fetus goes through a biochemical adaptation to the abnormal element. At delivery, abrupt removal of the drug is the catalyst needed to start the onset of symptoms. The newborn continues to metabolize and excrete the substance so that withdrawal signs occur when critically low tissue levels have been reached. Recovery from NAS is gradual and occurs as the infant's metabolism is reorganized to adjust to the absence of the offending drug.[14,23]

Prevention

Neonatal drug withdrawal is preventable if women do not use dependence-producing substances, licit and illicit, during pregnancy. Through intense educational efforts, the desirability and availability of drugs may be thwarted. Unfortunately, the psychosocial and socioeconomic milieu of our modern day society continues to propagate dysfunctional families, victimization of women, and an intergenerational cycle of substance abuse.

---

* References 14, 20, 25, 27, 38, 41.

Therefore our goals must be to provide prenatal care for the pregnant drug-dependent woman and her fetus to diminish or eliminate the sequelae of passive addiction. The medical community is challenged to become more astute in its assessment and intervention regarding problems of the drug-dependent parturient. More treatment is required for these women and their neonates through inpatient and residential care and outpatient interdisciplinary clinics that focus on the elimination, as well as the consequences, of addiction.

Franck and Vilardi, in addressing iatrogenic NAS, state that guidelines for effective weaning of neonates from opiate analgesics and sedatives are not yet well established. Researchers encourage dose reductions of 10% to 20% per day (see Chapter 11).[30] Further suggestions for the prevention of iatrogenic NAS include limiting total doses of fentanyl during ECMO by administering morphine boluses or using continuous morphine infusions to replace fentanyl.[30]

Diagnosis

History

A comprehensive prenatal medical and drug history, especially with respect to polydrug abuse, is of prime importance. All pregnant patients who are substance abusers, regardless of the drug used, are considered to be high risk because of the effects of the drug as well as complications arising from concomitant infections and lifestyle.[28,70] Fear of referral to child welfare agencies or the legal system has, in recent years, prompted women to conceal their drug abuse and/or pregnancy. This denial may prevent the parturient from seeking prenatal care. Thus she may appear at the emergency room of the hospital either in crisis or ready to deliver. In this instance, prenatal history is absent, making neonatal assessment more difficult.

Signs and Symptoms of NAS

At birth, most infants exposed to narcotics appear physically and behaviorally normal. Symptoms of withdrawal begin shortly after birth to 2 weeks of age, but the majority are exhibited within 72 hours.* Acute symptoms may persist for several weeks, whereas subacute symptoms (irritability, sleep problems, hyperactivity, feeding problems, and hypertonia) may persist for 4 to 6 months.[30,50,60] Mayes and Carroll report that infants of mothers who used cocaine in conjunction with their methadone had significantly higher first withdrawal scores on the NAS score sheet. However, they did not require more pharmacologic intervention nor did it lengthen the infant's number of days treated.[50]

The most common signs and symptoms of neonatal withdrawal are those of CNS hyperirritability, gastrointestinal dysfunction, respiratory distress, and autonomic instability. The NAS scoring system that is used in monitoring abstinence will be discussed later in the chapter. However, for the convenience of referencing, the signs and symptoms will be discussed here in the order in which they appear on an assessment sheet entitled Neonatal Abstinence Scoring System.

Initially, the infants appear only to be restless. Tremors develop, which are mild and occur only when the infants are disturbed, but progress to the point where they occur spontaneously without any external stimulation of the infant. High-pitched cry, increased muscle tone, and further irritability develop to the point of inconsolability. When examined, the infant tends to have increased deep tendon reflexes and an exaggerated Moro reflex.[5,21,22,24,26,27]

Infants undergoing narcotic withdrawal have seriously disturbed sleep patterns. Sisson et al studied electroencephalographic tracings and simultaneous electromyographic recordings of eye and mouth movements before, during, and after treatment of withdrawal in 10 infants.[62] REM and non-REM sleep patterns were correlated with muscular and respiratory activity. This study concluded that narcotics obliterate REM sleep in the neonate, withdrawal prevents normal adequate periods of deep sleep, proper therapy will cause the return of REM and sleep cycles, and maintenance of therapy can be best regulated by use of polygraphic recordings rather than observed absence of gross signs and symptoms of withdrawal. Schulman reported the absence of quiet sleep in

---

* References 20, 22, 24, 25, 27, 38, 41.

eight full-term infants whose mothers used heroin until delivery.[59] Recent studies by Pinto et al substantiate the findings of previous sleep studies.[55]

One of the most serious consequences of neonatal abstinence is the development of seizures. Seizures occur in about 1% to 2% of heroin-exposed neonates and approximately 7% of methadone-exposed neonates.[5,41] The relationship between maternal methadone dosage and the frequency or severity of the seizures has not been established. In addition, no significant differences were found between neonates with and those without seizures in birthweight, gestational age, occurrence of their withdrawal symptoms, day of onset of withdrawal symptoms, or the need for specific pharmacologic treatment.[25,26] The mean age of seizure onset was 10 days. Generalized motor seizures, or myoclonic jerks, are the principal seizure manifestation, although in some infants, the seizure manifestation can be complex. Seizures may occur even while the infant is being treated for NAS. Abnormal EEGs tend to occur only during the active seizure with normal interictal tracings.* The short-term prognosis for abstinence-associated seizures is favorable when compared with the prognosis after seizures associated with other causes. The authors suggest that this observed improvement in neurologic function may be based on the replenishment of neurotransmitters after transient depletion in the neonatal period.[24,25]

Infants experiencing NAS frequently exhibit respiratory distress symptoms such as rhinorrhea, a stuffy nose, tachypnea, nasal flaring, chest retractions, intermittent cyanosis, and apnea. Increased severity of these symptoms may occur when the infant regurgitates, aspirates, or develops aspiration pneumonia.

There is some evidence of transient abnormality of lung compliance and tidal volume in infants born to methadone or heroin-abusing mothers and tachypnea in the NAS, suggesting that opioids may alter the fetal development of the respiratory system.[66] Infants with acute heroin withdrawal have shown increased respiratory rates associated with hypocapnia and an increase in blood pH during the first week of life. The observed respiratory alkalosis was thought to have a beneficial role

in the binding of indirect serum bilirubin to albumin and possibly in the prevention of RDS, which is rarely observed in infants of opioid-abusing mothers. However, alkalosis can decrease the levels of ionized calcium and lead to tetany.[24,66]

The risk of SIDS should be considered when the neonate has an especially difficult course of NAS, when the mother supplemented her methadone with other substances (stimulants, nicotine), and when a combination of therapeutic agents is used for treatment since an increase in SIDS in these infants has been demonstrated to be 5 to 10 times over the general population. Bell and Lau report the risk of SIDS is increased in opiate-exposed infants and varies from 2.5% to 4%.[5] Wingkun et al and other researchers studied carbon dioxide sensitivity in infants of substance abusing mothers and found that these infants have abnormal sleep ventilatory patterns and "an impaired repertoire" of protective responses to hypoxia and hypercapnia during sleep cycles.[73]

Infants undergoing withdrawal have disturbed sleep patterns and exhibit excessive spontaneous generalized sweating, which may result from the predominantly central-neurogenic stimulation of sweat glands induced by heroin withdrawal.[24] Other autonomic nervous system signs include yawning, elevation of temperature, sneezing, and mottling.

The rooting reflex is exaggerated. It is not surprising then that infants frequently suck their fists or thumbs; yet when fed, their suck and swallow reflexes are uncoordinated and ineffectual. Therefore they tend to regurgitate or vomit in a projectile manner. The infant may also develop loose stools and is susceptible to dehydration and electrolyte imbalance.[20,24,27,41]

These symptoms are exhibited as a result of exposure to opioids as well as nonopioid CNS depressants. However, with nonopioid CNS depressant exposure, symptoms tend to begin at a later age with malnourishment at birth not a usual feature. In a study done by Shaw and McIvor, infants undergoing NAS treatment took up to 4 weeks to regain their birthweight and it was postulated that this may be due to their increased calorie requirement secondary to withdrawal.[60]

Since barbiturate withdrawal may not develop until an infant has been discharged from the

---

* References 16, 20, 24, 25, 27, 41, 45.

nursery, it may not be treated unless suspicion has been aroused by the mother's symptoms or actions. Furthermore, there is a greater risk of seizure activity in neonates withdrawing from barbiturates than those withdrawing from opioids.[20,22,24]

Symptoms exhibited by stimulant-exposed newborns differ markedly from those that are associated with maternal opioid use, unless the mother was using cocaine or amphetamines along with the opioids.

Recent literature describes cocaine-exposed infants as tremulous, irritable, lethargic, unable to respond appropriately to stimuli, and having abnormal state control and abnormal cry patterns.[1,5,11,35] Also described are abnormalities in orientation, motor ability, state regulation, muscular hypertonia, and abnormal reflexes. Infants may show symptoms of lethargy intermittently with irritability, poor sucking patterns, and sleep disturbances. When cocaine has been the primary drug of abuse, most clinicians have not seen symptoms severe enough to treat pharmacologically.[24] Most would not refer to the symptoms associated with cocaine as withdrawal, but instead, a manifestation of toxicity.[51]

Laboratory Data

Before the initiation of medication for abstinence, one must rule out common neonatal metabolic alterations that can mimic or compound withdrawal, such as hypocalcemia, hypomagnesemia, hypoglycemia, and hypothermia. Serum glucose and calcium tests may be indicated. If the mother has had no prenatal care, it would be prudent for the infant to have a thorough assessment at birth, including tests for occult disease, sepsis, and intracranial bleeding. A urine test for toxicology should also be obtained. Meconium testing, although expensive, and perhaps not readily available in all institutions, appears to be more accurate and has the ability to detect a longer period of drug exposure. Hair analysis of the mother and infant, although showing some promise, is still in the investigative stages, and problems exist with regard to hair color, texture, and acceptability to postpartum women. However, depending on the confidentiality laws of the state and whether the medical team is responsible by law to report the results of the urine

drug screen to child protection agencies, informed consent may be needed from the mother. Health care professionals caring for infants of mothers with no prenatal care will need to check their own state laws and institutional policies for clarification of this procedure.[32]

Treatment and Intervention

In order to determine if an infant will need pharmacologic treatment for withdrawal, appropriate assessment of symptoms is essential. Since only 50% to 60% of exposed infants have significant enough symptoms to require medication, an assessment tool is helpful.

We have used a scoring system to monitor the neonate in a comprehensive and objective way. With this score, one can assess the onset, progression, and resolution of symptoms. The score is also used to monitor the infant's clinical response to pharmacotherapy employed for the control of NAS symptoms. Titration of therapeutic pharmaceutic agents is thus based on the degree of withdrawal symptomatology that corresponds to a specific score (Fig. 8-1). The nurse is vital in the assessment of withdrawal symptoms since he or she will administer and record the score and any other activities that may affect the infant's progress. Therefore it is essential that interrater reliability be developed between all nurses responsible for the infant.

The abstinence scoring sheet lists 21 symptoms most commonly observed in the opioid-exposed neonate. Signs are recorded as single entities or in several categories if they occur in varying degrees of severity. Each symptom and its associated degree of severity has been assigned a score. Higher scores are assigned to symptoms found in infants with more severe withdrawal. The total score is determined by adding the score assigned to each symptom observed throughout the entire scoring interval. The scoring system is dynamic rather than static; all of the signs and symptoms observed during the 4-hour intervals at which infant symptoms are monitored are point-totaled for that interval. Infants are assessed 2 hours after birth and every 4 hours afterwards. If, at any time, the infant's score is 8 or higher, every 2-hour scoring is instituted and continued for 24 hours from the last total score of 8 or higher. If subsequent 2-hour

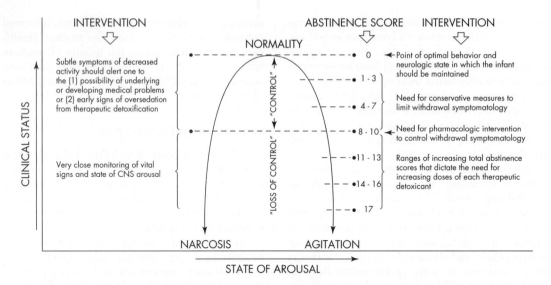

INTERVENTION   ABSTINENCE SCORE   INTERVENTION

NORMALITY

CLINICAL STATUS

Subtle symptoms of decreased
activity should alert one to
the (1) possibility of underlying
or developing medical problems
or (2) early signs of oversedation
from therapeutic detoxification

Very close monitoring of vital
signs and state of CNS arousal

"CONTROL"

"LOSS OF CONTROL"

0 ← Point of optimal behavior and
neurologic state in which the infant
should be maintained

1 - 3

4 - 7 ← Need for conservative measures to
limit withdrawal symptomatology

8 - 10 ← Need for pharmacologic intervention
to control withdrawal symptomatology

11 - 13   Ranges of increasing total abstinence
scores that dictate the need for
increasing doses of each therapeutic
detoxicant

14 - 16

17

NARCOSIS   AGITATION

STATE OF AROUSAL

Figure 8-1 Management of the neonatal abstinence syndrome (NAS). (From Finnegan LP: Neonatal abstinence syndrome. In Nelson N, editor: *Current therapy in neonatal-perinatal medicine,* ed 2, Ontario, 1990, BC Decker.)

scores continue to be 7 or less for 24 hours, then 4-hour scoring intervals may be resumed.

If medication is not warranted, the infant is scored for the first 4 days of life at the prescribed intervals. If the symptoms are severe enough to require medication, the infant is scored at 2- or 4-hour intervals, depending on whether the score is less than or greater than 8, as described previously, throughout the duration of the therapy. Once medication is discontinued, if there is no resurgence of the total score to 8 or higher after 3 days, scoring may be discontinued. If however, there is a resurgence of symptoms with scores consistently equaling 8 or higher, then scoring should be continued for a minimum of 4 days after discontinuation of medication to ensure that the infant is not discharged prematurely with the consequent development of symptoms at home.

A copy of the Neonatal Abstinence Scoring System can be seen in Figure 8-2. Symptoms are listed on the left, scores to the right. Times of each evaluation are listed at the top, and the total score is listed for each evaluation. A new sheet should be started at the beginning of each day. A "Comments" column has been provided for nursing and

medical staff to record important notes regarding the infant's progress.

Salient points to consider when using the scoring system are as follows:

- The first score should be recorded approximately 2 hours after admission to the nursery. This score reflects all infant behaviors from admission to that first point in time when the scoring interval is complete. The times designating the end of the scoring intervals (whether every 2 or 4 hours) have been left blank to permit the nursing staff to choose the most appropriate times for scoring intervals in relation to effective planning and implementation of nursing care.
- All infants should be scored at 4-hour intervals unless high scores indicate need for more frequent scoring.
- All symptoms exhibited during the entire scoring interval, not just a single point in time, should be included.
- The infant should be awakened to elicit reflexes and specified behavior, but if the infant is awakened to be scored, one should

NEONATAL ABSTINENCE SCORING SYSTEM

SYSTEM	SIGNS AND SYMPTOMS	SCORE	AM						PM							COMMENTS
CENTRAL NERVOUS SYSTEM DISTURBANCES	Excessive high pitched (or other) cry Continuous high pitched (or other) cry	2 3														Daily weight:
	Sleeps <1 hour after feeding Sleeps <2 hours after feeding Sleeps <3 hours after feeding	3 2 1														
	Hyperactive moro reflex Markedly hyperactive moro reflex	2 3														
	Mild tremors disturbed Moderate-severe tremors disturbed	1 2														
	Mild tremors undisturbed Moderate-severe tremors undisturbed	3 4														
	Increased muscle tone	2														
	Excoriation (specific area)	1														
	Myoclonic jerks	3														
	Generalized convulsions	5														
METABOLIC/VASOMOTOR/RESPIRATORY DISTURBANCES	Sweating	1														
	Fever <101 (99-100.8°F/37.2-38.2°C) Fever >101 (38.4°C and higher)	1 2														
	Frequent yawning (>3-4 times/interval)	1														
	Mottling	1														
	Nasal stuffiness	1														
	Sneezing (>3-4 times/interval)	1														
	Nasal flaring	2														
	Respiratory rate >60/min Respiratory rate >60/min with retractions	1 2														
GASTRO-INTESTINAL DISTURBANCES	Excessive sucking	1														
	Poor feeding	2														
	Regurgitation Projectile vomiting	2 3														
	Loose stools Watery stools	2 3														
	TOTAL SCORE															
	INITIALS OF SCORER															

Figure 8-2 Neonatal Abstinence Score Sheet. (From Finnegan LP: Neonatal abstinence syndrome. In Nelson N, editor: *Current therapy in neonatal-perinatal medicine,* ed 2, Ontario, 1990, BC Decker.)

not score him or her for diminished sleep after feeding. Sleeping should never be recorded for a scoring interval except when the infant has been unable to sleep for an extended period of time: more than 12 to 18 hours. If the infant is crying, he or she must be quieted before assessing muscle tone, respiratory rate, and the Moro reflex.
- Respirations are counted for 1 full minute.
- The infant is scored if prolonged crying is exhibited, even though it may not be high-pitched in quality.
- Temperatures should be taken (mild pyrexia is an early sign indicating heat production by increased muscle tone and tremors).
- If the infant is sweating solely because of conservative nursing measures (e.g., swaddling), a point should not be given. Medication is not indicated if consecutive total scores or the average of any three consecutive scores continues to be 7 or less during the first 4 days of life.

The total scores dictate the specific dose of the medication (e.g., paregoric morphine or phenobarbital), and all subsequent doses are determined by and titrated against the total score. In the phenobarbital loading dose approach, an initial dose of 20 mg/kg is administered in an attempt to achieve an expected therapeutic serum level with a single dose.

The need for medication is indicated when the total score is 8 or higher for three consecutive scorings (e.g., 9-8-10) or when the average of any three consecutive scores is 8 or higher (e.g., 9-7-9). Once an infant's score is 8 or higher, the scoring interval automatically becomes 2 hours, so that the infant exhibits symptoms that are out of control for no longer than 4 to 6 hours before therapy is initiated.

If the infant's total score is 12 or higher for two consecutive intervals or the average of any two consecutive scores is 12 or higher, therapy should be initiated at the appropriate dosage for that score before more than 4 hours elapse.

The longer the delay in initiation of an appropriate medication dose, the greater the risk of increased infant morbidity. Comfort mea-

sures employed for the infant should include the following:

- Swaddling
- Pacifier for nonnutritive, excessive sucking
- Nasal aspiration when needed
- Frequent diaper changes: exposure of hyperemic buttock in severe cases for air drying
- Soft sheets or sheepskin to decrease excoriations
- Position prone or right side-lying to reduce aspiration if vomiting or regurgitation is a problem
- Protect from face scratching by using mitten cuffs on the undershirt or tying a rubber band to the end of the shirt sleeves
- Consider demand feedings if weight change patterns are an issue
- Modification of the infant's environment (noise and light control); in severe cases, Oro and Dixon have recommended self-activated nonoscillating waterbeds as a useful adjunct to supportive care of narcotic-exposed neonates.[5,11,53]

Table 8-1 describes symptoms of withdrawal and appropriate nursing interventions.

The pharmacologic agents most commonly used in the treatment of withdrawal include paregoric (camphorated tincture of opium) and phenobarbital. A review of recent literature finds that some neonatal intensive care units treating NAS have switched from paregoric to an oral morphine solution because of their concerns over the contents of the paregoric mixture: morphine or opioid alkaloids, camphor, alcohol (46%), anise oil, and benzoic acid. Oral morphine solution contains only 10% alcohol.[30]

Table 8-2 outlines drug treatment for NAS. Any infant who exhibits a precipitous drop in a total score of eight points or higher should be monitored for vital signs immediately. It is important to determine whether any underlying medical problems are developing, such as sepsis, meningitis, hypocalcemia, or hypoglycemia. Detection of underlying medical problems may be difficult because poorly controlled abstinence may mimic and/or disguise many common neonatal conditions.

Table 8-1
Creating a Supportive Environment for the Drug-Exposed Neonate

Infant Behavior	Observations	Interventions

High-pitched cry	Note onset
	Note length of time the cry persists—is it continuous?
	Is it high pitched and piercing as though infant were in pain?
	Observe infant for other causes of abnormal crying patterns (meningitis, intracranial bleeding, pain, etc.)
	  • Is anterior fontanel full or bulging?
	  • Are cranial sutures widely separated?
	  • Is head circumference increased?
	  • Does infant stare without blinking and exhibit adder's tongue?
	  • Is cry aggravated or alleviated when infant is picked up?
		Soothe infant by swaddling, holding firmly and close to your body; soft-pack baby carrier; smooth, slow rocking
		Nonnutritive sucking
		Decrease feeding intervals and/or implement a demand-feeding schedule
		Reduce environmental stimuli (noise, light)
		Waterbeds, lambskin

Inability to sleep	Note how long infant sleeps after feeding Note general sleep and wake patterns If drug therapy has been initiated, note changes in sleep patterns, ability to rest, and whether there is decreased activity indicative of drug overdose	Decrease environmental stimuli (noise, light) Swaddle or use soft-pack baby carrier Feed small amounts at frequent intervals Waterbeds, lambskin Organize care to minimize handling
Frantic sucking of fists	Note onset and amount of fist sucking Observe for blisters on fingertips and knuckles If blistering occurs, observe sites for signs of infection	Use infant shirts with sewn-in sleeves for mitts to prevent skin trauma Offer pacifier for nonnutritive sucking Keep skin area clean; use aseptic technique
Yawning	Note onset and frequency	None
Sneezing	Observe onset and frequency	Aspirate nasopharynx prn
Nasal stuffiness	Note severity of nasal stuffiness and determine whether it hinders breathing and feeding; if mucus is excessive, consider possibility of other underlying problems, such as esophageal atresia, tracheoesophageal fistula, and congenital syphilis	Allow more time for feeding with rest between sucking Aspirate trachea if tracheal mucus is increased Check rate and character of respirations frequently Cardiorespiratory monitor with alarms set Daily weights
Poor feeding	Note sucking pattern—is infant uncoordinated in attempt to suck/swallow/breathe Observe for other possible causes of poor feeding (sepsis, hypoglycemia, immaturity, bowel obstruction, pyloric stenosis)	Decrease environmental stimuli Feed small amounts at close intervals Wrap securely Maintain fluid and caloric intake required for infant's weight Consider demand feedings Use alternative feeding methods (e.g., gavage) Avoid rocking; may be helpful for some babies Avoid talking or eye contact during feeding

Modified from Finnegan LP, MacNew BA: *Am J Nurs* 74(4):685, 1974.

Continued

Table 8-1
Creating a Supportive Environment for the Drug-Exposed Neonate—cont'd

Infant Behavior	Observations	Interventions
Regurgitation Vomiting Loose stools	Note when regurgitation or vomiting occurs—is there a precipitating factor (medication, handling, manipulation, position, etc.)? Observe for signs of dehydration • Specific gravity >1.015 • Urinary output <1 ml/kg/hr • Dry mucous membranes • Marked loss of weight • Poor skin turgor • Sunken anterior fontanel Note time, color, consistency, and quantity of vomitus and/or stool When stools are loose, estimate amount of water loss with stools Note whether vomiting is nonforceful or projectile Observe for electrolyte imbalance	Measure intake and output closely and correlate with infant's general condition, progress, and therapy Offer supplementary fluids if signs of dehydration appear Weigh frequently if weight loss, vomiting, and diarrhea persist Maintain IV at prescribed rate Maintain infant in prone or side-lying position to prevent aspiration of vomitus Head of bed may be elevated Give skin care to prevent excoriation of neck folds, buttocks, and perineum Frequent diaper changes, exposure of hyperemic buttocks for air drying Consider barrier dressings on knees, elbows, etc.
Hyperactive Moro reflex	Is reflex moderately or markedly exaggerated? If drug therapy has been started, note a diminished or absent Moro reflex Is there asymmetry of the reflex? Asymmetry may indicate underlying pathophysiology—Erb's palsy, fractured clavicle, intracranial hemorrhage	None
Hypertonicity	Note degree (mild, moderate, or severe) of increased muscle tone by • Attempting to straighten arms and legs and recording degree of resistance • Picking infant up by hands and noting body rigidity with degree of head lag (a withdrawing infant often exhibits trunk rigidity and holds the head on a plane with the body for a prolonged time) • Raising infant by arms and letting him or her stand (a withdrawing neonate exhibits marked leg rigidity and can support body weight for considerable periods) Correlate mother's obstetric history and delivery with infant's condition and observe baby for other pathophysiology—hypocalcemia, hypoglycemia, meningitis, asphyxia, and intracranial hemorrhage Observe for reddened areas over heels, occiput, sacrum, and knees Observe temperature frequently; increased activity may cause hyperthermia	Change infant's position often since prolonged or marked rigidity predisposes the infant to develop pressure areas Use sheepskin to reduce pressure, plus for relaxation and comfort Decrease environmental temperature if infant's temperature is >37.6° C (99° F)

Table 8-1

Creating a Supportive Environment for the Drug-Exposed Neonate—cont'd

Infant Behavior	Observations	Interventions
Tremors Convulsions	Note if tremors occur when infant is disturbed and/or undisturbed Note location of tremors • Upper extremities • Lower extremities • Generalized Note whether degree of tremors is mild, moderate, or severe Observe skin over nose, elbows, fingers, toes, knees, heels for excoriation Observe face for scratches Observe for underlying pathology mentioned under "Hypertonicity" Check temperature often for hyperthermia Observe for seizures; if they occur, note onset, length, origin, body involvement, whether tonic, clonic, or both, eye deviation, and infant's color	Change position frequently to prevent excoriation Give frequent skin care (cleansing, ointment, and exposure to air and/or a heat lamp) Use sheepskin Observe excoriations for healing, worsening, infection Decrease environmental temperature if infant exhibits hyperthermia If infant convulses, maintain patent airway and prevent self-trauma If infant is apneic after seizure, stimulate appropriately and be prepared to resuscitate Decrease environmental stimuli Organize nursing care to decrease handling Support movements during caregiving Swaddle as much as possible during caregiving

Table 8-2

Drugs Used for NAS*

Drug	Dosage	Comments
Paregoric	Starting dose: 0.8 ml/kg/day in 6 divided doses If score is ≥8, increase in increments of 0.4 ml/kg/day until control or signs of overtreatment occur Maintain dose for 72 hours Decrease dose: lower total daily dose 10% Adjust dose by weight gain or loss of ≥50 g Discontinue: when dose is 0.5 ml/kg/day Observe (depending on symptom severity) for 2-4 days after medication is discontinued	Signs of control: Scores are ≤8, infant is easily consoled, rhythmic sleep and feeding cycle, steady weight gain Signs of overtreatment: lethargy, hypotonia, irregular respirations, and/or bradycardia Advantages: diminishes bowel motility and loose stools; increases sucking coordination; controls symptoms in 90% of infants; reduces incidence of seizures Disadvantages: large doses often necessary; duration of therapy longer than with other drugs
Phenobarbital	Loading dose: 20 mg/kg to achieve an expected therapeutic level in a single dose If score ≥8, give 10 mg/kg every 12 hours until control or signs of toxicity appear Maintenance dose (once under control): 2-6 mg/kg/day for 3-4 days Decrease dose to 3 mg/kg/day Discontinue: serum levels <15 μg/ml	Daily serum levels can be obtained Advantages: drug of choice for polydrug use; especially effective in controlling irritability and insomnia; controls symptoms in 50% of infants Disadvantages: does not prevent loose stools Infant should be in a nursery where he or she is monitored closely

*Although clinicians have used laudanum, methadone, clonidine, and chlorpromazine in the treatment of NAS, there is very little data on outcomes.
NAS, Neonatal abstinence syndrome.

An infant may become increasingly depressed by a medication that is not specific for withdrawal. This situation may be reflected in the gradual development of depression with concomitant poorly controlled withdrawal, requiring reevaluation for appropriateness of the medication (Box 8-4).

Efficacy of the medication must always be assessed. Two common situations indicate the need for reassessment: (1) CNS depression and (2) failure to achieve "control" despite aggressive pharmacologic intervention and/or near-toxic serum levels of the agents. In these situations, the following measures are indicated:

- Evaluate the infant for metabolic derangements, sepsis, and CNS disturbances to detect an occult problem compounding the clinical picture. Evaluate laboratory data including serum calcium, electrolytes, glucose determinations, and blood cultures.

Box 8-4

Complications of Excessive Pharmacologic Treatment

- Diminished or absent reflexes: Moro, sucking, swallowing, Galant, Perez, tonic neck, corneal, grasp (palmar or plantar)
- Truncal (central) or circumoral cyanosis or persistent mottling not associated with ambient temperature decreases
- Decreased muscle tone with passive resistance to extension of extremities or decreased neck or trunk tone
- Altered state of arousal (e.g., obtunded or comatose)
- Diminished response to painful stimuli
- Failure of visual following
- Hypothermia
- Altered respirations: irregular (periodic breathing in full-term infants), shallow (decreased air entry), decreased respiratory rate (<20/min), apnea
- Cardiac alterations: irregular rate, distant heart sounds with weak peripheral pulses, heart rate of 80 to 100 beats/min, poor peripheral perfusion (pale, gray, mottled), cardiac arrest

---

- Review maternal drug history along with both maternal and infant urine toxicology results to ensure appropriate medication.
- If a single medication is ineffective, consider a combination of therapeutic agents.

Parent Teaching

It is important for primary caretakers to understand that infants exposed to narcotics because of maternal addiction have been found to be more irritable and less cuddly, exhibit more tremors, and have increased tone. They are also less responsive to visual stimulation and are less likely to maintain an alert state. Some symptoms of withdrawal may persist for 2 to 6 months, and the nurse should discuss this possibility with the caretakers well before discharge so that they may begin building the skills they'll need under the watchful eye of supportive staff. The infant may continue to feed poorly and regurgitate, yet vigorously suck fists and hands. Mothers frequently misread this continued, exaggerated rooting reflex as hunger and therefore may overfeed the infant. Loose stools may continue. The infants are easily disturbed by normal household sounds and do not sleep well. They sweat more than the other infants and, when crying, continue to have a high-pitched cry. Hypertonia may continue, and the mother may interpret this as a sign of rejection. Nursing support, including thorough descriptions of the potential symptoms and their management and the fact that they are time limited, is vital if maternal-infant attachment is to occur and potential neglect and abuse are to be avoided.

In recent studies the drug-dependent mother and her infant were assessed for patterns of interaction. Both drug-dependent mothers and their newborns demonstrated poor performance on a measure of social engagement. The drug-dependent mothers demonstrated significantly less positive affect and greater detachment, and the drug-exposed infants presented fewer behaviors promoting social involvement. Drug-exposed infants and their mothers experience a difficult early period during which both are less available, less likely to initiate, and less responsive to social involvement.[29] Therefore parents of the drug-exposed infant may need assistance in recognizing important symptoms that signal problems and cues necessary for caretaking.

All drugs of abuse pass through the breast milk. However, breastfeeding in the methadone-maintained mother need not be discouraged, for it does not appear to shorten or worsen the course of withdrawal.[41,46] On the other hand, women using stimulants and other drugs as well as those who are infected with the HIV virus should not be encouraged to breastfeed because of the potential toxic and negative effects on the neonate.

Finally, secondary crack smoke, crystal methamphetamine smoke, marijuana smoke, and tobacco smoke can be detrimental to the health of the newborn; therefore parents should be warned of the consequence of using these substances around their infant.

Prevention is the key and health-care providers need to be more diligent and vigilant in assessment and intervention.

References

1. American Academy of Pediatrics, Committee on Substance Abuse: Drug-exposed infants, *Pediatrics* 96(2)364, 1995.
2. Bandstra ES: Assessing acute and long-term physical effects of in utero drug exposure on the perinate, infant, and child. In Kibley MM, Asghar K, editors: *Methodological issues in epidemiological, prevention, and treatment and research on drug-exposed women and their children,* NIDA Research Monograph 117, Washington, DC, 1992.
3. Bandstra ES, Burkett G: Maternal-fetal and neonatal effects of in-utero cocaine exposure, *Semin Perinatol* 15(4):288, 1991.
4. Battin M, Albersheim S, Newman: Congenital genitourinary tract abnormalities following cocaine exposure in utero, *Am J Perinatol* 12(6)425, 1995.
5. Bell GL, Lau K: Perinatal and neonatal issues of substance abuse, *Pediatr Clin North Am* 42(2)261, 1995.
6. Bibb KW et al: Drug screening in newborns and mothers using meconium samples, paired urine samples, and interviews, *J Perinatol* 15(3):199, 1995.
7. Blinick G, Wallach RC, Jerez E: Pregnancy in narcotic addicts treated by medical withdrawal, *Am J Obstet Gynecol* 105:997, 1969.
8. Catanzarite VA, Stein DA: 'Crystal' and pregnancy: methamphetamine-associated maternal deaths, *West J Med* 162(5):454, 1995.
9. Chazotte C, Youchah J, Freda MC: Cocaine use during pregnancy and low birth weight: the impact on prenatal care and drug treatment, *Semin Perinatol* 19(4):293, 1995.
10. Connaughton LF, Reeser D, Schut J et al: Perinatal addiction: outcome and management, *Am J Obstet Gynecol* 729:679, 1977.
11. D'Apolito K: Can drug-exposed infants be rocked too much? *Neonat Net* 14(7):69, 1995.
12. Davis RC, Chappel JN: Pregnancy in the context of narcotic addiction and methadone maintenance, *Proc Fifth Nat Conf Methadone Treat* 2:1146, 1973.
13. Day NL, Robles N, Richardson G et al: The effects of prenatal alcohol use on the growth of children at three years of age, *Alcohol Clin Exp Res* 153:625, 1991.
14. Desmond MM, Wilson GS: Neonatal abstinence syndrome: recognition and diagnosis, *Addict Dis* 2:113, 1975.
15. Dickson PH et al: The routine analysis of breast milk for drugs of abuse in a clinical toxicology laboratory, *J Forensic Sci* 39(1):207, 1994.
16. Doberczak TM et al: One year follow-up of infants with abstinence-associated seizures, *Arch Neurol* 45(6):649, 1988.
17. Ehrlich S, Finnegan LP: Trends and changes in a treatment program for drug-dependent pregnant women: an 8-year study, *Pediatr Res* 21:1324, 1987 (abstract).
18. Gottbrath-Flaherty EK et al: Urinary tract infections in cocaine-exposed infants, *J Perinatol* 15(3):203, 1995.
19. Finnegan LP: Treatment issues for opioid-dependent women during the perinatal period, *J Psychoactive Drugs* 23(2):191, 1991.
20. Finnegan LP: Clinical perinatal and developmental effects of methadone. In Cooper JR Altman et al, editors: *Research on the treatment of narcotic addiction, state of the art,* US Department of Health and Human Services, National Institute of Drug Abuse, Washington, DC, 1983.
21. Finnegan LP: Influence of maternal drug dependence on the newborn. In Kacew S, Lock S, editors: *Toxicologic and pharmacologic principles in pediatrics,* Washington, DC, 1988, Hemisphere.
22. Finnegan LP: Neonatal abstinence syndrome: assessment and pharmacology. In Rubaltelli FF, Granati B, editors: *Neonatal therapy: an update,* New York, 1986, Elsevier.
23. Finnegan LP, Hagan TA, Kaltenbach K: Opioid dependence: scientific foundations of clinical practice, *Perspect Direct Bull NY Acad Med* 67(3):223, 1991.
24. Finnegan LP, Kaltenbach K: Neonatal abstinence syndrome. In Hoekelman RA, Nelson N: *Primary pediatric care,* ed 2, St Louis, 1992, Mosby.
25. Finnegan LP, Kaltenbach K: The assessment and management of neonatal abstinence syndrome. In Hoekelman RA, Friedman SB, Nelson NM et al, editors: *Primary pediatric care,* ed 3, St Louis, 1990, Mosby.
26. Finnegan LP, et al: Assessment and treatment of abstinence in the infant of the drug-dependent mother, *Int J Clin Pharmacol Biopharmacol* 12:19, 1975.
27. Finnegan LP, Macnew B: Care of the addicted infant, *Am J Nurs* 74(4):685, 1974.
28. Finnegan L, Wapner RJ: Drug use in pregnancy, In Neibyl JR, editor: *Narcotic addiction in pregnancy,* Philadelphia, 1987, Lea & Febiger.
29. Fitzgerald E, Kaltenbach K, Finnegan LP: Patterns of interaction among drug-dependent women and their infants, *Pediatr Res* 27(4):104, 1990.
30. Franck L, Vilardi J: Assessment and management of opioid withdrawal in ill neonates, *Neonat Net* 14(2):39, 1995.

31. Glass L, Evans HE: Narcotic withdrawal in the newborn, *Am Fam Physician* 6:75, 1972.

32. Horowitz RM: Drug use in pregnancy: to test, to tell: legal implications for the physician, *Semin Perinatol* 15(4):324, 1991.

33. Hanlonlundberg KM et al: Accelerated fetal lung maturity profiles and maternal cocaine exposure, *Obstet Gynecol* 87(1):128, 1996.

34. Hoyme HE et al: Prenatal cocaine exposure and fetal vascular disruption, *Pediatrics* 85:743, 1990.

35. Huffman DM, Price BK, Langel L: Therapeutic handling techniques for the infant affected by cocaine, *Neonat Net* 13(5):9, 1994.

36. Hurt H et al: Natal status of infants of cocaine users and control subjects: a prospective comparison, *J Perinatol* 15(4):297, 1995.

37. Jaffe JH: Drug addiction and drug abuse. In Gilman AG, Goodman LS, Gilman A, editors: *The pharmacological basis of therapeutics,* ed 8, New York, 1993, Pergamon.

38. Kaltenbach K, Finnegan LP: Prenatal opiate exposure: physical, neurobehavioral, and developmental effects. In Miller M, editor: *Development of the central nervous system: effects of alcohol and opiates,* New York, 1992, Wiley-Liss.

39. Kaltenbach K et al: The relationship between maternal methadone dose during pregnancy and infant outcome, *Pediatr Res* 27(4):227a, 1990.

40. Kandall S: Perinatal effects of cocaine and amphetamine use during pregnancy. Presented as part of a *Symposium on Pregnancy and Substance Abuse: Perspectives and Directions,* New York Academy of Medicine, 1990.

41. Kandall S: Drug abuse. In Sweet AY, Brown E, editors: *Fetal and neonatal effects of maternal disease,* St Louis, 1991, Mosby.

42. Kandall S, Gaines J: Maternal substance use: subsequent sudden infant death syndrome in offspring, *Neurotoxicol Teratol* 13(2):235, 1991.

43. Kandall SR et al: Differential effects of maternal heroin and methadone use on birth weight, *Pediatrics* 58:681, 1976.

44. Kandall SR et al: The narcotic-dependent mother: fetal and neonatal consequences, *Early Hum Dev* 1:159, 1977.

45. Kandall S, Gartner LM: Late presentation of drug withdrawal symptoms in newborns, *Am J Dis Child* 127:58, 1974.

46. Kreek MJ: Opioid disposition and effects during chronic exposure in the perinatal period in man. In Stimmel B, editor: *Advances in alcohol and substance abuse,* New York, 1982, Haworth.

47. Lester BM et al: Neurobehavioral syndromes in cocaine-exposed newborn infants, *Child Dev* 62:694, 1991.

48. Little B, Snell L, Gilstrap L: Methamphetamine abuse during pregnancy: outcome and fetal effects, *Obstet Gynecol* 72(4):541, 1988.

49. Little B et al: Patterns of multiple substance abuse during pregnancy: implications for mother and fetus, *South Med J* 83(5):507, 1990.

50. Mayes LC, Carroll KM: Neonatal withdrawal syndrome in infants exposed to cocaine and methadone, *Substance Use & Misuse,* 31(2):241, 1996.

51. Neuspiel DR, Hamel BC: Cocaine and infant behavior, *Dev Behavior Ped* 12(1):55, 1992.

52. Nora JG: Perinatal cocaine use: maternal, fetal, and neonatal effects, *Neonat Net* 9(2):45, 1990.

53. Oro AS, Dixon SD: Perinatal cocaine and methamphetamine exposure: maternal and neonatal correlates, *Pediatrics* 111(4):571, 1987.

54. Pietrantoni M, Knupple RA: Alcohol use in pregnancy, *Clin Perinatol* 18(1):93, 1991.

55. Pinto F et al: Sleep in babies born to chronically heroin-addicted mothers, a follow-up study, *Drug Alcohol Depend* 21(1):43, 1988.

56. Rosen TS, Pippenger CE: Pharmacologic observations on the neonatal withdrawal syndrome, *J Pediatr* 88:1044, 1974.

57. Rosen TS, Johnson HL: Children of methadone-maintained mothers: follow-up to 18 months of age, *J Pediatr* 101(2):192, 1982.

58. Schneider JW, Chasnoff IJ: Motor assessment of cocaine/polydrug exposed infants at age 4 months, *Neurotoxicol Teratol* 14(2):97, 1992.

59. Schulman L: Alteration of the sleep cycle in heroin addicted and "suspect" newborns, *Neuropaediatrie* 1(1):89, 1969.

60. Shaw NJ, McIvor L: Neonatal abstinence syndrome after maternal methadone treatment, *Arch Dis Child* 71:F203, 1994.

61. Silver H et al: Addiction in pregnancy: high-risk intrapartum management and outcome, *J Perinatol* 3(3):178, 1987.

62. Sisson TRC et al: Effect of narcotic withdrawal on neonatal sleep patterns, *Pediatr Res* 8:451, 1974.

63. Snodgrass RS: Cocaine babies: a result of multiple teratogenic influences, *J Child Neurol* 9(3):227, 1994.

64. Streissguth AP: Alcohol and motherhood: physiological findings and the fetal alcohol syndrome. In *Research Monograph No. 16, Women and Alcohol: Health Related Issues,* US Department of Health and Human Services, Washington, DC, 1986.

65. Streissguth AP, LaDue RA: Fetal alcohol syndrome: teratogenic causes of developmental disabilities. In Schroeder S, editor: *Toxic substances and mental retardation,* Washington, DC, 1987, American Association on Mental Deficiency.

66. Suguihara C, Bancalari E: Substance abuse during pregnancy: effects on respiratory function in the infant, *Semin Perinatol* (4):302, 1991.

67. Tronick EZ, Lester BM: The NICU network neurobehavioral scale: a comprehensive instrument to assess substance-exposed and high-risk infants. In Kibley MM, Asghar K, editors: *Methodological issues in epidemiological, prevention, and treatment research on drug exposed women and their children,* NIDA Research Monograph 117, Washington, DC, 1992.

68. Wallach RC, Jerez ME, Blinick G: Pregnancy and menstrual function in narcotic addicts treated with methadone, *Am J Obstet Gynecol* 105:1226, 1969.

69. Wapner R, Finnegan LP: Perinatal aspects of psychotropic drug abuse. In Bolognese RJ, Schwartz RH, Schneider I, editors: *Perinatal medicine,* Baltimore, 1981, Williams & Wilkins.

70. Weiner SM: Perinatal impact of substance abuse, *March of Dimes Continuing Education Module,* March of Dimes, Hamaroneck, NY, 1992.

71. Weiner SM: Substance abuse: alcohol and cocaine in pregnancy, *Unpublished manuscript,* 1996.
72. Wingert WE et al: A comparison of meconium, maternal urine and neonatal urine for detection of maternal drug use during pregnancy, *J Forensic Sci* 39(1):150, 1994.
73. Wingkun JG et al: Decreased carbon dioxide sensitivity in infants of substance-abusing mothers, *Pediatrics* 95(6):864, 1995.

74. Zuckerman B: Selected methodologic issues in investigations of prenatal effects of cocaine: lessons from the past. In Kibley MM, Asghar K, editors: *Methodological issues in controlled studies on affects of prenatal exposure to drug abuse,* NIDA Research Monograph 114, Washington, DC, 1991.

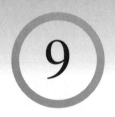

9

Pharmacology in Neonatal Care

M. Gail Murphy, Barbara S. Turner

Individual infants given an identical dosage regimen of a drug may exhibit a variety of clinical responses. There are many factors that influence either the intensity or the duration of a drug's effect. In some cases measurable characteristics that relate to the aging process (e.g., changes in maturation of the liver and kidney or changes in body weight and composition) result in predictable changes in drug disposition. Because some variability in drug response remains unexplained, it is critically important to monitor adequately for both desirable and toxic effects.

Physiology

Neonates show dramatic differences in the way they respond to drugs as compared with older children and adults. Variability in the dose-response relationship is attributed to differences in "what the body does to the drug" (*pharmacokinetics*) or "what the drug does to the body" (*pharmacodynamics*) (Fig. 9-1). Pharmacokinetics is the study of drug disposition (i.e., an overview of a drug's concentration in the body over time). *Disposition* can be classified into four processes: *drug entry* (absorption), *distribution, biotransformation,* and *elimination.* Pharmacodynamics refers to the study of the relationship between drug concentration and drug effect. Recognition of the essential role of drug concentration in linking dose to response enables an understanding of potential causes of variability in the dose-response relationship. The apparent increase in response, reflected in the statement, "Infants are more sensitive to the effects of drugs," might be attributed to differences in pharmacokinetics, pharmacodynamics, or both.

The drug-receptor theory is the unifying principle of drug therapy. At the site of action of a drug, the time course of drug concentration at the receptor strongly influences the time course of drug effect. Unfortunately, most drug receptors are in tissues that are clinically inaccessible for routine monitoring. For many commonly used drugs, after an initial short distribution phase, the rate of change of the plasma drug concentrations will parallel the rate of change of the drug concentration at the receptor.[24] This is the least complex model of drug movement in the body. Dose design and modification with drugs that follow this model are expressed mathematically in a straightforward fashion with disposition parameters, such as clearance, volume of distribution, and half-life, and can be solved with a four-function calculator.[21]

Initially, the clinician's choice of a dose regimen is based on data relating the dose with the incidence of therapeutic response and toxic effect in the average patient. Plasma drug concentrations can be a useful surrogate for drug effect when the relationship between concentration (C) and effect has been demonstrated in similar patients. Then the choice of dose regimen may be based on data relating to the dose with the target plasma concentration at steady state (Css). During maintenance therapy, steady state occurs when the input of a drug equals the elimination of the drug from the body. During this period a constant average plasma concentration (Css) is achieved with some variability around this value, which depends on the dose, dose interval, and drug disposition. As illustrated in Figure 9-2, the minimum effective concentration (MEC) is the concentration at which 50% of patients exhibit the desired response. The maximum safe concentration (MSC) is the concentration at which 50% of patients exhibit a toxic response. Toxicity may occur in some patients at concentrations close to the MEC and less than the MSC. For drugs whose MEC and MSC are close, rational drug

---

Box 9-1

Abbreviations

C	Drug concentration (plasma or serum)	mg/L
Css	Steady state concentration (average)	mg/L
MEC	Minimum effective concentration	mg/L
MSC	Maximum safe concentration	mg/L
F	Extent of drug availability (0 to 1); how much active drug gets to the systemic circulation	unitless
V	Volume of distribution; relates to loading dose	L/kg
Cl	Clearance: relates to maintenance dose	L/kg/hr
t½	Drug elimination half-life; relates to the time course of changes in drug concentration	hours

L = liter = 1000 milliliters
mg = milligram = 1000 micrograms

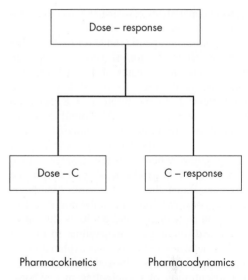

Figure 9-1   Variability in dose-response relationship can be the result of differences in pharmacokinetics or pharmacokynamics. *C,* Drug concentration (plasma or serum).

therapy includes monitoring of the patient for both desired and toxic effects.

The target Css is partly determined by the sensitivity at the drug receptor. Developmental differences in number and function of drug receptors may be critical for drug action. An example of the effects of aging on pharmacodynamics is the diminished sensitivity of the cardiovascular system to digitalis, which is associated with a decreased number of receptor sites in the newborn myocardium.[8]

The target Css is also influenced by the fraction of drug bound to plasma proteins. The goal of drug therapy is to achieve and maintain a free drug concentration at the site of action of the drug that will produce the maximum desired effect with a minimal risk of toxicity. However, the concentration that is measured is usually the total drug concentration in the serum, the sum of bound and free drug. The degree of plasma protein binding (which is often different in pediatric patients, especially newborns) will influence the relation-

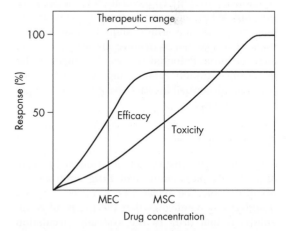

Figure 9-2   Percentage of patients with desired and toxic responses as a function of drug concentration. Therapeutic range is bounded by minimum effective and maximum safe concentrations. *MEC,* Minimum effective concentration; *MSC,* maxizmum safe concentration.

ship of total concentration measured to concentration at the active site.

The reported therapeutic range for theophylline in adults is 10 to 20 μg/ml versus a reported therapeutic range in neonates of 4 to 12 μg/ml.[24] Theophylline is reported to be 36% bound to plasma protein at a concentration of 8 μg/ml in newborns as compared with 70% bound in adults. A measured concentration in the serum of 10 μg/ml in an adult would be expected to represent 3 μg/ml free theophylline, whereas in the neonate a total concentration of 4.7 μg/ml consists of 3 μg/ml free theophylline. When the lower plasma binding is taken into consideration, the unbound effective concentration in neonates and adults is the same. The decreased binding of theophylline to plasma proteins in neonates could be one explanation of why therapeutic effect is achieved with lower total serum concentration of theophylline in newborns than in adults. An alternative explanation for the apparent difference in theophylline effect is that theophylline is metabolized to an active compound, caffeine, in newborns but not in adults.[20] **With the above age-related changes in the concentration-response relationship, a new way of directly monitoring drug response or a new target concentration is required. However, many age-related changes are the result of changes in the dose-concentration relationship, not the concentration-response relationship. When age-related changes occur in the dose-concentration relationship, the dose or dose interval is adjusted to achieve the original target concentration. Potential causes of changes in the dose-concentration relationship unique to newborns are described for each drug disposition process as follows.**

Absorption

The process of absorption determines the rate and the absolute amount of drug entering the blood-stream. The parameter F varies between 0 and 1; F = 1 indicates that the extent of availability of that drug to the systemic circulation is 100%.

Systematic studies of absorption of different drugs in sick newborns[11] are needed because differences in absorptive processes are anticipated between newborns and older patients and between well and critically ill newborns. Differences in newborns potentially affecting oral bioavailability include developmental changes in surface area and permeability of gastrointestinal mucosa, age-dependent changes in acid secretion in the stomach, and changes in total gastrointestinal transit time and in gastric emptying time.

Distribution

The volume of distribution of a drug is a useful but theoretical parameter that relates the total amount of drug in the body to the serum or plasma concentration. It may be used to estimate the size of a loading dose or a change in plasma concentration with a given loading dose:

$$\text{Loading dose} \times F = \text{change in C} \times V$$
$$\text{Change in C} = F \times \text{loading dose}/V$$

Volume of distribution is usually expressed as a function of body weight, with units of volume per kilogram. Major factors that affect distribution volume[8,14] are plasma protein binding and body composition. Changes in body composition occur throughout fetal and newborn life. Total body water (TBW) is increased (85% of body weight in preterm infants and 70% in term infants, compared with 55% in adults). Water-soluble drugs (e.g., sulfas, penicillins, aminoglycosides, and cephalosporin) will therefore be distributed in greater volume (i.e., higher TBW of the neonate), thus requiring a larger loading dose on a per kilogram body weight basis.

Premature and term infants have qualitatively and quantitatively different plasma proteins than older infants. Protein binding is decreased in the newborn because of a decreased concentration of albumin and a decreased capacity of fetal albumin to bind to drugs. Certain acidic drugs (e.g., salicylates, ampicillin, phenytoin, phenobarbital, and sulfa drugs) will bind less, thus increasing the free fraction of the drug (with resultant increase in their effect).

An issue of particular concern in newborn infants is the interaction between increased circulating bilirubin and drugs that are protein-bound.

A number of anionic compounds bind to albumin and may displace bilirubin and enhance bilirubin's neurotoxicity. Bilirubin may displace drugs (e.g., phenytoin) from albumin and increase bilirubin's pharmacologic effect. Binding to plasma proteins by drugs may also interfere with the transport of other endogenous substances such as fatty acids.

Biotransformation (Drug Metabolism)

Biotransformation (drug metabolism) usually occurs in the liver. Predicting the effect of aging on metabolism is difficult because of the variety of processes that occur in the liver, including oxidation, conjugation, and changing hepatic blood flow. **For example, oxidation and glucuronidation are decreased in newborns. Drugs that undergo oxidation (e.g., acetaminophen, phenobarbital, and phenytoin) will have a diminished clearance. Decreased glucuronidation of chloramphenicol has been cited as the cause of "gray baby" syndrome. Furthermore, age-related changes in the pathway of elimination occur. Theophylline is metabolized to an active compound, caffeine, in neonates. In adults, theophylline is metabolized to inactive metabolites. The clearance of certain drugs through the liver depends on the drug's free or unbound fraction. A decrease in plasma protein binding may increase the hepatic clearance of a drug.**

Clearance (Elimination)

Drug clearance (elimination) occurs by excretion or by biotransformation to an inactive metabolite. Most drug elimination pathways become saturated if the dose is high enough. Fortunately, the therapeutic dose for most drugs used in clinical practice is less than that which saturates elimination processes. **When disposition mechanisms are not saturated, then the Css in the plasma is proportional to the dose rate. Clearance equals the rate of drug elimination divided by the drug concentration. Just as volume of distribution relates to loading dose, clearance relates to maintenance dose at steady state:**

$$\text{(Dose/dose interval)} \times F = Cl \times Css \text{ or}$$
$$Cl = F \times \text{dose}/(\text{interval} \times Css)$$

Renal Excretion

Many common drugs (e.g., aminoglycosides, digoxin, penicillins) have the kidney as their primary route of excretion. Doses of drugs excreted in the urine are modified as a function of age. The GFR is low at birth and does not increase significantly until 1 week of age in term infants. In premature infants the GFR is even less, with a significant increase at a postconceptional age of 34 weeks or more. Aminoglycosides are examples of drugs excreted by glomerular filtration that demonstrate a decreased clearance and a longer half-life in newborns. In adults, dosages of these drugs might be reduced on the basis of creatinine clearance. However, creatinine is not an ideal marker for glomerular filtration in newborns, because newborn serum creatinine in the first week of life at least partly reflects the mother's creatinine. Complications such as acidosis and anoxia may also modify the infant's ability to eliminate a drug and therefore alter the pharmacokinetics of the drug.

Half-Life

The drug elimination half-life is the time required for the drug level to decline by 50%. Half-life is related to both V and Cl, so that

$$t_{1/2} = 0.7 \times V/Cl$$

The half-life is used to predict and interpret the time course of changes in plasma drug concentrations. For instance, the time to steady state is 4 to 5 half-lives. The half-life is useful in selecting dose intervals. The importance of considering the relationship of half-life and various dosing intervals is illustrated in Figure 9-3.

Prevention of Avoidable Therapeutic Mishaps

Even after the correct choice of therapeutic agents is made, attention to the following principles is necessary to ensure optimal drug treatment:

- Carefully consider predictable factors that may affect the intensity or duration of

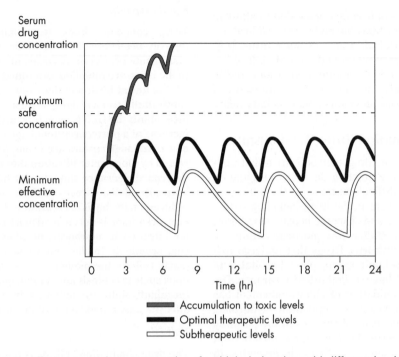

Serum drug concentration

Maximum safe concentration

Minimum effective concentration

Time (hr)

▬▬▬ Accumulation to toxic levels
▬▬▬ Optimal therapeutic levels
▭▭▭ Subtherapeutic levels

Figure 9-3   Effect on serum drug concentration of multiple dosing along with different time intervals between doses. *Curve 1,* Accumulation to toxic levels; *curve 2,* optimal therapeutic levels; *curve 3,* subtherapeutic levels. (From Roberts RJ: *Drug therapy in infants,* Philadelphia, 1984, WB Saunders.)

Box 9-2

The "Five Rights" of Drug Administration

Right drug
Right patient
Right route
Right dose
Right time

---

drug effect with the initial prescription of a given drug.
• Ensure certainty in patient dosing.
• Monitor the effect of therapy and modify the therapeutic plan based on clinical effects and, when warranted, blood concentrations.

Completing the "five rights" of medication administration (Box 9-2) becomes complicated when caring for the newborn because of small dosages and dosage adjustments based on infant weight or surface area. However, without meticulous attention to these issues, disasters can and will occur.

Drugs enter the body directly by injection into body fluids, such as the blood, and indirectly by absorption across membrane barriers of the gastrointestinal tract, skin, muscle, and pulmonary alveoli. The rate and extent of drug entry varies with different drug formulations. The administration of drugs to infants is further complicated because dosages are prescribed in amounts not commercially available. Drugs must be diluted from commercially available pediatric or adult dosage forms.

Errors in administration of medications to newborns are not unknown.[5,22] It has been reported that 8% of all drug doses calculated and administered by experienced neonatal intensive

NEONATAL RESUSCITATION MEDICATIONS

Name: _____   Weight: _____   Suction depth: _____

Date of birth: _____   ET tube size: _____

Drug	Strength	Dose	Route	Amount to administer
NaHCO$_3$	0.5 mEq/ml	1-2 mEq/kg	IV	_____
Epinephrine	1:10000	0.1 ml/kg	IV, ET	_____
Atropine	0.1 mg/ml	0.1 ml/kg	IV	_____

Other drugs and dosages could be added (see Table 5-2).

_____

Signature of preparer

Figure 9-4   Calculations for neonatal resuscitation medications.

care nurses are in fact at least 10 times greater or less than the dose ordered. Reports exist of infants having digitalis toxicity from receiving 0.09 mg of digoxin when 0.009 mg was ordered. Accuracy of dosage calculation, preparation, and administration of medications is crucial in the care of the neonate. Having two nurses calculate and check the dosage decreases errors.

Although pediatric dosing formulations exist, problems still are reported with such commonly used drugs as digoxin and morphine in 1 to 2 kg babies. The concentration of digoxin preparation available for intravenous (IV) use predisposes to errors in the amount of drug actually administered. A 1 kg newborn given digoxin (5 μg/0.05 ml) every 12 hours receives the dosage by a tuberculin (TB) syringe, which has a dead space sufficient to contain 10 μg of digoxin.[3,4] In a prospective study, preterm neonates given undiluted preparations of digoxin had an average serum level of digoxin of 4.5 ± 1.1 versus 1.9 ± 1.0 μg/ml (mean ± SD) in preterm infants given a diluted digoxin preparation.

In emergency situations the prompt and accurate preparation of emergency medications is critical. It is difficult to calculate medications both quickly and accurately when under the stress of a crisis. A better alternative, in anticipation of emergencies, is the calculation of emergency medications after the infant's admission. Calculations for the most commonly administered medications are posted at the bedside at all times (Fig. 9-4).

Data Collection

Desired effects and potential toxic effects of drug therapy should be recorded, along with the time, to monitor for these effects. The expected dose-effect relationship should be recorded, along with the expected dose-plasma concentration effect relationship when therapeutic drug monitoring is appropriate.

Dose recommendations and disposition parameters such as distribution volume, clearance, half-life, and bioavailability determined specifically in term or preterm infants should be recorded.

Factors that influence drug response, such as chronologic age, maturational age, birth weight, and current weight, should also be recorded. It is important to employ units correctly. It is important to overcome the problems associated with drug delivery in small infants.

Pharmacokinetic principles may be used to design a dose regimen as follows:

- In many clinical situations, drugs are administered in such a way as to maintain a steady state of the drug in the body. Therefore the dose input should equal the drug loss from the body. At steady state, dosing rate = (Cl × Css)/F. Thus if the clinician can specify the desired steady state plasma concentration and knows the clearance and bioavailability of that drug in a particular patient, the appropriate dosing rate can be calculated.

Example: Clearance for theophylline in preterm infants is reported as 0.017 L/kg/hr. If the desired average Css = 8 mg/L, then (assuming F = 1):

$$\text{Dose rate} = \text{Css} \times \text{Cl} = 0.136 \text{ mg/kg/hr or}$$
$$1.1 \text{ mg/kg every 8 hours}$$

- When the time to reach steady state is long, as it is with drugs with long half-lives, a loading dose may be desirable. The volume of distribution is the proportionality factor that relates the amount of drug in the body to the plasma concentration. For drugs with one-compartment distribution, the loading dose may be given as a single dose.

Example: Theophylline has a volume of distribution in preterm infants of about 0.7 L/kg. If 8 mg/L is the desired concentration, a loading dose (LD) can be calculated (assuming F = 1).

$$\text{LD} = (\text{Vd} \times \text{C})/\text{F} = 0.7 \text{ L/kg} \times 8 \text{ mg/L}$$
$$= 5.6 \text{ mg/kg or theophylline}$$

Laboratory Data

Even when predictable changes are taken into account, other nonpredictable factors may influence a drug's effect. Therefore clinical end points must be followed with the anticipation that dose regimens may require additional modification. For instance, the major short-term toxicity of indomethacin for patent ductus arteriosus (PDA) closure is transient, reversible renal dysfunction (i.e., oliguria, reduced GFR, and electrolyte imbalance). When signs of renal dysfunction are observed in infants receiving indomethacin, the next dose is withheld until renal function returns to normal.

Good data collection is essential for accurate timing of dosing and blood sampling. If the drug concentration in the blood has been related to the clinical response, then it is rational to follow blood concentrations in addition to clinical end points. To use measured blood levels optimally, one must calculate the expected blood concentration from the dosing history, measurable patient variables that might affect drug effect, and the timing of blood samples. Comparison of the expected value with the measured value[15,16] allows rational adjustment of future dosing. Potential explanations for differences between measured and expected concentrations are listed in Box 9-3.

If a suboptimal clinical response is noted in conjunction with a subtherapeutic target plasma concentration, then revised estimates of clearance may be cautiously made with one or two available plasma concentrations. If a single available concentration is drawn after absorption and distribution is complete or near steady state, then the maintenance dose formula can be rearranged to calculate a revised clearance. The common sense approach[15] suggests that if a patient has one half the expected concentration of a drug, then perhaps the clearance is twice the initial estimate. On the

---

Box 9-3

Potential Explanations for Discrepancies Between Measured and Expected Drug Concentration

Inadequate compliance
Inadequate medication delivery
Inappropriate timing of samples
Laboratory error
Revision in initial estimates of pK required

other hand, if the patient has twice the expected concentration of a drug, one explanation is that the clearance is only half the initial estimate. This technique will be misleading if steady state has not been reached. In response to twice the desired blood concentration, the drug should be discontinued until the blood concentration decays to the target concentration. Then, decreasing the dose rate by one half is anticipated to result in continued achievement of the desired target concentration.

If two concentrations are available after absorption and distribution, then a revised half-life is determined by plotting the concentrations on semilog paper. The revised clearance is then calculated by rearranging the half-life formula as follows:

$$Cl = 0.7 \times V/t_{1/2}$$

Practical Application

Following are some examples of simple pharmacokinetic calculations using the principles discussed above. These calculations should not be used unless meticulous attention has been given to the issues of delivery of medication and timing of dosing and blood sampling.

ASSIGNMENT 1: A 0.75 kg, 15-day-old premature infant is receiving an oral theophylline preparation diluted by the pharmacy for apnea of prematurity. He has been given 1.0 mg of theophylline every 8 hours for 5 days. At 8 AM on the fifth day and 4 hours after the patient's last dose of theophylline, the infant's heart rate is 180 beats/min, although apnea has abated. Clinical and laboratory evaluation of the tachycardia includes consideration of theophylline toxicity. The theophylline is discontinued, and blood samples for determination of theophylline and caffeine concentrations are sent to the laboratory. It will be 4 hours before the theophylline concentrations are run in the laboratory. Estimate what this concentration will be.

ASSIGNMENT 1 ANSWER: The data necessary to address this question include the following:

Total body weight = 0.75 kg
$V^{1,2} = 0.69$ L/kg = 0.53 L in this patient
$Cl^{1,2} = 0.017$ L/kg/hr = 0.013 L/hr in this patient
$t_{1/2} = 0.7 \times V/Cl = 28.5$ hr

Time to steady state $(Tss) = 4t_{1/2} = 114$ hr
Asume F = 1
MSC = 12 mcg/ml
MEC = 4 mcg/ml

Therefore:

Css = F × dose/(dose interval × Cl)
    = 1 × 1.0 mg/(8hr × 0.013 L/hr)
    = 9.6 mg/L

The Css was estimated based on average V and Cl values reported in similar infants and adjusted for this infant's weight. However, this infant may have diminished clearance relative to the "average" infant, resulting in possible toxicity with a standard dose. Toxicity might not have been noted until day 5 because of the estimated prolonged Tss (114 hr).

ASSIGNMENT 2: At 4 PM the theophylline concentration is reported to be 15 mg/L (caffeine <1 mg/L), confirming our suspicion of decreased clearance in this infant. Using this concentration, estimate the time at which the concentration will decline to 8 mg/L and determine an oral theophylline 12-hour dosage for maintaining that concentration.

The patient's tachycardia resolves 16 hours after the last dose.

ASSIGNMENT 2 ANSWER: A revised estimate of clearance is as follows:

Cl revised = F × dose/(interval × Css)
= 1 × 1 mg/(8 hr × 15 mg/L) = 0.008 L/hr

The revised estimate of $t_{1/2}$ is as follows:

$t_{1/2}$ revised = 0.7 × V/Cl revised
= 0.7 × 0.53 L/0.008 L/hr = 44.5 hr

Therefore the concentration 40 hours later should be approximately one half the measured 15 mg/L, or about 8 mg/L. To maintain this concentration of 8 mg/L:

Dose = (interval × Cl revised × Css)/F
     = 12 hr × 0.008 L/hr × 8 mg/L/1
     = 0.8 mg of theophylline PO every 12 hours

ASSIGNMENT 3: Before initiation of the oral regimen, another theophylline concentration is drawn 48 hours after the first and is reported to be 7.5 µg/ml. Since the patient has had no recurrence of apnea, an oral regimen that is based on the last two theophylline concentrations is begun to maintain a theophylline level of 7 µg/ml. Estimate the maintenance dose of theophylline.

ASSIGNMENT 3 ANSWER: The theophylline concentration fell 50%, from 15 to 7.5 mg/L in 48 hours, confirming our estimated half-life of approximately 45 hours.

This practical application section is not intended as a complete approach to the patient but merely as an example of the type of calculations useful in therapeutic drug monitoring. This exercise represents a small but important component of optimal care. The negligible serum caffeine concentration in the example is a simplification for the purpose of illustration of kinetic calculations. Therapeutic drug monitoring of theophylline therapy in infants may be complicated by measurable levels of the active metabolite, caffeine.

Methods of Administration

Oral Administration

When oral medications are being administered, the problem of how to get the medication into the infant arises. Oral administration of medication to newborns, especially premature infants, is complicated not only by variations in oral bioavailability but also by unanticipated loss of the drug. Loss of oral medication occurs when sick infants are unable to take or tolerate their feedings, have frequent and significant regurgitation, or require intermittent oral gastric suctioning and loss of residuals.

If the infant is receiving oral gastric or nasal gastric feedings, the medication is dropped into the center of the barrel of the syringe, which contains a small portion of the feeding. Medication that runs down the side of the barrel may adhere to the plastic and effectively decrease the amount of prescribed medicine delivered to the infant. The administration of the medication is documented on the chart, and any wet burps, emesis, or residual found is noted as to the color and the estimated or measured amount of the feeding lost. For infants receiving oral medications, the documentation of the color of the emesis or residual is important for determining if the color can be attributed to the medication or a pathophysiologic condition.

For infants receiving oral feedings by bottle, putting the medication into the full volume of feedings becomes problematic when the infant refuses to take the full amount of the feeding. The medication can be administered directly into the infant's mouth by gently introducing very small amounts of the medication into the cheek pouch and waiting for the infant to swallow. After this has been repeated several times, the infant will have taken the prescribed amount of medication. A second method is to put 5 to 10 ml of feeding into a Volufeed or bottle and let the infant take the entire amount before continuing with the remainder of the oral feeding. The medication can also be put into a nipple with some formula, and the infant allowed to consume this small volume early in the feeding. For infants who are breastfeeding, the medication can be administered into the mouth as described above, or it can be mixed with a small amount of the mother's breast milk and given to the infant. As with gavage feedings, the medication administration is documented, and the color and amount of any emesis is noted.

Intramuscular Injection

Unlike the adult who has sufficient muscle mass to receive intramuscular (IM) injections in numerous sites, the infant has relatively little muscle mass to receive injections. When IM injections are required, as with vitamin K, the anterior thigh is the site of choice. The area is cleaned with alcohol, and the medication is injected into the thigh using a 21- to 25-gauge needle. After injection, the area is massaged. For the infant weighing less than 1500 g, the volume of medication administered IM at one injection should not exceed 0.5 ml. The administration of the medication is documented, as is the site of the injection.

Intravenous Administration

IV medication is given to the infant in a newborn unit by a variety of methods, including push injection, antegrade injection, pump infusion, and retrograde injection.[7,12] Although drugs given IV do not have to cross a membrane barrier to enter the body, the time required to complete drug delivery is a function of dosage volume, IV flow rate, and injection site (with certain IV methods).[13,23] Failure to recognize potential time lags could easily result in inappropriate timing of expected physiologic responses or presumed peak-and-trough blood concentrations. The use of microbore IV tubing will partially facilitate the more rapid delivery of the drug, because the volume of the fluid contained in the tubing is greatly reduced. An example of one hospital's neonatal pediatric syringe infusion preparation and delivery chart for common neonatal drugs may be useful to the reader.[19]

Push Injection

The administration of IV push medications consists of preparing both the medication in an appropriate-size syringe and a flush solution (heparin with normal saline [NS], 10% dextrose in water [$D_{10}W$], 5% dextrose in water [D_5W], or sterile water). The IV tubing is inspected for a port that is close to the site of entry, the port is prepared, and the flush is used before and after the injection of the medication. The medication is given over 1 to 2 minutes, depending on the medication and the volume. If postinjection of flush is used, this should be given at the same rate as the medication; if not, then the medication may be delivered to the infant as a bolus, because it is pushed along by the flush. The use of flush after administering the medication will also remove any of the medication that may be left in the port of the IV tubing.

Certainly drugs can safely be given by rapid bolus infusion (IV push)—direct administration of medication into the venous circulation in less than 1 minute. *Slow IV push* is a term common to all nurses, but because interpretation varies widely, a specific rate of injection is preferable. Many drugs should not be administered by IV push because of the propensity to produce immediate adverse reactions when administered by rapid bolus injection to low-birth-weight infants.

Antegrade Injection

Antegrade injection of medication involves introduction of the medication into an entry port of the IV tubing. The medication is then carried in the tubing with the IV fluid at the same rate of infusion as the fluid. Because infusion rates in newborns are very low, marked delays in drug delivery may result. This method is not recommended for drug delivery to very-low-birth-weight infants.

Pump Infusion

To avoid delayed drug delivery times, an IV system employing a mechanical syringe infusion device allows control over the rate of drug delivery to the patient. The major drawback to these small pumps is their cost. The use of pumps for medication delivery has enhanced the consistency of the rate of delivery of the medication to the infant. The pumps vary by manufacturer and the principle by which they deliver fluids to the infant. Generally, pump infusion systems consist of a pump that can be regulated to deliver a specific volume over a specific time, a syringe or container of medication to be delivered, and connecting tubing and needles to connect the pump to the entry port for drug delivery.

There are two methods of using pumps to deliver medication to ensure that the infant receives the exact amount of medication ordered. Each newborn unit should have a unit policy to ensure that pump administration is carried out in the same manner by each staff member.

Method 1. The exact amount of medication is drawn into the syringe and diluted, if necessary, to bring the volume to that needed for the operation of the pump. This is then flushed through the connecting tubing and needle, and the syringe is placed in the pump. After the pump has finished the infusion, some of the medication remains in the connecting tubing and hub of the syringe. This medication needs to be flushed into the IV with a flush solution for the infant to receive the entire amount ordered.

Method 2. The medication is drawn into the syringe through the connecting tubing and needle until the medication volume desired is in the syringe. This is then put on the pump and infused. With this method the connecting tubing and needle is not flushed with a flush solution, because the infant has already received the entire dose ordered. If the medication is flushed through, then the infant receives more than the amount ordered. If the same care provider who starts the administration of the medication will be there to end it, there should not be a problem. But if a different care provider will end it, then the method used needs to be communicated. Setting a unit policy for one method over another would help alleviate any potential medication errors caused by lack of communication.

Retrograde Injection

Retrograde injection is the injection of medication in the opposite direction of the IV fluid flow. This system requires the injection of the medication into the IV tubing, resulting in displacement of a portion of the IV fluid in the tubing. The excess fluid is displaced into an upstream syringe. An alternate method is to use specifically developed retrograde tubing for administration of the medication or retrograde sets that contain a collection bag for the displaced fluid.

Retrograde injection as currently available is not recommended for premature infants. Reported disadvantages are that the amount of fluid injected is limited by the size of the tubing, syringe, or collection bag. There is increased risk of microbial contamination. There is also a total loss of calories, because the displaced fluid is replaced by the medication, which is calorie poor. Because there is no "catch up" on the fluids, the total caloric intake from IV fluids is reduced. In this system the drug delivery rate still depends on the IV infusion rate.

Other Considerations

The health-care provider must be attuned to additional considerations when administering IV medications. The use of filters, protection of certain medications from light sources (especially phototherapy lights), the preservatives used in some medications, and the specific gravity of the medication should be considered before administration of any medication.

A 0.22 μm filter may provide "cold sterilization" (i.e., remove particulate matter and bacterial contamination). There are some medications that cannot be administered using a filter, because the filter removes the active ingredient.

Medications with a lower specific gravity than the IV fluid have a tendency to accumulate at high points in the IV tubing, whereas those medications with higher specific gravity will settle into the low loops of the IV tubing. This can result in delay in the delivery of the medication to the infant.

Inserting Peripheral IV Lines. Peripheral IV access is often required for medication administration. Needles and catheters used in the neonate are necessarily small (22- to 27-gauge). The most commonly used are the "butterfly" needle and needles with catheter sheaths. Common IV placement sites include the hands, feet, legs, arms, or scalp veins. Extremity vessels that are difficult to visualize may be outlined by diffusing light through the extremity from a transilluminator placed under the extremity. CAUTION: Avoid burning the delicate skin of the premature infant by minimizing or avoiding direct contact of the transilluminator with the skin.

Equipment. The following equipment is required:

- Catheters, needles in sizes appropriate for the diameter of the vein
- Tape—clear or opaque
- Alcohol
- Gauze
- Syringe with 2 ml of flush solution
- Razor (if using head veins)
- Tourniquet (rubber band)
- Arm board or legboard
- Infant restraints
- Gloves

Procedure. Assemble equipment at the bedside or at a radiant warmer. Provide an adequate heat source throughout this procedure. Tear tape into two short pieces (1/2 inch by 2 inches) and three longer pieces (1/2 inch by 6 inches). Select a site for placement of an IV line by determining that the vessel is *not* arterial by palpating for a pulse. Determine the direction of blood flow—in the scalp arteries fill from below, veins from above; in the extremities veins fill distal to central.

Restrain the infant. If using vessels in the extremities, restrain the arm or leg on an armboard. Some care providers prefer to place the armboard after the vessel has been cannulated and the needle/catheter secured in position. If using scalp veins, shave the area and blot with a piece of tape to pick up the hair. Give the hair to the mother for the baby book.

Flush the needle/catheter and remove the syringe. Place the tourniquet around the extremity (optional: many IV lines are placed without a tourniquet). Prepare the site by cleaning with alcohol; allow to dry. After gloving, insert the needle/catheter into the vessel using the hand and fingers to anchor the skin surrounding the vessel. Insert into the vessel at an acute angle and in the direction of blood flow. Observe for blood return or flashback into the tubing or cannula of the catheter. Some vessels will not have a blood return. If there is not return and you feel the needle is in the vessel, a small amount of flush may be injected. If the needle is not in the vessel, a swelling of the tissue at the end of the needle will be obvious. If, with flushing, there is blanching of the skin distal to the insertion site, the vessel is most likely arterial (most common in scalp vein insertion). When there is a blood return, flush is injected to clear the needle and prevent clotting. If using a catheter, remove the needle while gently advancing the catheter.

Secure the IV line by placing a short piece of tape across the needle/catheter. Then cross a longer piece of tape over the needle/catheter, around the back of the catheter, and across the front. Check to see that the IV line is still positioned by disconnecting it from the syringe and watching for a blood return or by infusing a small amount of flush. If necessary, use gauze or a piece of cotton behind the needle for support. Secure this in place by using another long piece of tape. Cover the IV site with half a medicine cup or the clear needle package to protect the site. Infants who are inactive may not need an IV site protective cover. Restrain the extremity if this has not already been done.

If the medication is to be administered intermittently and the line is not needed for fluids and calories, it may be heparin locked and flushed every shift with a heparinized solution (0.2 units of heparin per 1 ml of solution).

Teaching Model. The use of a placenta as a teaching model for insertion of umbilical lines is discussed in Chapter 8. The fetal side of a placenta may also be used for teaching IV insertion of various needles and catheters.

Equipment and Supplies. The following equipment and supplies are required:

- Placenta
- Assorted sizes of needles and catheters
- Syringes filled with normal saline or flush solution
- Gloves
- Tape

Procedure. The placenta is placed on drapes with the fetal side up. The fetal membranes are removed, exposing the rich network of vessels. After gloving, insert both butterfly needles and catheters in the larger vessels first and then smaller vessels as the technique is perfected. Any skewering of the vessel is immediately apparent, because blood leaks out through the vessel wall. Tortuous vessels or those with branching patterns are used for various methods of cannulation. Once the catheters are in position, securing the needles/catheters by taping techniques is practiced. Two people may work on one placenta at a time.

Complications

Complications of IV therapy[18] include phlebitis, infiltration, hematomas, chemical burns, and emboli. Long-term complications of extravasation include disfigurement, contractions, and possible need for surgical repair. Frequent (hourly) assessment of the IV site helps prevent complications. Swelling and discoloration of the extremity or of the skin at the needle tip are signs to remove the needle/catheter. In the scalp, infiltration may be difficult to assess, because swelling is not only at the IV site, but also on the dependent side of the head. Scalp edema (on the dependent side) or a swollen eye are indicators of scalp vein infiltration. In the extremities, a swollen arm or leg, hand or foot, or fingers or toes indicates an infiltrated IV line.

Footdrop[10] has been associated with positioning a footboard along the lateral aspect of the fibula (caused by pressure on the peroneal division of the sciatic nerve). Use of rolled washcloths as footboards or extensive padding of IV boards with cotton, gauze, or washcloths may prevent excessive pressure.

Unnoticed infiltrations may result in skin burns

or sloughing and compromised circulation. Warm or hot soaks in an infiltrated site are contraindicated. When warm soaks are used, extravasated fluid is warmed to a temperature that results in burns, maceration, and necrosis. In addition, heat increases the oxygen demand in already compromised tissues.

Elevating the infiltrated area increases venous return and helps decrease edema. Hyaluronidase[9] destroys tissue cement and prevents or minimizes tissue damage by allowing rapid diffusion and absorption of the extravasated fluid. For best results, treat the area within 1 hour of injury. Inject hyaluronidase (15 units/ml) subcutaneously around the periphery of the extravasated area. The effectiveness of hyaluronidase has not been proved. It may not be effective if diagnoses and administration are delayed.

THEOPHYLLINE

Your baby is on a medication called *theophylline*. Other names for this drug include Slo-Phyllin, Theodyl, Theolair, and Aerolate. Theophylline is a very powerful drug that helps your baby breathe by relaxing the small air passages in the lungs.

It is very important that this medication be given on a strict schedule so that the right amount of the drug is in the baby's blood at all times. It is also important to give the right amount of medicine and to give it at the right time. Please be sure to keep all follow-up appointments so that the doctor can adjust the dose of theophylline to meet your baby's needs.

Theophylline can be upsetting to the baby's stomach. To prevent this, please be sure to give the medication with a feeding (formula or breast milk).

THE DOSE OF YOUR BABY'S THEOPHYLLINE IS: _____

THE TIMES TO GIVE THE MEDICATION ARE: _____

Be sure to give the amount of medication ordered by your doctor. Do not change the dose unless the doctor asks you to. Do not give this medication to any other person! Follow your doctor's orders carefully and follow these guidelines when giving this medication.

1. If your baby swallows some of the medicine but not all of it, do not repeat the dose.
2. If your baby vomits after the medication, do not repeat the dose.
3. If you forget to give a dose and it is less than 2 hours late, give the dose and keep the baby on the regular schedule. If the dose is more than 2 hours late when you remember it, give the dose and evenly space the doses over the next 24 hours. Then go back to the regular schedule.
4. If your baby is ill with a cold, flu, or fever; has loss of appetite, diarrhea, vomiting, wheezing, or trouble breathing; or is unusually irritable, CALL THE DOCTOR.
5. Be sure that any doctor seeing your baby knows all of the medicines your baby takes. Do not give other medicines to your baby unless a doctor tells you to.
6. Theophylline should be stored in a safe place. A locked cabinet out of reach of children is best.

IF SOMEONE ACCIDENTALLY TAKES THIS OR ANY OTHER MEDICATION OR POISON, CALL THE POISON CONTROL CENTER IMMEDIATELY!

Figure 9-5 Parent information sheet. (Courtesy University of Colorado Health Sciences Center, Denver, 1987.)

Parent Teaching

The presence of IV lines in newborns is frightening to parents, especially if the IV is in the infant's head. Without information, parents mistakenly believe the fluid is "going into the baby's brain." Reassuring the parents that the fluid is going into large veins in the head (and not into the brain) is important.

Even though their infant has an IV, parents are still encouraged to touch, hold, and feed their infant.

In answer to the question, "Does it hurt?" parents must be told the truth. "Yes, it hurts to have an IV placed, but once it is in, it doesn't hurt anymore." Parents are usually very cautious when handling their baby and do not want the infant "to get stuck again." The importance of frequent checks in noticing and discontinuing an infiltration should be explained, because some parents mistakenly believe this causes the infiltration. Venous fragility in the newborn, combined with relatively hypertonic solutions, make frequent restarting of IV lines commonplace, and these causes of infiltration should be explained to the parents.

A diagnosis of "rule out sepsis" is often very confusing to families who do not understand why antibiotics are started before the culture results are known. Explain to the parents that antibiotics can be stopped at 48 to 72 hours if cultures and latex agglutination are negative (in most cases), but that if cultures are positive, delaying the start of antibiotics markedly increases the morbidity and mortality.

Discharge teaching about medications that parents must administer is very important. Parents must know the name of the drug, dosage, frequency of administration, side effects, and any special instructions. Parents must be taught to administer medicines, must demonstrate their ability to do the same, and must receive written instructions (Fig. 9-5).

References

1. Aranda JV, Sitar DS, Parsons WP: Pharmacokinetics, aspects of theophylline in preterm infants, *N Engl J Med* 925:413, 1976.
2. Aranda JV, Turman T: Methylxanthines in apnea of prematurity, *Clin Perinatol* 6:87, 1979.
3. Berman W et al: Inadvertent overadministration of digoxin to low birth weight infants, *J Pediatr* 92:1024, 1978.
4. Berman W et al: Digoxin therapy in low birth weight infants with patent ductus arteriosus, *J Pediatr* 93:652, 1978.
5. Bleyer WA, Koup JR: Medication errors during intensive care, *Am J Dis Child* 133:366, 1979.
6. Boerth RC: Decreased sensitivity of the newborn myocardium to positive inotropic effects of ouabain. In Marselli PL, Garattine S, Sereni F, editors: *Basic and therapeutic aspects of perinatal pharmacology,* New York, 1975, Raven Press.
7. Burch SM, Chadwick JV: Use of a retroset in the delivery of intravenous medications in the neonate, *Neonat Net* 6:51, 1987.
8. Evans ME, Bhat R, Vidyasagar D: Factors modulating drug therapy and pharmokinetics. In Yeh TF: *Drug therapy in the neonate and small infant,* Chicago, 1985, Year Book Medical Publishers.
9. Few BJ: Hyaluronidase for treating intravenous extravasations, *MCN* 12:23, 1987.
10. Fischer AQ, Strasburger J: Footdrop in the neonate secondary to the use of footboards, *J Pediatr* 101:1003, 1982.
11. Giacoai GP, Yaffe SJ: Drugs and the perinatal patient. In Avery G, editor: *Neonatology, pathophysiology and management of the newborn,* Philadelphia, 1981, JB Lippincott.
12. Glass SM, Giacoia GP: Intravenous drug therapy in premature infants: practical aspects, *J Obstet Gynecol Neonat Nurs* 16:310, 1987.
13. Gould T, Roberts R: Therapeutic problems arising from the use of the intravenous route for drug administration, *J Pediatr* 95:465, 1979.
14. Hilligoss D: Neonatal pharmacokinetics. In Evans W, editor: *Applied pharmokinetics,* San Francisco, 1986, Applied Therapeutics.
15. Holford NHG: Clinical interpretation of drug concentrations. In Katzung BG, editor: *Basic and clinical pharmacology,* East Norwalk, Conn, 1987, Appleton & Lange.
16. Holford NHG, Sheiner LB: Understanding the dose effect relationship, *Clin Pharmacokinet* 6:429, 1981.
17. Kaufman RE: The clinical interpretation and application of drug concentration data, *Pediatr Clin North Am* 28:35, 1981.
18. MacCara ME: Extravasation: a hazard of intravenous therapy, *Drug Intell Clin Pharm* 17:71, 1983.
19. McCurdy DE, Arnold MT: Development and implementation of a pediatric/neonatal IV syringe pump delivery system, *J Neonatal Nurs* 16:9, 1995.
20. O'Donnel J: Theophylline misadventures. I, *J Neonatal Nurs* 13:35, 1994.
21. Ohning BL: Neonatal pharmacodynamics-basic principles II: drug action and elimination, *J Neonatal Nurs* 14:15, 1995.
22. Perlstein PH et al: Errors in drug computation during newborn intensive care, *Am J Dis Child* 133:376, 1979.
23. Roberts RJ: Intravenous administration of medication in pediatric patients: problems and solutions, *Pediatr Clin North Am* 28:23, 1981.
24. Roberts RJ: *Drug therapy in infants,* Philadelphia, 1984, WB Saunders.

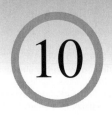

10 Acid-Base Homeostasis and Oxygenation

William H. Parry, Jan Zimmer

Examination of arterial blood gases and interpretation of acid-base balance are critical to the proper diagnosis, management, and outcome in the neonate. The measurement of arterial blood gases allows analysis of two interrelated but separate processes: acid-base homeostasis and oxygenation. This chapter describes the parameters that reflect oxygenation and acid-base balance, their measurements, and the effects of proposed treatment to maintain homeostasis. Common abbreviations and their meanings are listed in the Box 10-1.

Measurement of arterial blood gases involves (1) actual values (Pao_2, $Paco_2$ and pH) and (2) calculations from these values (oxygen saturation, base excess, and bicarbonate concentration). Some analyzer systems also estimate hemoglobin concentration. To assess acid-base homeostasis, one examines the pH, Pco_2, base excess, and bicarbonate components. The parameters used to assess the adequacy of oxygenation are Pao_2 saturation (Sao_2) and hemoglobin (Table 10-1).

Physiology

Acid-Base Homeostasis

An acid is a hydrogen ion donor, and a base is a hydrogen ion receptor. The pH (puissance hydrogen), which refers to the concentration of the hydrogen ion [H^+] in the blood, specifies the acid-base balance in the blood. The quantity of hydrogen ions is minute, amounting to approximately 0.0000001 moles/L. In logarithmic units this is 1×10^{-7} moles/L. The pH is the negative log

The opinions and assertions in this chapter are those of the authors and do not necessarily represent those of the Department of the Army or the Department of Defense.

of the hydrogen ion concentration (pH = 7) (equation 1). A pH of 7 represents a neutral solution, a pH of less than 7 represents increasing acidity, and a pH greater than 7 shows increasing alkalinity:

(1)

$$pH = -\log[H^+]$$
$$pH = -\log[0.0000001]$$
$$pH = -[-7]$$
$$pH = 7$$

The Henderson-Hasselbalch equation describes the pH as a constant (pK) plus the logarithm of the ratio of the base-to-acid concentration (equation 2). Thus if there is too much acid (an increase in the hydrogen ion reflected in the denominator), the blood pH value decreases. This condition is an acidemia. Conversely, if there is less acid or more base, the pH value increases. This is an alkalemia.

(2)

$$pH = pK + \log \frac{base}{acid}$$

The pK is the pH at which a substance is half dissociated (cations and anions) and half undissociated (conjugate pair). The pK of whole blood is 6.1, and therefore the pH of blood is:

(3)

$$pH = 6.1 + \log \frac{base}{acid}$$

Considering acid-base homeostasis is the first step in determining its status (pH). The suffix -*osis* denotes physiologic and pathophysiologic processes that tend to change the pH. Thus a process that tends to lower the pH is an acidosis, and the

Box 10-1

Abbreviations

pH	Negative log of hydrogen ion concentration
P	Partial pressure (tension, driving force)
a	Arterial
A	Alveolar
v	Venous
c	Capillary
C	Content
D	Difference
V	Volume
V̇	Volume per unit time
V_D	Volume of the dead space
V_T	Tidal volume
Q	Perfusion (flow)
Q̇	Flow per unit time
E	Expiration, expired
I	Inhalation, inspired
F	Fraction
ET	End tidal
tc	Transcutaneous

Combined abbreviations

Pa_{O_2}	Partial pressure of arterial oxygen
FI_{O_2}	Fraction of inspired oxygen
PET_{CO_2}	Partial pressure of carbon dioxide at the end of a tidal volume breath

Table 10-1
Normal (Arterial) Blood Gas Values

Blood Gases	Values
pH	7.35-7.45
Pa_{CO_2}	35-45 mm Hg
HCO_3^-	22-26 mEq/L
Base excess	(−4)-(+4)
Pa_{O_2}	60-80 mm Hg
O_2 saturation	92%-94%

process that tends to raise the pH is an alkalosis. The normal human pH is between 7.35 and 7.45; therefore a pH of less than 7.35 is acidemia, and the process that caused it is an acidosis.

Acid-base homeostasis refers to the physiologic mechanisms that maintain the pH in normal range. Pathophysiologic mechanisms result in pH changes that lead to acidemia or alkalemia. A "tendency" to change the pH, not the actual resultant change, connotes a pathophysiologic mechanism.

Arterial carbon dioxide and bicarbonate values in the blood gas analysis evaluate the processes of acidosis and alkalosis that affect the acid status of the body. These parameters assess separate components of the acid-base homeostasis: (1) respiratory contribution (Pa_{CO_2}) controlled by alveolar ventilation and (2) nonrespiratory or metabolic contribution (HCO_3^-) controlled primarily by renal excretion, retention, or manufacture of HCO_3^-.

Respiratory Contribution

Carbon dioxide, produced by each cell as a waste product of metabolism, is a gas and follows the laws of gas transport. As carbon dioxide is produced, it dissolves in the intracellular fluid and can be measured as the partial pressure (P) of the dissolved gas (CO_2). As the pressure of the dissolved gas increases in the cell, a pressure gradient develops between this pressure and the extracellular fluid. Accordingly, the dissolved carbon dioxide gas moves out of the cell and into the bloodstream (i.e., from the area of greater pressure to the area of lesser pressure). Blood transports the dissolved carbon dioxide gas to the lung, where the partial pressure in the pulmonary capillary is greater than that in the alveolus. The alveolus receives carbon dioxide according to the direction of the pressure gradient. Ventilation is the only method of excreting carbon dioxide. The amount of carbon dioxide in the blood is a consequence of the body's metabolism (production) and the alveolar ventilation (excretion). Because metabolism does not change greatly, the measurement of Pa_{CO_2} accurately reflects the alveolar ventilation.

Dissolved carbon dioxide is an acidic substance. A minute amount of dissolved carbon dioxide gas combines with water to form carbonic acid, which divides into a hydrogen ion and a bicarbonate ion:

(4)
$$H_2O + CO_2 \rightleftarrows H_2CO_1 \rightleftarrows H^+ + HCO_3^-$$

The ratio of the dissolved carbonic acid to the dissociated hydrogen cation and bicarbonate anion is 1000:1.

Elevated Paco2, resulting in too much "acid" in the blood, causes the pH to fall ($\uparrow$ Pco2, $\downarrow$ pH). Hypoventilation causes an increase in carbon dioxide. This process is an acidosis because the acid in the body increases. Because only the lung regulates the amount of carbon dioxide in the body, the process is a respiratory acidosis.

Depressed Paco2, resulting in less acid in the blood, causes the pH to rise ($\downarrow$ Pco2, $\uparrow$ pH). A pathophysiologic process that causes hyperventilation reduces the dissolved carbon dioxide. The result is a decreased amount of acid with a subsequent increase in the pH value. This process is an alkalosis. Because the parameter that is changing is controlled only by the lung, the process is a respiratory alkalosis.

Nonrespiratory (Metabolic) Contribution

Nonrespiratory (metabolic) factors involved in acid-base homeostasis are regulated mainly by generating fixed acid in the kidney but are also influenced by pathologic conditions of the gastrointestinal system and other organ systems. The bicarbonate ion is a base, that is, a hydrogen ion receptor. The calculated bicarbonate ion concentration, or its corollary, the "base excess," evaluates the nonrespiratory contribution to acid-base homeostasis.

The base excess primarily represents the actual excess or deficit of bicarbonate, but it also incorporates the buffering action of red blood cells. Multiplying the calculated bicarbonate by 1.2 and subtracting the normal bicarbonate value (24 mEq) from the product estimates the base excess. A positive value suggests a deficit of fixed acid or an excess of base; a negative value indicates an excess of fixed acid or a deficit of base.

Thus when there is a base excess or the bicarbonate ion increases above normal (normal = 21 to 24 mEq/L), too much base is in the blood, and the pH increases. Any process that raises the pH is an alkalosis. Because the bicarbonate ion or base excess is involved (and not carbon dioxide, the respiratory parameter), the process will be a nonrespiratory (metabolic) alkalosis. Conversely, when the bicarbonate ion is below normal, a base deficit or negative base excess is present, and because there is less base (or more acid) than normal, the pH decreases, reflecting an acidosis. Because bicarbonate is a nonrespiratory parameter, this represents a nonrespiratory (metabolic) acidosis.

In the Henderson-Hasselbalch equation discussed previously, the pH was equal to a constant, pK, plus the log of the base/acid ratio. We can substitute the bicarbonate ion concentration for the base, and substitute the dissolved carbon dioxide concentration for the acid.

The Henderson-Hasselbalch equation:

$$pH = pK + \log \frac{base}{acid}$$

Substituting:

(5)

$$pH = pK + \log \frac{[HCO_3^-]}{[Paco_2]}$$

The normal bicarbonate concentration is 24 mEq/L. Paco2 is 40 mm Hg. However, HCO_3^- units are in milliequivalents per liter and Paco2 is measured in millimeters of mercury.

Substituting:

(6)

$$pH = pK + \log \frac{24 \text{ mEq/L}}{40 \text{ mm Hg}}$$

Multiplying Paco2 by its solubility coefficient (0.03 mEq/L) can convert Paco2 to milliequivalents per liter:

(7)

$$pH = pK + \log \frac{24 \text{ mEq/L}}{40 \text{ mm Hg} \times 0.03}$$

Converting to common units: 40 mm Hg $\times$ 0.03 mEq/L = 1.2mEq/L.

Solving:

(8)

$$pH = pK + \log \frac{24 \text{ mEq/L} = 20}{1.2 \text{ mEq/L} = 1}$$

The ratio of base (bicarbonate) to acid (carbon dioxide) is 20:1. The pK of blood is 6.1. The log of 20 is 1.3. Therefore:

$$pH = 6.1 + 1.3 = 7.4$$

Changes in the 20:1 ratio accordingly have profound effects on the pH. For example, should some process occur causing hypoventilation (respiratory acidosis) of sufficient degree that the Pa_{CO_2} is doubled from 40 to 80, the mEq/L of carbon dioxide gas would be 2.4, and the ratio of bicarbonate to carbon dioxide gas becomes 24:2.4, or 10. The logarithm of 10 is 1, and the pH would be 6.1 + 1, or 7.1. Conversely, if a respiratory alkalosis, which results from hyperventilation, occurred, lowering the P_{CO_2} to 20 mm Hg, the resulting ratio would be (24 mEq/L):(0.6 mEq/L) or 40:1. The log of 40 is 1.6, and the subsequent pH would be 7.70. Similarly, if a metabolic acidosis reduced the bicarbonate ion from 24 mEq/L to 12 mEq/L, the ratio would be 12:1.2 or 10:1, and the pH value would be 7.1. If a metabolic alkalosis acutely raised the bicarbonate ion concentration from 24 mEq/L to 36 mEq/L, the ratio of bicarbonate to carbon dioxide gas would be 30:1, and the subsequent pH would be log 30 = 1.47 + 6.1 = pH 7.57.

Thus far, these derangements (Fig. 10-1) have been discussed as if they happened in isolation, but combined respiratory and nonrespiratory problems often occur, depending on pathologic processes in the body. Thus besides the four single acid-base derangements, there are combined acid-base derangements: (1) respiratory acidosis and metabolic acidosis, (2) respiratory acidosis and metabolic alkalosis, (3) respiratory alkalosis and metabolic acidosis, and (4) respiratory alkalosis and metabolic alkalosis. The combined acidoses or combined alkaloses have a cumulative effect on the pH, whereas an acidosis and alkalosis combination tends to negate the effects of each on the pH value.

Compensation

Acid-base homeostasis maintains the pH value near the normal range. Thus if either the respiratory or nonrespiratory acid-base system is "deranged," the other system will become "deranged" in the opposite direction in an attempt to balance the primary process. Compensation occurs when the body attempts to balance one pathophysiologic process with a second pathophysiologic process that opposes the pH effect of the primary process.

For example, any respiratory process that leads to retention of carbon dioxide (respiratory acido-

	Respiratory parameter pCO_2	Metabolic parameter HCO_3^-	Cause
Respiratory acidosis	⬆	↑	Hypoventilation
Respiratory alkalosis	⬇	↓	Hyperventilation
Metabolic acidosis	↓	⬇	Add acid or lose base
Metabolic alkalosis	↑	⬆	Add base or lose acid

Figure 10-1   Acid-base derangements. *Large arrow* indicates primary process that produces change in pH. *Small arrow* indicates compensatory process.

sis) activates a nonrespiratory system (i.e, the kidney retains bicarbonate) to return the pH to normal range. The nonrespiratory compensation is actually a second pathophysiologic process, and the retention of bicarbonate (metabolic alkalosis) counteracts the primary defect (respiratory acidosis). Thus a neonate with an increased $Paco_2$ and a compensating elevated bicarbonate is both acidotic and alkalotic but has a pH near the normal range.

Metabolic compensations to respiratory processes can go to remarkable extremes, but respiratory compensations to metabolic processes are limited. For example, hyperventilation cannot lower the $Paco_2$ much below 8 to 10 mm Hg. Similarly, hypoventilation (in the presence of an intact CNS) in compensation for a metabolic alkalosis is severely limited by the onset of hypoxemia. Hypoxemia, of course, stimulates the respiratory drive, overriding the compensatory hypoventilation, resulting in the alkalemia continuing unabated.

Correction

Correction of an acid-base disturbance occurs when the health-care provider detects the pathophysiologic process and directs therapy at the primary pathologic process, rather than counterbalancing it with a second pathologic process.

For example, if a respiratory acidosis is present, the clinician assesses the patient to discover the cause of the carbon dioxide retention and directs therapy at improving the ventilatory capacity of the lung, rather than attempting to increase the retention of bicarbonate.

Oxygenation

The remaining components of the blood gas analysis are the Po_2, hemoglobin, and oxygen saturation. Oxygenation is distinct from, although related to, ventilation. As previously stated, the $Paco_2$ correlates inversely to ventilation, whereas other factors besides ventilation influence oxygenation. What is important is the degree of oxygenation at the tissue level.

Many factors cause tissue hypoxia, including the inability of the lung to oxygenate the blood (arterial hypoxemia). Another cause of tissue hypoxia is interference with oxygen delivery to the tissue, such as that seen in congestive heart failure

(venous hypoxemia). In this situation the Pao_2 may be normal, but because of heart (pump) failure, oxygen is not delivered to the tissue. Treatment should be directed toward improving delivery by the pump (Chapter 23).

A third cause of tissue hypoxia may result from a decrease in oxygen content (which occurs with anemia). In this instance the heart and lungs work adequately, so the Pao_2 is normal, but there is insufficient hemoglobin to provide an adequate amount of oxygen to the tissues.

Finally, tissue hypoxia may result from an abnormal affinity of oxygen to the hemoglobin molecule. In this situation, the heart and lungs are performing properly, but the red blood cell releases inadequate oxygen amounts at the tissue level because of the abnormal affinity. Fetal hemoglobin has a greater affinity for oxygen than adult hemoglobin and thus requires a lower tissue Po_2 to release comparable amounts of oxygen molecules from the hemoglobin (see Fig. 7-1).

Because Pao_2 measures only partial pressure of oxygen in the arterial blood (i.e., measures the amount of dissolved oxygen gas in the blood), it reflects how the lung is working but does not measure tissue oxygenation. Despite oxygenation complexities at the tissue level, the Pao_2 taken with the clinical assessment of tissue perfusion is probably an adequate and accurate reflection of tissue oxygenation. In a few instances hemoglobin determination may be needed for assessing the etiology of tissue hypoxia.

Because respiratory disease is an important aspect of neonatal care, the Pao_2 or the Sao_2 is frequently measured. Most tissue oxygenation problems are directly related to a respiratory problem rather than to oxygen delivery, oxygen content, or hemoglobin affinity problems. A high Pao_2 can be as dangerous as a low Pao_2. Retinopathy of prematurity has been related to arterial oxygen tensions greater than 100 mm Hg and is directly related to Pao_2 but not to the Fio_2 (see Chapter 22).

Cyanotic congenital heart disease has a fixed shunt that does not allow the Pao_2 to rise when supplemental oxygen is given; thus a low Pao_2 is not related to lung disease. In respiratory distress, hypoxemia because of intrapulmonary shunting or ventilation and perfusion inequality can be overcome by increasing the inspired oxygen tension.

Theoretically, in the normal lung with matched ventilation and perfusion, the alveolar (PA_{O_2}) and the arterial oxygen tension (Pa_{O_2}) should be equal. The body never obtains this ideal situation, and a difference (gradient) in gas tension exists between the alveolar oxygen tension (Pa_{O_2}) and the arterial oxygen tension (Pa_{O_2}). An inequality in ventilation and perfusion creates the gradient, the functional intrapulmonary shunt and the anatomic shunt. The alveolar-arterial oxygen gradient $D(A-a)_{O_2}$ is useful in estimating the degree of pulmonary involvement in hypoxemia. The difference between the value of the alveolar oxygen and arterial oxygen tensions should be less than 20. The $D(A-a)_{O_2}$ will be greater than 20 in pulmonary disease.

To calculate the alveolar-arterial oxygen difference:

(9)

$$D(A-a)_{O_2} = Pa_{O_2} - Pa_{O_2}$$

Substitute the calculation of alveolar oxygen tension:

(10)

$$D(A-a)_{O_2} = \left(Fi_{O_2} - \frac{Pa_{CO_2}}{RQ} \right) - Pa_{O_2}$$

Substitute the calculation of inspired oxygen tension:

(11)

$$D(A-a)_{O_2} = \left[(P_B - 47)\, Fi_{O_2} - \frac{Pa_{CO_2}}{RQ} \right] - Pa_{O_2}$$

Blood gas analysis measures the arterial P_{O_2}. The alveolar (PA_{O_2}) is calculated as follows. First determine the inspiratory P_{O_2}, which is the barometric pressure minus the water vapor pressure multiplied by the fraction of the inspired oxygen.

To calculate the inspired oxygen tension:

(12)

$$Pi_{O_2} = (P_B - P_{H_2O})Fi_{O_2}$$

BUT

$$P_{H_2O} = 47$$

THUS

$$Pi_{O_2} = (P_B - 47)Fi_{O_2}$$

Thus the inspired oxygen pressure when one is breathing room air at sea level is $(760 - 47)(0.21) = 150$ mm Hg.

The alveolar oxygen is equal to the inspired oxygen minus the alveolar carbon dioxide divided by the respiratory quotient (RQ). Clinically, the alveolar carbon dioxide is equal to the arterial carbon dioxide, and RQ is 0.8.

To calculate the alveolar oxygen tension:

(13)

$$Pa_{O_2} = PI_{O_2} - \frac{Pa_{CO_2}}{RQ}$$

BUT

$$Pa_{CO_2} = Pa_{CO_2}$$

AND

$$RQ = 0.8$$

THUS

$$Pa_{O_2} = Pi_{O_2} - \frac{Pa_{CO_2}}{0.8}$$

Therefore when one is breathing room air at sea level with a Pa_{CO_2} of 40 mm Hg, the alveolar oxygen pressure is equal to the Pi_{O_2} (150 mm Hg) minus 40 divided by 0.8 (which is 50), or 100 mm Hg. The alveolar-arterial oxygen gradient in an infant with a Pa_{O_2} of 160 mm Hg and a Pa_{CO_2} of 40 mm Hg in an atmosphere of 40% oxygen at sea level is 75 mm Hg.

(14)

$$D(A-a)_{O_2} = \left[(760 - 47)\,0.4 - \frac{40}{0.8} \right] - 160 = 75$$

The alveolar-arterial oxygen gradient is useful in predicting the FI_{O_2} required to result in a desired Pa_{O_2}. Working from a known $D(A-a)_{O_2}$ and rearranging the equation 11:

(15)

$$Fi_{O_2} = \frac{D(A-a)_{O_2} + \dfrac{Pa_{CO_2}}{RQ} + Pa_{O_2}}{(P_B - 47)}$$

For example, to obtain a Pa_{O_2} of 90 mm Hg in an infant with an alveolar-arterial gradient of

75 mm Hg and a Pa_{CO_2} of 40 mm Hg at sea level the infant requires an atmosphere of 30% oxygen ($Fi_{O_2} = 0.3$).

(16)

$$Fi_{O_2} = \frac{75 + \dfrac{40}{0.8} + 90}{(760 - 47)} = 0.3$$

Knowledge of the $D(A\text{-}a)_{O_2}$ can help the clinician adjust the arterial oxygen concentration by working the equation backward (equation 15). Thus the alveolar-arterial gradient we can set an Fi_{O_2} on the ventilator that will predict a desired Pa_{O_2}.

Equation 15 can be simplified. The rule of seven states that the estimated percentage change in inspired oxygen is equal to the desired change in Pa_{O_2} divided by 7.

(17)

$$\%O_2 \text{ change} = \frac{\text{New } Pa_{O_2} - \text{Old } Pa_{O_2}}{7}$$

For example, to obtain a Pa_{O_2} of 90 mm Hg in an infant with a Pa_{O_2} of 160 mm Hg, a reduction of 10% inspired oxygen is required.

(18)

$$\%O_2 \text{ change} = \frac{90 - 160}{7} = \frac{-70}{7} = -10\%$$

Saturation

Saturation is the percentage of hemoglobin that is combined with oxygen. Oxygen binding with hemoglobin increases as the partial pressure of oxygen increases, but not linearly. The oxygen dissociation curve is a measure of the affinity that hemoglobin has for oxygen (Fig. 10-2).

The "30-60-90" rule is useful in remembering percent saturation and reconstructing the hemoglobin dissociation curve if required (see Fig. 10-2). At Pa_{O_2} of 30 mm Hg, the oxygen saturation is 60%; at a Pa_{O_2} of 60 mm Hg, saturation is 90%; and at 90 mm Hg Pa_{O_2} the hemoglobin is 95% saturated. At the normal venous oxygen tension of 40 mm Hg, the oxygen saturation is 75%.

Factors that affect this affinity include temperature, pH, and hemoglobin structure. Hypothermia,

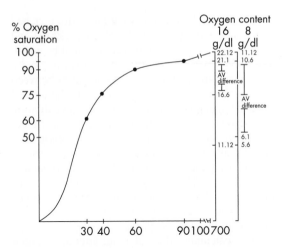

Figure 10-2 Oxygen hemoglobin dissociation curve; 30-60-90 rule is demonstrated. *Right,* oxygen content for hemoglobin concentration of 16 g/dl and 8 g/dl is given, demonstrating effect of anemia on venous saturation and tissue.

alkalemia, hypocapnia, and fetal hemoglobin increase the affinity of hemoglobin for oxygen (shift the curve to the left), whereas fever, acidemia, and hypercapnia decrease the affinity of hemoglobin for oxygen (shift the curve to the right). At a given tissue P_{O_2} an increased affinity for oxygen releases less oxygen at the tissue level, whereas a decreased affinity releases more oxygen to the tissue. Alternately, the P_{O_2} at which the hemoglobin is 50% saturated (the P_{50}) is low when the hemoglobin affinity is great and higher when the hemoglobin affinity is low.

Content

Oxygen content is calculated from the hemoglobin saturation and hemoglobin concentration. One gram of hemoglobin binds 1.39 ml of oxygen. The oxygen content in milliliters per deciliter is the product of the saturation percentage and the hemoglobin in grams per deciliter plus the amount of dissolved oxygen. For clinical purposes we can neglect the amount of dissolved oxygen in plasma because it is only 0.003 ml/dl/mm Hg.

Oxygen content becomes critical in anemia, which can cause a significant derangement in tissue oxygenation. An infant with a hemoglobin of 8 g/dl will have one half the oxygen content of an infant with a hemoglobin of 16 g/dl at an equivalent percentage saturation. In Figure 10-2, an infant with 16 g hemoglobin that is 95% saturated (Pa_{O_2} = 90 mm Hg) carries 21.1 ml/dl oxygen, whereas the infant with 8 g hemoglobin carries 10.6 ml/dl oxygen. Approximately 4 to 5 ml/dl oxygen is required by the tissues for metabolism. Therefore venous blood contains 4 to 5 ml/dl oxygen less than the arterial blood. The venous oxygen content in an infant with 16 g hemoglobin would be between 16 and 17 ml/dl (21.1 − 4.5 = 16.6), which corresponds to approximately 75% saturation (16.6/22.4 = 74.6%) or a Pv_{O_2} of 40 mm Hg. However, the venous oxygen content in the infant with 8 g hemoglobin would be 6.1 ml/dl oxygen (10.6 − 4.5 = 6.1). The saturation is 55% (6.1/11.12) which corresponds to P_{O_2} of less than 30, and suggests tissue hypoxia, as compared with the infant with 16 g/dl hemoglobin.

Blood Flow

The product of oxygen content (Ca_{O_2}) and the pulmonary blood flow determines the total amount of oxygen in arterial blood. The total blood flow ($\dot{Q}t$) can be divided into the amount of blood in the pulmonary capillaries ($\dot{Q}c$) and in the shunt ($\dot{Q}s$). Knowing the venous oxygen content, arterial oxygen content, and oxygen content in the pulmonary capillaries exposed to ventilated alveoli permits calculation of shunting.

(19)

$$\frac{\dot{Q}s}{\dot{Q}t} = \frac{Cc_{O_2} - Ca_{O_2}}{Cc_{O_2} - Cv_{O_2}}$$

A shunt occurs when blood passes from the systemic venous to the systemic arterial circulation without receiving oxygen, because of anatomic defects in the heart (such as cyanotic congenital heart disease) or because of blood perfusing alveoli that are not ventilated (such as intrapulmonary shunts). Shunts lower the final arterial oxygen saturation. The usual degree of shunt in the newborn is 15% to 20% of the cardiac output.

(20)

$$\frac{\dot{Q}s}{\dot{Q}t} = \frac{Sc_{O_2} - Sa_{O_2}}{Sc_{O_2} - Sv_{O_2}} \times 100$$

Venous and arterial saturation can be calculated from venous and arterial blood gases, and the pulmonary capillary saturation can be estimated from the calculated alveolar oxygen tension (see equation 13). Calculation of the shunt helps distinguish lung disease from congenital heart disease or helps document changes in the severity of lung disease.

Etiology

Acid-base homeostasis

Ventilation is usually defined as the amount of gas leaving the mouth per units of time (e.g., minute ventilation, $\dot{V}_E$). Minute ventilation is equal to the product of the tidal volume (V_T) and the respiratory frequency in breaths per minute:

(21)

$$\dot{V}_E = V_T \times f$$

The tidal volume can be divided into (1) the gas in the airway plus the gas in nonperfused alveoli (physiologic dead space, V_D), and (2) the gas in the alveolar space, which is involved in gas exchange (alveolar volume, V_A). Therefore:

(22)

$$\dot{V}_E = (V_D + V_A)f$$

OR

(23)

$$\dot{V}_E = \dot{V}_D + \dot{V}_A$$

Alveolar ventilation ($\dot{V}_A = \dot{V}_E - \dot{V}_D$) is measured by collecting the volume of expired gas (V_E) and measuring the concentration of carbon dioxide gas in the expired volume (FE_{CO_2}) and the arterial carbon dioxide tension (Pa_{CO_2}) and a constant:

(24)

$$\dot{V}_A = \frac{\dot{V}_E(FE_{CO_2})}{Pa_{CO_2}} \times K = \frac{V_{CO_2}(K)}{Pa_{CO_2}}$$

Thus the Pa_{CO_2} is inversely related to alveolar ventilation.

A disturbance in alveolar ventilation (a change in P_{CO_2}) causes an acid-base derangement. In a respiratory acidosis when carbon dioxide excretion is below normal, several conditions must be considered. The most common cause of carbon dioxide retention is obstructive lung disease. Meconium aspiration is a common cause of obstructive lung disease in the neonate, and transient tachypnea of the newborn is an obstructive lung disease. Obstructive lung disease is found in the recovery phase of uncomplicated respiratory distress syndrome and in bronchopulmonary dysplasia. Alveolar ventilation is decreased in these conditions from the increased physiologic dead space that occurs with (1) debris in the large and small airways, (2) inflammation in the large and small airways, and (3) ventilation and perfusion mismatch. An increase in dead space leads to carbon dioxide retention.

Another major cause of carbon dioxide retention is poor respiratory effort from (1) narcosis because of maternal anesthesia before delivery, (2) depressed respiratory drive because of sepsis, (3) severe intracranial hemorrhage, including intraventricular hemorrhage, or (4) metabolic disturbances, such as hypoglycemia, affecting the respiratory center.

The third cause involves injuries or changes in the thoracic cage, such as diaphragmatic hernia, phrenic nerve paralysis, or pneumothorax. These result in a decline in tidal volume, respiratory rate, or a combination of these.

In respiratory alkalosis the carbon dioxide excretion is greater than normal. The mechanism for this increased excretion is hyperventilation. Respiratory alkalosis because of hyperventilation may be (1) iatrogenic, resulting from vigorous ventilator therapy in a neonate with respiratory disease; (2) a result of restrictive lung disease, such as early RDS; (3) caused by CNS stimulation of the respiratory drive (e.g., high altitude and encephalitis); and (4) present in hypoxemia, which stimulates the respiratory centers through chemoreceptors.

In nonrespiratory (metabolic) acidosis the metabolic component results from either adding nonvolatile acid (an acid other than carbon dioxide) or losing base bicarbonate. Abnormal acids that are associated with diseases are lactic acid in hypoxia, organic acids in renal failure, and ketoacids in diabetic acidosis. Loss of base occurs in renal tubular acidosis (a defect in the ability of the renal tubules to reabsorb bicarbonate), diarrhea with loss of bicarbonate in the feces, or through urinary excretion resulting from the effects of certain drugs, such as acetazolamide (Diamox).

Nonrespiratory (metabolic) alkalosis is due to either a loss of acid or an addition of base, principally bicarbonate. A bicarbonate addition is most likely iatrogenic. Loss of acid occurs with nasogastric suctioning or severe vomiting, which may occur in pyloric stenosis. Acid loss also occurs from the kidney through the influence of certain drugs such as diuretics, digitalis therapy, and corticosteroids, which preferentially excrete sodium and potassium, causing depletion. A hydrogen ion is therefore substituted in the urine to conserve sodium or potassium. Acid is lost because the hydrogen ion is excreted, the base remains, and the body fluids become alkaline.

Oxygenation

Although delivery system failure (heart failure), anemia, abnormal hemoglobin affinity for oxygen, and a decreased Pao_2 may cause tissue hypoxia, hypoxemia results from only lung disease or cyanotic congenital heart disease. The most common abnormality of the lung leading to hypoxemia is mismatched ventilation and perfusion. Perfect matching of ventilation and perfusion takes place when an adequate amount of blood flows past oxygenated and ventilated alveoli, but this ideal situation rarely occurs. There is always some degree of ventilation and perfusion mismatch. Two extreme examples of mismatch are (1) ventilated and oxygenated alveoli without perfusion (e.g., pulmonary emboli) and (2) the well-perfused but nonventilated alveoli (atelectasis). The former is an example of wasted ventilation ($\dot{V}/\dot{Q} = $ infinity), and the latter is an example of a shunt ($\dot{V}/\dot{Q} = $ O). Either extreme of ventilation and perfusion abnormality is incompatible with life, and thus the degree of ventilation and perfusion mismatch is somewhere between the ends of the spectrum.

Hypoxemia because of ventilation and perfusion mismatch can be overcome by administering supplemental inspired oxygen. In spite of poorly ventilated alveoli, raising the inspired oxygen tension will wash nitrogen from the alveoli, resulting in a higher alveolar oxygen tension, which increases artery oxygen tension. In a shunt, however, no oxygen is exposed to any of the shunted blood, and the Pao_2 cannot increase.

To perform the "shunt test," place a neonate with hypoxemia in 100% oxygen; if the Pao_2 rises to more than 150 mm Hg pressure, cyanotic congenital heart disease is unlikely.

Central hypoventilation from narcosis may cause hypoxemia. As the alveolar carbon dioxide rises, the Pao_2 falls, and subsequently Pao_2 decreases. However, this condition should be clinically evident and should not be confused with lung or congenital heart disease. Other causes of hypoxemia are sufficiently rare in the infant that we need only mention them: decreased inspired oxygen tension, which may occur at high altitude, and oxygen diffusion limitations.

Most conditions that were thought to be diffusion limited are caused by ventilation and perfusion mismatch. The oxygen molecule must diffuse from the alveolus across the alveolar cell, interstitial space, the capillary endothelial cell, and the plasma to the red blood cell. A pathologic condition may occur that interferes with the diffusion process (e.g., thickening of the interstitial space). These processes, however, do not affect oxygen diffusion as much as they alter ventilation and perfusion relationships. Consequently, the abnormal ventilation and perfusion relationship causes the hypoxemia rather than diffusion limitation.

Prevention

Perinatal asphyxia has profound effects on neonatal oxygenation, involving the following factors: (1) decreased inspired oxygen tension, (2) an aggravated ventilation and perfusion mismatch (increased intrapulmonary shunt) and anatomic shunt through the ductus arteriosus and foramen ovale, (3) decreased cardiac output through asphyxic cardiomyopathy, and (4) decreased oxygen affinity by shifting the oxygen dissociation curve to the right during asphyxic acidemia that resulted from combined metabolic and respiratory acidosis.

Prevention of acid-base and oxygenation disturbances and maintenance of acid-base homeostasis require attention to detail. Prevention of premature births or transport of pregnant women who may deliver a high-risk infant to tertiary care centers for treatment can minimize perinatal asphyxia. Prompt and efficient resuscitation measures can also significantly improve the survival rate of premature infants with acid-base and oxygenation problems.

With respiratory disturbances, immediate assessment and prompt therapy, including supplemental inspired oxygen and assisted ventilation when indicated, minimize the respiratory component of acid-base and oxygenation disturbances (see Chapter 22). Careful monitoring of fluid intake and output, minimizing blood loss, observing for sepsis, and monitoring urine electrolytes for potential abnormalities will enable the clinician to control the continuous nonrespiratory conditions and ideally prevent development of nonrespiratory acid-base disturbances.

Monitoring inspired oxygen tensions and arterial oxygen tensions and supplying appropriate concentrations of additional inspired oxygen will prevent low arterial oxygen tensions (see Chapter 22). Monitoring may be accomplished intermittently through indwelling arterial catheters or continuously through transcutaneous oxygen monitors (see Chapter 7). Monitoring hemoglobin concentration and blood loss with replacement to an adequate hemoglobin concentration potentially ensures adequate oxygen content. Careful attention to fluids, electrolytes, and acid-base homeostasis minimizes adverse effects of asphyxic cardiomyopathy by reducing the strain of the heart.

Data Collection

History, physical examination, and laboratory data augment each other in assessing disturbances in acid-base homeostasis and oxygenation (Box 10-2).

History

An adequate obstetric and perinatal history may warn of potential acid-base and oxygenation disturbances:

- Premature delivery predisposes the infant to shock and respiratory distress.

Box 10-2

Evaluation of acid-base disturbances and oxygenation problems in the neonate

1. History
   a. Obstetric and perinatal
   b. Neonatal
   c. Family
2. Physical examination
   a. Vital signs
   b. General appearance
   c. Respiratory effort
   d. Pulmonary examination
   e. Cardiac examination
   f. Abdominal examination
   g. Neurologic examination
3. Laboratory
   a. Chest x-ray film
   b. Arterial blood gases
   c. Urinalysis
   d. In selected cases: sepsis evaluation, urine electrolytes, and serum electrolytes

- Meconium staining may portend respiratory difficulties.
- Prolonged rupture of membranes, infants of diabetic mothers, or abnormal maternal bleeding may be associated with either metabolic or respiratory acid-base disturbances and hypoxemia.
- A neonatal history of vomiting, diarrhea, or other gastrointestinal disturbances can cause acid-base disturbances.
- The infant's general appearance, feeding habits, and activity level may indicate sepsis or CNS injury, both of which promote acid-base disturbances and hypoxemia.
- Nosocomial infections and pneumonia may significantly influence acid-base and oxygen disturbances.
- A family history of inherited renal problems such as tubular acidosis may suggest an acid-base disturbance.
- A family history of salt-losing endocrinopathies may produce an acid-base disturbance.

Signs and Symptoms

Signs of acid-base disturbance vary widely and are often undetected. Vital signs that show hypothermia and low blood pressure imply metabolic derangements in acid-base homeostasis. Respiratory rate and pattern, grunting, flaring, and retractions indicate respiratory derangements of acid-base homeostasis and oxygenation. Abnormal auscultation of the chest or heart may suggest present or future acid-base or oxygenation disturbances, including possible congenital heart disease. Examining the abdomen, particularly for the proper number and size of kidneys, is important in assessing potential acid-base disturbances. Lethargy, seizures, generalized neurologic signs, or focal neurologic signs increase concern about either potential respiratory or metabolic acid-base disturbances or hypoxemia.

Laboratory Data

A chest x-ray examination may identify a respiratory cause for acid-base disturbance and hypoxemia.

Urinalysis

The routine urinalysis records urine specific gravity and demonstrates that urine is being produced.

Arterial Blood Gases

Interpretation of the arterial blood gases will point to the primary acid-base derangement and may reveal a secondary compensation and define the degree of hypoxemia. Presently, methods for monitoring of the components of acid-base analysis comprise both invasive and noninvasive techniques. Intermittant arterial punctures or indwelling catheters in various vessels (often the umbilical arteries or veins) supply the requisite data. However, we can continuously measure transcutaneous O_2 saturation. Monitors can continuously measure expired end-tidal CO_2, which corresponds to the alveolar CO_2. (We have seen earlier that alveolar and arterial CO_2 are equivalent.) Additionally, skin electrodes are available that measure Pa_{O_2} and Pa_{CO_2}. Although the pathophysiologic condition of the acid-base disturbance is determined through the analysis of arterial blood gases, further assessment of the infant is required:

- Respiratory alkalosis or acidosis should be evident from the physical examination, arterial blood gas analysis, and chest x-ray examination.
- Consider shock and sepsis in metabolic acidosis. Urine electrolytes may provide additional information to delineate causes. Blood pressure measurement, a complete blood cell count, serum and urine electrolyte and glucose determinations, and assessment of intake and output of fluids are necessary to assess a metabolic disturbance.
- Oxygenation disturbances may be analyzed from the preceding laboratory tests, and when indicated, electrocardiogram and arterial blood gas responses to increased inspired oxygen concentration are used to evaluate the possibility of cyanotic congenital heart disease.

Treatment

In respiratory acidosis the pathophysiologic condition is hypoventilation, which is associated with hypoxemia. Treatment is directed at the underlying cause. Where primary lung disease exists, we must provide ventilatory assistance. Hypoxemia, because of ventilation and perfusion mismatch in respiratory disease, is treated with increased inspired oxygen concentration or ventilatory support. Ventilatory techniques that may be of benefit include CPAP, standard ventilation, high-frequency ventilation, ECMO, and others (see Chapter 22).

Asphyxia often leads to a combined respiratory and metabolic acidosis. Ventilation will resolve the respiratory acidosis, and the improved oxygenation may allow the lactic acidosis to resolve without bicarbonate therapy. In narcosis, temporary ventilatory support may be required. The narcosis may be reversed with naloxone (Narcan) at a dose of 0.1 mg/kg. (Repeated doses may be required; see Chapter 4.)

The other acidoses and alkaloses must have a careful search for the causes, with therapy directed toward them. This may require drug therapy, replacement of losses, or surgical correction of abnormalities.

Complications

The outcome of unrecognized and untreated acid-base or oxygenation disturbances may be an increased mortality or an increased morbidity in the survivors. Complications of the correction of the acid-base and oxygenation disturbance vary according to the disturbance and treatment provided.

The major effect of acidosis on the body is CNS depression. In metabolic acidosis the rate and depth of respiration are increased, whereas in respiratory acidosis respiration is depressed. The major effect of alkalosis on the body is increased excitability of the CNS and tetany (often of the respiratory muscles).

Respiratory acidosis with treatment by assisted ventilation can produce all of the complications of assisted ventilation, including infection, trauma, oxygen toxicity, sepsis, air leak, subglottic stenosis, and others (see Chapter 22).

Complications of oxygen therapy include the risks of hypoxemia and hyperoxemia. Immediate effects of hypoxia include pulmonary vasoconstriction, a change from aerobic to anaerobic metabolism (with eventual metabolic acidosis), cyanosis, bradycardia, hypotonia, and decreases in CNS and cardiac functions. Prolonged high inspired oxygen concentrations increase pulmonary morbidity through pulmonary oxygen toxicity and contribute to retinopathy of prematurity. If ventilatory support is required to attain adequate oxygenation, the complications are those of ventilator therapy (see Chapter 22).

Parent Teaching

Obtaining blood for blood gas analysis by invasive techniques (arterial punctures and heelsticks) is stressful for parents and their infant. Explaining the rationale for the test, eliciting parental assistance (if they are present), and encouraging them to comfort their crying baby involves parents as primary care givers. **Explaining the results of the analysis and needed changes in therapy keeps parents appraised of their baby's progress. Many parents become quite adept at blood gas interpretation and are able to anticipate therapeutic alterations: "Did you change the Fio$_2$? The ventilator rate?" This helps parents master a difficult situation. Beyond sharing technical information, the care provider should also personalize the infant to his or her parents (see Chapter 28).**

References

1. Carl WA: Assessment of pulmonary function. In Fanaroff AA, Martin RS, editors: *Neonatal perinatal medicine,* ed 5, St Louis, 1992, Mosby.
2. Hanson T, Corbet A: Principles of respiratory monitoring and therapy. In Taeusch HW, Ballard RA, Avery ME, editors: *Schaffer and Avery's diseases of the newborn,* ed 6, Philadelphia, 1991, WB Saunders.
3. Mott SR, James SR, Sperhac AM: *Nursing care of children and families,* ed 2, Redwood City, Calif, 1990, Benjamin/Cummings.
4. Durand DJ, Philips BL: Blood gases: technical aspects and interpretation. In Goldsmith JP, Karotkin EH, editors: *Assisted ventilation of the neonate,* ed 3 Philadelphia, 1988, WB Saunders.
5. Gilbert HC, Vender JS: Arterial blood gas monitor *Crit Care Clin,* 11(1):233, 1995
6. Stork JE, Stork EK: Acid-base physiology and disorders in the neonate. In Fanaroff AA, Martin RS, editors: *Neonatal perinatal medicine,* ed 5, St Louis, 1992, Mosby.
7. Swartz MK: Assessment of the neonate and child. In Sexton, DL, editor: *Nursing care of the respiratory patient,* Norwalk, Conn, 1990, Appleton & Lange.
8. Weaver L: Issues in nursing care of the newborn. In Taeusch HW, Ballard RA, Avery ME, editors: *Schaffer and Avery's diseases of the newborn,* ed 6, Philadelphia, 1991, WB Saunders.
9. Whaley LR, Wong DL: *Nursing care of infants and children,* ed 4, St Louis, 1991, Mosby.

11 Pain and Pain Relief

Rita Agarwal, Mary I. Enzman Hagedorn, Sandra L. Gardner

Pain is a complex phenomenon that is at best elusive in the neonate. Rationalization for inadequate treatment of pain has resulted in unnecessary suffering for these fragile infants. **Research has shown that the "unchecked release of stress hormones by untreated pain may exacerbate injury, prevent wound healing, lead to infection, prolong hospitalization, and even [lead] to death."[86]** These fragile neonates are simply too sick to not have the pain treated. Health care professionals are responsible for influencing positive change in clinical practice regarding neonatal pain.[76]

In the past, neonates have not been given analgesia and/or anesthesia for surgery because of the controversy over whether they feel pain and whether they are physiologically stable enough to tolerate the effects of these drugs. The rationale for withholding analgesia and/or anesthesia included the following beliefs:

- Neonates have an immature CNS with non-myelinated pain fibers and are thus incapable of perceiving pain. Neonates have no memory of pain.
- Pain is a highly subjective experience that is difficult to objectively assess in nonverbal neonates.
- Anesthetics and analgesics are dangerous when administered to neonates, and neonates are safer being unmedicated.

There is increasing evidence from recent research that neonates, including preterm infants, have a CNS that is much more mature than previously thought.[3,4,35,36] Pain pathways are myelinated in the fetus during the second and third trimesters, and are completely myelinated by 30 to 37 weeks' gestation. Even thinly or nonmyelinated fibers carry pain stimuli. Incomplete myelination implies only a slower transmission, which is offset in the neonate by the shorter distance the impulse must travel.[4]

Even though pain is not expressed verbally in semiconscious patients, nonverbal adults (intubated, mute), or infants, this does not negate their experience of pain. In response to the question of whether the neonate's responses are reflexive or a perception of pain, research has focused on measuring the infant's pain experience. The infant's capacity for memory is far greater than previously thought,[3,49,83] and a neuropsychologic complex of altered pain threshold and pain-related behavior has been identified.[46-48,93]

Concern has been expressed that giving potent medications to an already critically ill infant might be dangerous. Local and systemic drugs now available, as well as new techniques and devices for monitoring, enable neonates (including preterm infants) to be safely anesthetized and provide safe and effective analgesia while maintaining a stable condition.[4]

Neonates, including premature infants, exhibit (1) physiologic, (2) hormonal, (3) metabolic, and (4) behavioral responses to surgical procedures that are similar to, but more intense than, adult responses.[4,7,8,44,51] Pain relief benefits the neonate by decreasing physiologic instability, hormonal and metabolic stress, and the behavioral reactions accompanying painful procedures.[4,7-9] The Committee on Fetus and Newborn of the American Academy of Pediatrics has recommended the administration of local and/or systemic drugs for anesthesia or analgesia to neonates undergoing surgical procedures.[3] The committee further states that any decision to withhold these drugs should not be based solely on the infant's age or perceived degree of cortical maturity but should be based on the same criteria used in older patients.[3]

Other national associations have promulgated standard of care guides and/or position statements regarding neonatal pain management.[1,74,75]

Physiology and Pathophysiology

"Pain is an unpleasant sensory and emotional experience associated with actual or potential tissue damage, or described in terms of such damage."[70] Although we are unable to assess the emotional experience associated with pain in these babies, the sensory pathways required are now better understood. **Neonates have a developing, incompletely myelinated nervous system at birth; however, all the components of the nociceptive (pain) pathways are present.**[35,36] To better understand neonatal responses and their differences from adults, the basic mechanisms of adult pain transmission are presented in Figure 11-1.

Neuroanatomy

Peripheral Nervous System

Peripheral nerves can be classified into three broad categories based on fiber diameter and velocity (Table 11-1). Pain receptors (nociceptors) are the A-delta fibers (A-δ) and C fibers that are widely spread in the superficial layers of the skin, periosteum, fascia, peritoneum, joints, muscle, pleura, dura, and tooth pulp. Most visceral tissues have fewer nociceptors, and these transmit to the spinal cord through the sympathetic, parasympathetic, and splanchnic nerves. **Tissue damage and inflammation cause the release of arachidonic acid and other chemicals that can sensitize nerve endings and cause vasodilatation and plasma extravasation. This causes pain, swelling, and hyperalgesia.**[29,30]

A-δ fibers are myelinated and therefore capable of fast impulse conduction. These nerves are

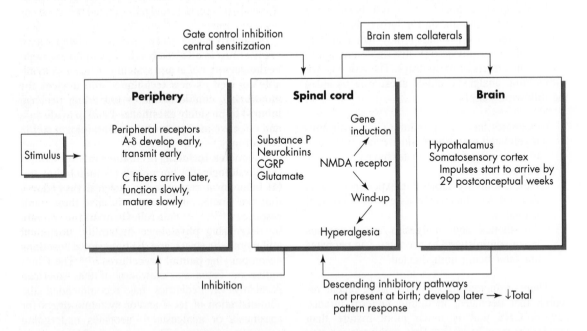

Figure 11-1   Schematic representation of transmission of noxious stimuli from the periphery to the brain.

responsible for "fast" or "first" pain. They are also known as high threshold mechanoreceptors (HTMs) because they respond to strong pressure or tissue injury. **The C fibers (polymodal nociceptors) are unmyelinated, conduct impulses more slowly, and are the main nociceptors for transmitting chemical, thermal, and mechanical *noxious* stimuli to the spinal cord.**[71] The A-δ fibers seem to develop ahead of the C fibers in the skin and the spinal cord. They start to function at initially lower thresholds than when they mature (i.e., less stimulation is required for conduction of what may be perceived as pain). Complete myelination occurs during the second and third trimesters. Lack of myelination had been thought to indicate the inability of a neonate to perceive pain; however,

incomplete myelination leads only to slower conduction, which is offset by the shorter distances traversed in the infant.[4]

Reflex responses to somatic stimuli begin at 7 ½ postconceptual weeks in the perioral skin and continue to develop in the palms of the hands before finally reaching the hindlimbs by 13½ to 14 weeks.[35] It is likely that both A-δ fibers (touching) and A-δ fibers (pinching) transmit painful stimuli in the human fetus. In rat pups the C fibers reach the spinal cord but do not start to stimulate dorsal horn cells until the end of the first postnatal week. They subsequently continue to mature for several weeks. This slow maturation in rats may be due to low levels of neuropeptides such as substance P (SP), neurotransmitters, or immature receptor sites. These changes in rat pups appear to correlate with the third trimester and the early neonatal period in humans.[35,36]

Spinal Cord

Once a noxious stimulus is detected by the nociceptors, the signal is transmitted via the primary afferents to the dorsal root ganglia and from there to the dorsal horn of the spinal cord.[29] Neurotransmitters and their receptors amplify or attenuate the signal in the dorsal horn before sending the signal to the brain.[30]

Excitatory neurotransmitters such as SP and other neurokinins are increased after acute inflammation and may be required for the transmission of painful stimuli to the brain. Glutamate and aspartame are amino acids that appear to be involved in central hypersensitivity and "wind-up."[29] **Wind-up is a phenomenon whereby repetition of the same noxious stimulus leads to an exaggerated response. This response can continue even after the stimulus has been stopped and may contribute to the development of chronic pain syndromes.** Wind-up may also be responsible for converting a low-level, pain-related activity to a high-level, pain-related activity.[29]

An additional factor in the development of hypersensitivity and hyperalgesia is the presence of nociceptive specific receptors, which respond only to pain. In the presence of peripheral inflammation, the threshold of these receptors is decreased so that they are capable of responding to other non-noxious stimuli.[29] For example, an in-

---

Table 11-1
Classification and Characteristics of Peripheral Nerves

Name/Characteristic	Function
A-alpha (A-α) d: 10-20 μ v: 70-120 m/sec myelinated	Innervate skeletal muscle
A-beta (A-β) d: 12-20 μg v: 30-70 m/sec myelinated	Light touch or pressure may be involved in peripheral sensitization and allodynia; in the premature and newborn infant, may be involved in the transmission of noxious stimuli
A-gamma (A-γ) d: 3-6 μ v: 15-30 m/sec myelinated	Muscle tone
A-delta (A-δ) d: 2-5 μ v: 12-30 m/sec myelinated	Fast, well localized pain; high threshold mechanoreceptors
B d: 3 μ v: 3-15 m/sec myelinated	Preganglionic autonomic fibers may be involved in sensory or sympathetic coupling
C d: 0.4-1.2 μ v: 0.5-2 m/sec unmyelinated	Slow pain, touch, temperature, postganglionic sympathetic fibers, polymodal nociceptors

d, Nerve diameter; *v*, nerve velocity.

fant whose heel has been repeatedly stuck for blood samples may demonstrate pain behavior even when the heel is merely touched. Many of these responses can be blocked by low doses of opioids. However, once these responses are established, a tenfold increased dose of opioids may be required to reverse them.[34]

The spinal cord also contains inhibitory neurotransmitters (γ-aminobutyric acid [GABA], glycine), which are activated by descending neural pathways (from the brain to the spinal cord) and decrease the intensity of pain transmission.[36] Descending inhibition is necessary to modulate the pain response and yet to allow for specific pain responses (i.e., withdrawal from a needle stick). Lack of inhibition produces exaggerated, generalized, but definite responses to pain such as body wriggling, facial grimacing, and excessive crying. These pathways, in contrast to the excitatory ones, are not fully developed at birth in rat pups and probably in humans.[36]

Neurotransmitters in the developing nervous system may be expressed early but are not necessarily located in areas normally found in an adult.[36] This is particularly true of SP and glutamate, which may contribute to the unorganized responses noted with pain stimuli in the newborn (i.e., the whole body moves when an IV is started).

Brain

Much less is known about the development of the pathways to the higher brain centers, such as the hypothalamus and cortex. Once again there is evidence of immaturity of the inhibitory pathways.[35,36] Development in the human cortex continues for many years after birth. **Contrary to prior beliefs that newborns do not feel pain, it appears that in fact cutaneous responses are exaggerated, occur at much lower thresholds, and reflex muscle contractions last longer in newborns when compared with mature individuals.[35] In summary, the newborn's nervous system, though still developing, is fully capable of transmitting, perceiving, responding to, and probably remembering noxious stimuli.**

Physiologic Responses

Acute pain in adults is associated with increased sympathetic stimulation, heart rate, respiratory rate, blood pressure, cardiac output, myocardial oxygen consumption, peripheral resistance, anxiety, emotional distress, hormonal imbalance, and greater morbidity and mortality.[26] **Numerous studies have shown that both premature and full term infants express the same physiologic responses to pain and noxious stimuli (e.g., intubation) as adults (Box 11-1).[2-7] Infants undergoing circumcision without the use of pain medication demonstrated increased irritability after the procedure, altered sleep-wake state, and abnormal feeding patterns for up to 22 hours. These responses can be attenuated or blocked with the appropriate use of analgesics.[15,37,89]**

Etiology

Invasive Procedures

Pain is produced with any invasive procedure (Table 11-2). One study found that the number of invasive procedures in 54 neonates during admission to the NICU was 3283.[13] The most common (56%) was heelstick followed by endotracheal suctioning (26%) and intravenous cannula insertion (8%). The most premature infants underwent the highest number of procedures with one infant undergoing 488 procedures!

A recent study examining the use of analgesics for "minor" procedures in NICUs and pediatric intensive care units (PICUs), found that analgesics were rarely used for the placement of intravenous catheters, suprapubic bladder aspiration, urinary bladder catheterization, venipuncture, arterial line placement, lumbar puncture, and paracentesis in NICUs. **Analgesics were used approximately 60% of the time in the NICU for the placement of chest tubes, central lines, and bone marrow aspiration.[14]** In contrast, analgesics were used in the majority of patients in the PICU undergoing arterial line placement, lumbar puncture, and paracentesis and in greater than 90% of chest tube insertions, central line placements, and bone marrow aspirations. **Possible reasons for these differences were that (1) neonates were more often critically ill and the use of analgesics may have prolonged the procedure or exacerbated the infants' medical problems, (2) the use of neuromuscular blocking agents prevented the physical response to pain, and (3) not**

Box 11-1

Neonatal Pain Response*

Physiologic

Increase in
  Heart rate
  Blood pressure
  Intracranial pressure, *which leads to higher risk for intraventricular hemorrhage*
  Respiratory rate
  Mean airway pressure
  Muscle tension
  Carbon dioxide ($\uparrow$ TcPCo$_2$; Pco$_2$)
Decrease in
  Depth of respirations (shallow)
  Oxygenation ($\downarrow$ TcPo$_2$; Po$_2$; Sao$_2$; *which leads to apnea/bradycardia*)
  Pallor or flushing
  Diaphoresis or palmar sweating
  Dilated pupils

Behavioral

Vocalizations
  Crying (higher-pitched, tense, and harsh)
  Whimpering
  Moaning
Facial expressions
  Grimacing
  Furrowing or bulging of the brow
  Quivering chin
  Eye squeeze
Bodily movements
  General diffuse body activity
  Limb withdrawal, swiping, thrashing

Changes in tone
  Hypertonicity, rigidity, fist clenching
  Hypotonicity, flaccidity
Touch aversion
States
  Sleep-wake cycle changes—wakefulness
  Activity level changes: increased fussiness, irritability, listlessness, lethargy
  Feeding difficulties
  More difficult to comfort, soothe, quiet
  Disrupts interactive ability with parents

Hormonal/Catabolic Stress Response

Increase in
  Plasma renin activity
  Catecholamine levels (epinephrine and norepinephrine)
  Cortisol levels
  Nitrogen excretion
  Release of
    Growth hormone
    Glucagon
    Aldosterone
  Serum levels of
    Glucose
    Lactate
    Pyruvate
    Ketones
    Nonesterified fatty acids
Decrease in
  Insulin secretion

* References 4, 7, 8, 10, 27, 42, 44, 45, 53, 78, 87, 96.

all infants respond to pain by crying loudly, withdrawing, or otherwise "protesting." This study indicates that considerable work needs to be done to educate practitioners about the benefits of appropriate pain management in neonates.

Endotracheal intubation, though not traditionally considered to be a "painful stimulus," is nevertheless associated with significant physiologic and hormonal perturbations and increased intracranial pressure that can be decreased with opioids. Using meperidine before tracheal suctioning in intubated, mechanically ventilated newborns can decrease the degree and duration of desaturation.[79] The use of morphine, meperidine, or alfentanil during mechanical ventilation in critically ill newborns significantly decreased plasma B-endorphin, cortisol, and blood glucose levels.[77]

Surgery

Painful stimuli, surgery, and traumatic injuries have been shown in adults to trigger the "stress response," which causes the release of a variety of hormones, including epinephrine, norepinephrine, corticosteroids, glucagon, and growth hormones.[25] These hormones prepare the body for a "fight or

Table 11-2
Common Causes of Pain in Neonates[13,14]

Invasive Procedures	Surgical Procedures	Others
Intravenous cannulation	Central line placement	Clavicle, rib fracture
Venipuncture	PDA ligation	Extremity fracture
Heelstick	TEF repair	Chest pain
Intramuscular injection	Gastroschisis repair	Central pain syndrome (i.e., pain derived from CNS damage)
Arterial line, blood gas	Omphalocele repair	
Umbilical catheterization	CDH repair	Spasticity
Chest tube insertion or removal	Inguinal hernia repair	Abdominal pain resulting from shortgut syndrome, multiple abdominal surgeries
Bone marrow aspiration	Cardiac surgery	
Lumbar puncture	Circumcision	
Paracentesis	Broviac catheter insertion or removal	Necrotizing enterocolitis
Endotracheal intubation	ECMO catheter insertion or removal	Bowel obstruction
Endotracheal suction		Prolonged and/or improper positioning
Mechanical ventilation		
Bladder catheterization		
Suprapubic aspiration		

PDA, Patent ductus arteriosus; *TEF,* tracheoesophageal fistula; *CDH,* congenital diaphragmatic hernia; *ECMO,* extracorporeal membrane oxygenation.

flight" response and cause, among other things, an increase in heart rate, respiratory rate, glucose production, muscle, and fat breakdown. This response in the short term allows the body to deal with an insult. If the insult continues or is untreated, the ongoing catabolic stress response may become deleterious to the body's well-being by promoting more tissue breakdown while preventing growth and tissue repair.[26] Both premature and full-term infants have a decreased stress response with the use of appropriate analgesia both during and immediately after surgery.[4-10] A special example of untreated operative pain is newborn circumcision. In addition to the previously mentioned short-term effects of not treating the pain associated with circumcision, male infants who have undergone circumcision without analgesia have an increased pain response to vaccination at 4 to 6 months of age.[93] It is possible, therefore, that newborns have a much greater capacity for memory than previously thought!

Other Etiologies

Rib, clavicular, and extremity fractures are not uncommon and should be considered in the presence of prolonged crying and failure to move the affected extremity.[39] Bronchopulmonary dysplasia is a common problem in infants who were premature and may cause chest pain, a syndrome known to occur in some older patients with chronic lung disease. Neurologic dysfunction can leave patients with ongoing pain from central pain syndrome or excessive spasticity. A recent study showed that 27% of former extremely-low-birth-weight (ELBW) infants who were now teenagers had neurosensory impairment, and 9% reported moderate or severe pain.[85]

Prevention

Prevention of pain in the neonate and preterm infant begins with a proactive plan of care aimed at preventing the pain cycle. The key approaches in this plan include (1) anticipation, (2) comprehensive and ongoing assessment of the variables, (3) distinguishing agitation and irritability from pain expressions and responses of the preterm infant, (4) ongoing communication among health care providers, utilizing input from the parents, (5) advocating and implementing timely and effective treatment for irritability, agitation, and pain (e.g., pharmacologic and comfort measures), and

(6) ongoing reevaluation of this proactive plan of care.[1]

Individualized behavioral and developmental care is another important area in preventing stress and sensory overload that often contribute to an ongoing pain cycle. These approaches help prevent disorganization in the neonate. In order to facilitate stability and self regulation before and during an invasive, painful procedure, (1) assess the infant's state and facilitate a change to an alert state, (2) contain extremities (see Chapter 12), (3) provide a pacifier and an opportunity to grasp (a finger, hand, or blanket), and (4) utilize another person (e.g., parent or care giver) to support, contain, and observe for stress. After the procedure, provide support, comfort, and slow withdrawal so that the infant remains calm.[96]

The suffering of neonates can be avoided. Needless suffering is prevented by an established plan of care for assessment, management, and evaluation of pain and attempts to relieve pain. Neonates depend on the skilled observations, assessments, and interventions of care providers for prompt, safe, and effective relief. A cooperative effort among health care providers and the parents in the form of pain management teams[16] and well established pain protocols prevents unnecessary suffering of both neonates and their families. Controlling environmental stimuli (e.g., dimming lights, controlling noise level, turning radios off, speaking softly when near the isolette or warmer, and performing rounds outside of the unit), although often difficult in the NICU, is crucial for decreasing stress and preventing unnecessary agitation. Quieting techniques are also a useful way to help control pain response in the neonate; these include nonnutritive sucking, containment interventions, and rocking[76] (see Chapter 12).

Data Collection

History

Neonates experiencing procedural, surgical, and/or chronic pain must be provided measures to alleviate pain. Neonatal irritability and agitation (Box 11-2) secondary to chronic conditions (e.g., BPD, necrotizing enterocolitis [NEC], short

bowel syndrome, neurologic deficits) and/or environmental overstimulation may also require a combination of environmental interventions and sedation.

Signs and Symptoms

Assessment of pain in neonates is often challenging because they cannot verbalize their experience. There are four objectives in the assessment of pain: (1) detection of the presence of pain, (2) impact of pain, (3) pain relieving interventions, and (4) effectiveness of interventions.[62,80] Expression of pain through behavior is one of the neonate's only means of communicating about pain. Behavioral cues may include diffuse or localized motor activity (e.g., pulling extremity away, hypotonia), facial grimacing, crying, agitation, and level of activity (see Box 11-1). Assessment of pain in the neonate is further complicated by the infant's state and level of neural development.[44] The younger the gestational age, the more immature the CNS and more limited the autonomic and self-regulatory abilities to deal with pain and stress and disorganized ineffective responses that make it more difficult to communicate pain.[2,27,96] A more immature, fragile neonate may manifest alterations in sleep-wake cycles and habituate to the overwhelming stimuli of the NICU (see Chapter 12) and thus be unable to exhibit any response to pain.

Behavioral expressions of pain by the neonate are further hampered by intubation, use of restraints, and neuromuscular blockers. Similarly, chronically ill infants who have developed what has been described as learned helplessness (see Chapter 12) have difficulty generating a pain response.[76]

Physiologic parameters may also indicate pain (e.g., increased heart and respiratory rates, elevated blood pressure, desaturation, apnea, palmar sweating). These symptoms are the result of sympathetic nervous system activation (see Box 11-1).

When pain is repetitive or persists for hours or days, there is a decompensatory response, resulting in hormonal and metabolic alterations (see Fig. 11-2 and Box 11-1). The fight or flight mechanism of the sympathetic nervous system is no longer able to compensate, so an adaptation syndrome begins with a return to baseline physiologic parameters.

Box 11-2

Indicators of Irritability and Agitation[19,21,38]

Physiologic

Increase in
    Heart rate and blood pressure only with activity
    Oxygenation ($\uparrow$ TcPo$_2$; Po$_2$; Sao$_2$)
    Respiratory rate and effort
Decrease in
    Oxygenation ($\downarrow$ TcPo$_2$; Po$_2$; Sao$_2$) after prolonged
        agitation
    Heart rate (bradycardia)
    Respirations (apnea)
Alterations in color: cyanosis, mottling, duskiness,
    pallor
Diaphoresis
Vomiting
Poor pattern of weight gain

Behavioral

Vocalizations
    Whining cry
    Intense, urgent cry
    High-pitched cry
    Resumes fussiness when consolation ceases
Facial expressions
    Frowning
    Worried facies
    Gaze aversion
    Closes eyes to tune out

Bodily movements
    Random movements of head and body
    Hypertonic, rigid posturing; arching; hyper-
        extended neck
    Flailing, thrashing, frantic activity of extremities
        during fuss or cry
    Decreased activity
    Tremulousness
States
    Hyperalert—easily aroused from sleep; startles
        easily
    Rapid and frequent state changes to fuss or cry
    Sleep-wake cycles unpredictable
    Feeding difficulties
    Difficult to console, soothe
    High level of persistence
    Needs environmental structure to fall asleep;
        takes a long time to fall asleep
    Ineffective in self-consoling; requires vestibular
        stimulation or body containment to console;
        responds inconsistently to consolation
    Noncuddly

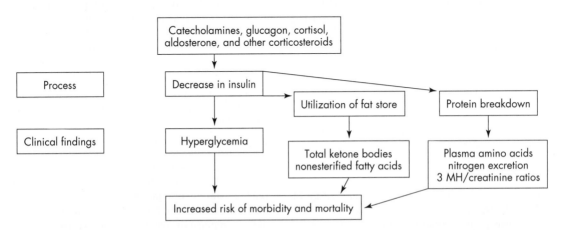

Figure 11-2 Hormonal response to pain in infants. (From Johnston C, Stevens B: Pain in infants. In
Watt-Watson J, Donovan M, editors: *Pain management, nursing perspective,* St Louis, 1992, Mosby.)

The return of the heart rate, respirations, and blood pressure to baseline parameters makes assessment of the infant's pain more difficult and does not mean that the infant has "adjusted" to or no longer is experiencing pain.[87]

The lack of an expression of pain through physiologic and behavioral responses does not mean that the neonate is not experiencing pain. Pain responses may be delayed, cumulative, or absent. In the preterm, sustained elevations in vital signs and decreased oxygenation confirm the persistence of physiologic alterations after painful stimuli.[27,90] Very critically ill neonates and immature preterms may be so weak and overwhelmed that they have completely exhausted their energy and are unable to respond.[40,91,97] The incidence of crying in response to painful or noxious stimuli is less than 50% in the preterm infant.[53,90] Depending on gestational age, a preterm infant's behavioral responses (e.g., facial changes and bodily movements) to pain are similar to the term infant. The responses of the very preterm infant are highly variable (a reflection of continuous maturation of the CNS) and less robust.[27,53,90] Preterm

infants exhibit significant variability in behavioral and physiologic responses to preparatory procedures and handling, making it unclear if these responses are related to stress, behavioral disorganization, or a conditioned response and/or pain perception.[54,90,91]

Differentiation between pain and agitation is a challenge (Fig. 11-3). Agitation is a behavioral symptom of many problems, including environmental overstimulation, respiratory insufficiency, neurologic irritability, and pain.[76] Causes of agitation other than pain should first be eliminated before pain management is initiated. Assessment of environmental stimuli should be a routine part of the neonate's care. The neonate may associate certain stimuli with unpleasant events over time, and repeated exposure (e.g., ventilator alarms, placement of heel warmer, the odor of an alcohol wipe) may trigger agitation. Although these stimuli are inevitable, identifying, avoiding, or limiting them will help prevent anticipatory decompensation in these fragile infants.[76]

Assessment of neonatal pain is influenced by the attitudes and beliefs of care providers, amount

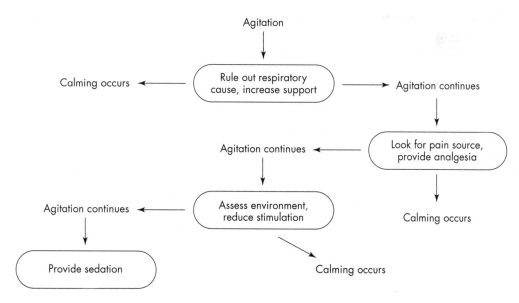

Figure 11-3 Decision tree for assessing and managing pain and/or agitation. (From Gordin P: Assessing and managing agitation in the critically ill infant, *MCN* 15:26, 1990.)

of time spent observing for and having knowledge of pain responses, discrepancy between attitudes and practice, and prioritization of pain recognition and relief in the NICU.[28,38,52,86,87] In an attempt to quantify and objectify the neonate's pain experience and to facilitate the health care professional's recognition of the presence and severity of pain in the neonate, ongoing research is aimed at tool development. Pain response is a multidimensional phenomenon, and pain assessment should include behavioral, physiologic,[91] and hormonal or metabolic indices. There has been development of research tools; however, limited reliability and validity have been established for these tools in clinical practice.[91]

The Postoperative Pain Score (Table 11-3) is an assessment tool developed to measure postoperative pain after minor surgical procedures in 1-

to 7 month-old infants. This scale has not been standardized or validated in the full-term or preterm neonate. The Neonatal Facial Coding System (Table 11-4) is an assessment tool based on nine facial expressions of term newborns in four sleepwake states while experiencing the discomfort of heel rub and the pain of heel lance. Quiet, awake neonates demonstrate the most facial activity, whereas those in quiet sleep demonstrate the least.[44,45] Facial activity also increases with gestational age, so that both infant state and gestational age must be considered when using this scale.[27,91] Because this tool is sensitive to changes in pain intensity, it is also useful for evaluating the effectiveness of interventions. There is recent evidence of reliable clinical use of this tool, although it is time consuming and requires experienced coders.[84]

Table 11-3
Postoperative Pain Score*

Behavior	0 (poor)	1 (mediocre)	2 (satisfactory)
1. Sleep during preceding hour	None	Short naps between 5 and 10 min	Longer naps ≥10 min
2. Facial expression of pain	Marked, constant	Less marked, intermittent	Calm, relaxed
3. Quality of cry	Screaming, painful, high-pitched	Modulated (can be distracted by normal sound)	No cry
4. Spontaneous motor activity	Thrashing around, incessant agitation	Moderate agitation	Normal
5. Spontaneous excitability and responsiveness to ambient stimulation	Tremulous, clonic movements; spontaneous Moro reflexes	Excessive reactivity (to any stimulation)	Quiet
6. Flexion of fingers and toes	Very pronounced, marked constant	Less marked, intermittent	Absent
7. Sucking	Absent or disorganized sucking	Intermittent (three or four) and stops with crying	Strong, rhythmic with pacifying effect
8. Global evaluation of tone	Strong hypertonicity	Moderate hypertonicity	Normal for age
9. Consolability	None after 2 minutes	Quiet after 1 minute of effort	Calm before 1 minute
10. Sociability (eye contact) reponse to voice, smile, real interest in face	Absent	Difficult to obtain	Easy and prolonged

Adapted from Attia J et al: Measurement of postoperative pain and narcotic administration in infants using a new clinical scoring system, *Anesthesiology* 67(3A): A532, 1987.
*Infants with a total score of 15 to 20 have arbitrarily been considered to have adequate postoperative pain management.

The Premature Infant Pain Profile (PIPP) (Table 11-5) is a multidimensional assessment tool intended for use within clinical practice.[92] The PIPP is a seven-item, four-point scale whose maximum score is dependent on the infant's gestational age. Having established beginning content and construct validity, the PIPP needs further validation in the clinical setting. Intrarater and interrater reliability has not yet been established.

The Neonatal Infant Pain Scale (NIPS) (Table 11-6) is a behavioral assessment tool for preterm and term neonates responding to a needle puncture. NIPS scores reveal an increase in behavioral response during the procedures and a decline in response scores after the procedure (Fig. 11-4). Thus NIPS provides a measurement of intensity of infant responses to painful procedure during and after the event.[60] NIPS scores have been correlated with gestational age (e.g., maturity and level of behavior) and Apgar scores. NIPS provides an objective measure of pain-relieving interventions and their effectiveness.[60] The NIPS scale is objective, nonintrusive, and assesses only behavioral response to pain; it has been used as a research tool and has not been used in clinical practice. Flow sheets have also been designed to facilitate the documentation of pain scores and behaviors.[60]

The CRIES assessment tool (Table 11-7), developed to measure physiologic and behavioral pain responses postoperatively is utilized hourly with vital sign assessment. CRIES utilizes a scoring system similar to the Apgar score: a score ≥4 indicates pain and requires intervention.[16] Validity and reliability to measure postoperative pain has been established,[57] whereas use of CRIES to measure procedural pain has not been validated.[16]

The National Practice Guidelines provides a list of assessment questions to ask when assessing pain management in the neonate (Box 11-3, p. 187). Lack of validated assessment tools may leave health care providers wondering if behaviors are indicators or responses to pain. The Acute Pain

Table 11-4
Neonatal Facial Coding System

Action	Description
Brow bulge	Bulging, creasing, and vertical furrows above and between brows occurring as a result of the lowering and drawing together of the eyebrows
Eye squeeze	Identified by the squeezing or bulging of the eyelids; bulging of the fatty pads about the infant's eyes is pronounced
Nasolabial furrow	Primarily manifested by the pulling upwards and deepening of the nasolabial furrow (a line or wrinkle that begins adjacent to the nostril wings and runs downward and outward beyond the lip corners)
Open lips	Any separation of the lips
Stretch mouth (vertical)	Characterized by a tautness of the lip corners coupled with a pronounced downward pull on the jaw; seen when an already wide open mouth is opened a fraction further by an extra pull at the jaw
Stretch mouth (horizontal)	Appears as a distinct horizontal pull at the corners of the mouth
Lip purse	Lips appear as if an "oo" sound is being pronounced
Taut tongue	Characterized by a raised, cupped tongue with sharp tense edges; the first occurrence of taut tongue is usually easy to see, often occurring with a wide open mouth; after this first occurrence, the mouth may close slightly; taut tongue is still scorable on the basis of the still visible tongue edges
Chin quiver	An obvious high frequency up-down motion of the lower jaw

From Grunau R, Craig K: Pain expression in neonates: facial action and cry, *Pain* 28(3): 399, 1987; Grunau R, Craig K: Facial activity as a measure of neonatal pain expression. In DC Tyler EJ Krane, editors, *Advances in pain, research and therapy*, vol 15, New York, 1990, Raven Press.

Table 11-5
Premature Infant Pain Profile (PIPP)

Infant Study Number: _____

Date/time: _____

Event: _____

Process	Indicator	0	1	2	3	Score
Chart	Gestational age	36 weeks and more	32-35 wk, 6 days	28-31 wk, 6 days	Less than 28 wk	
Observe infant 15 sec	Behavioral state	Active/awake; eyes open; facial movements	Quiet/awake; eyes open; no facial movements	Active/asleep; eyes closed; facial movements	Quiet/asleep; eyes closed; no facial movements	
Observe baseline Heart rate Oxygen saturation						
Observe infant 30 sec	Heart rate Max	0-4 beats/min increase	5-14 beats/min increase	15-24 beats/min increase	25 beats/min or more increase	
	Oxygen saturation Min	0-2.4% decrease	2.5-4.9% decrease	5.0-7.4% decrease	7.5% or more decrease	
	Brow bulge	None 0%-9% of time	Minimum 10%-39% of time	Moderate 40%-69% of time	Maximum 70% of time or more	
	Eye squeeze	None 0%-9% of time	Minimum 10%-39% of time	Moderate 40%-69% of time	Maximum 70% of time or more	
	Nasolabial furrow	None 0%-9% of time	Minimum 10%-39% of time	Moderate 40%-69% of time	Maximum 70% of time or more	
					Total Score	_____

Scoring method for the PIPP
1. Familiarize yourself with each indicator and how it is to be scored by looking at the measure.
2. Score gestational age (from the chart) before you begin.
3. Score behavioral state by observing the infant for 15 seconds immediately before the event.
4. Record baseline heart rate and oxygen saturation.
5. Observe the infant for 30 seconds immediately after the event. You will have to look back and forth from the monitor to the infant's face. Score physiologic and facial action changes seen during that time and record immediately after the observation period.
6. Calculate the final score.
From Stevens B et al: Premature Infant Pain Profile: development and initial validation, *Clin J Pain* 12(1):13, 1996.

Management Guideline suggests that "if care providers are unsure whether a behavior indicates pain, and if there is reason to suspect pain, an analgesic trial can be diagnostic as well as therapeutic."[1] Assessment of pain and delivery of effective pain relieving interventions in daily clinical practice must not be delayed while adequate, objective assessment tools are developed.[91] All health care providers must utilize their highly developed assessment skills, along with input from the parents, to gather information about infant behavioral, physiologic, and hormonal or catabolic

Table 11-6
Neonatal Infant Pain Scale (NIPS) Operational Definitions

Facial Expression

0-Relaxed Muscles	Restful face, neutral expression
1-Grimace	Tight facial muscles; furrowed brow, chin, jaw (negative facial expression—nose, mouth, and brow)

Cry

0-No Cry	Quiet, not crying
1-Whimper	Mild moaning, intermittent
2-Vigorous Cry	Loud scream; rising, shrill, continuous (Note: Silent cry may be scored if baby is intubated as evidenced by obvious mouth and facial movement.)

Breathing Patterns

0-Relaxed	Usual pattern for this infant
1-Change in Breathing	Indrawing, irregular, faster than usual; gagging; breath holding

Arms

0-Relaxed/Restrained	No muscular rigidity; occasional random movements of arms
1-Flexed/Extended	Tense, straight arms; rigid and/or rapid extension, flexion

Legs

0-Relaxed/Restrained	No muscular rigidity; occasional random leg movement
1-Flexed/Extended	Tense, straight legs; rigid and/or rapid extension, flexion

State of Arousal

0-Sleeping/Awake	Quiet, peaceful sleeping or alert and settled
1-Fussy	Alert, restless, and thrashing

From Children's Hospital of Eastern Ontario, 1989.

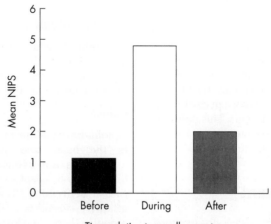

Figure 11-4   Mean NIPS scores over time in 22 infants. (From Lawrence J et al: The development of a tool to assess neonatal pain, *Neonat Net* 12:62, 1993.)

Table 11-7
CRIES: Neonatal Postoperative Pain Assessment Score

	Scoring Criteria for Each Assessment			
	0	1	2	Infant's Score
Crying	No	High-pitched	Inconsolable	_____
Requires O_2 for saturation >95%	No	<30%	>30%	_____
Increased vital signs*	HR and BP within 10% of preoperative value	HR or BP 11%-20% higher than preoperative value	HR or BP 21% or more above preoperative value	_____
Expression	None	Grimace	Grimace/grunt	_____
Sleepless	No	Wakes at frequent intervals	Constantly awake	_____
			Total score†	_____

From Krechel S, Bildner J: Neonatal pain assessment tool developed at the University of Missouri-Columbia.
*BP should be done last.
†Add scores for all assessments to calculate total score.

stress responses before, during, and after painful stimuli. These same assessment skills enable care providers and parents to evaluate the effectiveness of pharmacologic and comfort interventions and institute more and/or different interventions as necessary to relieve pain and suffering.

Laboratory Data

Hormonal and metabolic changes are listed in Box 11-1. Serum glucose levels and reagent test strips monitor for hyperglycemia, which may result in increased serum osmolality and increase the risk of intraventricular hemorrhage (IVH). Glucosuria, ketonuria, and proteinuria result in elevated specific gravity. Metabolic acidosis may result from increased serum levels of lactate, pyruvate, ketones, and nonesterified fatty acids. This data may also be indicative of other serious neonatal problems (e.g., sepsis, acute tubular necrosis).

Treatment

The neonate relies on the skilled observations, assessment, and interventions of care providers for prompt, safe, and effective relief. Limiting factors in providing adequate analgesia in these patients

has been an unfamiliarity with medication doses, regional techniques, and concern over increased drug sensitivity in neonates. Since routine care can be irritating to newborns, differentiating between agitation, which may respond well to comfort measures, and pain, which won't, is mandatory. Opioids are the mainstay of pharmacologic treatment; however, there are other useful medications and techniques that may be used for pain relief.

Pharmacologic

Absorption, metabolism, distribution, and clearance of drugs in the neonate differs from the older child and adult (see Chapter 9). These differences are summarized in Table 11-8.

Opioids

Opioids have their primary effect on the μ-receptor in the brain and spinal cord. High-affinity μ-receptors are associated with analgesia, and low-affinity μ-receptors are associated with respiratory depression. There may be fewer high-affinity μ-receptors in the newborn that are less sensitive to the analgesic effects of opioids. Higher initial doses of opioids may therefore be required for effect, which may in turn increase the risk of respiratory depression. Decreased protein binding, drug metabolism, and drug clearance may contribute to higher plasma and CNS concentrations and prolonged drug effect.[39]

All the opioids have similar mechanisms of action; however, there are a few important differences in side effects[98] (Table 11-9). Morphine commonly causes hypotension in dehydrated patients or when used in high doses. Fentanyl is the preferred drug in many NICUs because of its cardiovascular stability and its ability to decrease pulmonary vascular resistance. It can, however, cause chest wall rigidity and decreased lung compliance if administered too quickly. Neuromuscular blocking agents or slow administration of the drug will prevent this problem.[39,67,98] Fentanyl is also commonly used in patients on ECMO to provide sedation and analgesia and to prevent increases in pulmonary vascular resistance and pressure.[63] Sufentanil is 10 times more potent than fentanyl and significantly more expensive. It is shorter acting and can have even greater effects on lung and chest wall compliance.

Dosing by prn schedule may result in peaks and valleys of pain relief and increases in side effects. Since analgesia is most effective if given before the peak of pain (wind-up), continuous infusions or regular dosing can help prevent undue neonatal suffering.[87] Figure 11-5 on page 191 illustrates the variability in serum levels of analgesia with prn and continuous dose, loading dose, and breakthrough pain.

Local Anesthetics

Local anesthetics (LAs) have a variety of uses and provide analgesia by preventing the transmission of noxious stimuli either at the peripheral receptor site or the spinal cord. Bupivacaine and lidocaine are the two most commonly used LAs (see Table 11-9).

Bupivacaine is longer acting but more cardiotoxic than lidocaine. Both are more toxic in neonates than in adults because of increased organ sensitivity and free fraction of drug. The cardiovascular toxicity may be enhanced if epinephrine containing LAs is used.[32]

Regional Technique. Regional techniques provide good analgesia without the need for a lot of opioids (Table 11-10, p. 192). Advantages include

---

Box 11-3

Critical Questions to Ask About Pain Management in the Neonate

Is the infant being adequately assessed at appropriate intervals?

Are analgesics ordered for prevention and relief of pain?

Is the analgesic strong enough for the pain expected or the pain being experienced?

Is the timing of the drug administration appropriate for the pain expected or being experienced?

Is the route of administration appropriate (preferably PO or IV) for the infant?

Is the infant adequately monitored for side effects?

Are side effects appropriately managed?

Has the analgesic regimen provided adequate comfort and satisfaction from the family's perspective?

Questions to Consider Regarding Nonpharmacologic Strategies:

Is the strategy appropriate for the infant's developmental level, condition, and type of pain?

Is the timing of the strategy sufficient to optimize its effects?

Is the strategy adequately effective in preventing or alleviating the infant's pain?

Is the family satisfied with the strategy for prevention or relief of pain?

(From Acute Pain Management Guideline Panel: *Acute pain management: operative or medical procedures and trauma: clinical practice guideline,* AHCPR Pub No 92-0032, Rockville, Md, 1992, Agency for Health Care Policy and Research, Public Health Service, US Dept HHS.)

---

the following: (1) stress responses are significantly decreased, (2) normal respiratory patterns return more quickly, (3) the need for postoperative ventilation may be avoided or shortened, (4) intestinal motility recovers more quickly, and (5) morbidity decreases with the use of regional techniques,[26] particularly epidural blocks.[26,73]

Dorsal Penile Nerve/Ring Block. Dorsal penile nerve block is extremely easy to perform with

Table 11-8
Pharmacologic Differences Between Newborns and Adults[82]

Differences	Cause	Effect
Altered gastric acidity	Presence of alkaline amniotic fluids at birth Immature gastric mucosa Consumption of alkaline milk	Variable drug absorption
Decreased gastric emptying time		Increased absorption of some drugs
Decreased protein binding	Lower levels of albumin, a-acid glycoprotein Increased competition for binding sites by endogenous substances (bilirubin)	Increased levels of free drug (opioids, local anesthetics)
Increased volume of distribution	Larger volume of body water in the newborn	Larger initial dose may be needed for effect (neuromuscular blocking agents, local anesthetics)
Decreased drug metabolism	Immature liver enzyme systems	Prolonged effect of some medications (morphine, fentanyl, neuromuscular blockers)
Decreased drug clearance	Immature renal system and decreased glomerular filtration rate	Prolonged effect of some medications (morphine)

a high degree of success that can provide surgical anesthesia for circumcision. The block is performed by injecting 1% lidocaine 3 to 5 mm below the skin at the 2 o'clock and 10 o'clock positions on the dorsum of the penis (Fig. 11-6, p. 192).[67] In a full-term neonate, 0.5 ml/side is used, and 0.2 ml/kg/side is used in premature infants. An alternate technique less likely to cause hematoma is to inject a subcutaneous ring of 0.5% or 1.0% lidocaine around the base of the penis. All solutions should be *without epinephrine.*

Epidural Block. The epidural space is an area surrounding the dura of the spinal cord. This space can be accessed from the caudal, lumbar, or thoracic region. An epidural block is performed by a skilled pediatric anesthesiologist, often under general anesthesia.[31,68,73] A small catheter can be left in the space or a one-time dose of medication can be given. Local anesthetics act by anesthetizing either the local nerve roots or the spinal tracts at the level of the spinal cord where they are placed. The most commonly used medications are the local anesthetics lidocaine or bupivacaine. They are often used in combination with low doses of opioids, which have both a local and systemic action.

The major advantages of these techniques are the ability to provide continuous pain relief and the potential to minimize adverse effects and hasten recovery.

EMLA and Infiltration. Eutectic mixture of local anesthetic (EMLA) is a local anesthetic cream that anesthetizes the skin. It can be used for a variety of procedures (lumbar puncture, venipuncture).[56] Use of EMLA in circumcision is still under investigation, but at least one study has shown that it is more effective than placebo in decreasing tachycardia and facial grimacing.[15] Unfortunately, EMLA does not appear to alleviate pain resulting from heelsticks.[59,69] Infiltration of local anesthetic can also help decrease pain for such procedures as placement of percutaneous central lines, removal of broviac catheters, and circumcision.[12] Methemoglobinemia does not appear to be a problem in premature neonates, but studies are ongoing to address this issue.[59]

Other Medications

Acetaminophen and nonsteroidal antiinflammatory drugs can be helpful in providing mild to

Table 11-9
Analgesics and Sedatives for the Neonate

Drug	Dosage	Comments
Analgesics		
Narcotic		
Morphine	0.05-0.2 mg/kg/dose q2-4h prn IV, IM, or SC Continuous IV infusion: 10-15 µg/kg/h	CNS and respiratory depressant; bronchospasms; peripheral vasodilation with hypovolemic infants; hypotension; decreases intestinal motility; increases intracranial pressure; easily reversed with naloxone; slower onset but longer duration than fentanyl; withdrawal symptoms may occur.
Fentanyl (Sublimaze)	1-5 µg/kg/dose q1-2h prn IV or SC Continuous IV infusion: 1-5 µg/kg/hr	Same as morphine. Rapid onset of action; decreases motor activity; does not increase intracranial pressure in the absence of respiratory depression; easily reversed with naloxone; short duration of action; may cause bradycardia, hypotension, apnea, seizures, or rigidity if given too rapidly; withdrawal symptoms occur with prolonged use.
Sufentanil citrate (Sufenta)	0.5-1 µg/kg/dose q30min to 1 hr	Ten times more potent than Fentanyl; has a quicker onset and shorter duration of action than Fentanyl. Use with caution in neonates with IVH, hepatic or renal impairment, or pulmonary disease. Same side effects as in Fentanyl, above.
Nonnarcotic		
Acetaminophen (Tylenol)	10-15 mg/kg/dose q4-6h PO or PR	May cause hepatotoxicity in overdose. Potentiates effects of narcotics but alone does *NOT* relieve surgical pain. Do not use in G6PD deficiency patients.
Ibuprofen (Advil, Motrin)	4-10 mg/kg/dose q6-8hr PO	Gastric irritant—administer with or after feeding; use with caution in neonates with NEC, impaired renal function, hypertension, or compromised cardiac function.
Local		
Lidocaine	0.5%-1% solution (to avoid systemic toxicity, volume should be <0.5 ml/kg of 1% lidocaine solution—5 mg/kg)	Local infiltration anesthesia for invasive procedures; use solution *without epinephrine* to avoid vasoconstriction
Bupivicaine	2.5 mg/kg one time epidural dose Continuous IV infusion: 0.2 mg/kg/hr (max dose)	Monitor for CNS (i.e., seizures, irritability) and cardiotoxic (i.e., ventricular dysrhythmias) side effects. Monitor catheter site integrity. Epidural infusion is titrated to effect but *MUST NOT* exceed maximum dose.
EMLA (Lidocaine and Prilocaine)	2.5-5 g to site for at least 60 min	Vasoconstriction at the site. Site must be covered with water-impermeable dressing (i.e, Tegaderm), Prilocaine's metabolism may result in methemoglobinemia, which may decrease tissue oxygenation.
Sedatives/ Hypnotics *Barbiturates*		Do *not* provide pain relief; help reduce agitation precipitated by painful events. Frequently produce hyperalgesia and increased reaction to painful stimuli—contraindiated for neonates who have pain and also require sedation.

IV, Intravenously; *IM,* intramuscularly; *SC,* subcutaneously; *prn,* as needed; *PO,* per os; *PR,* per rectum; *G6PD,* glucose-6-phosphate dehydrogenase; *IVH,* intraventricular hemorrhage.

Continued

Table 11-9
Analgesics and Sedatives for the Neonate—cont'd

Drug	Dosage	Comments
Phenobarbital	Loading: 10-20 mg/kg IV to max 40 mg/kg Maintenance: 5-7 mg/kg in 2 divided doses beginning 12 hr after last loading dose	Prolonged sedation possible once therapeutic levels achieved (20-25 mg/ml); depresses CNS—motor and respiratory; slow onset of action; little or no pain relief; not easily reversed; withdrawal symptoms may occur; incompatible with other drugs in solution.
Nonbarbiturates		
Chloral hydrate	10-30 mg/kg/dose q6h prn PO to max daily dose of 50 mg/kg/day; PR	Gastric irritant—administer with or after feeding; paradoxic excitement; prolonged use associated with direct hyperbilirubinemia;[58] not to be used for analgesia; respiratory depressant.
Diazepam (Valium)	0.02-0.3 mg/kg IV, IM, or PO q6-8h	Do not dilute injection; venous sclerosing; may displace bilirubin and result in kernicterus; respiratory depression; hypotension; may cause agitation; induces sleep; relaxes muscles; withdrawal symptoms may occur; no analgesic effect; this drug should be used with caution in the neonate.
Lorazepam (Ativan)	0.05-0.1 mg/kg/dose IV (give over ≥3 min) q4-8h	Respiratory depressant, partial airway obstruction, drowsiness; respiratory depression potentiated when narcotics or barbiturates also being given; infuse slowly to avoid apnea, bradycardia, and hypotension.
Midazolam (Versed)	0.05-0.2 mg/kg/dose IV (give over ≥3 min) q4-8h prn Continuous IV infusion: 0.2-6 µg/kg/min	Same as above; continuous IV infusion enables precise titration until sedative effect obtained; calms agitated infant on ventilator.

IV, Intravenously; *IM,* intramuscularly; *SC,* subcutaneously; *prn,* as needed; *PO,* per os; *PR,* per rectum; *G6PD,* glucose-6-phosphate dehydrogenase; *IVH,* intraventricular hemorrhage.

moderate analgesia (see Table 11-9). These medications are more effective when administered on a regular schedule and can augment the effects of narcotics. Sedatives can help decrease agitation and improve comfort but do not by themselves provide analgesia.[12,39]

Comfort Measures

Comfort measures alone do not relieve pain; however, their use reduces agitation, which indirectly reduces pain by promoting behavioral organization, relaxation, general comfort, and sleep.[43,87] Nonnutritive sucking (e.g., on own fingers, hands, or a pacifier) soothes by reducing the infant's level of arousal and duration of cry while increasing the quiet alert state.[22,23,33,72] Distressed infants offered oral sucrose calmed quickly, stayed calm longer, and spent more time in quiet alert state than infants offered only a pacifier.[17,81,88] Sucking soothes, reduces heart and metabolic rates, induces hand-to-mouth behavior, and elevates the pain threshold through opioid and nonopioid systems.[18] Picking up, holding, and rocking provide tactile soothing, vestibular stimulation, and the soothing of rhythmic, repetitive movement.

Body containment of extremities in a flexed position (e.g., holding, swaddling, nesting; provision of opportunity to grasp a finger or pacifier) decreases gross motor movements that contribute to the infant's increased level of arousal, reduces physiologic and behavioral stress, and facilitates energy conservation in the preterm.[22,94] Improper body position contributes to discomfort and pain. Facilitated tucking, gentle containment of flexed extremities in the midline on the trunk while sidelying or supine, during a painful procedure (e.g., heelstick) results in lower heart rate, shorter crying time, less sleep disruption, and fewer sleep-state changes.[25] Motoric boundaries (e.g., containment of extremities) assist the preterm infant in maintaining a more secure, controlled response and facilitating self regulation. Therapeutic interventions include the use of positions that support flexion and restrain in physiologic position, periodic release of restraint and exercise of extremities, gentle change in body position, and positioning to guard operative sites. Along with comfort measures, minimizing stimulation in the NICU environment enables the neonate who is agitated and/or in pain to use internal and external resources in organizing his or her behavior and developing self-soothing strategies (see Chapter 12). Individualizing these techniques to the infant's likes and dislikes and listing these at the bedside helps to maintain consistency of care and builds trust in these developing neonates.[41,76]

Activation of cutaneous sensory nerves (transcutaneous electrical nerve stimulation [TENS] unit) and thermal (topical skin refrigerant) blocks inhibit transmission of peripheral pain impulses from procedural pain.[64,65] Low-frequency, monotonous sounds (e.g., heartbeat, vacuums) quiet and increase behavioral organization.[64] Use of music (see Chapter 12) and tape recordings of family voices soothe both term and preterm infants resulting in fewer state changes, less time in the arousal state, and increased behavioral organization.[24,55,61] However, during circumcision, music (with or without a pacifier) is not an effective distraction or soothing strategy for the pain of the procedure.[66]

Although comfort measures may prevent the intensification of pain (e.g., guarding an abdominal incision by positioning is less painful than four-point restraint), they may not relieve moderate to severe pain. Comfort measures are helpful but inadequate by themselves, considering the inten-

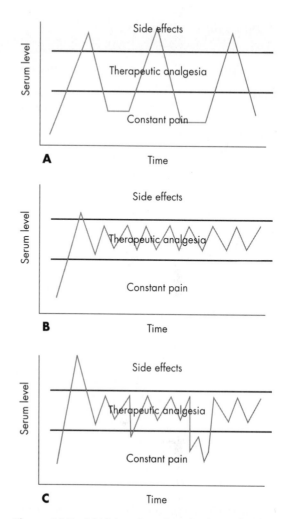

Figure 11-5 Administration of analgesic medication. **A,** Prn administration results in peaks and troughs in serum levels of analgesia. **B,** Continuous or around-the-clock administration produces effective pain relief with lower doses of analgesia and fewer side effects. **C,** Loading dose represented in first elevated serum level. Breakthrough pain (i.e., situational pain that "breaks through" baseline analgesia) requires additional analgesia and/or nonpharmacologic interventions. (From Hester N, Foster R: Integrating pediatric postoperative pain management into clinical practice, *Journal of Pharmaceutical Care in Pain & Symptoms Control* 1:5, 1993.)

Table 11-10
Types of Regional Blockade: Potential Uses and Complications

Block	Potential Uses	Complications
Spinal	Avoidance of general anesthesia for surgery below the umbilicus	Inability to access space, incomplete block or inadequate duration of anesthesia
Caudal/epidural	Intraoperative and postoperative analgesia for thoracic, abdominal, perineal, and lower extremity surgery	Inadequate block; local or opioid related toxicity; nerve damage, paralysis
Dorsal penile nerve/ ring block	Circumcision, analgesia for any penile surgery	Hematoma formation; end organ damage if epinephrine-containing solutions are used
Intercostal nerve block	Rib fractures, thoracic surgery	Pneumothorax; local anesthetic toxicity (highest rate of absorption)

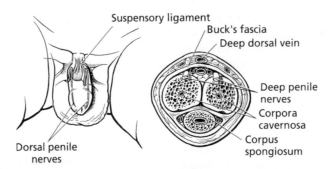

Figure 11-6   Anatomic landmarks for placement of a dorsal penile nerve block. (From McClain B, Anand KJS: Neonatal pain management. In Deshpande J, Tobias J, editors: *The pediatric pain handbook,* St Louis, 1996, Mosby.)

sity of the noxious stimuli causing moderate to severe pain.[25,66]

Complications

The neonate's complex behavioral response to pain has both short- and long-term ramifications. These behavioral changes may disrupt parent-infant interaction and attachment, adaptation to the postnatal environment, and feeding behaviors.[4] An alteration in brain development and maldevelopment of sensory systems can occur when distorted or inappropriate sensory input occurs during a critical period in development.[11] Because of a neonate's memory, painful experi-ences increase his or her sensitivity to subsequent medical encounters.[34,83,93] These initial experiences may affect the development of attitudes, fears, anxiety, conflicts, wishes, expectations, and patterns of interactions with others.[95]

As previously mentioned, unanesthetized surgery and/or unrelieved pain causes suffering that might itself be a risk to life.[4,28] Maintaining metabolic homeostasis by the appropriate use of anesthetics and analgesics improves postoperative outcome by preventing (1) protein wasting, (2) electrolyte imbalance, (3) impaired immune function, (4) sepsis, (5) metabolic acidosis, (6) pulmonary and cardiac insufficiency, (7) hypermetabolic state, and (8) death.[8,9,52]

Narcotic analgesics may produce respiratory

depression severe enough to require mechanical ventilation. Naloxone (0.1 mg/kg IV or IM) is the specific antidote for narcotic overdose. Lower doses of naloxone (0.001 to 0.01 mg/kg IV or IM) can be used for moderate respiratory depression. An ampule of neonatal naloxone should always be immediately available with the appropriate dose precalculated on the infant's emergency card. Respiratory depression may produce hypoxemia so that a pulse oximeter should be standard equipment along with cardiorespiratory monitoring. If available, TcP_{CO_2} monitors should also be used to watch for hypercapnia. All equipment for assisted ventilation should be at the bedside.

An overdose of local anesthetics can cause seizures, ventricular tachycardia, bradycardia, and cardiovascular collapse. Toxic doses for neonates should be carefully calculated, and lower doses should be administered. Benzodiazepines or phenobarbital can be used to treat refractive seizures; cardiopulmonary resuscitation (CPR) and defibrillation may be necessary to treat the cardiovascular complications.[32] Patients who are receiving epidural analgesia for postoperative pain control need to be monitored for signs of potential CNS toxicity (e.g., irritability, jitteriness, twitching, myoclonic jerking.) If an opioid is being administered with the local anesthetic infusion, then respiratory depression is also a possibility and patients should be monitored as described above. Other extremely rare complications of epidurals are nerve injury or paralysis.

Hematoma formation can occur (1.2%) with the placement of a dorsal penile nerve block.[37] Using a ring block usually avoids this problem. Epinephrine-containing solutions *must never be used,* since this can lead to compromise of the blood supply to the penis and severe tissue damage.

Tolerance and Withdrawal[39,98]

Tolerance is the need for escalating doses of drug to achieve the same effect. Physical dependence is the state wherein continued drug is needed to prevent the signs of withdrawal. Withdrawal arises when discontinuing the drug causes symptoms such as irritability, diarrhea, tachycardia, hypertension, insomnia, restlessness, diaphoresis, or palmar sweating and muscle twitches. Addiction oc-

curs when there is psychological as well as physical dependence, and is associated with active drug-seeking behavior and use (abuse) of the drugs for nonmedical conditions. Tolerance, dependence, and withdrawal can occur with opioids and benzodiazepines; however, addiction is exceedingly rare when these medications are used for medical purposes. Medications should not be restricted because of fear of addiction. Critically ill infants sometimes need long-term infusions of opioids or benzodiazepines to provide analgesia and sedation. ECMO and prolonged mechanical ventilation are two examples of this situation. Use of fentanyl for more than 5 to 7 days can lead to tolerance and withdrawal (also known as opioid abstinence syndrome). Opioid use should be decreased by no more than 10% to 20% every 1 to 3 days, depending on the duration of the medication's use and the infant's response to the changes. Shorter-acting medications such as fentanyl and midazolam can be switched to methadone and lorazepam, which have the advantage of being longer acting as well as being available in an oral form. In addition, minimal handling and a quiet, darkened environment help decrease external stimuli. A pacifier, swaddling, and holding are effective comfort measures.

Parent Teaching

Parents are excellent observers of their infant and often recognize when the infant is experiencing pain even before the care provider does.[76] The health care provider loses credibility when he or she does not acknowledge the infant's pain. Listening to parents' concerns about their infant's pain, including the parent's report of their assessment, communication of the plan of care regarding analgesia and/or sedation, and offering the rationale behind the medication decision-making help the parents become active participants in the management of their infant's pain. Parents of medically fragile infants have identified specific sources of stress in the NICU: (1) parental role alterations, especially inability to comfort the infant and (2) infant appearance and behavior, especially pain and difficulty breathing.[20] The most common fear expressed by parents is that their infant will experience undue pain while being cared for in the

NICU.[76] **The care provider's sensitivity to the neonate's pain and advocating for pain relief are comforting for parents.**[82] **Teaching parents to report their assessments and encouraging parents to comfort their infants will help them in the attachment process and foster a trusting relationship with the health care team. Comfort measures are ideally provided by parents who may then actively participate in their infant's pain relief.**

References

1. Acute Pain Management Guideline Panel: *Acute pain management: operative or medical procedures and trauma, clinical practice guideline,* AHCPR Pub No 92-0032, Rockville, Md, 1992, Agency for Health Care Policy and Research, Public Health Service, US Dept HHS.
2. Als H: Toward a synactive theory of development: promise for the assessment and support of infant individuality, *Infant Mental Health Journal* 3:299, 1982.
3. American Academy of Pediatrics, Committee on Fetus and Newborn, Committee on Drugs, Section on Anesthesiology and Section on Surgery: Neonatal anesthesia, *Pediatrics* 80:446, 1987.
4. Anand KJS, Hickey PR: Pain and its effect in the human neonate and fetus, *N Engl J Med* 317:1321, 1987.
5. Anand KJS, Sippel WG, Aynsley-Green A: Randomized trial of fentanyl anesthesia in preterm neonates undergoing surgery: effects on the stress response, *Lancet* 1:62, 1987.
6. Anand KJS, et al.: Does halothane anesthesia decrease the metabolic and endocrine stress responses of newborn infants undergoing operation? *Br J Med* 296:668, 1988.
7. Anand KJS, Carr DB: The neuroanatomy, neurophysiology and neurochemistry of pain, stress and analgesia in newborns and children, *Pediatr Clin North Am* 36:795, 1989.
8. Anand KJS: Neonatal stress response to anesthesia and surgery, *Clin Perinatol* 17(1):207, 1990.
9. Anand KJS, Hickey PR: Halothane-morphine compared with high-dose sufentanil for anesthesia and post-operative analgesia in neonatal cardiac surgery, *N Eng J Med* 326:1, 1992.
10. Anand KJS: Relationship between stress responses and clinical outcomes in newborns, infants and children, *Crit Care Med* 21:S358, 1993.
11. Anders T, Zeanah C: Early infant development from a biological point of view. In Call J, Galenson E, Tyson R, editors: *Frontiers of infant psychiatry,* New York, 1984, Basic Books.
12. Anderson C, Zeltzer L, Fanurik D: Procedural pain. In Schecter N, Berde C, Yaster M, editors: *Pain in infants, children and adolescents,* Baltimore, 1993, Williams & Wilkins.
13. Barker D, Rutter N: Exposure to invasive procedures in neonatal intensive care unit admissions, *Arch Dis Child* 72:F47, 1995.
14. Bauchner H, May A, Coates E: Use of analgesic agents for invasive medical procedures in pediatric and neonatal intensive care units, *J Pediatr* 4:647, 1992.
15. Benini F et al: Topical anesthesia during circumcision in newborn infants, *JAMA* 270:850, 1993.
16. Bildner J, Krechel S: Increasing staff nurse awareness of post operative pain management in the NICU, *Neonat Net* 15:11, 1996.
17. Blass EM, Hoffmeyer LB: Sucrose as an analgesic for newborn infants, *Pediatrics* 87:215, 1991.
18. Blass E: Behavioral and physiological consequences of suckling in rat and human newborns, *Acta Paediatr Suppl* 397:71, 1994.
19. Broome ME, Tanzillo H: Differentiating between pain and agitation in premature neonates, *J Perinat Neonat Nurs* 4(1):53, 1990.
20. Brunssen S, Miles M: Sources of environmental stress experienced by mothers of hospitalized medically fragile infants, *Neonat Net* 15:88, 1996.
21. Burdeau G, Kleiber C: Clinical indicators of infant irritability, *Neonat Net* 9(5):23, 1991.
22. Campos RG: Soothing pain-elicited distress in infants with swaddling and pacifiers, *Child Dev* 60:781, 1989.
23. Campos R: Soothing neonate's response to a stressful procedure, *Neonat Net* 12:93, 1993.
24. Collins S, Kuch K: Music therapy in the NICU, *Neonat Net* 9:23, 1991.
25. Corff K, et al: Facilitated tucking: a nonpharmacologic comfort measure for pain in preterm neonates, *J Obstet Gynecol Neonat Nurs* 24:143, 1995.
26. Cousins M: Acute and postoperative pain. In Wall P, Melzack R, editors: *Textbook of pain,* Edinburgh, 1994, Churchill Livingstone.
27. Craig K et al: Pain in the preterm neonate: behavioral and physiological indices, *Pain* 52:287, 1993.
28. Cunningham N: Ethical perspectives on the perception and treatment of neonatal pain, *J Perinat Neonatal Nurs* 4(1):75, 1990.
29. Devor M: Pain mechanism and pain syndromes. In Campbell J, editor: *Pain 1996. An updated review,* Seattle, 1996, IASP Press.
30. Dickenson A: Pharmacology of pain transmission and control. In Campbell J, editor: *Pain 1996. An updated review,* Seattle, 1996, IASP Press.
31. Ecoffey C, Dubousset A, Samii K: Lumbar and thoracic epidural anesthesia for urologic and upper abdominal surgery in infants and children, *Anesthesiology* 65:87, 1986.
32. Eyres R: Local anesthetic agents in infancy, *Paediatric Anaesthesia* 5:213, 1995.
33. Field T, Goldson E: Pacifying effects of non-nutritive sucking on term and preterm neonates during heelstick procedures, *Pediatrics* 74(6):1012, 1984.
34. Fitzgerald M, Millard C, Macintosh N: Hyperalgesia in premature infants, *Lancet* 1:292, 1988.
35. Fitzgerald M, Anand KJS: Developmental neuroanatomy and neurophysiology of pain. In Schector N, Berde C, Yastor M, editors: *Pain in infants, children and adolescents,* Baltimore, 1993, Williams & Wilkins.

36. Fitzgerald M: Neurobiology of fetal and neonatal pain. In Wall P, Melzad R, editors: *Textbook of pain.* Edinburgh, 1994, Churchhill Livingstone.

37. Fontaine P, Dittberner D, Scheltema K: The safety of dorsal penile nerve block for neonatal circumcision, *J Fam Prac* 39:243, 1994.

38. Franck LS: A national survey of the assessment and treatment of pain and agitation in the NICU, *J Obstet Gynecol Neonat Nurs* 16:387, 1987.

39. Franck L, Gregory G: Clinical evaluation and treatment of infant pain in the neonatal intensive care unit. In Schecter N, Berde C, Yastor M, editors: *Pain in infants, children and adolescents,* Baltimore, 1993, Williams & Wilkins.

40. Franck L: Identification, management, and prevention of pain in the neonate. In Kenner C, Brueggemeyer A, Gunderson L, editors: *Comprehensive neonatal nursing: a physiologic perspective,* Philadelphia, 1993, WB Saunders.

41. Grossman R, Lawhon G: Individualized supportive care to reduce pain and stress. In Anand KJS, McGrath P, editors: *Pain in neonates,* Amsterdam, 1995, Elsevier.

42. Goldstein R, Brazy J: Narcotic sedation stabilizes arterial blood pressure fluctuations in sick premature infants, *J Perinatol* 11:365, 1991.

43. Gruenwald P, Becker P: Developmental enhancement: implementing a program for the NICU, *Neonat Net* 9(6):29, 1991.

44. Grunau RVE, Craig KD: Pain expression in neonates: facial action and cry, *Pain* 28:395, 1987.

45. Grunau R, Johnston C, Craig K: Neonatal facial and cry responses to invasive and non-invasive procedures, *Pain* 42:295, 1990.

46. Grunau R et al: Extremely low birth weight (ELBW) toddlers are relatively unresponsive to pain at 18 mo. corrected age compared to larger birth weight children, *Abstract 18,* Proceedings of the Neonatal Society, 1993.

47. Grunau R, Whitfield M, Petrie J: Pain sensitivity and temperament in extremely low-birth weight premature toddlers and preterm and full term controls, *Pain* 58:341, 1994.

48. Grunau R et al: Early pain experience, child and family factors, as precursors of somatization: a prospective study of extremely premature and full term children, *Pain* 56:353, 1994.

49. Herzog JM: A neonatal intensive care syndrome: a pain complex involving neuroplasticity and psychic trauma. In Galenson E, Tyson RL, editors: *Frontiers in infant psychiatry,* New York, 1983, Basic Books.

50. Hester N, Foster R: Integrating pediatric postoperative pain management into clinical practice, *Journal of Pharmaceutical Care and Symptom Control* 1:5, 1993.

51. Johnston CC, O'Shaughnessy D: Acoustical attributes of pain cries: distinguishing features. In Dubner R, Gebbart GF, Bond MR, editors: *Advances in pain research,* New York, 1988, Raven.

52. 52. Johnston CC, Stevens B: Pain assessement in newborns, *J Perinat Neonat Nurs* 4(1):41, 1990.

53. Johnston C et al: Developmental changes in pain expression in premature, full term, two and four month old infants, *Pain* 52:201, 1993.

54. Johnston C, Stevens B: Experience in a neonatal intensive care unit affects pain response, *Pediatrics* 98:925, 1996.

55. Kaminski J, Hall W: The effect of soothing music on neonatal behavioral states in the hospital newborn nursery, *Neonat Net* 15:45, 1996.

56. Koren G: Use of eutectic mixture of local anesthetics in young children for procedure-related pain, *J Pediatr* 122:530, 1993.

57. Krechel S, Bildner J: CRIES: a new neonatal postoperative pain measurement score: initial testing of validity and reliability, *Pediatric Anaesthesia* 5:53, 1995.

58. Lambert GH et al: Direct hyperbilirubinemia associated with chloral hydrate administration in the newborn, *Pediatrics* 86:277, 1990.

59. Larsson B et al: Does a local anesthetic cream (EMLA) alleviate pain from heel lancing in neonates? *Acta Anaesthesiol Scand* 39:1028, 1995.

60. Lawrence J et al: The development of a tool to assess neonatal pain, *Neonat Net* 12:59, 1993.

61. Leonard J: Music therapy: fertile ground for application of research in practice, *Neonat Net* 12:47, 1993.

62. Lepley M et al: High-risk obstetrical care. In Gardner S, Hagedorn M, editors: *Legal aspects of maternal child nursing practice,* Menlo Park, Calif, 1997, Addison-Wesley.

63. Leuschen M et al: Plasma fentanyl levels in infants undergoing extracorporeal membrane oxygenation, *J Thorac Cardiovas Surg* 105:885, 1993.

64. Lynam L: Research utilization: nonpharmacological management of pain in neonates, *Neonat Net* 14:59, 1995.

65. Maikler V: Effects of a skin refrigerant/anesthetic and age on the pain response of infants requiring immunizations, *Res Nur Health* 14:397, 1991.

66. Marchette L et al: Pain reduction interventions during neonatal circumcision, *Nurs Res* 40(4):241, 1991.

67. McClain B, Anand KJS: Neonatal pain management. In Deshpande J, Tobias J, editors: *The pediatric pain handbook,* St Louis, 1996, Mosby.

68. McGown R: Caudal analgesia in children: 500 cases for procedures below the diaphragm, *Anaesthesia* 37:806, 1982.

69. McIntosh N, Van Veen L, Brameyer H: Alleviation of the pain of heel prick in preterm infants, *Arch Dis Child* 70:F177, 1994.

70. Mersky H: Clarification of chronic pain: disruption of chronic pain syndromes and definition of pain terms, *Pain* (Suppl)3:51, 1986.

71. Meyer R, Campbell J, Raja S: Peripheral neural mechanisms of nociception. In Wall P, Melzack R, editors: *Textbook of pain,* Edinburgh, 1994, Churchill Livingstone.

72. Miller H, Anderson G: Nonnutritive sucking: effects on crying and heart rate in intubated infants requiring assisted mechanical ventilation, *Nurs Res* 42:305, 1993.

73. Murrell D, Gibson P, Cohen R: Continuous epidural analgesia in newborn infants undergoing major surgery, *J Pediatr Surg* 28:548, 1993.

74. National Association of Neonatal Nurses: Position statement on pain management in infants, *Neonat Net* 14:54, 1995.

75. Nurses Association of the American College of Obstetricians and Gynecologists: *Standards for the nursing care of women and newborns,* ed 4, Washington, DC, 1991, Nurses Association of the American College of Obstetricians and Gynecologists.

76. Phillips P: Neonatal pain management: a call to action, *Pediatric Nursing* 21:195, 1995.

77. Pokela M: Effect of opioid-induced analgesia on B-endorphin, cortisol and glucose responses in neonates with cardiorespiratory problems, *Biol Neonate* 64:360, 1993.

78. Pokela M: Pain relief can reduce hypoxemia in distressed neonates during routine treatment procedures, *Pediatrics* 93:379, 1994.

79. Pokela M, Koivisto M: Physiological changes, plasma B-endorphin and cortisol responses to tracheal intubation in neonates, *Acta Paediatr* 83:151, 1994.

80. Porter F: Pain assessment in children and infants. In Schecter N, Bende C, Yaster M, editors: *Pain in infants, children and adolescents,* Baltimore, 1993, Williams & Wilkins.

81. Ramenghi L et al: Reduction of pain responses in premature infants using intraoral sucrose, *Arch Dis Child* 74:F126, 1996.

82. Reed M: Principles of drug therapy. In Behrman R, Kliegman R, Aruon A, editors: *Textbook of pediatrics,* ed 15, Philadelphia, 1996, WB Saunders.

83. Rovee-Collier C, Hayne H: Reactuation of infant memory: implications for cognitive development, *Adv Child Dev* 10:185, 1987.

84. Rushforth J, Levere M: Behavioral response to pain in healthy neonates, *Arch Dis Child* 70:F174, 1994.

85. Saigals S et al: Self-perceived health status and health related quality of life of extremely low birth weight infants at adolescence, *JAMA* 276:453, 1996.

86. Schecter N, Berde C, Yaster M: *Pain in infants, children and adolescents,* Baltimore, 1993, Williams & Wilkins.

87. Shapiro C: Pain in the neonate, *Neonat Net* 8(1):7, 1989.

88. Smith BA, Fillion RJ, Blass EM: Orally-mediated sources of calming in 1-3 day old human infants, *Dev Psychol* 26:731, 1990.

89. Snellman L, Stang H: Prospective evaluation of complications of dorsal penile block for neonatal circumcision, *Pediatrics* 95:705, 1995.

90. Stevens B, Johnston C, Hurton L: Factors that influence the behavioral pain responses of premature infants, *Pain* 59:101, 1994.

91. Stevens B, Johnston C, Gruanau R: Issues of assessment of pain and discomfort in neonates, *J Obstet Gynecol Neonat Nurs* 24:849, 1995.

92. Stevens B et al: Premature infant pain profile: development and initial validation, *Clin J Pain* 12(1):13, 1996.

93. Taddio A et al: Effect of neonatal circumcision on pain responses during vaccination in male infants, *Lancet* 345:291, 1995.

94. Taquino L, Blackburn S: The effects of containment during suction and heelstick on physiological and behavioral responses of preterm infants, *Neonat Net* 13:55, 1994.

95. Tyson P: Developmental lines and infant assessment. In Call JD, Galenson E, Tyson RL, editors: *Frontiers of infant psychiatry,* New York, 1984, Basic Books.

96. Van Cleve L et al: Pain responses of hospitalized neonates to venipuncture, *Neonat Net* 14:31, 1995.

97. Vogelpohl D, Evans J, Cedargren D: Behavioral pain response of the LBW premature neonate in the NICU, *Neonatal Intensive Care, Sept/Oct 1995,* p. 28, 1996.

98. Yaster M, Maxwell L: Opioid agonists and antagonists. In Schecter N, Berde C, Yaster M, editors: *Pain in infants, children and adolescents,* Baltimore, 1993, Williams & Wilkins.

Resources for Parents

American Association of Critical Care Nurses: It's critical that you know . . . what you should do when your baby is in the NICU, California, 1987, AACN.

Butler NC: Questions parents and concerned professionals might ask of their local health care institutions, *Birth* 15:40, 1988.

12 The Neonate and the Environment: Impact on Development

Sandra L. Gardner, Lula O. Lubchenco

For centuries the newborn baby has been considered a "tabula rasa"—a blank slate on which parents and the world "write" to create the individual. In the first half of this century, research emphasized the contributions of the environment in shaping the infant and child. Only recently has the individuality of the infant been recognized as a powerful shaper of the care giver, the care given, and thus the environment.

This chapter deals with the psychosocioemotional development of the term and preterm neonate. Infant development depends on the dynamic relationship between *endowment* and *environment.* Along the continuum of development, development of the infant is the beginning of the child and, ultimately, of adult competence in the world. Understanding the dynamic relationship between endowment and environment is enhanced by a review of the principles of development in Box 12-1. First, the developmental tasks of infancy are presented, along with the influences of endowment and environment on mastery. Home and family life, in which most infants are raised, is then contrasted with the experiences of babies in the NICU. Intervention strategies to normalize the NICU environment are then presented, along with strategies for parent teaching. The developmental and social outcomes of infants exposed to the NICU are then briefly discussed.

Developmental Tasks of the Neonate and Infant

Neonates begin extrauterine life able to attend with their sensory capabilities and communicate with their environment through a complex repertoire of behaviors. They are able to accumulate experience in memory. Infancy (birth to 12 months) is the time of further development and maturation of these capabilities through self-mastery and adaptation to the extrauterine environment.

Biorhythmic Balance: Primary Developmental Task of the Newborn

In utero the fetus depends on the mother's physiologic systems to regulate its own. At birth the neonate's basic physiologic needs (feeding, elimination, cleaning, heat balance, stroking, and communicating) are met in new and different ways. Emerging from a physiologically dependent fetus into a physiologically independent neonate introduces new variables for both mother and infant in the development of their extrauterine relationship.

The primary task of the newborn is to reestablish biorhythmic balance by stabilizing the function of sleep-wake cycles, respiratory and heart rates, blood chemistry levels, metabolic processes, and eating patterns.

Although biorhythmic balance is internally determined, care giving interaction between newborn and parent/care giver either facilitates or disturbs this transition. After birth, balance is facilitated by contact with familiar surroundings (i.e., the mother's body) (see Chapter 5).

When immediate recontact between the neonate and the mother is not possible (i.e., the mother refuses or is ill; or the neonate is preterm, sick, or anomalied and requires immediate emergency medical intervention or transport), the primary "mothering" role is temporarily transferred to professional (medical and nursing) care providers. Interactional dynamics necessary for reestablishing biorhythmic balance and fostering the psychosocioemotional development of the newborn are also transferred into the NICU.

Just as in a home or family setting, the infant's personality and behavioral development are affected by the nature and dynamics of the stimuli and relationships encountered with the staff in a nursery or NICU setting.[75] The level of function or dysfunction in the biorhythmic balance affects the neonate's long-range outcomes and is intrinsically interwoven with the development of a sense of self and a basic trust.

Sense of Self

In utero the preonate has continuous tactile-kinesthetic stimulation that develops and matures the CNS and establishes kinesthesis as the most natural pathway for growth and development. The interaction between infants and the extrauterine environment is also kinesthetic. Tactile contact and vestibular stimulation are essential for (1) the development of a physical identity (body image), (2) organization and sorting of stimuli, (3) coordination of sensory-motor skills, (4) a psychologic and social sense of self, (5) normal neurophysiologic development—mental and cognitive abilities, and (6) emotional stability and temperament.[25,105,135,141]

Daily caregiving and interaction (feeding, diapering, holding, playing, etc.) with the parent or care giver provide infants with reciprocal stimuli for further developing their identity. Through the manner in which the infant is handled, he or she receives messages about how the care giver feels about him or her. Response cues given by infants affect the care giver's response to and interaction with them.[8,25,65] Quieting and soothing by the infant in response to caregiving positively reinforces the parent to continue. Withdrawal, irritability, or continuous crying is perceived by the care giver as rejection and may result in parental frustration, withdrawal, and decreased interaction. Repeated exposure to the care giver's style and non-verbal messages thus enables the infant to adopt these patterns of care giving. The self of the infant is formed through interaction with people and objects within the environment.

Because the nature (amount and kind) of the kinesthetic interaction between infants and care givers determines how infants develop and mature, lack of appropriate stimulation has long-term consequences. Stimulus deprivation results in impairment, retardation, or deviancy in skill development for productive living. The degree or extent of impairment depends on the severity of the restrictions and limitations encountered. Studies have demonstrated that infants who were well cared for physically (fed, diapered, cleaned) either died or were seriously impaired (mentally, emotionally, and socially) because of lack of tactile or kinesthetic stimulation.[25,65,159]

Institutionally reared infants who had minimal contact and no social interaction with their care givers displayed significant developmental delays.[137] The effect of kinesthetic deprivation was seen in the minimal expression of social skills (cooing, babbling, crying), minimal interest in objects in the environment, increased self-stimulation (rocking), touch aversion, flat or withdrawn affect, and retarded mental and motor development. Environmental deprivation may also affect the physical growth of the infant.[65] Montagu[126] believes infants are able to overcome mental and nutritional deprivation as long as they are not deprived of tactile stimulation.

The Psychosocial Task: Trust versus Mistrust

Trust versus mistrust in oneself and the environment is solidified during infancy.[8] The response of the environment from the moment of birth is the means by which neonates continue to develop trust in themselves and decide on the reliability of their new environment. Two major factors influence the development of trust versus mistrust: (1) the infant's ability to communicate needs to the environment and (2) the reliability and constancy of the environment in responding.

In the course of routine care giving, the infant associates the care giver with either comfort and trust or with lack of need satisfaction and mistrust. The infant cries to communicate a need (e.g., "I'm hungry"; "I'm wet"). The care giver responds to the infant and meets the need—the infant is fed; the infant is changed. Thus the newborn learns to communicate when the need arises again, because the environment or care giver has responded and will respond. This contingent response of the care giver to the infant's need is the necessary reinforcement for the development of trust in self, in others, and ultimately in humankind. The infant develops a sense of mastery over his or her world and a sense that it is okay to have needs and to have them met.

Care giving that ignores or delays need gratification is noncontingent to the infant's cues for care. Need meeting that is externally defined by the care giver's agenda (e.g., feeding schedule, rigid or inflexible routines, medical or nursing procedures in the NICU) discourages the infant from being aware of and experiencing needs and communicating them. Such infants will eventually detach themselves (emotionally and kinesthetically) from the sensation of their needs, thus no longer experiencing or communicating them.[27,65]

As a result, these infants conclude that they and their needs (which they perceive as one and the same) are *not* important and that they have no effect on their environment. They do not cultivate their sense of self or of their own existence—physically (where their boundaries end and another's begin) or psychologically (their identity that exists independent of another). Some people with severe mistrust in themselves and their environment do not experience the sensation of hunger when hungry or express appropriate emotional responses to situations. They also do not kinesthetically feel where their body ends and another's begins when they are hugging—they totally merge and experience the two as one and the same person. Low self-concept and self-esteem and a sense of helplessness about succeeding in life are a result of lack of trust. Behaviorally this is manifested in touch aversion; avoidance of eye contact; flat, withdrawn, or depressed affect; or hyperactivity, restlessness, low frustration level, demanding behavior and perpetual dissatisfaction, and poor social relationships.[26,105,137,159]

Survival depends on the care giver meeting the newborn's needs. Need meeting is either contingent on the infant's cues or noncontingent on an external agenda. The degree of the mother's emotional investment and connectedness with the newborn will determine the nature and quality of the caregiving. Likewise, the temperament and responsiveness of the infant will affect the mother's feelings of competency, success, and emotional connectedness to her infant.[27,65] Parents who relate to the newborn as an individual (i.e., a person with feelings, wants, and needs; a person who knows what these are) will be sensitive and responsive to the infant's needs and interact with the baby during caregiving. This relationship facilitates the ongoing development of a good sense of self (esteem, confidence, and emotional security) and mastery of the world. Care givers who do not perceive infants as individuals do not respond to their need cry or interact with care giving. This style fosters the development of mistrusting, suspicious, helpless, emotionally insecure, and isolated children and adults.

Endowment

Infants possess innateness and individuality. Primitive reflex behaviors, higher cognitive abilities, temperament, and sensory-motor competencies are the *endowment* of the individual infant. Individual variation and utilization of these components of endowment are influenced by the environment of the newborn.

Even before conception, the genetic endowment of the parents and preceding generations affects the fetus or newborn. Everything that the individual will inherit from his or her parents is determined at the moment of conception. Of the vast number of possible combinations of chromosomes, chance determines which characteristics the individual receives. Thus each individual except monozygotic twins is genetically and biologically different from every other person. Either a faulty gene (e.g., sickle cell anemia) or an altered number of chromosomes (e.g., Down syndrome) is responsible for inherited defects (see Chapter 26).

Even though after the moment of conception hereditary endowment is never able to be changed, it is influenced by the intrauterine environment. Some birth defects are caused by teratogens—any environmental agent (drugs, virus, chemical, pollutant) that interferes with normal fetal development. The individual's potential for growth and development is limited by his or her genetic endowment. As Montagu[77] states, "Genetic endowment determines what we *can* do—environment what we *do* do."

The one exception to individual genetic endowment is identical twins, who share the same heredity. Identical twins have been extensively studied, because it is hypothesized that any differences between them are due to environmental effects. Identical twins raised apart have been found to be more similar in intelligence, temperament, and personality characteristics than are fraternal twins raised together.

Genetic endowment imposes limits on a child's potential. Studies show that children resemble their parents both physically and mentally more than they differ from them. Parental expectations that are unrealistic or beyond the child's capacity may set the child up for disappointment when he or she fails to meet these expectations. All too often abilities and potential are stifled within this environment, so that the child is unable to achieve what is within his or her capability.

The exact influence of genetics for most psychologic traits is unknown. Introverted (timid, shy, withdrawn) and extroverted (active, friendly, and outgoing) personality types may be partially genetically controlled. The degree to which intelligence is inherited is currently unknown, although the intelligence of children is most often similar to parental intelligence (i.e., intelligence is more similar between child and biologic mother than child and adopted mother).

Freedman[62] studied newborns of many ethnic groups to see if there were any similarities in disposition within the group or differences from other ethnic groups. He found that Chinese-American newborns were more adaptable, less irritable, and easier to console than Caucasian-American newborns. Maneuvers such as the Moro and covering the face with a cloth elicited very different responses, depending on the newborn's ethnic origin.

The same environmental stimuli elicit very different behavioral responses, which are individual and genetically influenced. These genetically influenced behaviors are also influenced by environment—both internal and external. Thus an individual may be more vulnerable to or more resilient in a specific environment. Therefore we are totally endowment and totally environment (100% endowment + 100% environment = an individual).[62]

Temperament

Parents often notice behavioral differences in their children from the first day. These differences are obvious in motor activity, irritability, and passivity. Some infants are quiet and placid, others are irritable and easily upset, and others are somewhere in between. Nine categories of behavior that describe individual temperament are outlined in Table 12-1. These temperamental qualities enable three basic types of infants to be identified:

- The "easy" child who is seen as regular, pleasant, and easy to care for and love
- The "difficult" child who is difficult to rear and reacts with protest and withdrawal to strange events or people
- The "slow to warm" child who reacts with withdrawal or passivity to new events

Table 12-1
Behavioral Categories Descriptive of Individual Temperament

Temperamental Quality	Rating
Activity level	*Low*—Decreased movement when dressed or during sleep
	High—Increased movement when asleep; increased wiggling and activity when diaper changed
Rhythmicity	*Regular*—Establishes own feeding; sleep and bowel movement pattern is fairly predictable
	Irregular—Amounts of sleep, feeding variable; "no two days are alike"; no pattern established
Approach and withdrawal	*Positive*—Eagerly tries new foods; interested in new surroundings and people
	Negative—Rejects new foods, new toys, and new environments; apprehensive, cries with new people
Adaptability	*Adaptive*—Little resistance to first bath; may enjoy bath
	Nonadaptive—Startles easily; resists diapering, bathing, and other manipulating
Quality of mood	*Positive*—Pleasant, easygoing disposition; easy to comfort; smiles
	Negative—Fussy; cries easily and is not easily comforted by external stimuli; unable to comfort self easily
Intensity of mood	*Mild*—No crying when wet; frets instead of crying when hungry
	Intense—Vigorously cries; rejects food
Sensory threshold (intensity of stimulus necessary to elicit a response)	*High*—Not startled or interrupted by noise or other stimuli
	Low—Noise, activity, or other stimuli enough to interrupt infant's behavior
Distractibility	*Distractible*—Rocking, pacifier, toy, voice, music will decrease fussing
	Nondistractible—No stimulus will decrease distress until need is met—food; stop changing diaper; bath over
Attention span and persistence	*Short*—Cries when awakened but stops immediately; mild objection if needs are not immediately met
	Long—Repeatedly rejects substitutions for perceived needs (no pacifier until diaper is changed; no water if milk is wanted)

Modified from Thomas A, Chess S: *The dynamics of personality development*, New York, 1980, Brunner/Mazel.

Neurologic Development

Brain growth of the fetus and newborn occurs in two stages.[49]

Stage I. Stage I occurs from 10 to 18 weeks of pregnancy. During this period the number of nerve cells that the individual has is developed. Any environmental occurrence (e.g., maternal malnutrition, medications, infections) that affects brain growth during this stage may also affect neonatal behavioral responses.

Stage II. Stage II occurs from 20 weeks' gestation to 2 years of age. This period marks a brain growth spurt and the most vulnerable period of growth of the dendrites of the human cortex.

The maturity of the infant is reflected in his or her behavior. Infants of a younger gestational age have less mature responses than infants of an older gestational age. A neurologic assessment of the newborn includes evaluation of (1) newborn reflexes, (2) neonatal states, (3) psychosocial interaction, and (4) sensory capabilities. The neonate is born with behaviors that are unlearned, instinctual, and of an adaptive and survival nature. They reflect the state of the nervous system and the level of neonatal maturation (see Fig. 5-4). Table 12-2 summarizes neonatal reflex behaviors, their significance, and the time of their integration into voluntary movement. Serial testing of reflex behavior gives more reliable data than one observation. Observations indicative of major deviations include asymmetry—total absence or no response on one side or in upper or lower extremities.

Table 12-2
Neonatal Reflex Behaviors

Behavior	Begins (in utero) (wk)	Integrates
Protection		
Moro	28	At 6-8 months to allow sitting and protective extension of the hands
Palmar grasp	28	At 5-6 months to allow voluntary grasping of objects
Plantar grasp	28	At 7-8 months with foot rubbing on objects; complete at 8-9 months for standing and walking
Babinski	28	(Same as plantar grasp)
Tonic neck	35	At 4 months, so rolling over and reaching or grasping may occur
Gag*	36	Protects against aspiration—does *not* disappear
Blink	25	Does *not* disappear
Crossed extension	28	Disappears around 2 months of age
Survival		
Rooting*	28	At 3 months; decreased response if baby is sleepy or with satiety
Sucking*	26-28	Not yet synchronized with swallowing
Swallowing*	12	32-34 weeks, stronger synchronization with sucking; perfect by 34-37 weeks

*Although isolated components of feeding behaviors are all present before 28 weeks' gestational age, they are not effectively coordinated for oral feedings before 32-34 weeks' gestational age. Coordination of respiration with sucking and swallowing during bottle feeding is consistently achieved by infants >37 weeks postconceptual age.[32]

Psychologic Interaction and Neonatal States

For years newborn behavior was thought to be only on a reflexive, instinctual level. Through the work of Brazelton[30] and others, newborns have been shown to have the ability to interact with and shape their environment. The Neonatal Behavioral Assessment Scale (NBAS)[30] enables the interactive behavior of the newborn to be observed and scored.

The NBAS enables assessment of the infant's individual capabilities for social relationships rated on the infant's best performance. Interest in the best performance is based on the belief that the newborn may briefly respond to external stimuli from higher centers of the nervous system (i.e., the cerebrum). Six categories of abilities are considered in evaluating the infant's performance: habituation, orientation to auditory and visual stimuli, motor maturity, state changes, self-quieting ability, and social behaviors.

Response decrement (i.e., habituation) is the protective mechanism by which the infant decreases responsivity to external stimuli. Habituation represents the cerebral behavior of memory— the infant stores the memory of the stimulus and with repeated presentation learns not to respond. Infants who are able to habituate are able to "tune-out" mild to moderate stimuli in the environment and protect themselves from overstimulation. An infant who is unable to habituate will continue to react vigorously to repeated stimuli. Infants who become "bored" with their toys have habituated to them—infants like variety. Dishabituation represents increasing attention to a new stimulus (new mobile, toy, face) after habituation to an old stimulus. The infant thus "recognizes" the novelty of the new stimulus and chooses to respond.

The neonate is able to imitate the facial and manual gestures of adults.[118] Infants as young as 12 days old imitate gestures such as mouth opening and tongue protrusion. Because the neonate has never seen his or her own face, this innate ability to match behaviors to those of another is a remarkable utilization of the cerebral cortex. Imitation may operate as a positive feedback mechanism to care givers; thus it is important in parent-infant reciprocity and represents early learning behaviors.

Table 12-3
Newborn States and Considerations for Care Giving

Newborn State	Comments
Sleep states	
Deep sleep (non-REM or quiet sleep)	Infant is very difficult if not impossible to arouse. Infant will not breastfeed or bottle-feed in this state, even after vigorous stimulation. Infant is unable to respond to environment; frustrating for care givers.
Slow state changes	
Regular breathing	
Eyes closed; no eye movements	
No spontaneous activity except startles and jerky movements	Term infants may exhibit a "slow" heart rate (80-90 beats/min), which may trigger heart rate alarms and result in unnecessary stimulation by NICU staff.
Startles with some delay and suppresses rapidly	At birth, preterm infants have altered states of consciousness:
Lowest oxygen consumption	Early dominant states are light sleep, quiet, and active alert. "Protective apathy" enables the preterm to remain inactive, unresponsive, and in a sleep state to conserve energy, grow, and maintain physiologic homeostasis.[100]
	As maturation occurs, there is an increase in quiet alert.
Light sleep (REM or active sleep)	Full-term infants begin and end sleep in active sleep; preterm infants are more responsive (than term infants) to stimuli in active sleep.
Low activity level	
Random movements and startles	
Respirations irregular and abdominal	Infant may cry or fuss briefly in this state and be awakened to feed before they are truly awake and ready to eat.
Intermittent sucking movements	
Eyes closed, REM	Lower and more variable oxygenation states.
Higher oxygen consumption	

Modified from Brazelton TB: *Neonatal behavioral assessment scale,* ed 2, Philadelphia, 1984, Spastics International Medical Publishers, JB Lippincott; Blackburn S: *JOGN Nurs* (Suppl) 805, 1983.

Continued

Learning, a function of the cerebral cortex, occurs with habituation and imitation. Early cognitive development is important to later learning and future cognitive development. Knowledge of the cognitive ability of the neonate enables care providers to provide opportunities for learning. Learning occurs in the context of experience[4] and influences structural development; there is increased CNS development during the first 2 years of life.[30,49]

The state of consciousness influences the reactions of the newborn to internal and external stimuli. The infant's state at the time of observation must be considered in interpretation of the findings. Table 12-3 shows the six states of the newborn and specific considerations for care giving in each state.

Clinical application of the NBAS includes evaluation of infant capabilities after illness, prematurity, or maternal medications. The most important application of the NBAS is in anticipatory guidance for parents. Demonstration of parts of the examination for parents enables them to become familiar with their infant's individual patterns of behavior, temperament, and states. Thus parents are able to more accurately assess and interpret their infant's cues for interaction and for distance.

Circadian Rhythms

Circadian rhythms are cyclic variations in function that occur daily at about the same time. Humans cycle their bodily functions (e.g., temperature, hormonal changes, blood pressure, urine volume, sleep-wake cycles) in a 24-hour period. These daily fluctuations are innately controlled by the individual's "biologic clock" in the hypothalamus. Environment does not cause cyclic variations; they are innate to the individual and persist despite environmental influences. In the infant the development of circadian rhythm is influenced by genetic

Table 12-3
Newborn States and Considerations for Care Giving—cont'd

Newborn State	Comments
Awake states	
Drowsy or semidosing	Infant may awaken further or return to sleep (if left alone).
Eyelids fluttering	Quietly talking and looking at the infant, or offering a pacifier or
Eyes open or closed (dazed)	an inanimate object to see and listen to may arouse the infant
Mild startles (intermittent)	to the quiet alert state.
Delayed response to sensory stimuli	Less mature infants (30 weeks) demonstrate a more drowsy than
Smooth state change after stimulation	quiet alert state than older infants (36 weeks).
Fussing may or may not be present	
Respirations—more rapid and shallow	
Quiet alert, with bright look	Immediately after birth, term newborns exhibit a period of quiet
Focuses attention on source of stimulation	alert, their first opportunity to "take in" their parents and the
Impinging stimuli may break through; may	extrauterine environment. Dimmed lights, quiet talking, and
have some delay in response	stroking optimize this time for parents.
Minimal motor activity	Best state for learning to occur, because infant focuses all of at-
	tention on visual, auditory, tactile, and sucking stimuli; best
	state for interaction with parents—infant is maximally able to
	attend and reciprocally respond to parents.
Active alert—eyes open	Infant has decreased threshold (increased sensitivity) to internal
Considerable motor activity—thrusting move-	(hunger, fatigue) and external (wet, noise, handling) stimuli.
ments of extremities; spontaneous startles	Infant may quiet self, may escalate to crying, or with consola-
Reacts to external stimuli with increase in	tion by caregiver may become quiet alert or go to sleep.
movements and startles (discrete reactions	Infant is unable to maximally attend to caregiver or environment
difficult to differentiate because of general	because of increased motor activity and increased sensitivity to
higher activity level)	stimuli.
Respirations irregular	
May or may not be fussy	
Crying—intense and difficult to disrupt with	Crying is infant's response to unpleasant internal or external
external stimuli	stimulation—infant's tolerance limits have been reached (and
Respirations rapid, shallow, and irregular	exceeded). Infant may be able to quiet self with hand-to-
	mouth behaviors; talking may quiet a crying infant; holding,
	rocking, or putting infant upright on caregiver's shoulder may
	quiet infant.

potential, brain maturation, and the environment.[68,169] Infant biorhythms have been studied in the areas of temperature, heart and respiratory rates, blood pressure, sleep-wake cycles, endocrine secretion, and feeding frequency.[169]

The term newborn sleeps from 16 to 19 hours a day. As sleep begins, the term infant enters active rather than quiet sleep and spends more time in active sleep than does the adult.[51] Active sleep durations vary from 10 to 45 minutes, whereas quiet sleep lasts about 20 minutes.[51] The infant's sleep cycle is 50 to 60 minutes, as compared with the adult's 90- to 100-minute cycle.[16] Infants exhibit a diurnal variation in the quality of their sleep—more quiet sleep occurs during afternoon naps.[157] As the infant matures, there is a decrease in active and an increase in quiet sleep.[16,51,177]

Infants have their own clock for sleep-wake, hunger, and feeding or fussy times. These often do not coincide with the family's rhythms and may cause disruption and conflict.[177] Sleep-wake states reflect the underlying status of the neurologic system.[16,51,86] The infant's maturity at birth greatly affects his or her rhythms and development of normal circadian rhythm. Early relationships with care givers provide the organization and stabilization necessary for sleep regulation as well as other biologic functions. A term newborn has innate rhythms and over a period of time (about 16 to 18 weeks) develops adult regularity (e.g., more sleep at night than in the daytime).[16] However, complete synchronization into a day-night pattern may not occur until 5 to 8 months of age.[86]

In preterm infants, active and quiet sleep are more poorly organized and of shorter duration (a sleep cycle is about 30 to 40 minutes).[50] Active sleep is "lighter" than quiet sleep—there is more response to stimuli in active sleep.[50] Quiet sleep is a more controlled state and occurs more frequently in term infants than in premature infants. Quiet sleep does not become significant in the preterm until approximately 36 weeks' gestation. Hence, a third sleep state, transitional sleep, has been identified for the premature infant.[130] This state is characterized by quiet sleep with periods of closed eyes, regular or periodic respirations, no bodily movements, and no REM. Prior to 36 weeks' gestation the preterm infant's predominant sleep state is transitional sleep. As the preterm infant matures, he or she spends progressively less time in transitional sleep, has more quiet than active sleep, and has more awake, alert time. However, the preterm who is 40 weeks' post-conceptional age does not have as well organized sleep patterns as the term newborn.[130,177] Preterms sleep more (>15%) than term infants because there is no decrease in sleep duration as exhibited by full-term infants, primarily during the day.

Sleep disruption may interfere with growth and development by altering neuronal maturation and growth hormone secretion. Human growth hormone has a rhythmic pattern associated with sleep-wake cycles. The highest peaks of growth hormone in infants occur during REM (active) sleep. The fetus (29 to 32 weeks' gestation) spends 80% of the time in utero in REM sleep; the term newborn's sleep is 50% REM sleep.[50,51] Because growth hormone secretion depends on the regular recurrence of sleep, any disturbance of the sleep-wake cycle results in irregular spikes of growth hormone during a 24-hour period.

An infant whose cycles are discrepant from his or her family's may be perceived as "difficult." Because this behavior does not fit parental expectations of regular eating, sleeping or eliminating, the parent-child interaction is off to a rocky start.[177] Gradually, through care giving, parents teach the infant synchronization with family rhythms. By 9 months of age the term infant has developed day-night fluctuations that are similar to adult patterns.

Sensory Capabilities

At birth, the neonate's senses are developed and functioning. Sensory development proceeds in a specific order: tactile/vestibular, olfactory/gustatory, and auditory/visual. The newborn is able to communicate—react to and initiate a reaction from those in the environment. As the neonate takes in the sensory information, he or she associates features of the environment that occur together (e.g., sound, smell, sight, touch of "mother" or "father"), demonstrating complex and intermodal abilities for handling the sensory input from the environment.[24]

Tactile/Kinesthetic

Touch is the major method of communication for neonates and infants. In utero, fetal existence has been primarily one of movement—floating within the amniotic fluid and rhythmic maternal movements. The sense of touch, temperature, and pressure are all well developed, and receptors lie in the newborn's skin. The sensitivity to touch is especially well developed in the face, around the lips (i.e., root reflex), and in the hands (i.e., grasp reflex). Because newborns are nonverbal, they pick up messages via the manner in which they are held and handled—by the adult's "body language." Infants are often barometers for adult feelings—if the adult is tired and irritable, the infant knows and may respond with irritability and crying.

Infants love to be held, rocked, and carried—note the soothing effects on the crying infant. Adults do *not* spoil infants by providing this important stimuli. Increased carrying of infants contributes to less crying at 6 weeks of age.[20] In response to being held, infants adjust their body posture to the body of the care giver. Adults describe infants as "cuddly" (comfortable, relaxed curl; snuggles to adult body and attempts to root or suck) or "noncuddly" (sprawls, tenses or stiffens, and "pushes away"). The most comforting position for a crying infant is upright on an adult's shoulder.[99] Responsiveness to tactile stimulation has been found to be greater in female than in male neonates.[99]

Hearing

The preonate in utero has heard the voices of mother, father, and siblings from the 5th week of intrauterine life.[158] These voices are "familiar" to the newborn, so that they "know" their family and are able to differentiate them from the voices of strangers.[46] Studies have suggested that fetuses and neonates exhibit memory.[46,47] Newborns who had been read a particular story while in utero responded to the story reread to them after birth with a recognition and attentiveness that was not exhibited in response to unfamiliar stories.[46,47] The ability to hear the outside world, particularly the spoken word, is a prerequisite to further verbal language development.

Neonates with an intact CNS are able to orient and respond to the auditory environment. In response to a sound, the neonate will

- Change motor activity (eye blink, decrease in activity, limb movements, head turn)
- Change heart rate and/or respiration—if the infant is quiet, the heart rate increases with stimuli; if the infant is crying, the heart rate decreases with stimuli; increase in respiratory rate, decrease, amplitude, or decrease in respiratory cycle rate
- Smile
- Startle or grimace
- Alert or arouse
- Cry or cease to cry
- Stop sucking

The response to sound depends on the sound's quality. When frequency and pitch are low, the infant is soothed and distress is decreased; high frequency and pitch alert, distress the infant and disturb sleep. Therefore monotonous low-frequency sounds are an auditory soother and induce sleep.

Frequencies below 4000 Hz (the range of human speech is 500-3000 Hz) produce the most newborn response.[127] Infants are maximally reactive to the human voice in typical speech patterns (rather than disconnected syllables). Infants prefer the high-pitched (such as female) voice over the low-pitched (such as male) voice. Note how adults and children instinctively pitch their voices higher when talking to an infant. Presented with a female and a male voice, the infant always turns toward the female voice. Parents who talk with their infants elicit increasing eye contact with the infant.

Stimuli presented for 5 to 15 seconds elicit the best reaction. Stimuli lasting longer than several minutes are less effective, because the term infant habituates to the sound and ceases responding. The ability to habituate to sound is indicative of an intact CNS. Infants will exhibit startle behavior if the stimulus rapidly reaches maximal loudness. A slower time to reach maximal loudness is associated with infant alerting and searching for the stimulus. Infant state is important in evaluation of response to auditory stimuli—light sleep is the optimal state. Infants quiet and soothe in response to rhythmic sounds (rather than disrhythmic ones). Neonates move their bodies in rhythmic synchrony (i.e., entrainment) with the spoken word.

Vision

Eye development begins 22 days after conception. The eyelids fuse at about 10 weeks and remain fused until about the twenty-sixth week of gestation. At birth, photoreceptors are developed, but maturation is not complete for several months. The fetus is able to distinguish light from dark and recoils from a bright light shone at the mother's abdomen. Even at term birth the visual system is immature, and significant development occurs over the next 6 months to a year. The ability to fix, follow, and alert is indicative of an intact CNS.[122] At birth, infants are able to see an object within 8 to 10 inches of the face (visual acuity of $20/140$).[56] Within seconds after birth, the neonate is able to recognize his or her mother's face.[24] The cradled-in-the-arms position of feeding is the exact distance from the adult's face that the newborn can see. In response to an interesting visual stimulus, neonates stop sucking to look, alert, and attend to the object, horizontally scan the object, and fix and follow a moving object in a 90-degree arc. Infants prefer the human face as a visual stimulus, prefer a patterned over a nonpatterned stimulus, and attend longer to larger patterns with more complex patterns and angles.[56] Infants prefer black and white because of the greater contrast and will focus on the outside of a figure where the contrast is the greatest.[122] Newborns are sensitive to bright light and will tightly close their eyes in its presence. They prefer moderate, diffuse lighting. Presentation of visual stimuli enables development of the neural pattern for vision. During the infant's first year of life, visual investigation of the environment is a primary mode of learning.

Smell/Taste[146]

The fetus increases its amniotic fluid consumption when saccharine is added to the fluid and decreases consumption with the injection of distasteful substances.[29] Taste may be a way the fetus monitors the intrauterine environment.[29] Olfaction is well developed at birth. Olfactory cues guide the full-term newborn to the maternal nipple.[175] At 5 days of age, the neonate is able to differentiate his or her mother's breast pad and demonstrates a preference for the smell over that of a "stranger." The infant's response to pleasant odors is to arouse and suck. After several presentations of the stimuli, the infant will habituate to the odor. Infants withdraw from unpleasant odors such as vinegar and ammonia. They are also able to differentiate tastes, preferring sweet solutions and refusing bitter, acid, and sour substances. Asphyxiated infants demonstrate a loss of olfaction that parallels the suppression of brainstem reflexes and activities.

Communication Skills

The neonate's ability to communicate is a naturally endowed survival skill. Crying is the infant's language to communicate needs. Crying may also be a response to the environment—noisy, cold, overstimulating, multiple care giving, or lack of synchrony. Because the cry brings someone to meet the need, the infant soon learns that the care giver gives attention and the world is a trustworthy place. The more responsive the care giver is to the infant's crying, thus the infant's needs, the less crying

behavior is necessary.[20] Learning occurs as the infant associates comfort with the care giver. The temperament of the individual infant and his or her ability to habituate to disturbing stimuli influence the amount of crying behavior. Tension of the care giver or the environment is communicated nonverbally to the infant and may potentiate or contribute to the infant's crying.

The amount and tone of the newborn's cry is influenced by birth weight, gestational age, and the events of birth. Types of cries include birth cry, hunger cry, pain cry, and pleasure cry.[36,37,167,182] Infants separated from their mothers in the first 90 minutes after birth exhibit a "separation distress call" (also seen in other mammal species) that ceases at reunion.[36,37] The newborn's cry physiologically affects the mother—her breasts change and prepare to nurse. Neonates possess a repertoire of self-quieting behaviors when in a fussy state: (1) hand-to-mouth efforts, (2) sucking on fist or tongue, and (3) use of visual and/or auditory stimuli from the environment.[30]

The neonatal cry may be diagnostic of existing conditions or trauma. CNS insult often results in a high-pitched, shrill cry. The pain cry of asphyxiated newborns differs significantly from that of healthy term infants[120] (see Chapter 5).

The smiling infant is a joy to the care giver. Smiling may be either spontaneous (from birth) or a response to the social human face (at 4 to 12 weeks of life). A smile is most easily elicited by the stimulus of a moving, smiling human face. The ability to smile begins before 40 weeks in the preterm infant as observed during REM sleep. The social implications of the smile include positive feedback to the care giver that the infant is happy and contented, which results in parental feelings of adequacy and competence.

Environment

Prenatal Environment

In utero, the fetus depends totally on its mother's emotional and physical health and well-being for their own. It is through her that they receive the nurturance, housing, and stimulation to develop their body, their sensory organs, and the rudiments of their personality and temperment.

Intrapartal Environment

Birth is a major transition from physiologic dependence to physiologic independence. At term, the neonate's physiologic systems are developed, sensory organs function, and the foundation of personality and temperment are established. Birth is disorienting and disruptive. The amount of disruption depends on the degree of trauma incurred during the labor and birth process. Not having a social support system compounds the stress, often escalating it beyond the mother's tolerance and coping skills. Anxious and fearful women have longer labors and more delivery complications than women who are confident about themselves and their infants. The recent shift toward family-centered birth enables mothers to receive support from their families, to be an active participant in the birth process, and to have immediate contact with their newborns.

The neonate is also influenced by medications and the events of labor and birth (see Chapter 2). Maternal medications for analgesia and anesthesia affect neonatal behaviors, resulting in decreased sucking ability, lethargy, and decreased habituation. Medicated infants are less able to evoke care giver behaviors such as smiling, touching, and vocalization. They also give less feedback to their parents than unmedicated infants. The parents may feel rejected, tend to stimulate the infant less, and thus begin a pattern of aberrant interaction.

Postnatal Environment

Home and family are the primary media through which newborns (1) reestablish their biorhythmic balance, (2) stabilize themselves in the extrauterine world, (3) develop a sense of self and mastery in the world, and (4) become socialized as human beings. Socialization teaches the adaptive psychosocial skills necessary for survival and functioning in society. Cultural and family values, behavioral expression, and ways of meeting social-emotional needs are learned within the family. Thus the home and family environment is considered to be a "normalized" environment for human development.

Care Giver Factors

The dyadic relationship continues postpartally between the care giver and the infant—the behavior of one reinforces the behavior of the other. The infant's physical and emotional needs are satisfied by care givers. The infant's response to the care giver depends on how he or she perceives and receives ministrations; this response affects the level of emotional satisfaction the care giver receives from the interaction. Parental expectations have a major effect on their perceptions and their behavior and ultimately affect the child's development. Parents must work out the discrepancy between the wished-for and the actual child, especially if the infant is preterm, ill, or has an anomaly. How attached the parents are to the infant influences their relationship to and ability to care for their infant (see Chapter 28). If the pregnancy has failed to produce a normal, healthy infant, the parents must grieve the loss of their expectations. Parents are unable to attach to and care for the infant until they have completed their grief work (see Chapter 29).

A care giver and infant have a reciprocal interaction when their cycles and signals are synchronized with each other. The biorhythmic cycle of the newborn has been in synchrony with one person (mother) while in utero, and the infant is accustomed to her cycles and rhythms for developing adaptive behavior. Consistent maternal care giving enables newborns to regulate their rhythms to the mother's and begin adapting to the postnatal environment.[87,98] From her, they expand their adaptation to the family and to the larger world of society.[58]

Experience in relating to infants does influence the care giver's efficiency in interpretation of and sensitivity to infant cues. Multiparous women have more sensitivity to infant cues than do primiparous mothers. Mothers with little or no experience exhibit more difficulty in quieting a crying infant.

Consistency in maternal responses is especially important as the infant continues to learn the accepted patterns of cues from the care giver. Cared for by one or two people, the infant is able to develop synchrony with and expectations of the parents. Single care giving improves establishment of biorhythms for sleep-wake cycles, feeding, and visual attentiveness. Consistent cues soon elicit a consistency of response from the infant. Consistency and promptness of maternal response result in less infant crying during the first year of life. A predictable and responsive environment enables the infant to progress to varied types of communication (not just crying). Care by parents provides for mutual cueing and mastery of the environment through interaction. Inconsistent cues distress and confuse the infant. Multiple care giving confuses the infant, increases distress with feeding, causes irritability, and upsets visual attention.

Regardless of how stable or unstable, consistent or inconsistent it is, family life has a rhythm, synchronicity, and predictability of its own. Through interaction with parents and siblings, infants further develop their ability to form relationships. From these primary relationships, the foundation and format for other relationships are established. The quality of subsequent relationships depends on the quality of the relationship experienced within the primary family from birth throughout infancy.[73]

Neonatal Factors

The neonate is not a passive recipient of the environment of the family but is an active participant in shaping that environment. Infants send cues about their ability and readiness for interpersonal interactions. Infants in the first 4 months of life interact differently with persons than with inanimate objects (Fig. 12-1). The excitement generated by interpersonal interaction is seen in the infant's arm and leg movements, bodily movement toward the other person, smiling, vocalizing, and increased visual attention. Because of the infant's immaturity, he or she is unable to maintain a continuous interaction. The infant attends for short periods and then turns away to decrease excitement, to protect himself or herself from bombardment by overwhelming stimuli, and to process the experience. Maternal or care provider sensitivity to the attention-withdrawal cycle of interaction enables the adult to modulate her behavior in synchrony with the infant's cues. Successful interaction with an infant includes reading the infant's cues, responding appropriately, and not overwhelming the infant with too much stimulation (thus overstepping the infant's tolerance for interaction). Overwhelming the infant results in his or her withdrawal for progressively longer periods of time in order to protect himself or herself from overstimulating and insensitive others.

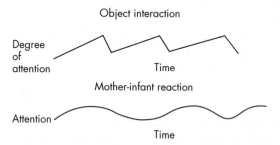

Figure 12-1 Interaction pattern with object and with mother. Object interaction is characterized by abrupt attention and excitement phases followed by sudden and abrupt looking away. Interaction with person is cyclical and involves initiation of interaction, orientation to person, acceleration of excitement, peak of excitement, deceleration of excitement, and withdrawal or turning away. (From Brazelton TB, Koslowski B, Main M: The origins of reciprocity: the early infant-mother interaction. In Lewis M, Rosenblum LA, editors: *The effect on the infant on its caregiver,* New York, 1974, John Wiley and Sons.)

Just as the parent has expectations, the infant also has expectations of the relationship. The infant expects relief or protection from painful experiences, maintenance of comfort, and homeostasis. Relief from the discomforts of hunger, cold, sleeplessness, and boredom enable the infant to respond positively to the care provider.

Care-eliciting behaviors are those neonatal cues used to signal the care giver that attention is needed. Crying, visual following, and smiling are care-eliciting. Newborn responses to care include quieting, suckling, clinging and cuddling, looking, smiling, and vocalizing. These social interactions positively reward the care provider and encourage and promote continued care. Infant characteristics that modify maternal attitudes include (1) a healthy or sickly infant; (2) an attractive, pretty infant or an infant with obvious congenital anomaly; (3) a premature infant; (4) a calm and contented or a fussy and irritable infant; (5) an infant responsive to or rejecting of maternal care. A maternal or care provider ability to soothe the infant reinforces a feeling of success (or failure) in her feelings of competence.

The infant's sex also affects the cues and the care giver's response. Male infants exhibit more startles, more muscle activity, and more physical strength. In response, they receive more holding from care givers as a means of soothing.[99] Females exhibit more tactile and oral sensitivity, more smiling, and more responsivity to sweet taste. As a result, girls are more often soothed by talking, eye-to-eye contact, and a pacifier.[99]

The infant's level of neurophysiologic development influences the appropriateness of maternal and care giving behaviors. The neurologically mature term infant who has already mastered autonomic, motoric, and state regulation is able to actively elicit and respond to care giving behaviors.[30,58] Because of the immaturity of the CNS, the preterm infant lags behind the term infant in care eliciting and responsivity to the care provider. Stages and characteristics of behavioral organization in preterm infants are described in Table 12-4. Because the young preterm infant's priority is mere survival, interaction with the environment and care providers is at the expense of physiologic stability.[171] Because the preterm infant sends cues

different from the term infant, knowledge of these stages enables care givers to modulate their behavior and the environment. Although overwhelming the term infant results in withdrawal from interaction, overwhelming the preterm infant first results in a real threat to physiologic survival, then to withdrawal from interaction.

Because preterm infants are not as neurologically mature as term infants, the NBAS has little value with this population. A behavioral assessment scale for preterm infants, Assessment of Preterm Infant's Behavior (APIB), has been developed that evaluates the preterm's behavioral organization along five subsystems of functioning: autonomic, motor, state, attentional-interactive, and self-regulatory.[9] Although subsystems are observed independently, they are interdependent since disorganization in one system affects other systems. This examination delineates the quality and duration of the preterm infant's response, the difficulty in eliciting the response, and the effort and cost to the preterm infant of achieving and maintaining a response. Because it, too, is an interactive test, the nature and amount of organization provided by the care provider is an indication of the preterm infant's lack of integrative skill. As the preterm infant matures and advances in development of organization, he or she is more able to interact with the environment (animate and inanimate). However, it must be remembered that this maturation process is "uneven"—as the preterm infant advances in one area of development, he or she may become, at least temporarily, more vulnerable (i.e., experience difficulties) in other areas such as physiologic stability.[73]

Interventions

Life in a special care nursery is characterized by sensory deprivation of normal stimuli that the preterm infant would have experienced in the womb and that term infants would experience at home with their families. However, the NICU is also an environment of sensory bombardment—constant noise, light, and tactile stimulation; intrusive, invasive procedures; upset of sleep-wake cycles; and multiple care givers; etc. Rather than

Table 12-4
Stages and Characteristics of Behavioral Organization in Preterm Infants

Als et al*	Gorski†
Physiologic homeostasis—stablizing and integrating temperature control, cardiorespiratory function, digestion, and elimination. Characteristics: becomes pale, dusky, cyanotic; heart and respiratory rates change—all symptoms of disorganization of autonomic nervous system.	"In turning"—physiologic stage of mere survival characterized by autonomic nervous system responses to stimuli (rapid color changes caused by swings in heart and respiratory rates); no or limited direct response; inability to arouse self spontaneously; jerky movements; asleep (and protecting the CNS from sensory overload) 97% of the time. Preterms (<32 weeks) are easily physiologically overwhelmed by stimuli.
Motor development may infringe on physiologic homeostasis, resulting in defensive strategies (vomiting, color change, apnea, and bradycardia). State development becomes less diffuse and encompasses full range: sleep, awake, crying. States and state changes may affect physiologic or motor stability.	"Coming out"—first active response to environment may be seen as early as 34-35 weeks (provided some physiologic stability has been achieved). Characteristics: remains pink with stimuli; has directed response for short periods; arouses spontaneously and maintains arousal after stimuli ceases; if interaction begins in alert state: maintains quiet alert for 5-10 min, tracks animate or inanimate stimuli; spends 10%-15% of time in alert state with predictable interaction patterns.
Alert state is well differentiated from other states; may interfere with physiologic or motor stability	"Reciprocity"—active interaction and reciprocity with environment from 36-40 weeks. Characteristics: directs response; arouses and consoles self; maintains alertness and interacts with both animate and inanimate objects; copes with external stress.

* Modified from Als H et al: *Am Acad Child Psychiatry* 2D:239, 1981.
† Modified from Gorski PA: *Semin Perinatol* 3:61, 1979.

too much or too little stimulation, infants in the NICU receive an inappropriate pattern of stimulation[73,75] (noncontingent, nonreciprocal, painful [rather than pleasant], multiple stimuli, etc). Because the immature CNS of the premature infant is unable to tolerate these stimuli, the easily overstimulated preterm infant protects himself or herself by physiologic and interactional defensive maneuvers that threaten survival and social ability and may lead to lifelong maladaptations. Research has shown medical, developmental, and cost benefits to low-birth-weight infants from individualized behavioral and environmental care in the NICU (Table 12-5). The most effective interventions (1) are contingent on the infant's responses, (2) balance protection from sensory overload with provision of enough stimulation to promote emerging capabilities, and (3) involve parents.*

Preterm infants are not the only infants at risk from the stress of overstimulation in the NICU. Sick or anomalied term infants and chronically ill infants with prolonged hospitalization also experience stress.[78] The term infant with persistent pulmonary hypertension (see Chapter 22) is particularly vulnerable to repeated handling, procedures, and interventions that decrease Pao_2. Thus these infants are managed on a minimal intervention regimen—care is organized, coordinated, and individualized to decrease noxious stimuli and physical manipulations. The chronically ill infant with BPD has been shown to improve when

* References 13, 31, 61, 73, 74, 138-140.

Table 12-5
Outcomes of Individualized Developmental Intervention in the NICU*

Physiologic Benefits	Developmental Benefits	Cost Savings

Decreases in
  Incidence of IVH or pneumo-
    thorax, and severity of BPD
  Ventilator/CPAP use
  Need for supplemental oxygen
  Need for gavage feedings
Increase in
  Daily weight gain
  Stability of cardiorespiratory
    function
  Sleep states
Significant electrophysiologic differ-
    ences in frontal, temporal, cen-
    tral, occipital, and parietal
    lobes of the brain.
	Improvement in
	  Behavioral organization of auto-
	    nomic, motor, attention modu-
	    lation, and self-regulatory
	    abilities.
	  Interactive capability
	  Quality of parent-infant interac-
	    tion
	  Cognitive function/IQ
	  Development of feeding skills
	    (earlier full oral feedings)
	Fewer behavioral problems and
	    attentional difficulties
	Continuation of maternal ability to
	    read and respond to infant
	    behavioral cues
		Shorter length of stay
		Earlier discharge at younger age
		Decrease in hospital charges

* References 11-13, 19, 31, 61, 138-140, 166.
CPAP, Continuous positive airway pressure; *IVH,* intraventricular hemorrhage.

behavioral or environmental changes were initiated.[11,12] The term SGA infant is sleepy and not alert in the first few weeks of life, which may result in the infant's being left alone or overstimulated to awaken for interaction.[10] After a few weeks, these infants become very irritable, fussy, and disorganized in spontaneous and social behaviors. Anticipatory guidance, reassurance that the disorganization is in the infant rather than a result of parental care, and practical intervention strategies enable the parents to shape the environment and the infant's response.[10,73]

The ultimate goal of intervention strategies in the NICU is to facilitate and promote infant growth and development and thus task mastery.[101] In the NICU, this goal is achieved by (1) altering the environmental and care giving stressors that interfere with physiologic stability, (2) promoting individual neurobehavioral organization and maturation by identifying and facilitating stable behaviors and reducing stressful behaviors, (3) conserving energy, (4) teaching parents to interpret infant behavior, and (5) promoting infant-parent interaction and care giving. Establishing biorhythmic balance and physiologic homeostasis is necessary

for survival and is enhanced by a sensitive, responsive NICU environment. An unresponsive environment may so stress the preterm infant that apnea, bradycardia, and other physiologic instabilities severely compromise and prolong recovery.* For the hospitalized infant, development of the sense of self and trust is undermined by noncontingent stimulation that prevents a sense of competence and control of the environment from being established.[75] When the ventilated infant experiences hunger or is wet, he or she is unable to signal the care provider with a cry because of the tube. Thus the infant experiences a need, but is unable to signal and bring care and relief. The infant soon learns that he or she is not in control of the situation. Another intubated infant may be quietly asleep and not experiencing a need; yet it is "care time," so the nurse moves, wakes, changes, and generally disturbs the infant. This infant also soon learns about not being in control of the situation.

Hospitalized infants, especially those with prolonged stays, may exhibit the classic signs of institutionalized infants or infants suffering from

* References 9, 54, 72, 73, 78, 103, 171.

maternal deprivation[65,159] (Box 12-2). It is the goal of "environmental neonatology"[75] to prevent this maladaptive behavior by altering the NICU to be more developmentally appropriate for infants. Normalizing the environment begins with an assessment of the stimulation to which the individual infant is exposed. The type (i.e., noxious versus pleasant; contingent versus noncontingent), amount, and timing of stimulation should be noted. To decrease noxious stimuli, no infant should have "routine" care (e.g., all infants are suctioned every 2 hours; all infants have a Dextrostix test every 4 hours)[11,73] Care should be individualized by asking the questions: "Why are we doing this procedure?" and "Is this procedure necessary for *this* infant's care?" Overstimulation in the NICU occurs when procedures (81% to 94% of all contacts are medical or nursing procedures, an average of 40 to 132 times per day) are performed[54]; it does *not* result from social interaction with parents.[75] Painful, invasive procedures that are not vital to the individual infant are stress-producing events that should be eliminated. Rest may be the most important environmental change.[77,88,89,103,162,171]

The fetus in utero and the term infant at home relate to a minimum of care givers and thus need to learn one or only a few sets of cues. Multiple caregivers in the NICU confuse the infant by providing many care-related cues for the infant to learn—many techniques of handling and many emotional, nonverbal messages to decode. Primary nursing minimizes the number of care providers, because the primary nurse and one or two associates always (or as much as possible) care for the infant; assess, revise, and write the care plan; and coordinate care. Primary nursing also adds consistency and continuity for parents.[11,19,78]

The infant's state or level of arousal provides an appropriate context for caregiving.[64] Some infants exhibit a low threshold to stimuli—they are easily overwhelmed and fatigued. Others, with a higher threshold, are quieter, more difficult to arouse, initiate less, and thus receive less interaction.[9] Organizing care to be reciprocal to the infant's state reinforces the infant's competence in signaling a need (sense of self) and having it met (sense of trust and mastery). As the infant matures, feeding on demand rather than on a schedule not only teaches this valuable lesson but also increases absorption

---

Box 12-2

Classic Signs of "Hospitalitis"

Asocial Affect

Gaze aversion—fleeting glances at care giver with inability to maintain eye contact

Flat affect—social unresponsiveness (little fixing and following; smiling) to care giver

Little or no quiet alert state—infant abruptly changes state and often is described as "either asleep or awake and crying" (crying is only "awake" state); out-of-control crying

Touch Aversion*

Becomes hypotonic or hypertonic with care giving or attempts at socialization

Fights, flails, and resists being cared for or held

Aversive responses (see Table 12-7) to care giving or holding persist

Feeding Difficulties

Have multiple origins, including delayed onset of oral feedings; touch aversion around mouth secondary to invasive procedures; multiple care givers; feeding on schedule, rather than demand

Rumination syndrome—voluntary regurgitation, a form of self-comfort and gratification when environment is not nurturing or gratifying[151]

Failure to Thrive

Poor or no weight gain despite adequate caloric intake

Develops mental delays (language, motor, social, emotional)

From Gardner LI: *Sci Am* 227(1):76, 1982; Spitz R: *Psychoanal Study Child* 1:53, 1945.
* Infant associates human touch with pain.

---

and utilization of caloric intake.[73,147] If the infant is asleep, ask: "Do we need to do this now? Would another time be better?" In some centers physicians make an appointment with the nurse to examine the infant—at a time that is optimal for the infant.

Because preterm infants exhibit short duration of state cycles until around 38 weeks, they have decreased tolerance for stimuli. Some preterm infants tolerate all care done at once and long periods of rest; others do not and need care spread out to decrease overstimulation and decompensation. Clustering care may not assure long rest periods since 50% of all rest periods in several NICUs were <10 min in length.[53] Even "premie growers" may be unable to tolerate more than one stimulus at a time—they feed best if visual, auditory, and social stimuli are not provided until *after* the feeding. As the infant matures and is able to tolerate integrated experience, multimodal stimuli are provided.[103]

Alterations in the individual infant's daily schedule are made to accommodate a more flexible or structured scheduled—whichever is better for the infant.[75] Assessing the infant before, during, and after an interaction or intervention guides the care provider in adapting care and the environment to the individual infant (Table 12-6). The organized infant is able to interact with the environment without disrupting his or her physiologic and behavioral functioning.[9,44] When the disorganized preterm interacts with the environment, signs of physiologic and behavioral stress may occur (Table 12-7), in which case the interaction should cease.[99,103] An intubated preterm infant cared for in an NICU with a strict suction "routine" every 2 hours responds with profound cyanosis, lowered $TcPo_2$ and pulse oximetery, and bradycardia, and requires bagging after every suction (with no secretions obtained)—an obviously unnecessary and stressful intervention. In a less rigid, more individualized care setting, that same infant may signal the need for suction by becoming restless, by a decrease in oxygenation, and/or by heart rate changes (tachycardia or bradycardia). Suctioning improves the infant's condition—the infant lies quietly and has improved oxygenation, and the heart pattern stabilizes. This infant has signaled his or her need, and the care providers have read the cues and responded with a stabilizing intervention—the infant has *not* been stressed by an unnecessary procedure.

Knowledgeable professionals are able to role model for and teach parents how to relate to their premature infant.[138] Parents are taught to recognize and use infant states to maximize interaction.[9,39,103,138] The drowsy premature infant may be unable to engage in eye-to-eye contact with the parents or be able to sustain it for too short (for the

parents) a period of time. Waiting until the infant is more awake to initiate eye contact will be more rewarding to the parent and less stressful to the infant. Role model for parents that this infant is an individual and, even though premature, is able to signal for more or less stimulation (Table 12-7).

The preterm infant who is lightly touched may startle, jerk, or withdraw from parental touch. In response, the parent suddenly and sadly pulls his or her hand away and is reticent to touch the infant again. Intervention includes helping parents read cues and learn appropriate responses to their infant. The infant may be interpreted to the parents: "Jamie likes firm touch . . . like this." Teach parents how to recognize a stressed infant and how to intervene. The prime rule of relating to infants is: the infant leads; the adult follows.

Feeding the premature infant may be difficult, because the infant "goes to sleep" or "gets lazy" during feedings. The usual parental ministrations of talking to the infant, soothing with touch, or holding upright on the shoulder may not work with a fussy, irritable preterm infant. The preterm infant's behavior may be so disorganized, unpredictable, or misunderstood by the parents that an appropriate response is not possible.[8,73] Thus parents often become exhausted, bewildered, and frustrated in their encounters with their preterm infant's behavioral response to their care as rejecting and unloving: "My baby doesn't like me."[58] Teach parents that their infant's disorganization with stimuli is due to prematurity (i.e., an immature CNS) and *not* to parent ministrations. Reassure them that as the premature infant grows and evidences maturational changes, he or she will be able to tolerate more stimulation and will be more responsive to their care.

Just as parent-infant interaction is responsible for normal development of the term infant, parent-infant interaction is crucial in the development of at-risk infants.[138,140] Many parents of premature infants have been observed making heroic efforts, over long periods of time, to interact with their less alert, active, and responsive infants.[72,73] "Setting parents up to succeed" involves placing parents in situations where they will experience positive feedback from their infants. Suggesting and role modeling intervention strategies shows parents what and how to play and interact with their infants.

Table 12-6
Parameters for Assessing Interaction and Intervention with Neonates

Time Frame	Assessment

Before
Gather baseline data *before* touching the infant
	Gestational age and postconceptual age
	Diagnosis
	Level of physiologic homeostasis
	  Previous vital signs
	  Oxygenation state—(continuous pulse oximetry or transcutaneous monitor)
	Neonatal state
	  Sleep—deep, light, drowsy
	  Awake—quiet, active alert, crying
	Self-regulatory vs stress behaviors (Table 12-7)

During
Gently and as nonintrusively as possible assess physiologic and behavioral signs *during* intervention
	Level of (current) physiologic homeostasis: vital signs and changes
	  Observation (without touching infant)—color, posture, general appearance, respiratory rate, temperature (skin, incubator), blood pressure (transducer), oxygenation (from continuous monitor)
	  Quiet (with minimal disturbance)— ausculate heart, lungs, and abdomen; axillary temperature, blood pressure (cuff); head-to-toe assessment; oxygenation (saturation decreases with stressful, disturbing stimuli)
	Neonatal state change
	  Sleep—deep, light, drowsy
	  Awake—quiet alert, active alert, crying
	Self-regulatory vs stress behaviors (Table 12-7)

After
Assess physiologic and behavioral signs *after* intervention (delayed reactions may occur minutes after care)
	Level of physiologic homeostasis
	  Vital signs—returned to baseline values? More or less stable than baseline values?
	  Neonatal state change—return to baseline state? To a higher state? Unstable to be consoled? More consolable left alone?

Parent participation in intervention strategies is assured by stressing how important it is to infant development, that professionals are too busy to provide all necessary interventions, and that parents are in a unique position to provide developmental care in the hospital and at home after discharge. Parents (with help from professionals) are the ideal planners and providers of developmentally appro-priate intervention strategies. Beneficial effects of parent involvement in developmental care of VLBW infants include better interaction with and perception of the infant and improved cognitive development.[18,138,140]

Rooming-in of parents and their at-risk newborns is the best environment for cues to be learned and care given according to these cues. Unlimited

Table 12-7
Self-Regulatory versus Stress Behaviors

Organization	Disorganization
Physiologic	
Cardiorespiratory: stable heart and/or respiratory rate; regular, slow respirations	Cardiorespiratory: increase or decrease in respiratory rate; irregular respirations; apnea; gasping; bradycardia; blood pressure instability; sneezing, hiccoughs, coughing, sighing
Color: pink, stable	Color: mottling, duskiness; cyanosis—central or generalized; pallor or plethora
Gastrointestinal: tolerates feedings	Gastrointestinal: abdominal distention; spitting up; vomiting; gagging; stooling
Behavioral	
Body movements smooth and synchronous: consistent tone of all body parts; arms and legs flexed with smooth movements	Tremors, jittery and jerking movements; hypotonia or hypertonia (flaccid trunk, extremities; arching, flailing, extended extremities; finger splays, fisting)
States; well-defined sleep-wake	Unable to modulate states: sudden state changes; more active than quiet sleep; awake states with gaze aversion, frowning, grimacing, staring, irritability, wide-eyed "help me" look
Self-quieting behaviors: hand-to-mouth, hand or foot clasping, finger folding or grasping, sucking, foot or leg bracing	Limited use of self-quieting behaviors (may need assistance from caregiver)
Attentive behaviors: alert gaze; fixes and follows visual stimuli; ceases to suck or slows suck rate, turns toward auditory stimuli, smiles; imitates: mouth opening, tongue extension; vocalizes: cooing, babbling, habituates to stimuli	May demonstrate any of above stress signals when attempting to interact with one or more modes of stimuli (e.g., rocking and talking) simultaneously in environment (either animate or inanimate)

Modified from Als H et al: *J Am Acad Child Psychiatry* 20:239, 1981; Gorski PA: *Semin Perinatol* 3:61, 1979.

and unrestricted contact of parents and newborns should be the policy in every normal, medium, and high-risk nursery (see Box 28-2). Providing a "family room," "bonding room," or "apartment" where parents and their soon-to-be discharged newborn can room in helps the transition from hospital to home care.

Intervention Strategies

Because infants experience their environment through sensory capabilities, intervention strategies are based on tactile/kinesthetic, auditory, visual, olfactory/gustatory, and communication skills. Interventions must be individualized according to the

infant's state, sensory threshold, physiologic homeostasis, and stability or stress cues.[7,54,171]

Circadian Rhythms

In utero, the states of the fetus are regulated by the sleep-wake cycles of the mother. In the NICU multiple intrusions disrupt regulation; how this affects the infant is not fully known, although limited energy may be drained and the infant subjected to further stress.[11,75,78] To minimize interruptions and excessive handling, infants should not be awakened when asleep; if they must be awakened for care, it should be during active sleep by talking softly and gentle stroking.[38,50,173] Appointments for examinations should be made before feeding to decrease unnecessary disturbance of sleep but with enough rest time (if needed) before actual feeding.

Adequate numbers of care-giving encounters—physical assessment, vital signs, diaper or linen change, procedures—must be balanced against constant manipulations.[11,73] Because essentially all NICU (level II and III) infants are continuously monitored, "laying on of hands" every 1 to 2 hours is often unnecessary. Thorough physical assessment and vital sign recording every 4 hours is easily alternated with recordings from the monitors every 4 hours—thus the infant is evaluated every 2 hours but *not* disturbed that often. An acutely ill infant may need closer observation, but alternating "hands on" with monitor readings accomplishes the goal without overwhelming an infant with few reserves.

Day-night cycles are facilitated by afternoon nap time and nighttime in which the dimming of lights or covering of incubators and cribs with blankets and quieting of NICU noise enables infants to sleep.[21,22,110,162] Deep, quiet sleep is facilitated by quiet and dark, soft (classical) music, gentle stroking of the head, and self-regulated task (self-sought proximity of infant to breathing bear).[168] Maintaining daily nap time and night-time hours helps infants reset their diurnal rhythms and become accustomed to sleeping in dim light and a quiet environment[21,10] (something that babies discharged from the hospital for even short stays have difficulty doing). Among convalescing preterms (<34 weeks' gestational age), four standard rest periods/day resulted in (1) increased daily weight gain, (2) increased sleep, (3) less active states during nap time, and (4) by 3 weeks, less quiet waking time and longer uninterrupted sleep episodes.[88,89,157,159] Uninterrupted sleep and diurnal rhythmicity is also associated with improved state organization in VLBW infants.[55]

Tactile/Kinesthetic Intervention

Because the sense of touch is highly developed in utero, even the very immature preterm has acute tactile sensitivity. For the newborn, human touch is the most important tactile stimulation. Tactile sensation both arouses and quiets—gentle but firm handling quiets infants, because they feel more secure; light, uncertain touch often results in agitation and withdrawal.[101,106] Excessive handling of preterm or sick neonates results in significant physiologic consequences such as (1) blood pressure changes, (2) alterations in cerebral blood flow, and (3) hypoxia and other stress behaviors.[49,107]

In the NICU, infants who are repeatedly subjected to painful, intrusive procedures develop touch aversion—the association of human touch with pain. These infants cry uncontrollably, squirm away, flail arms and legs, and recoil when touched, knowing that pain will soon follow. The infant who was ventilated may have touch aversion around the mouth; the infant is averse to facial stroking and rooting, has a hypersensitive gag reflex, and refuses to nipple feed. Painful procedures should be minimized to those absolutely (medically) indicated—*no* infant should be subjected to "routine" painful procedures. During those necessary procedures, providing body containment, comfort measures (like a pacifier), and adequate pain relief (see Chapter 11) is essential.

Noncare-giving touch (i.e., social contact) should be provided by parents and professionals when the preterm infant is aware, alert, and receptive.[35,103] Kangaroo care, skin-to-skin contact between parents and infant by placing the infant in a vertical position between the maternal or paternal breasts, benefits both parents and neonates (Table 12-8).

Nonpainful touch such as stroking (the head, trunk, or hands) during care may calm, soothe, and prevent touch aversion. Stroking of physiologically stable preterm infants has been associated with increased activity, a faster regaining of birth weight, less crying, and better social scores.[18,148,178] However, in preterm infants (26 to 30 weeks' gestation) who are not physiologically stable, stroking results in decreased oxygen saturation and signs of behavioral stress (e.g., grasping, grunting, and gaze aversion).[128] If the preterm becomes agitated with stroking, a hand firmly placed on the head or trunk often quiets. Hand placement without stroking does not decrease oxygen saturation or alter heart rate and has a soothing effect (i.e., decreases active sleep, increases quiet sleep, decreases motor activity and behavioral distress) in small preterm infants.[84,85,124,170] Handle gently to avoid stressful reactions, (e.g., flailing, arching, oxygen desaturation) and enable the infant to become calm and rest between care giving.

As the preterm infant matures, head-to-toe massage at the rate of 12 to 16 strokes/min (for respiratory homeostasis)[94] soothes, provides for tension release, and stimulates respiration, circulation, and gastrointestinal function. Confidence in parenting skills and tactile communication between parent and infant are encouraged when parents massage their infant. Parents may also tub bathe the premature grower, which provides a relaxing, tension-relieving experience of multiple textures (water, water temperature, soap, washcloth). However, sponge bathing critically ill preterm infants (28 to 34 weeks' gestational age) results in significant increases in behavior state and activity levels (i.e., motor stress behavior, stability, and reorganization), stress cue frequency, increase or decrease in heart rate, and decrease in oxygen saturation.[132,133] These detrimental effects were exhibited most frequently by neonates of the younger gestational ages.

Varying sensation and touch pattern keeps the infant interested in stroking and massaging. As the preterm infant matures and is able to tolerate

---

Table 12-8
Benefits of Kangaroo Care/Skin-to-Skin Contact[2,3,17,63]

Parental	Neonatal
Activates maternal processes of search for meaning and mastery of the experience of premature birth	Thermal synchrony—mother's body temperature rises and falls to maintain infant in neutral state (see Chapter 6)
Increases maternal self-confidence, competence, and self-esteem	Cardiopulmonary
Enhances parent-infant attachment	Adequate or improved oxygenation
Initiates and maintains maternal behavior	Fewer episodes of periodic breathing, apnea, and bradycardia
Positive and personally beneficial experience	Breastfeeding
Positively impacts parental identity and knowledge of infant	Increased incidence and length
Increases confidence in meeting infant's needs	Increased milk supply
More frequent visiting	Behavioral
Parental eagerness for infant's discharge	Increased alert activity
	Increased deep sleep
	Decreased or no crying[36,37]
	Increased enface positioning
	Earlier discharge
	Increased weight gain
	No increased infection
	Out of incubator earlier
	Regulatory interaction[87]
	Behavioral
	Sucking
	Neurochemical
	Metabolic
	Sleep-wake cycles
	Cardiovascular
	Endocrine
	Immune
	Circadian

variety, he or she should be introduced to different textures (e.g., lambskins, stuffed toys, cotton, satin). Baby clothes provide various textures, make the infant more attractive ("He looks like a real baby!" "She looks like a girl, since her shaved head is covered."), and decrease heat loss (especially hats).

Consoling hand-to-mouth behaviors are observed more frequently during care giving (by nurses, rather than parents) and before and after feeding (especially in gavage-fed infants).[22] Hand to-midline behaviors are encouraged by cradling the infant for feedings (for both bottle and gavage feedings if the infant tolerates it) with both arms in the midline. If the premature infant needs an oxygen hood, using one large enough so that the infant's whole upper body will fit inside encourages hand-to-mouth quieting (Fig. 12-2). VLBW preterms whose whole body was not inside the oxygen hood have been videotaped expending energy in persistent attempts (30 to 40 minutes) to self-

console and reduce stress by trying to get their hands to their mouths.[22] Use arm restraints only when necessary and immobilize the extremity in a physiologic position. Release and exercise the restrained extremity with each care-giving encounter. Avoid restraining both arms so that one is free for hand-to-mouth behaviors. If both must be restrained (e.g., the infant pulls out the orogastric tube), give the infant a pacifier.

Positioning. Preterm infants display different motor development from term infants. A continuous assessment of muscle tone, response to positioning and handling, oral-motor function, and response to sensory stimuli provide data for individualizing intervention.[59] The goal of intervention is to provide opportunities for normal development and organization of the sensory systems, to detect early developmental problems, and to educate parents about stimulation, handling, and positioning. Although some studies have shown

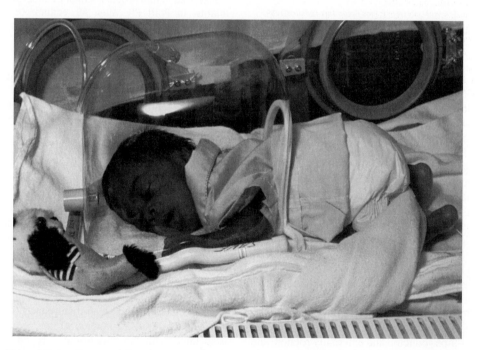

Figure 12-2.   Preterm infant in oxygen hood that is large enough to accommodate upper body to facilitate hand-to-mouth behavior. Note sling that helps maintain flexion without frog-leg position.

Table 12-9
Development of Tone*

Gestational Age (wk)	Development
28	Completely hypotonic and lacks all physiologic flexion
32	Hips and knees begin to show some flexion while arms remain extended
34	Flexor tone apparent in legs
36	Loose flexion of arms and legs evident and grasp reflex present
40	Develops tone in utero and develops flexed position in intrauterine space; after birth, reflex activity and CNS maturity help term infant to unfold and extend; term infant holds all four limbs in flexed position

*Muscle tone develops in caudocephalic and centripetal (distal to proximal) directions and interacts with simultaneous cephalocaudal development of movement to help affect posture. Although knowledge of normal development before term helps detect signs of abnormality, variability of ±2 weeks' gestational age must be taken into consideration.[5]
From Anderson J, Auster-Liebhaber J: *Phys Occup Ther Pediatr* 4(1):89, 1984; Dubowitz L et al: *J Pediatr* 77:1, 1970; Palisano R, Short M: *Phys Occup Ther Pediatr* 4(4): 43, 1984.

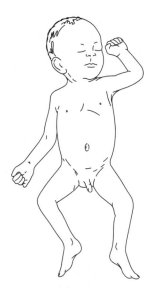

Figure 12-3 Premature infant resting posture exhibiting shoulder retraction and abduction and frog-leg position: hips abducted and externally rotated and ankle and feet everted. (From Pelletier-Sehnar J, Palmeri A: High-risk infants. In Pratt PN, Allen AS, editors: *Occupational therapy for children,* ed 2, St Louis, 1989, Mosby.)

that specific positioning for premature infants does not significantly affect development,[1] others have shown that a developmental approach to care of VLBW infants greatly reduces the long-term effects of prematurity.[19]

Preterm infants usually have less developed physiologic flexion in the limbs, trunk, and pelvis than term newborns (Table 12-9). Even at term conceptual age, preterms have less flexion than their full-term counterparts.[83] For preterm infants, long periods of immobilization without a positioning device, on a firm mattress with the influences of gravity, result in a number of abnormal characteristics: (1) increased neck extension with a right-sided head preference, (2) shoulder retraction and abduction (reduces forward rotation and ability to reach midline), (3) increased trunk extension with "arching" of the neck and back, (4) frog-leg position—hips abducted and externally rotated, and (5) ankle and feet eversion[172] (Fig. 12-3). These characteristics interfere with development of eye-hand coordination, cognitive development, and

equilibrium[77] Box 12-3 lists the reasons for proper positioning in the NICU.

To prevent overstretching of the joints and to facilitate development of flexor tone, the infant should be provided with a variety of positions. Side lying (Fig. 12-4) is used to improve visual awareness of hands, to encourage hands-to-midline movement, and to discourage the frog-leg position. In this position the infant is able to bring the hands to the mouth for sucking and self-comforting.

Acutely ill preterms are often positioned supine with the head to the side or in the midline to accommodate their ventilators, umbilical catheters, and other devices. Supine positioning does not promote flexion and may be stressful to acutely ill infants.[7,28] Placed supine, infants experience more startle behaviors and sleep disturbance from environmental stimuli. Prolonged supine positioning is associated with the hypertonic "arched" position (hyperextension of head, neck, and shoulder girdle) of many chronically ventilated infants. Supine positioning should promote as much flexion as

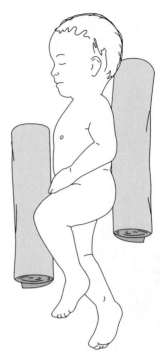

Figure 12-4   Side-lying is obtained by using a rolled blanket behind infant's head and trunk; additional support is added by placing another roll in front of infant's chest and abdomen with infant's top leg over it. Placing a blanket over the infant and tucking it under the mattress helps hold this position. Placing the rolled blanket in a stockinette helps provide a firm boundary for the roll. To avoid neck flexion or hyperextension, the infant's head should be monitored and the position of the neck changed as necessary. Blanket roll at the feet gives the infant a boundary on which to brace the feet.

possible (Fig. 12-5). Use of a positioning device of foam with the middle cut out sloping under the scapulae is another method of obtaining supine flexion. Pillows filled with polystyrene beads (i.e., premie bean bags) require skill for optimal positioning and close infant monitoring[95] but are useful in providing positioning for very small premature infants (1000 to 1500 g).

Body containment increases the infant's feeling of security, promotes quieting and self-control, enhances physiologic stability, promotes energy conservation, reduces physiologic and behavioral stress, and enables stress to be better endured.[164] Many premature infants "travel" (no matter how many times they are moved) to the sides or bottom of their incubator. Just as premature infants are able to seek proximity to a breathing bear[168] they are able to seek out security. Parents and professionals are inclined to move the uncomfortable-looking infant back to the middle of a "boundaryless" world. Leave infants where they feel safe and comfortable—if they become uncomfortable they will let you know. Providing boundaries (e.g., blanket rolls) often stops this migration.

Small, acutely ill premature infants who are positioned supine are often extremely agitated, thrashing arms and legs, tachycardic, and expending precious energy and calories. Instead of medications, these infants are often calmed by providing a "nest" of blankets on either side and at the head and feet. The infant's limbs are then flexed inside the "artificial womb," and the infant quietly rests

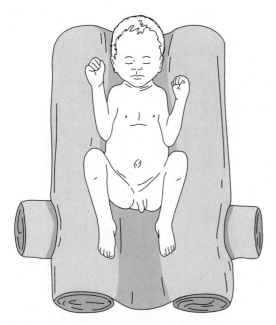

Figure 12-5 Supine positioning with rolled blankets or pads on either side of body and under knees to provide secure boundaries and promote flexion. *NOTE:* Supine positioning should be used with caution. Preterm infants who have not developed gag reflex (<36 weeks gestation) are at particularly high risk for aspiration. Supine position should not be used until most of a feeding has been absorbed (at least 1 to 1 1/2 hours after feeding). (From Pelletier-Sehnar J, Palmeri A: High-risk infants. In Pratt PN, Allen AS, editors: *Occupational therapy for children,* ed 2, St Louis, 1989, Mosby.)

(Fig. 12-6). If agitation recurs, a limb (usually a leg) has extended outside the infant's secure boundary—flexing and returning it to the "womb" quiets the infant.[7,173]

Body containment maneuvers such as swaddling, holding onto a finger or hand, and crossing the infant's arms in the midline and holding them securely help with self-regulation during feeding, procedures, or other stressful manipulations[34,41,164] Because being wrapped in a blanket with extremities flexed simulates in utero position, swaddling (1) improves flexed posture and flexor muscle tone, (2) facilitates behavioral responses, and (3) improves the development of primitive reflexes.[152]

Picking the preterm infant up from a supine position often produces startles, apnea, or head hyperextension.[57] A better technique is to roll the infant prone, which flexes the head, and then flex the limbs onto the trunk and pick the infant up.[173] If the infant has difficulty breathing in prone position, swaddle or contain the extremities before picking the infant up.

Prone positioning encourages the infant to work on using neck extension and promotes flexion of the extremities. This position does not require the use of any device—it merely encourages knee and arm flexion; a small hiproll or sling (see Fig. 12-2) assists in maintaining flexion.[57] Prone (versus supine) positioning has numerous benefits and is the position of choice for many NICU infants (Box 12-4). Use of a sheepskin or lambskin helps to further facilitate flexion and prevents skin abrasion, especially on the knees.

A combination of vestibular and tactile stimulation increases quieting behaviors, decreases apneic and bradycardic episodes, entrains respirations, increases visual and auditory fixation, and increases brain growth.[99,100,104] Waterbeds provide contingent stimuli, because they move in response to the infant's movement; oscillating waterbeds provide rhythmic motion. Kinesthetic stimulation is provided by rocking chairs, hammocks, baby swings, and baby carriers whose effects have not been investigated. Upright positioning in a car or infant seat encourages symmetry and spatial orientation. Soft rolls or foam padding maintains flexion while a rolled blanket in a horseshoe configuration around the infant's head and shoulders prevents lateral slouching.[131] Carrying quiets the infant, provides sensory communication with the care giver, changes the infant's environment, and provides visual and auditory as well as tactile stimuli. A nasal cannula (see Chapter 22) and portable tank enable mobility for the infant receiving oxygen.

Rather than standardized protocols, tactile interventions must be individualized by assessing each infant's physiologic and behavioral responses before, during, and after touch (see Table 12-6). While acutely ill, tactile intervention should include (1) minimal handling, (2) containment, and (3) gentle touch (without stroking). As the infant matures and becomes physiologically stable, strok-

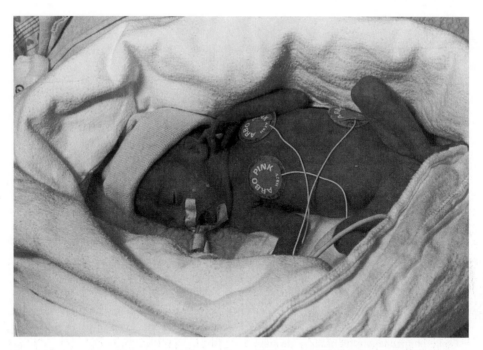

Figure 12-6 Very small premature infant resting quietly in a "nest" of pads and blankets.

ing, rocking, and holding are integrated based on the individual infant's tolerance and preferences.

Auditory Intervention

The NICU is a noisy environment that has no diurnal rhythm—it is as noisy at night as in the daytime[48,75,162] (Table 12-10). The NICU infant is exposed to an onslaught of noise 24 hours a day for days, weeks, or months. At follow-up, preterm infants exhibit a lower threshold for sound.[90] Neonatal illnesses, drug therapies, and possibly acoustic insult account for the increased risk (i.e., 10% to 12% of LBW) for sensorineural hearing loss in NICU infants (regardless of gestational age).[151] Institution of a quiet time or rest period through reduction of (1) noise from talking, equipment, telephones, etc.; (2) light by dimming overhead light; and (3) procedures to only emergency treatment has resulted in enhanced infant sleep and less parental and care giver stress.[162]

Box 12-4

Effects of Prone Positioning

1. Improves oxygenation by 15% to 25%[111,149,176]
   a. Increased TcP_{O_2} values
   b. Increased Pa_{O_2} values
2. Improves lung mechanics and lung volumes[176]
   a. Increased lung compliance
   b. Increased tidal volume
3. Decreases energy expenditure[112,149]
   a. Increased quiet sleep
   b. Decreased awake time
   c. Decreased caloric expenditure (median difference supine versus prone: +3.1 kcal/kg/day)
   d. (?) Decreased heat loss
4. Decrease in gastric reflux in prone position with head of bed elevated 30 degrees[129]

Table 12-10
Noise Levels in the NICU

Level (dB)	Comments
50-60	Normal speaking voice
50-73.5*†	Incubator (motor noise)
45-85‡	Noise in NICU (talking, equipment alarms, telephones, radio)
48-69	Humidifiers and nebulizers[123]
65-80†	Life support equipment (ventilator, IV pumps)
85	Noise level at which hearing damage is possible for adult; (?) neonatal effects
90§	Adult exposure for 8 hours requires protective device and hearing conservation program
92.8†	Opening incubator porthole
96-117†	Placing bottle of formula on top of incubator
110-116†	Closing one or both cabinet doors
114-124†	Closing one or both portholes
130-140†	Banging incubator to stimulate apneic premature infant
160-165	Recommendations for peak, single noise level not to exceed to prevent (adult) hearing loss; (?) neonatal effects

Modified from Mitchell SA: *Semin Hear* 5(1):17, 1984.
*American Academy of Pediatrics recommends incubator noise not to exceed 58 dB (Modern incubators generate 51-52 dB).[23]
†Measures from inside the incubator.
‡Noise levels do not vary from morning to night.
§Occupational Safety and Health Administration (OSHA) standard. (No safety standards for neonates have been established.)

Box 12-5

Effects of Loud Noise*

Increase in stress behaviors
 State lability
 Arousal state
 Avoidance behaviors—more fussy, more startles, etc. (see Table 12-7)
Decrease in approach behaviors (see Table 12-7)
Cardiorespiratory changes
 Increased heart rate
 Increased respiratory rate
 Increased apnea or bradycardia
 Increased hypoxemia (decreased pulse oximeter)
 Increased peripheral and arterial vasoconstriction
 Increased systemic blood pressure
 Increased intracranial pressure
Alters development of sleep-wake cycles

* References 35, 72, 73, 92, 108, 145, 154, 179, 184.

The first goal in auditory intervention is to assess the current level of noise in the NICU and to decrease the noise decibels wherever possible. Increased environmental noise levels are a stressor to all NICU infants—the preterm, as well as the ill term infant (e.g., persistent pulmonary hypertension of the newborn [PPHN]; drug withdrawal) (Box 12-5). The sudden high-pitched, shrill, dysrhythmic noise of equipment alarms alerts the care provider but it also results in infants manifesting an extreme hypersensitivity to sound (as a learned conditioned response).[90]

Strategies to minimize external auditory stimuli include quieting alarms with suction (and remembering to reset them); not taking a shift report over, or allowing medical rounds near, the infant's incubator; having noisy equipment repaired immediately; emptying sloshing water in ventilator or nebulizer tubing; and maintaining cardiac monitors in a quiet state with alarms on. Choosing heated humidifiers (48 dB) rather than nebulizers (69 dB) and keeping the containers full (rather than low) of water decrease noise from respiratory equipment.[123] Nursery design changes include smaller cubicles rather than one large room, soundproofing materials, lights for phones and alarm systems, and minimizing equipment noise. Placing a blanket on top of the incubator or using an incubator cover muffles the noise of equipment placement; gentle, considerate (to the infant) placement of equipment on or in the incubator muffles sound; and closing portholes and drawers gently decreases the structural noises of care giving. Prohibiting placement of equipment (e.g., clipboards, stethoscopes, formula bottles) on top of the incubator prevents such noises.

No tapping (by parents or siblings) or banging (by medical, nursing, or ancillary personnel) on the incubator Plexiglas should ever be permitted. This (along with a brisk startle reflex from the infant) is an opportunity to teach about the noise levels generated by such activity. Infants should be kept in incubators as long as necessary to maintain heat balance. The incubator does *not* protect the infant from noise—a well-managed NICU environment may be much quieter than the continuous noise of an incubator. However, the noise in modern incubators (see Table 12-10) is below the recommended 58 dB and, in one study, noise in the incubator was significantly lower than measured in an open crib.[179] Prolonged stays in an incubator *do* expose the infant to repeated care giving noises, as well as to a dearth of kinesthetic stimulation (e.g., carrying, holding, rocking, swinging, and sitting upright in an infant seat) and socially relevant speech patterns.

Conductive hearing loss is attributed to endotracheal intubation, poor Eustachian tube function, and increased otitis media in preterms.[158] Noise levels in the NICU may interfere with development of other sensory systems and influence the development of hearing and language delay.[158] Radios have been banned in many NICUs. If music is played, it should be on a low volume (below the dB range of normal speech), should *not* be rock music, and preferably should be classical (infants prefer Brahms, Bach, and Beethoven). Agitated, intubated preterms who received music therapy (i.e., in utero sounds and female voice) improved their oxygen saturations and behavioral states,[40,102] whereas full-term newborns exposed to soothing music spent less time in high arousal states and had fewer behavioral state changes.[93] Day-night cycles (nap time; nighttime) when auditory stimulation is decreased should be established in the NICU.[21] On discharge, NICU infants often will not sleep in a quiet room—softly playing a radio facilitates sleep, and the infant is gradually weaned from it. Signs such as: "Quiet . . . baby sleeping" or "Do not disturb—I'm asleep (talk to my nurse)" ensure undisturbed sleep—provided they are heeded.

The "in turning" premature infant (see Table 12-4) of less than 34 weeks' gestation probably receives enough auditory input from the NICU—auditory enhancement at this stage is probably overstimulation. Just as high-frequency sounds arouse, low-frequency ones—like the heart beat, respiratory sounds, and vacuum cleaners—quiet and facilitate sleep.[50,82] Music boxes with a repetitious lullaby and tape recordings of mother's,

father's, or siblings' voices (reading stories, poems, or singing) soothe the infant.[35,40] Watch for the infant's reaction and use only if the infant is soothed. If the infant becomes restless, turning the volume lower or placing the device on the outside, rather than inside, of the incubator may be more relaxing. However, since preterms are less able to habituate to sound than term babies, they may be unable to tolerate any added sound and may become exhausted by such stimuli.[158]

The human voice is the most preferred sound.[60] Teach parents the neonatal preference for high-pitched voices speaking in typical speech patterns (not baby talk). Role model and teach parents to gently talk to the infant while touching and giving care. Teach parents to talk to their infant while presenting their faces in the infant's range of vision. Watch for infant tolerance and increase or decrease talk time to avoid overload. Imitate the infant's coos and babbles—this reinforces and encourages vocalizations.

For the neonate, hearing may initially be more important than vision for attachment and bonding to the parents. Within seconds after birth, newborns are able to discriminate and prefer their mother's face—they have connected her familiar voice with her unfamiliar face.[24] A high index of suspicion regarding hearing loss is warranted if care givers do not observe normal responses to sound stimulation. All newborns, especially those with a history of familial hearing loss, hyperbilirubinemia (>15 mg in preterm infant; >20 mg in term infant), congenital viral infections, defects of the ear, nose, and throat, small preterm infants (<1500 g); those with bacterial sepsis or meningitis, severe asphyxia at birth, prolonged (>10 days) mechanical ventilation, stigmata, and other syndromes, and those receiving ototoxic drugs should have a hearing screening before discharge.[15]

Visual Intervention

The NICU is lit with bright cool-white fluorescent lights 24 hours a day to enable immediate and ongoing visibility of all infants. The American Academy of Pediatrics recommends 60 foot candles for adequate observation and 100 foot candles for procedures.[14] Although there is no neonatal research on the hazards of this type of lighting, there is abundant animal, child, and adult research documenting negative biochemical and physical effects (change in endocrine function, increased hypocalcemia, cell transformations, immature gonadal development, and chromosome breakage.)[25] Exposure to bright lights in the NICU is associated with (1) decreased oxygenation, (2) increased incidence of retinopathy, (3) poorer circadian rhythms, (4) altered sleep patterns, (5) skin changes (e.g., tanning, rashes), and (6) alteration of nutrients in total parenteral nutrition (TPN) solution, formula, and breastmilk.* Rapid increase in the intensity of ambient light causes younger, more immature preterms to decrease their oxygen saturation.

The first goal in visual intervention is to assess the current level of light and decrease it wherever possible. The very immature preterm infant is accustomed to the muted light of the uterus—light filtered through the abdominal and uterine walls— and has fused (if <26 weeks' gestation) eyelids. Draping blankets on top of the incubator or using a commercial incubator cover[164] decreases the light at the infant's level but allows immediate maximal illumination when the cover is pulled back. Because infants are continuously monitored, not all infants need to be maximally illuminated at all times.[75] Cycled light, dimming the lights in day-night cycles, is associated with positive effects (Box 12-6). Use of indirect full-spectrum light may require color assessment adjustments (at each bedside) but does not have the side effects of coolwhite light and can be individually controlled.[75]

Visual attentiveness is correlated with birth weight and gestational age—the more mature the infant, the more the infant is able to fix and follow. The infant at 28 weeks gestation fixes and follows but may become apneic as a result. Visual stimulation is very tiring and taxing (increases the heart rate) to the immature infant—those of less than 34 weeks' gestation probably receive enough stimulation from the NICU environment. When these infants reach the "coming out stage" (see Table 12-4) they may signal their readiness for visually enhancing activities.

Infants receiving phototherapy are visually sensory deprived because of their protective eye pads. These should be removed during care and

---

* References 21, 69, 75, 110, 153, 154, 169, 174.

Box 12-6
Effects of Cycled Light*

Behavior
  Decreases movement or motor activity
  Increases motor coordination
  Increases sleep time
  Decreases crying
Cardiorespiratory changes
  Decreases heart rate
  Decreases respiratory rate
Feeding behavior
  Quicker progression to oral feedings
  Feeds more efficiently and in less time
  Increased weight gain
Circadian rhythm development
  Temperature
  Heart rate
Decreased cortisol levels
Decreased incidence and severity of retinopathy of prematurity (ROP)
Decreased parental or care provider stress

* References 21, 45, 69, 76, 110, 121, 153, 162, 165.

---

feeding and interaction with parents and professionals. Providing interesting visual stimuli includes inanimate (e.g., toys, black and white faces and patterns, pictures of family members, artwork from siblings, mobiles) and animate (faces of parents, siblings, and professionals) objects (Fig. 12-7). Infants prefer the human face as a visual stimulus, especially the talking face, which stimulates both visual and auditory pathways. Parents often need to be encouraged that *their* faces, rather than all the infant's toys, are what their infant prefers to listen to and watch.

Teach parents the abilities of the infant and appropriate methods of visual stimulation:

- Place mobiles, pictures, and faces within the visual range of the newborn—8 to 12 inches for term infants, a little closer for preterm infants.
- Quiet alert is the best state for visual encounters—after feedings, if awake; swaddle infant to quiet or unwrap infant to arouse; hold infant upright.

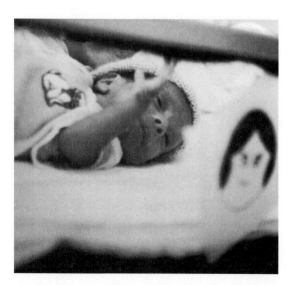

Figure 12-7 Premature infant fixing on black and white face.

- Place infant on abdomen with objects of various sizes and shapes within visual range.
- Change toys and visual stimuli—infants become bored with the same thing.
- When the preterm infant tolerates multiple stimuli, hold infant in en face position (see Chapter 28) to feed, talk to, and rock. Whether the infant is nipple or gavage fed, alternate sides so the infant sees both sides of the care provider's face (especially important if the preterm infant exhibits the common preference for right-sided head turning).
- Place infant at varied heights (in baby carrier, crib, swing, infant seat, on floor) so the infant sees the world from various angles.
- Place infant so that he or she is able to bring hands to midline and can see hands and fingers and eventually reach for toys.

Infants who exhibit gaze aversion should not be "pursued" by the face of the parent or professional, because this only potentiates the time "spent away" with their gaze to protect themselves from overload. Gaze aversion, flat facial affect, and absence of a smile may cast doubt on the ability of these infants to see, because there is no eye language or care giver feedback of preference, recognition, and delight. These infants *do* see, but they fix only fleetingly. Minimizing care providers is crucial so that the infant deals with as few care giver cues, styles, and ways of being handled as possible.

Smell/Taste Intervention

The neonate's well-developed sense of smell is not stimulated in the NICU with pleasant odors. The high-risk infant is stimulated by the smell of forgotten alcohol, skin prep, or povidine-iodine (Betadine) pads inside the incubator. Because the premature infant is unable to respond by crying or moving away, the infant responds to noxious smells by a decrease in respiratory rate, transient apnea, and/or an increase in heart rate. Removal of noxious odors from the incubator is as critical as removal of sharp instruments after a procedure.

Enhancing the olfactory environment includes having parents hold the infant or sit close if the infant cannot yet be held. The smell of the mother's breast milk is especially pleasant and may elicit a suckling reflex. Placing one drop on the infant's lips with a cotton ball or gauze sponge helps the infant to recognize the mother's smell and to associate that smell with food and feeding when the infant is able to nipple feed.

Nonnutritive suckling (during gavage and between feedings) is associated with better oxygenation, quieter, more restful behavior and improved behavioral organization, increased readiness for nipple feedings, and better weight gain.[134,183] Sucking on a pacifier satisfies the infant's sucking needs and may facilitate early learning that satiety and sucking are associated. However, nutritive and nonnutritive suckling are *not* alike (see Chapter 18); because the infant vigorously sucks on a pacifier does not mean the infant will be able to suckle nutritively, because the expressive and swallow phases have not been present in nonnutritive suckling. This is very confusing to most parents and many professionals.

High-risk infants often undergo prolonged periods of nothing by mouth (NPO) when their sensation of hunger is not relieved. Although pacifiers are soothing, these infants may learn that sucking and satiety are not related. NICU infants also undergo many aversive stimuli around and within the mouth (i.e., oral intubation, oral and endotracheal tube suction, intermittent gavage) that result in touch aversion of the mouth and a hypersensitive gag reflex. Feeding difficulties may be the result of (1) neurologic damage (e.g., IVH); (2) structural abnormalities (e.g., cleft palate or submucous cleft, recessed chin); (3) prematurity—infant is too neurologically immature and tires easily with "work" of feeding. Neural maturation (34 to 35 weeks' gestation) is the developmental guideline for initiation of oral feedings[96] (see Table 12-2), although some infants are ready at an earlier age (32 to 34 weeks' gestation).[33,115-117] However, preterm infants may exhibit periods of apnea and tachypnea with bottle feeding because consistent coordination of breathing with sucking and swallowing occurs >37 weeks[32] (see Table 12-2). (4) aversive feeder (acquired or developmental sucking defect, psychologic—"hospitalitis," rumination); or (5) a combination of these types.[66,67] Preterm infants are not at risk for chronic feeding problems if they are changed from nonoral methods (TPN and tube feeding) to oral methods by the end of the first month of life.[96]

The goals of intervention include (1) a safe feeding (i.e., diminished risk of aspiration); (2) a functional feeding (i.e., adequate caloric intake with minimal energy expenditure); and (3) a pleasant, social interactive experience for infant and parents or care givers. Box 12-7 outlines intervention strategies to facilitate oral feeding.

A feeding plan must be individualized for each infant and posted at the bedside. All care providers must adhere to the plan for consistency of stimuli and to promote infant learning.

Tommy was a 28-week preterm infant with severe RDS, prolonged ventilation, and now BPD. He is now 38 weeks' postconceptual age, receiving hood and nasal cannula oxygen, and trying to learn to nipple feed. In the morning report, the night nurse says that Tommy "has bradycardia with tube passage so that 24 hours ago he had a cardiorespiratory arrest that required resuscitation. He also has bradycardia and tachypnea with bottle feeding."

Tommy's nurse evaluated his initial attempts to bottle feed (after waiting for him to demand) and wrote the care plan (Box 12-8) after feeding him 45 ml in 20 minutes without tachypnea, cyanosis, or bradycardia.

Crying/Smiling Intervention

Crying is the infant's innate care-eliciting behavior—a signal that the infant needs attention. Immediate response decreases the infant's physiologic stress, increases the infant's trust in the environment, and enhances the sense of self and of control over the world. The infant's need to escalate to "out of control" crying is decreased with immediate response, so that infants are easier to soothe. Consoling the crying infant also helps the infant change states so he or she is able to attend to and interact with the environment.

Term infants vocalize, cry, and look at their care giver more than do preterm and ill infants.[75] NICU infants exhibit fewer care-eliciting behaviors (some preterm infants in one study never cried, vocalized, or looked at their care giver).[75] Preterm infants are thus less responsive to the care givers (both parents and professionals), who receive less positive feedback from the infant and hence are less rewarded. In one study those NICU infants who were able to cue the care provider (cry, look, vocalize) were consistently responded to 80% to 100% of the time.[75]

Intubated infants who are unable to produce an audible cry signal their needs by agitation, heart rate changes, and changes in oxygenation. Preterm infants (<32 weeks) may recover better from agitation when left alone, because active consolation is overstimulating.[73] How care givers attempt to soothe a crying infant (while giving NICU care) includes no response to cries (58.1% of the time), response by talking (29.2% of the time), response by social touching (5.5% of the time), and response by talk and social touching (7.2% of the time).[75]

Parents and staff should use graduated interventions in quieting a crying infant by:

- Soothing with gentle high-pitched talking (loud enough that the infant is able to hear it above his or her crying).
- Placing the palm of the hand across the infant's chest or holding arms on chest with the palm of the care provider's hand.
- Swaddling with blankets to decrease self-upsetting startles.
- Picking up infant, holding (upright is the most soothing position), and rocking.
- Offering a pacifier.

Box 12-7

Strategies to Facilitate Oral Feeding

I. Minimize noxious stimuli to the mouth
   A. Suction *only* as needed (*not* routinely)
   B. Consider indwelling gastric tube rather than intermittent gavage (an infant fed every 2 hours would have gavage tube passed 12 times a day)
   C. Pass intermittent gavage tube
      1. Down mouth through hole in pacifier nipple
      2. If infant has hypersensitive gag, passing smaller tube down nose stimulates gag reflex less than passing tube down mouth
   D. Perioral and intraoral stimulation techniques
      1. Are only *more aversive,* rather than therapeutic, on babies with touch aversion at mouth area
      2. When performing oral exercises, do so with care—do *not* stimulate aversive reflexes (e.g., gag reflex)
II. Enhance pleasant stimuli to the mouth (first experiences with suckling have lasting neurobehavioral effects[15])
   A. Have infant smell or taste breast milk
   B. Provide nonnutritive suckling with tube feeding
   C. Facilitate hand-to-mouth behaviors
   D. Firm nipple—a nipple that is too soft increases flow, stimulates anxiety and/or gag reflex, and causes bradycardia
   E. Perioral and intraoral stimulation—(?) facilitates development of normal sucking behaviors
   F. Use Lact-Aid nursing supplementer (see Chapter 18)
      1. Never frustrate infant with a dry breast
      2. Positive reinforcement for infant to nurse
      3. Calorically and energy efficient method
      4. Oral therapy—teaches infant proper nutritive suckle
   G. For infants with difficulty in coordination of respiration with suck or swallow (prevents stress of apnea and hypoxia and enhances pleasure of feeding experience)
      1. Assess feeding pattern, pulse oximeter, muscle tone, and breathing pattern
      2. Remove nipple from mouth to enable infant to beathe
III. Positioning—use proper position to facilitate swallow and improve suction
   A. Hold with feedings (even gavage) as much as possible
   B. Consistent caregivers—parents, primary nurses, foster grandparents
   C. Swaddle
      1. Decreases startles
      2. Infant may become too warm and sleepy
   D. Facilitate swallowing
      1. Position with chin tucked
      2. If breastfeeding, turn infant's whole body toward mother so head and trunk are in alignment (infant is not trying to swallow with head turned to one side)
      3. Upright position with neck, shoulders, and back supported—slows gravitational flow of formula from nipple (as when infant is in semireclined position)
      4. Cuddling, semireclined position—increases flow of formula by gravity—may be too fast, regardlless of nipple chosen; results in increased gags, choking, and bradycardia
      5. Prone with neck extended (slightly)
         a. Keeps tongue forward and airway unobstructed
         b. Good for aversive feeder who chokes
      6. Gentle, upward pressure under chin or at base of tongue facilitates swallowing, because it mimics upward thrust of tongue with swallowing
   E. Improve formation of suction
      1. Semireclining (>45-degree angle) on lap of care giver—frees both hands to work with infant on oral control
      2. Cupping both cheeks with fingers of free hand (i.e., hand not holding bottle) improves lip closure and suction formation
      3. Gentle tugging at nipple (as if to take it out of mouth) causes infant to begin or continue suckling
IV. Timing
   A. Do not allow infant to cry to exhaustion before feeding—infant will be too tired to eat
   B. Keep external stimuli to a minimum in immature preterm infants (<34 weeks) for optimal intake and weight gain
   C. If satiated, infant will not suck
      1. Feed on demand or when alert[91] (demand feeding reinforces sleep-wake cycle)[189]

continued

Box 12-7

Strategies to Facilitate Oral Feeding—cont'd

2. If feeding on schedule, note whether infant gives cue of hunger: fussiness/crying, hand-to-mouth behaviors and/or rooting, hiccups. Infants as young as 32 to 33 weeks can provide cues so that feeding can be individualized.[33]
3. If feeding on schedule, space time and see whether infant exhibits cues of hunger (as above.)
4. First, nipple what infant is able to feed; than tube feed (Presence of an indwelling nasogastric tube may result in compromised respirations, oxygen desaturation, and bradycardia in the VLBW infant)[155]

D. Try to nipple feed for no longer than 20 minutes (infant becomes too tired and uses up energy and calories to feed instead of to grow)
E. Infants of advanced age (around 6 months) may be unable to nipple if they have never had the opportunity; it may be more developmentally appropriate to cup or spoon-feed infant

---

Box 12-8

Tommy's Feeding Plan

1. *Sit upright.* This decreases the flow of formula from the bottle and thus decreases
   a. His gag reflex, which causes the bradycardia
   b. His anxiety caused by a bolus of formula in his mouth
2. *Use a blue nipple.* This is the shortest nipple and decreases stimulation of his hypersensitive gag reflex, which causes his bradycardia. (All other nipples stimulated him to gag.)
3. *Gently push up under his chin when he gets a mouthful of formula.* This pushes his tongue upward against his palate, the same way the tongue moves during swallowing. (Reader, swallow and watch your tongue motion.) He becomes frightened (i.e., eyes wide open and fearful; increased respiratory rate; arching and struggling) when he has a mouthful of formula, because he is used to only sucking on a dry pacifier and having nothing to swallow. His fear raises his heart rate, his respiratory rate, and his gag reflex, which causes bradycardia.
4. *Talk to him.* Softly and gently, tell him he can swallow and praise him when he does.
5. *Nipple.* Have him do this as much as possible (he will only get better with practice) and supplement feeding with the *indwelling* NG tube (no more intermittent tube passage).

Most stimulation in the NICU is procedural. The lack of social stimulation in the NICU not only affects the infant, but also teaches parents that their infant is too weak for, too fragile for, uninterested in, or incapable of social interaction. Again, social stimulation must be paced according to the stage of development and stability of the infant[35,103] (see Table 12-4). Enhancing the infant's social environment includes presenting the smiling, moving, talking care provider's face to the alert infant; touching and stroking; and soothing and consoling the distressed infant.

In many busy NICUs, parents and a foster grandparent program provide this sensory integrated social experience. If the infant has been transported to a referral center, parents may live some distance away and be unable to visit daily. The chronically ill 4- to 5-month-old infant who begins to recognize the foster grandmother may smile, relax, and feed better for her and is often fussier and more irritable on her day off. A foster grandparent program benefits both infants and seniors—the infant receives love and socialization, and the senior "has a reason to get up in the morning."

If at all possible, parents should be encouraged to perform the "firsts" with their infant (e.g., first nipple feeding, first bath, first time out of the incubator). Because parents are not always present, they will miss some important milestones for their infant (e.g., extubation). Many NICUs have developed baby diaries (or calendars) where the nurses, physicians, and foster grandparents write important information about the infant's day (as if the infant were the author). The text is accompanied by self-developing pictures with humorous captions (e.g., "Look at me—I've got my tube out!"). Staff are very creative in relating "what's been happening" so that the parents not only have a verbal report (that over time will be forgotten) but also a keepsake of NICU progress.

Long-Term Care in the NICU

Because smaller, more immature preterm infants are now surviving, some infants spend months in the NICU. To facilitate the development of these chronically hospitalized infants, parents and professionals must have realistic expectations of their developmental levels. A preterm infant who reaches 40 weeks' postconceptual age is not as mature in sleep-wake cycles, attentiveness, or soothability as a 40-week term infant.[73] In evaluating the developmental performance of a preterm infant, one must correct for the weeks of prematurity. For example: Susie is chronologically 8 months old; she was 32 weeks' gestation at birth, so her developmental age would be calculated as follows:

$$8 \text{ months} - 8 \text{ weeks (2 months)}$$
$$\text{preterm} = 6 \text{ months}$$

Susie will be developmentally appropriate in performance if she functions at a 6-month level; developmental delay would be functioning below the 6-month level.

Table 12-11 outlines developmental expectations for infants from birth to 6 months. Remember to correct for prematurity.

Outcome

Even though the survival rate of preterm infants, including VLBW preterm infants, has dramatically improved as a result of education of care providers, regionalization of care, and improved technology, there has not been a corresponding change in neonatal morbidity.* These infants are still at increased risk for physical and psychosocial emotional disabilities (Table 12-12, p. 236) despite recent NICU advances. Low birth weight, intraventricular hemorrhage, the need for assisted ventilation, and chronic lung disease are the risk factors associated with the highest risk of sequelae.†

There is an increased incidence of failure to thrive and child abuse and neglect in preterm infants.[104] Separation of infants and parents at birth disrupts the parent-infant attachment process and increases the risk of parenting disorders (see Chapters 28 and 29). In the first year of life, preterm infants are often more "difficult" and less "easy" to care for: are difficult to soothe, less adaptive, less able to habituate, state labile, negative in mood, and withdrawn.[64,113,114,181] Many families (40% to 45%) of VLBW infants experience feeding difficulties in the first years of the infant's life.[136,181] The parent who finds the preterm infant "too difficult" may become less responsive to and involved with the infant and thus escalate the infant's difficult behavior. Although an unsupportive environment may increase the difficult behavior, a supportive parent-infant interaction benefits the infant (i.e., the infant makes developmental gains). The impact on the family of VLBW infants is long lasting and includes financial burden, familial and social impact, personal strain, and mastery.[42]

The increased risk of cognitive impairment with decreasing birth weight may diminish with time and a supportive environment or may persist until school age.‡ Preterm infants are more likely to function below their genetic potential because of increased incidence of mental retardation, cerebral palsy, and learning disabilities.[79,80,81,91,97,142] Children who were preterm infants require more special education, repeat grades, and do less well on reading and math achievement tests than children who were born at term. Even when NICU graduates perform well on developmental tests, they may have neurosensory difficulties (e.g., problems with visual-motor integration, spatial relationships, and speech and language development) and passive, withdrawn behavior that negatively affects school accomplishment.[97] Early identification of cognitive

Text continued on p. 236

---

* References 6, 71, 79, 80, 81, 91, 97, 163, 180.

† References 6, 79, 80, 81, 97, 142, 163, 180.
‡ References 79, 80, 81, 91, 97, 142, 143.

Table 12-11
Neonatal and Infant Development (0-6 months)*

Age (mo)	Auditory	Language	Visual
0-1	Reacts to vocal sounds (recognizes and is soothed by mother's or caregiver's voice) Smiles when spoken to by mother Locates sound by turning head toward it Distinguishes volume and pitch; prefers high voice Distinguishes mother's or caregiver's voice from other female voices Stops crying with music	Produces crying or mewing sounds Communicates with body movements and cries Quiets when picked up	Sees within 8-10 in from face—watches and recognizes mother's face Fixes—follows moving objects, lights; stops sucking to look Sense of location or direction established by 1 mo Imitates facial expressions
1-2	Vocally responds to and imitates sounds of mother or caregiver Babbling accompanied by motor activity (1-6 mo) Quiets to voice	Imitates sounds of others Babbles or coos and repeats sounds with intention Deliberately cries for assistance	Binocular vision begins (6 wk) Gives equal time and concentration to familiar or unfamiliar objects (6-8 wk) Prefers linear patterns over curves; prefers people over objects Discriminates horizontal and vertical patterns Quiets to face
2-3	Sound has stimulus-response effect Stops sucking to listen; searches for sound with eyes	Refines intonation through interaction with caregiver Coos one-syllable sounds—ooh, ah, ae; gurgles, chuckles Cries less Vocalizes when talked to	Prefers looking at new things Begins facial differentiating with focus on eyes (2 mo) Color vision begins functioning Prefers curves to lines (2-6 mo)

*This table represents a generalized/normative grouping of developmental ages in which an infant accomplishes these tasks. Because some infants develop faster and some slower, this table is to be used as a guideline and not a literal interpretation of the milestone age for accomplishing a developmental task.

Tactile motor	Cognitive-mental	Social-emotional

Primitive reflexes
  Hands fisted—random grasp with intention
  Prone—tucked position
  Supine—tonic neck position
Pulled to sit: head lags—back is rounded with head rolled forward
Tactile contact aids in reestablishing biorhythmic balance and developing sense of self and confidence
	Reflex reactions (i.e., grasp, Moro, root, suckle, etc.)
	Organizes incoming stimuli
	Internal and external world are not differentiated—all are experienced as a part of the self
	Actions done with little indication of purpose or intention
		Task-development of trust versus mistrust through constancy and reliability of environment; response to infant's cries is essential
		Spends two thirds of time sleeping (7-8 short naps/day)
		Shuts out noxious stimuli

Rolls from supine to side-lying position Hands open or loosely closed—manipulative play with hands and fingers (6 wk) Deliberate holding grasp when finger placed in hand (8 wk) Raises head to vertical position (45-degree angle) when prone Begins unfolding body, extending and kicking legs (6-12 wk)	Attracted to unfamiliar and novel stimuli (0-6 mo) Converting reflexes into intentional responses through movement (i.e., body exploration) (1-4 mo) Developing rudimentary problem-solving skills (begins 5th-12th wk and evolves throughout infancy); expects feeding at certain time; associates people with behaviors (e.g., mother with food)	Accepts or tolerates care giver Begins formulating sense of mastery through interaction with environment Sleeps 2-4 long periods/day (6 wk), awake 10 hr/day Responds positively to comfort and care; negatively to pain and need Smiles at familiar voice or face—mother, father, and siblings Does not discriminate odd elements in a matrix Swipes at objects Tears when crying
Prone position favored—raises head 90 degrees and holds for several seconds; turns from prone to side-lying position Supine—slight head lag when pulled to sit; sits supported with head erect and bobbing Reciprocal kicking (precursor to crawling) Discovers hands (3 mo); grasp reflex decreasing (3 mo); reaches for object with both hands	Learning is sensory-kinetic (physical through movement) Engages in purposeful activity—repeat actions; associates action with result Distinguishes near from distant objects Begins to exhibit memory Begins to become aware of self	Gives different response to emotions expressed by others Duplicates mother in facial movements and sometimes affect Is developing a sense of mastery Cries when mother leaves Attracts mother's attention

Continued

Table 12-11—cont'd
Neonatal and Infant Development (0-6 months)*

Age (mo)	Auditory	Language	Visual
3-4	Turns head toward sound immediately	Organizes behaviors into expressive acts—coos are pitch-modulated and sustained for 15-20 min Makes sounds and recreates them to recapture experience Smiles, squeals, coos when talked to	Discovers hands (3 mo) Differentiates patterns and shapes (3 mo) Color vision same as adult's Binocular vision well established; sees 15-inch distance Differentiates aberrant facial features Raises and moves hand toward object seen Smiles and vocalizes at mirror image
4-5	Locates sound to the side but cannot locate sound above or below (4-7 mo) Turns head and looks for speaker Understands name	Utters vowel sounds and a few consonant sounds (d, b, l, m) Spontaneously vocalizes to self, toys Stops crying when talked to Protests if another tries to take toy	Sees but is unable to pick up small objects Visually directed movement (contacts object) Differentiates facial features (more refined)—focuses on mouth and oval head shapes Smiles and vocalizes to mirror image Looks for fallen objects
5-6	Discriminates p/t; b/g; i/a	Enjoys playing vocal games—attempts to repeat sounds Combines vowel and consonants—sounds contain intonation patterns Imitates and differentiates p/t; b/g; i/a	Distinguishes live, animated faces from no expression or affect Responds to or ignores familiar objects and focuses on new or less familiar objects

Tactile motor	Cognitive-mental	Social-emotional
Hand-to-mouth relationship well coordinated Tonic neck and Moro reflex decreasing Attempts to grasp from visual cues; transfers toy from one hand to the other On tummy may rock like an airplane, arching back and extending limbs Sits supported, head erect and steady, back firm	Is refining perceptual abilities (e.g., awareness of facial features, including differentiating unfamiliar faces; aware of differences in depth and distance; stares at place from which object drops) Is aware of strange situations Is aware of self from others and objects Discriminates—may prefer one object or person over others	Regulation of patterns of eating, sleeping, alert Takes several naps of a couple hours' duration (in morning and afternoon); sleeps 10 hr a night Laughs when socializing Shows anticipation Responds to and enjoys handling; not content to lie alone in bed
Head and hand activities at midline—grasps bidextrously Voluntarily reaches for and bats objects; raises arms to be picked up Sits supported with upper back erect and head steady—no head lag when pulled to sit Prone—lifts head at 90-degree angle; lifts head and chest, supporting weight on forearms Prefers novel to known stimuli	Discovers actions have effect on environment Is developing intentional behavior (4-8 mo)—objects exist only in relation to infant; they have no meaning or existence separately Indicates existence of memory	Solidifies attachment with mother or primary caregiver who is base from which to explore world Is becoming aware of others as separate beings and that needs are met by another Responds to differing emotions in people Smiles and vocalizes for social contact
Uses hands and mouth to learn about world Supine—holds head upright; reaches for objects; can hold bottle independently; shakes and pounds objects on surface and in air; releases object in one hand while grasping with the other ("mirror reflex"); sits supported with head steady and lower back erect; full head control in supine and prone positions Prone—supports weight on palms with arms extended; rolls from prone to supine to prone position (5-7 mo)	Endows mental representations with meaning and attributes Organizes and develops schema of world Watches actions as a spectator and gestures to have act repeated Directs visual attention to unfamiliar objects Is surprised when encounter is unexpected	Eats pureed foods Distinguishes or discriminates mother or primary caregiver from others (i.e., unfamiliar from familiar)—is beginning to prefer the familiar and known; resents strangers

Table 12-12
Sequelae Associated with Prematurity

Physical

1. Failure to thrive[43,72,157,178]
   a. Organic (i.e., physiologic cause)
   b. Nonorganic (e.g., attachment problems; neglect)
2. Child abuse and neglect[104,109,160]—psychologic sequelae ("the unattached child")
   a. Feelings of powerlessness—learned helplessness
   b. Poor ego development—low self-esteem, insecurity, oriented outside the self for cues and guidance
   c. Lack of trust in self and others
   d. Needy dependence
   e. Increasingly prone to depression
   f. Difficulty or inability in establishing and maintaining initmate relationships with others
   g. Increased irritability
3. Developmental delay in gross motor skills[19,77,83,161]
   a. Neurologic impairment (e.g., IVH, cerebral palsy)
   b. Nursery-acquired positioning malformations
   c. Difficulty in balance

Psychosocioemotional

1. Cognitive impairment—decrease in intelligence quotient (IQ) and development quotient (DQ)*
2. Learning disorders†
   a. Visual and/or auditory perceptual difficulties[81,161]
   b. Visual and/or auditory motor incoordination

   c. Normal or delayed acquisition of speech or language
   d. Visual disorders including poor visual acuity, astigmatism, myopia, strabismus.
3. Difficult behavioral style[81,113,114,143,161]
   a. Difficult to soothe
   b. Less adaptive—difficulty with habituation; state lability; dysrhythmicity
   c. Negative mood
   d. Withdrawn or highly active
4. Emotional sequelae—(the "unattached child")[109,135,141,160]
   a. Feelings of powerlessness—learned helplessness
   b. Poor ego development—low self-esteem, insecurity, oriented outside the self for cues and guidance
   c. Lack of trust in self and others
   d. Needy dependence
   e. Prone to depression
   f. Difficulty or inability in establishing and maintaining intimate relationships with others
   g. Increased irritability
5. Social sequelae[81,109,135,141,160]
   a. Lack of social conscience: violent or aggressive behaviors toward self and others; no guilt or remorse for behavior
   b. Difficulty or inability in developing intimate relationships with others

*References 79, 80, 81, 91, 97, 142, 143, 160, 163, 180.
†References 80, 91, 97, 142, 150, 160, 163, 180.

or learning difficulties enables the infant, toddler, and preschool years to be the optimal time for intervention.[166]

Graduate preterms are at increased risk for motor impairment, particularly gross motor skills (e.g., rolling over, sitting, crawling, standing, and walking). Rather than neurologic impairment, some of these deficits may be due to abnormal positioning and handling in the NICU.[19,57,77,83]

Just as the ability of parents to attach to and care for their infant is disrupted by illness and hospitalization (see Chapters 28 and 29), the ability of the newborn to form a symbiotic attachment to the parents is disrupted by the NICU experience. The unattached child results when the infant internalizes the rage associated with unmet needs.[109,160] Because of a lack of contingent, reliable, and consistent care giving, these infants do not develop a

sense of trust in parents, self, or humankind. Unmet needs may be a result of (1) lack of parental attachment and care giving; (2) asynchrony between care givers and infant, so that the infant's cues are not interpreted and responded to appropriately; (3) neglect and abuse; or (4) multiple care giving.

The emotional disruptions of the unattached child are the same as the psychologic outcomes of the battered child.[109,135,141,160]

- The infant's ego development is derived primarily from sensations from the body surface.
- When the body suffers pain, there is a decrease in the pleasure principle as a guide to development and an increase in violent, aggressive tendencies, because the care giver, who should comfort, is inflicting pain.

- The infant identifies with and incorporates the abusive care giver into the infant's own ego development.
- The care giver's control in the relationship negates the needs, feelings, and states of the infant, who also learns to discount himself or herself and inhibits self-initiated activity—is passive with learned helplessness.

Unattached and battered children exhibit poor self-esteem, difficulty or inability in developing close, intimate relationships, lack of a social conscience, and a preoccupation with or increase in violent tendencies.[109,135,141,160]

NICU infants are at risk for being unattached because (1) they have multiple care givers; (2) the parents are not always present and after a prolonged stay of the infant may be "strangers" to the infant; (3) the needs of the multiple care givers and infant may be asynchronous (e.g., it is "care time," but the infant is asleep); (4) lifesaving care in the NICU is intrusive, noxious, and painful; and (5) these experiences give the infant a history independent of his or her parents. Rather than receiving the soothing, pleasurable nurturing of family, the NICU infant is constantly bombarded with painful touch, handling, and stimuli. From the infant's perspective, the altruistic pain of lifesaving care is indistinguishable from the pain of child abuse.[160] The infant is cognitively unable to distinguish or be taught the difference—he or she merely subjectively experiences the pain. As one mother stated, "To Joshua, cauterizing his gastrostomy site with a silver nitrate stick was no different than if I'd burned him with a cigarette. To him, his mother was causing him pain.[7,52]

It is unclear whether developmental delays are due totally to organic insults, the effect of the NICU environment on an immature CNS, or a combination of insults. Because the NICU environment does not, by itself, ensure optimal developmental outcome, research into the environmental characteristics of the NICU and strategies to minimize its negative effect continue.[74]

The effect on the neonate's experience of hospitalization may be ameliorated or exacerbated by such variables as maturity at birth, severity of illness, length of hospital stay, primary nursing, genetic endowment, temperament, maternal socioeconomic group, education and care giving, and

postdischarge follow-up and interventions. Because keeping parents involved is so important to outcome, parents need anticipatory guidance about "taking their premie home." Instead of telling parents that preterm infants are "more difficult," a more positive "preterm infants need more help from parents in the first year of life" is warranted. Concrete techniques to soothe, feed, and interact with *their* infant and "rooming-in" practice help parents be more confident in care giving. Absolving parental guilt (i.e., "What am I doing wrong?") by teaching parents that the *infant* has a problem, helps keep parents involved with the infant. Teaching appropriate play activities assists parents in enjoying their infant while providing the infant with vital sensory and social experience for development.

Care of preterm infants began with a minimal handling policy. Research and knowledge of the unique anatomy and physiology of the neonate preceded the development of high-technology devices and high touch to manage both machines and newborns. Observation and research has documented the effect of the NICU environment on its vulnerable inhabitants. Individualized developmental interventions in the NICU and beyond have resulted in decreased developmental delay as well as medical benefits and cost savings (see Table 12-5). Since individualized developmental care improves outcomes, several recommendations have been proposed: (1) third party reimbursement may favor NICUs that are cost-effective, (2) NICUs choosing not to utilize developmental care should have clear reasons and consider randomized trials to disprove its effectiveness, and (3) the American Academy of Pediatrics should critically evaluate developmental care and make recommendations regarding its use.[119]

References

1. Aebi V et al: Outcome of 100 randomly positioned children of VLBW at two years, *Child Care Health Dev* 17(1):1, 1991.
2. Affonso D, Wahlberg V, Persson B: Mother's reactions to kangaroo method of prematurity care, *Neonat Net* 7:43, 1989.
3. Affonso D et al: Reconciliation and healing for mothers through skin-to-skin contact provided in American tertiary level intensive care nursery, *Neonat Net* 12:25, 1993.
4. Alberts J: Learning as adaptation of the infant, *Acta Paediatr Suppl* 397:77, 1994

5. Allen MC, Capute AJ: Tone and reflex development before term, *Pediatrics* 85:393, 1990.

6. Allen M et al: The limit of viability-neonatal outcome of infants born at 22-25 weeks gestation, *NEJM* 329:1597, 1993.

7. Als H: Toward a synactive theory of development: promise for assessment and support for infant individuality, *Infant Ment Health J* 3(4):229, 1982.

8. Als H: Infant individuality: assessing patterns of very early development. In Call JD, Galenson MD, Tyson R, editors: *Frontiers of infant psychiatry,* New York, 1983, Basic Books.

9. Als H et al: Toward a research instrument for the assessment of preterm infant's behavior (APIB). In Fitzgerald HE, Lester BM, Yogman MW, editors: *Theory and research in behavioral pediatrics,* vol 1, New York, 1982, Plenum Press.

10. Als H et al: The behavior of the full-term yet underweight newborn infant, *Dev Med Child Neurol* 18:590, 1976.

11. Als H et al: Individualized behavioral and environmental care for the VLBW preterm infant at high risk for BPD: neonatal intensive care unit and developmental outcome, *Pediatrics* 78(6):1123, 1986.

12. Als H et al: Individualized behavioral and environmental care for the VLBW preterm infant at high risk for BPD & IVH. Study II: NICU outcome. Paper presented at the annual meeting of The New England Perinatal Association, Woodstock, Vt, 1988.

13. Als H et al: Individualized developmental care for VLBW preterm infants, *JAMA* 272:853, 1994.

14. American Academy of Pediatrics and American College of Obstetricians & Gynecologists: *Guidelines for perinatal care,* ed 3, Elk Grove Village, Ill, 1992.

15. American Academy of Pediatrics, Joint Committee of Infant Hearing: Position Statement: *Policy reference guide,* ed 6, Elk Grove Village, Ill, 1993.

16. Anders TF, Keener M: Developmental course of night-time sleep-wake patterns in full term and preterm infants during the first year of life, *Sleep* 8:173, 1985.

17. Anderson G: Current knowledge about skin-to-skin (kangaroo) care for preterm infants, *J Perinatol* 11:216, 1991.

18. Barnard KE, Bee HL: The impact of temporally patterned stimulation on the development of preterm infants, *Child Dev* 54:1156, 1983.

19. Becker PT et al: Outcomes of developmentally supportive nursing care for VLBW infants, *Nurs Res* 40(3):150, 1991.

20. Bell SM, Ainsworth MD: Infant crying and maternal responsiveness, *Child Dev* 43:1171, 1972.

21. Blackburn S, Patteson D: Effects of cycled light on activity state and cardiorespiratory function in preterm infants, *J Perinat Neonatal Nurs* 4:47, 1991.

22. Blackburn S: The use of orally directed behaviors by VLBW infants, *Neonat Net* 12:61, 1993.

23. Boone O et al: Sound levels in incubators: a laboratory and clinical evaluation. Abstract: *The physical and developmental environment of the high risk infant,* Orlando, Fla, 1995, University of S. Florida College of Medicine.

24. Bower TGR: *The rational infant: learning in infancy,* New York, 1989, WH Freeman.

25. Bowlby J: *Attachment,* New York, 1973, Basic Books.

26. Bowlby J: *Separation,* New York, 1973, Basic Books.

27. Bowlby J: *Loss,* New York, 1980, Basic Books.

28. Bozynski ME et al: Lateral positioning of stable VLBW infant: effect on transcutaneous oxygen and carbon dioxide, *Am J Dis Child* 142:200, 1988.

29. Bradley RM, Mistretta CM: Fetal sensory receptors, *Physiol Rev* 3:353, 1975.

30. Brazelton TB: *Neonatal behavioral assessment scale,* ed 2, Philadelphia, 1984, Spastics International Medical Publishers/JB Lippincott.

31. Buehler D et al: Effectiveness of individualized developmental care for low-risk preterm infants: behavioral and electrophysiologic evidence, *Pediatrics* 96:923, 1995.

32. Bulock F, Woolridge M, Baum J: Development of coordination of sucking, swallowing, and breathing: ultrasound study of term and preterm infants, *Dev Med Child Neurol* 32:669, 1990.

33. Cagan J: Feeding-readiness behavior in preterm infants, *Neonat Net* 14:82, 1995.

34. Campos R: Soothing pain-elicited distress in infants with swaddling and pacifiers, *Child Dev* 60:781, 1989.

35. Catlett AT, Holditch-Davis D: Environmental stimuli of the acutely-ill premature infant: physiologic effects and nursing implications, *Neonat Net* 8(6):19, 1990.

36. Christensson K et al: Temperature, metabolic adaptation and crying in healthy full term newborns cared for skin-to-skin or in a cot, *Acta Paediatr* 81:488, 1992.

37. Christensson K et al: Separation distress call in the human neonate in the absence of maternal body contact, *Acta Paediatr* 84:468, 1995.

38. Cole JG: Infant stimulation reexamined: an environmental- and behavioral-based approach, *Neonat Net* 3(5):24, 1985.

39. Cole JG et al: Changing the NICU environment: the Boston City Hospital model, *Neonat Net* 9(2):15, 1990.

40. Collins SK, Kuch K: Music therapy in the NICU, *Neonat Net* 9(6):23, 1991.

41. Corff K et al: Facilitated tucking: a non-pharmacologic comfort measure for pain in preterm neonates, *JOGNN* 24:143, 1995.

42. Cronin C: Impact of VLBW infants on the family is long-lasting, *Arch Pediatr Adolesc Med* 149:151, 1995.

43. Daily D et al: Growth patterns of infants weighing <801 gms at birth to 3 years of age, *J Perinatol* 14:454, 1994.

44. D'Apolito K: What is an organized infant? *Neonat Net* 10(1):23, 1991.

45. D'Souza S et al: Skin temperature and heart rate rhythms in infants of extreme prematurity, *Arch Dis Child* 67:784, 1992.

46. DeCasper AJ, Fifer WP: Of human bonding: newborns prefer their mother's voices, *Science* 208:1175, 1980.

47. DeCasper AJ, Spence MJ: Prenatal maternal speech influences newborn's perception of speech sounds, *Infant Behav Dev* 9:133, 1986.

48. DePaul D, Chambers S: Environmental noise in the NICU: implications for nursing practice, *J Perinat Neonat Nurs* 8:71, 1995.

49. Dobbing J, Sands J: Quantitative growth and development of the human brain, *Arch Dis Child* 48:757, 1973.

50. Dreyfus-Brisac C: Organization of sleep in preterms: implications for caretaking. In Lewis M, Rosenblum LA, editors: *The effect of the infant on its caregiver,* New York, 1974, John Wiley & Sons.

51. Dreyfus-Brisac C: Ontogenesis of brain bioelectric activity and sleep organization in neonates and infants. In Faulkner F, Tanner JM, editors: *Human growth,* vol 3, New York, 1979, Plenum Publishing.

52. Eickner S: Personal communication, 1987.

53. Evans J: Comparison of two NICU patterns of caregiving over 24 hours for preterm infants, *Neonat Net* 13:87, 1994.

54. Eyler FD et al: Effects of developmental intervention on heart rate and transcutaneous oxygen levels in LBW infants, *Neonat Net* 8(3):17, 1989.

55. Fajardo B et al: Emergence of state regulation in VLBW premature infants, *Infant Behav Dev* 13:287, 1990.

56. Fantz RL, Fagan JF, Miranda SB: Early visual selectivity as a function of pattern variables, previous exposure, age from birth and conception and expected cognitive deficit. In Cohen L, Salaptic P, editors: *Infant perception,* vol 1, New York, 1975, Academic Press.

57. Fay MJ: The positive effects of positioning, *Neonat Net* 6(5):23, 1988.

58. Field TM: Interaction patterns of preterm and term infants. In Field TM, editor: *Infants born at risk,* New York, 1979, Spectrum Books.

59. Field TM et al: Tactile/kinesthetic stimulation effects on preterm neonates, *Pediatrics* 77(5):654, 1986.

60. Fifer W, Moon C: The role of mother's voice in the organization of brain function in the newborn, *Act Paediatr Suppl* 397:86, 1994.

61. Fleisher B et al: Individualized developmental care for very-low-birth-weight premature infants, *Clin Pediatr* 34:523, 1995.

62. Freedman DG: Ethnic differences in babies, *Hum Nature* 2(1):36, 1979.

63. Gale G, Franck L, Lund C: Skin-to-skin (kangaroo) holding of the intubated premature infant, *Neonat Net* 12:49, 1993.

64. Garcia-Coll C: Behavioral responsivity in preterm infants, *Clin Perinatol* 17(1):113, 1990.

65. Gardner LI: Deprivation dwarfism, *Sci Am* 227(1):76, 1982.

66. Gardner S, Hagedorn M: Physiologic sequalae of prematurity: the nurse practitioner's role. Part V. Feeding difficulties and growth failure (pathophysiology, cause and data collection), *J Pediatr Health Care* 5:122, 1991.

67. Gardner S, Hagedorn M: Physiologic sequalae of prematurity: the nurse practitioner's role. Part VI. Feeding difficulties and growth failure (prevention, intervention, parent teaching, and complications), *J Pediatr Health Care* 5:306, 1991.

68. Gemelli M et al: Circadian blood pressure pattern in full term newborn infants, *Biol Neonate* 56:315, 1989.

69. Glass P et al: Effects of bright light in the hospital nursery on the incidence of ROP, *NEJM* 313:401, 1985.

70. Glass P: The vulnerable neonate and the neonatal intensive care environment. In Avery G, Fletcher M, MacDonald M, editors: *Neonatology,* ed 4, Philadelphia, 1994, JB Lippincott.

71. Goldson E: The micropreemie: infants with birth weight less than 800 gms, *Inf Young Children* 8:1, 1996.

72. Gorski PA: Premature infant behavioral and physiological responses to caregiving interventions in the intensive care nursery. In Call JD, Galenson E, Tyson RL, editors: *Frontiers in infant psychiatry,* New York, 1983, Basic Books.

73. Gorski PA, Davison MF, Brazelton TB: Stages of behavioral organization in the high risk neonate: theoretical and clinical considerations, *Semin Perinatol* 3:61, 1979.

74. Gorski PA: Developmental intervention during neonatal hospitalization—critiquing the state of the science, *Pediatr Clin North Am* 38(6):1469, 1991.

75. Gottfried AW, Gaiter JL: *Infant stress under intensive care: environmental neonatology,* Baltimore, 1985, University Park Press.

76. Grauer T: Environmental lighting, behavioral state, and hormonal response in the newborn, *Sch Inq Nurs Pract* 3:53, 1989.

77. Grunwald P, Becker P: Developmental enhancement: implementing a program for the NICU, *Neonat Net* 9(6):29, 1991.

78. Gunderson LP, Kenner C: Neonatal stress: physiologic adaptation and nursing implications, *Neonat Net* 6(1):37, 1987.

79. Hack M, Fanaroff A: Outcomes of extremely LBW infants between 1982 and 1988, *N Engl J Med* 321:1642, 1989.

80. Hack M: Follow-up for high-risk neonates. In Fanaroff AA, Martin RJ, editors: *Neonatal-perinatal medicine,* vol 1, St Louis, 1992, Mosby.

81. Hack M et al: School age outcomes in children with birth weights <750 gm, *NEJM* 331:753, 1994.

82. Hall B, Ballweg D, Howell R: Infant acute response to ambient noise and light in the NICU—a preliminary report, Abstract: *The physical and developmental environment of the high-risk infant,* Orlando, Fla, 1995, University of S. Florida School of Medicine.

83. Harris MB et al: Joint range of motion development in premature infants, *Pediatr Phys Ther* 2(4):185, 1990.

84. Harrison L et al: Effects of gentle human touch on preterm infants: results of a pilot study, *Infant Behavior Special ICIS Issue* 15:12, 1992.

85. Harrison L et al: Effects of gentle human touch on preterm infants: results of pilot study, *Neonatal Network* 15:35, 1996.

86. Hellbrugge T: The development of circadian rhythms in infants, *Cold Spring Harb Symp Quant Biol* 25:311, 1960.

87. Hofer M: Early relationships as regulators of infant physiology and behavior, *Act Paediatr Suppl* 387:9, 1994.

88. Holditch-Davis D et al: Effect of standard rest periods on convalescent preterm infants, *JOGNN* 24:424, 1995.

89. Holditch-Davis D et al: Standardized rest periods affect the incidence of apnea and rate of weight gain in convalescent preterm infants, *Neonat Net* 15:87, 1996.

90. Hyde BB, McCown DE: Classical conditioning in neonatal intensive care nurseries, *Pediatr Nurs* 12(1):11, 1986.

91. Johnson A et al: Functional abilities at age 4 yrs of children born before 29 weeks gestation, *Br Med J* 306:1715, 1993.

92. Jurkovicova J, Aghova L: Evaluation of the effects of noise exposure on various body function in LBW newborns, *Acta Nerv Super* 31:228, 1989.

93. Kaminski J, Hall W: The effect of soothing music on neonatal behavioral states in the hospital newborn nursery, *Neonat Net* 15:45, 1996.

94. Kattwinkel J et al: Apnea of prematurity, *J Pediatr* 86:588, 1975.

95. Kemp J, Thach B: Sudden death in infants sleeping on polystyrene filled cushions, *N Engl J Med* 324:1858, 1991.

96. Kennedy C, Lipsitt L: Temporal characteristics of non-oral feedings and chronic feeding problems in premature infants, *J Perinat Neonat Nurs* 7:77, 1993.

97. Klein N et al: Children who were very low birthweight: developmental and academic achievement at nine years of age, *J Dev Behav Pediatr* 10:32, 1989.

98. Klinnert M, Bingham R: The organizing effects of early relationships, *Psychiatry* 57:1, 1994.

99. Korner AF: The effect of the infants state, level of arousal, sex and ontogenetic stage on the caregiver. In Lewis M, Rosenblum LA, editors: *The effect of the infant on its caregiver,* New York, 1974, John Wiley & Sons.

100. Korner AF: The use of waterbeds in the care of preterm infants, *J Pediatr,* 6:142, 1986.

101. Korner AF: Infant stimulation: issues of theory and research, *Clin Perinatol* 17(1):173, 1990.

102. Leonard J: Music therapy: fertile ground for application of research in practice, *Neonat Net* 12:47, 1993.

103. Lester BM, Tronick EZ: Guidelines for stimulation with preterm infants, *Pediatr Clin North Am* 17(1):31, 1990.

104. Leventhal J et al: Identification during the postpartum period of infants who are at high risk of child maltreatment, *J Pediatr* 114:481, 1989.

105. Lewis M, Michalson L: The socialization of emotional pathology, *Infant Ment Health J* 3:125, 1984.

106. Litovsky R: Stimulus differentiation by preterm infants can guide caregivers, *Prenat Perinat Psychol J* 5(1):41, 1990.

107. Long J, Philip A, Lucey J: Excessive handling as a cause of hypoxemia, *Pediatrics* 65:203, 1980.

108. Long JG et al: Noise and hypoxemia in the intensive care nursery, *Pediatrics* 65:143, 1981.

109. Magid K, McKelvey CA: *High risk: children without a conscience,* New York, 1989, Bantam Books.

110. Mann N et al: Effect of night and day on preterm infants in a newborn nursery: randomized trial, *Brit Med J* 292:1265, 1986.

111. Martin RJ et al: Effect of supine and prone positions on arterial oxygen tension in the preterm infant, *Pediatrics* 63:528, 1979.

112. Masterson J et al: Prone and supine positioning effects on energy expenditure and behavior of low birth weight neonates, *Pediatrics* 80.689, 1987.

113. Medoff-Cooper B, Schraeder BD: Developmental trends and behavioral styles in VLBW infants, *Nurs Res* 31(2):68, 1982.

114. Medoff-Cooper B: Temperament in VLBW infants, *Nurs Res* 35(3):139, 1986.

115. Medhoff-Cooper B: Changes in nutritive sucking patterns with increasing gestational age, *Nurs Res* 40:245, 1991.

116. Medoff-Cooper B, Verklan T, Carlson S: The development of sucking patterns and physiologic correlates in VLBW infants, *Nurs Res* 42:100, 1993.

117. Meier P: Bottle- and breast-feeding: effects on transcutaneous oxygen and temperature in preterm infants, *Nurs Res* 37:36, 1988.

118. Meltzoff AN, Moore MK: Imitation of facial and manual gestures by human neonates, *Science* 198(4312):74, 1977.

119. Merenstein G: Individualized developmental care; an emerging new standard for neonatal intensive care units? *JAMA* 272:890, 1994.

120. Michelson K, Sirvio P, Wasz-Hockert O: Pain cry in full term asphyxiated newborn infant correlated with late finding, *Acta Paediatr Scand* 66(5):611, 1977.

121. Miller C et al: The effects of cycled and noncycled lighting on growth and development in preterm infants, *Infant Behavior and Development* 18:87, 1995.

122. Miranda SB, Fantz RL: Visual abilities and pattern preference of preterm infants and full term neonates, *J Exp Child Psychiatry* 10:189, 1970.

123. Mishoe S et al: Octave waveband analysis to determine sound frequencies and intensities produced by nebulizers and humidifiers used with hoods, *Neonat Int Care* 9:20, 1996.

124. Modrein-McCarthy M: The physiological and behavioral effects of a gentle human touch nursing intervention on preterm infants. Doctoral dissertation, U of Tennessee, Knoxville. *Dissertation Abstracts Int,* AAC9319218.

125. Montagu A: *Prenatal influences,* Springfield, Ill, 1962, Charles C Thomas, Publisher.

126. Montagu A: *Touching,* New York, 1971, Harper & Row.

127. Northern J, Downs MA: *Hearing in children,* ed 4, Baltimore, 1991, Williams & Wilkins.

128. Oehler J: Examining the issue of tactile stimulation of preterm infants, *Neonat Net* 4:24, 1985.

129. Orenstein SR, Whitington PF: Positioning for prevention of gastroesophageal reflux, *J Pediatr* 103(4):534, 1983.

130. Parmalee AH: Sleep states in premature infants, *Dev Med Child Neurol* 9:70, 1967.

131. Pelletier-Sehnar J, Palmeri A: High-risk infants. In Clark-Pratt PN, Allen AS, editors: *Occupational therapy for children,* ed 2, St Louis, 1989, Mosby.

132. Peters K: Dinosaurs in the bath, *Neonat Net* 15:71, 1996.

133. Peters K: Selected physiologic and behavioral responses of the critically ill premature neonate to a routine nursing intervention, *Neonat Net* 15:74, 1996.

134. Pickler R, Frankel H: The effect of non-nutritive sucking on preterm infant's behavioral organization and feeding performance, *Neonat Net* 14:83, 1995.

135. Prescott J: Body pleasure and the origins of violence, *Futurist* 2:64, 1975.

136. Pridham KF et al: Parental issues in feeding young children with BPD, *J Pediatr* 4:177, 1989.

137. Provence S, Lipton RC: *Infants in institutions,* New York, 1962, International Universities Press.

138. Rauh VA et al: The mother-infant transaction program, *Pediatr Clin North Am* 17(1):31, 1990.

139. Renaud M et al: Neonatal outcomes in a modified NICU environment, *Neonat Net* 15:6, 1996.

140. Resnick MB et al: Developmental intervention program for high-risk premature infants: effects on development and parent-infant interactions, *J Dev Behav Pediatr* 9:73, 1988.

141. Rice R: Infant stress and the relationship to violent behavior, *Neonat Net* 5:39, 1985.

142. Saigal S et al: General health, cognitive ability and school performance of extremely LBW children and matched controls at eight years: a regional study, *J Pediatr* 118:751, 1991.

143. Saigal S et al: Comprehensive assessment of the health status of VLBW children at 8 years of age: comparison with a reference group, *J Pediatr* 125:411, 1994.

144. Sammon M, Darnell R: Entrainment of respiration to rocking in premature infants: coherence analysis, *Appl Physiol* 77:1548, 1994.

145. Sampers J: The effect of noise on the behavior of preterm infants in a neonatal intensive care unit, Abstract: *The physical and developmental environment of the high-risk infant,* Orlando, Fla, 1995, University of S. Florida College of Medicine.

146. Sarnat HB: Olfactory reflexes in newborn infants, *J Pediatr* 92(4):624, 1978.

147. Saunders RB, Friedman CB, Stramoski PR: Feeding preterm infants: schedule or demand? *JOGN* 20(3):212, 1991.

148. Scafidi FA et al: Effects of tactile/kinesthetic stimulation on the clinical course and sleep-wake behavior of preterm neonates, *Infant Behav Dev* 9:91, 1986.

149. Schwartz R: Effect of position on oxygenation, heart rate, and behavioral state in the transitional newborn infant, *Neonat Net* 12:73, 1993.

150. Scott DT: Premature infants in later childhood: some recent follow up results, *Semin Perinatol* 11:191, 1987.

151. Sheagren TG et al: Rumination—a new complication of neonatal intensive care, *Pediatrics* 66(4):551, 1980.

152. Short M et al: The effects of swaddling v. standard positioning on neuromuscular development in VLBW infants, *Neonat Net* 15:25, 1996.

153. Shiroiwa Y et al: Activity, cardiac and respiratory responses of blindfolded preterm infants in a neonatal intensive care unit, *Early Hum Dev* 14:259, 1986.

154. Shogan M, Schumann L: The effect of environmental lighting on the oxygen saturation of preterm infants in the NICU, *Neonat Net* 12:7, 1993.

155. Shyang-Yun P et al: Nasogastric tube placement: effects on breathing and sucking in VLBW infants, *Nurs Res* 44:82, 1995.

156. Smotherman W, Robinson S: Milk as the proximal mechanism for behavioral change in the newborn, *Act Paediatr Suppl* 397:64, 1994.

157. Sostek AM, Anders TF, Sostek AJ: Diurnal rhythms in two to eight week old infants: sleep-wake state organization as a factor of age and stress, *Psychosom Med* 38(4):250, 1976.

158. Sound Study Group: The effects of sound, noise, and vibration in the environment of the high risk infant, University of S. Florida, Tampa, Fla (in press).

159. Spitz R: Hospitalism, *Psychoanal Study Child* 1:53, 1945.

160. Steele BF: The effect of abuse and neglect on psychological development. In Call JD, Galenson E, Tyson RL, editors: *Frontiers of infant psychiatry,* New York, 1983, Basic Books.

161. Stjernquist K, Svenningsen N: Extremely LBW infants less than 901 gm: development and behavior after four years of life, *Acta Paediatr* 84:500, 1995.

162. Strauth C, Brandt S, Edwards-Beckett J: Implementation of a quiet hour: effect on noise levels and infant sleep states, *Neonat Net* 12:31, 1993.

163. Symes A et al: Perinatal outcomes of a large cohort of extremely low gestational age infants (23-28 wks), *Pediatrics* 125:952, 1994.

164. Taquino L, Blackburn S: The effects of containment during suction and heelstick on physiological and behavioral responses of preterm infants, *Neonat Net* 13:55, 1994.

165. Tenreiro S et al: The development of ultradian and circadian rhythms in premature babies maintained in constant conditions, *Early Hum Dev* 27:33, 1991.

166. The Infant Health and Development Program: Enhancing the outcome of low birth weight premature infants: a multisite randomized trial, *JAMA* 263:3035, 1990.

167. Thoden C, Koivisto M: Acoustic analysis of the normal pain cry. In Murry M, Murry J, editors: *Infant communication: crying and early speech,* Houston, 1980, College Hill Press.

168. Thoman EB, Ingersol EW, Acebo C: Premature infants seek rhythmic stimulation and the experience facilitates neurobehavioral development, *Dev Behav Pediatr* 12(1):11, 1991.

169. Thomas K: Biorhythms in infants and role of the care environment, *J Perinat Neonat Nurs* 9:61, 1995.

170. Treas L: Incubator covers: health or hazard? *Neonat Net* 12:50, 1993.

171. Tribotti S: Effects of gentle touch on the premature infant. In Gonzenhauser N, editor: *Advances in touch: new implications in human development,* Skillman, NJ, 1990, Johnson & Johnson.

172. Tronick EZ, Scanlon KB, Scanlon JW: Protective apathy: a hypothesis about the behavioral organization and its relation to clinical and physiologic status of the preterm infant during the newborn period, *Clin Perinatol* 17(1):125, 1990.

173. Updike C et al: Positional support for premature infants, *Am J Occup Ther* 40(10):712, 1986.

174. Vandenberg KA: Revising the traditional model: an individualized approach to developmental interventions, *Neonat Net* 3(5):32, 1985.

175. VanZoeren-Grobben D et al: Lipid perioxidation in human milk and infant formula: effect of storage, tube feedings, and exposure to phototherapy, *Acta Paediatr* 82:645, 1993.

176. Varendi H, Porter R, Winberg J: Does the newborn baby find the nipple by smell? *Lancet* 344:989, 1994.

177. Wagaman MJ et al: Improved oxygenation and lung compliance with prone positioning of neonates, *J Pediatr* 94:787, 1979.

178. Watt JE, Strongman KT: The organization and stability of sleep states in full term, preterm and SGA infants: a comparative study, *Dev Psychobiol* 18:151, 1985.

179. White-Traut RC, Pate CM: Modulating infant state in premature infants, *J Pediatr Nurs* 2:96, 1987.
180. White-Traut R et al: The relationship of sound levels to apnea, bradycardia, and arterial oxygen saturation in the special care nursery. Abstract: *The physical and developmental environment of the high-risk infant,* Orlando, Fla, 1995, University of S. Florida College of Medicine.
181. Whyte H et al: Extreme immaturity: outcome of 568 pregnancies of 23-25 weeks gestation, *Obstet Gynecol* 82:1, 1993.
182. Wingert WA et al: Pediatric nurse practitioners in follow up care of high risk infants, Am J Nurs 80:1485, 1980.
183. Wolff P: The natural history of crying and other vocalizations in early infancy. In Foss B, editor: *Determinants of infant behavior,* ed 4, London, 1969, Metheum.
184. Woodson R et al: Effects of non-nutritive sucking on state and activity: term-preterm comparisons, *Infant Behav Dev* 8:435, 1985.
185. Zahr L, Balian S: Responses of premature infants to routine nursing interventions and noise in the NICU, *Nurs Res* 44:179, 1995.

Resources for Parents

Dorner A: *Prematurely yours* (video), Boston, 1983, Polymorph Films.
Dorner A: *To have and not to hold: helping parents cope* (video), Boston, 1983, Polymorph Films.
Flushman B et al: *My special start: a guide for parents in the neonatal intensive care unit,* Palo Alto, Calif, VORT.
Healy T: *Guiding your child through preterm development,* Alexandria, Va, 1988, Parent Care.
Hussey B: *Understanding my signals,* Palo Alto, Calif, 1988, VORT.
Institute for Family-Centered Care: *Newborn intensive care: changing practice, changing attitudes* (video), Bethesda, Md, 1996, Institute for family-centered care.
Ludington-Hoe S, Golant S: *Kangaroo care: the best you can do to help your preterm infant,* New York, 1993, Bantam Books.
Rosenberg S: *Kangaroo care: a parent's touch* (video), Chicago, 1996, Prentice Women's Hospital.

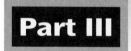

Part III *Metabolic and Nutritional Care of the Neonate*

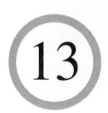

13 # Fluid and Electrolyte Management

Eugene W. Adcock III, Carol Ann Consolvo, David D. Berry

Although advances in management of specific neonatal disorders have contributed to a remarkable decline in morbidity and mortality, fluid and electrolyte therapy, thermal regulation, and maintenance of oxygenation remain the central features of modern, supportive neonatal intensive care. It is assumed, therefore, that all infants requiring tertiary care (and most infants requiring so-called intermediate, level II, or secondary care) will receive parenteral fluid and electrolytes initially. Much useful information has accumulated about full-term infants, but some crucial information is still missing, especially about VLBW infants. For example, it is now clear that the restrictive fluid policies of the 1950s (which were aimed at reducing the observed postnatal diuresis) were misguided efforts that eventuated in hyperosmolality, hyperbilirubinemia, and hypoglycemia. On the other hand, the degree to which initial fluid, electrolyte, and glucose administration should be "liberalized" remains unsettled,[1,5,6] largely because of suggestions that in VLBW infants patent ductus arteriosus, necrotizing enterocolitis, BPD, IVH, and hyperglycemia are associated with larger volumes of fluid, electrolyte, and glucose administration.[3] At best, approximations for therapy are necessary in many clinical situations. This chapter is based on the following fundamental principles: (1) rapidly assessing the infant's initial condition, (2) developing a short-term, time-oriented, management plan, (3) initiating therapy, and (4) monitoring the infant and modifying the plan based on clinical and biochemical data.

Physiology

Neonates show dramatic physiologic differences when compared on a per kilogram basis with older children and adults: (1) their basic metabolic rate is at least double; (2) their water requirements are four or five times greater; and (3) their sodium excretion is only 10% of that in older children and adults. The subdivisions of total body mass (TBM) are illustrated in Fig. 13-1.[10] TBW as a percentage of TBM demonstrates a curvilinear decline with increasing age (Fig. 13-2).[10] Intracellular fluid (ICF) and extracellular fluid (ECF) as percentages of TBM change in opposite directions as gestation advances.

These physiologic and body composition phenomena result in a narrow margin of safety in calculating fluids and electrolytes for small infants, especially those weighing less than 1250 g. Care givers should calculate independently all requirements and compare calculations with each other. IV fluid should be administered by a special infusion pump that can regulate fluid at rates of 1 ml/hr or less. The intake should be measured hourly, and the output should be quantitated as soon as it occurs. Intake and output should be balanced at least every 8 to 12 hours using a standard form (Fig. 13-3). Once clinical signs of fluid overload or

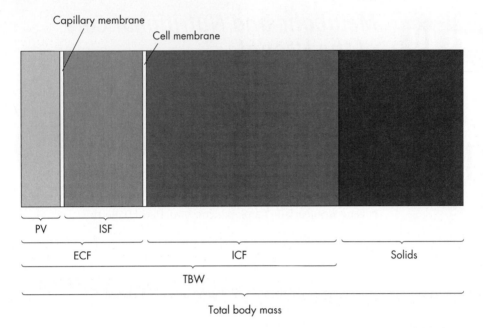

Figure 13-1 Major subdivisions of total body mass. *PV,* Plasma volume; *ISF,* interstitial fluid; *ECF,* extracellular fluid; *ICF,* intracellular fluid; *TBW,* total body water.(From Winters RW, editor: *The body fluids in pediatrics,* Boston, 1973, Little, Brown.)

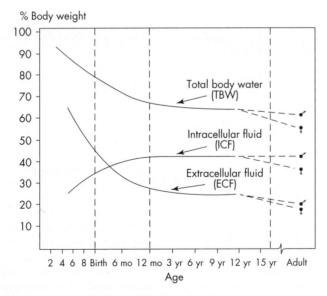

Figure 13-2 Effects on age on TBW, ICF, and ECF. Note curvilinear changes that are maximal during perinatal period. (From Winters RW, editor: *The body fluids in pediatrics,* Boston, 1973, Little, Brown.)

Output

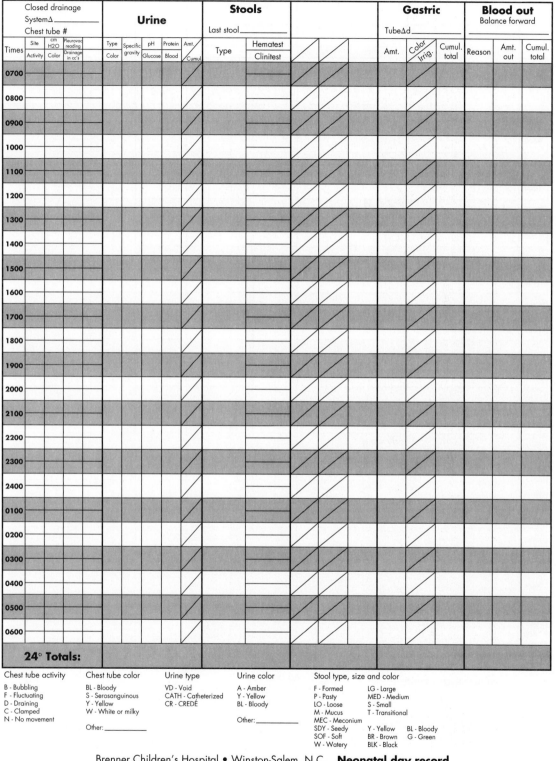

Brenner Children's Hospital • Winston-Salem, N.C. **Neonatal day record**

Continued

Figure 13-3 Model intake and output sheet. (Courtesy Brenner Children's Hospital, Winston-Salem, North Carolina.)

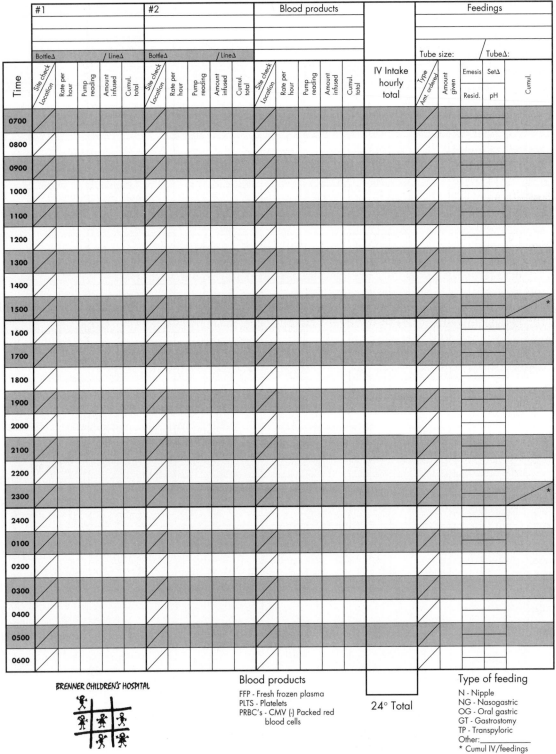

Figure 13-3, cont'd Model intake and output sheet.

deficit occur, it may be extremely difficult to regain balance. **Fluid balance should be viewed prospectively. A similar procedure should be a part of every initial care plan.**

The effect of gestational age on body composition is striking (Fig. 13-4).[7] Because gestational age is an important determinant of the percentage and distribution of TBW, accurate assessment is important. Changes in distribution and percent of body water may also depend on intrauterine growth, maternal fluid balance, postnatal age, diet, daily water intake, and changing metabolism. Furthermore, it now seems clear that at least part of the initial (first 1 to 3 days) weight loss of both healthy term (up to 5% to 10% of TBM) and preterm (up to 10% to 15% of TBM) infants should be considered a normal physiologic loss of fluid from the interstitial fluid (ISF), rather than a pathophysiologic catabolism of body tissues.[2]

The maternal history and the intrapartum course may be helpful in calculating the infant's fluid and electrolyte requirements. For example, if the mother received large amounts of electrolyte-free fluids in the intrapartum period, the neonate may be hyponatremic and have expanded ECF at birth. Because SGA infants have reduced amounts of fat, body water (as a percentage of TBM) increases. Conversely, LGA infants have a smaller percentage of TBW because of an increased amount of body fat.

Electrolyte composition of ISF and plasma is similar but strikingly different from ICF (Fig. 13-5).[10]

Sodium is the major cation in ECF (both ISF and plasma) and is easily measured. Potassium, the major cation in ICF, cannot be measured readily, because ICF is not clinically accessible. Because 90% of the total body potassium is intracellular, when plasma potassium is low, it is assumed that the total body potassium is invariably low.

Osmotic force or pressure is a phenomenon that is a colligative property of any solution. Osmotic phenomena depend on the number (N) of particles (regardless of size or charge) in a solution and are measured in milliosmoles, according to the equation:

$$mOsm = (mM) \times (N)$$

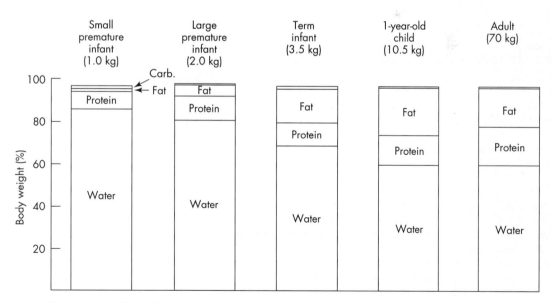

Figure 13-4 Effects of gestational age on body composition compared with older children and adults. (From Heird WC et al: *J Pediatr* 80:352, 1972.)

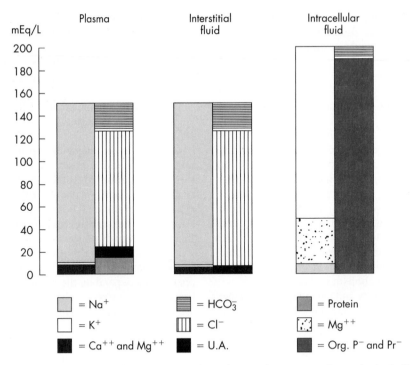

Figure 13-5 "Gamblegram" of plasma ISF and ICF. (From Winters RW, editor: *The body fluids in pediatrics,* Boston, 1973, Little, Brown.)

Table 13-1
Examples of Osmotic Force

	mM	N	mOsm
NaCl	1	2	2
Glucose	1	1	1
CaCl$_2$	1	3	3

Table 13-1 shows three examples. **Unfortunately, two physical chemistry terms are used interchangeably in clinical medicine: (1) osmolality (milliosmole per kilogram of water) and (2) osmolarity (milliosmole per liter of solution). In most laboratories, osmotic forces are determined by the technique of freezing point depression, so osmolality is the correct term (normally 280 to 300 mOsm/kg water). The difference in terms is usually** unimportant, because the total solid content per liter of plasma is small.

Osmotic forces can be satisfactorily estimated (Fig. 13-6)[10] in many clinical settings by the following formula:

$$2(\text{Na}^+) + \frac{\text{BUN (mg/dl)} \times 10}{28} \times \frac{\text{Glucose (mg/dl)} \times 10}{180}$$

The molecular weights of two nitrogen atoms and glucose are 28 and 180, respectively, and BUN is blood urea nitrogen.

Osmotic forces are responsible for apparently low plasma electrolyte concentrations in some common clinical settings.

In hyperglycemia, the plasma sodium concentrate reported by the laboratory is usually low, but

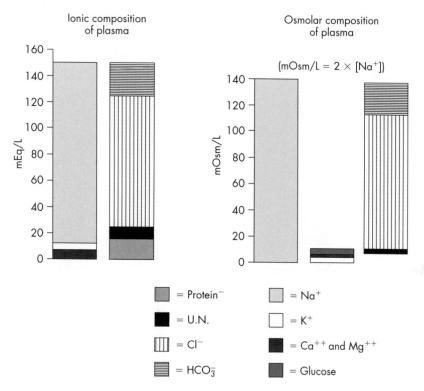

Ionic composition of plasma

Osmolar composition of plasma

$(mOsm/L = 2 \times [Na^+])$

mEq/L

mOsm/L

 = Protein$^-$

 = U.N.

 = Cl$^-$

 = HCO$_3^-$

 = Na$^+$

 = K$^+$

 = Ca^{++} and Mg^{++}

 = Glucose

Figure 13-6   Ionic and osmolar composition of plasma. (From Winters RW, editor: *The body fluids in pediatrics,* Boston, 1973, Little, Brown.)

the total effective osmolality may be normal, as seen in this example:

$$Glucose = 720 \text{ mg/dl}$$
$$(Na^+) = 120 \text{ mEq/L}$$
$$mOsm/L = 280$$
$$\frac{720 \times 10}{180} + 120 \times 2 = 280$$

Although hyperlipidemia is less frequent, an analogous situation exists (Fig. 13-7).[10] Low laboratory values for plasma sodium occur because the increase in plasma solids (lipids) causes a lower plasma water content and hence a lower sodium concentration per liter of whole plasma. In this case the plasma water sodium concentration may be normal.

Osmotic forces largely determine shifts in the internal redistribution of water in hydration disturbances.

Four pure disturbances of hydration exist: (1) too much electrolyte, (2) too little electrolyte, (3) too much water, and (4) too little water. Combinations of these disturbances may also occur.

Neonatal renal "immaturity" influences fluid and electrolyte needs. Various renal functions do not develop at the same rate.

GFR is low at birth and, despite the initial gestational age, characteristically rises rapidly during the first 6 weeks of life. A VLBW infant in satisfactory condition at 6 weeks may have an adequate GFR. These observations correlate with the infant's obtaining a full complement of nephrons (about 34 weeks' gestation) and the continued

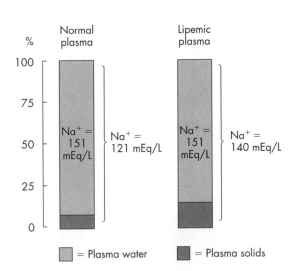

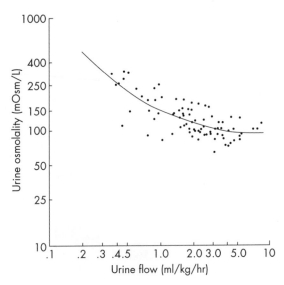

Figure 13-7 Effects of hyperlipemia on plasma water and plasma sodium concentration. (From Winters RW, editor: *The body fluids in pediatrics,* Boston, 1973, Little, Brown.)

Figure 13-8 Normal urine flow rates. (From Jones MD, Gresham EL, Battaglia FC: *Biol Neonate* 22:324, 1972.)

increase in glomerular surface area (beyond 40 weeks' gestation).[5,6]

Urinary sodium excretion increases slowly during the first 2 years of life.

Measuring the urine sodium concentration should be considered part of the routine assessment of fluid and electrolyte balance. All neonates tend to retain sodium if it is given in large amounts.

Urine sodium losses are influenced by sodium intake and gestational age.

Urine sodium may rise when moderately increased amounts of sodium are given to more mature infants. VLBW infants, however, tend to lose urine sodium, which may be greater per kilogram than that of term infants, when receiving the normal (1 to 4 mEq/kg) sodium intake.

The capacity to dilute and concentrate the urine appears limited but can be influenced by nutrient intake.

In summary, the immature concentrating ability (maximum of approximately 600 mOsm/L, Fig. 13-8) coupled with the inability to excrete rapidly either an acute water or sodium load results in a narrow margin of safety in prescribing fluid and electrolytes, especially in the VLBW infant.[1,2,5,6]

Urea is usually the major component of urine osmolality (and hence specific gravity), whereas electrolytes quantitatively contribute less. When total parenteral nutrition is being provided, urine specific gravity may rise because of the low renal threshold for glucose and amino acids. When specific gravity rises, therefore, the cause must be ascertained before altering the fluid infusion rate. A diagnostic test (Bili-Labstix or Chemstrip) can screen for glucose and protein but misses amino acids, which must be detected by amino acid chromatography when necessary.

Neonatal urinary acidification is limited, and the bicarbonate threshold is reduced.

Both physiologic and pathophysiologic factors can contribute to an alkaline urine. For example, VLBW infants have a limited capacity for hydrogen ion excretion, whereas other infants may have acute illnesses such as bicarbonate-losing tubular necrosis or urinary tract infection.

The roles of hormones, such as antidiuretic hormone, aldosterone, atrial natriuretic factor, and parathormone, in regulating neonatal fluid and electrolyte balance are not well defined.

Hormonal influences can be primary, such as in

Table 13-2
Factors That Influence IWL

Decrease IWL	Increase IWL
Heat shield or double-walled incubators	Inversely related to gestational age and weight
Plastic blankets	Respiratory distress
Clothes	Ambient temperature above thermoneutral
High relative humidity (ambulator ventilator gas)	Fever
	Radiant warmer
	Phototherapy
	Activity

the syndrome of inappropriate secretion of antidiuretic hormone and in some cases of hypocalcemia. Secondary hormonal influences can be caused by certain drugs, such as spironolactones, which are aldosterone antagonists.

IWL occurs via both pulmonary and cutaneous routes and is influenced by the factors listed below. Because clinical states and environmental factors influence water needs, there is normally a wide range (30 to 60 ml/kg/24 hr) of IWL in healthy term infants.

Factors that decrease IWL may do so by as much as one third in VLBW infants and should be given consideration in each patient (Table 13-2). When operative concomitantly, several of these factors can increase IWL by as much as 300%, such as when phototherapy is used and a VLBW infant is under a radiant warmer.[5,6] For every 1°C rise in body temperature, metabolism and fluid needs increase approximately 10% ("Q-10 effect"). These expected increases must be recognized in calculating fluid requirements.

Etiology

The causes of common electrolyte problems and common clinical syndromes are discussed in the section on treatment.

Prevention

Prevention of fluid and electrolyte imbalance in the neonate begins with knowing the proper calculation of fluid and electrolyte requirements. The estimated metabolic rate forms the reference base for all calculations. The metabolic rate (and hence oxygen consumption) normally increases steadily over the first weeks of life, so increases in water and probably electrolyte needs should be anticipated.

If the caloric requirement is approximately 100 cal/kg/day, the physiologic basis of metabolic rate may be used in calculating needs; however, most settings use the 100 ml/kg basis, which will be modified by factors that influence IWL and adjusted depending on body weight, clinical composition, and urine volume and composition (Fig. 13-9 and Table 13-3).

Preterm infants usually have slightly lower metabolic rates per kilogram than term infants. SGA infants may have higher metabolic rates than preterm infants of similar weight, which is thought to be related to their relatively large brain/body mass ratio. Both SGA and preterm infants, especially VLBW infants, are expected to require more frequent modification of requirements.

Preterm infants, however, often are subject to other problems that may make this physiologic fact less crucial in calculating needs. SGA infants may require more water per kilogram than either preterm or term, normally grown infants. Input should be recorded every hour, and output should be recorded as it occurs. VLBW infants require frequent monitoring of fluid balance, so that if output is unusually large, intake must be adjusted immediately. If fluid intake decreases, critically ill infants may not tolerate "catching up." Continuous monitoring is necessary to ensure that fluid is infusing in appropriate amounts. Infusion pumps that accurately register 1 ml/hr or less must be used.

Requirements for fluid and electrolytes can be divided into maintenance and deficit needs. Maintenance needs keep the organism in a zero balance state and can be subdivided into (1) normal loss, which consists of water and electrolyte loss through sweat, stool, urine, and insensible (lung and skin) routes and (2) abnormal or ongoing losses, such as diarrhea, ostomy, or chest tube drainage.

All diapers should be preweighed on a gram scale and marked with dry weight. After each stool or void, the diaper is reweighed, and the difference equals the amount of loss. For example, if the dry weight is 20.7 g and the "wet" weight is 26.4 g, the

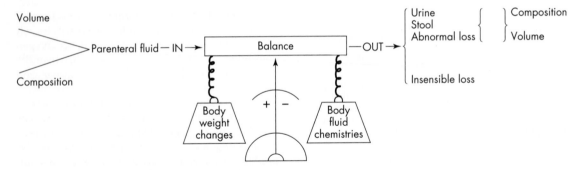

Figure 13-9 Basic scheme for monitoring and modifying therapy.

Table 13-3
Guidelines for Fluid (ml/kg/day) and Solute Provision by Patient Weight and Days of Age

Weight (g)	Ranges of Water Loss		Day 1*	Day 2-3*	Day 4-7*
<1250	IWL†	40-170			
	Urine	50-100			
	Stool	5-10			
	TOTAL	95-280	120	140	150-175
1250-1750	IWL†	20-50			
	Urine	50-100			
	Stool	5-10			
	TOTAL	75-160	90	110	130-140
>1750	IWL†	15-40			
	Urine	50-100			
	Stool	5-10			
	TOTAL	70-150	80	90	100-120

Increment for phototherapy: 20-30 ml/kg/day
Increment for radiant warmer: 20-30 ml/kg/day
Maintenance solutes: Glucose: 7-12 g/kg (4-8 g/kg in VLBW infants)
　　　　　　　　　　　　Na: 1-4 mEq/kg (2-8 mEq/kg in VLBW infants)
　　　　　　　　　　　　K: 1-4 mEq/kg
　　　　　　　　　　　　Cl: 1-4 mEq/kg
　　　　　　　　　　　　Ca: 1 mEq/kg

*Adjustment based on a urine flow rate of 2 to 5 ml/kg/hr with a specific gravity of 1.002 to 1.010 and stable weight.
†May be reduced by 30% if the infant is on a ventilator.
IWL, Insensible water loss; *VLBW,* very-low-birth-weight.

difference is 5.7 g or 5.7 ml of stool or urine. All losses should be calculated to the nearest milliliter. IV volumetric chambers or small urine collection cups can be used as collection chambers for tube drainage.

Deficit needs refer to previously incurred losses. These should be extremely rare in the newborn but are common in older neonates with disorders that have an insidious or delayed onset,

such as renal tubular dysfunction or nonvirilizing congenital adrenal hyperplasia.

Deficits are best estimated by body weight comparisons. A weight loss greater than 10% to 15% in 1 week should be considered excessive. VLBW infants are particularly difficult to maintain within 10% to 15% of birth weight during the first week of life.

The initial choice of parenteral solutions depends on the weight and postnatal age of the infant (Table 13-3). Another important consideration is whether the infant is in an incubator or under a radiant warmer without a plastic blanket or heat shield. IWL of 170 ml/kg/day has been demonstrated in VLBW infants under radiant warmers.[5] Maintenance of water needs in larger infants on the first day of life can usually be met by a 7.5% to 10% glucose solution infused at 80 ml/kg/day. The infusion rate should be increased gradually to 100 to 120 ml/kg/day using principles of monitoring discussed later.

All sick infants require IV access for fluid administration.[9] The IV equipment should include (1) a needle or catheter, (2) connecting tubing, (3) a volumetric chamber to measure small volumes, and (4) an infusion pump. IV infusions should never be given without a volumetric chamber and infusion pump.

Electrolytes such as sodium and potassium are usually omitted the first day and then added as chloride salts in amounts of 1 to 4 mEq/kg. Mildly acidotic and VLBW infants may be given their sodium requirements as sodium bicarbonate or acetate. Hypocalcemia also may be frequent in tertiary care patients.

Potassium should never be added to IV fluid until urine flow and renal function have been assessed. The maintenance requirement for calcium is 0.5 to 1 mEq (100 to 200 mg)/kg given as calcium gluconate. This maintenance is most important in VLBW infants and those who are severely ill.

Factors that influence IWL must be identified early and maintenance needs adjusted appropriately to prevent problems with water and electrolyte balance.

VLBW infants present special problems because data on their management are incomplete. Our recent experience (unpublished) with 30 infants weighing 1250 g or less can be summarized as follows:

- **Water requirements should start at 110 to 120 ml/kg at birth and often need to be increased by 20 to 40 ml/kg/day over days 2 to 4 of life, at which time they plateau at 150 to 175 ml/kg/day.**
- **Sodium requirements (including medications) were 2 to 3 mEq/kg/day after 12 hours**

of age and reached a maximum of 7 mEq/kg/day on days 5 and 6, which was required to prevent hyponatremia.
- **Cumulative weight loss plateaued at 10.8% to 12.7% of birth weight (95% confidence limits) by day 3.**
- **Maintenance of normal serum glucose concentrations (<150 mg/dl) required relatively less glucose (4 to 8 g/kg/day) than term infants. As anticipated, infants weighing 900 g or less were the most difficult to manage without causing either excessive weight loss or hyponatremia.**

VLBW infants, especially those under radiant warmers, may have greatly increased IWL. They also commonly receive phototherapy. Hence their fluid requirements may be 175 to 200 ml/kg/day. By the end of the first week of life, as the epithelium becomes more cornified, the requirements decrease toward 120 to 150 ml/kg/day.

Neonates requiring maintenance fluids when significant oral caloric intake is low (<50 kcal/kg/day) for more than 3 to 5 days should be given parenteral nutritional support with increased glucose, amino acids, lipids, vitamins, and micronutrients (see Chapter 16).

Data Collection

All parenteral therapy should be based on the following principles: (1) assessing the patient, including maintenance needs, factors that modify IWL, and specific medical or surgical disorders; (2) calculating short-term (12 to 24 hours) fluid and electrolyte needs; (3) initiating therapy at the proper site and rate; and (4) monitoring and modifying based on clinical and biochemical data.

History

A history of factors that influence IWL (see Table 13-2) includes gestational age, birth weight, and postnatal age.

Signs and Symptoms

Weight and urine output are the best overall clinical guide to assessing the adequacy of therapy.

Weight is the most sensitive index of IWL and must be accurately determined at least every 24 hours. Accurate daily weights in VLBW infants require special nursing efforts and often the use of electronic bed scales.

Urine output should be 2 to 5 ml/kg/hr with a specific gravity of 1.002 to 1.010 (60 to 300 mOsm) (Fig. 13-10 [note nonlinear relationship as specific gravity exceeds 1.010] and 13-8). Blood pressure and peripheral perfusion may reflect changes in vascular volume and cardiac output. Normal capillary refill occurs within 3 seconds, but hypothermia may falsely delay capillary refill.

Loss of skin turgor is a late and variable sign and is usually not helpful in assessing therapy, but vital signs (heart and respiratory rate and skin and core temperature) provide helpful clues about metabolic rate and stress. Drainage from ostomy sites, chest tubes, and nasogastric or other tubes must be quantitated accurately. These types of drainage represent abnormal or ongoing maintenance requirements that must be added to the calculation of normal maintenance needs (abnormal + normal = total maintenance).

Laboratory Data

Tests for concentrations of electrolytes (Na^+, K^+, Cl^-, Ca^{++}), red blood cells (hematocrit), glucose, BUN or creatinine, and acid-base status should be performed serially. Occasionally, serum osmolality and protein concentrations are helpful in assessing the neonate's condition.

Urine specific gravity and volume must be measured as soon as voiding occurs. Urine osmolality and electrolyte concentration help clarify fluid and electrolyte balance when glucose, protein, or unusual solutes appear in the urine.

The water content of urine evaporates rapidly under a radiant warmer. Glucosuria and proteinuria (>2+) cause modest elevations in specific gravity, whereas radiographic dyes excreted in the urine cause extreme increases in the specific gravity. All urine should be screened with a diagnostic test (BiliLabstix or Chemstrip).

All drainage must be collected and measured, so that the concentration of solutes can be determined. Collections every 4 to 6 hours are preferable to a single "spot" collection, which is commonly misleading. Occasionally, determining trace elements, hematocrit, and protein content of urine or drainage can be crucial to management.

Treatment

Techniques of IV Therapy

Peripheral veins are the most easily accessible and have the least adverse effects for parenteral therapy. Scalp vein infusion sets are most commonly used in the foot, hand, or scalp veins. However, the advent of extremely small catheter and introducer sets (Quick-Cath, Angiocath, and others) has permitted prolonged (5 to 7 days) use of a single peripheral infusion site.

Often, a rubber band is the most effective tourniquet for the extremity of a small infant. The area of skin should be cleaned with an antiseptic, and efforts should be made to avoid shaving the head, because parents often find this upsetting. Before puncturing the skin, have the "setup" (as described previously) and the appropriate fluid ready.

It is important to recognize the high potential of

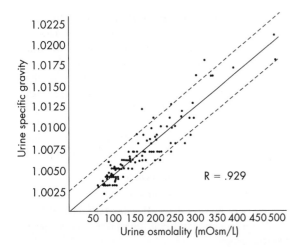

Figure 13-10   Urine specific gravity compared with osmolality. *Solid line* represents mean; *broken line* represents 95% confidence limits. (From Jones MD, Gresham EL, Battaglia FC: *Biol Neonate* 21:322, 1972.)

infiltration and skin sloughs with peripheral IVs. The risk is greatest in the foot, less with the hand, and the least on the scalp. Calcium-containing solutions present an added risk. Although the needle or catheter must be taped in place, the tape must not prevent adequate visualization. At least every hour record the fluid administered, and observe the site for any sign of infiltration. The arm or leg can be positioned on a padded tongue blade (armboard or footboard) to prevent needle displacement. A "flap" of tape can be made at the end of the board, which can be pinned or tied to the bed for further immobilization. Padded sandbags can be used to hold an infant's head or extremity still for a period of time but must be removed regularly to allow some movement. The need for immobilization is less with catheters than with scalp vein sets. However, the board may need to be removed after several hours for additional assurance of no infiltration, as well as mobilization of the limb.

Deep and central veins can be approached by two techniques. Percutaneous insertion using silastic catheters can be accomplished readily only after much experience. Saphenous or antecubital insertion while advancing the catheter to a deep vein is a relatively simple technique (long lines), and even subclavian cannulation of VLBW infants can be accomplished with appropriate training and experience.[4] The risk of infection and thrombosis is probably no greater than with peripheral infusion, but the consequences may be much more serious (see Chapter 16).

The second technique, venesection or cutdowns, can also be performed readily with appropriate training. Catheterization for total parenteral nutrition, however, requires special consideration (see Chapter 16). The catheter is advantageous because patient mobility is greater, but the risks of infection and thrombosis may be greater than those with percutaneous techniques.

Umbilical vessel catheterization should not be performed for fluid infusion only, except in emergencies (see Chapter 7).

Common Problems

In NICUs virtually all patients initially receive IV fluid therapy, so that conventional rules of pediatric fluid therapy, which estimate losses and project deficit replacement, are not completely satisfactory. Weight, urine output and concentration, and the concentration of various solutes in serum and other body fluids are usually known. The correct diagnosis usually rests on clinical and laboratory measurements (not estimates), which are supported by the clinical setting. A pure disorder of hydration is rarely encountered, but mixed disorders or syndromes usually are.

For example, one can compute the amount of sodium required to correct a deficit by the following formula:

$$\text{Sodium required} = (\text{Sodium desired} - \text{Sodium observed}) \times ECF$$

This calculation considers that the sodium will be given as a "dry salt." The total amount and the rate given is a matter of clinical judgment. In practice, the care giver usually begins sodium deficit therapy, measures serum (and preferably urine) sodium, and modifies the IV solution. The cause of the deficit must be identified while these conditions are being corrected, or it is likely to recur.

Common Electrolyte Disorders

Hypocalcemia (Infants with <7 mg/dl)

Clinical findings may correlate poorly with biochemical data (total or ionized calcium). Jitteriness and twitching are nonspecific, and serum calcium (and probably glucose) should be measured.

Hypocalcemia is strongly associated with infants of diabetic mothers, asphyxia, and prematurity (especially the VLBW infant). "Early" (<72 hours) hypocalcemia can be prevented by the inclusion of 18 mg/kg of elemental calcium as 200 mg/kg of calcium gluconate in maintenance IV solution (1 mEq = 2 ml of 10% calcium gluconate).

Bolus infusion (also associated with dysrhythmias) and slow infusion for 2 to 3 minutes are not as successful as more gradual attempts to correct hypocalcemia. Either repeated (every 6 hours), slow infusion or continuous infusion is best. Additional elemental calcium should be given intravenously at 18 to 75 mg/kg for 4 to 6 hours if seizures or biochemical abnormality persists. "Late" (>7 days) hypocalcemia usually has a specific cause, such as high phosphate intake, malabsorption and postdiarrhea state, hypomagnesemia, hypoparathyroidism, or rickets and should be evaluated in detail.

Care should be taken in administering the IV calcium: (1) place the infant on a cardiac monitor to detect bradycardia, (2) immediately discontinue calcium administration if bradycardia occurs, and (3) check the peripheral IV site for patency before and during administration because of sloughing, calcification, and necrosis caused by infiltrated calcium.

Hypernatremia (Infants with >150 mEq/L)

Clinical signs of hypernatremia are rare, except for seizures that occur late. The most common causes of hypernatremia are (1) dehydration (usually caused by too little "free water" administration), (2) injudicious use of sodium-containing solution (sodium bicarbonate bolus infusion and sodium-containing medications can be overlooked), and (3) congenital reduction in antidiuretic hormone. Both nephrogenic and central diabetes insipidus are uncommon. Cerebral palsy and intracranial bleeding correlate strongly with hypernatremia. Management is directed toward the causes, and serum sodium should be reduced slowly to prevent seizures.

Hyponatremia (Infants with <130 mEq/L)

Hyponatremia is usually asymptomatic because of chronic rather than acute development of imbalance, but a late clinical sign is seizures. Most common causes include (1) overhydration as a result of maternal or neonatal administration of electrolyte-free solutions, (2) renal loss of sodium (commonly in VLBW infants) in any neonate receiving diuretic therapy, and (3) a syndrome of inappropriate antidiuretic hormone secretion that is suspected clinically when decreased serum sodium and increased urine specific gravity occur. This syndrome is associated with CNS and lung pathologic conditions. Criteria include (1) low serum sodium, (2) continued urine sodium loss, (3) urine osmolality greater than plasma, and (4) normal adrenal and renal function. Management is by water restriction until diuresis follows and is directed toward the etiology.

Hyperkalemia (Infants with >7 mEq/L)

Causes of hyperkalemia include (1) acidosis with or without tissue destruction, (2) renal failure (water overload may limit management), and (3) adrenal insufficiency (relatively uncommon). Table 13-4 outlines clinical signs and ECG changes. Management is directed toward the causes and nonspecific treatment, depending on the severity of the hyperkalemia:

- Stop all potassium administration.
- Infuse 100 to 200 mg of calcium gluconate to lower the cell membrane threshold (this is transient but may be lifesaving).
- Infuse sodium bicarbonate, 1 to 2 mEq/kg, diluted at a 1:2 ratio with water, which is another transient therapy aimed at enhancing intracellular sodium and hydrogen exchange for potassium.
- Administer 1 g/kg cation exchange resin (sodium polystyrene-sulfonate [Kayexalate]) as an oral or rectal solution. Little experience has been reported in neonates, and technical problems of retention can be substantial.
- Perform peritoneal dialysis, but frequently sodium bicarbonate must be added to dialysate to prevent acidosis.

Hypokalemia (Infants with <3.5 mEq/L)

Clinical signs of hypokalemia are related to muscular weakness and cardiac dysrhythmias. Ileus may occur also. Electrocardiographic changes include a decreased T wave and ST depression. The most common causes of hypokalemia are (1) increased gastrointestinal losses from an ostomy and a nasogastric tube and (2) renal losses common in diuretic therapy.

Table 13-4
Hyperkalemia (Infants With >7 mEq/L)

Clinical Signs	Electrocardiographic Changes
Muscular weakness	Short QT interval
Cardiac dysrhythmias	Widening QRS
Ileus	Sine wave QRS/T

About 90% of total potassium is intracellular. Management is directed toward the causes: (1) low serum potassium always implies significant intracellular depletion, (2) intracellular potassium can be low with normal serum potassium, and (3) IV solutions should not exceed 40 mEq/L potassium.

Common Clinical Syndromes

Acute renal failure is most often caused by (1) extrinsic factors such as asphyxia, shock, and heart failure; (2) intrinsic factors, such as congenital or acquired lesions; and (3) obstructive uropathy, including urethral or extragenitourinary mass. Oliguria or anuria usually occurs initially. Electrolyte-free glucose infusion should be limited to IWL and urine output. Elevations of BUN often do not occur, because protein intake is commonly low. Recovery is usually associated with natriuresis and osmotic diuresis. This may develop rapidly, and sodium loss as high as 20 mEq/kg/day may occur. Body weight and fluid losses must be carefully and frequently measured, at least every 12 hours. Nonrenal losses, such as gastrointestinal drainage, must also be measured. Ideally, balance treatment is directed toward no weight gain or 1%/day weight loss until recovery is nearly complete. Any weight gain demands careful reevaluation of the fluid plan.

Asphyxia is frequently associated with the following:

- Hypotension
- Renal failure (tubular necrosis is suggested by proteinuria and hematuria)
- Respiratory failure (ventilators reduce IWL from lungs)
- Myocardial ischemia (echocardiography can often assess ventricular function)
- Syndrome of inappropriate antidiuretic hormone secretion (early or late in the clinical course)
- Cerebral edema (usually after 24 hours)

The asphyxiated neonate should be managed by prospectively reducing the initial fluid estimates by 30% to 60%. IWL and urine output may be the best initial plan, although volume expansion to treat hypotension may be a greater priority.

Major surgery

Surgical trauma is superimposed on the normal metabolic responses of the neonate and determined by both gestational and postnatal age. In healthy term infants, negative balance of water, electrolytes, nitrogen, and calories with associated weight loss occurs during the first 3 to 5 days, with transition to positive balance and weight gain by 7 to 10 days. Similar transition times for preterm infants vary enormously. Deficits may exist as a result of delayed diagnosis, with external loss or internal loss. "Third space" (especially peritoneal) loss is a notorious source of deficit underestimation.

The exactness of the metabolic response to surgery is not resolved and varies widely among individual patients, even with similar lesions. Perhaps too many uncontrollable variables exist to define a normal postoperative physiologic response of neonates, especially those weighing less than 2 kg. Negative nitrogen balance always occurs postoperatively but is considerably less than in adults. The control of this tendency to minimize nitrogen loss is unknown. Thermal regulation is almost never controlled as well in the operating room as in the intensive care unit, but transport incubators, warmed operating rooms, radiant warmers, and prewarmed solutions should be used in an attempt to achieve thermoneutrality. Intraoperative fluid balance is rarely precise despite the best efforts. Blood loss on sponges, drapes, and other objects should be measured, but IWL from open body cavities is difficult to estimate.

The principles of postoperative management are (1) serial monitoring of clinical and chemical variables, and meticulously and frequently (every 4 to 6 hours) watching fluid balance, including drainage; (2) providing 30 to 40 kcal/kg as glucose and planning a zero balance of water and electrolytes for 1 to 3 days; and (3) using total parenteral nutrition if significant enteral feedings (<50 kcal/kg) cannot be achieved by 3 to 5 days. Gastrointestinal motility returns rapidly in term infants as compared with adults. Almost all VLBW infants require total parenteral nutrition after surgery.

Water intoxication (hypotonicity) is common in neonates because of small volumes of urine and relatively high volumes per kilogram of infusates. A high index of suspicion and meticulous attention to the details of IV therapy prevent hypotonicity. Increased antidiuretic hormone secretion commonly occurs and may progress to a syndrome of inappropriate antidiuretic hormone. Water intoxication may be hard to distinguish from hypotonic dehydration. Water restriction and continued sodium administration should be instituted only after the diagnosis is established. Fresh frozen plasma (10 to 20 ml/kg) given with a diuretic (1 to 2 mg/kg furosemide [Lasix]) may be used to make the diagnosis, because a good diuresis suggests dehydration or decreased plasma volume.

Complications

Increased fluid administration (>180 ml/kg) has been associated with (1) BPD, (2) necrotizing enterocolitis, and (3) PDA. Reduced fluid administration (to prevent increased fluid administration) has been associated with (1) hypertonicity; (2) CNS damage, including bleeding and cerebral palsy; and (3) renal failure and tubular damage.

Parent Teaching

The need for and presence of an IV line in the newborn may be frightening for parents. Clear, physiologically sound explanations of the need for fluid and electrolyte support in the sick neonate allay their fears. Scalp vein IVs are particularly of concern (1) if the hair must be shaved and (2) because a common fantasy is that the needle is in the infant's brain. Explain to parents that scalp vein IVs are in the large veins of the head and not the brain and that an IV in the head stays in longer, thus decreasing the need for multiple vein puncture and allowing more mobility. In answer to the question: "Does it hurt?" a truthful answer is "Yes, when it is put in, but not after it is in the vein."

Infiltrates at peripheral IV sites should be addressed prospectively with parents. Erythema and edema are expected. Sloughing of the skin is not infrequent in VLBW infants and is more common on the feet and hands than on the scalp. Topical therapy similar to thermal burn management is indicated, whereas skin grafting is rarely needed.

Including parents in the care of their sick neonate requires an explanation about the importance of measuring intake and output. Inadvertent disposal of diapers and giving fluids that are not recorded are prevented by emphasizing the importance of saving them for the infant's nurse. "A little spitting up" after feeding may seem insignificant if parents are not instructed in the importance of telling the nurse and saving it for inspection or testing.

References

1. Aiken CGA et al: Mineral balance studies in sick preterm intravenously fed infants during the first week after birth; a guide to fluid therapy, *Acta Pediatr Scand* suppl 355, 1989.
2. Bauer K et al: Body composition, nutrition, and fluid balance during the first two weeks of life in preterm neonates weighing less than 1500 grams, *J Pediatr* 118:615, 1991.
3. Bell EF et al: Effect of fluid administration on the development of symptomatic patent ductus arteriosus and congestive heart failure in premature infants, *N Engl J Med* 302:598, 1980.
4. Chathas MK et al: Percutaneous central venous catheterization, *Am J Dis Child* 144:1246, 1990.
5. Costarino AT et al: Sodium restriction versus daily maintenance replacement in very low birth weight premature neonates: a randomized, blind, therapeutic trial, *J Pediatr* 120:99, 1992.
6. El-Dahr SS, Chevalier RL: Special needs of the newborn infant in fluid therapy, *Pediatr Clin North Am* 37:323, 1990.
7. Heird WC et al: Intravenous alimentation in pediatric patients, *J Pediatr* 80:351, 1972.
8. Jones MD, Gresham EL, Battaglia FC: Urinary flow rate and urea excretion rates in newborn infants, *Biol Neonate* 21:322, 1972.
9. Wilson D: Neonatal IVs: practical tips, *Neonat Net* 2(2):49, 1992.
10. Winters RW: *The body fluids in pediatrics,* Boston, 1973, Little, Brown.

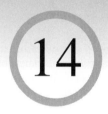

14 Glucose Homeostasis

Jane E. McGowan, Mary I. Enzman Hagedorn, William W. Hay, Jr.

During intrauterine life the fetus depends on the constant transfer of glucose across the placenta to meet its glucose requirements. After birth, neonates must maintain their own glucose homeostasis by producing and regulating their own glucose supply. This requires activation of a number of metabolic processes, including gluconeogenesis and glycogenolysis, as well as intact regulatory mechanisms and an adequate supply of metabolic substrates.

Physiology

Throughout gestation, maternal glucose provides the principal source of energy for the fetus via facilitated diffusion across the placenta. Fetal glucose concentration varies directly with maternal concentration and is usually approximately 70% of the maternal value. Changes in maternal metabolism, including increased caloric intake and decreased sensitivity of the maternal tissues to insulin, provide the additional substrate necessary to meet fetal energy demands. During maternal normoglycemia the fetus produces little, if any, glucose, although the enzymes for gluconeogenesis are present by the third month of gestation.[36] If fetal energy demands cannot be met, however, as is the case in maternal starvation with resultant maternal hypoglycemia, the fetus is capable of adapting both by using alternate substrates, such as ketone bodies, and by "turning on" its endogenous glucose production. There is additional evidence that even in the basal state the fetus relies on fuels other than glucose to meet some of its energy demands. These include both lactate and amino acids.

Fetal glycogen synthesis begins as early as the ninth week of gestation. Most fetal glycogen is synthesized from glucose, directly or via three-carbon intermediates such as lactate. The major sites of glycogen deposition are liver, lung, heart, and skeletal muscle. Rates of hepatic glycogen deposition vary with different species depending on the length of gestation; in the human, with a relatively long gestation, hepatic glycogen increases slowly throughout the first two trimesters of pregnancy, with a more rapid rate of deposition during the third trimester.[43] By 40 weeks' gestation, hepatic glycogen stores are two to three times adult levels. Skeletal muscle glycogen content also increases during the third trimester to as much as five times adult levels. In contrast, lung and cardiac muscle glycogen stores decrease as the fetus approaches term, although they are still of physiologic significance. Survival after asphyxia, for example, has been shown to be directly related to cardiac glycogen content. The decrease in lung glycogen, which begins at 34 to 36 weeks, may be related to ongoing developmental processes that require utilization of stored energy (e.g., synthesis of surfactant).

Several factors can affect rates of glycogen accumulation. Decreased availability of substrate as in maternal malnutrition, placental insufficiency, or multiple gestations has been associated with a decreased rate of glycogen synthesis. Acute intrauterine hypoxia does not appear to produce a measurable change in glycogen content, but chronic hypoxia, as seen in maternal preeclampsia, does result in lower tissue glycogen content as compared with normoxic fetuses.

In addition to glycogen, the human fetus also stores energy as adipose tissue. Most triglyceride synthesis occurs during the third trimester. By 40 weeks the human fetus has a fat content of about 16%, making it the fattest of all terrestrial newborn mammals. The human placenta transports some free fatty acids, although the amount transported has not been well quantified. Preliminary studies suggest that the maternal fatty acids transported to the fetus are not sufficient to account for the amount of adipose tissue present; therefore the fetus must also synthesize triglycerides directly from glucose. Again, conditions in which fetal glucose supply is reduced will result in less adipose tissue accumulation.

Insulin, considered a major stimulus for fetal growth, is present in the fetal pancreas by 8 to 10 weeks. Pancreatic insulin content increases in late gestation, exceeding adult levels by the time the infant reaches term.[27] However, the fetal pancreas seems to be less sensitive than the adult pancreas to the insulin secretion–stimulating effects of increased glucose concentration. Nevertheless, insulin secretion is augmented by higher glucose concentrations; increased concentrations of amino acids add to this effect, although this may only be true for pharmacologic concentrations, not physiologic concentrations, of amino acids. The elevated insulin concentration increases both fetal glucose utilization and glucose oxidation rates without increasing total fetal oxygen consumption.[14,19] This implies that other substrates (e.g., amino acids) become available for nonoxidative metabolism, which may promote tissue accretion and growth. Animal studies have demonstrated increased rates of protein synthesis and glucose uptake with increased insulin concentration and, conversely, decreased cell numbers and DNA content with insulin deficiency, supporting insulin's role as a growth-promoting factor. The fetuses of diabetic mothers who have very unstable plasma glucose concentrations during late gestation have an increased islet cell response to hyperglycemia compared with controls, releasing more insulin than normal fetuses at any given blood glucose concentration.[27] The higher insulin levels, in turn, lead to increased growth, primarily of adipose tissue, producing the macrosomia typically seen in IDMs.

The related pancreatic hormone glucagon, which, like insulin, does not cross the placenta, has been detected as early as 15 weeks' gestation. The role of glucagon in regulating fetal glucose metabolism remains unclear. The concentration of glucagon in fetal blood is relatively low, even though pancreatic content is higher than in the adult. The high insulin-to-glucagon ratio in the fetus may be important in preferentially maintaining glycogen synthesis and suppressing gluconeo-

genesis, because glucagon is a potent inducer of gluconeogenic enzymes.[36]

At birth the infant is removed abruptly from its glucose supply, and blood glucose concentration falls. Several hormonal and metabolic changes occur at birth that facilitate the adaptation necessary to maintain glucose homeostasis. Catecholamine levels increase markedly at birth, possibly as a response to the decrease in environmental temperature, as well as the loss of the placenta, which in utero may remove as much as 50% of circulating fetal epinephrine. Glucagon concentrations also increase, reversing the relatively low fetal glucagon/insulin ratio.[45] The elevated glucagon and norepinephrine levels activate hepatic glycogen phosphorylase, which induces glycogenolysis; simultaneously the falling glucose concentration and the perinatal surge in fetal cortisol secretion stimulate hepatic glucose-6-phosphatase activity. Together, these changes lead to an increase in hepatic glucose release.[11] Increased catecholamines also stimulate lipolysis, providing substrate for gluconeogenesis. The reversal of the insulin/glucagon ratio induces synthesis of phosphoenolpyruvate carboxykinase (PEPCK), which is considered the rate-limiting enzyme in hepatic gluconeogenesis. The concentrations of PEPCK and other gluconeogenic enzymes continue to increase with postnatal age during the first 2 weeks of life regardless of gestational age.[11,35] These changes act in concert to provide glucose to replace the supply previously received via the placenta.

Studies in normal infants using several different methods have determined that the steady state glucose production/utilization rate in the term neonate is 3.5 to 5.5 mg/min/kg[12]—approximately twice the weight-specific rate measured in adults. As in the fetus, it appears that approximately half of this glucose is oxidized to CO_2 during normal metabolic processes, whereas the remainder is used in nonoxidative pathways such as glycogen and fat synthesis.

Maintenance of glucose homeostasis depends on the balance between hepatic glucose output and peripheral glucose utilization. Hepatic glucose output is a function of rates of glycogenolysis and gluconeogenesis, which are regulated by the factors discussed above. Peripheral glucose utilization varies with the metabolic demands placed on the neonate. Some circumstances in which peripheral utilization is increased include hypoxia, because anaerobic metabolism of glucose is less efficient than aerobic glycolysis; hyperinsulinemia, which increases glucose uptake by the insulin-sensitive tissues, including muscle and liver; and cold stress, under which the infant must increase the metabolic rate to maintain body temperature. If rates of glycogenolysis and gluconeogenesis do not match the rate of glucose utilization because of failure of the hormonal control mechanisms or variability of substrate supply, then disturbances of glucose homeostasis occur. These disturbances are recognized clinically by the presence of hypoglycemia or hyperglycemia.

Etiology

Hypoglycemia

Hypoglycemia during the first 72 hours of life was defined previously as a whole blood glucose concentration of less than 35 mg/dl in the term infant or less than 25 mg/dl in the preterm infant, or alternatively as a plasma concentration of less than 40 mg/dl or less than 30 mg/dl, respectively. Although arbitrary and based only on a statistical cross-sectional analysis, these definitions did point out the increased risk of hypoglycemia among all preterm and all SGA infants. These definitions were based on statistical analysis of glucose concentrations measured in large groups of neonates. The definition of hypoglycemia was based on the glucose concentration two standard deviations (2 SD) below the mean for the group. Based on such definitions the overall incidence of hypoglycemia has been estimated at 1.3 to 4.4/1000 live births; differences in incidence figures probably reflect the difference between those studies that reported only symptomatic infants and those that evaluated data from screening measurements on all infants, thus including those with asymptomatic hypoglycemia. In preterm infants the incidence of hypoglycemia is increased, with estimates ranging from 1.5% to 5.5% (Fig. 14-1).

More recently with changes in nursery care,

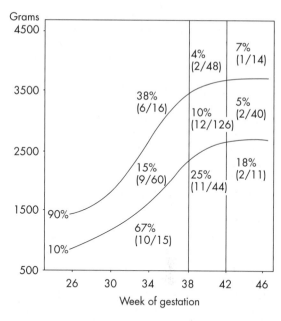

Figure 14-1   Incidence of neonatal hypoglycemia (blood glucose <30 mg/dl) by birth weight and gestational age. (From Lubchenco LO, Bard H: *Pediatrics* 47:831, 1971.)

including earlier feeding and the use of IV dextrose infusions, average glucose concentrations in newborns appear to be increased compared with earlier data. As a result, several authors have suggested redefining hypoglycemia based on current data. For example, a recent study[21] of blood glucose levels in 65 normal term neonates found that 95% had values greater than 30 mg/dl in the first 24 hours of life and greater than 45 mg/dl after 24 hours of life (Fig. 14-2). Similarly, Srinivasan et al found that in infants who received the first feeding by 3 hours of age, subsequent plasma glucose values were higher than previously reported "normal" values; in addition, several infants with plasma glucose concentrations within 2 SD of the study mean had symptomatic hypoglycemia. Additionally, measurements of cord blood glucose concentrations in normal human fetuses show that even at midgestation as well as late gestation, fetal glucose concentration is normally above 50 mg/dl.[35] Such data indicate that the normal fetal brain develops in the presence of glucose

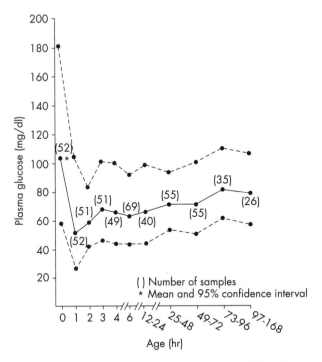

Figure 14-2   Plasma glucose concentrations during the first week of life in healthy appropriate-for-gestational age (AGA) term infants. (From Srinvasan G et al: *J Pediatr* 109:114, 1986.

concentrations that are higher than lower limit values for the range of glucose concentrations accepted as "normal." In support of this concern is the data from Lucas et al,[33] which showed decreasing neurodevelopment scores (mental and motor) with an increased incidence of hypoglycemia (<2.6 mm or <47 mg/dl) in preterm infants over several weeks of life. These data suggest that the definition of hypoglycemia should be revised to reflect both changes in newborn care and the higher "normal" glucose concentrations that have now been documented in the fetus and after the first to second days of life in normal newborns. This should apply to preterm as well as term infants.

A further consideration when evaluating blood glucose concentrations is that significant metabolic derangements, including decreases in cerebral glucose supply, may occur at glucose concentrations above the "hypoglycemic" level as defined by large population studies. The infant with polycythemia, for example, may have a normal blood glucose

concentration but may have decreased cerebral delivery of glucose because of reduced plasma flow. Additionally, preterm infants have much lower plasma concentrations of alternate brain energy substrates such as ketones, increasing the vulnerability of such infants to the potential for cerebral energy deficiency when glucose concentrations in their plasma are decreased. Thus an infant may have "physiologic hypoglycemia" in the presence of a statistically normal blood glucose concentration if glucose delivery to the brain or other organ does not meet demand. Such cases underscore the importance of assessing the history and clinical presentation rather than relying only on results of laboratory tests and statistical definitions for normal and abnormal concentrations of glucose.

The causes of hypoglycemia can be partitioned into several broad categories based on the mechanisms producing the hypoglycemia. These include inadequate substrate supply, abnormal endocrine regulation of glucose metabolism, and increased rate of glucose utilization. There are also a number of etiologies whose mechanisms are not well defined.

Inadequate Substrate Supply

If substrate availability is inadequate, the hepatic glucose output will not meet metabolic demands. Most often this is due to subnormal fat and glycogen stores, which therefore do not provide enough energy to maintain glucose homeostasis until gluconeogenesis reaches adequate levels. Because most hepatic glycogen is accumulated during the third trimester, infants born prematurely will have diminished glycogen stores. The infant with IUGR secondary to placental insufficiency is also at risk for decreased glycogen accumulation, presumably because of diminished transfer of precursors across the placenta. The limited supply is then used for oxidative metabolism and tissue growth, rather than fat or glycogen accretion. Postnatally, catecholamine- and glucagon-stimulated lipolysis and glycogenolysis rapidly deplete the already less-than-adequate supplies at a time when gluconeogenesis is still impaired because of low levels of PEPCK and other gluconeogenic enzymes. Hypoglycemia results. These infants may be asymptomatic with the initial episode of hypoglycemia, but they can become symptomatic if the hypoglycemia persists.

Although inadequate stores of glycogen and lipid have been cited as the major etiology of hypoglycemia in the premature and SGA infant, a number of other factors may also play a role. The preterm infant with RDS, for example, has increased metabolic demands because of the increased work of breathing. Infants with IUGR and hypoglycemia have been shown to have an increased rate of glucose disappearance when receiving an IV glucose infusion, as well as reduced fat mobilization in response to hypoglycemia, when compared with normoglycemic SGA newborns. Because of the increased brain weight/liver weight ratio in the infant with asymmetric growth restriction cerebral glucose requirements are high relative to the liver's capacity to respond, even if glycogen stores are normal for size[28] (Fig. 14-3). Inappropriately elevated insulin/glucose ratios have also been observed in some SGA infants. These findings

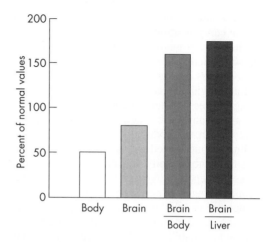

Figure 14-3 Differences in organ/body/weight ratios in small-for-gestational age (SGA) infant compared with appropriate-for-gestational age (AGA) counterpart. (From Lafeber HN, Jones CT, Rolph TP: Some of the consequences on intrauterine growth retardation. In Visser HKA, editor: *Nutrition and metabolism of the fetus and infant,* Boston, 1979, Martinus Nijhoff.)

suggest that other disturbances in glucose metabolism in addition to lower-than-normal energy stores may be present in some growth-restricted infants.[26]

A much rarer, but related, problem occurs in several types of glycogen storage disease. In these inherited disorders hypoglycemia is due not to inadequate glycogen stores, but rather to the inability to utilize stored glycogen as a result of one of several enzyme deficiencies.[36]

Abnormalities of Endocrine Regulation

Hyperinsulinemia is the most common endocrinologic disturbance resulting in neonatal hypoglycemia and may be the most common cause of persistent hypoglycemia in the first year of life even though such conditions are relatively uncommon. Excessive insulin secretion in the newborn increases glucose utilization by stimulating cellular glucose uptake in insulin-dependent tissues. At the same time, the high circulating insulin concentration promotes continued glycogen synthesis and inhibits both glycogenolysis and gluconeogenesis, impairing the infant's glucogenic response to the

increased glucose demand and decreasing plasma glucose concentration.

The most common clinical situation in which hyperinsulinemia occurs is in the IDM. In utero the fetus becomes hyperglycemic because of increased transfer of glucose across the placenta from the hyperglycemic mother. The fetal pancreatic beta cells are stimulated by the increased fetal glucose concentration to produce increased quantities of insulin. As mentioned previously, the islet cells seem to be abnormally sensitive to this stimulus because of repeated hyperglycemia stimuli as well as time-averaged hyperglycemia. Before delivery the increase in cellular glucose uptake in response to the increased insulin secretion is matched by the increased availability of glucose from the mother. After delivery, however, the source of glucose is abruptly removed while the hyperinsulinemia persists, producing hypoglycemia. The decrease in glucose concentration postpartum is a result of insulin-stimulated peripheral glucose uptake, as well as inhibition of gluconeogenesis and glycogenolysis by the high insulin concentrations. Although some studies have reported other abnormalities in glucose kinetics in the IDM, Cowett et al[9] found no difference in glucose kinetics in IDMs versus controls. This may reflect the fact that maternal diabetic control was maintained during pregnancy in the group studied, although a large review of pregnancies in diabetic mothers found no association between the incidence of neonatal hypoglycemia and the number of episodes of maternal hyperglycemia (a reflection of the degree of control) late in pregnancy.[18] The incidence of hypoglycemia in IDMs ranges from 15% to 75%; these infants are frequently asymptomatic. The incidence of a number of other complications is increased in these infants as well, including polycythemia, which may add to disturbances of glucose homeostasis, hypocalcemia, dystocia secondary to macrosomia, and congenital anomalies. Infants of mothers with severe diabetic vasculopathy, in contrast to most IDMs, may have IUGR caused in part by decreased placental blood flow.

Like IDMs, infants with Beckwith-Wiedemann syndrome are also macrosomic and hyperinsulinemic; in addition, they have other associated anomalies, including macroglossia, which may cause airway obstruction, and omphalocele. Up to 50% have symptomatic hypoglycemia in the first few days of life. As in the IDM, the hyperinsulinemia is due to pancreatic beta-cell hyperplasia; however, in these infants, maternal or fetal hyperglycemia has not been documented, and the etiology of the islet cell hyperplasia is unknown.

Islet cell hyperplasia is also seen in some infants with severe erythroblastosis fetalis.[3] The mechanism responsible for the hyperplasia is unknown, but glutathiones released from erythrocytes during hemolysis may indirectly stimulate islet cell hyperplasia by inactivating circulating insulin. Regardless of the etiology, infants with erythroblastosis may exhibit symptomatic or asymptomatic hypoglycemia. The incidence ranges from 2% to 20%, increasing with decreasing umbilical cord hemoglobin concentrations. Exchange transfusion, often required to treat severe anemia or hyperbilirubinemia, may further contribute to hyperinsulinemia.[42] The high dextrose content of the common blood preservative agents used for the exchange transfusion stimulates insulin release from the hyperplastic beta cells. When the transfusion is completed, glucose entry rates return to baseline but insulin levels remain high, causing "rebound" hypoglycemia.

A number of infants have been described as having persistent hyperinsulinemia caused by islet cell dysplasias such as nesidioblastosis (diffuse increase in beta-cell number) or discrete islet cell adenomas. Seventy percent of infants with these disorders manifest refractory hypoglycemia in the first 3 days of life. If the hyperinsulinemia begins in utero, these infants, like the others described above, also can be macrosomic at birth.

Hypoglycemia has been noted after the use of beta-agonist agents for tocolysis. Both animal[39] and human[41] studies have documented increased insulin concentrations in infants whose mothers received such drugs before delivery; the risk of developing hypoglycemia may be inversely related to the duration of therapy as well as the length of time between the last dose received by the mother and delivery. Acute hyperinsulinemia may also be induced by maternal infusion of IV solutions containing dextrose if the total infusion just before delivery exceeds 25 g of glucose.[13]

In addition to hyperinsulinemia, global endocrine disturbances can also result in hypoglycemia.

These disturbances include a range of abnormalities of the hypothalamic-pituitary axis, with the most severe being panhypopituitarism. Such infants frequently have growth hormone deficiency and hypothyroidism in addition to severe hypoglycemia. If pituitary dysfunction is due to a structural CNS lesion, other neurologic problems, including abnormal muscle tone and neonatal seizures, may be present. Adrenal failure and hypoglycemia can occur as a result of adrenal hemorrhage, often in association with neonatal sepsis. Isolated endocrine defects, including primary hypothyroidism and cortisol deficiency, may also be associated with hypoglycemia.

Increased Glucose Utilization

Some term infants may have normal energy stores at birth and intact regulating mechanisms but may be stressed by one of several conditions so that the available supplies do not meet the neonate's energy requirements. The asphyxiated newborn is one common example. After asphyxia and subsequent tissue ischemia, the neonate relies largely on anaerobic metabolism for energy production. Because this process is relatively inefficient, more glucose is metabolized to produce the amount of energy required than would be used under aerobic conditions. As a result, glucose produced by lipolysis and glycogenolysis is rapidly consumed. Hypoxic-ischemic damage to the liver may further impair synthesis of gluconeogenic enzymes and thus delay the normal postnatal onset of gluconeogenesis. Elevated insulin levels may also be present, providing an additional etiology for the hypoglycemia.

Hypothermia may result in hypoglycemia through rapid depletion of brown fat stores for nonshivering thermogenesis and secondary breakdown and exhaustion of glycogen stores. Hypothermia is most often seen in infants born at home, but milder degrees may occur in the delivery room. Hypoglycemia also has been observed in some infants with sepsis. A study done in several such infants found that they had an increased rate of glucose disappearance in response to an IV glucose infusion, suggesting an increased rate of glucose utilization.[29] Stimulation of glucose utilization may be a result of circulating endotoxins, which increase the rate of glycolysis. In addition, increased catecholamine levels in response to the stress of acute infection may play a role.

Hyperglycemia

Hyperglycemia in the newborn is usually defined as a blood glucose concentration of greater than 125 mg/dl in the term infant or greater than 150 mg/dl in the preterm infant. Incidence is difficult to determine; estimates range from 5.5% of all infants receiving IV infusions of 10% $D_{10}W$ to as high as 40% in infants weighing less than 1000 g.

Most often the neonate with hyperglycemia is a low birth weight (LBW) infant (<32 weeks' gestation and <1200 g birth weight) who cannot tolerate an IV glucose infusion at the usual rate of 4 to 8 mg/kg/min (i.e., $D_{10}W$ at 60 to 100 ml/kg/day). This relative glucose intolerance is probably due to general immaturity of the usual regulatory mechanisms, including decreased insulin release in response to glucose.[25] Some investigators have also reported that unlike fetuses and adults, preterm as well as some term infants fail to suppress endogenous glucose production despite the administration of an adequate exogenous supply (e.g., IV infusion)[9]; however, other investigators did not measure any glucose production in premature infants receiving IV glucose at a rate of more than 2 mg/kg/min.[53] The risk of developing hyperglycemia is significantly increased with decreasing birth weight, as well as with an increasing rate of glucose infusion, even within the accepted range of glucose infusion rates.[31] Delay in initiating enteral feedings may be an additional risk factor, because the incidence of hyperglycemia is higher in LBW infants receiving all of their nutrition parenterally than in those who receive at least a part of their nutrition enterally. The rate at which the glucose concentration is increased in IV solutions, including hyperalimentation, may also play a role. The presence of RDS with its requirement for mechanical ventilation is also associated with an increased risk of developing hyperglycemia. This may be due to increased circulating catecholamines, leading to increased lipolysis and glycogenolysis.

Although SGA infants are more likely to be hypoglycemic, a few cases of what has been termed *transient diabetes mellitus* have been reported in growth-retarded infants.[44] In these cases hyperglycemia is thought to be a result of partial insulin insensitivity, but increased levels of catecholamines and other stress-related hormones may play an important role. Unlike true diabetes mellitus, ketosis does not develop. Most cases are self-resolved or respond to decreasing the glucose administration rate; occasionally insulin therapy may be required, but this should be reserved for those infants with severe hyperglycemia that is persistent, over 400 mg/dl, and that produces clinically significant hyperosmolality and glucosuria.

There are several other etiologies that must be considered in infants with hyperglycemia. Increased blood glucose concentrations have been reported in association with gram-negative sepsis.[23] **IV lipid infusions may also produce hyperglycemia if given rapidly at rates of more than 0.25 g/kg/hr; however, this exceeds the rate at which lipids are usually given.**[50] Methyl xanthines are frequently used to treat apnea in the preterm infant and may be a cause of hyperglycemia.[47] This problem has been well documented after theophylline overdose; one study also measured increased blood glucose concentrations in infants with therapeutic theophylline levels, including concentrations in the hyperglycemic range in two infants.[47] Neonates undergoing surgical procedures are also at increased risk for hyperglycemia, probably because of a combination of the large quantities of glucose-containing fluids and blood products that may be administered during the procedure and the effects of stress-related hormones.

Prevention

Recognition of those infants at risk for disturbances in glucose homeostasis is the most important step in preventing both hypoglycemia and hyperglycemia. In infants with conditions predisposing to hypoglycemia, such as the SGA infant or the IDM, early feeding and hourly monitoring of blood glucose concentrations until the infant is stable may prevent a decrease in blood glucose or at least reduce the severity of the hypoglycemia. Maintenance of a neutral thermal environment is especially critical to minimize energy expenditure in those infants at risk for hypoglycemia.

Other conditions associated with hypoglycemia, such as asphyxia and hypothermia, may be avoidable through appropriate obstetric and neonatal intervention.

Hyperglycemia occurs most often in premature infants receiving IV glucose. In the VLBW infant, hyperglycemia may be avoided by starting IV glucose infusions at rates of 2 to 3 mg/kg/min and checking blood glucose concentrations frequently (as often as every 3 to 4 hours) while these infants continue to receive IV glucose. However, hyperglycemia may be unavoidable in the very immature infant.

Data Collection

History

The history of any neonate must include a detailed prenatal and family history. Important maternal risk factors are listed in Box 14-1. Other important data include a history of family members with hypoglycemia or metabolic disease and previous unexplained stillbirths.

The most important information to be obtained from the infant's history is gestational age, Apgar scores, and details of events in the delivery room, especially any findings that would suggest the presence of significant perinatal asphyxia. An infant with a history of any of the conditions listed in Table 14-1 or Box 14-2 should be considered at high risk for developing a problem with glucose homeostasis.

Box 14-1

Neonatal Hypoglycemia: Maternal Risk Factors

Diabetes or abnormal glucose tolerance test
Pregnancy-induced or essential hypertension
Previous macrosomic infants
Substance abuse
Treatment with beta-agonist tocolytics[40]
Antepartum administration of IV glucose

Physical Examination

Careful measurement of birth weight and head circumference in combination with accurate gestational age assessment will establish whether the infant is preterm, LBW, SGA, or LGA and thus at increased risk for hypoglycemia. IDMs frequently have small heads relative to their general macrosomia and have been described as having "tomato facies" because of plethora and increased buccal fat. The physical findings associated with Beckwith-Wiedemann syndrome have already been described.

Signs and Symptoms

Signs of neonatal hypoglycemia are nonspecific and extremely variable. They include general findings, such as abnormal cry, poor feeding, hypothermia, and diaphoresis; neurologic signs, including tremors and jitteriness, hypotonia, irritability, lethargy, and seizures; and cardiorespiratory disturbances, including cyanosis, pallor, tachypnea, periodic breathing, apnea, and cardiac arrest.

These findings may also be seen in prematurity, sepsis, intraventricular hemorrhage, asphyxia, hypocalcemia, congenital heart disease, and structural CNS lesions, among other etiologies. In the presence of any of the above signs, however, hypoglycemia should always be considered, because the diagnosis can be made relatively easily and prompt treatment is essential.

Box 14-2

Etiologies of Neonatal Hyperglycemia

Iatrogenic (e.g., during IV glucose infusion)
Decreased insulin sensitivity (e.g., VLBW Infant or transient diabetes mellitus)
Sepsis
Methylxanthine side effect

Table 14-1
Neonatal Hypoglycemia: Etiologies and Time Course

Mechanism	Clinical Setting	Expected Duration
Decreased substrate availability	Intrauterine growth restriction	Transient
	Prematurity	Transient
	Glycogen storage disease	Prolonged
	Inborn errors (e.g., fructose intolerance)	Prolonged
Endocrine disturbances		
Hyperinsulinemia	Infant of diabetic mother	Transient
	Beckwith-Wiedemann syndrome	Prolonged
	Erythroblastosis fetalis	Transient
	Exchange transfusion	Transient
	Islet cell dysplasias	Prolonged
	Maternal beta-agonist tocolytics	Transient
	Improperly placed umbilical artery catheter	Transient
Other endocrine disorders	Hypopituitarism	Prolonged
	Hypothyroidism	Prolonged
	Adrenal insufficiency	Prolonged
Increased utilization	Perinatal asphyxia	Transient
	Hypothermia	Transient
Miscellaneous/multiple mechanisms	Sepsis	Transient
	Congenital heart disease	Transient
	CNS abnormalities	Prolonged

Hyperglycemia is usually asymptomatic and is most often diagnosed on routine screening of the infant at risk.

Laboratory Data

When the diagnosis of hypoglycemia is suspected, the plasma glucose concentration must be determined. Ideally, this determination should be made using one of the preferred enzymatic methods, such as the glucose oxidase method, but even bedside reagent test strip glucose analyzers (i.e., glucometers) can be used if done carefully and with respect for their more limited accuracy. The sample should be obtained from a warmed heel or by venipuncture and transported in a sample tube containing a glycolytic inhibitor. If a standard serum chemistry tube is to be used (i.e., one without a glycolytic inhibitor), the sample must be processed promptly, because the erythrocytes in the sample will continue to metabolize glucose and may falsely reduce the value obtained.

In the clinical setting, early and rapid determination of glucose concentrations in the high risk or symptomatic neonate is essential.[16] Prompt detection of hypoglycemia permits early treatment and potentially avoids long-term neurologic sequelae.[8,39] The most effective method for early detection of hypoglycemia in neonates remains the appropriate standard, although laboratory measurements of glucose concentrations may require up to 1 hour, far longer than appropriate for diagnosing hypoglycemia (Fig. 14-4), which could delay critical intervention and treatment. Rapid

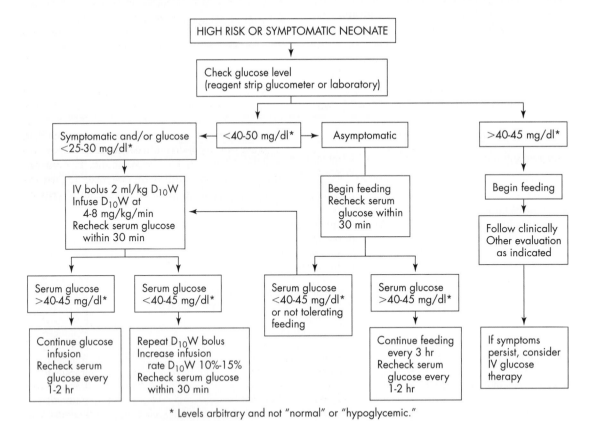

Figure 14-4   Decision tree for management of neonate with hypoglycemia.

measurement available to the clinician at the bedside includes several different enzyme/chromogen test strips. These test strips produce a color change that varies with the glucose concentration in the drop of blood applied to the pad surface, which can be assessed with visual interpretation by the clinician against a color chart or with a reflectance colorimeter, which measures the color and amount of light reflected from the strip and converts the results to a glucose concentration.[6,20] The two most commonly used test strips are Dextrostix and Chemstrips BG. Of these two test strips, the Chemstrip BG was found to most accurately reflect the actual serum glucose.[3,4,8] The sample of blood can be obtained from a warmed heelstick or venipuncture specimen.

These methods can be useful in screening infants in whom abnormal glucose concentrations are suspected, provided that the user is aware of their limitations. Accuracy of test strip results depends in part on the technique used. An adequate sample must be placed on the test strip pad, and timing of reading the result is critical. With proper technique, test strip results demonstrate a reasonable correlation with actual blood glucose concentrations but with a range of variation around the actual blood glucose concentration as much as ±10-20 mg/dl.[6,7,20,22] Recently, the glucometer (e.g., the One Touch II) has shown somewhat improved accuracy and is not subject to observer bias.[1,14] Regardless of the test strip or the instrument, however, correlations with actual blood glucose concentrations are lowest at the lower glucose concentrations at which neonatal hypoglycemia must be accurately determined. Several studies have shown that use of test strips alone, without the more accurate laboratory glucose concentration measurement, may fail to detect as much as 11% to 67% of infants with statistically defined hypoglycemia.[7,20,37]

Because of the limitations of these methods, a diagnosis of hypoglycemia or hyperglycemia suggested by test strip or glucometer results should be confirmed by a specimen sent to the chemistry laboratory with a request for prompt ("stat") determination and reporting. Treatment of suspected hypoglycemia should not be postponed until confirmation is obtained from the laboratory, since this could mean a delay of more than 1 to 2 hours. Hospital personnel should be trained and certified in the use of test strip methods and the bedside instruments used to quantify glucose concentration.[1,3,4,9,10]

Similarly, if hypoglycemia is suspected on the basis of clinical symptoms, initial treatment should be instituted even if the test strip result is "normal." If the actual value is abnormal, a delay in therapy could be harmful; if the actual value is within the normal range, therapy can be stopped without serious side effects.

Most cases of neonatal hypoglycemia will have an identifiable etiology (e.g., the IDM, the SGA infant). In the term infant with no known risk factors for hypoglycemia, sepsis must be considered as the most likely etiology for hypoglycemia and appropriate evaluation should be performed. Of those infants without an identifiable etiology, most will have idiopathic hypoglycemia, which will resolve spontaneously within 2 to 5 days, and no further evaluation in needed. However, in rare cases hypoglycemia will persist beyond the first week of life with no obvious cause detected. The diagnostic evaluation of these infants should include simultaneous determination of glucose and insulin concentrations; evaluation of pituitary function, including measurement of TSH, thyroxine (T_4), adrenocorticotropic hormone (ACTH), cortisol, and growth hormone levels; pancreatic ultrasound (if hyperinsulinemia is present); and appropriate studies to diagnose inborn errors of metabolism, such as lactate and pyruvate concentrations.

Treatment

Hypoglycemia

Anticipation and prevention are the key elements of intervention and management. Early identification of the infant at risk for developing hypoglycemia and institution of prophylactic measures to prevent its occurrence constitute the best treatment for this disorder. In those infants in whom hypoglycemia does occur, the treatment goals are twofold: to return the glucose concentration to normal levels and, once normalized, to maintain it within the normal range.

A decision tree suggesting guidelines for management of infants with hypoglycemia is shown in Figure 14-4. Although some asymptomatic infants can be managed with frequent formula feedings, most asymptomatic and all symptomatic neonates will require IV therapy using the "minibolus" plus dextrose infusion regimen originally described by Lilien et al.[30] Advantages of the minibolus regimen include the following: (1) there is a lower incidence of hyperglycemia immediately after the bolus, (2) the slower rate of administration decreases the insulin response to glucose infusion, thus lowering the risk of rebound hypoglycemia after the bolus, and (3) glucose concentration reaches the normal range more quickly than if continuous infusion is started without a preceding bolus (Fig. 14-5). The suggested infusion rates cover the range of hepatic glucose production in normal term newborns. In IDMs the initial "minibolus" and the infusion rate should be kept at the minimum necessary to produce and maintain normal blood glucose concentrations to prevent an excessive insulin response. When glucose infusion rates are being calculated, it is important to remember that commercially prepared glucose solutions actually contain glucose in its hydrated form (MW 198 versus MW 180 for anhydrous glucose), which lowers the actual glucose content of the solution by approximately 8%. Thus $D_{10}W$ contains approximately 9.2 g of glucose per deciliter.

Once the infant's glucose requirement has been determined, the glucose infusion should be maintained at that level until blood glucose concentrations are stable. If the infant was being fed before instituting IV therapy, feedings may be continued. However, the calculated minimum glucose requirement should be provided by the IV infusion alone rather than by the combination of glucose infusion and feedings. In infants who were not previously fed, feedings can be instituted when clinically indicated. There are several advantages to feeding the hypoglycemic infant during treatment with IV glucose. In the hyperinsulinemic infant, galactose (one of the components of lactose) stimulates less insulin release than glucose and therefore helps stabilize blood glucose concentrations. Continuation of oral feedings also aids in the process of weaning off IV glucose. When feedings are well tolerated, the IV infusion generally can be slowly tapered, provided the glucose concentration and clinical status remain stable.

Adjunctive Therapy

Glucagon.   Glucagon, 30 µg/kg IV or IM, will release glycogen from hepatic stores. Its administration may be useful diagnostically, because failure to respond to glycogen administration with an increase in serum glucose concentration suggests depletion of hepatic glycogen stores. IDMs may require much larger doses, up to 300 µg/kg, to produce a response. Glucose infusion should be maintained after glucagon administration, because there is a risk of increased insulin secretion in response to the glucagon-produced surge in glucose production. In addition, the rapid, but transient, increase in glucose concentration immediately after glucagon injection may produce a false sense that the hypoglycemia has resolved, even though the underlying etiology still exists.

Other Agents.   Steroids, somatostatin, and diazoxide have been used to treat hypoglycemia in refractory cases. Use of steroids to reduce peripheral glucose utilization and increase gluconeogenesis should be limited to those infants requiring

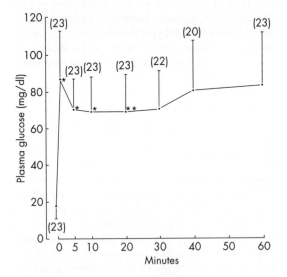

Figure 14-5   Plasma glucose response to glucose "minibolus" followed by continuous glucose infusion (8 mg/min/kg) as therapy for neonatal hypoglycemia. (From Lilien LD et al: *J Pediatr* 97:295, 1980.)

more than 15 to 18 mg/kg/hr glucose infusion to maintain normal glucose concentrations. Somatostatin and diazoxide, which suppress insulin release, are most often used in infants with islet cell dysplasias who have persistent hypoglycemia after partial pancreatectomy.

Miscellaneous.   In those infants with hypoglycemia caused by a specific medical problem, therapy should be directed toward alleviating the underlying illness. This includes administration of antibiotics to treat sepsis, partial exchange transfusion to relieve hyperviscosity, hormone replacement in cases of hypopituitarism, and dietary intervention for metabolic disorders. Surgery is usually required in cases of nesidioblastosis and islet cell adenomas because these are relatively unresponsive to medical therapy alone.

Hyperglycemia

Glucose.   Most cases of hyperglycemia can be treated by reducing the neonate's glucose intake. Many LBW infants will tolerate glucose infusions at rates of up to 4 mg/kg/min, although Zarif et al[52] reported that more than 40% of infants weighing less than 1000 g had a blood glucose concentration higher than 125 mg/dl while receiving glucose at an average rate of 4.4 mg/kg/min. In addition, the VLBW infant, with high fluid requirements resulting from large IWLS through the skin, may require a combination of water and glucose intake that could only be administered by using a hypotonic solution such as $D_{2.5}W$. The use of a low glucose concentration necessitates the addition of sodium (e.g., $D_{2.5}W$ has approximately 130 mOsm/L, requiring the addition of sodium chloride to produce an isotonic solution with 280 mOsm/L), which may further complicate management of fluids and electrolytes. The VLBW infant needs adequate caloric intake (50 to 60 kcal/kg/day) to avoid a negative nitrogen balance and tissue catabolism. These needs often cannot be met without resultant hyperglycemia. If the glucose is only mildly elevated (e.g., concentrations of 150 to 200 mg/dl) and the infant has no evidence of adverse effects such as osmotic diuresis, there may be no indication for reducing the rate of IV glucose administration.

Insulin Infusion.   Because of the above considerations, some authors[5,37] have suggested the use of a continuous insulin infusion in the infant who cannot tolerate infusion of glucose solutions with concentrations greater than 5 g/dl (i.e., D_5W). Infusion of insulin at rates of 0.2 to 0.8 mU/kg/min (0.01 to 0.05 units/kg/hr) for 12 to 24 hours may result in improved glucose tolerance. Hypoglycemia can be avoided by starting with a low infusion rate and increasing the rate by 10% to 20% every 60 to 90 minutes until the glucose concentration is less than 150 mg/dl. Blood glucose concentrations should be monitored every 15 to 20 minutes during initiation of the insulin infusion, and an IV glucose infusion should be maintained to avoid any abrupt changes in blood glucose.

Use of insulin infusion has been reported to improve tolerance to glucose infusion, resulting in increased carbohydrate intake and weight gain. However, this therapy has not been evaluated in a randomized prospective study and must be used cautiously given the role of insulin as a potent fetal and neonatal growth hormone.

Miscellaneous.   Galactose infusion has been substituted for glucose on an experimental basis in glucose-intolerant VLBW infants[45] and has resulted in a 65% to 80% increase in total carbohydrate intake as well as resolution of hyperglycemia. Further studies are needed before galactose can be considered an appropriate alternative for glucose.

In addition to specific measures to lower the blood glucose concentration, close attention must be paid to fluid balance in the hyperglycemic infant, because hyperglycemia can induce an osmotic diuresis. However, this is rarely seen at blood glucose concentrations less than 400 mg/dl. Finally, as in hypoglycemia, efforts should be made to treat any underlying etiology, such as sepsis.

Complications

Hypoglycemia

The outcome for infants with neonatal hypoglycemia appears to be related to the duration and severity of the hypoglycemia, as well as the underlying etiology. Those with asymptomatic hypoglycemia usually have a normal neurodevelopmental outcome, although minor abnormalities such as learning disabilities and abnormal electroencephalograms (EEGs) without seizure disorder occasionally have been reported at long-term follow-up. Symptomatic infants have a poorer prognosis, with abnormalities ranging from learning disabilities to cerebral palsy and seizure disorders, as well as mental retardation of varying degree.[15] Prompt initiation of treatment is thought to be associated with a more positive outcome, although this has not been well documented.

In the preterm infant, however, recent data[33] suggest that hypoglycemia may adversely affect long-term outcome. A follow-up study of more than 600 former preterm infants found significantly lower mental and motor indices in those infants with five or more documented episodes of moderate hypoglycemia (defined as a blood glucose concentration <45 mg/dl) during the neonatal period. This difference remained significant even when confounding factors such as IVH, need for ventilator support, and asphyxia were taken into consideration.

The incidence of neurodevelopmental abnormalities in IDMs ranges from 0% to 35%; the lower figures are from more recent studies and may represent improvement in obstetric and neonatal care. None of the long-term follow-up studies has shown an association between the presence of neonatal hypoglycemia and later neurodevelopmental impairment.[18,39] Instead, outcome has been related to such factors as prematurity, presence of congenital anomalies, and degree of control of maternal disease.

Infants with islet cell dysplasias, who are more likely to have recurrent and prolonged episodes of hypoglycemia, generally have poor outcomes,[2] possibly because these infants do not generate ketone bodies, which could serve as an alternative source of energy for cerebral metabolism during periods of hypoglycemia. Hypoglycemia secondary to hypopituitarism is also associated with a poor outcome; often this is due to other CNS or endocrine dysfunction rather than the hypoglycemia itself.

Hyperglycemia

Although there is little direct evidence, it has been postulated that hyperglycemia in the preterm infant

may increase the risk of IVH by causing rapid changes in osmolarity with resultant rapid fluid shifts within the brain and germinal matrix. One study did report an increased mortality in hyperglycemic premature infants as compared with their normoglycemic counterparts, although hyperglycemia may have been a marker for those infants with more severe illness rather than a direct cause of the increased mortality. Increased morbidity may be seen in the form of greater difficulty with fluid and electrolyte management, as well as problems establishing adequate nutrition.

Infants with transient diabetes mellitus usually recover spontaneously within the first week; persistent insulin resistance is extremely rare. No neurologic sequelae have been directly attributed to the presence of transient hyperglycemia in these neonates.

Parent Teaching

Parent teaching should begin before delivery, with emphasis placed on good nutrition and early and regular prenatal care. Teaching also should include information about those conditions that increase the risk of hypoglycemia (e.g., IUGR associated with maternal cigarette smoking and poor maternal nutrition). Regular prenatal care assures the early detection of potentially serious problems, including preeclampsia, gestational diabetes, and abnormal fetal growth.

Prenatal teaching is especially important in the woman with known diabetes mellitus, because overall outcome (although not necessarily the incidence of hypoglycemia) is directly related to the degree of control before and during pregnancy. In addition, the possibility of neonatal hypoglycemia and requirement for IV therapy can be discussed with the parents before delivery so that they will be aware that the infant may require a longer hospital stay even if delivered at term.

If IV therapy is selected to treat neonatal hypoglycemia, regardless of etiology, a thorough explanation of the treatment plan must be given to the parents at the time therapy is instituted. Frequent progress reports should be provided to resolve unanswered (and often unasked) questions and relieve parental anxiety. Parents of children with islet cell dysplasias need to be aware of the symptoms of hypoglycemia and emergency treatment measures that can be instituted, because recurrent hypoglycemia may occur in these cases. Parents of infants with inborn errors of metabolism also need counseling with regard to prognosis, as well as genetic counseling about risks of recurrence in future pregnancies.

Acknowledgments

Supported by NIH grants HD20761 and RR000690

References

1. Altimier L, Roberts W: One touch II hospital system for neonates: correlation with serum glucose values, *Neonat Net* 15(2):15, 1996.
2. Aynsley-Green A: Nesidioblastosis of the pancreas in infancy, *Dev Med Child Neurol* 23:372, 1981.
3. Barrett CT, Oliver TK: Hypoglycemia and hyperinsulinism in infants with erythroblatosis fetalis, *N Engl J Med* 278:1260, 1968.
4. Bernbaum M et al: Laboratory assessment of glucose meters does not predict reliability of clinical performance, *Lab Med* 25(1):32, 1994.
5. Binder N et al: Insulin infusion with parenteral nutrition in extremely low birth weight infants with hyperglycemia, *J Pediatr* 114:273, 1989.
6. Brown M, Nelson S, Stewart B: Detection of neonatal hypoglycemia: a comparison of three reagent strips, *Nurse Pract* 13(10):32, 1988.
7. Conrad P et al: Clinical application of a new glucose analyzer in the neonatal intensive care unit: comparison with other methods, *J Pediatr* 114:281, 1989.
8. Cornblath M, Schwartz R: Hypoglycemia in the neonate, *J Pediatr Endocrinol* 6(2):113, 1993.
9. Cowett RM, Oh W, Schwartz R: Persistent glucose production during glucose infusion in the neonate, *J Clin Invest* 71:467, 1983.
10. Cowett RM et al: Glucose kinetics in infants of diabetic mothers, *Am J Obstet Gynecol* 146:781, 1983.
11. Dawkins MJR: Biochemical aspects of developing function in newborn mammalian liver, *Br Med Bull* 22:27, 1961.
12. Denne SC, Kalhan SC: Glucose carbon recycling and oxidation in human newborns, *Am J Physiol* 251:E71, 1986.
13. DiGiacomo JE, Hay WW Jr: Disorders of metabolic adaptation: abnormal glucose homeostasis. In Sinclair JC, Bracken MB, editors: *Effective care of the newborn infant*, New York, 1992, Oxford University Press.
14. DiGiacomo JE, Hay WW Jr: Effect of hypoinsulinemia and hyperglycemia on fetal glucose utilization, *Am J Physiol* 259:E506, 1990.
15. Fluge G: Neurological findings at follow-up in neonatal hypoglycemia, *Acta Paediatr Scand* 64:629, 1975.
16. Gardner S, Hagedorn M: High risk neonatal care: level III nursery. In Gardner S, Hagedorn M, editors: *Legal aspects of maternal-child nursing practice*, Menlo Park, 1997, Addison Wesley.
17. Grazaitis DM, Sexson NR: Erroneously high Dextrostix values caused by isopropyl alcohol, *Pediatrics* 66:221, 1980.
18. Haworth JC, McRae KN, Dilling LA: Prognosis of infants of diabetic mothers in relation to neonatal hypoglycemia, *Dev Med Child Neurol* 18:471, 1976.
19. Hay WW Jr et al: Effect of insulin and glucose concentrations on glucose utilization in fetal sheep, *Pediatr Res* 23:381, 1988.
20. Hay WW Jr, Osberg IM: The "Eyetone" blood glucose reflectance colorimeter evaluated for *in vitro* and *in vivo* accuracy and clinical efficacy, *Clin Chem* 29:558, 1983.
21. Heck LF, Erenberg A: Serum glucose levels during the first 48 hours of life in the healthy full-term neonate, *Pediatr Res* 17:317A, 1983.
22. Herrera A, Ying-Hui H: Comparison of various methods of blood sugar screening in newborn infants, *J Pediatr* 102(5):769, 1983.
23. James T III, Blessa M, Boggs TR Jr: Recurrent hyperglycemia associated with sepsis in a neonate, *Am J Dis Child* 133:645, 1979.
24. Karp T, Scardino C, Butler L: Glucose metabolism in the neonate: the short and sweet of it, *Neonat Net* 14(8):17, 1995.
25. King RA, Smith RM, Dahlenburg GW: Long term postnatal development of insulin secretion in newborn dogs, *Early Hum Dev* 13:285, 1986.
26. Kliegman RM: Alterations of fasting glucose and fat metabolism in intrauterine growth-retarded newborn dogs, *Am J Physiol* 256:E380, 1989.
27. Ktorza A et al: Insulin and glucagon during the perinatal period: secretion and metabolic effects in the liver, *Biol Neonate* 48:204, 1985.
28. Lafeber HN, Jones CT, Rolph TP: Some of the consequences of intrauterine growth retardation. In Visser KHA, editor: *Nutrition and metabolism of the fetus and infant*, Boston, 1979, Martinus Nijhoff Publishers.
29. Leake RD, Fiser RH, Oh W: Rapid glucose disappearance in infants with infection, *Clin Pediatr* 20:397, 1981.
30. Lilien LD et al: Treatment of neonatal hypoglycemia with minibolus and intravenous glucose infusion, *J Pediatr* 97:295, 1980.
31. Louik C et al: Risk factors for neonatal hyperglycemia associated with 10% dextrose infusion, *Am J Dis Child* 139:783, 1985.
32. Lubchenco LO, Bard H: Incidence of hypoglycemia in newborn infants classified by birth weight and gestational age, *Pediatrics* 47:831, 1971.
33. Lucas A, Morely R, Cole TJ: Adverse neurodevelopmental outcome of moderate neonatal hypoglycaemia, *Br Med J* 297:1304, 1988.
34. Maisels M, Lee C: Chemstrip glucose test strips: correlation with true glucose values less than 80 mg/dl, *Crit Care Med* 11(4):293, 1983.
35. Marconi A et al: An evaluation of fetal glucogenesis in intrauterine growth retarded pregnancies: steady state fetal and maternal enrichments of plasma glucose at cordocentesis, *Metabolism* 42:860, 1993.
36. Marsac C et al: Development of gluconeogenic enzymes in the liver of human newborns, *Biol Neonate* 28:317, 1976.

37. Ostertag SG et al: Insulin pump therapy in the very low birth weight infant, *Pediatrics* 78:625, 1986.
38. Perelman RH et al: Comparative analysis of four methods for rapid glucose determination in neonates, *Am J Dis Child* 136:1051, 1982.
39. Persson B, Gentz J: Follow-up of children of insulin-dependent and gestational diabetic mothers, *Acta Paediatr Scand* 73:349, 1984.
40. Pildes R, Pyatti S: Hypoglycemia and hyperglycemia in tiny infants, *Clin Perinatol* 13(2):351, 1986.
41. Procianoy RS, Pinheiro CEA: Neonatal hyperinsulinemia after short-term maternal beta-sympathomimetic therapy, *J Pediatr* 101:612, 1982.
42. Schiff D et al: Metabolic effects of exchange transfusions, II. Delayed hypoglycemia following exchange transfusion with citrated blood, *J Pediatr* 79:589, 1971.
43. Shelley HJ: Glycogen reserves and their changes at birth and in anoxia, *Br Med Bull* 17:137, 1961.
44. Sodoyez-Goffant F, Sodoyez JC: Transient diabetes mellitus in a neonate, *J Pediatr* 91:395, 1977.
45. Sparks JW et al: Parenteral galactose therapy in the glucose-intolerant premature infant, *J Pediatr* 100:255, 1982.
46. Sperling MA et al: Fetal-perinatal catecholamine secretion: role in perinatal glucose homeostasis, *Am J Physiol* 247:E69, 1984.
47. Srinivasan G et al: Plasma glucose changes in preterm infants during oral theophylline therapy, *J Pediatr* 103:473, 1983.
48. Srinivasan G et al: Plasma glucose values in normal neonates: a new look, *J Pediatr* 109:114, 1986.
49. Tenenbaum D, Cowett RM: Mechanisms of beta-sympathomimetic action on neonatal glucose homeostasis in the lamb, *J Pediatr* 107:588, 1985.
50. Vileisis RA, Cowett RA, Oh W: Glycemic response to lipid infusion in the premature neonate. *J Pediatr* 100:108, 1982.
51. Wilkins B: Renal function in sick very low birth weight infants part IV: glucose excretion, *Arch Dis Child* 67(10):1162, 1982.
52. Zarif M, Pildes S, Vidyasagar D: Insulin and growth-hormone responses in neonatal hyperglycemia, *Diabetes* 25:428, 1976.
53. Zarlengo KM et al: Relationship between glucose utilization rate and glucose concentration in preterm infants, *Biol Neonate* 49:181, 1986.

Selected Readings

Aynsley-Green A: Glucose: a fuel for thought, *J Paediatr Child Health* 27:21, 1991.
Cornblath M et al: Hypoglycemia in infancy: the need for a rational definition, *Pediatrics* 85:834, 1990.
Cowett RM: Neonatal glucose metabolism. In Cowett RM, editor: *Principles of perinatal-neonatal metabolism,* New York, 1991, Springer Verlag.
DiGiacomo JE, Hay WW Jr.: Disorders of metabolic adaptation: abnormal glucose homeostasis. In Sinclair JC, Bracken MB, editors: *Effective care of the newborn infant,* Oxford, 1992, Oxford University Press.
Garland J et al: Clinical utility of a glucose reflectance meter for screening neonates for hypoglycemia, *J Perinatol* 16:25, 1996.
Giep TN et al: Evaluation of neonatal whole blood versus plasma glucose concentration by ion-selective electrode technology and comparison with two whole blood chromogen test strip methods, *J Perinatol* 16:244, 1996.
Hay WW Jr.: Reliability of blood glucose analysis. In Schwartz R, Cornblath M, editors: *Hypoglycemia in infancy: the need for a rational definition,* 1990, Ciba Symposium Report.
Koh THHG, Eyre JA, Aynsley-Green A: Neonatal hypoglycemia: the controversy regarding definition, *Arch Dis Child* 63:1386, 1988.
Ogata ES: Carbohydrate metabolism in the fetus and neonate and altered glucoregulation, *Pediatr Clin North Am* 33:25, 1986.
Pildes RS, Pyati SP: Hypoglycemia and hyperglycemia in tiny infants, *Clin Perinatol* 13:35, 1986.

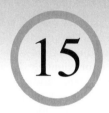

15 Enteral Nutrition

Susan F. Townsend, Cynthia B. Johnson, William W. Hay, Jr.

Providing adequate nutritional support to the sick newborn in the intensive care unit is an important challenge: maturational, functional, and physical disturbances to the normal postnatal transition may result if this challenge is not met. Optimal nutrition after birth enhances future neurodevelopmental outcome in preterm infants.[26] Good nutrition improves surgical outcome, decreases morbidity, and shortens hospital stays. Thus it is critical to adapt feeding practices and the composition of feedings to achieve optimal nutrition in the hospitalized neonate. Special attention must be given to the unique needs of individual patients, such as infants, with extremely low birthweight (ELBW), congenital heart disease, short bowel syndromes, or chronic lung disease. To meet the requirements for metabolic homeostasis, growth, and development, a combination of parenteral and enteral nutritional support is often provided. A goal of any nutritional support strategy must also be parental involvement, both to facilitate and encourage eventual breast-feeding, as well as to initiate educational interventions promoting healthy long-term nutrition practices. The authors currently view nutrition support of the newborn in the hospital as part of a continuum of care from birth through the first months at home after discharge, where ongoing attention to optimal nutrition may further enhance long-term outcome.

This chapter provides an overview of the physiology of nutrition and growth, with a brief discussion of gastrointestinal maturation and function. Fundamentals of neonatal nutritional requirements and monitoring are elaborated. The chapter discusses techniques and strategies for enteral nutrition in the hospitalized term and preterm infant, with emphasis on those infants requiring unique or special attention. Finally, the chapter discusses elements of enteral nutrition after hospital discharge in recovering infants.

Physiology

Growth

Fetal growth is regulated by complex genetic, nutritional, hormonal, and physical factors. Maternal nutritional factors exert some influence: weight gain during pregnancy is well correlated with fetal growth rate[22,37]; and the quality of the maternal diet (protein, energy, vitamins, and minerals) directly affects fetal growth.[22,32] However, there is a large maternal reserve of nutrients available to the fetus in most circumstances, and in general, maternal diet is not the rate-limiting factor in fetal growth. Many aspects of placental function are important determinants of fetal growth. For example, there are strong correlations between placental size, uteroplacental blood flow, and fetal size. Provision of oxygen and essential nutrients by the placenta is largely responsible for determining the rate of tissue accretion and composition in the fetus over the course of gestation.[39]

In addition to maternal nutritional factors and placental function, certain hormones and growth factors play increasingly recognized roles in regulating intrauterine growth. Insulin is one of the most influential growth-promoting hormones in the fetus.[18] Apancreatic infants are among the most severely growth restricted of all newborns (Fig. 15-1), whereas IDMs who respond to increased maternal-fetal glucose delivery with increased insulin secretion are among the fattest (Fig. 15-2). Other peptide growth factors have been implicated in fetal growth and maturation, including the insulin-like growth factors, epidermal growth factor, transforming growth factors, and fibroblast growth factors.[39] Some of these factors may, in turn, be nutritionally regulated. Infants with other endocrine disturbances, such as those resulting from anencephaly, panhypopituitarism, or hypothyroidism, are near normal in age-specific size at birth. Thus there is a complex interplay between provision of nutrients across the placenta to the fetus and the fetal endocrine milieu that influences intrauterine growth.

Understanding intrauterine growth is important for developing a standard by which to judge postnatal growth in preterm infants. In the absence of other standards, it is generally accepted as a

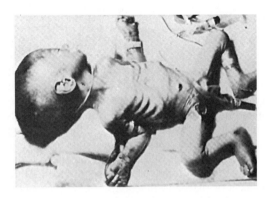

Figure 15-1 Term newborn (birth weight 1280 g) with pancreatic agenesis confirmed at autopsy. Plasma insulin was absent. Note marked deficiency of adipose tissue and muscle development. (From Hill D: *Semin Perinatol* 2:319,1978.)

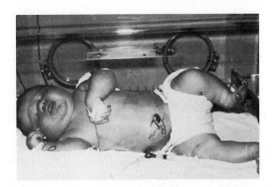

Figure 15-2 Characteristic large-for-gestational age (LGA) infant of diabetic mother. (Courtesy Newborn Service, University of Health Sciences Center, Denver, 1981.)

nutritional goal to seek a postnatal growth rate approximating normal intrauterine growth (Fig. 15-3). For the average infant, this translates into an expected weight gain of approximately 15 g/ kg/day in a growing preterm infant. However, it may be inappropriate to apply these intrauterine reference standards to extrauterine life, given that after birth, in most infants, there are marked changes in metabolic state, body composition, and environmental influences on energy utilization and metabolic rate. Important environmental factors influencing infant energy expenditure include varying temperature and humidity and exposure to radiant and convective heat losses. In addition, the transition from the continuous delivery of elemental nutrients by the placenta to the intermittent provision of complex nutrient mixtures to the gut requires maturation and adaptation of gastrointestinal function. Infants facing the increased energy-consuming demands of temperature maintenance, breathing, resistance to gravity, and so on can be expected to lose weight initially. Because

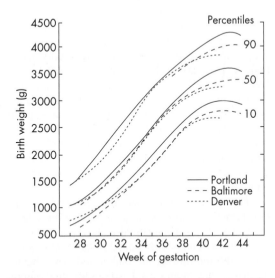

Figure 15-3 Comparisons of fetal weight curves for different populations in the United States. These growth curves suggest that maternal socioeconomic status and race may influence fetal growth rate as much as altitude. (From Babson SG, Behrman RE, Lessel R: *Pediatrics* 45:937, 1970.)

of the excretion of excess extracellular salt and water after birth resulting in marked shifts in body water content, infants born at all gestational ages can be expected to lose weight initially. Up to 1% per day weight loss reaching as much as a 5% loss of birthweight by the third day of life in term infants and 6% to 8% in ELBW (<1000 g) infants is normal. In healthy term infants who are exclusively bottle-fed, this weight loss may not be evident. It is therefore critically important to assess and evaluate the infant's growth.

Growth Monitoring

The normal intrauterine growth rate of 15 to 20 g/kg/day usually is not seen in the first 1 to 2 weeks of life in the sick preterm infant in the intensive care nursery. Similarly, stressed and sick term infants will not gain weight at a rate comparable to their healthy peers. Nonetheless, increase in body length can be documented in the early newborn period without increase in weight, demonstrating new tissue accrual and the need for adequate provision of nutrients.[3] Early provision of adequate calories to sustain optimal nutrition is difficult without the addition of some parenteral nutrition for sick infants of all gestational ages as the gastrointestinal tract begins to function in the early newborn period (see Chapter 16).

Assessment of Nutritional Status and Response to Feeding (Box 15-1)

We lack good methods to assess nutritional adequacy in very small infants. Rates of change in anthropometric measurements provide some post-hoc information, but they do not tell us what an infant needs at any one time. All too often they simply document the failure to provide adequate nutrition for the previous days to weeks. Indirect calorimetry offers some advantage, but instruments that are physically practical and sufficiently accurate to quantify nutrient metabolism in tiny infants are not yet available. This is particularly true for infants who are on ventilators and receiving high mixtures of oxygen. Similarly, application of stable isotope methodology to measure utilization and oxidation rates of individual nutrients remains confined to large medical centers with expensive and sophisticated mass spectrometry facilities. Evaluation of an individual infant's immediate

nutrient requirements and responses to the administration of different mixtures and amounts of nutrients remains an elusive but still necessary goal.

Gastrointestinal Development and Function

The gastrointestinal tract must adapt in the immediate postnatal period to meet the nutritional and metabolic needs of extrauterine life. In utero, the gut has been somewhat prepared for this role through the passage of large volumes of amniotic fluid (up to 300 ml/day at term) that contains enzymes, immunoglobulins, growth factors, and hormones.[46] The human gastrointestinal tract is fully developed anatomically by 20 weeks' gestation, but many functional abilities develop later (Table 15-1). Thus infants delivered prematurely will have some limitations in gastrointestinal function. After birth at term, gastrointestinal function also continues to develop; for example, full pancreatic function is limited until late infancy. Some gastrointestinal functions may be "switched on" at birth (such as decrease in intestinal permeability, increase in mucosal lactase activity) regardless of gestation. However, others seem to be intrinsically "programmed" to occur at a certain postconceptional age (such as the onset of peristalsis at 28 to 30 weeks and the coordination of suck and swallow at 33 to 36 weeks).[46] Environmental influences, including colonization of the gut by bacteria and introduction of nutrients into the gut, also affect postnatal gastrointestinal development. Initiation of enteral feedings in the hospitalized infant must take all these diverse factors into account.

The gastrointestinal tract of the preterm newborn handles multiple nutrients in a variety of ways. Protein digestion and absorption are remarkably efficient in the preterm infant despite the fact that enterokinase, the rate-limiting enzyme in the activation of pancreatic proteases, has only 10% of the adult activity. Carbohydrate absorption is limited by a relative deficiency of lactase, which splits lactose into glucose and galactose. Lactase in the infant of less than 34 weeks' gestation is present at only about 30% of the activity found in the normal term infant. Preterm infants may malabsorb

Box 15-1

Growth Monitoring

I. Weight is subject to large variations based on fluctuations in fluid balance (e.g., presence or absence of edema, congestive heart failure, renal failure), as well as attached equipment (e.g., peripheral IV lines, endotracheal tubes). Infant weight should be measured daily as follows:
   A. Use the same scale, minimal (or no) clothing, and weigh separately or remove, when possible, attached "equipment." In-bed scales are useful for the ELBW infant, or infants who become unstable with handling. An electronic scale that averages several measurements reduces movement artifacts and may be useful in very active infants.
   B. Reference standards for the weights of nursery equipment (such as diapers, IV boards, tubing, endotracheal tubes) should be available for nursery use.
   C. Weigh the infant at the same time daily, preferably before feeding.
   D. Record the time the infant was weighed and the scale used in addition to the weight. Daily weight should be plotted on available preterm or term growth charts. Energy (calories) and fluid intake can often be recorded on the same chart. This information, combined with biochemical parameters such as serum electrolytes, hemoglobin, and albumin, as well as the physical examination, provides the best overview of an infant's status. Weekly assessments of the infant's change in weight often provide a useful overview of the infant's nutritional support and can document trends in weight gain (or loss) that may be overlooked in the daily charting.
II. Length and head circumference are measured and recorded on admission and at least weekly, although accurate length measurements are difficult to obtain without special equipment (a stadiometer). Increase in head circumference is used as an indicator of brain growth. The following guidelines are useful:
   A. To measure length, place the infant flat with the legs extended and ankles flexed 90 degrees. Measure length from the top of the head (crown) to the bottom of the heel.
   B. Head circumference is obtained with a paper tape measure, using the largest measurement around the frontoparietooccipital axis.
III. Other indices of growth include the ponderal index (or weight-length index) to assess "quality" of growth. The ponderal index is calculated as the weight in grams times 100, divided by the cube of the length measured in centimeters. True organ growth and tissue accretion is accompanied by increases in both weight and length and can partly be evaluated using this index. The triceps skinfold thickness or mid-arm (mid-thigh) circumference may be used as an index of fat accretion, although standards for growing preterm infants are poorly defined.
IV. Biochemical monitoring may include weekly measurements of serum electrolytes and periodic evaluations of serum calcium, phosphorus, alkaline phosphatase, total protein, albumin, and blood hemoglobin. These data can be used to help prevent specific deficiencies in the diet, such as hyponatremia in growing preterm infants with excessive renal solute losses or hypophosphatemia associated with development of rickets. An elevated alkaline phosphatase also is seen with osteopenia. Hypoalbuminemia must be assessed against the shifts in body water content frequently seen in sicker infants in the nursery and also against the frequent use of albumin-containing solutions used for intravascular volume expansion.

Table 15-1
Development of the Gastrointestinal Tract in the Human Fetus: First Appearance of Developmental Markers

	Developmental Marker	Weeks of Gestation
Anatomic Part		
Esophagus	Superficial glands	20
	Squamous cells	28
Stomach	Gastric glands	14
	Pylorus and fundus	14
Pancreas	Differentiation of endocrine and exocrine tissue	14
Liver	Lobules	11
Small intestine	Crypt and villi	14
	Lymph nodes	14
Colon	Increased diameter	20
	Villi	20
Functional Ability		
Sucking and swallowing	Mouthing only	28
	Immature suck-swallow	33-36
Stomach	Gastric motility and secretion	20
Pancreas	Zymogen granules	20
Liver	Bile metabolism	11
	Bile secretion	22
Small intestine	Active transport of amino acids	14
	Glucose transport	18
	Fatty acid absorption	24
Enzymes	Alpha-glucosidases	10
	Dipeptidases	10
	Lactase	10
	Enterokinase	26

From Lebenthal E: *Pediatr Ann* 16:211, 1987.

10% to 30% of dietary fat because of a small bile acid pool size and relative lack of pancreatic lipase. Nonetheless, despite relative deficiencies in many enzymes important in nutrient processing, the preterm infant is usually able to digest and absorb complex nutrient mixtures such as human milk quite effectively.

Despite anatomic and functional shortcomings in gastrointestinal function in the premature newborn, early (day 2 to 3) initiation of slow, careful feeding is recommended. Enteral feedings are associated with surges in gut hormone production that may mediate trophic effects on gastrointestinal growth and mucosal maturation.[46] In fact, provision of only small quantities of milk into the neonatal gastrointestinal tract ("minimal enteral feeding" or "hypocaloric feeding") promotes increases in gut

hormones, such as gastrin, enteroglucagon, and motilin, that are thought to be very important for normal intestinal maturation. Minimal enteral feedings have been shown to improve nutritional outcome (weight gain, bone mineralization) in preterm infants.[10] Failure to provide any enteral nutrition for prolonged periods of time to the newborn infant should be avoided, unless there is a specific contraindication for feeding (e.g., necrotizing enterocolitis).

In addition to growth of the intestine and maturation of intestinal absorption, motile function of the gut changes during gestation and after birth. Coordination of suck and swallow patterns is absent before about 34 weeks' gestation, gastroesophageal sphincter pressure increases from 28 weeks' gestation through the first week of life, and peristalsis of the small intestine improves during the third trimester of gestation. The rate of gastric emptying is slowed in preterm infants.[30] A measure of gastrointestinal motility is provided by the passage of stool within 24 hours of birth in over 95% of full-term infants. However, the more premature the infant, the greater the delay in passing the first stool. Enteral feeding promotes gastric emptying and the release of hormones that may improve peristalsis in both the term and preterm infant.

Nutritional Requirements

Nutritional requirements may be considered in three general categories: **energy (or calories), minerals and solutes, and vitamins.** Water requirements also must be considered when designing nutrition support strategies. The source, complexity, and constituents of these nutrients are important, as well as the route of administration. Enteral nutritional requirements are discussed here. See Chapter 16 for parenteral nutrition and Chapter 18 for breast-feeding.

Energy

Energy requirements are determined by an infant's total energy expenditure, energy excretion, and energy stored in new tissue as growth. Total energy expenditure can be subdivided into contributions of basal metabolic rate, activity, requirements for thermoregulation, and the energy costs of digestion and metabolism. Energy excretion is composed of fecal and urinary losses. Estimates of energy requirements for growing preterm infants are shown in Table 15-2.[2,7] The large variability of these estimates reflects largely the variability of infant activity and environmental conditions. It is important, therefore, to adjust nutrient delivery to individual requirements. For example, if an infant is particularly active and is showing poor growth, nutrient delivery should be adjusted upward accordingly. Estimates of caloric requirements for the healthy term infant are slightly lower than those of preterm infants, averaging 110 kcal/kg/day.[33] Increased energy requirements can be anticipated during recovery from surgery, sepsis, and respiratory distress. **Daily caloric intake should be calculated for each infant growing or recovering from illness in the nursery. Useful approaches for calculating caloric intake are shown in Box 15-2. Major components of energy (calorie) delivery are derived from protein, carbohydrate, and fat.**

Protein.　Protein accretion is critical for normal growth. The amount and type of protein necessary for optimal growth in preterm infants have been

Table 15-2
Estimated Daily Energy Requirement (kcal/kg) for Premature Infants

Factor	American Academy of Pediatrics	European Society of Gastroenterology and Nutrition	
		Average	Range
Energy expenditure			
Resting metabolic rate	50	52.5	45-60
Activity	15	7.5	5-10
Cold stress	10	7.5	5-10
Energy cost of digestion	8	17.5	10-25
Energy stored	25	25	20-30
Energy excreted	12	20	10-30
TOTAL REQUIREMENTS	120	130	95-165

Modified from American Academy of Pediatrics, Committee on Nutrition: *Pediatrics* 112:622, 1988; Committee on Nutrition of the Preterm Infant, European Society of Pediatric Gastroenterology and Nutrition: *Nutrition and feeding of the preterm infant,* Oxford, UK, 1987, Blackwell Scientific Publications.

difficult to establish. Metabolic balance studies support a need for higher protein intakes in the growing preterm infant than in the term infant. Human milk provides adequate protein to meet the recommended goals of 2.0 to 2.5 g/kg/day for term infants, but it is inadequate to meet the goals of 3.0 to 3.5 g/kg/day for preterm infants.[25] Preterm infants receiving both protein and energy supplementation during enteral feedings (to as much as 3.6 g/kg/day protein and 149 kcal/kg/day) had increased gains in weight, length, head circumference, and triceps skinfold thickness compared with infants receiving 2.24 g/kg/day protein and 115 kcal/kg/day energy (Fig. 15-4).[19] **Studies of preterm infants maintained on diets fortified in protein and energy have shown improved neurodevelopmental outcome at 9 months of corrected age.[1] Neurodevelopmental outcome appears to be even better when human milk is supplemented with protein and energy compared with an enriched**

Box 15-2

Calculating Daily Caloric Intake (kcal/kg/day)

Conversion Factors

Full Strength	*Half Strength*
20 kcal/oz = 0.67 kcal/ml	(= 0.33 kcal/ml)
24 kcal/oz = 0.80 kcal/ml	(= 0.40 kcal/ml)
1 kcal = 1 Calorie	
1 oz = 30 ml	

Calculations

1. Add up total daily intake (in milliliters) of feedings.
2. Divide total ml intake by the infant's weight in kg. This equals total ml/kg/day intake.
3. Multiply ml/kg/day formula calories (kcal/ml). This equals enteral kcal/intake/kg/day.

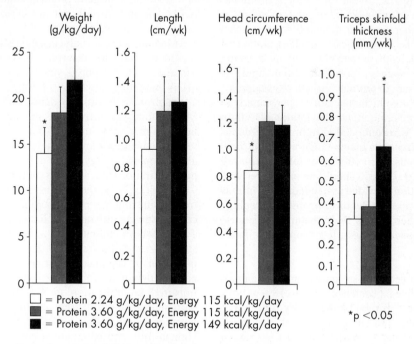

Figure 15-4 Growth rates with varying protein and energy intakes. (From Kashyap S et al: *J Pediatr* 113:713, 1988; Kennaugh JM, Hay WW Jr: *Western J Med* 147:435, 1987.

cow's-milk-based formula.[1] **Because of this and other benefits of human milk feeding in preterm infants, including provision of antimicrobial factors and improved feeding tolerance, protein and energy supplementation (e.g., from Human Milk Fortifier, Mead Johnson) of human milk at reasonable milk volumes is recommended.**

The type of protein in the newborn diet is as important as the amount provided. Human milk is a whey-predominant food (whey/casein ratio of 80:20), whereas cow's milk has a whey/casein ratio of 18:82. Whey protein is particularly rich in essential amino acids and contains more cysteine than cow's milk. Because of developmental immaturity of metabolic pathways, cysteine is more important for the preterm and term infants than for adults. Human milk is also rich in taurine, but cow's milk contains little. Taurine is thought to be an essential nutrient for the newborn; experiments in animals suggest an important role for taurine in brain and retinal development.[14]

Human milk from an infant's own mother is the preferred source of protein for the preterm infant. Milk expressed from mothers of preterm infants is somewhat higher in protein than milk from mothers of term infants. Nonetheless, supplementation of maternal milk with protein (as well as calcium, phosphorous, sodium, potassium, and lipid) is usually necessary to promote growth rates approximating that of normal human fetuses, particularly in the VLBW preterm infant. **An intake of 3.0 to 3.5 g/kg/day is recommended in preterm infants. Protein requirements may be higher (4 g/kg/day) in ELBW infants (i.e., ≤1000 g) or infants who are extremely SGA. Growth should be monitored and supplementation provided as needed. Term infants in general will not require protein or energy supplementation unless their dietary fluid is restricted because of illness, (e.g., congestive heart failure).**

Fat. Human neonates are unique among animals in having a white fat content of 16% to 18% of body weight at term.[40] Brown fat, necessary for thermogenesis, is also present at term. Fat deposition occurs predominantly during the last 12 to 14 weeks of gestation. Thus infants born prematurely will be significantly deficient in fat stores, both for use as energy and for thermogenesis. In addition,

deposition of specific lipids is deficient in VLBW infants. An example is docosahexaenoic acid, or DHA, a long chain polyunsaturated fatty acid (22 carbons with 6 double bonds) necessary for normal brain and retinal development.[6]

Newborn infants absorb fat less efficiently than older children. Preterm infants demonstrate even greater deficiencies in fat digestion and metabolism. Pancreatic lipase and bile acids are less available for fat digestion and absorption. Lingual and gastric lipases, present in newborn secretions, compensate for deficient pancreatic lipase, as does mammary gland lipase, if the infant is receiving breast milk.[17] **Current recommendations for dietary fat consist of provision of 30% to 54% of total calories (3.3 to 6.0 g/100 kcal), with at least 3% of total calories as linoleic acid.** Human milk also contains considerable quantities of linolenic acid, the precursor to DHA and other long chain fatty acids that are important for normal brain development and nerve function. The preterm infant may not be able to synthesize DHA from its precursor linolenic acid. Small amounts of DHA are present in human milk but not currently in commercially available formulas.

Medium chain triglycerides (MCTs) do not require bile salts for absorption and can be directly absorbed into the portal venous circulation. This offers theoretical advantages for the preterm infant, although there is little evidence that inclusion of MCTs improves growth of the healthy preterm infant. The routine use of MCTs is therefore not recommended, although they can improve fat absorption and energy intake in infants with hepatic dysfunction or short bowel syndromes.

Carnitine is synthesized in the liver and kidney from lysine and methionine and is essential for the catabolism and utilization of long chain fatty acids. The newborn infant has a limited ability to synthesize carnitine and may depend on exogenous provision of adequate carnitine to maintain fatty acid oxidation. Carnitine deficiency may lead to impaired fat utilization in sick preterm infants, particularly in those who are maintained on IV nutritional support that does not contain carnitine.[17] Human milk and commercial cow's-milk–derived formulas contain sufficient carnitine to maintain plasma carnitine levels after birth.

Although there is concern that overfeeding of

infants may lead to adult obesity and therefore fat intake should be restricted, it is important to remember that fats are essential for normal infant growth. Fats provide a concentrated source of energy and also important components of cell membranes, particularly significant for the developing nervous system. **Therefore there is no place for "fat restriction" in the nutritional support of preterm or term infants, within the guidelines given above.** Areas of ongoing research include the supplementation of preterm formulas with fish oil emulsions to provide n3 and n6 long chain polyunsaturated fats necessary for optimal brain and retina development in animals and the relationship of neonatal fat composition to the development of atherosclerosis in later life.

Carbohydrate. Carbohydrate reserves begin to accumulate as glycogen in the developing fetus as early as the start of the second trimester. This glycogen serves local organ needs, and hepatic glycogen is used by other glucose-dependent tissues, primarily the brain. Immediately after birth, with cessation of glucose supply from the placenta, the neonate must use this stored glycogen for energy. **The newborn can exhaust this supply of stored glucose within 12 hours of birth if food or IV glucose is not provided. The normal glucose utilization rate in the term newborn is 4.0 to 6.0 mg/kg/min, with the brain accounting for most of the glucose use, especially in preterm and asymmetrically growth-restricted infants who have a larger than normal brain/body weight ratio.**

The predominant carbohydrate in human milk is lactose, a disaccharide composed of glucose and galactose. Although preterm infants have only 30% of the lactase activity of term infants, they tolerate lactose quite well in most circumstances.[28] Glucose has a central role in energy metabolism. Galactose provides 50% of the calories derived from lactose; its major metabolic role is in energy storage, because the newborn liver readily incorporates galactose from the portal circulation into hepatic glycogen.[20]

Provision of 40% to 60% of total caloric intake as carbohydrate (12 to 14 g/kg/day) will prevent accumulation of ketone bodies and other adverse metabolic effects (e.g., hypoglycemia) in the newborn. This amount of carbohydrate is generally supplied as lactose in human milk or commercial formulas. If there are signs of lactose intolerance, such as frequent loose stools, abdominal distention or cramping, or positive stool reducing substances (Clinitest), then a portion of the carbohydrate may be given as sucrose or as glucose polymers. Glucose polymers have the added advantage of keeping formula osmolality low. Lactose–free infant formulas are commercially available (e.g., LactoFree, Bristol-myers Squibb Co. See Table 15-6).**

Vitamins

Vitamins are organic substances, present in trace amounts in natural food sources, that are essential to normal metabolism. Lack of vitamins in the diet produces well-recognized deficiency states in adults. The biological roles of many of these vitamins are incompletely understood, and recognition of clinical deficiency states in infants is often difficult. Because vitamins have a central role in many metabolic processes, signs of vitamin deficiency can be nonspecific, such as lethargy, irritability, and poor growth. Table 15-3 is a summary of the recommended vitamin intake for enterally and parenterally fed infants. **For comparison, the average vitamin content of human milk and commercial infant formulas is given in Table 15-4.[34] Certain vitamins have received close attention in neonatology, in particular vitamin C for its role in enhancing iron absorption from the gastrointestinal tract, vitamin K for prevention of hemorrhagic disease of the newborn, and vitamins A and E as antioxidants. Routine supplementation above recommended levels cannot be advised at present because of possible toxicity and lack of clearly demonstrated benefits. Supplementing vitamin D above the recommended dose of 400 IU/day does not prevent osteopenia in preterm infants.[12]**

Minerals and Trace Elements

Mineral requirements for the preterm infant have been largely estimated from in utero accretion rates. Published recommendations for daily intakes in healthy, enterally fed preterm infants are shown in Table 15-5. Supplementation with calcium and phosphorus to achieve the recommended intakes (with a Ca/P ratio of 2:1) has been shown to decrease the incidence of metabolic bone dis-

Table 15-3
Recommended Daily Vitamin Intake for Infants

Vitamin	Enteral		Parenteral	
	FDA Minimum (units/100 kcal)	RDA: 0-6 mo (units/day)	Preterm (units/kg/day)	Term (units/day)
C (mg)	8	30	25	80
Thiamine (µg)	40	300	350	1200
Riboflavin (µg)	60	400	150	1400
B_6 (µg)	35	300	180	1000
Niacin (mg)	0.25	5	6.8	17
Biotin (µg)	1.5	10*	6	20
Pantothenic acid (mg)	0.3	2	2	5
B_{12} (µg)	0.15	0.3	0.3	1
Folate (µg)	4	25	56	140
A (IU)	250	1250	1665	2330
D (IU)	40	300	400†	400
E (mg)	0.5	3	2.8	7
K (µg)	4	5	80	200

Modified from Lucas A, Hudson G: *Arch Dis Child* 59:831, 1984.
*Estimated safe and adequate intake.
†Units/day.

Table 15-4
Vitamin Content of Human Milk and Commercial Infant Formulas

Vitamin	Human milk* (units/100 kcals)	Standard Milk-based Formulas† (units/100 kcals)	Preterm Formulas‡ (units/100 kcals)
C (mg)	6-7.8	8.1-9	10.5-37
Thiamine (µg)	13.4-31	78-100	120-250
Riboflavin (µg)	40.1-60	150-156	190-620
B_6 (µg)	9.3-30	60-63	75-250
Niacin (mg)	0.22-0.31	0.75-1.25	0.93-5
Biotin (µg)	0.6-1.0	2.2-4.4	2-37
Pantothenic acid (mg)	265-340	315-470	530-1900
B_{12} (µg)	0.03-0.15	0.2-0.25	0.3-0.55
Folate (µg)	4-7.4	7.5-15.6	15-37
A (IU)	73-323	300-310	475-1200
D (IU)	3-12	60-63	75-270
E (IU)	0.2-0.6	1.4-3.1	2.2-4.6
K (µg)	0.3-3	8-8.6	10.5-13

Modified from Reidel BD, Greene HL: Vitamins. In Hay WW Jr, editor: *Neonatal nutrition and metabolism,* St Louis, 1991, Mosby.
*Human milk composition varies greatly (with gestation, stage of lactation, individually, etc.).
†20 kcal/oz, Enfamil (Mead Johnson), Similac (Ross Laboratories).
‡20 kcal/oz, Enfamil Premature, Similac Special Care.

Table 15-5
Minerals and Trace Elements in Neonatal Nutrition

Mineral or Element	Biologic Role	Deficiency State	Recommended Oral Intake for Rapidly Growing Preterm Infants
Sodium	General growth and tissue accretion, body fluid equilibrium, cellular energy, and electrical charge balance	Poor growth, fluid imbalance, neurologic dysfunction, lethargy, seizures	3-5 mEq/kg/day
Potassium	General growth and tissue accretion, acid-base balance, cellular energy, and electrical charge balance	Myocardial damage, dysrhythmia, hypotonia, muscle weakness	2-3 mEq/kg/day
Chloride	General growth and tissue accretion, cellular energy, and electrical charge balance	Failure to thrive, muscle weakness, vomiting	3-5 mEq/kg/day
Calcium	Bone and tooth formation, fat absorption, nerve conduction, muscle contraction	Bone demineralization, tetany, dysrhythmias, seizures	200 mg/kg/day
Phosphorus	Bone and tooth formation, energy transfer compounds	Bone demineralization, weakness	100-140 mg/kg/day
Magnesium	Metalloenzymes, cellular electrical charge balance	Neurologic dysfunction, anorexia, diarrhea, renal disease	5-10 mg/kg/day
	Hemoglobin formation, metalloenzymes	Anemia, pallor, apathy, intellectual dysfunction	2 mg/kg day after 1-2 months of age
	Metalloenzymes, DNA-RNA synthesis, wound healing, host defenses	Growth restriction, dermatitis, alopecia, diarrhea, delayed wound healing	1.2-1.5 mg/kg/day
Copper	Metalloenzymes, protein metabolism	Neurologic dysfunction, anemia, neutropenia, bone demineralization	100-200 µg/kg/day
Manganese	Metalloenzymes, carbohydrate metabolism, antioxidants, hemostasis	Neurologic dysfunction, defects in lipid metabolism, reduced coagulants, animals—growth restriction	10-20 µg/kg/day
Chromium	Carbohydrate metabolism, component of nucleic acids	Impaired glucose tolerance, impaired growth	2-4 µg/kg/day
Selenium	Metalloenzymes, antioxidants	Cardiomyopathy	1.5-3.0 µg/kg/day
Iodine	Thyroid hormone synthesis	Hypothyroidism	1 µg/kg/day
Fluoride	Bone and tooth formation	Dental caries	100 µg/kg/day
Molybdenum	Metalloenzymes, purine metabolism	Neurologic and visual dysfunction, animals—growth restriction	2-3 µg/kg/day

Modified from Forbes GB: *Pediatric nutrition handbook,* Elk Grove Village, Ill, 1985, American Academy of Pediatrics; Tsang RC, editor: *Vitamin and mineral requirements of preterm infants,* New York, 1985, Marcel Dekker.

ease in preterm infants. Mineral supplementation of human milk or use of an enriched pretermformula is usually necessary to achieve the intakes recommended in Table 15-5.

Feeding Techniques and Strategies

Formula and Milk Composition

Human Milk

The preferred enteral diet for the term newborn infant is human milk, providing sufficient energy, protein, fat, carbohydrate, micronutrients, and water for normal growth. In addition, human milk, unlike formulas, provides a variety of antimicrobial factors that may protect against infection, such as secretory immunoglobulins (IgA), leukocytes, complement, lactoferrin, and lysozyme. Human milk also contains hormones and growth factors such as epidermal and nerve growth factors, insulin-like growth factor I (somatomedin C), erythropoietin, prolactin, calcitonin, steroids, TRH, and thyroxine.[39] The role of these milk hormones and trophic factors has not clearly been established, but they may play a role in organ maturation and growth. Taurine is present in high concentrations in human milk and is an essential amino acid in the newborn. The protein and fat components of human milk are readily digestible, and human milk contains large numbers of enzymes that may aid in nutrient digestion and processing (e.g., lipase). Finally, there are obvious psychological benefits to a mother who provides her own milk for her sick infant (see Chapter 18).

The preterm infant may not grow as fast on human milk alone because of the special nutritional requirements addressed previously. Recommended daily requirements for energy, protein, calcium, sodium, phosphorus, magnesium, iron, zinc, and several vitamins necessary to meet the normal rate of in utero growth will not be achieved in the growing "healthy" preterm infant who is fed with unsupplemented human milk. The preterm infant with respiratory distress, infection, excessive heat losses, or increased activity will have even greater

nutritional needs. Nonetheless, milk from mothers of preterm infants has more protein and sodium than milk obtained at term, and occasionally will provide for adequate growth in larger and healthier preterm infants.[40] The nutrient content of term (mature) human milk is compared with standard and "preterm" formulas in Table 15-6. Commercially available supplements to human milk that provide additional energy, protein, vitamins, and minerals are shown in Table 15-7 on page 290. The nutritional composition of preterm human milk is compared with term human milk in Table 15-8 on page 290.

Formula

Cow's-milk–derived formulas have been engineered to provide biologically available protein mixtures with appropriate protein/energy ratios for normal growth. In general, formulas designed for term infants contain 20 kcal/oz and are adequate to meet the needs of term and larger preterm infants (>1800 g) with an intact gastrointestinal tract and "normal" fluid requirements. A whey and casein mixture approximating that of human milk is usually preferred. Preterm formulas all contain whey/casein ratios of 60:40 and have a higher protein content than term formulas. Preterm formulas also contain less lactose as a carbohydrate source, and substitute glucose polymers to provide approximately 50% of the calories derived from carbohydrate. Most preterm formulas provide some of the fat in the form of medium chain triglycerides because of the ease with which they are absorbed. Calcium and phosphorus content is increased, with a Ca/P ratio of 2:1, which provides for improved bone mineralization. Other minerals and vitamins are also present in higher concentrations in preterm formulas to reflect the special nutritional need of the VLBW infant. Preterm formulas are available in 20, 22, and 24 kcal/oz preparations, with similar osmolalities and renal solute loads.

Soy protein formulas should be reserved for infants with a strong family history of allergy who are not being fed human milk. Soy-derived formulas should not be used for long periods in the VLBW infant because of the poorer quality of protein and lower calcium accretion rates seen with these formulas. Formulas derived from protein hydrolysates should be reserved for infants who are clearly allergic to cow's milk proteins and are not breast fed or do not tolerate soy-derived formulas. In general, families with a strong history of cow's-milk-protein allergy should be strongly encouraged to breast feed. For infants requiring soy or protein hydrolysate formulas, careful attention should be paid to monitoring long-term growth, and amino acid, vitamin, and trace mineral balance.

Elemental formulas are used in infants with malabsorption, abnormal gastrointestinal tracts, or severe protein allergy. The protein source in these formulas is derived from casein hydrolysates, and the fat is largely from MCT oil. The composition of Pregestimil (Mead-Johnson) is shown as an example of an elemental formula in Table 15-6. Use of elemental formulas is generally indicated in the infant with severe liver disease and fat malabsorption, with short-bowel syndrome (such as after necrotizing enterocolitis with surgical resection), or with dysmotility syndromes (such as in gastroschisis). Occasionally, formulas derived from protein hydrolysates are useful after a severe episode of infectious gastroenteritis with mucosal injury and resulting protein or lactose intolerance. A lactose free formula may also be used in this setting. It is not necessary to use an elemental formula in the routine care of VLBW infants. A variety of other modified formulas are available for infants with special needs (lactose-free, protein-free, etc.).

In some circumstances, infants require fluid restriction (e.g., because of pulmonary edema, congestive heart failure, or renal failure) while on full enteral feedings. Caloric delivery and nutritional support can be maintained by increasing caloric density of feedings. This can be done by adding powdered formula, milk fortifiers, glucose polymers, corn oil, microlipids (a lipid emulsion, Sherwood), or MCT oil to the formula or milk as desired to achieve acceptable concentrations and intakes of these nutrients. Caloric densities of 27 to 30 kcal/oz can be achieved in this fashion, although infants tolerate these supplements in a highly individual fashion and should be monitored for signs of feeding intolerance (e.g., abdominal distention, increased stooling, presence of fat or sugar in the stool). Increasing caloric density of feedings necessitates less water delivery to the infant and generally leads to an increase in formula

osmolality as well. Careful monitoring of feeding tolerance and fluid balance (renal function) is therefore necessary on a high-calorie-density feeding regimen.

Future formulas engineered for preterm infants are likely to include a more complex mixture of fatty acids, including long-chain polyunsaturated fatty acids important for brain and retinal development. Immunoglobulins, such as IgA, may be added to decrease the incidence of NEC, and trophic factors, such as epidermal growth factor (EGF) or other hormones may be added after their role in human milk has been established. Taurine (and other amino acids), cysteine, carnitine, nucleotides, and other complex organic compounds may be supplemented or provided at unique rates as our understanding of gastrointestinal maturation and optimal growth-promoting substrates for the developing preterm infant evolves.

The Preterm Infant

There is an urgent need to address the nutrition of ELBW (<1000 g) and VLBW (<1500 g) preterm infants. The nutritional requirements of these very small infants are marked, unique, poorly understood, and inadequately provided for, including both the quality and the quantity of nutrients in currently used IV and enteral nutrient regimens (Box 15-3, p. 291). Also, many of these infants are growth restricted at birth, thus their nutritional needs for "catch up" growth and for normal rates of metabolism and growth are very likely to differ from those of normally grown infants. Furthermore, in spite of increasingly aggressive in hospital nutritional management, the majority of these infants are growth restricted and they are SGA at the time of discharge.[23] In fact, the fraction of these infants who are SGA at discharge is several fold greater at birth. There is increasingly strong evidence that inadequate nutrition of preterm and growth-restricted infants can have lasting consequences resulting in neurologic and developmental impairment.[23] Many previous studies in humans and animals have documented that prolonged postnatal undernutrition and malnutrition add far greater insult than does prenatal undernutrition alone. Such observations have important implications.

Table 15-6
Formula Comparison (Amounts per Deciliter)

	Mature Human Milk	Cow's Milk			
		Similac 20	Enfamil 20	Lacto Free 20	NeoCare 22
Protein source					
Whey/casein	80:20	18:82	60:40	—	60:40
Amount (g)	1	1.45	1.5	1.5	1.5
Calories (%)	6	9	9	9	9
Fat source (%)					
Medium-chain triglycerides	—	—	8.1	—	—
Polyunsaturated (linoleate [olive])	16	37	29	—	—
Saturated (coconut)	38	45	47.3	—	—
Monounsaturated (oleate [safflower])	42	18	15.5	—	—
Amount (g)	4.5	3.6	3.8	3.7	4.1
Calories (%)	55	48	50	49	49
Cholesterol (mg)	14.5	1.1	1.1	—	—
Vitamin E/PUFA (mg/g)	0.4	1.1	1.9	—	—
Carbohydrate source (%)					
Lactose	100	100	100	—	Lactose
Glucose polymers	—	—	—	100	Corn syrup
Amount (g)	7.1	7.2	6.9	7	7.7
Calories (%)	39	43	41	42	41
Calories	73	68	68	68	74
Minerals					
Calcium (mg)	33	49	53	55	78
Phosphorus (mg)	15	38	36	37	46
Ca/P ratio	2.2:1	1.3:1	1.5:1	1.5:1	1.7:1
Sodium, mg (mEq)	16 (0.7)	18 (0.8)	18.1 (0.8)	20 (0.9)	25 (1.1)
Potassium, mg (mEq)	51 (1.3)	71 (1.8)	72 (1.84)	74 (1.9)	105 (2.7)
Chloride, mg (mEq)	39 (1.1)	43 (1.2)	42 (1.19)	45 (1.3)	56 (1.6)
Magnesium (mg)	4	4.1	5.4	5.4	6.7
Zinc (mg)	0.16	0.5	0.7	0.7	0.9
Iron (mg)	0.021	1.2	1.2	1.2	1.3
Iodine (µg)	30	6.1	6.8	10.1	11.2
Copper (µg)	25-40	61	51	50.7	89.3
Manganese (µg)	7-15	3.4	10.5	10.1	7.4
Osmolality (mOsm/kg)	300	300	300	200	290
Estimated renal solute load (mOsm/L)	71	96.3	95.5	100	130.8

*24 kcal/oz preterm formulas.

	Cow's Milk* Preterm			Casein Hydrolysate	Soy	
	Similac Special Care 24	**Enfamil Premature 24**	**Premie SMA 24**	**Pregestimil 20**	**Prosobee 20**	**Isomil 20**
	60:40	60:40	60:40			
	2.4	2.4	2	1.9	2	1.7
	11	12	10	11	12	10
	50	40	11	3	—	—
	21	23	15.4	36.2	29.1	37
	66	25.7	48	9.1	47.3	46
	13	11.7	35	17.1	15.5	17
	4.4	4.1	4.4	3.8	3.6	3.6
	47	44	48	48	48	49
	2.5	—	2-4	—	0	0
	2.5	3.9	1.6	1.6	0.5	1.1
	50	40	50	—	Sucrose	Sucrose
	50	60	50	100	Corn syrup	Corn syrup
	8.6	8.9	9.0	6.9	6.8	6.96
	42	44	42	41	40	41
	81	81	81	68	68	68
	146	134	75	63	71	71
	73	68	40	42	56	51
	2.0:1	2.0:1	1.9:1	1.5:1	1.3:1	1.4:1
	35 (1.5)	32 (1.4)	32 (1.4)	32 (1.4)	24 (1.0)	30 (1.3)
	105 (2.7)	90 (2.3)	75 (1.9)	74 (1.9)	82 (2.1)	73 (1.9)
	66 (1.9)	69 (1.9)	53 (1.5)	58 (1.6)	54 (1.5)	42 (1.2)
	10	6.1	7	7.4	7.4	5.1
	1.2	1.27	0.8	0.6	0.8	0.5
	1.5	1.52	0.3	1.3	1.2	1.2
	5	6.4	8.3	4.8	10	10
	203	130	70	63	51	51
	10	10.6	20	21	16.9	20
	280	300	280	320	200	230
	149	230	128	125	127	110

First, we cannot now think of "early" nutrition of these small infants simply in terms of providing immediate nutrient needs just for metabolic maintenance (such as glucose to prevent hypoglycemia); we must consider that early nutrition has biologic effects that have lasting or lifelong significance. Second, we can no longer regard nutritional practices in preterm infants as simply a matter of personal choice. The major impact on long-term outcome should be a stimulus to new research that defines consistent approaches to the nutrition of ELBW, preterm infants to optimize their future health and development. Early, low-calorie enteral feedings ("minimal enteral foods") may improve gastrointestinal function of the VLBW infant[10] and protect against infection and the development of chronic lung disease.[43] During the acute phase of a preterm infant's illness, aggressive nutrition should be provided by the parenteral route (see Chapter 16). The transition to enteral feedings can then proceed slowly, with continuous assessment of feeding tolerance to avoid complications such as NEC. Human milk is fed initially, then supplemented to provide adequate nutrient composition. Preterm formula is used as an alternative.

Few controlled trials support any given feeding strategy, although rapid advances to large feeding volumes are poorly tolerated by preterm infants. Feeding dilute formula or human milk may improve feeding tolerance and hasten achievement of full enteral feedings.[8] Similar growth is achieved whether infants are fed intermittently or continuously.[35] The following guidelines reflect just one approach to enteral feedings; caution and flexibil-

Table 15-7
Nutrient Composition of Human Milk Fortifier and Natural Care*

	Human Milk Fortifier† (amount per four packets)	Natural care‡ (amount per 124 ml)
Calories (kcal)	14	100
Protein (g)	0.7	2.7
Fat (g)	0.05	5.4
Carbohydrate (g)	2.73	10.6
Calcium (mg)	60	210
Phosphorus (mg)	33	105
Sodium (mg)	7	43
Chloride (mg)	17.7	81
Vitamin A (IU)	780	680
Vitamin D (IU)	260	150
Vitamin C (mg)	24	37

*This table lists the major constituents; refer to product for complete listing of vitamins, minerals, and trace elements.
†Mead Johnson, Evansville, Ind.
‡Ross Laboratories, Columbus, Ohio.

Table 15-8
Nutritional Composition of Preterm and Term Breast Milk

Nutrient	7 days Preterm	7 days Term	14 days Preterm	14 days Term	28 days Preterm	28 days Term	>56 days Preterm	>56 days Term
Calories (kcal/dl)	73.86 ± 1.81	73.62 ± 3.32	74.59 ± 1.96	71.81 ± 3.57	73.33 ± 2.14	72.71 ± 1.88	70.10 ± 1.424	76.33 ± 2.34
Protein nitrogen (g/L)	2.76 ± 0.18	2.55 ± 0.18	2.39 ± 0.16	1.97 ± 0.14	1.90 ± 0.09	1.76 ± 0.08	1.99 ± 0.10	1.96 ± 0.10
Sodium (mEq/L)	17.23 ± 1.88	9.54 ± 1.30	12.36 ± 1.42	9.37 ± 1.95	9.56 ± 0.70	7.04 ± 0.96	8.85 ± 0.80	7.14 ± 0.51
Calcium (mg/L)	293 ± 16	293 ± 8	266 ± 15	274 ± 13	282 ± 12	267 ± 13	310 ± 16	314 ± 12
Fat (g/dl)	3.1 ± 0.71	2.98 ± 0.28	3.42 ± 0.18	3 ± 0.26	3.24 ± 0.16	3.07 ± 0.21	3.43 ± 0.16	3.46 ± 0.32
Lactose (g/dl)	6.38 ± 0.22	6.43 ± 0.13	6.86 ± 0.16	6.63 ± 0.23	6.79 ± 0.17	6.92 ± 0.36	7.21 ± 0.11	6.68 ± 0.22

Modified from Lemons JA et al: *Pediatr Res* 16:113, 1982.

ity must be used in following any feeding schedule. In general, the smaller the infant, the greater attention must be paid to feeding tolerance, although large infants can certainly develop serious feeding intolerance and NEC.

Initial feedings for the less than 1000 g infant may be "half-strength" dilutions of human milk or preterm infant formula on the first day, to provide about 15 to 20 ml/kg/day, divided into bolus gavage feedings of 1 to 2 ml/kg every 2 hours. Feedings are advanced by no more than 15 to 20 ml/kg/day until full feedings of dilute milk or formula (approximately 150 ml/kg/day) are achieved over 7 to 10 days. Feedings can then be advanced to full strength over the next 2 to 3 days and then fortified by gradual addition of liquid or powdered human milk fortifiers (see Table 15-7). Thus progression to full enteral feedings of fortified human milk or 24 kcal/oz preterm infant formula occurs over a minimum of 2 weeks. During this time, parenteral nutritional support is tapered. Larger preterm infants (>1000 g) may tolerate advancing to full-strength feedings before achieving full volume. Breast milk should be fed to the infant in the order in which it is collected, with the colostrum given first.[1] Infants weighing less than 1500 g are fed every 2 hours, and more than 1500 g every 3 hours if bolus feedings are tolerated without emesis or residuals. Additional feeding guidelines are presented in Table 15-9.

Procedure

Gavage Feeding (Box 15-4)

Intragastric feedings provide a method of feeding an infant who is too immature to allow for safe nipple feeding or who is too sick to take adequate nourishment. Intragastric feedings are preferred to the transpyloric route because the transpyloric route may have increased mortality without proven benefits.

Precautions.   Aspiration is of major concern in any infant of gestational age who does not have a neurologically mature swallow, gag, or cough reflex (<34 to 36 weeks). Any tachypneic infant with labored respirations or with an endotracheal tube is also at increased risk for aspiration. Gavage tube position must be carefully checked,

Box 15-3
Special Nutritional Conditions in ELBW Infants

1. Minimal energy reserves (both carbohydrate and fat)
2. Intrinsically higher metabolic rate (greater relative mass of more metabolically active organs: brain, heart, liver)
3. Higher protein turnover rate (especially when growing)
4. Higher glucose needs for energy and brain metabolism
5. Higher lipid needs to match the in utero rate of fat deposition
6. Excessive evaporative rates (immature skin)
7. Occasionally very high urinary water and solute losses (depending on intake and renal maturation)
8. Low rates of gastrointestinal peristalsis
9. Limited production of gut digestive enzymes and growth factors
10. Higher incidence of stressful events (hypoxemia, respiratory distress, sepsis)
11. Metabolic effects of medications used frequently (steroids, antibiotics, sedatives, catecholamines)
12. Abnormal neurologic outcome if not fed adequately

Modified from Thureen P, Hay WW Jr.: Conditions requiring special nutritional management. In Tsang RC et al, editors: *Nutritional needs of the preterm infant,* Baltimore, 1993, Williams & Wilkins.

feedings should run in slowly, and these infants should not be overfed. *Gavage feeding should never be pushed.*

Passage of the gavage tube should be done gently, because it can cause trauma, and may stimulate the vagus nerve, causing apnea or bradycardia. Tactile stimulation usually will cause the infant to breathe. However, the tube may have to be withdrawn if the symptoms persist.

Feeding intolerance may be the first symptom of illness (e.g., hypoxia, dyspnea, congestive heart failure, sepsis, and NEC). At first symptoms may be subtle, so the care giver should be constantly aware of any change in the infant's overall condition and feeding intolerance.

Nipple Feeding

Development of appropriate neuromuscular coordination is necessary to successfully initiate nipple feedings. Criteria for initiating nipple feeding must be individualized. Coordination of suck, swallow, and breathing emerges at about 34 weeks' gestation, regardless of postnatal age.[46] Respiratory illness leads to energy depletion. Nipple feeding is not usually possible unless respiratory rate is less than 60 breaths/min and the oxygen required is less than 40%.

The ability to suck on a pacifier, fingers, or a gavage tube *does not* ensure the infant's ability to perform nutritive sucking. A preterm infant without a gag is at risk for aspiration with nipple feedings. An infant who is successful at nipple feeding should exhibit an active suck, coordinated swallow, minimal fluid loss around the nipple, and completion of feeding within 15 to 30 minutes.[35] The preterm infant hospitalized in the NICU has usually been exposed to many unpleasant oral sensations, such as endotracheal tubes, suction catheters, gavage tubes, and facial tape. These infants often become "disorganized feeders."[45]

When nipple feedings are initiated in the recovering ill preterm infant, they may last only minutes. Coordination of sucking with breathing is the first lesson for the premature infant. Stress behaviors (e.g., increase or decrease in respiratory or heart rate, decreased oxygen saturation, color change, gagging, choking, emesis, fatigue, irritability, or a "panicked look") should result in a rest period or cessation of the feeding.

An infant receiving supplemental oxygen should be monitored by pulse oximetry to determine oxygen requirement during nipple feedings. Different types of nipples may be used for different infants. Strategies to facilitate oral feedings include a relaxed care giver, a quiet environment with subdued light, and a snugly wrapped infant (see Chapter 12).

Nipple feedings should begin slowly at one feeding per day, then increase as tolerated to once every 8 hours, then once every third feeding, then every other feeding, and finally all feedings should be nipple feedings. Scheduling nipple feedings for parent visits enables them to actively participate in their infant's care. A too-rapid change to nipple feeding results in weight loss; the infant tires with feedings and is unable to take in caloric requirements or needs gavage supplementation after nippling to meet caloric needs (with inherent danger of vomiting the nippled feeding and aspiration). Diligent attention is warranted, and a decrease in nipple feedings is necessary to prevent dehydration, malnutrition, and a worsening of the infant's condition.

Many premature infants are still preterm when they are discharged, and most are small for their corrected gestational age despite aggressive in-hospital nutrition. Continued attention to increased nutrient requirements in these infants after hospital discharge seems appropriate and represents a continuum of support. Therefore efforts to wean infants to 20 kcal/oz formula before discharge may be counterproductive. In fact, providing premature infants with a formula containing a higher energy and protein content after discharge until a corrected age of 9 months has resulted in improved growth.

The ideal composition of feedings in "recovering" premature infants has yet to be determined; however, efforts to continue feeding with a 22 or 24 kcal/oz infant formula with a higher protein and mineral content for several months after hospital discharge are supported by such studies, even for premature infants who do not have significant chronic illness. Infants with a significant chronic lung disease and home oxygen are particularly likely to need 24 kcal/oz formula after discharge to maintain adequate growth at home. Oxygen supplementation itself also improves growth in these infants when normal oxygen saturation is maintained.[16] Infants who are discharged on breast feedings can be supplemented with a 24 kcal/oz formula or fortification of mother's milk if growth is suboptimal. Demand feeding should be initiated to document adequate growth on the feeding regimen chosen before discharge.

Effect of Disease on Nutritional Requirements

Many diseases unique to preterm infants, either directly or by enhancing the effects of stress on the metabolism of such infants, provide important

Table 15-9
Suggested Guidelines for Feeding the Preterm Infant

Weight	Day of Feeding	Type of Food	Volume	Frequency
<1000 g	1.2	Human milk or half-strength preterm formula (10 kcal/oz)	2 ml	q 2 hr
	3-4	Human milk or half-strength preterm formula (10 kcal/oz)	4 ml	q 2 hr
	5-7	Human milk or half-strength preterm formula (10 kcal/oz)	6-8 ml	q 2 hr
	8-10	Human milk or full-strength preterm formula (20 kcal/oz)	8-10 ml	q 2 hr
	11-12	Human milk or full-strength preterm formula (20 kcal/oz)	10-14 ml	q 2 hr
	13-15	Fortified human milk or preterm formula (22 kcal/oz)	14 ml	q 2 hr
	16 on	Fortified human milk or preterm formula (24 kcal/oz)	14 ml	q 2 hr
1001-1500 g	1	Human milk or full-strength preterm formula (20 kcal/oz)	2 ml	q 2 hr
	2-3	Human milk or full-strength preterm formula (20 kcal/oz)	4 ml	q 2 hr
	4-5	Human milk or full-strength preterm formula (20 kcal/oz)	6 ml	q 2 hr
	6-10	Human milk or full-strength preterm formula (20 kcal/oz)	8-12 ml	q 2 hr
	9-11	Fortified human milk or preterm formula (22 kcal/oz)	12 ml	q 2 hr
	12-14	Fortified human milk or preterm formula (24 kcal/oz)	12-14 ml	q 2 hr
1501-2000 g	1-2	Human milk or full-strength preterm formula (20 kcal/oz)	4-5 ml	q 2-3 hr
	3-5	Human milk or full-strength preterm formula (20 kcal/oz)	6-10 ml	q 2-3 hr
	6-8	Human milk or full-strength preterm formula (20 kcal/oz)	11-20 ml	q 3 hr
	9-12	Human milk or preterm formula (±fortifier to 22 or 24 kcal/oz)	21-40 ml	q 3 hr

changes in the requirements for nutrients.[44] The overriding observation from all studies, however, is that ELBW and VLBW preterm infants are underfed during the early postnatal period and that this undernutrition, combined with additional stresses from various diseases, increases the risk of long-term neurologic sequelae. The value of achieving a specific body composition and growth rate is less certain. There remains a critical need for determining the right quality as well as quantity of nutrients for these infants.

Similarly, disease states that prompt intensive care for term infants will have important effects on their nutrient requirements and may influence the timing, route, and composition of feeds provided. For example, infants with sepsis may have increased protein requirements in excess of increased energy needs. Infants with congenital heart disease will have increased energy requirements but may or may not require restriction of free water. The effects of common disease states on elements of the nutrient requirements in preterm and term infants are shown in Table 15-10.

The Sick Term Infant

Any infant recovering from asphyxia or shock should probably not receive enteral feedings for 24 to 72 hours to allow recovery of the bowel from the ischemic injury and decrease the risk for NEC.

The surgical neonate is at increased risk for nutritional deficiencies resulting from the stresses of illness and surgery and possible abnormal nutrient and water losses. In these infants, enteral feedings are preferred because they are safe and more economical, preserve the integrity of the intestinal mucosa, and promote continued development of the GI tract.[11,31] After an operative procedure, the infant is often NPO for 3 to 14 days until the return of intestinal motility and function (e.g., stooling, lack of abdominal distention, decreased gastric aspirates, and absence of bilious aspirates).[31] The method of feeding chosen, rapidity of feeding advancement, formula composition, and type of feeding depend on the infant's general medical condition, gastrointestinal function, and type of surgery.

Nipple feedings should be started postopera-

Box 15-4

Gavage Feeding Procedure

Equipment

I. Prepackaged gavage set with no. 8 Fr catheter, 20 ml syringe, and medicine cup
   A. Use of 3.5 or 5 Fr feeding tube for infants less than 1500 g.
   B. Use an 8 Fr feeding tube for larger infants.
II. Stethoscope

Steps

I. Intermittent gavage feeding
   A. Before starting a feeding, make sure the infant tolerated the previous feeding.
      1. Determine the amount of formula according to the infant's size, gestational age, physical condition, amount of previous feeding, and feeding regimen.
      2. Alter the amount of formula depending on how the infant tolerated the last feeding. It may be necessary to decrease the amount of formula given based on the following:
         a. Vomiting between feedings
         b. Unusual abdominal distention
         c. Residuals of previous feeding in the stomach
            (1) Gently aspirate all stomach contents into the syringe. Note amount, color, and appearance. Immediately report bloody or "coffee grounds" (heme positive), green or yellow (test these for bile), or fecal-appearing aspirates. Withhold feeding pending a decision about the feeding plan.
            (2) Unless residuals are mostly mucous, return them to the stomach to prevent loss of electrolytes. Subtract this amount from the total given. For example, if an infant is to receive 30 ml and 5 ml of residual is aspirated, return the 5 ml and give only 25 ml of additional formula. (Large aspirates may indicate overfeeding and may necessitate a decrease in formula. Large aspirates may also indicate partial ileus or early signs of sepsis, necrotizing enterocolitis, or obstruction.)
      3. Increase the amount of feeding with great care. Following orders for advancing feeds without constantly evaluating the infant is dangerous.
   B. Insert the feeding tube (oral placement).
      1. Oral is preferred to nasal tube placement for infants because they are obligatory nose breathers. However, because it produces less stimulation of the gag reflex, nasal tube passage may be chosen in certain situations (e.g., older preterm infant who needs supplementation after nippling but who fights, gags, and vomits with oral tube passage). Small (3.5 or 5 Fr) indwelling nasogastric tubes can be placed for gavage feedings, and the infant learns to nipple with the tube in place.
      2. Measure tube length by holding one end of the tube at the back of the earlobe and drawing the tubing to the mouth and down to the tip of the xiphoid process. Observe this point in relation to the black marking on the tube.
      3. Use the natural bend of the tube to follow the natural curves of the mouth and throat for easier insertion.
      4. Insert the tube in the mouth and toward the back of the throat, gently pushing it down the esophagus until reaching the premeasured mark on the tubing.
   C. Check tube position
      1. Verify the exact position of the gavage tube on insertion and before every feeding. During insertion, the tube may go into the trachea instead of the esophagus causing fighting, coughing, and cyanosis.
      2. Attach the syringe to the gavage tube. Aspirate gently on the tube while rotating the tube between the thumb and index finger. This helps prevent aspirating stomach mucosa. Usually a few curds of formula or mucus may be aspirated.
      3. Inject a small amount (2-3 ml) of air into the tube while listening with a stethoscope over the stomach.
      4. If the infant is very active or vigorous, wrap in a blanket to prevent pulling on the tube.
      5. Tape the tube in place or always keep one hand on the tube at the premeasured mark to prevent the tube from slipping.

continued

Box 15-4

Gavage Feeding Procedure, cont'd

D. Begin feeding.
  1. After determining that the tube is in position and it is safe to feed the infant, begin feeding by removing the plunger from the syringe and affixing the syringe to the gavage tube. Pour the predetermined amount of formula into the syringe. (Flow down the tube may begin spontaneously or require a gentle nudge with the plunger.) *Allow feedings to run by gravity.* (The higher the tube is held, the faster the milk will flow.) Let the formula run at a slow, steady pace to prevent the infant from vomiting. Always observe the infant through the entire gavage feeding.
  2. Offering the premature infant a pacifier for nonnutritive sucking during bolus gavage feeding improves gastrointestinal function[40] and produces earlier nipple feedings and earlier hospital discharge.[13]
  3. When all the formula has run in, pinch the gavage tube to prevent drops on the end from falling into the infant's throat and being aspirated. Withdraw the tube.

II. Continuous gavage feeding
  A. An indwelling gavage tube should be used for infants who need maximal total intake but cannot tolerate a bolus of formula at any one feeding; for example:
    1. Very small immature infants may tolerate continuous gavage feedings better than bolus feedings and may have improved weight gain.[42] Continuous feedings are associated with lower energy expenditure in preterm infants compared with bolus feedings.[15]
    2. Infants of diabetic mothers—to stabilize blood glucose
    3. Some bowel surgery patients with short gut or dumping syndrome
  B. Normally, use the oral route. The nasal route may be chosen for greater stability of the tube and if the infant has increased gagging, apnea, and bradycardia with an oral tube. Ascertain the correct position of the tube. Once in position, secure the tubing with tape.
  C. Run continuous gavage feedings into a sterile, measured container such as a large syringe or a Buretol (Travenol, inline burette) *without* a membrane. To control the rate of flow, attach the container to a volumetric or syringe pump.
  D. Because of the danger of infection, change continuous drip feeding and gavage tubes (syringe, tubing, and milk) depending on institutional studies of bacterial growth.[9,21]
  E. Carefully watch the infant for emesis or abdominal distention. Check stomach residuals every 2 to 4 hours. Every hour check the amount of formula infused and record it in the same manner as an IV.
  F. Potential complications of low-flow continuous human milk feedings include separation of milk fat with loss of fat calories in the gavage tubing and syringe and bacterial contamination when milk is maintained at room temperature for extended periods. If the syringe pump is positioned below the infant or placed in a vertical position with use of mini bore tubing[5] some of the fat loss can be avoided, because the milkfat will rise toward the infant. As the infant grows, gastric capacity and motility increase, and feedings can be changed to intermittent boluses.

III. After any feeding, position the infant to prevent aspiration. Should regurgitation occur:
  A. Elevate the head of the bed 35 to 45 degrees.
  B. Place the infant prone or on the right side to prevent aspiration.

tively if the infant is awake, hungry, and able to suck, swallow, and gag and has normal intestinal motility and no respiratory distress. To evaluate nippling ability and risk of aspiration, sterile water may be given for the first feeding. Daily and weekly growth should be monitored and assessed relative to caloric intake, Inadequate growth may be treated with increased volumes, increased caloric density, or a less stressful method of feeding (e.g., a combination of nipple and gavage feedings). Neo-

Table 15-10
Impact of Disease on Selected Nutrient Requirements in Preterm and Term Infants

Nutrient	Preterm			Term			Both
	RDS	CLD	NEC/SBS	Cyanotic CHD	CHF	Sepsis	IUGR
Free H$_2$O	↓	↓	↑	←→	↓	←→	↑
Energy	↑	↑↑	↑↑	↑	↑↑	↑	↑
Fat	←→	↑	↑↑*	↑	↑	←→	↑
CHO	↑	↓	↑	↑	↑	↑	↑
Protein	←→	↑	↑	↑	↑	↑↑	↑
Calcium	←→	↑†‡	↑*	↑§	↑‡§	←→	↑
Iron	←→	↑↑†	↑	↑	←→	↓	↑

RDS, Respiratory distress syndrome; *CLD*, chronic lung disease; *NEC*, necrotizing enterocolitis; *SBS*, short bowel syndrome; *CHD*, congenital heart disease; *CHF*, congestive heart failure; *IUGR*, intrauterine growth restriction; *CHO*, carbohydrate.
*Particularly with loss of the terminal ileum.
†In <1500 g preterm infants.
‡Particularly with calciuric diuretics such as furosemide.
§Particularly if postoperative.

nates with craniofacial malformation (e.g., cleft lip or palate, choanal stenosis or atresia, mandibular hypoplasia) are at greatly increased risk for aspiration. Use of different nipple shapes and sizes and sitting the infant in the upright position facilitates safe oral feeding. Gastrostomy tube placement may be necessary if oral feedings are not adequately established.

Gavage feedings are indicated in term infants requiring endotracheal intubation or those with a weak or absent suck, swallow, or gag reflex. Gavage feedings are begun at 3 to 5 ml/kg every 3 to 4 hours and advanced over 3 to 5 days as tolerated. Continuous feedings may be initiated in infants recovering from NEC, with short bowel syndrome, or with intolerance of bolus feedings. The care giver should monitor the number and consistency of stools or stoma output. Stools should be tested (e.g., Clinitest) for blood or reducing substances (to detect undigested or partially digested carbohydrate) when feeding intolerance or malabsorption are suspected. If short bowel syndrome is present, transition from continuous to bolus feedings should proceed slowly and cautiously. This may be accomplished by infusing feedings over gradually shorter periods of time, with increasing intervals between feedings until bolus feedings every 3 to 4 hours are tolerated. Prolonged oral or nasal gastric tube feedings may cause adverse oral stimulation

and promote gastroesophageal reflux.[31] After certain surgical procedures, some term neonates will require gastrostomy tube placement (see Chapter 27).

Feeding Intolerance and Complications

Assessment for signs of feeding intolerance is imperative because, although some feeding complications can be mild and respond to nursing interventions, others are more serious and require medical intervention.[4]

Residuals

The feeding tube is aspirated every 4 to 6 hours before a feeding to determine whether gastric emptying is adequate. Incompletely digested aspirates of 2 ml/kg or a 1 hour volume if on continuous feedings is considered normal and should generally be returned to the infant. Increasing residuals are a sign of feeding intolerance and may necessitate decreasing feeding volumes or slowing the rate of feeding advance. Occasionally, medications (e.g., metoclopramide or cisapride to accelerate bowel motility) improve feeding tolerance.[29]

The presence of bile or blood in the gastric aspirate warrants further investigation and consideration of NEC.

Emesis

Emesis may be due to an overdistended stomach, gastroesophageal reflux, gastric irritation from enterally administered medications, infection, obstruction, metabolic disorders, increased intracranial pressure, drug withdrawal, or overstimulation in a very small infant. Interventions include allowing the feeding to flow more slowly by use of a smaller gavage tube, decreasing feeding volumes, prone positioning, giving medications at the end of the feeding, or modifying a stressful environment (see Chapter 12).

Gastroesophageal reflux may be suspected in an infant with irritability, emesis, apnea and bradycardia, respiratory deterioration, refusal to eat, or otherwise unexplained blood in the stools. Postoperative emesis and abdominal distention may be indicative of a stricture, partial obstruction, or inflammatory abcess (see Chapter 27).

Abdominal Distention

Abdominal distention with or without palpable or visible loops of bowel may be a sign of poor gastric motility, ileus, constipation, or "gas." If the abdomen remains soft and nontender, prone positioning and gentle rectal stimulation with a glycerin sliver may be helpful to relieve gas and enable stooling. Persistent abdominal distention can be a sign of pathology (e.g., anatomic obstruction or infection), and requires investigation. An abdominal x-ray examination is indicated in these patients. Abdominal girth is measured every 4 to 8 hours to document increased distention. Place paper or cloth tape around the abdomen at a consistent point marked on the abdomen.

Diarrhea

Diarrhea, or frequent water-loss stools, should be investigated. Stool Clinitest of 1% or greater may signify lactase deficiency (transient), or other pathology. Stool culture for bacterial or viral pathogens may also be obtained. In lactose malabsorp-

tion, short-term use of a non–lactose-containing formula should result in return to normal stools.

Apnea and/or Bradycardia

Apnea and/or bradycardia caused by abdominal distention with compromise of lung volumes or airway obstruction, or caused by vagal stimulation from passage of the tube, stomach distention, or gastroesophageal reflux, may occur during or after gavage feeding. Interventions to decrease vagal stimulation include changing to an indwelling gavage tube, decreasing feeding volume, and feeding more slowly.

Poor Growth

The first response to poor growth may be to increase feeding volume and calories. Factors that increase caloric expenditure (e.g., thermal instability or overstimulation) should also be considered.

When one is feeding the postsurgical neonate, the choice of formula depends on bowel integrity. An infant recovering from mild NEC may be started on human milk or a dilute (half-strength) regular formula. With serious or surgically treated NEC, dilute human milk, dilute formula, or in the most severe cases an elemental formula is preferred.[31] As feeding volumes are slowly advanced, feeding tolerance must be closely assessed. Use of a heat shield, plastic wrap, hat or other clothing, supportive positioning, and grouping of care to conserve energy may result in better growth. Although these interventions intuitively make sense, convincing data supporting success for these maneuvers is hard to find.

Danger Signs

Bile in the gastric aspirate is generally a sign of significant ileus or obstruction. The presence of blood in the stools or gastric aspirate, a tense or tender abdomen, and abdominal wall erythema are more ominous signs of feeding intolerance and may indicate frank NEC. Presence of these signs and symptoms warrants a careful physical examination and usually further investigation including x-ray examinations. Feedings should be postponed while these signs and symptoms are being investigated. Other useful studies include a complete blood count with differential to evaluate extent of blood loss, presence of thrombocytopenia (a marker of necrotic bowel), and change in white blood cell count as evidence of infection. Although feeding of human milk may protect against developing NEC, 5% to 10% of cases of NEC occur in infants who have never been fed enterally. Therefore abnormal abdominal distention or bilious or bloody gastric aspirates should be investigated in any infant regardless of feeding status.

Parent Teaching

Holding and feeding an infant are two of the most important and enjoyable aspects of parenting. Unfortunately, such practices are often denied to parents of sick, preterm infants. Parents are already overwhelmed by guilt and fear. Parents who are prevented from providing care and nurturing to their infant will also experience feelings of helplessness, frustration, and isolation. It is essential that care providers involve parents in the care, and especially the feeding, of their infant (see Chapter 28).

Feeding is an excellent way to involve parents in their infant's care. The mother who provides milk for her infant is involved in care giving (see Chapter 28). A nonnursing mother, and the father, can also be involved with the infant's feeding in other ways. Parents should be involved in discussions of feeding practices and formula choices. Parents should be taught (1) the signs of feeding intolerance, (2) the slow progress and routine "ups and downs" of feeding prematures, and (3) how to follow daily weight and caloric intake. During gavage feedings parents may hold their infant and support the pacifier to encourage nonnutritive sucking.[13,47] Finally, parents should be supported and encouraged to nipple feed their infant. Nothing encourages parents to bond with their infant quite as well as holding, feeding, and watching the growth of their infant.

References

1. Adamkin DH: Nutrition in very very low birthweight infants, *Clin Perinatol* 13:419, 1986.

2. American Academy of Pediatrics, Committee on Nutrition: Nutrition needs of low-birthweight infants, *Pediatrics* 112:622, 1988.

3. Bishop JH, King FJ, Lucas A: Linear growth in the early neonatal period, *Arch Dis Child* 65:707, 1990.

4. Bragdon DB: A basis for the nursing management of feeding the premature infant, *JOGN* 12(suppl 3):51, 1983.

5. Brennan-Behan M et al: Calorie loss from expressed mother's milk during continuous gavage infusion, *Neonat Net* 13:27, 1994.

6. Carlson SE: Very long chain fatty acids in the developing retina and brain. In Polin RA, Fox WW, editors: *Fetal and neonatal physiology,* Philadelphia, 1992, WB Saunders.

7. Committee on Nutrition of the Preterm Infant, European Society of Paediatric Gastroenterology and Nutrition: *Nutrition and feeding of the preterm infants,* Oxford, UK, 1987, Blackwell Scientific Publications.

8. Currao WJ, Cox C, Shapiro DL: Diluted formula for beginning the feeding of premature infants, *Am J Dis Child* 142:730, 1988.

9. Dodd V, Freman R: A field study of bacterial growth in continuous feedings in a NICU, *Neonat Net* 9:17, 1991.

10. Dunn L et al: Beneficial effects of early hypocaloric enteral feeding on neonatal gastrointestinal function: preliminary report of a randomized trial, *J Pediatr* 112:622, 1988.

11. Duffy B, Pencharz P: The effect of feeding route (I.V. or oral) on the protein metabolism of the neonate, *Am J Clin Nutr* 43:108, 1986.

12. Evans JR et al: Effect of high-dose vitamin D supplementation on radiographically detectable bone disease of very low birthweight infants, *J Pediatr* 115:779, 1989.

13. Field T et al: Nonnutritive sucking during tube feedings: effects on preterm neonates in an intensive care unit, *Pediatrics* 70:381, 1982.

14. Gaull GE: Taurine in milk: growth modulator or conditionally essential amino acid? *J Pediatr Gastroenterol Nutr* 2(suppl 1):266, 1983.

15. Grant J, Denne SC: Effect of intermittent versus continuous enteral feeding on energy expenditure in premature infants, *J Pediatr* 118:928, 1991.

16. Groothuis J, Rosenberg A: Home oxygen promotes weight gain in infants with bronchopulmonary dysplasia, *Am J Dis Child* 141:992, 1987.

17. Hamosh M: Lipid metabolism. In Hay WW Jr, editor: *Neonatal nutrition and metabolism,* St Louis, 1991, Mosby.

18. Hill D: Effect of insulin on fetal growth, *Semin Perinatol* 2:319, 1978.

19. Kashyap S et al: Growth, nutrient retention, and metabolic response in low birthweight infants fed varying intakes of protein and energy, *J Pediatr* 113:713, 1988.

20. Kliegman RM, Morton S: Sequential intrahepatic metabolic effects of enteric galactose alimentation in newborn rats, *Pediatr Res* 24:302, 1988.

21. Lemons PM et al: Bacteria in human milk during continuous feedings, *Am J Perinatol* 1:76, 1983.

22. Lin CC, Evans MI: *Intrauterine growth retardation: pathophysiology and clinical management,* New York, 1984, McGraw Book Co.

23. Lucas A, Bishop NJ, Cole TJ: Randomised trial of nutrition for preterm infants after discharge, *Arch Dis Child* 67:324, 1992.
24. Lucas A et al: A multicenter trial on feeding low birthweight infants: effects of diet on early growth, *Arch Dis Child* 59:722, 1984.
25. Lucas A, Hudson G: Preterm milk as a source of protein for low birthweight infants, *Arch Dis Child* 59:831, 1984.
26. Lucas A et al: Early diet in preterm babies and developmental status in infancy, *Arch Dis Child* 64:1590, 1989.
27. Lucas A et al: Early diet in preterm babies and developmental status at 18 months, *Lancet* 335:1477, 1990.
28. MacLean WC, Fink BB: Lactose malabsorption by premature infants: magnitude and clinical significance, *J Pediatr* 97:383, 1980.
29. Meadow WL et al: Metoclopramide promoted enteral feeding in preterm infants with feeding intolerance, *Dev Pharmacol Ther* 13:38, 1989.
30. Milla PJ, editor: *Disorders of gastrointestinal motility in childhood,* New York, 1988, John Wiley & Sons.
31. Periera GR, Ziegler E: Nutritional care of the surgical neonate, *Clin Perinatol* 16:233, 1989.
32. Phillips C, Johnson NE: The impact of quality of diet and other factors on birthweight of infants, *Am J Clin Nutr* 30:215, 1977.
33. Prentice AM et al: Are current dietary guidelines for young children a prescription for overfeeding? *Lancet* 2:1066, 1988.
34. Reidel BD, Greene HL: Vitamins. In Hay WW Jr, editor: *Neonatal nutrition and metabolism,* St Louis, 1991, Mosby.
35. Shaker CS: Nipple feeding premature infants: a different perspective, *Neonat Net* 8:9, 1990.
36. Silvestre MA et al: A prospective randomized trial comparing continuous versus intermittent feeding methods in very low birth weight neonates, *J Pediatr* 128:748, 1996.
37. Simpson JW, Lawless RW, Mitchell AC: Responsibility of the obstetrician to the fetus. II. Influence of pre-pregnancy weight gain on birthweight, *Obstet Gynecol* 45:481, 1975.
38. Sparks JW, Girard J, Battaglia FC: An estimate of the caloric requirements of the human fetus, *Biol Neonate* 38:113, 1980.
39. Sparks JW, Cetin I: Intrauterine growth. In Hay WW Jr, editor: *Neonatal nutrition and metabolism,* St Louis, 1991, Mosby.
40. Steichen JJ, Krug-Wispe SK, Tsang RC: Breast-feeding the low birthweight preterm infant, *Clin Perinatol* 14:131, 1987.
41. Thureen P, Hay WW Jr: Conditions requiring special nutritional management. In Tsang RC et al, editors: *Nutritional needs of the preterm infant,* Baltimore, 1993, Williams & Wilkins.
42. Toce SS, Keenan WJ, Homan SM: Enteral feeding in very low birthweight infants, *Am J Dis Child* 141:439, 1987.
43. Unger A et al: Nutritional practices and outcome of extremely premature infants, *Am J Dis Child* 140:1027, 1986.
44. VandenBerg KA: Nippling management of the sick neonate in the NICU: the disorganized feeder, *Neonat Net* 9:9, 1990.
45. Wahlig TM, Georgieff MK: The effect of illness on neonatal metabolism and nutritional management, *Clin Perinatol* 22:77, 1995.
46. Weaver LT, Lucas A: Development of gastrointestinal structure and function. In Hay WW Jr, editor: *Neonatal nutrition and metabolism,* St Louis, 1991, Mosby.
47. Widstrom AM et al: Non-nutritive sucking in tube fed preterm infants: effects on gastric motility and gastric contents of somatostatin, *J Pediatr Gastroenterol Nutr* 7:517, 1988.

16 Total Parenteral Nutrition

Howard W. Kilbride, Kathy Bendorf, Nancy Allen

TPN support for the critically ill newborn was first reported 3 decades ago.[11] Currently, LBW infants comprise the largest group of pediatric patients receiving TPN. For preterm infants, duration of TPN therapy is inversely related to birth weight, with those less than 1500 g receiving, on average, about 3 weeks of TPN.[13] This chapter familiarizes the reader with the nutritional needs of the newborn, specific indications for TPN, and guidelines for formulation and administration of IV nutritional solutions. Mechanical, infectious, and metabolic complications are discussed with emphasis on prevention and early identification.

Physiology

Fuel Stores

During periods of fasting, tissue stores of energy provide the major source of fuel for the body. Carbohydrate is stored in the liver and muscle as glycogen. Stable blood sugar levels are maintained by hormonal regulation of glycogen production (glycogenesis) and breakdown to glucose (glycogenolysis). Newborns, particularly those who are growth retarded or preterm, have low glycogen stores and, often, insufficient regulation mechanisms.

The greatest body energy stores are in the form of fat, which provides a calorie yield of 9 kcal/g when metabolized. In addition to normal deposits of adipose tissue, newborns (and hibernating adult animals) have unique stores termed brown fat. These stores, which are anatomically located between the scapulae, in the axillae and mediastinum, and around the adrenals, protect the body from hypothermia through nonshivering thermogenesis (see Chapter 6).

Protein makes up lean body mass. Although protein is not used as an energy store, it may be oxidized for this purpose during periods of starvation. Catabolism usually leads to some bodily dysfunction as noted later.

Effects of Starvation

The brain during the last trimester of gestation, as well as through the first 2 years of life, will grow rapidly with increases in glial and neuronal cell numbers, myelinization, synaptic connections, and dendritic arborization. An infant who receives inadequate nutrition prenatally or postnatally may have an interruption of brain growth and is at risk for permanent brain injury. Autopsy studies of brains of malnourished infants have shown diminished cell numbers and deficiencies in lipid and phospholipid content. Additionally, preterm infants with microcephaly or slow postnatal head growth have worse neurodevelopmental outcome than those with normal head growth.[17]

Malnutrition may cause immediate clinical problems. These include muscle wasting, hypotonia, loss of ventilatory drive, apnea, and difficulty weaning from the ventilator. Immune responses may be depressed with increased susceptibility to infection (see Chapter 21).

Nutritional Requirements of the Neonate

Caloric

Caloric requirements for the growing preterm infant are 105 to 120 kcal/kg/day (see Chapter 15). These estimates are based on enteral intake. Parenteral requirements are about 20% less, or approximately 85 to 100 kcal/kg/day.

Basal values of caloric requirements must be adjusted according to the patient's activity, body temperature, and degree of stress. An elevation of body temperature increases the caloric expenditure by approximately 12% for each degree centigrade above 37.8° C (100.2° F). Metabolic demands of surgery or severe cardiac or pulmonary distress may increase caloric requirements by 30% and chronic failure to thrive by 50% to 100%. In addition, postnatal dexamethasone therapy will diminish protein and micronutrient retention.[32]

Water

Water requirements vary with gestational and postnatal age (postconceptual age) and environmental conditions (e.g., care in an incubator versus radiant heat warmer, use of phototherapy).

Mineral

Sodium requirements are minimal for the first days of life. After 1 week, the average requirement is 2 to 3 mEq/kg/day. Large renal losses (>5 mEq/kg/day) may occur in very immature infants (<28 weeks' gestation) in the first weeks of life.

Potassium and chloride requirements are approximately 2 mEq/kg/day and 3 to 4 mEq/kg/day, respectively. Glucosuria with resulting osmotic diuresis may increase sodium and potassium urinary losses.

Calcium is an important cofactor in hemostasis, enzyme function, and cell membrane stability. In the newborn, 98% of calcium is stored in the bone. The initial calcium requirement is 0.5 to 1 mEq/kg/day to maintain calcium homeostasis and to avoid irritability and tetany associated with low serum ionized calcium levels. In utero, the accretion rate is 4 to 5 mEq/kg/day, which the growing preterm infant should receive in addition to adequate phosphorus and vitamin D to avoid osteopenia, rickets, and bone fractures.[20] Excess calcium intake may cause CNS depression or signs of renal toxicity.

The phosphorus requirement for the growing preterm infant is 40 to 60 mg/kg/day (31 mg = 1 mmol). Bone contains 80% of the body's phosphorus. Low phosphorus intake will cause increased renal calcium excretion and a depletion of bone calcium phosphate. Low phosphorus intake or chronic furosemide diuretic therapy may also lead to hypercalciuria and nephrolithiasis.[9] Because phosphorus is a major constituent of cellular energy function (adenosine triphosphate, 2,3-disphosphoglycerate, creatinine phosphate), severe depletion may result in muscle paralysis, respiratory failure, and interruption of important cellular functions such as the hemoglobin-oxygen dissociation curve and leukocyte activity.

Magnesium is essential for intracellular enzyme systems. The requirement is 0.25 to 0.5 mEq/kg/day. Magnesium deficiency states mimic hypocalcemia, manifesting as irritability, tremulousness, tetany, and cardiac dysrhythmias.

Carbohydrate

During parenteral nutrition, at least 40% to 45% of caloric requirements should be provided as carbohydrate, generally as dextrose (calculated as 3.4 kcal/g of hydrated carbohydrate). A glucose infusion rate (GIR) of 6 to 8 mg/kg/min is generally sufficient to meet metabolic needs of the infant. Requirements are greater for infants who are stressed (e.g., sepsis, hypothermia) or hyperinsulinemic (e.g., IDMs, infants with Beckwith-Wiedemann syndrome).

Protein

The quantity of daily nitrogen required by a term newborn infant based on estimates from breast milk intake is approximately 325 mg/kg/day (approximately 2 g/kg/day of protein).[13] **Requirements for preterm infants are much higher as indicated by in utero accretion rates during the latter half of pregnancy. At 28 weeks' gestation the fetus requires 350 mg/kg/day of nitrogen. This figure declines to 150 mg/kg/day by term gestation. When the estimated accretion rate is added to the obligatory postnatal nitrogen excretion, the requirement for a 28-week gestation preterm may be calculated to be approximately 495 mg/kg/day (3.1 g/kg/day of protein). If one assumes parenterally administered amino acids are converted to body proteins at 75% efficiency, the estimated parenteral amino acid requirement would be as high as 3.7 g/kg/day.**[21]

Nitrogen retention and body growth have been shown to be greater when high quantities of protein are provided with adequate calories.[20] For example, in a study in which caloric intake was held constant, weight gain and linear growth were greater with protein intake of 3.5 g/kg/day compared with 2.24 g/kg/day.[25] Other investigators have demonstrated that protein intake in excess of 4 g/kg/day does not result in greater nitrogen retention.[18] **Excessive quantities of protein may be associated with hyperaminoacidemia, hyperaminoaciduria, azotemia, and hyperaminemia, all of which have implications for long-term neurodevelopmental outcome.**

Provision of specific amino acid requirements for the growing preterm infant is perhaps more important than the total protein quantity.[1] An essential amino acid is one that cannot be synthesized in adequate quantity to meet the requirements for normal growth and development. The differentiation between essential and nonessential amino acids is not clear in newborn infants, because the ability to synthesize some amino acids may vary with clinical situation or stage of maturity. Lysine and threonine are essential in their entirety. The requirement for other amino acids may be met by providing ketoanalogues, which may accept a nitrogen group during transamination. There is a high requirement for branched amino acids (leucine, isoleucine, and valine) in the growing newborn. These are primarily metabolized in skeletal muscle. Administration of branched amino acids during parenteral nutrition may be advantageous since the metabolic function of the liver is in part bypassed compared with enteral feedings, which pass through the portal circulation.

Methionine is an essential sulfur-containing amino acid that is metabolized to cysteine and taurine. For preterm infants less than 32 weeks' gestation, cystathionase activity is insufficient for cysteine synthesis.[34] Thus, at least for these high risk infants, cysteine should be added to parenteral amino acid infusions. Taurine is a nonprotein amino sulfonic acid that is converted from cysteine by cysteine sulfonic acid decarboxylase. Taurine concentrations are low in infants provided with non-supplemented TPN infusions. Recent evidence suggests taurine may prevent cholestasis in newborns by more effectively conjugating bile salts and creating soluble end-products.[22] Although phenylalanine is an essential amino acid for protein synthesis, if given in excess it may be neurotoxic (as evidenced in classic phenylketonuria). Histidine is considered to be an essential amino acid for newborns, with the lowest levels evident in preterm infants. Arginine may be essential only for

the newborn with reduced arginine synthetase activity. This amino acid is thought to facilitate clearance of nitrogenous waste products by "priming the urea cycle." Use of amino acid infusates with deficient arginine has been associated with hyperammonemia.[18]

Nonessential amino acids make up the largest percentage of the amino acid pool in the fetal body. Although, as with essential amino acids, the desired quantities of these amino acids are not known, it is thought they should be provided in parenteral solutions in a balanced formulation rather than with overrepresentation by one amino acid.

Fat

Long-chain fatty acids are essential in the newborn for brain development. Essential fatty acids (EFA) include linoleic and arachidonic acids. Biochemical evidence of EFA deficiency may be seen in less than a week in VLBW infants receiving a deficient diet, and the administration of parenteral glucose and amino acids may accelerate these abnormalities. EFA deficiency results in an imbalance in fatty acid production with an overproduction of nonessential fatty acids. **These biochemical changes are measured as an elevated triene/tetraene ratio (>0.4).[12] Clinical manifestations appearing at variable times after biochemical changes of EFA deficiency include scaly dermatitis, poor hair growth, thrombocytopenia, failure to thrive, poor wound healing, and increased susceptibility to bacterial infection. Clinical manifestations of EFA deficiency can be avoided if 3% to 4% of caloric intake is supplied as linoleic acid.**

In addition to preventing EFA deficiency, lipid emulsion is a concentrated source of non-protein calories, which promotes nitrogen retention. Preterm infants appear to have limited capability to oxidize fatty acids. This limitation may be related to deficiency of carnitine, which in the form of acyl-carnitine promotes transfer of fatty acids into mitochondria, where oxidative metabolism occurs.[5]

Vitamins

The biologic role of the vitamins, signs and symptoms of deficiency states, and recommended oral requirements are available in Chapter 15. The American Society for Clinical Nutrition (ASCN) has suggested that preterm infants receive 40% to

65% of the daily recommended vitamin doses for term infants and children.[16] These guidelines may result in excessive intakes of some water-soluble vitamins, particularly pyridoxine and riboflavin. Although preterm infants have limited stores of lipid-soluble vitamins because of low body fat, potential toxicity from excess administration is a concern. Vitamin A is a lipid-soluble vitamin important for tissue growth, protein synthesis, and epithelial differentiation. Additional supplementation will result in increased serum retinol levels and has been associated with a decreased incidence of BPD in some studies.[33] Vitamin A may be more effectively administered in lipid emulsion rather than dextrose amino acid solutions.[2,7] Formulations that provide greater Vitamin A intake than indicated in the ASCN guidelines may be appropriate for sick, preterm infants.[15]

Vitamin E is a lipid-soluble, biologic antioxidant that is deficient in preterm infants. However, daily parenteral intake of 2 to 3 mg/kg has been associated with serum levels generally in the recommended range of 1 to 2 mg/dl. Pharmacologic doses have been tried unsuccessfully for prevention of BPD and ROP. Recent experience suggests that Vitamin E supplementation to achieve serum levels as high as 4 to 5 mg/dl may be used in combination with cryotherapy to decrease the sequelae of ROP.[23] Vitamin K production by intestinal flora is impaired by insufficient enteral feedings and use of broad spectrum antibiotics in infants on long-term TPN. Vitamin K is provided at the recommended dosage through parenteral pediatric multivitamin solutions.[15]

Trace Minerals

Although trace minerals are relatively scarce (less than 0.01% of the weight of the human body by definition), they play an important role in normal growth and development. Deficiencies of both zinc and copper have been identified in infants on long-term TPN. Manifestations of deficiency and recommendations for intake are provided in Chapter 15. Parenteral recommendations are lower than oral based on physiologic requirements. For infants not receiving frequent blood transfusions, iron therapy may be necessary by 2 months of age. Infants on erythropoietin therapy may need earlier iron supplementation, given either orally or intravenously.[27]

Etiology

Clinical indications for parenteral nutrition include any situation in which there will be a delay in establishing adequate oral nutrition. When parenteral nutrition is administered through a peripheral vein, caloric intake is limited by the concentration of carbohydrate (usually <12.5% dextrose) and amino acids (≤2%) or required fluid volume. Using lipid emulsions, a caloric intake of 70 to 100 kcal/kg/day and a protein intake of 2.5 g/kg/day may be realized. This intake will prevent catabolism and, in some cases, result in moderate growth. Peripheral parenteral nutrition is usually adequate for term newborns with transient bowel disease (such as may be seen after the repair of a small omphalocele) or for preterm infants whose enteral feedings are delayed for 1 to 2 weeks. Peripheral TPN is also commonly used to supplement nutrition in newborns who are receiving partial enteral feedings. When caloric needs can be met by peripherally administered TPN, this route is preferred to the central route because the catheter insertion risks are avoided and generally the risk of infection is less. The placement of a central line for parenteral nutrition allows a higher carbohydrate load to be used, giving more calories with less fluid. In preterm infants at risk for a patent ductus arteriosus and pulmonary edema, diminishing fluid intake and improving nutritional status may be important aspects of management. TPN by a central catheter should be considered in the following:

- **ELBW infants (<1000 g birth weight) and others who do not tolerate oral feedings after a week of age or who cannot receive adequate caloric intake by peripheral parenteral nutrition (PPN)**
- **Infants who have had gastrointestinal surgery and will have a significant delay in enteral nutrition, such as an infant with a gastroschisis, bowel resection after NEC, or meconium peritonitis**
- **Infants with chronic gastrointestinal dysfunction, such as intractable diarrhea**

Data Collection

Monitoring Growth

Weight loss or insufficient weight gain is the initial effect of inadequate caloric intake. Linear growth, although less affected, will be diminished after long periods of poor nutrition. Because of "brain-sparing," head circumference growth is the least affected.

Fetal weight gain in utero at each week of gestation is currently used as the standard to assess adequacy of postnatal growth. Although absolute weight acquisition in utero increases from approximately 20 g/day at 28 weeks' gestation, the percentage of weight-specific gain decreases during the latter half of gestation. Growth curves are available to allow comparison of postnatal weight gain with expected weight acquisition.[36]

Adequacy of nutrition is probably better assessed by evidence of fat and muscle acquisition in the neonate. Triceps skinfold thickness is used to estimate fat accretion, and the midarm circumference measurement is used to approximate muscle acquisition.[14] The need for these measurements should be weighed against the importance of protecting the fragile skin of the preterm infant. **Minimum monitoring of growth should consist of the following:**

- **Weight measured daily, twice a day (bid), or three times a day (tid) in ELBW infants with rapidly changing extracellular fluid states**
- **Length measured weekly**
- **Head circumference measured weekly**

These measurements should be obtained in a standardized fashion and recorded weekly using the same equipment each time and the appropriate growth curve for premature infants.

Biochemical Monitoring

In addition to anthropometric measurements, biochemical parameters may be monitored to assess nutritional adequacy. Tests for protein malnutrition have included serum total protein, albumin, transferrin, retinol-binding protein, and prealbumin, the latter two suggested primarily for preterm infants.[13] Routine clinical use of these measurements awaits greater definition of normal variation and independent effects of systemic illness and medications.

Biochemical monitoring of the infant's physiologic status is necessary to avoid complications of TPN. Usefulness of the laboratory data should be balanced with the economic costs and risks from iatrogenic blood losses for the infant (Table 16-1).

Treatment

Central Catheter Placement

Although many materials have been used, silicone elastomer catheters (Silastic) are preferred for central venous placement because of their pliability and low incidence of thromboembolic complications. Percutaneous placement of a small diameter (2 Fr) catheter is routinely performed in even the smallest of neonatal patients by trained nurses and physicians.[26,31] The catheter is usually placed in the antecubital or axillary veins in the arms; however, leg, scalp, or external jugular veins may be used to achieve central access. Veins that may be needed for percutaneous central line placement should not be sites for routine venipuncture.

Percutaneous line placement involves stabili-

Table 16-1
Metabolic Monitoring for Infants Receiving Parenteral Nutrition

Variable	Frequency	
	Acute Phase	Stable
Electrolytes (Na, K Cl, CO$_2$)	daily	2 × per week
Calcium, phosphorus	weekly	biweekly
Alkaline phosphatase	—	biweekly
Serum glucose screen	q8h	daily
Urine glucose	q8h	daily
Hemoglobin/hematocrit	daily	weekly
Liver function		
Bilirubin	2 × per week	prn
Transaminases	weekly	biweekly
Triglyceride*	—	weekly

*When on lipid emulsion.

zation of the vein, maximal sterile barriers, and antiseptic preparation of the skin with providone-iodine and alcohol.[31] Fully equipped, prepackaged kits are available for this procedure from a number of manufacturers. In most kits, an 18- or 19-gauge "break away" needle is used to puncture and tunnel through the subcutaneous tissue before entering the vein. Once the needle is within the vein, the catheter, which has been flushed with heparinized saline, is passed through the needle into the vein and advanced a premeasured distance to the approximate location of the superior vena cava (if the basilic vein is used, turn the infant's head to face the insertion site to minimize the risk of the catheter entering neck vessels). The catheter tip position should be documented radiographically. The needle is carefully removed from the skin, separated, and discarded. A Steri-Strip should be placed over the catheter insertion site to maintain its position before the dressing is completed. Heparinized flush solution should be periodically instilled to maintain patency.

The length of tubing outside the infant's body should be measured and recorded. Excess may be carefully curled at the site of insertion and covered with a sterile, transparent dressing. If an armboard was used for stabilization, it may be removed. Arm restraints should not be necessary.

Large-bore silastic catheters (Broviac) are placed surgically in infants in whom the percutaneous method is not technically possible and long-term access is anticipated. Generally the catheters are placed in the internal or external jugular veins or common facial vein by cutdown and threaded to a central venous site. The distal end is tunneled subcutaneously and exited through the anterior chest wall. The catheter must be secured and dressed sterilely. Other sites that may be used for TPN infusion, on a short-term basis, include subclavian, jugular, or femoral veins. Some centers use a UVC for short-term parenteral nutrition when another site is not feasible.

Composition of Infusate

Carbohydrate

The prime source of calories is usually dextrose given peripherally as a 10% to 12% solution. Centrally, a 15% to 30% solution may be used. The glucose load will be increased if either the infusion rate or glucose concentration of the infusate is increased. Too rapid an increase in glucose load may exceed an infant's carbohydrate tolerance and result in hyperglycemia. A rapid decrease in the infusion rate or the glucose concentration of the infusate may result in hypoglycemia.

When calculating caloric intake, use the following:

$$1 \text{ g dextrose} = 3.4 \text{ kcal}$$

or

$$100 \text{ ml/kg of } D_{10}W = 34 \text{ kcal/kg}$$

or

$$100 \text{ ml/kg of } D_{30}W = 102 \text{ kcal/kg}$$

The glucose infusion rate (GIR) can be calculated:

$$\text{GIR (mg/kg/min)} = \frac{\text{g glucose/day} \times 100}{1440 \text{ (min/day)}} \div \text{weight (kg)}$$

Generally, a newborn of 28 weeks' or greater gestation (>1000 g birth weight) will initially tolerate a GIR of about 6 mg/kg/min. Daily increases in dextrose concentration or fluid volume to increase carbohydrate administration by 1.5 to 2.0 mg/kg/min usually are tolerated. ELBW infants may be carbohydrate intolerant, and initial GIR should be lower for these infants.

Blood sugar determinations and screening for glucosuria should be performed several times each day when glucose delivery is initiated or altered.

Lipids

One gram per day of lipid emulsion per 100 kcal is sufficient to prevent EFA deficiency; however, additional lipids may be provided to supplement nonprotein caloric intake and support growth. Lipids should never make up more than 50% to 60% of total caloric intake. Fat emulsions should be given cautiously, beginning with 0.5 g/kg/day and advanced 0.5 g/kg every 1 to 2 days as tolerated to 3 g/kg/day maximum. Lipids should be infused over a 24 hour period, since this usually results in a well tolerated infusion rate.[29] There appears to be no advantage to a rest period to allow for lipid clearance.[2] Fat emulsions are available as either 10% or 20% concentrations (Table 16-2). The 20% concentration may be beneficial for VLBW infants because its lower phospholipid concentration may result in lower plasma levels of triglyceride and cholesterol.[19]

Emulsified fat particles are similar in size and metabolic rate to naturally occurring chylomicrons. Most are cleared through passage in the adipose and muscle tissue. The capillary endothelial lipoprotein lipase hydrolyzes triglycerides and phospholipids, generating free fatty acids (FFAs), glycerol, and other glycerides. Most of the FFAs diffuse into the adipose tissue for reesterification and storage. A small portion circulates to be used by other tissues for fuel or for conversion by the liver into very low-density lipoprotein. Extremely immature and SGA infants with decreased adipose tissue have delayed clearance of fat emulsion. Rates of administration should be slowest in these infants. The rate-limiting step for lipid clearance is the metabolism by lipoprotein lipase. The use of heparin stimulates the release of this enzyme and may enhance clearance of IV lipids. The use of 0.5 to 1.0 μ heparin/ml of TPN is common in many nurseries. Carbohydrate must also be administered with fat to provide the necessary substrates for fatty acid oxidation and to promote FFA clearance.[6]

Amino Acid Solution

The compositions of four crystalline amino acid solutions available for neonatal parenteral use and one formulated for renal failure are presented in Table 16-3. The maximum concentration of the amino acid solution is generally 2% for peripheral use and 3% for central use. Each solution supplies an excess of nonessential amino acids, although more recently available solutions have sought to balance the nonessential amino acid profile.

Cysteine, which may be an essential amino acid in preterm infants, is not stable in solution. This amino acid is commercially available to be added immediately before the solution is administered. Trophamine and Aminosyn-PF include taurine, which is not available in other solutions.

To allow for safe and effective use of parenteral nitrogen, the maximum quantity provided should be guided by the nonprotein calories infused. A calorie/nitrogen ratio of approximately 150 to 200 nonprotein calories/1 g nitrogen (1 g nitrogen = 6.25 g protein) is a general guideline.

Table 16-2
Composition of Fat Emulsions

Composition	Intralipid (Clinitec)		Liposyn II (Abbott)	
	10%	**20%**	**10%**	**20%**
Fatty acid distribution (%)				
Linoleic acid	50	50	65.8	65.8
Oleic acid	26	26	17.7	17.7
Palmitic acid	10	10	8.8	8.8
Linolenic acid	9	9	4.2	4.2
Stearic acid	3.5	3.5	3.4	3.4
Components (%)				
Soybean oil	10	20	5	10
Safflower oil	—	—	5	10
Egg phospholipid	1.2	1.2	1.2	1.2
Glycerin	2.25	2.25	2.5	2.5
Caloric contents (kcal/dl)	110	200	110	200
Osmolarity (mOsm/L)	260	260	276	258

Based on the ratio of 200 calories/1 g nitrogen, if an infant received 2 g of protein (.31 g N), at least 62 nonprotein calories should be provided to promote protein sparing.

Electrolytes

Sodium is given in an estimated maintenance quantity (3 to 4 mEq/kg/day) as long as the serum sodium is 135 to 140 mEq/L and there are no excessive losses. Potassium is given in maintenance amounts (2 to 3 mEq/kg/day) unless there are excessive losses or renal dysfunction. Potassium needs may increase with anabolism. Sodium and potassium requirements may be further evaluated by monitoring urinary electrolyte levels (i.e., if sodium were depleted, low urine concentration would be expected).

Sodium and potassium may be supplied with chloride, acetate, or phosphate anions. The daily chloride requirement is approximately 3 mEq/kg/day and should be balanced with acetate to avoid alkalosis or acidosis (acetate is converted to bicarbonate). Amino acid preparations also supply anions that must be recognized to calculate a balanced anion solution. For example, Trophamine supplies 6.1 mEq of acetate per gram of nitrogen.

Minerals

Phosphorus may be provided as sodium or potassium phosphate. Calcium may be provided as 10% calcium gluconate (9.7 mg of elemental calcium/100 mg of salt). When one is preparing a solution with both calcium and phosphate, care must be taken to avoid calcium phosphate precipitation. Magnesium is supplied as magnesium sulfate.

Table 16-3
Concentrations (mg/dl) of Amino Acids Adjusted to 3% Solution

Amino Acid	Solutions				
	Travasol (Clintec)	Freamine III (Kendall McGaw)	Aminosyn-PF (Abbott)	Trophamine (Kendall McGaw)	Aminosyn-RF* (Abbott)
Essential					
L-Leucine	185	272	356	420	413
L-Phenylalanine	184	168	128	144	413
L-Methionine	176	160	54	101	413
L-Lysine	174	219	204	246	305
L-Isoleucine	143	208	228	244	263
L-Valine	137	198	194	235	300
L-Histidine	133	85	95	146	244
L-Threonine	126	121	155	126	188
L-Tryptophan	53	45	52	59	94
Nonessential					
L-Alanine	624	212	211	161	
L-Arginine	310	285	368	364	342
L-Proline	127	339	247	207	
L-Tyrosine	12	—	19	69	
L-Cysteine	—	—	†	<10†	
L-Serine	150	177	142	165	
L-Glycine	623	421	116	110	
L-Glutamine	—	—	—	—	
L-Taurine	—	—	196	70	

*Amino acid formulation for renal failure.
†Cysteine hydrochloride supplement may be added.

When one is using a potassium phosphate solution at pH 7.4, 4.4 mEq of potassium supplies 93 mg of elemental phosphorus. When a solution of sodium phosphate is used at pH 7.4, 4.0 mEq of sodium is given with each 93 mg of elemental phosphorus.

Calcium

- Because of increased risk of precipitation, calcium chloride should not be used.
- An elevation in ambient temperature, increased storage time, rise in pH, and decrease in protein or glucose concentration may increase the likelihood of precipitation. The addition of cysteine, which lowers solution pH, may enhance calcium and phosphate solubility.
- When one is preparing the solution, calcium and phosphate salts should be added separately, but not in sequence, during the last stages of solution mixing. The solubility of the added calcium should be calculated from the volume at the time the calcium is added, not the final volume.
- The use of a physiologic ratio of calcium to phosphorus, which is 1.8 : 1, in the TPN solution should allow for increased concentration of these minerals.[28]

Vitamins

A preparation approximating the AMA's recommended formulation of IV vitamins is available (MVI-Peds). The daily recommended dose is 1 vial for infants greater than 3 kg, 65% vial for infants 1 to 3 kg, and 30% vial for infants less than 1 kg.

Trace Elements

Commercially available amino acid solutions contain trace elements as contaminants, but variability even within the same brand means they cannot be relied on to meet trace element requirements.

Generally, zinc is supplied as zinc sulfate. Serum zinc levels usually approximate the maternal levels at birth and decline over the first week of life. By the second week of life, neonates not receiving dietary zinc should have supplementation. It may be necessary to initiate zinc intake earlier in neonates with intestinal loss, such as after gastrointestinal surgery.

Copper may be supplied as cupric sulfate. Approximately two thirds of stored copper is accumulated during the last trimester. Therefore the preterm infant may need early supplementation, but the term infant will have adequate hepatic stores for at least several weeks. Copper is lost through biliary secretion; therefore IV copper should be given with caution to an infant with biliary obstruction.

Manganese, chromium, selenium, molybdenum, and iodide salts should be provided for long-term parenteral nutrition. Manganese supplementation should not be provided to infants with cholestasis. The chromium dose may be reduced or discontinued with impaired renal function.

Aluminum is a contaminant in parenteral solutions with no known physiologic role.[24] Aluminum toxicity has been associated with bone disease, encephalopathy, anemia, and hepatic cholestasis. Renal elimination of aluminum is incomplete in newborn infants. Therefore levels should be monitored in infants on long-term TPN, especially those with renal failure.

Table 16-4 outlines a suggested composition for a TPN solution (guideline only).

Case Study

The following case example serves to illustrate the preceding points regarding writing orders for TPN:

History A male infant born at 29 weeks' gestation at 1300 g is now 14 days old and unable to be fed because of bowel resection after NEC. Because there will be a prolonged delay in oral alimentation, a central vein catheter is placed for TPN. He is currently receiving $D_{10}W$ at 120 ml/kg with maintenance electrolytes. He appears cachectic and weighs 1100 g. Serum electrolytes and blood glucose are normal. The approach to calculating TPN requirements is as follows:

Caloric Requirement Because this patient has already had a significant postpartum period without adequate nutrition, achieving caloric intake necessary for growth is a very important part of his care. The infant will probably require 120 kcal/kg or more for tissue repair and growth. We will begin with

60 kcal/kg and advance daily to reach this level.

Carbohydrate Initially, a dextrose load just above what has been previously tolerated should be used. Thus the patient should receive $D_{12.5}W$ at perhaps 130 ml/kg/day, depending on the fluid requirements of the infant. Overhydration with risks of cardiovascular and pulmonary complications should be avoided.

This represents

12.5 g glucose/dl × 130 ml/kg =

16.2 g glucose/kg

16.2 g glucose/kg ×

3.4 kcal/g glucose = 55.1 kcal/kg

Lipid emulsion may be added to increase the caloric intake, starting with 0.5 g/kg/day.

2.5 ml/kg 20% lipid emulsion (0.5 g) ×

2.0 kcal/ml = 5 kcal/kg/day

Thus the total nonnitrogen calories on the first day of TPN will be 60 (55 + 5).

Protein Calculate the quantity of protein by using the ratio 200 kcal/1 g nitrogen; 0.3 g of nitrogen/kg may be given with 60 calories: (60/200 × 1 g). This quantity of nitrogen represents 1.9 g protein/kg (0.3 g/nitrogen × 6.25 g protein/g nitrogen).

Electrolytes The patient should receive maintenance sodium ion (3 mEq/kg) and potassium ion (2.5 mEq/kg) unless there are excessive renal or gastrointestinal losses.

Anions Balancing anions is the next consideration. The 0.3 g/kg of nitrogen, if given as Trophamine, will add approximately 1.8 mEq of acetate/kg to the solution (6.1 mEq acetate/1 g nitrogen). If 2.8 mEq/kg of sodium is provided as sodium chloride and 0.2 mEq/kg as sodium acetate, the solution will have balanced anions. Giving 2.5 mEq/kg of potassium as potassium phosphate will provide approximately 53 mg/kg of elemental phosphorus:

$$(2.5 \text{ mEq K}^+/\text{kg}) \times \frac{93 \text{ mg (P)}}{4.4 \text{ mEq Na}^+}$$

Table 16-4
Suggested Composition for Intravenous Nutrition Regimen

Component	Daily Amount
Calories	
Dextrose 3.4 kcal/g	10-20 g/kg
Lipids 2.0 kcal/ml (20%) solution	1-3 g/kg
Nitrogen	0.32-0.48
Protein (6.25 g protein = 1 g N₂)	2-3 g/kg
Electrolytes	
Sodium	3 mEq/kg
Potassium	2-3 mEq/kg
Chloride	3-4 mEq/kg
Acetate	3 mEq/kg
Phosphate	2 mM/kg
Calcium	1 mEq/kg
Magnesium	0.8 mEq (20 mg)/kg
Vitamins	
MVI = Ped	1.0 vial*
Vitamin A	700 µg
Thiamine (B₁)	1.2 mg
Riboflavin (B₂)	1.4 mg
Niacin	17 mg
Pyridoxine (B₆)	1.0 mg
Ascorbic Acid (C)	80 mg
Ergocalciferol (D)	400 IU
Vitamin E	7.0 IU
Pantothenic acid	5.0 mg
Cyanocobalamin	1.0 µg
Folate	140 µg
Vitamin K	200 µg
Trace elements	
Zinc (zinc sulfate)	400 µg/kg
Copper (cupric sulfate)	20 µg/kg
Manganese sulfate	1.0 µg/kg
Chromium chloride	0.2 µg/kg
Selenium	2.0 µg/kg
Molybdenum	0.25 µg/kg
Iodide	1.0 µg/kg

*Reduced amount provided for VLBW infants (see text).

Minerals, Vitamins, and Trace Elements

Calcium, magnesium, vitamins, and trace elements should be ordered at this point. Calcium initially should be started at 1 mEq/kg/day but should be increased as tolerated with growth to 4-5 mEq/kg/day.

Volume Calculating the concentration of each ingredient in a 250 ml bottle of TPN solution is the next step. Because the per kilogram figure of each additive is to be delivered in 130 ml, the amount of each to be put in the 250 ml bag should be calculated by multiplying by 1.92 (250/130). Based on the 1.3 kg weight, the total volume calculated for this infant will be 169 ml.

TPN Orders Thus the TPN orders would be written for this patient as follows:

- $D_{12.5}W$ with the following per 250 ml to run 7 ml/hr:
    - 0.58 g nitrogen (3.7 g protein)
    - 5.3 mEq sodium as sodium chloride
    - 0.4 mEq sodium as sodium acetate
    - 4.8 mEq potassium as potassium phosphate
    - 102 mg phosphorus as potassium phosphate
    - 3.5 mEq acetate (Trophamine nitrogen)
    - 1.9 mEq calcium
    - 1.5 mEq magnesium
    - 1.25 vials MVI-Ped
    - 768 µg zinc
    - 58 mg copper
    - 1.9 µg manganese
    - 0.4 µg chromium
    - 3.8 µg selenium
    - 0.5 µg molybdenum
    - 1.9 µg iodide
    - 148 mg L-cysteine
- 20% lipid emulsion to run .13 ml/hr × 24 hr (3.1 ml)

Progression On subsequent days the dextrose concentration and lipids would be advanced slowly to increase the caloric intake to requirement as tolerated. The quantity of protein would also be increased to about 3.0 g/kg/day.

Solution Preparation

Solutions should be prepared in the hospital pharmacy under a laminar flow hood in a work area isolated from traffic and contaminated supplies. There should be quality control checks to monitor for sterility breaks in equipment, personnel, environment, and solutions.

Because many additives potentially can be insoluble in combination, a mixing sequence should be established that separates the most incompatible ingredients. Storage increases the risk of microbial contamination; therefore TPN solutions should be prepared on the day they are needed.

Administration of the TPN Solution

Proper administration of the TPN solution is as important as its preparation in preventing complications. The solution label should always be checked for correct patient identification and current formulation order.

Routine procedures must be established to avoid infectious complications from solution contamination. A standardized schedule should be maintained. Bottles and bags should be changed and initiated at the same time each day.

Solutions on the nursing units may be returned to the pharmacy for additives before hanging, but no additives should be placed in the solution once it is hanging.

Infections may occur from contamination of the solution or by breathing or touching during tubing changes. Good handwashing is critical before changing bags, filters, and other support equipment.

Changes in TPN infusion rates result in changes in glucose delivery to the newborn and may lead to hypoglycemia or hyperglycemia if the glucose homeostatic mechanisms do not adjust fast enough. Reactive hypoglycemia may occur if the glucose load is abruptly discontinued.[4] Parenteral nutrition solutions must infuse at a constant rate via an infusion pump. Attempts to rush or slow down solutions should not occur. If the parenteral nutrition infusion is suddenly discontinued because of a clotted catheter or accidental removal, an appropriate solution with dextrose should be infused via a peripheral vein, and blood glucose should be monitored.

Use of parenteral nutrition may increase an infant's risk of hyperglycemia during surgery. Because rapid fluid infusions may be necessary during operative procedures, the TPN solution should be discontinued and replaced with a physiologic infusate during the perioperative period. After surgery, TPN should be resumed when the patient is euglycemic.

Tapering of the TPN solution may occur as the infant begins to tolerate oral feedings. When the patient is taking approximately two thirds of the required calories orally, the central line may be removed. The length of the indwelling portion of the percutaneous catheter should be measured and compared with that stated in the original procedure note, and a slightly beveled tip should be observed. Careful attention to this detail will alert the clinician to the unlikely occurrence of catheter fragmentation, in which a portion is left in the tissue or vessel.

Administration of Fat Solution

Lipids should be given through a Y-tube to bypass the filter in the TPN line. Fat emulsions are never given proximal to a filter.

Rapid infusion of the fat emulsion may exceed its clearance rate from the body and accentuate complications; therefore fat emulsions should not be infused faster than 0.15 g/kg/hr.

Complications

Mechanical Complications

Pneumothorax, hemothorax, hydrothorax, air embolism, thromboembolism, catheter misplacement, or cardiac perforation are generally recognized complications of Broviac, subclavian, and/or jugular catheter insertions. Potential mechanical complications of percutaneous central lines include catheter occlusion, accidental dislodgment, erythematous tracking, phlebitis, and catheter migration. Chest x-ray examination for documentation of catheter placement is necessary before instilling a hypertonic solution.

The preceding complications may occur at any time as long as the catheter is present. Documentation of catheter position should be repeated if there is any history of pulling or tension on the catheter or any apparent change in its external position.

If the line is malfunctioning, it must be properly checked to avoid the possibility of complications from release of a clot into the bloodstream. If a clotted line is suspected, the line may be aspirated using strict sterile technique. If a good blood return

occurs or a clot is aspirated and removed, the catheter may be irrigated with sterile, dilute heparin solution.

Some clinicians will flush a partially occluded line with a thrombolytic agent, such as urokinase.[35] The risk of this practice must be weighed against the benefits of maintaining the central line. In most cases, if the catheter is a temporary line, it may be better to remove it and place a new line in another site.

A pleural effusion may be blood or chyle or may signal that the catheter has eroded into the pleural space. The effusion may be the infusate.

Superior vena cava syndrome and thrombophlebitis may also occur with continued use of a catheter.

Infectious Complications

Contaminated Solution Preparation

Rigid criteria for sterile preparation of the solutions are mandatory (see previous section on solution preparation).

An in-line, 0.22 μm membrane filter is capable of trapping bacteria and fungi (although not endotoxin) and should be helpful in minimizing the risk of septicemia from a contaminated IV bag. However, a filter provides a break in the line and another potential place for contamination. Additionally, filters lessen the risk of an air embolism.

There should be nothing added to the TPN after it leaves the pharmacy.

Contamination of the IV Line from Misuse

General guidelines to avoid IV contamination are as follows:

- Blood should not be drawn or given through the catheter because it increases formation of a fibrin sleeve and clots.
- Stopcocks should never be used.
- Generally, medications should not be injected nor "piggy backs" given through the central venous line.
- When changing IV fluids, one should take care to avoid bleeding back into the catheter.

The source of an infection is usually contamination with an organism that has colonized on the skin.

Dressings are not routinely changed on percutaneous central lines. If the dressing becomes non-occlusive or moistened, the site should be cleaned according to hospital protocol and redressed with a sterile transparent dressing. This should be performed using sterile gloves. The exposed catheter should be remeasured to ensure that it was not inadvertently moved during this process. Dressings are changed routinely on Broviac, subclavian, jugular, and femoral catheters. Dressing changes are recommended every 48 to 72 hours when using sterile gauze dressings and every 5 to 7 days when using sterile transparent dressings.

Evaluating the Infant for an Infectious Disease Complication

Although thermal instability is frequently present in infants with catheter-induced sepsis, this sign may be less evident in newborns than in the older child. Sepsis must be suspected when nonspecific findings such as lethargy or apnea occur.

Of the catheters removed on suspicion of catheter sepsis, 75% are removed unnecessarily. Other sources of infection must be investigated. Catheter removal is not routinely required unless the infant is extremely ill.

Some guidelines for management of an infant on TPN with temperature instability or other signs of suspected sepsis are as follows:

- The infant should be evaluated for potential sources of infection, including a general physical examination looking for non-TPN related sources and inspection of peripheral and central venous sites for erythema.
- Laboratory aids should include (1) complete blood count including platelet count, (2) aerobic and anaerobic bacterial cultures of blood (drawn from a peripheral site and from the catheter), (3) urine culture, (4) cerebrospinal fluid culture, (5) wound culture if indicated, and (6) stool cultures if indicated.
- Chest x-ray examination should be obtained to rule out pneumonia.
- Consider discontinuing lipid infusion for 24 to 48 hours to avoid interfering with the infant's nonspecific immune responses.
- If no source for the fever is found and it persists for 8 to 12 hours, septicemia should be

suspected. If the infection responds to treatment but a positive blood culture was present, there is risk that the catheter is the focus for continued seeding of the blood. Follow-up blood cultures obtained through the catheter and close clinical monitoring are important if the catheter is to be left in place.

- If the infant is stable, the bacteremia may be treated using appropriate antibiotics through the catheter, thus prolonging the life of the TPN line. Choose antibiotics that are compatible with TPN to avoid stopping the TPN during antibiotic infusion (consult the pharmacist). Quantitative blood cultures may be helpful in determining whether catheter-related sepsis is being adequately treated. If the patient is critically ill, the catheter should be removed immediately, and appropriate antibiotic therapy should be initiated.

Catheter removal should be performed according to the following steps:

- Prepare the skin site as for surgery.
- Obtain a blood culture specimen through the catheter and remove catheter.
- Obtain a peripheral blood culture.

If a central line is pulled because of sepsis, a new central line should not be placed for 48 to 72 hours.

Metabolic Complications

Glucose Metabolism

Hyperglycemia may occur with increased carbohydrate load, especially in ELBW infants who may have inadequate endogenous insulin production or decreased sensitivity to insulin. Elevated blood sugar may lead to hyperosmolality and osmotic diuresis, resulting in hyperosmolar dehydration. Manifestations include polyuria, glucosuria, and dry, hot, flushed skin. Serum sodium is not a reliable measure of serum osmolality if there is hyperglycemia. Direct measurement or estimate by use of the following formula is necessary:

Serum osmolality =
$$(1.86)Na^+ + BUN/2.8 + glucose/18$$

Transient glucose intolerance may be seen with stress. If hyperglycemia occurs without apparent change in glucose infusion, the possibility of sepsis, pain, hypoxemia, IVH (especially if infant is less than 34 weeks' gestation), or inadvertent increase in carbohydrate administration (mistake in preparation or rate of infusion) should be considered. Glucose intolerance may also be accentuated during infusions of lipid emulsion, especially in the ELBW infant. Discontinuation of the lipid infusion without alteration of the carbohydrate load will often eliminate hyperglycemia in this situation.

Hypoglycemia may result from an abrupt interruption of glucose infusion or excessive exogenous insulin administration. Manifestations of hypoglycemia include tachycardia or apnea, lethargy, jitteriness, and seizures. If these occur immediately after an interruption of the TPN infusion, an IV glucose infusion must be initiated at once, followed by close monitoring of the blood glucose to allow appropriate glucose administration. The glucose concentration of the infusate may usually be safely decreased by 5 g/dl every 12 hours. Blood glucose values should be monitored hourly until stable after each change.

Amino Acid Metabolism

Hyperammonemia may be seen in preterm infants given excessive protein loads. Hyperammonemia will also occur in an infant with a congenital metabolic disturbance, such as a urea cycle defect, when challenged with an amino acid load. Hyperammonemia may be manifested as somnolence, lethargy, seizures, and coma. Biochemical screening is necessary to identify this complication before there are symptoms.

Azotemia may occur before hyperammonemia, depending on the hepatic ability to convert ammonia to urea. Azotemia may also be a sign of dehydration.

Initially the BUN should be monitored daily. When there are no further changes in amino acid administration and the BUN is stable, monitoring two times per week is adequate.

Approximately 30% of infants receiving TPN for more than 2 weeks will develop cholestatic jaundice (direct bilirubin greater than 2 mg/dl).[10] The risk appears greatest for the least mature infants and those receiving the longest period of TPN without enteral feeding. It occurs earliest and

is most severe in those infants with the highest protein intakes and is possibly accentuated by hypertonic dextrose loads. The etiology appears to be multifactorial, including lack of bile flow stimulation, malnutrition, and amino acid toxicity or deficiency. Fat emulsions have been associated with cholestasis, but objective evidence of an etiologic role has not been provided. An increase in serum bile acid concentration usually precedes elevated conjugated bilirubin levels. Serum amino transferases are often normal early in the clinical course. Serum albumin and prealbumin levels usually remain normal. An abnormality in hepatic synthetic function or early rise in isoenzyme levels should lead the clinician to investigate other forms of liver disease. The differential of cholestatic jaundice includes the following:

- Bacterial sepsis
- Congenital viral infection
- Postpartum acquisition of cytomegalovirus
- Neonatal hepatitis
- Bile duct obstruction, such as biliary atresia or choledocal cyst
- Galactosemia
- Cystic fibrosis
- Alpha-1-antitrypsin deficiency

Management of cholestatic jaundice should include (if possible) the following:

- Reduction of parenteral protein to 1 g/kg/day
- Reduction of dextrose concentration to 10%
- Enteral feedings

Lipid Metabolism

Infants with decreased adipose tissue may demonstrate intolerance to fat emulsions infusions. Lipids may be poorly tolerated by SGA infants and extremely premature infants in the first week of life. Parenteral fats should be used cautiously in these infants. Hyperlipidemia may result, causing elevation of triglyceride, FFA, and lipoprotein levels. Serum may be checked daily for evidence of visible lactescence (increased plasma turbidity) by observation of plasma such as in a spun hematocrit tube. If plasma is turbid, the fat emulsion dose should be lowered or discontinued until resolved. Triglyceride and fatty acid levels should be obtained at least weekly, and doses should be adjusted accordingly. Transient hyperglycemia may result from lipid infusion. This complication is usually dose related and rarely requires treatment.[6]

Hyperlipidemia is responsible for the known and theoretical complications of fat emulsion infusions. Competitive displacement of bilirubin by FFA may increase the risk of kernicterus in infants with hyperbilirubinemia, particularly those of less than 30 weeks' gestation. Therefore hyperbilirubinemia requiring therapy is a theoretical contraindication to lipid infusion, although risks appear minimal when lipids are infused slowly and total dose is no more than 3g/kg/day.

Altered immune function by lipid deposition in macrophages and the reticuloendothelial system must be considered in infants with sepsis. Malassezia furfur is a lipophilic fungus that is increasingly reported as an opportunistic organism in infants receiving long-term lipid infusions.[8] Discontinuation of the central line and lipid infusion eliminates the infection.

Parent Teaching

In Hospital

Clinicians caring for an ill newborn must be attentive to the involvement and emotional state of the parents. There is a higher incidence of child abuse, subsequent foster placement, and relinquishment among infants who have been cared for in the NICU compared with healthy, "normally treated" newborns.

Bonding problems may be worsened by the early separation from parents that may occur in the NICU. When a newborn infant cannot be fed orally, an important, normal part of the infant's care is no longer available for the parents. The placement of a central line may be frightening to parents and result in less handling and caregiving on their part.

A neonatal service that uses TPN has the best results if there is an experienced "nutritional team," including pediatrician, surgeon, nutritional support nurse, pharmacist, dietitian, and social worker, with each member playing a vital role to make TPN a safe and effective therapy.

Infants requiring continuous care including TPN should have primary nursing (one regular nurse) and one physician who communicates regularly with the parents. Care providers should attempt to keep the parents involved in other parts of the infant's care, because the parents are unable to feed the infant. Parents should be fully informed regarding the purpose and appropriate care of the infant's central line so they will feel comfortable handling their infant with the line in place.

Home TPN

Home parenteral nutrition has been used in infants with congenital intestinal anomalies or after massive bowel resection for NEC.

TPN is initiated in the hospital. If growing and otherwise well, the infant may be a candidate for TPN at home. Issues to be addressed include ability and willingness of parents to care for the infant at home, available financial support, adequate home setting, and additional skilled nursing care needed at home. The infant should have a more permanent central line placed as early in the discharge process as possible. Parent teaching should begin early, including verbal, written, and hands-on demonstrations. Teaching sessions cover sterile technique, central line care, TPN administration, and potential complications and their management. Potential complications the parents need to know include catheter infections (sepsis, site infection), catheter occlusion, catheter breakage, air embolus, hypoglycemia or hyperglycemia, and dehydration or fluid overload. Parents must know what to do and who to call if a complication occurs. They also need to know that there is always someone on call 24 hours a day to help with any questions or concerns.

Parents also need to understand the importance of continuing to give the infant a pacifier at home. The infant on TPN, with no oral stimulation, uses the pacifier not only for comfort but also to strengthen muscles that will eventually be necessary for sucking, eating, and speech.

Administration of TPN at home is different from hospital administration of TPN. Infants often go home on cyclic TPN (12 hours per day). An ambulatory pump improves the mobility and flexibility of the parent and infant and allows for a more normal lifestyle.

Three-in-one TPN, when appropriate, allows

for one pump and tubing and decreases the workload of the parents. The three-in-one solution, or "total nutrient admixture" (TNA), in which the glucose, amino acids, and lipids are mixed in the same bag, has been successfully used in neonates and young infants at home.[30] A 1.2 μm filter is used to filter the TPA. This filter removes precipitate, air, and Candida, but it is not effective in removing bacteria. The decision to use TNA should be approached with caution in infants for the following reasons:

- The recommended pH of the amino acid solution for home TPN is 5.4 to 6.5, which is higher than the pH of Trophamine or Aminosyn-PF.
- Lipid emulsions increase the pH of the TPN solution.
- Calcium and phosphorus are more compatible in a solution with a low pH.

Compliance with home TPN is greatly increased when the parents understand TPN, the need for the TPN, and the need for strict adherence to sterile technique.

References

1. Adamkin DD et al: Comparison of a neonatal versus general-purpose amino acid formulation in preterm neonates, *J Perinatol* 15:108, 1995.
2. American Academy of Pediatrics Committee on Nutrition. In Barnes LA, editor: *Pediatric nutrition handbook,* ed 3, Elk Grove Village, Ill, 1993, American Academy of Pediatrics.
3. Baeckert PA et al: Vitamin concentration in very low birthweight infants given vitamins intravenously in a lipid emulsion—measurement of vitamins A, D, and E and riboflavin, *J Pediatr* 113:1007, 1988.
4. Bendorf K et al: Glucose response to discontinuation of parenteral nutrition in patients less than 3 years of age, *JPEN* 20(2):120, 1996.
5. Bonner CM et al: Effects of parenteral L-Carnitine supplementation on fat metabolism and nutrition in premature neonates, *J Pediatr* 126(2):287, 1995.
6. Cooke RJ et al: Soybean oil emulsion administration during parenteral nutrition in the preterm infant: effect of essential fatty acid, lipid, and glucose metabolism, *J Pediatr* 11:767, 1987.
7. Dahl GB et al: Stability of vitamins in soybean oil fat emulsion under conditions simulating intravenous feeding neonates and children, *JPEN* 18(3):234, 1994.
8. Danker WM et al: Malassezia fungemia in neonates and adults: complications of hyperalimentation, *Rev Infect Dis* 9:743, 1987.
9. Downing GJ et al: Kidney function in very low birth weight infants with furosemide-related renal calcifications at ages 1 to 2 years, *J Pediatr* 120:599, 1992.
10. Drongowski RA, Coran AG: An analysis of factors contributing to the development of total parenteral nutrition-induced cholestasis, *JPEN* 13:586, 1989.
11. Dudrick SJ et al: Long term total parenteral nutrition with growth, development, and positive nitrogen balance, *Surgery* 64:134, 1968.
12. Farrell PM et al: Essential fatty acid deficiency in premature infants, *Am J Clin Nutr* 48:220, 1988.
13. Fomon SJ: Requirements and recommended dietary intake of protein during infancy, *Pediatr Res* 30:391, 1991.
14. Georgieff MK et al: Determinants of arm muscle and fat accretion during the first postnatal month in preterm newborn infants, *J Pediatr Gastroenerol Nutr* 9:219, 1989.
15. Greene HL et al: Evaluation of a pediatric multiple vitamin preparation for total parenteral nutrition. II. Blood levels of vitamins A, D, and E, *Pediatrics* 77:539, 1986.
16. Greene HL et al: Guidelines for use of vitamins, trace elements, calcium, magnesium, and phosphorus in infants and children receiving total parenteral nutrition, *Am J Clin Nutr* 48:1324, 1988.
17. Hack M et al: Effect of very low birthweight and subnormal head size on cognitive abilities at school age, *N Engl J Med* 325:231, 1991.
18. Hanning RM, Zlotkin S: Amino acid and protein needs of the neonate: effects of excess and deficiency, *Semin Perinatol* 13:131, 1989.
19. Haumont D et al: Plasma lipids and plasma lipoprotein concentrations in very low birthweight infants given parenteral nutrition with twenty or ten percent lipid emulsion, *J Pediatr* 115:757, 1989.
20. Hay WW: Nutritional needs of the extremely low birthweight infant, *Semin Perinatol* 15:482, 1991.
21. Heird WC: Amino acid and energy needs of pediatric patients receiving parenteral nutrition, *Ped Clin NA* 42:765, 1994.
22. Howard D, Thompson DF: Taurine: an essential amino acid to prevent cholestasis in neonates? *Ann Pharmaco Ther* 26:1390, 1992.
23. Johnson L et al: Severe retinopathy of prematurity in infants with birth weights less than 1250 grams: incidence and outcome of treatment with pharmacologic serum levels of vitamin E in addition to cryotherapy from 1985 to 1991, *J Pediatr* 127:632, 1995.
24. Klein GL: Aluminum in parenteral solutions revisited—again, *Am J Clin Nutr* 61:449, 1995.
25. Kushyap S et al: Effects of varying protein and energy intakes on growth and metabolic response in low birthweight infants, *J Pediatr* 108:955, 1986.
26. Leick-Rude MK: Use of percutaneous silastic intravascular catheters in high risk neonates, *Neonat Net* 9:17, 1990.
27. Meyer MP et al: A comparison of oral and intravenous iron supplementation in preterm infants receiving recombinant erythropoietin, *J Pediatr* 129:258, 1996.

28. Pelegano JF et al: Simultaneous infusion of calcium and phosphorus in parenteral nutrition for premature infants: use of physiologic calcium phosphorus ratio, *J Pediatr* 114:115, 1989.

29. Phelps ST et al: Effect of the continuous administration of fat emulsion on the infiltration of intravenous lines in infants receiving peripheral parenteral nutrition solutions, *JPEN* 13:628, 1989.

30. Rollins CJ et al: Three-in-one parenteral nutrition: a safe and economical method of nutritional support for infants, *JPEN* 14:290, 1990.

31. Ryder M et al: Peripherally inserted central venous catheters, *Nurs Clin North Am* 28:937, 1993.

32. Schanler RJ et al: Parenteral nutrient needs of very low birthweight infants, *J Pediatr* 125:961, 1994.

33. Shenai JP et al: Clinical trial of vitamin A supplementation in infants susceptible to bronchopulmonary dysplasia, *J Pediatr* 111:269, 1987.

34. Viña J et al: L-Cysteine and glutathione metabolism are impaired in premature infants due to cystathionase deficiency. *Am J Clin Nutr* 61:1067, 1995.

35. Winthrop AL, Wesson DE: Urokinase in the treatment of occluded central venous catheters in children. *J Ped Surg* 19:536, 1984.

36. Wright K et al: New postnatal grids for very low birthweight infants, *Pediatrics* 91:922, 1993.

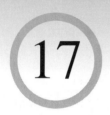

17 Skin and Skin Care

Carolyn Houska Lund, David J. Durand

The skin is a large organ in premature and term infants, comprising at least 13% of body weight in contrast to 3% of the body weight in adults.[37] Skin functions include thermoregulation; barrier against toxins and infections, water and electrolyte excretion, fat storage and insulation, and tactile sensation.

Like many other organs, the skin of the premature infant is immature. The combination of immaturity with the need for intensive care monitoring and procedures places premature infants at risk for skin trauma and loss of skin integrity. Skin trauma, as well as skin immaturity, has serious consequences for infants in the NICU, including problems in thermoregulation, fluid and electrolyte balance, diversion of calories for tissue repair, discomfort, potential toxicity from absorbed substances, and increased risk for infection.

This chapter reviews the physiology of both term and premature infants' skin, the differences in structure and function related to skin immaturity, and both prevention and treatment strategies to promote optimal skin integrity for infants in the NICU.

Physiology

There are three layers to the skin: the epidermis, the dermis, and the subcutaneous layer (Fig. 17-1). The epidermis is comprised of the stratum corneum, a nonliving layer, and the basal layer. The stratum corneum is formed of lipids and protein in "brick and mortar" configuration. The basal layer of the epidermis replaces the stratum corneum with cells; approximately every 26 days, cells migrate from the basal layer to the exfoliated layers of the stratum corneum. Both keratinocytes and melanocytes are also found in the basal layer.

The dermis, a woven layer of collagen and elastin fibers, is 2 to 4 mm thick at birth. It contains nerves, blood vessels, and hair follicles. Sensations of heat, touch, pressure, and pain originate in the dermal layer. Both sebaceous glands and sweat glands are located in the dermis, as well as in the subcutaneous layer of the skin. Sweat glands become mature in term infants during the first week of life, whereas maturation in premature infants occurs between 21 and 33 days and perhaps even longer in extremely premature infants. Full adult sweat gland function does not occur until 2 to 3 years of age.[20]

The subcutaneous layer is comprised of fatty connective tissue, with fat deposition occurring primarily during the last trimester of pregnancy. This layer provides heat insulation and functions as a calorie reservoir.

The skin of a normal term infant is covered with vernix caseosa, a cheesy substance composed of sebum from sebaceous glands, broken off lanugo, and desquamated cells from the amnion that accumulate during the last month of pregnancy to protect against maceration from the amniotic fluid and chafing caused by crowding in utero.[55] After delivery the vernix is either worn off or removed, and a desquamation process begins that results in visible peeling over the first week of life. Since vernix is both protective to the stratum corneum and has bacteriocidal activity, it should be allowed to wear off gradually and should not be actively or vigorously removed.

The skin of premature infants is thinner than that of term infants and may appear transparent or even gelatinous in extremely immature infants. There is usually a ruddy, red appearance caused by the underdeveloped stratum corneum, making skin color a poor tool for assessing the oxygenation status of very immature infants. There are fewer wrinkles on skin surfaces, and the skin is covered by lanugo to varying degrees depending on matu-

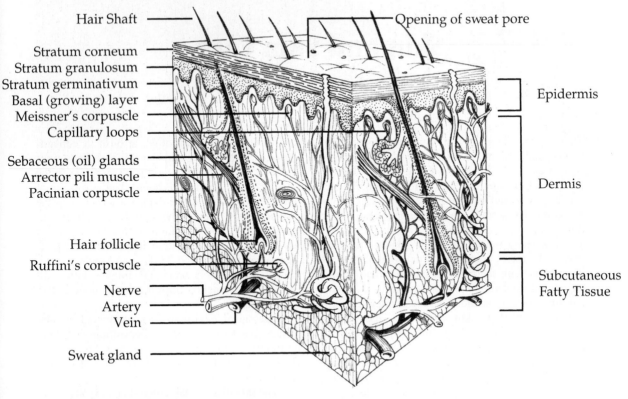

Figure 17-1   Cross section of skin layers and anatomic structures. (From *Principles of infant skin care*, Skillman, NJ, 1994, Johnson & Johnson.)

rity; these fine hairs cover the upper back, arms, and forehead. The subcutaneous layer in premature infants is often edematous because of an excess of cutaneous water and sodium (Fig. 17-2) (see Chapter 13).[69]

Etiology

Term Newborn Skin Variations

Although the basic skin structures are the same in all term newborns without dermatologic disease, there may be cutaneous variations seen on physical examination. These variations (Table 17-1) are not considered pathologic, but it is useful for clinicians

to know them, since many parents will ask the significance of physical variations as they examine their newborn.

Physiologic and Anatomic Differences in Premature Skin

There are, however, developmental differences in skin physiology and anatomy in premature infants. In this section these differences are discussed, and implications for care are identified.

Underdevelopment of the Stratum Corneum

The stratum corneum, the nonliving layer of the epidermis that is responsible for controlling evapo-

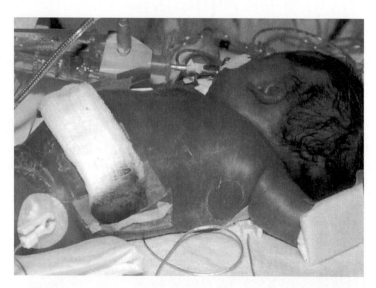

Figure 17-2   Edema in a premature infant caused by excess cutaneous water and sodium.

Table 17-1
Normal Variations of Term Newborn Skin

Linea nigra	Line of increased pigmentation from umbilicus to genitalia
Mongolian spots	Irregular, blue-gray, bruise-like spots
	Usually seen over sacrum and buttocks, may extend over back and shoulders
	Caused by pigmented cells in dermis
	Most common in infants with darker pigmentation
Lanugo	Fine, downy hair over back, shoulders, and face
	Shed at 32 to 36 weeks' gestation
Milia	White, pinhead-sized bumps over chin, cheeks, nose, and forehead
	Tiny, epidermal cysts
	If on palate, called Epstein's pearls
Miliaria	Caused by retention of sweat from edema in stratum corneum that blocks sweat glands
	Most common is rubra (prickly pear), but there are clear versions as well
Harlequin sign	Color of one half of body turns deep red while the other half is pale
	Caused by immature autoregulation of blood flow
Vernix caseosa	Gray-white, cheesey substance that protects fetal skin in utero
	Gradually diminishes near term
Cutis marmorata	Mottling caused by vasomotor immaturity
Erythema toxicum	Small, firm white or yellow pustules with erythematous margin
neonatorum	Most often seen on trunk, arms, and perineal area
	Benign condition seen in 30% to 70% of newborns
Acne neonatorum	Acne-like rash seen in newborns at several weeks of age
	Caused by stimulation of sebaceous glands by maternal hormones
	More common in males
	Instruct care givers not to use creams, lotion, or ointments since they can worsen the rash
Transient neonatal	Resembles miliaria but present at birth
pustular melanosis	Most frequently found on face, palms of hands, soles of feet
	Not infectious or contagious
Cafe au lait spots	Irregularly shaped oval lesions
	If large size (>4 × 6 cm), or if greater than 6 in number, associated with neurofibromatosis

rative heat loss and transepidermal water loss (TEWL), contains 10 to 20 layers in adults and term infants. **Premature infants have fewer layers of stratum corneum depending on their gestational age; at less than 30 weeks, it may contain only 2 to 3 layers (Fig. 17-3), and the extremely premature infants less than 24 weeks may have virtually no stratum corneum.**[31,57] Another function of the stratum corneum, protection against toxins and in-

fectious agents such as bacteria and viruses, is minimal in premature infants, leaving them vulnerable to transcutaneously transmitted infections and toxicity from topically applied substances.

The transition from the aquatic, intrauterine environment to the atmospheric, external environment has been thought to result in accelerated maturation of the stratum corneum and more mature function after the first 10 to 14 days of

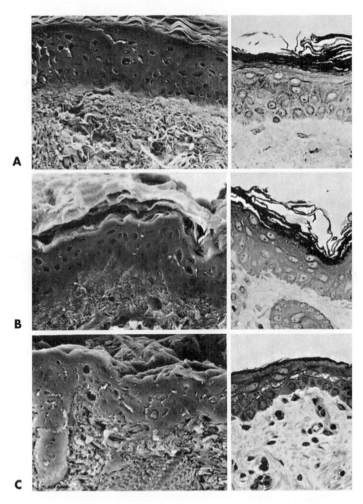

Figure 17-3   Photomicrograph of stratum corneum in adult (**A**), term newborn (**B**), and premature infant (**C**) of 28-week's gestation. Note fewer layers of stratum corneum in premature. (From Holbrook KA: A histological comparison of infant and adult skin. In Maibach HI, Boisits EK, editors: *Neonatal skin: structure and function,* New York, 1982, Marcel Dekker.)

life.[24,30] However, other authors cite a slower process in premature infants less than 27 weeks' gestation, with rates of TEWL nearly double adult levels even at 28 days of life.[66] Our own research,[36] involving daily TEWL and impedance spectroscopy measurements of the thickness of the stratum corneum, found that adult levels of maturation were evident at 30 to 32 weeks postconceptional age regardless of the postnatal age. Thus the maturation process can take as long as 8 weeks in an infant of 23 weeks' gestation, or 3 weeks in an infant of 28 weeks' gestation.

Dermal Instability

Collagen deposition in the dermis increases with advancing gestational age and results in less edema. Thus extremely premature infants tend to become more edematous because they have less collagen and fewer elastin fibers in the dermis.[20] They may be prone to more necrotic injury because edema in the dermis reduces blood flow, and they may need protection from pressure and ischemic injury including routine turning and the use of surfaces to minimize pressure points such as water beds and gelled mattresses or pads.

Diminished Cohesion between Epidermis and Dermis

Numerous fibrils connect the epidermis to the dermis at the epidermodermal junction. These fibrils are more widely spaced and fewer in number in the premature infant[31] (Fig. 17-4) but become stronger with advancing gestational and postnatal age. Genetically abnormal fibrils at this junction result in the dermatologic disorder epidermolysis bullosa, a blistering skin condition that occurs with

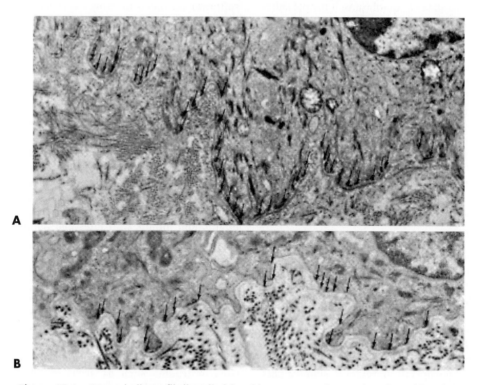

Figure 17-4 Arrows indicate fibrils called hemidesmosomes, that anchor the epidermis to the dermis. They are fewer in number and more widely spaced in the premature infant (**B**). (From Holbrook KA: A histological comparison of infant and adult skin. In Maibach HI, Boisits EK, editors: *Neonatal skin: structure and function*, New York, 1982, Marcel Dekker.)

even minimal trauma. **Premature infants are also prone to blistering from injury, although this decreases as they mature. This diminished cohesion places premature infants at risk for injury from adhesive removal as well. Particularly if extremely aggressive adhesives are used, there may be a stronger bond of the adhesive to the epidermis than of the epidermis to the dermis, and epidermal stripping may result during adhesive removal.**

Skin pH

The ability of the skin surface to form and maintain an acid surface is a function of various chemical and biologic processes. Acid skin surfaces with a pH less than 5 have been documented extensively in adults and children.[6] This "acid mantle" has protective qualities against some pathogens and other microorganisms. Since microbial colonization begins with delivery, the acid skin surface helps to keep a state of equilibrium; if the pH shifts from acidic to neutral, there may be an increase in total numbers of bacteria and a shift in species.[67] There may also be an increase in TEWL when skin pH rises.[73]

Term newborns are born with a relatively alkaline skin surface, measuring a mean pH of 6.34. Within 4 days the pH declines to a mean of 4.95. Skin pH measurements have been reported in premature infants of varying gestational ages and found to have a mean pH of 5.04 on the ninth day of life.[6] Bathing and other skin care practices alter skin pH; it may take an hour or longer to regenerate the acid mantle after bathing with an alkaline soap.[59]

Nutritional Deficiencies

Both fat and zinc accumulate in the fetus during the last trimester of pregnancy. Since these nutritional components are necessary for maintaining an intact, healthy skin surface, premature infants born before the last trimester may develop skin problems caused by deficiencies in either of these nutrients. Problems may also be seen in infants who are unable to receive adequate enteral nutrition unless appropriate parenteral supplements are employed.

EFA deficiency can be seen in premature and postmature infants because of decreased fat stores (see Chapter 15). In this condition, there is a superficial scaling and occasionally desquamation and irritation in the neck, groin, or perianal areas. There may be decreased serum levels of EFAs, thrombocytopenia, and impaired platelet aggregation since EFAs are needed to promote platelet function.[26]

Providing adequate EFA prevents skin manifestations of EFA deficiency. In infants who are receiving small amounts of enteral nutrients or none at all, administration of IV lipid solutions at a total dose of 0.5 g/kg/day can prevent EFA deficiency (see Chapter 16). Once EFA deficiency occurs, IV lipids can reverse the process in 1 to 2 weeks. Dietary replacement takes longer and is effective only if gastrointestinal function is good. **Topical therapy with sunflower seed oil rich in linoleic acid promotes transdermal absorption of EFA and raises serum levels but is variable in the rate of absorption. In a study of topical application, safflower oil failed to show improvement in EFA deficiency.[32]**

Zinc, an essential trace mineral, is a cofactor in many areas of metabolism, including lymphocyte transformation and metabolism of protein, nucleic acids, and mucopolysaccharides of skin and subcutaneous tissues, and is required for normal wound healing.[21] Two thirds of the transfer of zinc from mother to fetus occurs in the last 10 weeks of pregnancy.

Zinc deficiency occurs when there are abnormal losses of zinc in stool or urine, when there are low or absent stores as in premature birth, or during increased demands such as during rapid growth, stress, or tissue healing. Thus premature infants and infants with intestinal pathology (including chronic diarrhea, short bowel syndrome, intestinal diversions such as ileostomy, or intestinal resection) are at increased risk for zinc deficiency. In addition, any infant receiving total parenteral nutrition should receive trace minerals to prevent zinc deficiency (see Chapter 16).

Symptoms of zinc deficiency include erythematous, scaly skin and excoriations of the groin and perianal areas, neck folds, circumoral area, and at sites of trauma such as areas of adhesive removal.[23] Other clinical features include lethargy, poor growth; alopecia, and diarrhea. Serum zinc levels of less than 68 μg/ml accompanied by a low alkaline phosphatase and clinical symptoms are diagnostic of zinc deficiency. Prevention of zinc deficiency for infants on total parenteral nutrition includes zinc supplementation with 150 to 350 µg/kg/day.[77] Premature infants have also been reported to develop zinc deficiency while fed breastmilk; they may require an oral zinc sulfate supplement.[76]

Prevention

During daily skin care practices such as bathing, lubrication, antimicrobial skin disinfection, and adhesive removal, the skin of newborns is at risk for trauma or disruption of normal barrier function. This is particularly true of newborns in the neonatal intensive care nursery, who may be critically ill, require surgery, or born prematurely. In this section, basic skin care practices are reviewed in terms of impact on skin integrity, and recommendations are presented for preventing trauma, protecting immature barrier function, and promoting skin integrity.

Bathing

Among the purposes of bathing the newborn are removal of waste materials, general aesthetics, and reduction of microbial colonization. Studies of antimicrobial bathing practices have shown that, although hexachlorophene does reduce numbers of *Staphylococcus aureus* strains, there is toxicity associated with absorption, especially in premature infants.[2,39,64] Chlorhexidine, another antimicrobial soap, has proven effective in reducing colonization for up to 4 hours[18] but is also absorbed.[17] Although toxicity has not been identified, many nurseries do not use chlorhexidine for routine bathing because of the potential risk.

Other soaps selected for routine bathing of newborns include regular soaps such as adults use, neutral pH soaps (Neutrogena, Dove), superfatted soaps (Basis, Oilatum), and "baby soaps" (Johnson & Johnson). Some use deodorant soaps (Dial) since they contain antimicrobial properties.[56] All soaps are at least mildly irritating and drying to skin surfaces,[27,67,70,71] and the degree to which the skin is irritated depends on the length of contact and the frequency of bathing. In addition, although not extensively studied, there is concern about bathing disrupting the normal skin surface pH.

The wisest route is to select soaps that have a neutral pH and minimal dyes and perfumes to reduce risk of future sensitization to these products and to bathe only 2 to 3 times per week. The use of superfatted soaps is probably not necessary unless an underlying dermatologic disorder is diagnosed. For extremely premature infants (<26 weeks' gestation) plain water may be the safest choice. When clinically feasible, immersion bathing may be beneficial. Immersion bathing has been described as more soothing to the infant from a developmental perspective[1] and may have positive effects on skin integrity.[50]

Emollients

Preventing dry, scaly skin involves improving the hydration of the stratum corneum. The skin surface of term newborns is drier than that of adults but becomes gradually better hydrated as the eccrine sweat glands mature during the first year of life.[54,63] Products used to counteract dryness are called moisturizers, emollients, or lubricants. Common emollients include mineral oils, petrolatum, and lanolin and its derivatives. Emollients are sometimes divided into oil-in-water or water-in-oil emulsions.

Recent studies of emollients in premature infants offer encouraging information about how routine application may improve skin integrity. In one report,[40] premature infants 29 to 36 weeks' gestation were treated with Eucerin cream daily and had less dermatitis as measured by a visual grading scale but no differences in TEWL as measured by evaporimeter. In a later study, premature infants of both younger gestation and postnatal age were treated with Aquaphor ointment, a water miscible oil-in-water preparation that contains neither dyes nor perfumes. In this study, there was improvement in both TEWL and visual scale dermatitis. In addition, both studies obtained cutaneous cultures and found no increase in bacterial or fungal colonization on skin treated with emollients. There was also a statistically significant smaller number of treated infants with positive blood or cerebrospinal fluid cultures compared with controls.[58]

Routine use of an emollient such as Aquaphor ointment can prevent excessive drying, skin cracking, and fissures. Avoiding products with perfumes or dyes is prudent since these can be absorbed and are potential contact irritants.[14]

Skin Disinfection Solutions

Decontamination of skin before invasive procedures such as venipuncture and placement of umbilical catheters and chest tubes is common practice in neonatal intensive care nurseries. However, there are anecdotal reports of skin injury including blistering, burns, and sloughing from both isopropyl alcohol and povidone-iodine use in premature infants.[29,65] There have also been case reports of high iodine levels, iodine goiter, and hypothyroidism associated with povidone-iodine use in premature infants.[15,35,60] Two prospective studies of routine povidone-iodine use, one in an intensive care nursery[68] and another in presurgical skin preparation of infants under 3 months of age,[53] also found alterations in iodine levels and potential thyroid effects from povidone-iodine exposure.

Another important aspect of skin disinfection is the efficacy of the solutions used. A study comparing isopropyl alcohol with povidone-iodine found less microbial colonization with povidone-iodine.[16] A comparison of povidone-iodine with chlorhexidine in premature infants during IV catheter placement found no differences;[49] however, the number of infants was small.[12] The authors recommended longer periods of cleansing (>30 seconds) or two consecutive cleansings for maximum reductions of colonization. In adults with central venous catheters, a comparison of isopropyl alcohol, povidone-iodine, and chlorhexidine for disinfection of 668 insertion sites during routine dressing changes showed chlorhexidine to be more effective.[48] In addition, there was residual antibacterial activity from chlorhexidine that lasted for several hours after application.

Recommended skin disinfection practices for newborns include using povidone-iodine or chlorhexidine solutions (although there is not a commercially available chlorhexidine product available in pledget form in the USA). The solutions should be applied and allowed to dry for at least 30 seconds before the procedure. Any solution should then be completely removed using sterile water to

prevent any further absorption. Disinfection with isopropyl alcohol is questionable in the neonatal intensive care nursery since it is less efficacious than either povidone-iodine or chlorhexidine and can be irritating and drying to skin surfaces.

Adhesive Application and Removal

One of the most common practices in the neonatal intensive care nursery is the application and removal of adhesives that secure endotracheal tubes, IV devices, and monitoring probes and electrodes. Using the measurement of TEWL to determine reduced barrier function and skin disruption, changes are seen in adults after 10 consecutive removals of adhesive tape[45] and after one removal of adhesive tape in a premature infant.[30]

Solvents are sometimes used to prevent discomfort and skin disruption from adhesive removal. However, the danger of toxicity from such products (Whisk, Dermasol, Detachol) remains, especially in premature infants with their underdeveloped stratum corneum and increased skin permeability. There has also been at least one report of a toxic epidermal necrosis resulting from the use of a solvent in a premature infant.[34] Other substances such as mineral oil may be helpful in removing adhesives but cannot be used if the site must be used again for reapplication of adhesives, such as with the retaping of an endotracheal tube.

Skin barriers include liquid preparations such as Benzoin, Mastisol, or plastic polymers, which promote adherence and protect skin from adhesives. Both Benzoin and Mastisol, unfortunately, may create a stronger bond between adhesive and epidermis than the fragile cohesion of the epidermis to the dermis; when removed, epidermal stripping may result. Plastic polymers have been studied and are reported to reduce skin trauma.[25] There is a nonalcohol version now commercially available (3M) that is less irritating to skin surfaces of adults; no studies are yet available on its use in infants or newborns.

Skin barriers such as karaya rings and pectin products have been used to protect the peristomal skin in adult ostomy patients. A comparison of regular adhesive electrodes and karaya electrodes found less skin disruption, as measured by TEWL, from the karaya electrodes in premature infants.[13] However, some premature infants developed skin irritation from the karaya electrodes, and they are no longer available. Pectin barriers (Hollihesive, Duoderm, Comfeel) have been used beneath adhesives in premature infants and are reported as leaving less visible skin trauma when removed.[22,47,52] However, more recently a controlled trial of pectin barrier (Hollihesive), plastic tape (Transpore), and hydrophilic gelled adhesive found that significant skin disruption, as measured by TEWL and visual inspection, occurred after removal of both the pectin barrier and plastic tape.[46] Since the adhesives were left in place 24 hours before removal in this study, there may be a time effect of peak adhesive aggressiveness that was reached. It is interesting to note that significant changes were identified after a single adhesive removal in all three weight groups studied (<1000 g, 1001 to 1500 g, >1501 g), indicating that even larger premature infants are at risk for skin injury from tape removal.

Prevention of skin trauma from adhesive removal includes minimizing tape use when possible by using smaller pieces, backing the adhesive with cotton, and delaying tape removal until at least 24 hours after application. Pectin barriers may prove helpful because they mold and adhere well to body contours and often stay better in moist conditions. As with tape, pectin barriers should not be removed until more than 24 hours after application if possible. Soft gauze wraps to secure probes and the use of hydrophilic gelled adhesives for ECG electrodes and tape are helpful. Adhesives should be removed with warm water and cotton balls slowly and carefully. Mineral oil or an emollient may facilitate adhesive removal if reapplication of adhesives at the site of removal is not necessary.

Data Collection

History

The gestational age and postnatal age of neonates in the NICU are both important considerations for determining appropriate skin care practices. Premature infants of lower gestational ages have underdeveloped skin layers and function. With advancing postnatal age and maturation, skin integrity and skin barrier function results.

Reviewing the maternal history for any derma-

tologic diseases is also important. Many of the most severe skin diseases such as forms of congenital ichthyosis or epidermolysis bullosa are inherited disorders; a positive family history will alert the clinician to the potential for developing these rare disorders.[3,33,42,44]

Signs and Symptoms

A thorough examination of all skin surfaces on a daily basis will reveal the state of skin integrity for neonates in the NICU. In the first week of life in ELBW infants (<30 weeks, <1000 g), there may be problems with thermoregulation (see Chapter 6) and dehydration (see Chapter 13) because of the large evaporative heat losses and transepidermal water losses through the immature stratum corneum. Early signs such as skin abrasions or small excoriations may call for either diagnostic or treatment procedures.

Laboratory Data

With the many skin excoriations in both small and large neonates that result from traumatic events such as adhesive removal or pressure necrosis, there is the potential for infection through this portal of entry in the skin. In VLBW infants, it may be useful to obtain a skin culture, gram stain, or KOH prep[4,5] for early detection of microorganisms that can lead to systemic illness in these immune compromised patients. A skin surface culture is helpful if the skin breakdown cannot be traced to a traumatic injury, since the etiology of the breakdown is often linked to infection, especially with fungal infections[62] or Staphylococcal scalded skin syndrome. A more comprehensive workup for infection may be indicated if there is evidence of clinical deterioration in infants with extensive skin breakdown (see Chapter 21).

Treatment

Skin Excoriations

Skin excoriations are cleansed with warmed sterile water and may be covered with either an ointment or a dressing. Ointments are sometimes useful because of their antibacterial or antifungal properties and also because covering the wound with a semiocclusive layer promotes healing by facilitating the migration of epithelial cells across the surface. Only if extensive bacterial colonization is suspected, Polysporin, Bacitracin, or Bactroban ointment is used sparingly, every 8 to 12 hours. Many dermatologists recommend against the use of Neosporin because of the potential for developing later sensitization to this ointment. Overuse of antimicrobial ointments can be a problem in promoting more resistant strains of bacteria. If fungal infection is suspected, Nystatin ointment is used and it can also be applied to surrounding intact skin to prevent extension of the infection. In general, ointments are preferable to creams in this application, because of better adherence and healing properties.

Other types of dressings used to treat excoriations involving the epidermal and dermal layers include transparent adhesive dressings (OpSite, Tegaderm, Bioclusive). These products are made from a polyurethane film backed with adhesive that is impermeable to water and bacteria but allows air flow. There must be a rim of intact skin around the wound to attach the dressing. Uses include wound care, dressings for IV devices including central venous lines and percutaneous silastic catheters, and prevention of friction injuries to areas such as the knees or sacrum.

When used for wound care, transparent adhesive dressing promotes "moist healing" that allows the rapid migration of epithelial cells across the site. These dressings should only be used on "clean wounds" (uninfected) since bacteria and fungus can proliferate under the dressing. When placed over a clean wound, there is often a serous or milky exudate that forms that is composed of leukocytes that actually aid in the prevention of infection. The dressings can be left in place for days at a time or until they become loose. Removing and reattaching the dressings on a daily basis is not recommended since the adhesive can injure the intact skin around the wound and further impede healing.

Another use of transparent adhesive dressings in the NICU is the prevention of excessive TEWL in premature infants.[11,38,51,72] TEWL, as measured by an evaporimeter, can be reduced by as much as 50% by the creation of this "second skin." In one study,[51] a nonadhesive transparent dressing (not commercially available) was used, and the skin un-

der the dressing not only had a lower TEWL while covered but actually had lower TEWL when removed, suggesting that perhaps a faster maturation of the skin barrier function had occurred. Cultures were obtained both on covered and uncovered skin and showed no increase in either bacterial or fungal colonization under the dressings. Unfortunately, nonadhesive dressings are not available, and the use of transparent dressings remains difficult, particularly when the dressings must be removed in less than 2 weeks since a significant amount of skin trauma will occur with dressing removal. Alternative ways to reduce TEWL in VLBW infants can be used, including double-walled incubators, heated humidity (see Chapter 6), and emollients such as Aquaphor ointment.

Other strategies to treat excoriations include frequent irrigation with sterile normal saline or half-normal saline solutions using a 20 to 30 ml syringe and a 20-gauge blunt needle or Teflon catheter. This technique is effective in flushing out debris and dead tissue from an infected or "dirty" wound, allowing a better surface for healing. The moistening of tissue every 4 to 6 hours aids in the healing process since drying of tissue actually impedes the migration of cells. Once the wound surface is clear, other dressings or ointments can be used.

Dressings used in wound management include hydrophilic dressings (Vigilon) and hydrocolloid, pectin dressings (Duoderm), both of which promote moist healing. Hydrophilic dressings can be used after irrigation of the wound and in conjunction with either antibacterial or antifungal ointment if the wound is infected. These dressings must be changed every 8 to 12 hours since they can dry out. There is no adhesive that attaches these dressings. It is best to avoid placing hydrophilic dressings on intact skin surfaces, because they can macerate the skin and actually reduce barrier function. Hydrocolloid dressings are used over uninfected wounds and can be left in place for 5 to 7 days while healing takes place.

Surgical wounds that open or dehisce are infrequent but require expert wound management. Nutrition is often a part of the process in getting these wounds to heal, as is the prevention of infection.[28] Often the surgeon or enterostomal therapist will design the appropriate wound management program for these situations.

Intravenous Extravasations

Prevention of tissue injury from IV extravasations includes taping IV devices with transparent dressings or plastic tape so that the insertions site is clearly visible (Fig. 17-5) and observing the site with appropriate documentation every hour. If the IV device is placed in a limb, the tape that secures it to the rigid board should be placed loosely over a bony prominence, such as the elbow or knee, and not on skin in close proximity to the insertion site. This allows extravasated fluid and medications to expand over a larger surface and not remain in a small, constricted area that can result in greater tissue injury. It may be wise to avoid poorly perfused extremities in favor of scalp veins, except the forehead. Using central venous lines such as percutaneous catheters to infuse highly irritating solutions and medications is also recommended. Many nurseries limit the glucose concentrations in peripheral lines to 12.5% and the amino acid concentrations to 2%; calcium and potassium concentrations are also more dilute than those used in central lines.

If IV fluid has extravasated into surrounding tissue, the IV device should be removed and the extremity elevated. Use of moisture or heat is not recommended since the tissue is vulnerable at this point to further injury from moist heat.[9] Hyaluronidase (Wydase) can be extremely helpful if administered within an hour of extravasation (see Chapter 9). This medication is an enzyme that causes a breakdown of interstitial barrier and allows the diffusion of the extravasated fluid over a larger area to prevent tissue necrosis.[41,74] The dose of hyaluronidase is 15 units diluted to 1 ml, although in one study using an animal model, 150 units was used without harmful effects.[41] It is administered in five injections, inserted subcutaneously around the periphery of the extravasation site (Fig. 17-6), and should be administered within 1 to 2 hours of the extravasation. Extravasations that may benefit from the administration of hyaluronidase include any with evidence of blanching, discoloration, blistering, or extravasations involving hypertonic or calcium-containing solutions, even if the site appears relatively undisturbed. Calcium-containing solutions may cause deep tissue injury even when epidermal tissues are not involved.

Hyaluronidase is not recommended in the ex-

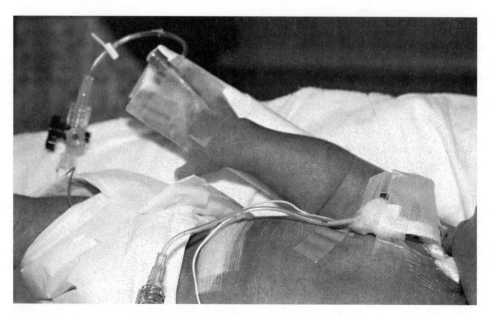

Figure 17-5 Appropriately taped peripheral intravenous catheter with insertion site clearly visible and arm anchored at joint to prevent obstruction of venous return.

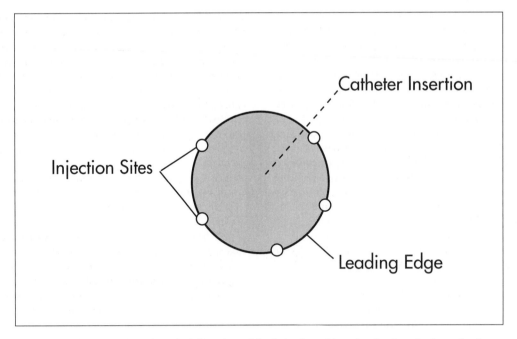

Figure 17-6 Technique for administration of both hyaluronidase (Wydase) and phentolamine (Regitine). Total volume of 1 ml is administered at five sites subcutaneously (0.2 ml each) around the periphery of the intravenous extravasation.

travasation of vasoconstrictive medications such as dopamine since the vasoconstriction could extend with its use. Phentolamine (Regitine) is used in this case, because it directly counteracts the action of dopamine. The method of delivery is the same as hyalurondiase, with the total dose (0.5 mg) diluted to 1 ml, injected in 5 sites subcutaneously around the periphery of the extravasation.[75]

When tissue injury occurs after extravasation, the use of antibacterial ointment is helpful. For deeper wounds, irrigation in conjunction with either ointments or dressings may be used. In the most severe cases, surgical or plastic surgical consultation is necessary, and skin grafts may be required. In all cases of tissue injury, open wounds should be considered a portal of entry for infection, and topical or systemic treatment should be considered.

Diaper Dermatitis

Diaper dermatitis, which has a multitude of causes in infants, affects the perineum, groin, thighs, buttocks, and anal regions. The underlying skin condition of the infant contributes to the degree of diaper dermatitis that occurs.

Another factor that influences the development of diaper dermatitis is the degree of wetness of the skin, because skin that is moist and macerated becomes more permeable and susceptible to injury.[7] In addition, skin that is moisture laden becomes more heavily colonized with microorganisms. Skin pH also has an effect; when exposed to urine, the pH can rise from acid to alkaline ranges and become more vulnerable to injury and penetration by microorganisms.[8,43] The alkaline pH can also activate enzymes found in stool, protease, and lipase, which break down protein and fat, the building blocks of the stratum corneum.[10] This is the primary mechanism for direct contact dermatitis from exposure to stool, the most common form of diaper dermatitis.

Strategies for the prevention of diaper dermatitis include maintaining a skin surface that is dry and has a normal (acidic) skin pH. Super-absorbent gelled diapers have been introduced that keep

skin surfaces dry by "wicking" the moisture away from the skin.[12,19] Use of powders is discouraged because of the risk of inhalation of particles into the respiratory tract.

After skin injury from diaper dermatitis has occurred, protection of injured skin to prevent reinjury is the primary goal of treatment. Generous application of protective skin barriers that contain zinc oxide can prevent further injury while allowing skin to heal. Keeping skin open to air may not be effective since there may be reinjury with fecal contact to the already impaired tissue as well as the fact that dryness is counterproductive to healing. It is not necessary or desirable to completely remove skin barriers with diaper changes since this may disrupt healing tissue. Instead, remove as much waste material as possible, and reapply the barrier generously to the affected areas with each diaper change.

If Candida albicans is involved in the diaper dermatitis, it is necessary to use an antifungal ointment or cream. In older infants (>3 months of age), it may be helpful to add a steroid cream to reduce inflammation; in younger and premature infants, there is concern over absorption. Antifungal preparations include Mycostatin, miconazole, chlortrimazole, and ketoconozale in ointment, cream, or powder forms. If the dermatitis is both fungal and a contact irritant dermatitis, it may be necessary to layer the ointment with the antifungal preparation. In this case, Mycostatin powder is preferable since it causes a dry surface on which the barrier cream can adhere.

Occasionally, infants may experience extremely severe diaper dermatitis from intestinal malabsorption syndromes or if there is constant dribbling of stool, as in the case of infants with spina bifida. In the case of malabsorption, the stool may have a pH that is higher than normal because of rapid transit from the small bowel, and there may be significant amounts of undigested carbohydrates and stool enzymes, as well as increased stool frequency. Severe diaper dermatitis in this case can be a symptom of more severe nutritional deficiency, or even dehydration, and needs thorough medical evaluation. Stools in these infants should be regularly tested for pH, carbohydrates, and occult blood in addition to measuring their number and total volume.

While optimal nutritional therapy is being addressed with special diets or parenteral nutrition, skin protection from injury should be initiated. Products such as pectin-based powders or pectin paste without alcohol (such as Ilex nonalcohol pectin paste) are often better barriers for these infants than are zinc oxide preparations. The skin should be thoroughly cleansed before a very thick application of the pectin paste. It is then necessary to apply a greasy ointment over this, because the pectin-based paste may adhere to the diaper. When the infant has a stool, it is not necessary to completely remove the barrier paste; the stool can be wiped away as much as possible before reapplying the thick paste barrier. The skin will heal under this protective covering as long as it is protected from reinjury. If fungal infection is a component of the dermatitis, antifungal therapy must be instituted in addition to the protective barriers. A thin paste of Mycostatin powder can be applied to the clean skin surface and allowed to dry before application of the pectin-based paste.

Complications

The improper handling of newborn skin (and injudicious use of products) can cause damage, prevent healing, and interfere with normal maturation processes. Compromised skin integrity can lead to infection, pain and discomfort, and diversion of calories for tissue repair. Other dangers include toxicity from topically applied substances that are readily absorbed by small infants with large surface-area/body-weight ratio as well as immature renal and hepatic function that cannot detoxify chemicals readily.

Injury from infiltrated IV solutions can cause skin injury and, occasionally, deep tissue necrosis with both muscle and nerve damage. Factors that increase the risk of injury from IV extravasations include length of time between extravasation and treatment; hypertonic solutions, such as those with high calcium, potassium, amino acids or glucose solutions; medications such as nafcillin that are irritating to veins; and the use of mechanical pumps for infusions. There may be an added risk for injury in patients with poor perfusion to extremities and in limbs that have been secured with restricting adhesives that obstruct venous return.

If the epidermis has been injured, it can easily

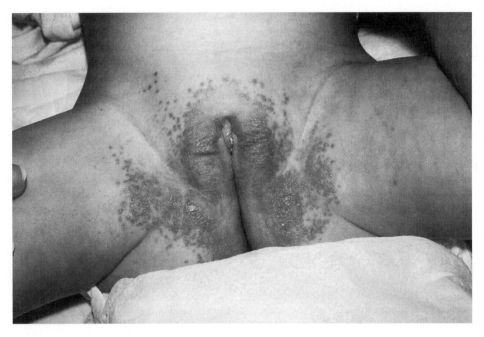

Figure 17-7   Diaper dermatitis caused by candida albicans infection. Red pustular satellite lesions extend into periphery.

become a portal of entry for infection. Thus a contact irritant diaper dermatitis can progress to a fungal or staphylococcal infection. *Staphylococcus aureus* can cause pustule formation at hair follicles and be a complication of diaper dermatitis. The mechanism for fungal diaper dermatitis is still debated. Some researchers believe that Candida albicans is a secondary invasion to skin that has been previously injured, whereas others see this organism as a primary cause of skin disruption.[61]

Candida albicans diaper dermatitis causes an intense inflammation that is bright red and sharply demarginated in the inguinal folds, buttocks, thighs, abdomen, and genitalia, often with satellite lesions that extend the rash over the trunk (Fig. 17-7). Candida albicans can be harbored in the gastrointestinal tract, necessitating oral therapy if lesions are found in the mouth.

Parent Teaching

It is the responsibility of professionals to teach parents informally during care giving procedures such as bathing and diaper changes and to prepare written materials regarding appropriate skin care practices for their infant after discharge from the NICU. Helping parents to understand that minimal use of skin care products is optimal and may prevent later contact sensitization to chemicals. It is also extremely useful to educate parents about the mechanisms that are involved in diaper dermatitis so that prevention is stressed and appropriate interventions are selected depending on the underlying cause.

Developmental differences in the anatomy and physiology of neonatal skin affect skin integrity for term and premature infants in the NICU. Prevention is the primary focus of care, and decisions about the best way to provide basic skin care and hygiene based on current research are essential for care providers, both professionals and parents.

References

1. Als H et al: Individualized behavioral and environmental care for the very low birth weight preterm infant at high risk for bronchopulmonary dysplasia: neonatal intensive care unit and developmental outcome, *Pediatrics* 78:1123, 1986.

2. American Academy of Pediatrics: *Standards and recommendations for hospital care of newborn infants,* Evanston, Ill, 1977, American Academy of Pediatrics.

3. Artnak K, Moore L, Clements C: Epidermolysis bullosa: an inherited skin disorder, *Am J Nurs* 81(10):1837, 1981.

4. Baley J, Silverman R: Systemic candidiasis: cutaneous manifestations in low birth weight infants, *Pediatrics* 82(2):211, 1988.

5. Baley J et al: Fungal colonization in the very low birth weight infant, *Pediatrics* 78:225, 1986

6. Behrendt H, Green M: *Patterns of skin pH from birth through adolescence,* Springfield, Ill, 1971, Charles C Thomas.

7. Berg R: Etiologic factors in diaper dermatitis: a model for development of improved diapers, *Pediatrician* 14(1):27, 1987.

8. Berg R, Buckingham K, Stewart R: Etiologic factors in diaper dermatitis: the role of urine, *Pediatr Dermatol* 3:102, 1986.

9. Brown A, Hoelzer D, Piercy S: Skin necrosis from extravasation of intravenous fluids in children, *Plast Reconstr Surg* 64(2):145, 1979.

10. Buckingham K, Berg R: Etiologic factors in diaper dermatitis: the role of feces, *Pediatr Dermatol* 3:107, 1986.

11. Bustamante S, Steslow J: Use of a transparent adhesive dressing in very low birthweight infants, *J Perinatol* 9(2):165, 1989.

12. Campbell R et al: Clinical studies with disposable diapers containing absorbent gelling materials: evaluation on infant skin condition, *J Am Acad Dermatol* 17:978, 1987.

13. Cartlidge P, Rutter N: Karaya gum electrocardiographic electrodes for preterm infants, *Arch Dis Child* 62:1281, 1987.

14. Cetta F, Lambert G, Ros S: Newborn chemical exposure from over-the-counter skin care products, *Clin Pediatr* 30:286, 1991.

15. Chabrolle J, Rossier A: Goiter and hypothyroidism in the newborn after cutaneous absorption of iodine, *Arch Dis Child* 53:495, 1978.

16. Choudhuri J et al: Efficacy of skin sterilization for a venipuncture with the use of commercially available alcohol or iodine pads, *Am J Infect Control* 18:82, 1990.

17. Cowen J, Ellis S, McAinsh J: Absorption of chlorhexidine from the intact skin of newborn infants, *Arch Dis Child* 54:379, 1979.

18. Davies J, Babb J, Ayliffe A: The effect on the skin flora of bathing with antiseptic solutions, *J Antimicrob Chemother* 3:473, 1977.

19. Davis J et al: Comparison of disposable diapers with fluff absorbent and fluff plus absorbent polymers: effects on skin hydration, skin pH, and diaper dermatitis, *Pediatr Dermatol* 6:102, 1989.

20. Dietel K: Morphological and functional development of the skin. In Stave U, editor: *Perinatal physiology,* New York, 1978, Plenum Press.

21. Dixon A: Think zinc, *Neonat Net* 5(4):29, 1987.

22. Dollison E, Beckstrand J: Adhesive tape vs. pectin-based barrier use in preterm infants, *Neonat Net* 14:35, 1995.

23. Esterly N, Spraker M: Neonatal skin problems. In Moschella S, Hurley H, editors: *Dermatology,* vol 2, ed 2, Philadelphia, 1985, WB Saunders.

24. Evans N, Rutter N: Development of the epidermis in the newborn, *Biol Neonate* 49:74, 1986.

25. Evans N, Rutter N: Reduction of skin damage from transcutaneous oxygen electrodes using a spray on dressing, *Arch Dis Child* 61:881, 1986.

26. Friedman Z: Essential fatty acids revisited, *Am J Dis Child* 134:397, 1980.

27. Frosch PJ, Kligman AM: The soap chamber test, *J Am Acad Dermatol* 1:35, 1979.

28. Garvin G: Wound healing in pediatrics, *Nurs Clin North Am* 25(1):181, 1990.

29. Harpin V, Rutter N: Percutaneous alcohol absorption and skin necrosis in a preterm infant, *Arch Dis Child* 57(6):825, 1982.

30. Harpin V, Rutter N: Barrier properties of the newborn infant's skin, *J Pediatr* 102(3):419, 1983.

31. Holbrook KA: A histological comparison of infant and adult skin. In Maibach HI, Boisits EK, editors: *Neonatal skin: structure and function,* New York, 1982, Marcel Dekker.

32. Hunt C et al: Essential fatty acid deficiency in neonates: inability to reverse deficiency by topical applications of EFA-rich oil, *J Pediatr* 92:603, 1978.

33. Hymes D: Epidermolysis bullosa in the neonate, *Neonat Net* 1(4):36, 1983.

34. Ittman P, Bozynski ME: Toxic epidermal necrolysis in a newborn infant after exposure to adhesive remover, *J Perinatol* 13:476, 1993.

35. Jackson H, Sutherland R: Effect of povidine-iodine on neonatal thyroid function, *Lancet* 2:992, 1981.

36. Kalia Y, Nonato L, Lund C: *Development of the stratum corneum of extremely low birth weight infants as measured by transepidermal water loss and impedance spectroscopy techniques* 1996, (unpublished).

37. Klaus MH, Fanaroff AA: *Yearbook of perinatal/neonatal medicine,* Chicago, 1987, Year Book.

38. Knauth A et al: Semipermeable polyurethane membrane as an artificial skin for the premature neonate, *Pediatrics* 83:945, 1989.

39. Kopelman AE: Cutaneous absorption of hexachlorophene in low-birth weight infants, *J Pediatr* 82:972, 1973.

40. Lane A, Drost S: Effects of repeated application of emollient cream to premature neonates' skin, *Pediatrics* 92:415, 1993.

41. Laurie S et al: Intravenous extravasation injuries: the effectiveness of hyaluronidase in their treatment, *Ann Plast Surg* 13(3):191, 1984.

42. Lawlor F: Progress of a Harlequin fetus to nonbullous ichthyosiform erythroderma, *Pediatrics* 82:870, 1988.

43. Leydon J: Urinary ammonia and ammonia-producing micro-organisms in infants with and without diaper dermatitis, *Arch Dermatol* 113:1678, 1977.

44. Lin A, Carter DM: Epidermolysis bullosa: when the skin falls apart, *J Pediatr* 114:349, 1989.

45. Lo J et al: Transepidermal potassium, ion, and water flux across delipidized and cellophane tape-stripped skin, *Dermatologica* 180:66, 1990.

46. Lund C et al: *Comparison of the effects of removal of three adhesives on barrier-function in premature infants,* 1996.

47. Lund C et al: Evaluation of a pectin-based barrier under tape to protect neonatal skin, *J Obstet Gynecol Neonat Nurs* 15(1):39, 1986.

48. Maki D, Ringer M, Alvarado C: Prospective randomized trial povidone-iodine, alcohol, and chlorhexidine for prevention of infection associated with central venous and arterial catheters, *Lancet* 338:339, 1991.

49. Malathi I et al: Skin disinfection in preterm infants, *Arch Dis Child* 69:312, 1993.

50. Malloy-McDonald M: Skin care for high-risk neonates, *J Wound Ostom Cont Nurs* 22:177, 1995.

51. Mancini A et al: Semipermeable dressings improve epidermal barrier function in premature infants, *Pediatr Res* 36:306, 1994.

52. McLean S et al: Three methods of securing endotracheal tubes in neonates: a comparison, *Neonat Net* 11:17, 1992.

53. Mitchell I et al: Transcutaneous iodine absorption in infants undergoing cardiac operation, *Ann Thorac Surg* 52:1138, 1991.

54. Mize M, Vila-Coro A, Prager T: The relationship between postnatal skin maturation and electrical skin impedance, *Arch Dermatol* 125:647, 1989.

55. Moore K: *The developing human*, ed 4, Philadelphia, 1988, WB Saunders.

56. Morelli J, Weston W: Soaps and shampoos in pediatric practice, *Pediatrics* 80:634, 1987.

57. Nonato L, Guy R: *Light and transmission electron microscopy: developmental changes in neonatal skin structure,* 1995.

58. Nopper AJ et al: Topical ointment therapy benefits premature infants, *J Pediatr* 128:660, 1996.

59. Peck S, Botwinick J: The buffering capacity of infants' skin against an alkaline soap and neutral detergent, *J Mt Sinai Hosp* 31:134, 1964.

60. Pyati S et al: Absorption of iodine in the neonate following topical use of povidone-iodine, *J Pediatr* 91(5):825, 1977.

61. Rasmussen J: Classification of diaper dermatitis: an overview, *Pediatrician* 14(1):6, 1987.

62. Rowen J et al: Invasive fungal dermatitis in the <1000-gram neonate *Pediatrics* 95:682, 1995.

63. Saijo S, Tagami H: Dry skin of newborn infants: functional analysis of the stratum corneum, *Pediatr Dermatol* 8:155, 1991.

64. Sarkany I, Arnold L: The effect of single and repeated applications of hexachlorophene on the bacterial flora of the skin of the newborn, *Br J Dermatol* 82:261, 1970.

65. Schick JB, Milstein JM: Burn hazard of isopropyl alcohol in the neonate, *Pediatrics* 68:587, 1981.

66. Sedin G et al: Measurements of transepidermal water loss in newborn infants, *Clin Perinatol* 12:79, 1985.

67. Shalita A:*Principles of infant skin care,* Skillman, NJ, 1981, Johnson & Johnson.

68. Smerdely P, et al: Topical iodine-containing antiseptics and neonatal hypothyroidism in very-low-birthweight infants, *Lancet* 16:661, 1989.

69. Solomon L, Esterly N: Neonatal dermatology. In Schaffer A, editor: *Major problems in clinical pediatrics,* vol 9, Philadelphia, 1973, WB Saunders.

70. Tupker RA, Pinnagoda J, Nater JP: The transient and cumulative effect of sodium lauryl sulphate on the epidermal barrier assessed by transepidermal water loss: interindividual variation, *Acta Derm Venererol* 70:1, 1990.

71. Tupker RA et al: Evaluation of detergent-induced irritant skin reactions by visual scoring and transepidermal water loss measurement, *Dermatol Clin* 8:33, 1990.

72. Vernon H et al: Semipermeable dressing and transepidermal water loss in premature infants, *Pediatrics* 86:357, 1990.

73. Wilhelm K, Maibach H: Factors predisposing to cutaneous irritation, *Dermatol Clin* 8:17, 1990.

74. Zenk K: Management of intravenous extravasations, *Infusion* 5(4):77, 1981.

75. Zenk K, Sills J: Management of dopamine-induced perivascular blanching and extravasation in LBW infants, *J Perinatol* 6(1):82, 1986.

76. Zimmerman A: Acrodermatitis in breast-fed premature infants: evidence for a defect in mammary gland zinc secretion, *Pediatrics* 69:176, 1982.

77. Zlotkin S, Buchanan B: Meeting zinc and copper intake requirements in the parenterally fed preterm and full-term infant, *J Pediatr* 103:441, 1983.

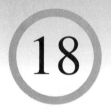

18

Breastfeeding the Neonate with Special Needs

Sandra L. Gardner, B.J. Snell, Ruth A. Lawrence

Human milk has been recognized as the gold standard for the human infant for centuries. Early published studies, from 1918 on, have confirmed that problems develop when human milk is replaced with artificial formulas made from the milk of other species. Milk of other species that is fed to the human infant has been known to contribute to increased mortality in infancy. Over the years, increasing research has confirmed the presence of antiinfective properties of human milk, which provide protection against not only gastrointestinal but upper and lower respiratory tract infections, otitis media, and even urinary tract infections.[27,29,50] In the case of the preterm infant, human milk also provides both short and long term advantages (Table 18-1).

Because of a lack of experience and knowledge about breastfeeding, a new mother, discharged early (24 to 48 hours) (see Chapter 5) from the hospital, may be challenged in initiating breastfeeding for her healthy newborn infant. The mother of a newborn with special needs (i.e., preterm infant, sick term newborn, infant with a congenital anomaly) may have even more difficulty in establishing breastfeeding because of the stress of separation and concerns about the infant's well-being. The tremendous benefits of providing human milk for all infants, but especially the premature, outweigh any apparent difficulties.

Healthy People 2000,[104] the health policy statement for the United States, states the following goal regarding breastfeeding: 75% of women leaving the hospital breastfeeding and at least 50% still breastfeeding their infant at 6 months. In addition, a report published by the Institute of Medicine from the Subcommittee on Nutrition during Lactation[41] states that all infants in the United States, under ordinary circumstances, should be breastfed. Furthermore, all women's milk is quality milk, even

though the mother's diet is not perfect. The goal of this chapter is to give the health care provider the skill and knowledge to support the breastfeeding dyad, especially when it involves the neonate with special needs.

Physiology[33,44,50,106]

Nutritional Value of Breast Milk

The components of breast milk vary with the (1) stage of lactation, (2) time of day, (3) sampling time during a feeding, (4) maternal nutrition, and (5) variation among individuals.

Colostrum is produced immediately at delivery and over 5 to 7 days, gradually changing to transitional and finally mature milk. It contains a higher ash content and higher concentrations of sodium, potassium, chloride, protein, fat-soluble vitamins, and minerals than mature milk. Colostrum has a lower fat content, especially of lauric and myristic acids, than mature milk. This milk is yellowish, thick, and rich in antibodies, has a specific gravity between 1.040 and 1.060, and contains 67 kcal/dl. Multipara and women who have previously breastfed have more colostrum during the first few days than women who have not.

Transitional milk is produced between 7 and 10 days postpartum, remains high in protein and lower in fat, and has a dramatic increase in water content compared with colostrum. Among mothers, the high variability of transitional milk accounts for 67 to 75 kcal/dl. Mature milk is produced after 10 days postpartum and contains 75 kcal/dl. During a feeding, the relative content of protein and the absolute content of fat increase. Morning feedings have a higher fat content than afternoon and evening feedings. Foremilk is lower in fat than

333

Table 18-1
Advantages of Breastfeeding and Human Milk Intake for Preterm Infants

Benefit	Comment
Protection from necrotizing enterocolitis (NEC)	Formula-fed infants developed NEC 6-10 times more often than infants receiving only human milk. Infants ≥30 weeks' gestation: incidence of NEC 20 times more in formula-fed than human milk-fed infants.[56]
Protection from infection or sepsis	Lowered incidence and severity of infections in hospitalized LBW infants fed human milk. Decreased protection if formula feeding added to human milk feedings.[104] Increased rehospitalizations: 7 for formula-fed compared with 0-1 for breastfed (both partially and completely) infants.[36]
Increased feeding tolerance	Whey protein in human milk is more easily digested, which results in more rapid gastric emptying and less gastric residual.[18] Achievement of complete enteral feedings by 6 weeks of age in VLBW infants fed own mother's milk (as compared with donor milk and formula feeding).[103] Formula-fed infants: increased vomiting, gastric residuals, and longer time to achieve complete enteral feedings.[55]
Decreased risk of later allergy	Lower incidence of allergic symptoms (especially eczema) at 18 months in human milk-fed preterm infants.[56]
Improved retinal function	Better retinal function depending on omega-3 fatty acid concentration (found in human milk, but not previously in formula) in enteral feedings.[102]
Improved neurocognitive development	Long-term advantages: higher intelligence quotients (IQ) at 7-8 years of age[57] and better developmental outcomes at 18 months of age.[58]

Adapted from Meier P, Brown L: Breastfeeding for mothers and low birth weight infants, *Nurs Clin North Am* 31:351, 1996.

hindmilk. Severely malnourished mothers have been shown to produce less milk, and water-soluble vitamins may be affected by deficient diets (e.g., strict vegetarians).

Cow's Milk Versus Human Milk

Cow's milk has significant differences from human milk. Cow's milk has 18 parts whey to 82 parts casein, whereas human milk has 60 parts whey to 40 parts casein. Casein is composed of proteins with ester-bound phosphate, high proline content, and low solubility at a pH of 4 to 5. Casein forms curd by combining with calcium caseinate and calcium phosphate. The cysteine and taurine content is low in cow's milk but high in human milk, whereas the methionine content is high in cow's milk and low in human milk (the human infant lacks the enzyme to digest methionine). Human milk also has lower aromatic amino acids, phenylalanine, and tyrosine. Human milk contains 6.8 g of lactose/dl, and cow's milk contains 4.9 g of lactose/dl. Sodium, phosphorus, calcium, magnesium, citrate, and total ash content are higher in cow's milk, but potassium and the calcium/phosphorus ratio are higher in human milk. Formula attempts to mimic milk but still lacks cholesterol, omega-3 fatty acids, enzymes, antibodies, lactoferrin, and other protective anti-infective properties.

Human milk contains more iron than unsupplemented cow's milk but less iron than supplemented cow's milk. Only 10% of iron is absorbed from formula, whereas about 80% is absorbed from human milk. Iron in formula encourages the growth of *E. coli* and inactivates lactoferrin. Cow's milk has a mean pH of 6.8, osmolality of 350 mOsm, and 221 mOsm renal osmolar load. Human milk has a mean pH of 7.1, osmolality of 286 mOsm, and 79 mOsm renal osmolar load.

Cow's milk forms curd much easier and thus delays gastric emptying. The newborn cannot handle certain proteins well because of lack of specific enzymes required for metabolism. Iron is more bioavailable in human milk, and iron absorption from human milk is more efficient, but cow's milk has a higher concentration of zinc

and contains more flourine than human milk. Human milk contains a ligand specific to zinc absorption and has been used as a therapy in zinc deficiency. (See also Chapter 15 for other human milk components.)

Preterm Versus Term Breast Milk

Significant evidence exists that there are many differences in preterm and term breast milk: (1) increased protein content in preterm breast milk,[7,8] (2) types of protein, predominantly whey, have a more physiologic balance of amino acids and contain many antiinfective properties, (3) lipid content in preterm breastmilk is more specific for the preterm neonate (i.e., increased supply of long-chain polyunsaturated fatty acids),[59] and (4) lactose, the major carbohydrate in breast milk, has increased absorption in the preterm infant (see Chapter 15 for comparison of preterm and term breast milk).

Immunologic Value of Breast Milk[22,29]

Because human milk protects neonates through its many antiinfective properties, breastfed infants have decreased morbidity compared with bottle-fed infants. Immune properties of breast milk are divided into cellular and humoral factors (Table 18-2). Since the highest concentration of some of these factors is found in colostrum, this early milk should be pumped, preserved, and fed to the neonate with special needs. Reduction of antiinfective activity occurs with the addition of formula but not breast milk fortifier to the diet.[50,81]

Normal Lactation

Breast development during pregnancy is stimulated by luteal and placental hormones, lactogen, prolactin, and chorionic gonadotropin. Estrogen stimulates growth of the milk collection (ductal) system, whereas progesterone stimulates growth of the milk production system. There is great variation in breast growth during pregnancy, and it is unclear how much breast tissue is necessary to support full lactation. Many factors other than breast size affect milk production, such as stress and fatigue, both of which are increased when a preterm infant is born.

If women should abort as early as 16 weeks, their breasts will secrete colostrum. Therefore mothers are capable of breastfeeding any viable infant.

The estrogen and progesterone function as inhibitors to actual milk production. Therefore stimulation of the breast before delivery will not create milk. Once the infant and placenta are delivered, stimulation of the nipple becomes effective in producing milk.

Stimulating the nipple by the infant's sucking action causes an increase in the prolactin released in the bloodstream and induces the synthesis and release of oxytocin (Fig. 18-1).[45,66] The amount of prolactin is directly related to the quantity and quality of nipple stimulation; because prolactin stimulates the synthesis and secretion of milk, the surges in prolactin levels are related to the quantity of milk. A decrease in the quality of stimulation causes a decrease in prolactin production and thus a decrease in milk production.

Adequate prolactin secretion controls the maintenance of milk supply. The sooner the infant nurses, the sooner the milk comes in and becomes established. Initially, production of milk is on a more consistent basis because the basal level of prolactin is very high immediately after birth. Maintenance of milk is dependent on the adequate stimulation of the breast on a regular and frequent basis. Initially, a newborn needs to nurse for a longer time in order to stimulate milk production and letdown. As the infant grows, sucking becomes more efficient with the infant stimulating sequential letdowns early in the nursing period, thereby shortening the length of nursing. Establishing a generous milk supply is critical in long-term maintenance. Research has demonstrated that for mothers who are separated from their infants, pumping both breasts simultaneously stimulates a higher prolactin surge with increased milk supply than single breast pumping.

Psychologic Values of Breastfeeding

The short-term advantage of breastfeeding is early mother and infant contact. The "en-face" position of breastfeeding enhances this contact. In the sick neonate, early contact, whether it is breastfeeding

Table 18-2
Immune Benefits of Breast Milk

Component	Action
White Blood Cells	
B lymphocytes	Synthesize IgA and other antibodies targeted against specific pathogens
Macrophages	90% of cells in breast milk; phagocytize microorganisms and kill bacteria in neonatal intestine; produce lysozyme, lactoferrin, and complement
Neutrophils	Phagocytize bacteria in neonatal gastrointestinal tract
T lymphocytes	Phagocytosis against organisms in gastrointestinal tract; mobilizes other host defenses; antigens introduced into maternal respiratory and/or gastrointestinal systems stimulate development of antibodies in breast milk; incorporation into neonatal tissue bestows short-term adoptive immunity[50]
Molecules	
Antibodies-Secretory IgA (sIgA)	Attaches to mucosal epithelium of digestive tract, thus preventing attachment of pathogens; sIgA against enteric, respiratory, and viral pathogens, as well as specific pathogens to which the mother has been exposed; highest concentration in colostrum, peaks during first 3-4 days postpartum, present in mature milk through first year of life;[49] antiallergic properties—inhibits absorption of macromolecular antigens from neonatal small intestine
B_{12} binding protein	Reduces amount of B_{12} available for bacterial growth (e.g., *E. coli* and bacteriodes)
Bifidus factor	Promotes growth of lactobacillus bifidus, the normal intestinal flora for breastfed infants and inhibits pathogens (e.g., staphylococcus, *E. coli,* Shigella, protozoa); by one month of age, bifidobacterium level in infants fed human milk is 10 times that of formula-fed infants
Fatty acids	Disrupt and destroy lipid-enveloped virus (e.g., herpes, influenza)[50]
Fibronectin	Enhances antimicrobial activity of macrophages; assists in repair of intestinal tissue damaged by immune reactions
Gamma-interferon	Enhances antimicrobial activity of immune cells
Hormones and growth factors	Stimulates neonatal gastrointestinal maturation that renders gastrointestinal tract less vulnerable to invasion by microorganisms
Lactoferrin	Binds iron and thwarts growth of pathogens (e.g., *E. coli,* staphylococcus); highest levels in colostrum; present in mature milk through first year of life[49]
Lysozyme	Destroys pathogens (e.g., enterobacteriacae and gram-positive bacteria) by cell wall lysis; human milk contains three hundred times the lysozyme found in cow's milk[50]
Mucins	Adheres to bacteria or viruses, thus preventing pathogens from attaching to mucosal surfaces
Oligosaccharides	Bind to microorganisms, thus preventing pathogens from attaching to mucosal surfaces

Modified from Newman J: How breast milk protects newborns, *Sci Am* 273(6):76, 1995.

or another physical means, sometimes must be delayed or modified.

The long-term psychologic effect for the mother of unrestricted nursing appears to be a more even mood cycle as a result of elevated prolactin levels, which enhance coping mechanisms associated with caring for a new family member.

Providing maternal milk, including pumping and gavaging breast milk and eventual feeding at the breast, enhances maternal attachment and maternal behaviors[88] and enables the mother to contribute to her infant's care (see Chapter 28).[75] Proximity of mother and infant, as well as the infant's initial experience at the breast contribute to ma-

Ejection Reflex Arc or Let-Down Reflex

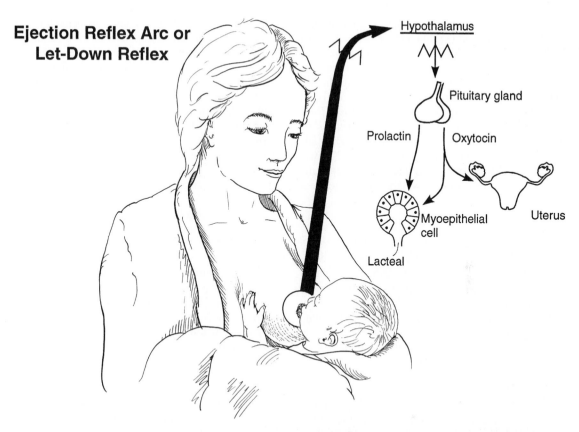

Figure 18-1   Ejection reflex arc. Infant suckling stimulates mechanoreceptors in the mother's nipple and areola that send the stimuli along the nerve pathways to the hypothalamus. Stimulation of the posterior pituitary releases oxytocin that (a) stimulates myoepithelial cells of the breast to contract and eject milk and (b) stimulates the uterus to contract. Stimulation of the anterior pituitary releases prolactin, which is responsible for milk production in mammary alveoli. (Adapted from Lawrence R: *Breastfeeding, a guide for the medical profession,* ed 4, St Louis, 1994, Mosby.)

ternal and infant regulation and the establishment of innate behaviors and emotional and social ties between mother and infant.[19,39,51,88,97]

All referring physicians and nursing personnel who admit infants to the intensive care unit should support and assist mothers who wish to breastfeed their infant. Use of kangaroo care (see Chapter 12) in the NICU facilitates early initiation of breast feeding, increased maternal confidence, competence, and breastfeeding duration.[6,15,38,39] If the infant is able to take oral nourishment, he or she can be breastfed at 1000 to 1200 g and about 32

weeks' gestational age.[17,34,65,69-72,98] (See Strategies to Facilitate Oral Feeding, Chapter 12.)

Etiology

Although breastfeeding is a normal, natural function, it is not a reflex, but rather a highly complex interaction and interdependence between mother and infant. To be successful, the breastfeeding dyad must synchronize their behavior and physiology and receive support from their environment. Delayed breastfeeding may be as successful as immediate feeding when (1) problems are prevented, (2) mothers receive support and encouragement in maintaining their milk supply, and (3) everyone is patient and knowledgeable about teaching the infant to suckle. Initiating breastfeeding as early as possible is important to prevent problems. However, thorough evaluation of the effectiveness of the nursing couple is important in achieving adequate nutrition and breastfeeding success. Knowledgable health care providers and lactation consultants or specialists, where available, perform these evaluations.

Sucking

Sucking is a primitive reflex appearing as early as 15 to 16 weeks' gestation. Although isolated components of feeding behaviors (e.g., root, suck, swallow, gag) are all present early in gestation, they are not effectively coordinated for oral feedings before 32 to 34 weeks' gestational age (see Table 12-2).[34] Two distinct types of sucking, nonnutritive and nutritive, develop in the human infant.

Nonnutritive Sucking

Nonnutritive sucking refers to sucking activity when no fluid or nutrition is delivered to the infant. Characterized by short bursts of rapid motion, pauses, and few swallows, nonnutritive sucking has a stabilizing effect on physiologic responses (e.g., better oxygenation, quieter, more restful behavior, improved behavioral organization, better weight gain, improved readiness for oral feedings).[82,109] In addition, nonnutritive sucking, in both term and preterm infants results in increased insulin and gastrin secretion, which may stimulate digestion and storage of nutrients.[60]

Nutritive Sucking

Nutritive sucking, used by an infant when fluid or nutrition is available, is characterized by an organized, rhythmic pattern that is about half the rate of nonnutritive sucking (i.e., one per second).[108] During nutritive sucking, each milk expression is followed by a reflexive swallow and an occasional brief pause. In the term neonate, rates of sucking range from 40 to 100/min.[80] Nutritive sucking provides the neonate with positive reinforcement,

which encourages a steady level of behavior.[67] A variety of factors affect nutritive sucking including (1) maternal anesthesia and/or analgesia, (2) length of labor, (3) type of delivery, (4) gestational age, (5) birth weight, (6) type of fluid, (7) disorders of the CNS, and (8) individual variations.[26,30,48,53,108] Although nutritive sucking is associated with faster heart rate,[26,53] little information is available describing energy requirements of nutritive sucking. The findings of one study suggest that during bottlefeeding, preterm infants expend significantly less energy to suck the same volume than does the full term infant.[42]

An increasing level of organization of nutritive sucking occurs with increasing gestational age and maturity.[22,61,68,108] By 32 to 34 weeks' postconceptual age, there is a change in sucking bursts (i.e., increase in number of sucks, number of suck bursts and pressure, decrease in time between sucking bursts). This developmental maturation enables nutritive sucking to take less time and is less tiring. Nutritive sucking requires coordination between suck, swallow, and breathing. During coordinated sucking bursts, suck/swallow/breathing occur in a 1:1:1 sequential pattern.[22] Although suck/swallow is achieved by 32 weeks,[34,68] respiration may still not be well coordinated so that the preterm may develop apneic episodes, especially with bottle feeding.[22] With increasing postconceptual age and neuromuscular maturity *consistent* coordination of suck/swallow/breathing (with bottle feeding) occurs by 37 weeks' postconceptual age.[22]

Human nutritive suckling is composed of five separate yet interrelated processes: (1) rooting, (2) orienting, (3) suction, (4) expression, and (5) swallowing[20] (Fig. 18-2). Rooting, the tactile stimulating of the infant's face and lips, elicits the head to turn toward the stimulus. Stimulation of the center of the lower lip enables the infant to root by coming forward and latching on, rather than turning the head to one side.[51] Orienting, or latching on, occurs when the tongue draws the nipple and areola into an enlongated teat and compresses it against the hard palate.[96] The lactiferous sinuses, located behind the nipple and areola, must be stimulated by the infant's mouth for milk to be extracted (Fig. 18-3).

Suction, the application of negative pressure in the infant's mouth, holds the nipple and areola in

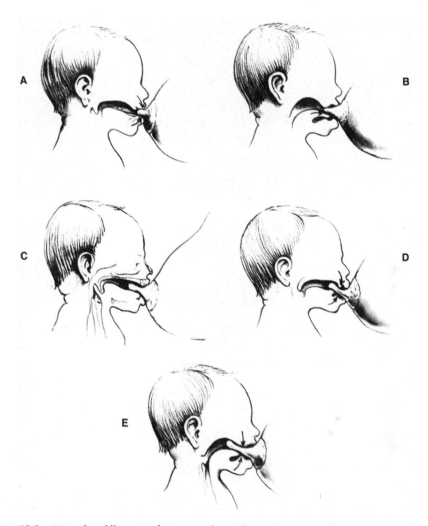

Figure 18-2   Normal suckling. **A,** Infant grasps breast (note *arrows* showing jaw action). **B,** Tongue moves forward to draw nipple in. **C,** Nipple and areola move toward palate as glottis still permits breathing. **D,** Tongue moves along nipple, pressing it against hard palate, creating pressure. **E,** Ductules under areola are milked, and flow begins because of peristaltic movement of tongue. Glottis closes and swallow follows. (From Lawrence RA: *Breastfeeding, a guide for the medical profession,* ed 3, St Louis, 1985, Mosby.)

place.[96] At the beginning of breastfeeding, a strong suction stretches and shapes the nipple, but only moderate suction is required to maintain adequate grasp of the nipple. During the feeding, occasional bursts of suckling enable milk to be expressed. Expression of milk occurs when the peristaltic motion of the tongue stimulates the myoepithelial cells surrounding the milk ducts (see Fig. 18-3) to contract, and milk is ejected from the ducts. As peristaltic motion of the tongue stimulates milk ejection, the lips should be flanged out to create a seal. After maximal compression of the nipple[96] with peristaltic motion, milk is expressed from the lactiferous sinuses. Swallowing milk occurs as the

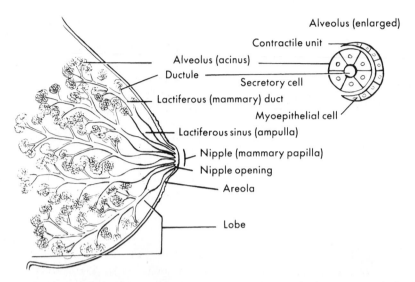

Figure 18-3   Structure of human breast during lactation. (From Riordan J: *A practical guide to breastfeeding,* St Louis, 1983, Mosby.)

peristaltic motion of the tongue triggers peristaltic motion of the posterior pharynx (reflexive swallowing)[79,80] and propulsion down the esophagus (which also shows peristalsis). These peristaltic motions coordinate suck and swallow so breastfeeding infants do not choke, unless letdown reflex is excessive. Swallowing milk also reflexively initiates the expression cycle of jaw and tongue movements. Therefore nutritive suckling is primarily expression and swallowing of milk. During nursing, just enough suction to keep the nipple in proper position is used, even during the expressive phase of suckling. Breastfeeding is an infant-regulated system; milk flow is dependent on the active suckling by the infant. When an infant pauses to regain physiologic stability, flow of milk from the breast ceases.

Ultrasound studies of full-term infants breastfeeding note (1) an elongation to twice the resting size of the maternal nipple, (2) formation of a passive seal by the neonatal oral cavity, and (3) milk ejection coinciding with the downstroke of the tongue and jaw, creating negative pressure by oral cavity enlargement.[96] Ultrasound studies of full-term infants bottlefeeding note (1) less elasticity and less elongation of artificial nipples (compared with human nipple) (2) similar mechanisms used

to suckle artificial nipples as used to breastfeed, and (3) milk expression dependent on vacuum phenomenon by oral cavity enlargement rather than by nipple compression.[22,79,80] Artificial nipples have also been shown to vary in their rate of milk flow,[62-64] so that fluid flows into the posterior oropharynx by gravity (Fig. 18-4). Artificial nipples and bottles are gravity-regulated systems requiring the infant to actively inhibit milk flow to permit swallowing and breathing. In an attempt to regulate milk flow and prevent choking or gagging, infants may clench their jaws or obstruct the nipples' holes with their tongues.[22]

Prevention

Problems with breastfeeding may be a maternal problem, a neonatal problem, or a combination of these. Lack of information regarding common problems in the early weeks of breastfeeding is a common reason for breastfeeding failure.[85,91] In descriptive studies addressing breastfeeding problems, mothers have frequently identified concerns related to sore nipples, breast discomfort, and inadequate milk supply.[14,18] Breastfeeding problems should be prevented. To solve a breastfeeding

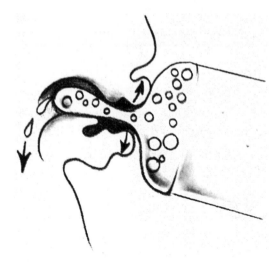

Figure 18-4 Artificial nipple. (From Lawrence RA: *Breastfeeding, a guide for the medical profession,* ed 3, St Louis, 1985, Mosby.)

problem, the mother must be observed feeding the infant.

Maternal Problems

Inadequate Milk Supply

Inadequate milk supply, a major problem for both mother and infant is the most commonly cited reason for discontinuation of breastfeeding in the NICU and after discharge.[38,47,73,74] Initially, some neonates with special needs are unable to breastfeed. In this common situation, the most compelling breastfeeding issue is establishing an adequate milk supply without the neonate's assistance (Table 18-3). Developing a very early program of education and support for the mother will provide early establishment of milk supply and prevent low milk volume.

Initiating, establishing, and maintaining a milk supply must be accomplished mechanically when the infant is unable to breastfeed. Since milk production is dependent upon adequate and frequent expression, maternal education is the key to establishing an adequate supply (see Table 18-3). The mother who desires to breastfeed should be given instruction about initiating and maintaining a milk supply until the infant can breastfeed. In general, instruction includes information about pumping, which is individualized to the mother's situation. Milk production through pumping should be encouraged early and regularly in order to (1) collect colostrum, rich in antiinfective properties, (2) ease initial engorgement associated with lack of regular stimulation, (3) provide quality nutrition for the neonate, and (4) alleviate concerns about available volume once the infant begins breastfeeding. The early postpartal period in the hospital is the optimal time to teach pumping methods, while support and encouragement are readily available.

Breast Discomfort

Maternal problems include engorgement, painful nipples, and cracked nipples.[86] A primipara is at high risk for developing engorgement. Frequent emptying of the breast is the best prevention.

Engorgement occurring in the early postpartum period is characterized by general discomfort, usually in both breasts in a well, afebrile woman. Areolar engorgement blocks the nipple and makes grasping the areola difficult for the infant. Gentle breast massage and manual expression of a small amount of milk softens the areola so the infant is able to "latch on." When the body of the breasts and the areola are affected, the goal of management is to make the mother comfortable so that nursing may continue. Supporting the breasts is crucial, and the mother should wear a well-fitting but adjustable brassiere 24 hours a day.[50] Applying cold packs decreases pain, and pain relievers may be prescribed. Applying heat (packs or a warm shower) and expressing some milk is good preparation for feeding. A nursing infant, manual expression, or an effective pump helps initiate and maintain milk flow. After feeding or pumping, application of cold packs may be comforting and help decrease breast edema.

Prenatally, stimulation of the nipple by pulling or rolling is not recommended because of the possibility of initiating uterine contractions and premature labor.[50,76]

Sore nipples are another major discomfort and concern for the new mother. The initial grasp of the nipple by the infant or with pumping can be painful. Poor positioning of the infant causes painful and eventually cracked nipples. Prevention and treatment involve educating the mother about careful

Table 18-3
Factors that Influence Maternal Milk Supply and Successful Breastfeeding of the Preterm Infant

Enhances	Reduces	Comments
Early initiation of pumping, preferably with a double-pumping set up	Immediate separation at birth,[49] delayed initiation of pumping or feeding at the breast	Initiate within 2-3 hours of birth, if possible; pumping both breasts simultaneously is associated with higher prolactin levels, milk yield, fat concentration, and maternal preference[12,111]
Frequent milk expression with complete breast emptying at each session[40]	Failure to express frequently and/or incomplete emptying of the breasts	5-8 expressions/day (every 3-4 hr); duration of pumping >100 min/day (about 15-20 min with double-pump set up); longest nonpumping interval ≤6 hours[13,40,92,99]
Rest, relaxation, and stress management[32] (see Chapters 28 and 29)	Fatigue, anxiety, stress (i.e., maternal illness; return to work; more commitments in and outside the home)	Inverse relationship between maternal anxiety scores and milk volume for mothers of preterms; uninterrupted sleep of at least 6 hours[21,50]
Adequate nutrition	Inadequate nutrition	At least 60% of recommended daily allowances produces milk of adequate quantity and quality to promote infant growth[83]
Medications: Metoclopramide Oxytocin Reserpines Phenothiazines	Bromocriptine Antihistamine Oral contraceptives (especially estrogen and progesterone combination)	Knowledge of maternal medication use enables effective counseling
Positive feedback to mother regarding infant growth; infant's condition improving	Worsening infant's condition	Mothers report feeling rewarded by infant's growth while receiving expressed mother's milk by gavage[74]
Skin-to-skin contact (kangaroo care) (see Chapter 12)	Parental separation	Maternal reinforcement of lactation, maternal behaviors, confidence, and attachment; assures maternal exposure to pathogens in NICU so that her immune system is stimulated to produce environmentally-specific antibodies that will be passed in maternal milk and protect the preterm[92]
Educational information (e.g., video, brochure) readily available	No verbal or written information for parents	Decision about type of pump, frequency; written instructions on collection and storage per NICU protocol; information about maternal rest, fluid intake, and nutrition
Knowledgeable professional careproviders (e.g., nurses, lactation specialists, physicians) who educate, support, and assist through consistent, practical advice	Nonsupportive care providers and/or inconsistent advice and information	Prevention of maternal problems (e.g., inadequate supply, sore nipples, engorgement) through self-education and professional interaction and education enhances success and prevents discontinuation of breastfeeding

Modified from Schanler R, and Hurst N: Human milk for the hospitalized preterm infant, *Semin Perinatol* 18:476, 1994.

Table 18-3
Factors that Influence Maternal Milk Supply and Successful Breastfeeding of the Preterm Infant—cont'd

Enhances	Reduces	Comments
Initiation of breastfeeding *before* bottlefeeding	Initiation of bottle feeding before breastfeeding	Early breastfeeding is less stressful than early bottlefeedings[17,70-72,74,98] because of differences in the patterns of sucking and breathing; during bottlefeedings, preterms alternate short bursts of sucking with breathing and do not breathe within sucking bursts; during breastfeeding, breathing is integrated within sucking bursts[72]
		Test weighing (i.e., weighing before and after breastfeeding with differences in weight representing milk intake [1 g = 1 ml]) using electronic scales is a reliable method of documenting milk intake in preterm infants[75]
		For specific problems, maximizing milk intake may be assisted by lactational support devices and/or breast pump stimulation of the opposite breast during infant feeding[50,74]

positioning of the infant facing the mother, looking directly at the breast, and tummy-to-tummy with her (Fig. 18-5). Compression of the areola behind the nipple extracts milk from the sinuses[86] (see Fig. 18-3). Changing the infant's position on the nipple several times during the feeding may also be helpful but may be too confusing for mother or baby who are just learning to breastfeed.

Positioning the infant correctly at the breast will assist in the prevention of sore nipples. There are three positions that can be used with breastfeeding: the cradle hold, the football hold, and lying down (see Figs. 18-5 to 18-7). Initially, the cradle and/or football hold will allow the most control for the mother and infant to learn breastfeeding. Breastfeeding in the lying down position becomes easier once latch-on techniques are developed.

Nipple care involves keeping nipples clean and dry. Clear water (no soap or alcohol) is all that is necessary to keep the nipples clean. Drying nipples well, not using plastic nursing pads, and exposing nipples to air and dry heat (sunlight, light bulb sauna, or a low setting on a hair dryer) is comforting. Using ointments may not be helpful, because they prevent exposure to air and drying, but if used, a small amount (i.e., one drop) should be

gently massaged into the nipple. Lanolin (if there is no allergy to wool), A and D ointment, or vitamin E may be used to treat but will not prevent sore nipples. Nipple shields are not recommended because they are awkward for the mother, confusing for the infant, and decrease milk production by 50%.

Flat or inverted nipples may be difficult for the infant to grasp and result in maternal engorgement and infant frustration (Fig. 18-8). Inverted nipples may be treated by wearing plastic breast cups or shells, which apply pressure to the areola, everting the nipple. (Fig. 18-9).

Neonatal Problems

Ideally, no term or preterm infant who will be breastfed should ever be fed with an artificial nipple, but this is not always possible, especially for the sick premature infant who requires prolonged hospitalization. However, teaching the premature infant to suck often starts long before nutrition is obtained from a nipple. When the premature infant is gavage fed, giving a pacifier teaches the infant to equate satiety with sucking. Using a pacifier provides nonnutritive sucking that calms and soothes

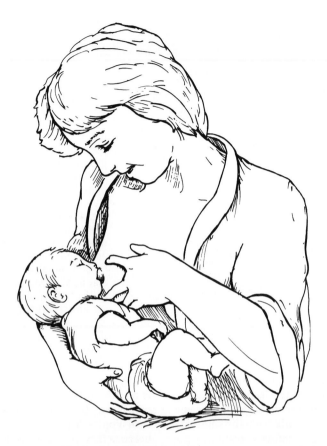

Figure 18-5   Proper positioning for breastfeeding infant tummy-to-tummy facing the mother.

the preterm infant, as well as providing the opportunity to develop sucking skill. When the mother is present for gavage feeding, the infant can be given the breast instead of an artificial nipple. If it is necessary to avoid swallowing any fluid, the breast can be prepumped. Placing the infant in direct skin-to-skin contact with the mother's breast enables nuzzling and licking behaviors and teaches that relief from hunger and the breastfeeding position are associated. Because increased stimulation creates an increased milk supply, it is possible to breastfeed multiple infants.[101] In the early weeks it will be difficult and time consuming, but eventually it can become faster and more convenient than bottle feeding. Two infants can be fed

at the same time, in the cradle position or in the football hold position (see Fig. 18-7). The infants should change breasts with each feeding, because one may have a stronger suck than the other and each breast should receive an equal amount of stimulation.

Understanding the mechanisms of suckling is essential to preventing, assessing, and intervening in neonatal suckling problems. "Nipple confusion" describes the difficulty of infants who have been fed with artificial nipples before learning to breastfeed. The infant who has learned to feed from a bottle nipple often sucks incorrectly at the breast, preventing milk flow. The infant's confusion creates frustration and crying, which may inhibit

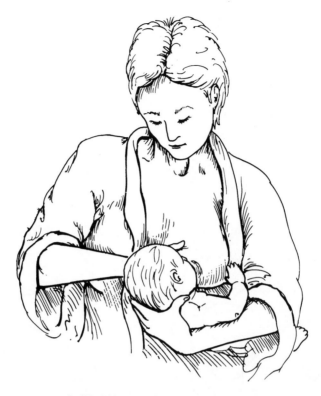

Figure 18-6   Football hold in breastfeeding. Pillows may be used for support.

milk letdown. The best prevention of nipple confusion is to enable the infant to learn breastfeeding *before* bottle feeding is established.

Assessment of the problem includes evaluation of the method of feeding and possibly using alternative nutritional methods (gavage feedings) until the cause is determined. If the infant is bottle-fed, choking may be a result of a soft nipple, a fast flow that the infant cannot control, or a nipple that is too long for the infant's (particularly the preterm infant's) mouth. If the mother is breastfeeding and the ejection is strong, the first rush of milk could cause choking, which may be prevented by manual expression of a small amount (several spurts) of milk before offering the nipple to the infant.

Some suckling problems result from the sequelae of perinatal events (i.e., low APGARS, preterm low birth weight, SGA, LGA, IDM, multiple births)[78] or of physical disorders (i.e., hyperbilirubinemia, hypoglycemia, cardiorespiratory conditions, sepsis, neuromotor/developmental problems, structural abnormalities of the oral cavity)[77] and represent developmental delays. These suckling difficulties require diagnostic evaluation and appropriate intervention into the underlying cause.

Some mothers may not establish or have difficulty maintaining an adequate milk supply while some infants with problems require an easily obtainable milk supply. The Lact-Aid Nursing Trainer system addresses a variety of breastfeeding problems, including suckling defects[9-11] (Fig. 18-10). Expressed breast milk or formula is contained in a presterilized, disposable bag suspended between the mother's breasts by a cord, and the liquid is delivered by a thin, flexible tube attached to the

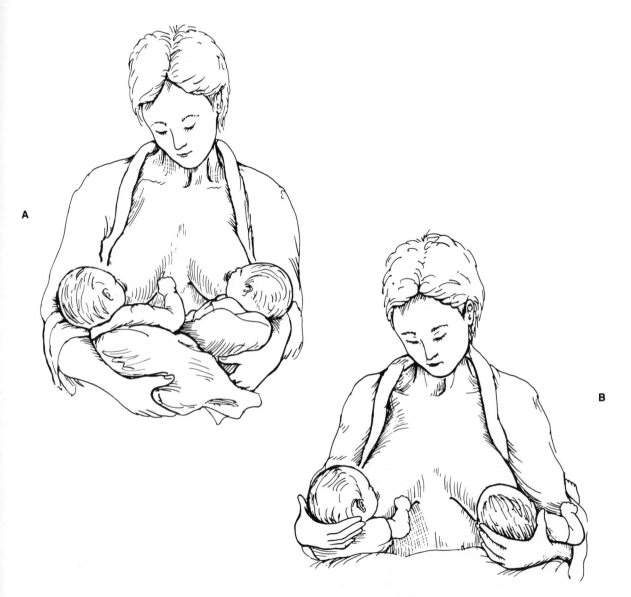

Figure 18-7   Breastfeeding twins. **A,** Cradle position. **B,** football hold position.

bag. The end of the tube is placed against the mother's nipple to enable the infant to suckle the tube and nipple at the same time. This device provides the correct rate of flow and volume of liquid that elicits the reflexes of swallowing and expression. The Lact-Aid trainer provides oral therapy and nutritional supplement for the infant and mammary therapy that enhances the mother's lactation.[14] It is effective in managing low milk production in the mother caused by separation, delayed breastfeeding, poor technique, or other correctable problems and in giving nutritional and oral

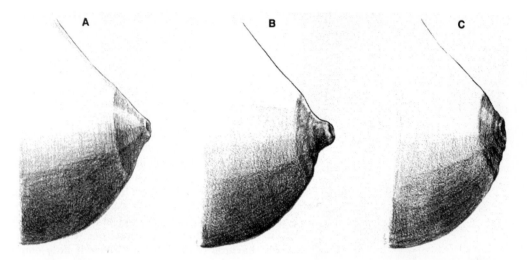

Figure 18-8 Inverted nipples. **A,** Normal and inverted nipples may look similar when nipple is not stimulated. **B,** Normal nipple protrudes when stimulated. **C,** Inverted nipple retracts when stimulated. (Courtesy Jimmy Lynne Scholl Avery.)

therapy to the infant who is slow in gaining weight or has a suckling dysfunction. CAUTION: To prevent the spread of serious infections, Lact-Aid should never be borrowed, rented, or loaned from another mother. The Lact-Aid STARTrainer Nursing System (Fig. 18-11) is an economic "starter" breastfeeding supplementer introduced in 1997. It was developed especially for use when the infant needs assistance latching onto the breast, when supplementing is needed for a brief period, a trial period is desired, or a semi-disposable unit is needed. The Lact-Aid® trainer converts any standard infant feeding bottle, including Volufeed, Accufeed and similar feeders, to create a breastfeeding supplementer system that is equivalent in function, safety, and effectiveness as the original Lact-Aid Nursing Trainer System. Should a mother need to switch to the original model for longer-term use, she will be able to use most of the STAR-Trainer components with it.

Problems with the letdown reflex may be maternal, neonatal, or a combination of these. The mother's emotional state may interfere with letdown. A tense mother will not have a letdown reflex. Often, especially in breastfeeding a prema-

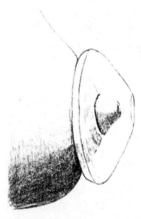

Figure 18-9 Breast shell. Special breast shells may be worn under bra during last 3 to 4 months of pregnancy. Gentle pressure at edge of areola gradually forces nipple through center opening of shell to help increase nipple protractility. It may be used after childbirth if needed. NOTE: Milk can leak from breasts into shells. Since maternal body warmth can foster rapid bacterial contamination, such milk should be discarded. (Courtesy Jimmy Lynne Scholl Avery.)

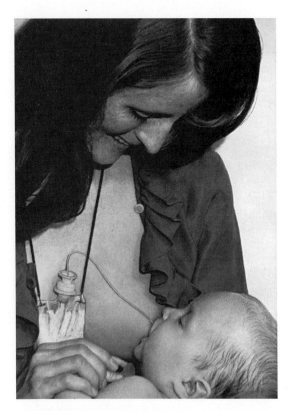

Figure 18-10 Lact-Aid Nursing Trainer. (Courtesy Lact-Aid International, Inc.)

ture infant, this is because of fear of failure or lack of privacy. Knowledge of the mechanisms of lactation can help avoid a fear of failing. It is important to give the mother as much privacy and the least stressful environment as possible when pumping her breasts and while breastfeeding. If a mother experiences a weak or delayed letdown, she should massage the colostrum or milk down to the nipple before putting the infant to the breast. Infants with a poor suck (i.e., preterm infants or infants with Down syndrome or a neurologic deficit) understimulate the breast and do not trigger the letdown reflex. Use of the Lact-Aid Nursing Trainer provides oral therapy, improves these infants' suckling ability, and enables a successful nursing relationship. The breast can also be stimulated with a good pump between feedings to increase the milk supply.

Data Collection and Intervention

Establishment of Breastfeeding

Available Feeding and Suckling Neonate

Infants who have been admitted to an NICU often present a dilemma to care providers regarding the most favorable time to begin putting the infant to the breast. The infant's present physical status coupled with considerations regarding nutrition and energy expenditure provide data for arriving at such decisions. In a national survey, criteria used to determine readiness for oral feedings included the following: (1) 75% used gestational age (e.g., 34 weeks' by 60%), or weight (e.g., 1500 g by 50%) and (2) infant behavioral cues (e.g., sucking behaviors) (Table 18-4).[94] There is little empirical data to support the contention that either weight or gestational age affects the ability of the preterm infant to coordinate suck/swallow. In the same survey, a majority (85% to 93%) responded that bottle feeding is started first, before breastfeeding.[94] Professional care givers believe and teach parents that breastfeeding is too stressful and requires more energy and exertion than bottle-feeding.[65] Traditionally, progression of nutritional support for the preterm has proceeded from IV fluids→total parenteral nutrition→gavage (continuous→intermittent)→bottlefeeding (at 1500 to 1800 g or 34 to 35 weeks' postconceptual age,→breastfeeding (after bottle feeding without distress). Problems arising from this approach include (1) delay in initial oral feedings, (2) establishing a sucking method that may not easily transfer to breastfeeding, and (3) initiation of breastfeeding when discharge is imminent so that the mother receives little, if any, breastfeeding assistance and support.[65,75]

Studies show that the preterm infant may be able to breastfeed far earlier (<1500 g or 28 to 36 weeks) than previously thought.[17,69-72,98] A comparison of studies of breastfeeding and bottle feeding shows (1) less oxygen desaturation, (2) warmer skin temperature, (3) no bradycardia, and (4) better coordination of sucking and breathing with breastfeeding versus bottlefeeding (see Table 18-4). According to these research data, the ability of the preterm to breastfeed without alterations in homeostasis occurs *before* the ability to safely bottle feed.

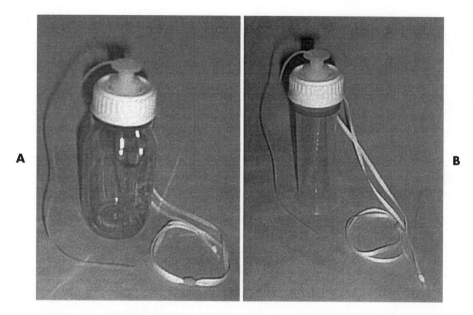

Figure 18-11   Lact-Aid STARTrainer Nursing System. **A,** With standard infant feeding bottle. **B,** With metered feeding bottle. Lact-Aid STARTrainer Unit replaces nipple of infant bottle cap to make an infant feeding bottle a Lact-Aid breastfeeding supplementer and suckling aid for short term use or whenever a semidisposable is desired. The adjustable neck strap raises or lowers unit to adjust flow rate. Tip of the Nursing Tube fits notch of bottle holder to stop flow when not in use. Lact-Aid STARTrainer Nursing System includes STARTrainer Unit (Body/Nursing Tube, STARTrainer Ring, Extension Tube), STARTrainer Adjustable Neck Strap and Notched Bottle Holder, and STARTrainer Instructions. (Courtesy Lact-Aid International.)

Skin-to-skin (kangaroo) care provides a safe, effective alternative method of caring for premature infants[6]. During skin-to-skin contact, the infant may initiate nonnutritive suckling at the breast. Nonnutritive time at the breast is used to accustom both mother and baby to each other and the pleasant sensory stimuli at the breast. As the preterm matures, nonnutritive suckling is replaced by hunger cues, latching on, and effective nutritive suckling. Both AGA and SGA (700 to 2450 g) infants experience benefits from early (sometimes starting at birth) and sustained breastfeeding: (1) more mothers breastfeed and are more confident, (2) more frequent feedings are given, (3) more milk is produced, (4) infants breastfeed longer, (5) there is less bradycardia than with gavage or bottle feeding, and (6) there is better weight gain and earlier discharge (see Chapter 12).[6]

Both maternal and neonatal responses to breastfeeding should be monitored. Adequate milk volume is available when the milk ejection (letdown) reflex occurs. Breast massage may assist in bringing down the milk, thus making it easier for the infant to obtain. Let-down may be felt by the mother and/or observed as a change in the rhythm of infant sucking and audible swallowing. After let-down is established, the infant expends little energy in sucking. He or she only needs to coordinate swallowing and breathing with an occasional burst of sucking. The nurse should be available during the initial breastfeeding to provide support to the mother, to assure that the infant exhibits no signs of distress (e.g., color changes, bradycardia, oxygen desaturation, drop in temperature), and to provide guidance for the mother if the infant chokes with letdown. The nurse also needs to reinforce to the mother that the infant's sucking pattern will be a pattern of bursts and pauses. The pauses are present in all infants and provide rest periods for the infant.

Table 18-4
Readiness for Initiation of Oral Feedings: Research Basis

Breastfeeding	Criteria	Bottlefeeding
Preterm: 28-36 wk: Better able to coordinate suck, swallow, and breathing[69-72,98] <1500 g: Better able to coordinate sucking, swallowing, and breathing[17,69-72,98]	**Gestational/post-** ←**conceptual**→ **age (PCA)** ←**Weight**→	**Preterm:** 34-35 wk: PCA is developmental guideline;[47] some infants are ready at an earlier age (i.e., 32-34 wk)[34,68] 1500-1800 g: traditional criteria without research basis
Full Term: Ultrasound study shows human nipple elongates to twice its resting length; neonatal cheeks act as a passive seal for the oral cavity[96]	**Mechanics of** ←**sucking**→	**Full Term:** Higher maximum pressure and number of sucks or bursts; greater suck widths[67] **Preterm:** Burst width (interburst and intersuck width) similar to full-term infant[67]
Full Term: 50% of feeding obtained in first 2 min; 80%-90% by 4 min; last 5 min minimal obtained from each breast[55] **Premature:** • After 34 wk: 70%-80% of feeding ingested in first 6 min, then intake sluggish, rest periods increase, and sucking and nourishment decrease[61] • At 36-37 wk: sucking standards are similar to mature neonate[61] • The younger the gestational age the higher the variability[61] • Longer duration of breast than bottlefeeding[69-71] • No difference in duration of breast vs bottlefeeding[17]	←**Energy**→ **expenditure**	**Full Term:** 86% of feeding obtained in first 4 min of sucking[55] **Preterm:** 40% of total volume ingested in first min;[61] less energy to suck same volume as full-term infant[42]
Preterm: • Skin temperature higher (than when bottlefeeding) because of bodily contact with mother[69-71,98] • No temperature change before (ac) or after feeding (pc)[17]	←**Temperature**→	
Preterm: Less weight gain after breastfeeding compared with bottlefeeding[17]	←**Weight gain**→	

Table 18-4
Readiness for Initiation of Oral Feedings: Research Basis—cont'd

Breastfeeding	Criteria	Bottlefeeding
	←Heart rate→	**Preterm:** Bradycardia occurred with bottlefeeding but not breastfeeding; bradycardia possibly related to faster milk flow and interference with breathing;[69-71,98] apnea and bradycardia with bottlefeeding in otherwise healthy preterms[35]
Preterm: Different patterns of sucking bursts and better coordination, breathing is integrated within sucking bursts[72]	←**Coordination**→ **of sucks** **swallow and** **breathing**	**Preterm:** • Effective coordination by 32-34 weeks[34] • High flow nipples result in apnea or bradycardia[62-64] • Do not breathe within sucking bursts but alternate short bursts of sucking with breathing[72] • Consistently achieved by infants 37 wk PCA[22]
Full term: No desaturation with feeding[94] 18% pc saturations <90%	←**Oxygen**→ **saturation**	**Full term:** No desaturation with feeding[93] 29% of pc saturations <90%
Preterms: No difference in oxygenation with breast vs bottlefeeding;[69-71,98] no pc decline of oxygenation; oxygenation more stable than with bottlefeeding Desaturation (<90%) in 21% of breast feedings[17] With BPD, saturations higher than with bottlefeeding[17]		**Preterms:** Decreased oxygenation during initial sustained sucking but oxygenation increased as sucking pattern modulated[93] 32-36 wk: range of 94%-97% with feeding;[69] with sucking decreased saturation from 2.5%-16% (range 80%-100%)[68] Fluctuations and sharper decrease in saturation with bottlefeedings vs breastfeeding;[69-71,98] 10 min pc saturation 50% below baseline[70,71] Desaturation (<90%) in 38% of bottle feedings[17]
	←**Hypercapnea**→ ($\uparrow$ P_{CO_2})	**Preterm:** 34-35 wk: $\uparrow$ P_{CO_2} depresses sucking and swallowing so that respirations may supercede feeding in preterms with increased respirator drive[100] (i.e., BPD)
Preterm: 32 wk: increased feeding in active/alert and quiet/alert[5]	←**Behavioral**→ **cues**	**Full term and Preterm:** Motor behavior: a change in arm posture (i.e., flexion) with feeding[28]

The infant's respiratory status should be reviewed. Infants requiring supplemental oxygen can breastfeed. If the infant requires 35% oxygen or less, oxygen may be delivered via a nasal cannula to ensure adequate and consistent oxygenation. This will eliminate another source of concern for the mother (i.e., having to worry about juggling the blow-by oxygen line). If the infant has not previously been placed on a nasal cannula, the nurse should initiate the cannula and then assess oxygenation using a pulse oximeter. After oxygenation has been documented, the pulse oximeter may be discontinued, and the breastfeeding experience may begin. The infant should be assessed by using a pulse oximeter before the feeding begins. The line should be anchored securely near the infant's nose or held in place by the nurse or the father. The infant's temperature status requires review. Attention should be directed toward preventing hypothermia with infants who require significant thermal support. The infant should be swaddled, and a hat should be placed on the infant's head to prevent heat loss. Duration of breastfeeding should be based on cues of satiety (e.g., sucking cessation, falling asleep) or cues of physiologic instability and/or fatigue.[65] Frequency of breastfeeding can be progressed as can frequency of bottle feeding: one breastfeeding per day to one per shift to every other breastfeeding. If the mother is available with this progression, bottle feeding may be deferred until breastfeeding is well established or avoided altogether. When the infant is taking all nutrition orally, the mother can be encouraged to breastfeed as often as possible and to institute an "ad lib" schedule.[65] If the mother is available, the infant should breastfeed as often as is necessary and supplementation should not be provided. However, if the breast milk supply is insufficient, using a Lact-Aid Nursing Trainer provides nutritional supplementation and mammary stimulation to increase maternal milk supply.

In skin-to-skin contact, such as kangaroo care, the warmth of the mother's body maintains the baby's temperature (see Chapter 6). Families and staff often fear that the infant will not get enough during a breastfeeding. This concern is especially predominant when infants have been hospitalized for prematurity and fluids and calories have been scrutinized closely. Health professionals need to be sensitive to such concerns and refrain from employing methods such as weighing infants before and after feedings or using gavage tubes to attempt to determine the exact amount of breast milk ingested during the feeding. With today's electronic NICU scales, test weighing (before and after feeding; see Table 18-3) is accurate, if really necessary. However health professionals need to focus on cues that can be used during and after hospitalization by both care givers and the family. These cues include the infant's satisfaction after the feeding (i.e., asleep or fussy), the frequency of feedings, voiding pattern (minimum of six to eight wet diapers per day, weighing diapers and checking specific gravity) and palpation of maternal breasts before and after feeding. Trends in weight gain can also demonstrate the success of the mother and infant in breastfeeding.

The small infant may have difficulty taking a large nipple into the mouth. The mother should shape her nipple by compressing behind the areola to allow more of the nipple to be placed in the infant's mouth. The thumb and index finger or the first two fingers should be parallel to the infant's nose and chin. The breast must be soft enough to be compressed in this manner. It is important that the mother hold the infant closely for the comfort of both with the infant's entire body, not just the head, turned toward the mother's body (see Fig. 18-5).

A nipple shield allows the infant to get a nipple in the mouth but increases the amount of sucking required to obtain milk and decreases the amount of stimulation received at the nipple. Therefore using a nipple shield is never recommended and does not provide a rewarding experience for the mother or the infant. Preventing maternal and neonatal problems associated with breastfeeding is essential in making this a successful experience for both mother and infant (see section on prevention).

Because nonnutritive suckling does not stimulate prolactin secretion and milk production, infants should not be placed on an empty breast to feed. Without positive reinforcement (i.e., milk) for their efforts, infants soon learn that the breast does not give milk, become frustrated, and refuse to feed. The Lact-Aid Nursing Trainer may be used to initiate proper suckle and supplement intake in the small premature infant able to nurse (see section on prevention).

Supplementing breastfeedings with bottle-fed formula is energy and calorically inefficient, because the infant expends energy, thus calories, to feed twice. More energy and calorically efficient methods of initiating breastfeeding include feeding more often (i.e., smaller, more frequent feeds), supplementing by gavage feeding, or use of a Lact-Aid Nursing Trainer. Breast milk fortifiers (see Chapter 15) should be used when the mother is unavailable for feedings since use in a nursing trainer may "clog the system."

Nonavailability of a Feeding or Suckling Neonate

If premature birth or neonatal or maternal illness delays the onset of breastfeeding, the mother experiences a decrease in her milk production. Depending on how long breastfeeding has been delayed, mammary involution and the return of menstrual hormonal cycles may inhibit breastfeeding. The ill or preterm infant may be weak and tire easily, so that adequate lactation is not established.

It is important that the mother and infant be comfortable while breastfeeding. A comfortable chair with armrests or a pillow often helps, and the mother should be assured of privacy during breastfeeding and breast pumping.

If a neonate is unable to feed at the breast, breast milk can be produced through artificial stimulation of the breast. The mother should establish a regular routine of breast massage and pumping soon after the infant's birth. It is often necessary for the care provider to help the mother start and encourage her routine. Each breast should be pumped every 2 to 4 hours, preferably with a double pumping system in order to enhance milk supply. Mothers should increase pumping time up to 15 to 20 minutes as her milk comes in, with the suction pressure increased as the mother tolerates. Early in pumping the mother should awaken to pump at night in order to establish a good milk supply. Sleep and rest are necessary for good milk supply; however, the mother should not sleep when breasts are engorged since this will decrease the supply. Mothers need to be advised that if their infant were with them, they would be feeding every 2 to 4 hours around the clock and therefore should develop that pattern in order to establish an adequate supply. CAUTION: Mothers should be counseled regarding the potential risks

of using breast shells or breast pump kits that have been used by other women. Breast shells, pumps, and lactation aids are intimate care items and are meant for use with one mother and one baby.

Induction Aids. Various induction aids using tactile and mechanical principles are available to assist the mother in lactating and relactating. Knowledge of the different systems and their advantages and disadvantages enables the health care provider to help the mother choose the most helpful aid.

Breast massage (gentle, tactile, stimulus usually in a circular motion using increasing pressure) before breastfeeding or pumping may help unplug breast ducts and enable milk to flow more easily. Breast massage during pumping provides the important tactile stimulation that is missing without the infant's nursing and facilitates prolactin release and yields milk.[13]

Hand Expression. Once breast milk supply has been established, hand expression (Fig. 18-12) is the simplest and most cost-effective way to collect milk; however, prolactin secretion and milk yields

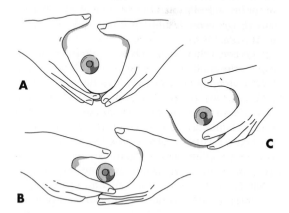

Figure 18-12 Breast massage. **A,** Place hands with palms toward chest at breast. Encircle breast with fingers and thumbs. **B** and **C,** Applying pressure, move hands forward, overlapping as they near nipple. Stop posterior to areola. Continue for 1 to 2 minutes or until milk is on nipple. Repeat on opposite breast. (From Bowman J, Hill R: *Pediatrics* 35:815, 1965; *Breastfeeding,* Evanston, Ill, 1981, American Academy of Pediatrics.)

are less than with a pulsative breast pump.[111] Some mothers find hand expression aesthetically unsatisfactory, and they should use other methods.

Mechanical Devices.   There are many different breast pumps costing from a few dollars to more than $1000. Available pumps include (1) automatic electric, (2) semiautomatic electric, (3) battery operated, and (4) hand operated. Serum prolactin levels and increased milk yield more closely approximate those of natural infant suckling when an intermittent, pulsative pump is used.[111] Just as nursing twins simultaneously results in a greater prolactin response, pumping both breasts simultaneously provides higher prolactin release (and higher milk yield).[95,111] Electric pumps are available in many NICUs and are available for rent for home use. For mothers whose infants will not be able to nurse at the breast for the first month of life, the automatic electric pump is the easiest and most efficient.

Breast pumps provide stimulation to initiate and maintain a milk supply until the infant is able to suckle. Beginning on the low or normal pump setting and carefully breaking the suction at the breast with a finger helps to prevent sore nipples. Painful maternal engorgement is relieved by pumping each breast just enough to obtain relief. Nipple or areolar engorgement must be relieved so that the infant is able to grasp and suckle the nipple.

To increase milk supply, the pump should be used frequently (see Table 18-3). Because the breast pump is not as efficient as the suckling infant, prior to initiating pumping tactile stimulation and breast massage may help increase the milk supply. Looking at the infant's picture or listening to a tape recording of the infant's cry stimulates milk production with a pump. To decrease engorgement, the pump should be used only as necessary to relieve discomfort, and only enough milk to make the breast more comfortable should be removed.

Complications

There are many complications other than prematurity that may pose difficulties with breastfeeding.

Information on perinatal complications and breastfeeding is contained in Table 18-5.[2] Due to the significant benefits of breast milk, infants with special needs should be encouraged and mothers assisted in breastfeeding. Many principles used with the preterm and other variations of feeding styles and techniques may be helpful in facilitating these infants and their mothers in enjoying a successful breastfeeding experience. Consultation with and/or referral to a lactation consultant or specialist may also be helpful.

Drugs in Breast Milk

Information about specific drugs excreted in breast milk is provided in Table 18-6.[3,50] Protein binding, degree of ionization, molecular weight, and solubility of drugs influence the passage of drugs into milk. Protein-bound drugs and drugs of large (>200) molecular weight are less likely to pass into milk. Conversely, lipid-soluble drugs pass more easily into the milk. Because breast milk is slightly acidic as compared with plasma, weakly alkaline compounds are equal or greater in breast milk than in plasma. Weakly acidic compounds have a higher concentration in plasma than in breast milk.

Several factors influence the drug effect on the infant. Most drugs appear in milk, but drug levels usually do not exceed 1% of the ingested dose and do not depend on the milk volume.[50] Many variables, such as gastric emptying, pH, and effects of intestinal enzymes, affect absorption. Finally, the chronologic and gestational ages of the infant affect the maturity of the systems involved in excretion and detoxification (see Chapter 9).

Parent Teaching

Parent teaching has been discussed throughout this chapter because it is so essential to a successful breastfeeding experience for both mother and infant.

Before a premature or sick infant is actually nursed at the breast, the colostrum and breast milk are pumped and fed to the infant. If the mother's production is adequate, no supplement is neces-

Table 18-5
Perinatal Complications and Breastfeeding

Complications	Breastfeed Yes	Breastfeed No	Comments
Maternal Complications			
Cesarean section	X		Regional anesthesia enables contact and feeding in recovery room. Pain medication is best given after feeding so levels peak before next feeding.
Pregnancy-induced hypertension	X		Preterm or SGA infants may be delivered, making delayed breastfeeding and pumping necessary. Maternal drugs may affect infant (see Table 18-6).
Venous thrombosis and pulmonary embolism	X		Depending on mother's ability; radioactive materials may be used for diagnosis, and anticoagulants may be used for therapy (see Table 18-6).
Bacterial Infections			
Urinary tract	X		Choice of antibiotics is important (see Table 18-6)
Mastitis	X		Continued emptying of breast (i.e., nursing baby or breast pump), bed rest, antibiotic therapy that is safe for infant, application of heat and cold, and use of analgesics are therapeutic.
Sexually transmitted diseases	X		No contraindication once mother is treated appropriately.
Tuberculosis		X	Culture-positive mothers must be separated from their infants regardless of mode of feeding.
	X		After therapy, when it is safe for mother to contact infant, then it is safe to breastfeed.
Diarrhea	X		Proper hand washing should be done and breastfeeding continued.
Viral Infections			
Cytomegalovirus	X		Both virus and protective antibodies occur in breast milk.
Rubella	X		Isolate infected infant from other infants and susceptible personnel. Mother is not contagious postpartum and need not be isolated from infant. Rooming-in may be considered.
Rubella immunization	X		There is no known adverse effect on infant.
Herpes simplex (HSV)	X	X	May breastfeed if there is no active lesion on breast. Strict hand washing, as well as covering of genital lesions, is necessary. Rooming-in supports breastfeeding while isolating infant from others in nursery.
Varicella (chickenpox)	X	X	If mother has chickenpox within 6 days of delivery, isolate mother and do not allow her to breastfeed until she is no longer contagious. Infant should be separated regardless of mode of feeding.
Measles (rubeola)	X	X	If infant has measles, may isolate mother and infant together and allow breastfeeding. Mothers with measles portpartum have breastfed, and neonates have acquired mild disease. Secretory antibodies are probably present in milk in 45 hr. Mother exposed before delivery without active disease should be isolated from infant, because 50% of infants contract disease.

Modified from American Academy of Pediatrics: *Report of the committee on infectious disease,* ed 23, Evanston, Ill, 1994, American Academy of Pediatrics; Lawrence RA: *Breastfeeding: a guide for the medical profession,* ed 4, St Louis, 1994, Mosby.

Continued

Table 18-5
Perinatal Complications and Breastfeeding—cont'd

Complications	Breastfeed		Comments
	Yes	No	
Viral Infections—cont'd			
Hepatitis	X	X	Hepatitis B antigen has been found in breast milk, but transmission by this route is not well documented. Both infants of chronic HBsAg carriers, and those with acute hepatitis should receive high titer hepatitis B immunoglobulin and hepatitis vaccine and breastfeeding is permitted.
HIV, AIDS		X	Breastfeeding is absolutely contraindicated in mothers who are HIV positive and living in developed countries where *safe* alternatives are available.[6,16,39]
Parasitic Infections			
Toxoplasmosis	X		No transmission of toxoplasmosis has been demonstrated in humans. Antibodies are present in breast milk.
Other Infections			
Trichomoniasis		X	Metronidazole is contraindicated for infant; milk may be pumped and discarded until therapy is completed. Mother's dose can be modified so she can pump and discard milk for 24-48 hours.
Other Maternal Complications			
Diabetes	X		Lactation is antidiabetogenic. Lactosuria must be differentiated from glycosuria.
Thyroid disease	X	X	Radioisotopes and thiouracil are found in breast milk and may adversely affect infant. Mother who is taking propylthiouracil can breastfeed. Neither hypothyroidism nor hyperthyroidism is contraindication alone.
Cystic fibrosis	X	X	May cause nutritional drain on mother. Milk composition is normal. The Cystic Fibrosis Association has guidelines for lactation.
Smoking	X	X	Nicotine interferes with letdown and is excreted in milk. Of mothers who smoke, breastfed infants are healthier than bottlefed infants.
Neonatal Complications			
Medical			
Diarrhea	X	X	Maintain breastfeeding in infectious diarrhea unless milk is source of infection. Congenital lactase deficiency is rare but requires lactose-free formula.
Respiratory disease	X	X	Breast milk by gavage may be used if infant's condition permits.
Galactosemia		X	Galactose (lactose) free diet is required.
Inborn errors of metabolism (such as PKU)	X	X	Combination of breast milk and special formula may sometimes be used. Careful monitoring of blood and urine levels of the amino acid is required.

Table 18-5
Perinatal Complications and Breastfeeding—cont'd

Complications	Breastfeed Yes	No	Comments
Neonatal Complications—cont'd			
Acrodermatitis enteropathica	X		Low plasma zinc levels are corrected by human milk and zinc sulfate supplementation.
Down syndrome	X		Hypotonia and poor suck reflex contribute to poor let-down and inadequate supply. Proper positioning, manual expression to begin feeding, and supporting the breast so infant does not lose nipple are helpful. Support from another mother with Down syndrome infant is helpful.
Hypothyroidism	X		Enough T_3 may be ingested to avoid serious symptoms.
Hyperbilirubinemia	X		May have slightly higher bilirubin than bottle-fed infant. There is no evidence that supplements are beneficial (see Chapter 20).
Breast milk jaundice	X	X	Uncommon occurrence; diagnosis of exclusion; if all other causes are excluded, a temporary cessation of breast milk may be indicated (see Chapter 20).
Cystic fibrosis	X		Increased losses of and lower electrolyte content of breast milk may cause electrolyte imbalance, which is less likely than with formulas.
Surgical			
Cleft lip and/or palate	X		Associated lesions, size, and position of defect influence successful feeding. Positioning and stabilizing breast in infant's mouth may help seal defect. Expressed milk in bottle with special nipple may be used. Consult plastic surgeon.
Gastrostomy	X		If gastrostomy feedings are used, expressed breast milk is appropriate.
Partial obstruction (meconium plug, ileus, Hirschsprung's disease)	X		If oral feedings are indicated, breast milk is feeding of choice because of digestibility and mild cathartic effect.
Necrotizing enterocolitis	X		Breastfeeding may be partially protective and may be used when feedings resume.
Gastrointestinal bleeding	X		Most common cause is maternal bleeding from nipple. Perform Apt test to differentiate fetal from adult hemoglobin.
CNS malformations	X		Weak suck and uncoordinated suck and swallow may be problems; however, may breastfeed more effectively than bottlefeed.

sary. Before collecting the mother's milk, perform the following:

- Screen (by history) mother for disease.
- Screen (by history) mother for maternal drugs.
- Instruct mother in sterile technique.

Proper collection and storage must be discussed with each family so that stored milk does not cause infections. Often the mother pumps and collects the milk, and the father transports it to the NICU (see Chapter 28). Methods of treatment and storage are listed in Box 18-1 on page 362. Rewarming techniques include placing frozen

Table 18-6
Drugs Excreted in Breast Milk

Drugs	Breast Milk	Infant
Analgesics		
Heroin,* codeine, meperidine, fentanyl, pentazocine, dextropropoxyphene, and diazepam	Appears in variable amounts.	Symptoms of depression and floppiness have been associated with these drugs.
Aspirin	Safe on a single-dose schedule, although it passes into milk.	In a deliberate overdose, metabolic acidosis resulted from an accumulation in the infant.
Acetaminophen	Appears in small amounts.	Well tolerated.
Ibuprofen	Appears in small amounts.	Well tolerated.
Antibiotics and Sulfa Drugs		
Sulfa drugs	Appear in breast milk and may interfere with bilirubin binding in neonate; infants with G6PD deficiency may develop hemolysis.	Should not be used for breastfeeding mother in the first month if infant is jaundiced or if infant has G6PD deficiency.
Chloramphenicol	Appears in breast milk.	Contraindicated in nursing mother because infant may accumulate it and develop "gray baby syndrome."
Tetracycline	Appears in breast milk at 50% of serum level.	Infants may develop stained and mottled teeth when therapy exceeds 10 days; should only be given for life-threatening maternal infections. Negligible absorption in infant—no contraindication to breastfeeding.
Metronidazole/Tinidazole	Appears in breast milk in levels equal to serum levels.	Side effects include decreased appetite, vomiting, blood dyscrasia, and animal evidence of tumorigenicity. Mother's dose can be modified (i.e., 2 g single-dose therapy) so she can pump and discard milk for 24 hours.
Cephalexin, cephalothin, oxacillin, chloroquine, and para-amino-salicylic acid	Very small amounts appear in breast milk.	Rash and sensitization are possible. May also affect bacterial flora.
Anticholinergics		
Atropine, scopolamine, synthetic quaternary ammonium derivatives	Atropine appears, but quaternary ammonium derivatives do not appear in breast milk.	The neonate of a nursing mother receiving atropine should be observed for tachycardia, constipation, and urinary retention.
Cimetidine	Appears in higher concentration than in serum.	No reported effects, although may suppress gastric activity, inhibit drug metabolism, and produce CNS stimulation. Use with caution until more information about antiandrogenic effects.

Modified from Lawrence RA: *Breastfeeding: a guide for the medical profession,* ed 4, St Louis, 1994, Mosby; American Academy of Pediatrics, Committee on Drugs: *Pediatrics* 93:137, 1994.
*Drug of abuse, contraindicated during breastfeeding—hazardous to both mother and infant.

Table 18-6
Drugs Excreted in Breast Milk—cont'd

Drugs	Breast Milk	Infant
Anticoagulants		
Heparin and warfarin (Coumadin)	Do not appear in breast milk.	
Antithyroidal Drugs		
Iodide	Passes into milk.	May affect thyroid activity and cause goiters. Not contraindicated during breastfeeding.
Thiouracil	Higher concentration in maternal milk than in blood.	Neonatal problems include suppression of thyroid activity and agranulocytosis. If breastfed, infant should be given thyroid supplement and thyroid function should be followed.
Propylthiouracil	Appears in small amounts.	No reported effects on infant. Follow with T_3, T_4, and TSH.
Anticonvulsants		
Phenobarbital, phenytoin, carbamazepine (Tegretol), and valproic acid (Depakene)	All appear in small amounts.	Sedation is possible, but rarely are clinical symptoms significant enough to cause adverse effects. Due to long half-life of valproic acid, accumulation may occur.
Cardiovascular Drugs		
Digitalis and propranolol	Appear only in small amounts.	Digitalis and propranolol appear to be safe.
Reserpine	Appears in breast milk.	Symptoms include diarrhea, lethargy, nasal stuffiness, bradycardia, and respiratory difficulties; contraindicated in breastfeeding.
Cathartics		
Aloin, cascara sagrada, and anthraquine preparations	Appear in breast milk.	Colic and diarrhea are possible side effects.
Contraceptives		
Birth control pills (combined; progestin only; mini pill)	Appear in breast milk with peak levels 2 hours after intake.	Combined: may alter the quality and quantity of milk—suppress lactation, shorter breastfeeding, and slower weight gain. Progestin only or mini pill—no alteration of milk volume or infant weight gain.
		Unknown long term risk of cancer—no evidence in last 30 years.[50]

Continued

Table 18-6
Drugs Excreted in Breast Milk—cont'd

Drugs	Breast Milk	Infant
Contraceptives—cont'd		
Medroxyprogesterone (Depo-Provera)	Increased prolactin levels before/after sucking.	No adverse effects—3 month injection (increased protein and quantity of milk); 6 month injection (increased quantity but decrease in protein, fat, calcium).[50]
Norplant	Steroid appears in small amount in breast milk.	No effect on milk production or infant growth and development.
Intrauterine devices	No chemicals to be excreted into breast milk.	No effects on infant.
Barrier methods (diaphragm, condoms, foams, cervical cap).	No chemicals to be excreted into breast milk.	No effects on infant.
Diagnostic Radioactive Compounds		
^{67}Ga, ^{125}I, ^{131}I, and ^{64}Cu	Appear for 24-48 hr.	Check half life of specific compound. Pump and discard, then resume breastfeeding.
Diuretics	May suppress lactation.	Inadequate milk; no significant risks are present.
Psychotherapeutics		
Lithium	Appears in breast milk; infant serum level is 10%-50% of mother.	Contraindicated in pregnancy and lactation. Cyanosis, hypotonia, ECG changes. Inhibits cyclic 3'-5' AMP, a substance significant to brain growth.
Phenothiazines	Appear in small amounts.	Evaluate each drug separately.
Diazepam (Valium)	Appears in breast milk and may accumulate in infant, because it is detoxified in liver.	Poor feeding, weight loss, hypoventilation, and drowsiness may be seen.
Tricyclic antidepressants	Appear in minimal amounts.	Careful considerations to select the safest for the infant.
Stimulants		
Caffeine	Appears in small amounts but may accumulate in infant.	Symptoms include jitteriness, wakefulness, and irritability.
Theophylline	Appears in moderate amounts.	Irritability, jitteriness, and wakefulness may be seen in infant.
Cocaine*	Appears in breast milk.	Cocaine intoxication: neurotoxicity, (e.g., irritability, hyperactive reflexes, tremulousness, and mood lability) and seizures have been reported[23,24] (see Chapter 4).

Modified from Lawrence RA: *Breastfeeding: a guide for the medical profession,* ed 4, St Louis, 1994, Mosby; American Academy of Pediatrics, Committee on Drugs: *Pediatrics* 93:137, 1994.
*Drug of abuse, contraindicated during breastfeeding—hazardous to both mother and infant.

Table 18-6
Drugs Excreted in Breast Milk—cont'd

Drugs	Breast Milk	Infant
Other		
Methadone	Appears in breast milk.	Management depends on maternal dosage—under 20 mg/24 h probably safe.
Ethanol (alcohol)	Quick equilibration between serum and breast milk levels.	Large quantities associated with lethargy, drowsiness, and affected motor development.[54] May inhibit milk let-down reflex and suppress lactation. Avoid nursing within 1-2 hours of alcohol intake.
Marijuana*	May reach high concentrations.	May decrease prolactin levels, milk supply, and motor development. Exposure to secondary smoke. Avoid breastfeeding for several hours after use.[49]
Nicotine	Appears in breast milk in proportion to number of cigarettes smoked.	Irritability; failure-to-thrive may result because of suppression of lactation. Effects of secondary smoke: increased incidence of upper respiratory infections, otitis media, bronchitis, and pneumonia. Avoid smoking in the same room with the infant.
Herbal tea mixtures (containing anise, fennel, liquorice, galega) used to stimulate lactation (i.e., mother's milk tea).	Essential oils found in anise and fennel appear in breast milk.	Difficulty feeding; growth failure; hypotonia; lethargy; vomiting; weak cry; poor suck; decreased reaction to painful stimuli.[89]
Silicone breast implants	Intact implants—not necessary to check milk for silicone. Leaking or ruptured implants—amount in breast milk unknown without silicone testing of milk and urine.	Abnormal results of motility studies of esophagus, recurrent abdominal pain, vomiting, and dysphagia, decrease wt/ht ratio.[52] No absolute contraindication to breastfeeding by women with silicone implants.[16]

milk in (1) a room temperature water bath, (2) a hot water bath, (3) a microwave oven, or (4) under cold running water and then tepid water. Slow room temperature rewarming is a concern because of bacterial overgrowth, especially if thawing is prolonged. Most nurseries use room temperature water bath rewarming to avoid exposure to the high temperatures of the hot water bath and the microwave. Microwaving is contraindicated because of the destruction of antiinfective properties (e.g., lysozyme and secretory IgA), re-

sulting in an overgrowth of bacteria.[35,43,95] Fresh breast milk is preferable for feedings because of its immunologic properties. If the mother visits the infant at feeding time, she may pump her breasts and the breast milk immediately fed to the infant.

Human milk banks that collect, store, and distribute milk to infants other than those of the donating mother exist around the world. This support is not available to some NICUs; others intentionally choose not to store donor milk. The reservations

---

Box 18-1

Treatment and Storage of Breast Milk

Treatment

1. Heat—Significant loss of lysozyme, lactoferrin, immunoglobulins, lactoperoxidase, lymphocyte function, complement, phagocytosis, and macromolecules may occur.
2. Lyophilization—Effects are similar to those of heat treatment.
3. Freezing—Limited information; cells are not viable, but there is no effect on IgA content.

Storage

1. Use sterile glass or polypropylene containers (amount for one feeding/bag); polyethylene bags change immunologic properties of breast milk and are more difficult for mothers to handle.
2. Label with name, date, and time of collection.
3. Store in refrigerator for 24 hours (at 0° C-4° C) or freeze (at −18° C) for longer periods.

---

about storing donor milk generally involve questions concerning adequate nutrition and immunologic benefit versus harm to the high-risk infant. Adequate screening of human milk donors (for cytomegalovirus [CMV], human immunodeficiency virus [HIV], etc.) is essential, as is informed consent. Because of the possibility of milk-borne pathogens (e.g., HIV, Hepatitis C) all donor milk must be pasteurized. Milk banks ship human milk when necessary. Contact the North American Association of Milk Banks (Box 370464, West Hartford Conn., USA, 06137-0464; phone (203)232-8809) for milk bank locations. Many nurseries do not give human milk other than the mother's.

A mother may be so concerned about the welfare of her infant that she spends most of her time at the hospital and receives inadequate rest, which is a common cause of milk production problems. The care plan includes encouraging, educating, and giving a mother permission to go home and rest, which may require someone to assist with the care of siblings. The stress of having a sick infant and the time spent at the hospital may preclude adequate maternal nutrition.

It is necessary to add about 600 kcal to the non-pregnant diet and to replace elements, such as calcium, minerals, and fat-soluble vitamins, used in producing milk. The recommended dietary increases are similar to those during pregnancy. Adequate fluid intake, 6 to 8 glasses of water, skim milk, or other noncaffeine liquids, should be consumed every day. Certain components of breast milk, such as quantity, protein, and calcium content, do not vary with maternal diet, whereas others (e.g., fatty and amino acids, lysine, methionine, and water-soluble vitamins) vary with maternal intake.

A mother's diet does not have much effect on the quality of the breast milk (unless malnutrition intervenes) but affects the mother's overall health. She should be reminded to eat a balanced diet. Vegetarian diets should be supplemented with about 4 mg of cyanocobalamin per day.

Anticipatory guidance for the mother breastfeeding a preterm infant is essential. The mother must be informed in the beginning that her milk supply may dwindle, even though she closely adheres to the pumping schedule. This is normal, because no pump stimulates the breast as efficiently and physiologically as the suckling infant. When the pumping regimen begins, explaining and drawing the mother a picture (Fig. 18-13) of what is commonly experienced helps alleviate guilt caused by a dwindling milk supply. A rather sparse supply of milk does not mean she cannot nurse the infant, because the milk supply will build in response to the infant's nutritive suckle. The parent should be taught that there is no correlation between the amount of breast milk expressed and the amount of milk a mother actually lets down when the infant is at the breast.

Breastfeeding problems may be particularly detrimental to the mother's perception of breastfeeding success. Disappointment with the breastfeeding experience may be due to unrealistic expectations regarding breastfeeding the preterm infant. Establishing realistic parental expectations for the first time the infant breastfeeds decreases disappointment from unattainable goals. Breastfeeding, like parenting, is not instinctual but is a learned behavior for both the mother and the infant. No one, including the health care provider, should expect immediate latch-on and vigorous sucking. The first several attempts at breastfeeding may consist only of direct skin contact, nuzzling,

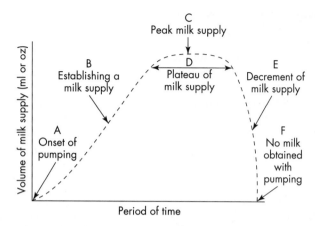

Figure 18-13 Establishing and maintaining milk supply by pumping. **A,** Pumping begins. **B,** Milk supply is established and increases. **C,** Peak or maximum volume of milk is established and plateaus. **D,** Gradually, supply begins to dwindle and may totally cease (**E**). **F,** Volume of milk and time period for decline in supply to begin and end in no milk production is an individual process. Some women begin and end cycle in days or weeks; others are able to pump for months. Even if supply dwindles to no milk, nutritive suckle of infant with Lact-Aid Nursing Trainer in place (see Fig. 18-10) will reestablish supply.

and licking behaviors by the infant, and cuddling and positioning by the mother. Any actual sucking is an "extra" reward but should not be anticipated.

Emotional support during breastfeeding of a normal or sick infant facilitates a successful experience for both the mother and the infant.[87,107] In one NICU without formalized support, only 10% of mothers were still breastfeeding 2 weeks after discharge. After a breastfeeding support group was instituted, 80% of mothers continued breastfeeding 2 weeks after discharge.[107] Support groups with mothers who have had similar experiences are helpful in supplementing support obtained from significant others and professionals.[87]

In the United States in 1989, only 32% to 38% of mothers of LBW infants initiated breastfeeding compared with 52% of all mothers.[90] There is an inverse relationship between gestational age and duration of breastfeeding, with most mothers (>50%) abandoning breastfeeding before their infants are discharged from the hospital.[38,65,74,75] The most common reason cited by mothers for discontinuation of breastfeeding (both in the hospital and after discharge) is inadequate milk supply (or "not getting enough").[46,65,75] Early initiation and establishment of adequate feeding at the breast before discharge encourages both mothers and

professionals that exclusive breastfeeding is successful. However, the early postdischarge period may be significantly stressful for mothers since the breastfeeding preterms feeding pattern may (1) predispose to underconsumption (i.e., inability to compensate for inadequate intake in one feeding by increasing the number or intake of subsequent feedings), (2) result in behaviors indicative of inadequate intake, and (3) require nutritional supplementation.[46,75]

Medical and nursing staff need to receive education and training regarding the many facets of the breastfeeding experience.[1,107,110] Staff attitudes and behaviors are important to breastfeeding families and provide input into the breastfeeding experience. A multidimensional approach to such education includes having manuals, guides, and other educational materials available for staff as well as scheduling routine classes, in-services, and workshops. Moreover, professionals with clinical expertise should be identified.[110] These reliable resource personnel can increase the staff's competency in counseling and assisting breastfeeding families.

Protocols addressing breastfeeding can outline a consistent approach for staff, as well as provide resource material that addresses successful strategies for handling common problems. Protocols can also serve to diminish the amount of incorrect information that is disseminated.[110]

Breast milk is the best milk, especially for the sick or premature infant. By understanding normal lactation, the health care provider can support the breastfeeding dyad when breastfeeding is delayed or disrupted.

References

1. American Academy of Pediatrics, Taskforce on the promotion of breastfeeding: The promotion of breastfeeding, *Pediatrics* 69:654, 1982.
2. American Academy of Pediatrics: *Report of the Committee on Infectious Disease,* ed 23, Evanston, Ill, 1994, American Academy of Pediatrics.
3. American Academy of Pediatrics, Committee on Drugs: The transfer of drugs and other chemicals into human breastmilk, *Pediatrics* 93:137, 1994.
4. American Academy of Pediatrics, Committee on Pediatric AIDS: Human milk, breastfeeding, and transmission of human immunodeficiency virus in the United States, *Pediatrics* 96:977, 1995.
5. Anderson G et al: Self-regulatory gavage-to-bottle feeding for preterm infants: effects on behavioral state, energy expenditure, and weight gain. In Fink S et al, editors: *Key aspects to recovery,* New York, 1990, Sprigle Publishing Company.
6. Anderson GC: Current knowledge about skin-to-skin (kangaroo) care for preterm infants, *J Perinatol* 11:216, 1991.
7. Atkinson S et al: Human milk: comparison of the nitrogen component in milk from mothers of premature and full-term infants, *Am J Clin Nutr* 33:811, 1980.
8. Atkinson S, Kaufman K: Lactational performance and milk composition in relation to duration of pregnancy and lactation. In Hamosh M, Goldman A, editors: *Human lactation 2: maternal and environmental factors,* New York, 1986, Plenian Press.
9. Auerbach K, Avery JL: Relactation after an untimely weaning: report from a survey, *Resources in Human Nurturing* (monograph 2), 1979.
10. Auerbach K, Avery JL: Relactation and the premature infant: report from a survey, *Resources in Human Nurturing* (monograph 3), 1979.
11. Auerbach K, Avery JL: Relactation after a hospital-induced separation: report from a survey, *Resources in Human Nurturing* (monograph 4), 1979.
12. Auerbach K: Sequential and simultaneous breast pumping: a comparison, *Int J Nurs Study* 27:257, 1993.
13. Auerbach K, Walker M: When the mother of a premature infant uses a breast pump: what every NICU nurse needs to know, *Neonat Net* 13:23, 1994.
14. Avery JL: Relactation and induced lactation. In Riordan J, editor: *A practical guide to breastfeeding,* St Louis, 1983, Mosby.
15. Bell E, Geyer J, Jones L: A structured intervention improves breastfeeding success for ill or preterm infants, *MCN* 20:309, 1995.
16. Berlin C: Silicone breast implants and breast feeding, *Pediatrics* 94:547, 1994.
17. Bier J et al: Breastfeeding of very low birth weight infants, *J Pediatr* 123:773, 1993.
18. Billeaud C, Guillet J, Sandler B: Gastric emptying in infants with our without gastro-esophageal reflux according to the type of milk, *Eur J Clin Nutr* 44:577, 1990.
19. Blass E: Behavioral and physiological consequences of suckling in rat and human newborns, *Acta Paediatr Suppl* 397:71, 1994.
20. Bosma JF, editor: *Oral sensation and perception,* Department of Health, Education & Welfare Pub No. (NIH) 73-546, Bethesda, Md, 1973, US Department of Health, Education and Welfare.
21. Brown L, Hollingsworth A, Armstrong C: Factors affecting milk volume in mothers of VLBW infants. In Programs and Abstracts of the 1991 Scientific Sessions of the 31st Biennial Convention, 1991.
22. Bulock F, Woolridge M, Baum J: Development of coordination of sucking, swallowing, and breathing: ultrasound study of term and preterm infants, *Dev Med Child Neurol* 32:669, 1990.
23. Chaney NE, Franke J, Wadlington WB: Cocaine convulsions in a breastfeeding baby, *J Pediatr* 112:134, 1988.
24. Chasnoff IJ, Lewis DE, Squires L: Cocaine intoxication in a breastfeeding infant, *Pediatrics* 80:836, 1987.
25. Cowett R et al: Aberrations in sucking behavior of low birth weight infants, *Dev Med Child Neurol* 20:710, 1978.
26. Crook C, Lipsitt L: Neonatal nutritive sucking: effects of taste stimulation upon sucking rhythm and heart rate, *Child Dev* 47:518, 1976.
27. Cunningham A, Jelliffe D, Jelliffe E: Breastfeeding and health in the 1980s: a global epidemiologic review, *J Pediatr* 118:659, 1991.
28. Daniels H, Casaer P: Development of arm posture during bottle feeding in preterm infants, *Infants Behav Dev* 8:241, 1985.
29. Dewey K, Heinig J, Nommsen-Rivers L: Differences in morbidity between breastfed and formula fed infants, *J Pediatr* 126(5):696, 1995.
30. Dubignon J et al: The differences between laboratory measures of sucking, food intake, and perinatal factors during the newborn period, *Child Dev* 40:1118, 1969.
31. European Collaborative Study: Risk factors for mother-to-child transmission of HIV-1, *Lancet* 339:1007, 1992.
32. Fehrer S et al: Increasing breast milk production for premature infants with a relaxation/imagery audiotape, *Pediatrics* 83:57, 1989.
33. Freier S, Eidelman AI: Human milk, its biological and social value, *Excerpta Medica,* International Congress Series 518, 1980.
34. Goldson E: Nonnutritive sucking in the sick infant, *J Perinatol* 9(1):30, 1987.
35. Guilleminault C, Coons S: Apnea and bradycardia during feeding in infants weighing >2,000 grams, *J Pediatr* 104:932, 1984.

36. Hagan R et al: Breastfeeding and very low birthweight (VLBW) infants, Abstract #1284, *Neonatology General,* 1991.
37. Hammerman C, Kaplan M: Oxygen saturation during and after feeding in healthy term infants, *Biol Neonate* 67:94, 1995.
38. Hill P, Anderson J, Ledbetter R: Delayed initiation of breastfeeding the preterm infant, *J Perinat Neonat Nurs* 9(2):10, 1995.
39. Hofer M: Early relationships as regulators of infant physiology and behavior, *Acta Pediatr Suppl* 397:9, 1994.
40. Hopkinson J, Schanler R, Garza C: Milk production by mothers of premature infants, *Pediatrics* 81:815, 1988.
41. Institute of Medicine, Committee on Nutritional Status During Pregnancy and Lactation: *Nutrition during pregnancy and lactation: an implementation guide,* Washington DC, 1992, National Academy Press.
42. Jain L et al: Energetics and mechanics of nutritive sucking in the preterm and term neonate, *J Pediatr* 111:894, 1987.
43. Jason JM, Jones BM, Haff BC: The effects of microwave on human milk immune components. *Pediatr Res* 20:390A, 1986.
44. Jelliffe DM, Jelliffe EFP: *Human milk in the modern world,* London, 1978, Oxford University Press.
45. Johnston JM, Amico JA: A prospective longitudinal study of the release of oxytocin and prolactin in response to infant suckling in longterm lactation, *J Clin Endocrinol Metab* 62:653, 1986.
46. Kavanaugh K et al: Getting enough: mother's concerns about breastfeeding a preterm infant after discharge, *JOGNN* 24:23, 1995.
47. Kennedy C, Lipsitt L: Temporal characteristics of non-oral feedings and chronic feeding problems in premature infants, *J Perinat Neonatal Nurs* 7(3):77, 1993.
48. Kron R, Stein M, Goddard K: Newborn sucking behavior affected by obstetric sedation, *Pediatrics* 37:1012, 1966.
49. Lawrence P: Breast milk: best source of nutrition for term and preterm infants, *Pediatr Clin North Am* 41(5):925, 1994.
50. Lawrence RA: *Breastfeeding: a guide for the medical professional,* ed 4, St Louis, 1994, Mosby.
51. Lawrence R: The clinician's role in teaching proper infant feeding techniques, *J Pediatr* 126:5112, 1995.
52. Levine J, Ilowite N: Scleroderma like esophageal disease in children breastfed by mothers with silicone breast implants, *JAMA* 271:213, 1994.
53. Lipsitt L et al: The stability and interrelationships of newborn sucking and heart rate, *Dev Psychobiol* 9(4):305, 1976.
54. Little R et al: Maternal alcohol abuse and infant motor development at one year, *NEJM* 321:425, 1989.
55. Lucas A, Lucas P, Baum J: Differences in the pattern of milk intake between breast and bottlefed infants, *Early Hum Dev* 5:195, 1981.
56. Lucas H, Cole T: Breast milk and neonatal necrotizing enterocolitis, *Lancet* 336:1519, 1990.
57. Lucas A et al: Breast milk and subsequent intelligence quotient in children born premature, *Lancet* 339:261, 1992.
58. Lucas A et al: A randomized multicenter study of human milk versus formula and later development in preterm infants, *Arch Dis Child* 70:F141, 1994.
59. Luukkainen P, Salo M, Nikkani T: Changes in fatty acid composition of preterm and term human milk from one week to six months of lactation, *J Pediatric Gastroenterol Nutr* 18:355, 1994.
60. Marchini G et al: The effect of non-nutritive sucking on plasma insulin, gastrin, and somatostatin levels in infants, *Acta Paediatr Scand* 76:753, 1987.
61. Martell M et al: Suction patterns in preterm infants, *J Perinat Med* 21:363, 1993.
62. Matthew O: Nipple units for newborn infants: a functional comparison, *Pediatrics* 81:688, 1988.
63. Matthew O: Determinants of milk flow through nipples, *Am J Dis Child* 144:222, 1990.
64. Matthew O: Science of bottle feeding, *J Pediatr* 119:511, 1991.
65. McCoy R et al: Nursing management of breastfeeding for preterm infants, *J Perinat Neonat Nurs* 2(1):42, 1988.
66. McNeilly AS et al: Release of oxytocin and prolactin in responses to suckling, *Br Med J* 286:257, 1983.
67. Medoff-Cooper B, Weininger S, Zukowsky K: Neonatal sucking as a clinical assessment tool: preliminary findings, *Nurs Res* 40:245, 1991.
68. Medoff-Cooper V, Verklan T, Carlson S: The development of sucking patterns and physiologic correlates in very-low-birth-weight infants, *Nurs Res* 42:100, 1993.
69. Meier P, Pugh EJ: Breastfeeding behavior of small preterm infants, *Matern Child Nurs J* 10:396, 1985.
70. Meier P, Anderson GC: Responses of small preterm infants to bottle and breastfeeding, *Matern Child Nurs J* 12:97, 1987.
71. Meier P: Bottle and breastfeeding: effects on transcutaneous pressure and temperature in preterm infants, *Nurs Res* 37:36, 1988.
72. Meier P: Suck-breathe patterning during bottle and breastfeeding for preterm infants. In *Programs and Abstracts of the 1993 council of nurse researchers,* Washington DC, 1993.
73. Meier P et al: Breastfeeding support services in the neonatal intensive care unit, *JOGNN* 22:338, 1993.
74. Meier P, Mangurten H: Breastfeeding the preterm infant. In Riordan J, Averback K, editors: *Breastfeeding and human lactation,* Boston, 1993, Jones and Bartlett.
75. Meier P, Brown L: Breastfeeding for mothers and low birth weight infants, *Nurs Clin North Am* 31:351, 1996.
76. Melnikow J, Bedinghaus J: Management of common breastfeeding problems, *J Fam Pract* 39(1):56, 1994.
77. Neifert M, Lawrence R: Nipple confusion: toward a more formal definition, *J Pediatr* 126:5125, 1995.
78. Newman J: How breast milk protects newborns, *Sci Am* 273(6):76, 1995.
79. Nowak A, Smith W, Erenberg A: Imaging evaluation of artificial nipples during bottlefeeding, *Arch Pediatr Adolesc Med* 148:40, 1994.
80. Nowak A, Smith W, Erenberg A: Imaging evaluation of breastfeeding and bottlefeeding systems, *J Pediatr* 126:5130, 1995.
81. Orlando S: The immunologic significance of breast milk, *JOGNN* 24:678, 1995.
82. Pickler R, Frankel H: The effect of non-nutritive sucking on preterm infant's behavioral organization and feeding performance, *Neonat Net* 14:83, 1995.

83. Position of the American Dietetic Association: Promotion and support of breastfeeding, *J Am Diet Assoc* 93:467, 1993.

84. Quan R et al: Effects of microwave radiation on anti-infective factors in human milk, *Pediatrics* 89(4):667, 1992.

85. Rentschler D: Correlates of successful breastfeeding, *Image: J Nurs Scholar* 23(3):151, 1991.

86. Riordan J: *A practical guide to breastfeeding,* St Louis, 1983, Mosby.

87. Riordan J: Social support and breast feeding, *Breastfeeding Abstracts* 8:13, 1989.

88. Rosenblatt J: Psychobiology of maternal behavior: contribution to the clinical understanding of maternal behavior among humans, *Acta Paediatr Suppl* 397:3, 1994.

89. Rosti L et al: Toxic effects of herbal tea mixture in two newborns, *Acta Paediatr* 83(6):683, 1994.

90. Ryan A et al: A comparison of breastfeeding data from the national surveys of family growth and the Ross Laboratories' mothers surveys, *Am J Public Health* 81:1049, 1991.

91. Samuels SE, Margen S, Schoen EJ: Incidence and duration of breastfeeding in a health maintenance organization population, *Am J Clin Nutr* 42:504, 1985.

92. Schanler R, Hurst N: Human milk for the hospitalized preterm infant, *Semin Perinatol* 18(6):476, 1994.

93. Shivpuri C et al: Decreased ventilation in preterm infants during oral feeding, *J Pediatr* 103:285, 1983.

94. Sidell E, Froman R: A national survey of neonatal intensive care units: criteria used to determine readiness for oral feedings, *JOGNN* 23:783, 1994.

95. Sigman M et al: Effects of microwaving human milk: changes in IgA content and bacterial content, *J Am Diet Assoc* 89:690, 1989.

96. Smith WL, Erenberg A, Nowak A: Imaging evaluation of the human nipple during breastfeeding, *Am J Dis Child* 142:76, 1988.

97. Smotherman W, Robinson S: Milk as the proximal mechanism for behavioral changes in the newborn, *Acta Paediatr Suppl* 397:64, 1994.

98. Snell BJ: Physiologic response of the preterm infant during the early initiation of breastfeeding versus bottlefeeding, Doctoral dissertation, 1991, Oregon Health Sciences University.

99. Stine M: Breastfeeding and the premature newborn: a protocol without bottles, *J Hum Lact* 6(4):167, 1990.

100. Timms B, et al: Increased respiratory drive as an inhibitor of oral feeding of preterm infants, *J Pediatr* 123:127, 1993.

101. Tyson JE: Nursing and prolactin secretion: principal determinants in the mediation of puerperal infertility. In Crosignani PG et al, editors: *Prolactin and human reproduction,* New York, 1977, Academic Press.

102. Uauy R et al: Effect of dietary omega-3 fatty acids on retrieval function of very-low-birth-weight neonates, *Pediatr Res* 28:415, 1990.

103. Urzizee F, Gross S: Improved feeding tolerance and reduced incidence of sepsis of very low birth weight infants fed maternal milk (abstract), *Pediatr Res* 25:298A, 1989.

104. US Public Health Service: *Healthy people 2000,* Washington, DC, 1989, Government Printing Office.

105. Van de Perre P et al: Infective and anti-infective properties of breastmilk from HIV-infected women, *Lancet* 341:914, 1993.

106. Vorherr H: Human lactation, *Semin Perinatol* 3(3):191, 1979.

107. Woldt EH: Breastfeeding support group in the NICU, *Neonat Net* 9(5):53, 1991.

108. Wolff P: The serial organization of sucking in the young infant, *Pediatrics* 42:943, 1968.

109. Woodson R et al: Effects of non-nutritive sucking on state and activity: term-preterm comparison, *Infant Behav Dev* 8:435, 1985.

110. Ziemer MM, George C: Breastfeeding the LBW infant, *Neonat Net* 9(4):33, 1990.

111. Zinamen MJ et al: Acute prolactin and oxytocin responses and milk yield to infant suckling and artificial methods of expression in lactating women, *Pediatrics* 89(3):437, 1992.

Resource Materials for Parents

Danner, S: *Nursing your premature infant, nursing the neurological impaired infant; nursing the infant with cleft lip and cleft palate,* 1994, Childbirth Graphics.

Harrison H: *The premature baby book,* New York, 1983, St Martin's Press.

Huggins K: *The nursing mother's companion,* Boston, 1990, The Harvard Common Press.

Lact-aid, International, P.O. Box 1066, Athens, TN 37303; (615) 744-9090.

LaLeche League International: *The womanly art of breastfeeding,* Danville, Ill, 1987, The Interstate Printers and Publishers.

Lauwers J, Woessner C: *Counseling the nursing mother,* ed 2, New York, 1990, Avery Publishing Group.

Olds SW, Eiger MS: *The complete book of breastfeeding,* New York, 1987, Workman Publishing.

Renfrew M, Fischer C, Arms S: *Breastfeeding, getting breastfeeding right for you,* California, 1990, Celestial Arts.

Tomaselli KM: *Guide to breastfeeding,* New York, 1991, Childbirth Graphics.

Walker M, Watson J: *Breastfeeding your premature or special care baby: a practical guide for nursing the tiny baby,* ed 2, Boston, Mass, 1989, Lactation Associates.

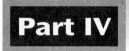

Part IV — Infection and Hematologic Diseases of the Neonate

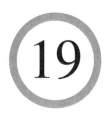

19 Newborn Hematology

Marilyn Manco Johnson, Donna J. Rodden, Shannon Collins

Red Blood Cells

Physiology

Red blood cells transport and deliver oxygen to vital organs and body tissues. Red blood corpuscles are simple cells composed of membrane encasing hemoglobin with an energy system to fuel the cells. Hemoglobin is the protein in red cells that carries oxygen, binding and releasing it based upon concentration differences. Ex utero, red cells absorb oxygen by diffusion in the lungs, where the oxygen tension of the alveolar air is higher than that of the capillary blood, and release it from the systemic capillaries, where the oxygen tension is now higher than that of surrounding tissues. In utero, oxygen diffuses to the fetus from the placental venous circulation. Fetal red cells contain a unique hemoglobin (fetal hemoglobin) in which the two beta chains of adult hemoglobin (called hemoglobin A1) are replaced by two gamma chains. Fetal hemoglobin (called hemoglobin F) has a higher affinity for oxygen than does adult hemoglobin, allowing fetal red cells to compete successfully for available oxygen. Normal fetal red cells are characterized by an increased mean corpuscular hemoglobin (MCH), mean corpuscular volume (MCV), hemoglobin, and hematocrit. After birth with the transition to air breathing and a higher blood oxygen tension, the hypoxic stimulus driving fetal red cell production in the bone marrow is removed. The plasma concentration of erythropoi-etin, the hormone that stimulates bone marrow production of red blood cells, falls. The number of circulating reticulocytes, which are young red blood cells in the circulation, decreases. Subsequently, the hemoglobin and hematocrit diminish until a new equilibrium is reached. Postnatal changes in red cell production include an increase in the ratio of hemoglobin A to hemoglobin F and an increase in levels of the red cell enzyme 2,3-diphosphoglycerate (2,3-DPG). 2,3-DPG promotes the release of oxygen to tissues by decreasing hemoglobin affinity to oxygen within tissues. Oxygen delivery in the neonate is a function both of the ratio of hemoglobin F to A and of the red cell concentration of 2,3-DPG.

The production of embryonic and fetal hematopoieic cells is first seen within the yolk sac in the 14-day embryo and disappears by the eleventh week of gestation.[13] Hematopoiesis in other tissues results from colonization by stem cells derived from the yolk sac.[6] By the fifth to sixth week, embryonic erythropoietic activity is present in the liver. The liver becomes the primary source of red cell production by 8 to 9 weeks.[9] Between the eighth to twelfth week the spleen and lymph nodes are involved in erythropoiesis.[11] Other tissues and organs involved in erythropoiesis include the kidney, thymus, and connective tissue. There is no evidence of erythropoietin production before the tenth week.[48] After the tenth week of gestation, erythropoietin production rises and seems to be

involved in red cell production in the bone marrow during the third trimester.[12] Initially, production of erythropoietin is in the fetal liver, and by the last trimester, production is in the kidneys. The level of erythropoietin gradually rises to significant levels after the thirty-fourth week of gestation.[11] Elevated erythropoietin levels can be found when the fetus is hypoxic.[9] Erythropoiesis is found in the bone marrow at 10 to 11 weeks. This activity increases rapidly until the twenty fourth week when bone marrow erythropoiesis replaces liver erythropoiesis. **Changes in the blood count at the time of birth are shown in Table 19-1.**[10,11]

In more than 90% of healthy term infants the **hematocrit range is 48% to 60% and the hemoglobin range is 16-20 g/dl.**[11] **Normally after term birth, hemoglobin concentrations fall from a mean of 17 g/dl to approximately 11 g/dl by 2 to 3 months of age. This nadir in red blood cell values is termed** *physiologic anemia of the newborn* **and is a normal process in the adaptation to extrauterine life.**

Several factors need to be considered in the interpretation of hematocrit values in the newborn, including age of the infant (both in hours and days), site of blood collection, and method of analysis. Hematocrit changes significantly during the first 24 hours of life; it peaks at 2 hours of age and then progressively drops with decreases occurring at 6 and 24 hours of age.[41] **This is due to transudation of fluid out of the intravascular space. The** method used to determine hematocrit can significantly affect the value. **Capillary hematocrit measurements are highly subject to variations in blood flow.**[20,30] **Prewarming the site minimizes the artifactual increase in the hematocrit. When obtaining blood counts, it is important to note that in both term and preterm infants there can be as much as a 20% difference between the hematocrit obtained from a capillary puncture (commonly termed heel stick) and the hematocrit drawn from a central vein. Capillary, arterial, and venous blood reveal notably decreasing values in that order, thereby underscoring the importance of same source serial measurements. Finally, it is crucial that a microcentrifuge or spun hematocrit be obtained rather than a hematocrit determination in an automated blood cell counter (Coulter Counter) because the latter frequently gives falsely low hematocrit values in the newborn.**[44]

Adult red cells circulate for an average of 120 days. Normal neonatal red blood cells have a circulating half-life reduction of 20% to 25% compared with older children or adults. Survival of red cells of premature infants is reduced by approximately 50%.

Pathophysiology of Anemia

Anemia is a deficiency in the concentration of red cells and hemoglobin in the blood and results in tissue hypoxia and acidosis. Anemia is defined by a hemoglobin or hematocrit value that is greater than two standard deviations below the mean for postconceptual and postnatal age.

Determination of the cause of anemia is important to direct treatment. Anemia in the newborn results from one or more of the following basic mechanisms:

- **Blood loss (acute or chronic)**
- **Decreased red cell production**
- **Shortened red cell survival**

Blood Loss

Acute and chronic blood loss is the most common cause of anemia in the neonate. Blood loss can occur intrauterine, perinatally, or postnatally. Some form of fetomaternal hemorrhage occurs in 50% of all pregnancies.[10] Blood loss is usually

Table 19-1
Changes in Erythropoiesis Around the Time of Term Birth

	In Utero	Postdelivery
Oxygen saturation (%)	45*	95
Erythropoietin levels	High	Undetectable
Red cell production	Rapid	<10% (by day 7)
Reticulocyte count (%)	3-7	0-1 (by day 7)
Hemoglobin (g/dl)	16.8	18.4
Hematocrit (%)	53	58
MCV (fl)	107	98 (by day 7)
MCHC (g/dl)	31.7	33 (by day 7)

*Mean values represented. *MCV,* Mean corpuscular volume; *MCHC,* mean corpuscular hemoglobin concentration.[4,7]

insignificant; however, in 1% of pregnancies, blood loss can be greater than 40 ml.[22] The blood volume of the fetus is approximately 90 ml/kg. Large blood loss can cause profound anemia, asphyxia, and death. Anemia caused by chronic blood loss is better tolerated as the neonate is able to compensate for the gradual loss in red cell mass. There is a large differential for blood loss in the neonate (Box 19-1).

Fetomaternal transfusion is a common cause of occult blood loss in the fetus. The Kleihauer-Betke acid elution test is the method used to confirm the presence of fetal blood cells in the maternal circulation.[47] The volume of fetal blood in the maternal circulation is estimated by counting fetal red cells on the maternal blood smear under light microscopy. Fetal cells retain red staining of hemoglobin after fixing, whereas adult cells are very pale because hemoglobin has been eluted (also called ghost cells). Ten fetal cells per 30 fields viewed under high power are equal to 1 ml of fetal blood.

Twin-to-twin transfusion is another cause of occult blood loss and is seen in 15% to 30% of all monochorionic twins with abnormalities of placental blood vessels.[42] The anemic twin is on the arterial side of the placental vascular malformation. The clinical significance of twin-to-twin transfusion depends on the duration of blood transfer. With chronic transfusion, a 20% weight discordance similar to that observed with placental insufficiency can be found.[32]

Intracranial bleeds associated with prematurity, later birth order of multiple gestation delivery, rapid delivery, breech delivery, and massive cephalhematoma can cause anemia. Other sites of neonatal hemorrhage include umbilical, retroperitoneal, adrenal, renal, and gastrointestinal bleeding, as well as ruptured liver or spleen.

Swallowed maternal blood may be confused

Box 19-1

Etiologies of Blood Loss in the Neonate

I. Hemorrhage before birth
  A. Fetomaternal
    1. Traumatic amniocentesis or periumbilical blood sampling
    2. Spontaneous
    3. Chronic gastrointestinal
    4. Blunt trauma to the maternal abdomen
    5. Postexternal positioning
  B. Twin-to-twin
  C. External
    1. Abruptio placenta
    2. Placenta previa
II. Hemorrhage during birth
  A. Placental malformation
    1. Chorangioma
    2. Chorangiocarcinoma
  B. Hematoma of the cord or placenta
  C. Rupture of a normal umbilical cord
    1. Precipitous delivery
    2. Entanglement
  D. Rupture of an abnormal umbilical cord
    1. Varices
    2. Aneurysm
  E. Rupture of anomalous vessels
    1. Aberrant vessel
    2. Velamentous insertion of the cord
    3. Communicating vessels in the multilobular placenta
  F. Incision of placenta during cesarean section
III. Internal fetal or neonatal hemorrhage
  A. Intracranial
  B. Giant cephalohematoma, caput succedaneum
  C. Pulmonary
  D. Retroperitoneum
  E. Subcapsular liver or spleen
  F. Renal or adrenal
IV. External neonatal hemorrhage
  A. Delayed clamping of the umbilical cord
  B. Gastrointestinal
  C. Iatrogenic from blood sampling

Modified from Luchtman-Jones L, Schwartz A, Wilson D: Hematologic problems in the fetus and neonate. In Fanaroff A: *Neonatal-perinatal medicine,* vol 2, 1997.

with gastrointestinal bleeding. The Apt test is used to distinguish swallowed maternal blood from neonatal blood and is based upon alkali resistance of fetal hemoglobin.[2] A 1% solution of sodium hydroxide is added to 5 ml of diluted blood. Fetal hemoglobin will remain pink, but adult hemoglobin will become yellow.

Iatrogenic blood loss results from blood sampling with inadequate replacement. A survey performed in the intensive care nursery of the University of California at San Francisco found that an average of 38.9 ml of blood was removed for laboratory tests during the first week of life.[38] For premature infants whose blood volume can be as little as 50 ml, anemia is commonly caused by blood draws. **The majority of red cell transfusions given in nurseries is directly related to frequent blood sampling.[28]**

Decreased Red Cell Production

Anemia caused by decreased production of red cells tends to develop slowly, allowing time for physiologic compensation. Affected infants may have few signs of anemia other than pallor. The reticulocyte count will be low and inappropriate for the degree of anemia.

Iron deficiency is the leading cause of anemia in infancy and childhood worldwide. Iron deficiency anemia can occur at any time when growth exceeds the ability of the stores and dietary intake to supply sufficient iron for erythropoiesis. Iron storage at birth is directly related to body weight. A term infant should have sufficient iron stores for 4 to 6 months of life.[31] Infants who are fed exclusively breast milk or iron-enriched formula and cereal are less likely to develop iron deficiency anemia.

Premature infants have iron stores adequate for less than 3 months postnatally because of low birth weight, faster rate of growth, and iatrogenic blood losses. Iron supplementation is required early in preterm infants to prevent anemia (Table 19-2).

Iron deficiency causes a hypochromic, microcytic anemia. The peripheral smear shows small, pale red cells with a large variety of shapes and sizes resulting in an increased relative distribution of width (RDW). The platelet count is increased and may be greater than 1,000,000/μl.

Table 19-2
Recommended Iron Supplementation for the Neonate

Group	Dose (mg/kg/day)	Initiation, Duration
Full term	1	4 mo to 3 yr
Preterm, low birth weight	2	2 mo to 1 yr, then
	1	1 yr to 3 yr
Very low birth weight	4	2 mo to 1 yr, then
	1	1 yr to 3 yr

Mild forms of iron deficiency may be confused with other causes of anemia, including infection and thalassemia. A therapeutic trial of iron can be used to diagnose iron deficiency. After 1 month of ferrous sulfate, 6 mg/kg/day, the hemoglobin should rise at least 1 g/dl, in the absence of ongoing blood loss.[22]

Anemia of prematurity is common in infants born at less than 35 weeks' gestation. This is a normocytic, normochromic anemia appearing between 2 and 6 weeks characterized by a low reticulocyte count and an inadequate response to erythropoietin.[39] If hemoglobin levels drop below 10 g/dl, the infant may display decreased activity, poor growth, tachypnea, and tachycardia. Randomized, placebo-controlled studies that include supplemental iron demonstrate a reduction in the amount of blood transfused in infants treated with erythropoietin.[29]

Hypothyroidism, deficiency of transcobalamin II, and inborn errors of cobalamin utilization cause macrocytic anemia because of decreased and ineffective bone marrow production.

Constitutional pure red cell aplasia is also known as Blackfan-Diamond anemia.[21] This normocytic or macrocytic anemia presents at birth in 10% and by 1 month in 25% of affected infants. Signs and symptoms include pallor, anemia, and reticulocytopenia. In red cell aplasia the platelet count may be moderately elevated and the leukocyte count may be slightly decreased. Bone marrow examination is normocellular with few erythroid precursors. Thirty percent of affected infants demonstrate congenital anomalies primarily of the head, face, eyes, and thumb. The syndrome can have autosomal dominant or recessive inheritance. As infants grow older, characteristics of fetal erythropoiesis persist, including elevations in fetal hemoglobin, i antigen, and red cell adenosine deaminase (ADA), as well as fetal patterns of red cell enzymes. Seventy percent of affected infants respond to corticosteroids, particularly if they are initiated early in infancy. Infants who do not respond to steroids require chronic red cell transfusion therapy and are at risk for subsequent iron overload. Il-3 infusions may be effective in some patients.

Fanconi's anemia is a congenital syndrome of progressive bone marrow failure with autosomal recessive inheritance.[1] At birth, infants may be recognized by one or more of the associated congenital defects, which include microcephaly; short stature; absent or abnormal thumb; and other cutaneous, musculoskeletal, and urogenital abnormalities. Thrombocytopenia and an elevated MCV are usually the first hematologic abnormalities, but they are seldom recognized in the neonatal period. The underlying defect in Fanconi's anemia is an inability to repair damaged DNA. Chromosomal breakage analyses and specific molecular diagnosis have been used for prenatal diagnosis.

B19 parvovirus exerts an inhibitory effect on bone marrow production of red cells.[46] Infection with B19 parvovirus during pregnancy can cause hydrops fetalis, a syndrome of congestive heart failure, massive skin edema, and severe anemia, especially during the first two trimesters. Early detection of parvovirus infection in pregnant women and serial examinations with ultrasound are important to diagnose and monitor the condition. Affected fetuses have been successfully supported with intrauterine transfusions of red blood cells. Parvovirus effects on the bone marrow are insufficient to cause anemia in most infants with a normal red cell life span but may cause symptomatic anemia in infants with hemolytic anemia or immunodeficiency. Infants with congenital or acquired immunodeficiency may become anemic because of an inability to clear parvovirus.

Infants with genetic hemoglobin mutations of alpha or gamma chains, resulting in production of hemoglobins with decreased oxygen affinity, will have lower hemoglobins without signs of tissue hypoxia.

Shortened Red Cell Survival

Senescent red cells are removed from the circulation by the reticuloendothelial system. Bilirubin is produced by degradation of the heme moiety of hemoglobin, and red cell iron is recycled. Many conditions accelerate removal of red cells from the circulation. Hemolysis is a term for premature red cell destruction relative to expected life-span for postconceptual age. Hyperbilirubinemia is evident in most cases of hemolysis. Reticulocytosis is usually found. However, in the presence of chronic illness, nutritional deficiency, or congenital infection, the reticulocyte count may be lower than expected for the degree of anemia. In the most severe case of intrauterine hemolysis the outcome is hydrops fetalis, a syndrome of severe anemia with congestive heart failure and diffuse skin edema (Box 19-2).

Isoimmune hemolytic anemia occurs when fetal cells, bearing antigens of paternal origin that the mother does not possess, enter the maternal circulation and stimulate production of IgG antibodies. The IgG antibodies are transferred across the placenta, coat fetal red cells, and mediate their removal from the circulation through the reticuloendothelial system.

The major fetal red cell antigens responsible for isoimmune hemolytic anemia include the Rh (also called D) antigen in an Rh negative mother and the blood group A and B antigens in a group O mother. Kell, Duffy, and Kidd antigens can also cause isoimmune hemolytic anemia. Sources of maternal sensitization to fetal red cell antigens include chorionic villus sampling, amniocentesis, abortion, rupture of an ectopic pregnancy, maternal blood transfusion, and fetomaternal transfusion. Anti-Rh antibodies derived from plasma of previously sensitized donors are given to Rh negative mothers at 28 weeks' gestation, at delivery, and at the time of any of the above mentioned events. These antibodies coat any fetal red cells present in the maternal circulation and prevent them from initiating the maternal immune response. Thus they provide a form of passive immunization. With widespread use of Rh immune globulin (Ig) to Rh negative mothers, the rate of anti-Rh Ig formation dropped from 17% to 9% to 13%.[3,45] The rate of Rh hemolytic disease in the United States is 10.6 per

Box 19-2

Etiologies of Shortened Red Cell Survival in the Neonate

I. Isoimmune-mediated hemolysis
  A. Rh incompatibility
  B. ABO incompatibility
  C. Minor blood cell antigen incompatibility
II. Infection
  A. Bacterial sepsis
  B. Campylobacter jejuni
  C. Clostridium welchii
  D. Rubella
  E. Cytomegalovirus
  F. Epstein-Barr virus
  G. Disseminated herpes
  H. Malaria
  I. Toxoplasmosis
  J. Syphilis
III. Microangiopathic and macroangiopathic
  A. Cavernous hemangioma (Kasabach-Merritt)
  B. Renal vein thrombosis
  C. Disseminated intravascular coagulation
  D. Severe coarctation of the aorta
  E. Renal artery stenosis
IV. Vitamin E deficiency

V. Congenital red cell membrane disorders
  A. Hereditary spherocytosis
  B. Hereditary elliptocytosis
    1. Hereditary poikilocytosis
    2. Hereditary pyropoikilocytosis
    3. Hereditary stomatocytosis
  C. Infantile pyknocytosis
VI. Congenital red cell enzyme disorders
  A. G6PD deficiency
  B. Pyruvate kinase deficiency
VII. Congenital hemoglobinopathies
  A. Alpha and fetal chain defects
    1. Alpha and gamma thalassemia
    2. Alpha and gamma structural abnormalities; unstable hemoglobin
VIII. Metabolic
  A. Galactosemia
  B. Organic aciduria; orotic aciduria
  C. Prolonged or recurrent acidosis
IX. Liver disease

G6PD, Glucose-6-phosphate dehydrogenase

10,000 live births.[8] The persistence of Rh isoimmunization may be attributed to failures in administering Rh Ig to all women at risk and incorrect dosing. Women who receive no prenatal care and women who develop silent antenatal sensitization comprise two populations that are difficult to reach with prevention strategies.

ABO hemolytic anemia is more common than Rh hemolytic disease but less severe. Unlike Rh disease, hemolysis secondary to ABO incompatibility can occur during the first pregnancy because A- and B-antigens are ubiquitous in foods and bacteria, causing sensitization.

Most isoimmune hemolytic diseases that are not related to ABO or Rh incompatibility are caused by sensitization to minor blood group antigens Kell, Duffy, Lewis, Kidd, M, or S. Mothers should be screened at 34 weeks for antibodies to these minor blood group antigens.

Congenital bacterial and viral infections may cause hemolytic anemia and bone marrow suppression with reticulocytopenia. Microspherocytes may be very prominent.

The microangiopathies and macroangiopathies are characterized by red cell fragmentation, shortened red cell survival, and thrombocytopenia. Coagulation proteins are also consumed in cavernous hemangiomas and disseminated intravascular coagulation (DIC).

Vitamin E is a fat-soluble vitamin that functions as an antioxidant. Deficiency of vitamin E manifests with hemolytic anemia, reticulocytosis, thrombocytosis, and edema of the lower extremities.[39] Diets high in polyunsaturated fatty acids and iron increase requirements for vitamin E. Although infant formulas contain vitamin E, neonates with birth weight less than 1500 grams may benefit from supplementation with 5 mg/day of a water soluble form of tocopheral.

Shortened red cell survival secondary to an

intrinsic red cell defect is a rare but important cause of shortened red cell survival in the neonate. Affected infants usually present with anemia and hyperbilirubinemia. Splenomegaly develops later in infancy or early childhood. A preliminary diagnosis of constitutional red cell defect is made by family history and careful inspection of the peripheral smear. Abnormalities of red cell shape, including spherocytes, eliptocytes, pyknocytes, "bite cells," target cells, and other bizarre morphology, are often characteristic of the specific red cell defect.

Constitutional defects in red cell membranes cause life-long hemolytic anemia. Because even normal neonates have shortened red cell survival and hyperbilirubinemia, the presentation of these syndromes in the neonate is often more severe than in older affected family members. Hereditary spherocytosis is the most common red cell membrane defect and is usually inherited as an autosomal dominant trait.

Glucose-6-phosphate dehydrogenase (G6PD) is the first rate-limiting enzyme in the pentose phosphate pathway of red cell energy metabolism. This enzyme is important in the production of NADPH, which maintains cellular systems in a reduced state. G6PD deficiency is the most common inherited disorder of red blood cells and is transmitted as an X-linked recessive. There are many isoforms of abnormal G6PD enzymes. The Mediterranean type produces severe hemolysis, whereas the form found in African-Americans is usually mild. Infants are asymptomatic until challenged with oxidant stresses from infections or drugs. Agents associated with hemolysis in G6PD deficient infants are shown in Box 19-3.

Hemoglobinopathies are inherited disorders resulting from defects in the quantity or function of the hemoglobin proteins. The clinical expression of a hemoglobinopathy is dependent upon the affected globin chain, the developmental state of globin synthesis, and the amount and function of alternate hemoglobins. Beta chains of hemoglobin are not produced until 3 months of postnatal age; therefore defects of beta chains, including beta thalassemia and sickle cell anemia, do not present in the nursery. Hemoglobinopathies presenting at birth affect either the alpha or gamma chains of hemoglobin.

The thalassemias are disorders manifested by absence or decrease of specific globin proteins. Because there are four genes controlling alpha globin synthesis, clinical signs may range from asymptomatic (absence of hemoglobin production from one alpha hemoglobin gene) to incompatible with life (absence of production from all four alpha hemoglobin genes). Alpha globin is an essential component of both hemoglobin F and hemoglobin A. Compensatory hemoglobins include hemoglobin Barts in the neonatal period, which is composed of four gamma chains, and later hemoglobin H, which is composed of four beta chains. These hemoglobins are poor carriers of oxygen.[43] Homozygous thalassemia of the gamma chain is incompatible with life. Heterozygotes may have a moderately severe microcytic hemolytic anemia at birth.[18] In Western societies, there has been a dramatic decline in the incidence of new births with severe thalassemia syndromes because the widespread use of molecular diagnostic techniques by couples at risk.

Methemoglobin contains an oxidized form of heme iron, ferric Fe^{+++} which renders it incapable of reversible binding to oxygen. Constitutional methemoglobinemia is caused either by deficiency of the red cell enzyme methemoglobin reductase or by an M hemoglobinopathy. Infants with either of these disorders present with cyanosis of the skin and mucous membranes but are otherwise asymptomatic. Normal newborn infants are susceptible to acquired methemoglobinemia from oxidative stresses because neonatal red blood cells contain lower levels of the enzyme NADH-methemoglobin reductase.

Data Collection

History

Information obtained should include maternal history of illness and dietary intake during pregnancy, delivery type, hemorrhage, transfusion or iron therapy, and any abnormal occurrences during birth. A careful family history includes specific questioning regarding anemia, iron or transfusion therapy, pallor, jaundice, splenomegaly, splenectomy, gall stones, cholecystectomy, or congenital malformations in the parents, grandparents, siblings, aunts, uncles, and cousins of the infant.

Box 19-3

Some Agents Reported to Produce Hemolysis in Patients with G6PD Deficiency

Drugs and Chemicals Clearly Shown to Cause Clinically Significant Hemolytic Anemia in G6PD Deficiency:

Acetanilid
Methylene blue
Nalidixic acid (NegGram)
Naphthalene
Niridazole (Ambilhar)
Phenylhydrazine
Primaquine
Pamaquine

Pentaquine
Sulfanilamide
Sulfacetamide
Sulfapyridine
Sulfamethoxazole (Gantanol)
Thiazolesulfone
Toluidine blue
Trinitrotoluene (TNT)

Drugs Probably Safe in Normal Therapeutic Doses for G6PD-Deficient Individuals (Without Nonspherocytic Hemolytic Anemia):

Acetaminophen (Paracetamol, Tylenol, Tralgon, Hydroxyacetanillid)
Acetophenetidine (Phenacetin)
Acetylsalicylic acid (aspirin)
Aminopyrine (Pyramidone, Amidopyrine)
Antazoline (Antistine)
Antipyrine
Ascorbic acid (vitamin C)
Benzhexol (Artane)
Chloramphenicol
Chlorguanidine (Proguanil, Paludrine)
Chloroquine
Colchicine
Diphenhydramine (Benadryl)
L-Dopa
Menadione sodium bisulfite (Hykinone)
Menaphtone
p-Aminobenzoic acid
Phenylbutazone

Phenytoin
Probenecid (Benemid)
Procaine amide hydrochloride (Pronestyl)
Pyrimethamine (Daraprim)
Quinidine
Quinine
Streptomycin
Sulfacytine
Sulfadiazine
Sulfaguanidine
Sulfamerazine
Sulfamethoxypyriazine (Kynex)
Sulfisoxazole (Gantrisin)
Trimethoprim
Tripelennamine (Pyribenzamine)
Vitamin K

G6PD, Glucose-6-phosphate dehydrogenase. From Beutler: *Hemolytic anemia in disorders of red cell metabolism.* Plenum, 1978.

Signs and Symptoms

When performing a physical examination of a newborn with anemia, attention should be paid to the infant's cardiovascular function, general vigor, and signs of pallor, jaundice, skin lesions, hepatosplenomegaly, lymphadenopathy, and congenital malformations (Box 19-4).

Laboratory Data

The diagnosis of anemia is based upon the hemoglobin and hematocrit in comparison with normal values established for postconceptual and postnatal age. The peripheral blood smear should be carefully examined in all cases of abnormal hemoglobin and hematocrit, and the red cell indices

Box 19-4

Signs and Symptoms of Anemia in the Neonate

I. Acute anemia (with hemorrhage anemia may not be present initially; hemodilution will develop over 3-4 hours)
  A. Hypovolemia, hypotension
  B. Hypoxemia, tachypnea
  C. Tachycardia
II. Chronic anemia (may be well compensated)
  A. Pallor, metabolic acidosis, poor growth
  B. High output congestive heart failure
  C. Persistent or increased oxygen requirement
  D. Iron deficiency with hypochromia, microcytosis

should be evaluated. A clinical decision tree in the evaluation of anemia is shown in Figure 19-1. The characterization of anemia is dependent upon additional laboratory testing (Table 19-3).

Treatment

If acute blood loss is suspected and the infant is pale and limp at birth, blood pressure should be obtained and monitored, IV fluids started at 20 ml/kg, and oxygen administered. A catheter should be inserted into the umbilical artery to measure blood gases. Blood should be obtained for complete blood count (CBC), reticulocyte count, Coombs' test, blood type, and serum screen for blood group antibodies. Since infants less than 4 months of age rarely produce antibodies against blood group antigens, maternal serum can be used in the antibody screen.

Once the infant's condition stabilizes, a decision can be made regarding transfusion based on clinical status. If the infant is anemic with signs of hypoxemia or has underlying pulmonary or cardiac disease, transfusion of 10 ml/kg of red blood cells over 2 to 3 hours may be given to increase oxygen carrying capacity. Normally, larger quantities of blood should not be given in one transfusion. If the antibody screen in the infant (or mother) is

negative, major cross-matching need not be done provided that red cells used for transfusion are either type O or ABO type compatible with both infant and mother, and Rh compatible.[33] Blood used for transfusion should be less than 7 days old and negative for syphilis, hepatitis B and C, cytomegalovirus (CMV), and human immunodeficiency virus (HIV). Irradiation of red blood cells and other blood cell products to prevent graft-versus-host disease is recommended for intrauterine transfusions or neonatal exchange transfusion and for infants with congenital or acquired immune deficiency. For infants with continuing hemorrhage requiring massive transfusion exceeding one blood volume, transfusions of fresh frozen plasma are required to replace clotting factors and prevent the consumptive coagulopathy that results from massive transfusion of stored blood. Platelet transfusions may also be needed.

An order from a physician or nurse practitioner is required for any blood transfusion. Parental consent should be obtained by the physician before transfusion. In the neonatal intensive care nursery a policy of "double checking" blood is essential to ensure that the proper blood is being administered to the infant. Blood should be warmed and administered through a blood filter of at least 40 µm. Fresh blood can be administered through a 25-gauge needle without significant hemolysis.

Directed donor programs are becoming more widely used in hospitals for nonemergent blood transfusions. In most cases, biological parents are able to serve as directed donors for their neonates. At this time there is no scientific data that suggests directed donor programs increase blood safety. Some immunologic incompatibilities may exist between maternal and paternal donors; therefore the following guidelines should be considered for parental donors:

1. Mothers should not provide blood components containing plasma. If maternal red cells are transfused, they should be washed.
2. Fathers are not recommended as blood cell (red, white, or platelet) donors for their newborns unless maternal serum is shown to lack cytotoxic antibodies.
3. All parental blood components should be irradiated before transfusion to the infant.[11]

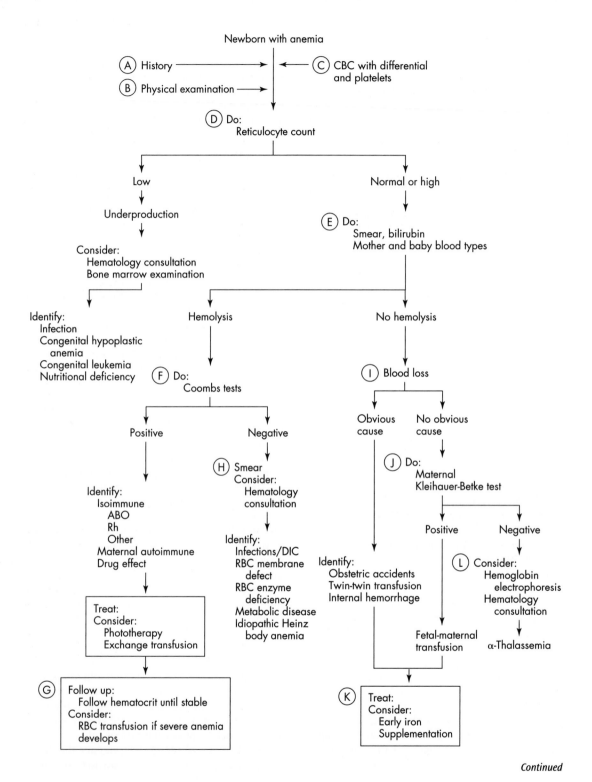

Continued

Figure 19-1 Clinical decision tree in evaluation of anemia.

A. In the history, document any prenatal infections or drug use. Also note any history of maternal vaginal bleeding, placenta previa, abruptio placentae, or umbilical cord rupture, constriction or velamentous insertion, as well as cesarean, breech, or traumatic delivery. Obtain a family history of neonatal jaundice, anemia, splenomegaly, and unexplained gallstones.

B. In the physical examination, note tachypnea, tachycardia, peripheral vasoconstriction (acute blood loss), and hepatosplenomegaly (chronic anemia, intrauterine infection, congenital malignancy). Jaundice appearing before 24 hours of age suggests significant hemolysis.

C. A hematocrit less than 45% during the first 3 days of life is abnormal and requires explanation. The mean corpuscular volume (MCV) at birth is normally above 95. An MCV below 95 suggests α-thalassemia or chronic intrauterine blood loss (as with fetal maternal transfusion). Rarely, a low MCV may be seen with hemolytic disease caused by hereditary elliptocytosis or pyropoikilocytosis. The presence of neutropenia or thrombocytopenia suggests the possibility of infection. Except in an emergency, no anemic newborn should receive a blood transfusion before adequate diagnostic studies.

D. Normal reticulocyte values are 3% to 7% during the first day of life and 1% to 3% during the second and third days. A low reticulocyte count in the face of significant anemia suggests bone marrow failure.

E. An indirect hyperbilirubinemia, abnormal peripheral blood smear, or ABO or Rh incompatibility between the mother and infant suggests hemolysis.

F. Perform direct and indirect Coombs tests. ABO isoimmunization is usually associated with a negative direct and a positive indirect Coombs test.

G. Infants with immune hemolysis have varying degrees of hemolysis, which may continue for 3 months. Severe, life-threatening anemia may develop in infants with Rh sensitization; such infants require close follow-up with serial hematocrits until the hemolysis resolves.

H. Examine the peripheral blood smear. Spherocytes suggest ABO isoimmunization, hereditary spherocytosis, or infection (e.g., cytomegalovirus). Red cell fragmentation suggests intravascular hemolysis (infection, disseminated intravascular coagulation [DIC]). Consider infection or DIC in any ill newborn with hemolysis, particularly if thrombocytopenia is also present.

I. Review the obstetric history and examine the placenta for clues to the cause of fetal blood loss.

J. Perform a Kleihauer-Betke test to detect fetal red cells in the maternal circulation. False-negatives occur when an ABO incompatibility results in the rapid clearance of the infant's red cells from the maternal circulation.

K. Newborns with significant prenatal or perinatal blood loss are at risk for iron deficiency during the first 6 months of life.

L. Anemic infants without evidence of hemolysis or blood loss whose mothers have a negative Kleihauer test may have α-thalassemia, especially if the MCV is below 95. Ethnic groups affected most often include South and Southeast Asians, Mediterraneans, and Africans. The diagnosis of α-thalassemia may be confirmed with a hemoglobin electrophoresis that shows Bart's hemoglobin.

References

Ballin A, Brown EJ, Zipursky A: Idiopathic Heinz body hemolytic anemia in newborn infants, *Am J Pediatr Hematol Oncol* 11:3, 1989.

Blanchette VS, Zipursky A: Assessment of anemia in newborn infants, *Clin Perinatol* 11:489, 1984.

Oski FA: Anemia in the neonatal period. In Oski FA, Naiman JL, editors: *Hematologic problems in the newborn*, ed 3, Philadelphia, 1982, WB Saunders.

Oski FA: The erythrocyte and its disorders. In Nathan DG, Oski FA, editors: *Hematology of infancy and childhood*, ed 4, Philadelphia, 1993, WB Saunders.

Figure 19-1, cont'd   Clinical decision tree in evaluation of anemia.

Table 19-3
Characterization of Anemia

Characterization	Test
Blood loss	Kleihauer-Betke on maternal sample
	Apt test on gastric blood from infant as indicated
Bone marrow production	Reticulocyte count
	Platelet and white blood cell count
	Erythropoietin level
	T3, T4, TSH
	Bone marrow aspirate and biopsy
	Fetal hemoglobin, I antigen, MCV
Iron deficiency	Ferritin, iron, and iron-binding capacity
Antibody mediated	Maternal and infant blood type
	Direct and indirect Coombs' test
Hemolysis	Bilirubin
	Coagulation tests (if sepsis or liver disease is suspected)
	Osmotic fragility, specific determiantions of red cell membrane proteins, enzymes, hemoglobin, and ceruloplasmin as indicated
Infection	Culture and serologies as appropriate
Microangiopathy, macroangiopathy	DIC screen
Vitamin E deficiency	Vitamin E level
Metabolic disorder	pH, Lactate, Pyruvate
	Galactosemia screen

TSH, Thyroid-stimulating hormone; *MCV,* mean corpuscular volume; *DIC,* disseminated intravascular coagulation.

Equipment required for blood transfusion includes a filter, extension tubing, and a pump. Except in extreme emergencies, blood should be administered through a peripheral catheter rather than through a UAC. It is essential to confirm that the unit of blood infused matches the typed blood bank form and assigned number, patient name, and patient hospital number. The expiration date and time must be respected. IV tubing used for blood transfusion should be flushed with 0.45% normal saline before infusing blood products.

Blood bags should not be used for more than 4 to 6 hours after opening. Vital signs should be obtained and recorded every 15 minutes during blood transfusion. Careful observations should be made for reactions including increased temperature, diaphoresis, irregular respiration, bradycardia, restlessness, and pallor. Transfusions should be stopped promptly in the face of any of these signs. All materials used for blood transfusion should be disposed of properly.

Infants who are anemic as a result of chronic blood loss or acute blood loss not requiring trans-

fusion therapy should be treated with iron replacement: 6 mg/kg/day until blood count is normal and 2 additional months to replace stores.

Infants who are born with isoimmune hemolytic anemia are often treated with exchange transfusion. In this procedure, catheters placed in central and peripheral veins are used to remove the infant's blood in small aliquots and replace it with packed red cells usually reconstituted with fresh frozen plasma. General guidelines for aliquot volumes are as follows:

3 kg	20 ml per aliquot
2 kg	15 ml per aliquot
1 kg	5 ml per aliquot

Infants who are treated for isoimmune hemolytic anemia with intrauterine transfusions may be born with normal or near normal hematocrit and bilirubin. Exchange transfusion is often used early after delivery to remove antibody and decrease postnatal hemolysis. Hyperbilirubinemia can be managed using phototherapy.

Prevention

Many forms of neonatal anemia are preventable. Improved fetal monitoring and obstetric care may prevent anemia caused by blood loss during delivery.

Administering Rh Ig to Rh negative mothers within 72 hours of delivery of an Rh positive infant prevents most cases of hydrops fetalis in subsequent pregnancies. For previously sensitized Rh negative mothers carrying Rh positive fetuses, amniocentesis performed between 20 and 22 weeks' gestation may allow for intrauterine transfusion of Rh negative red blood cells and possible early delivery of a nonhydropic infant. For severe thalassemia syndromes and sickle cell anemia, prenatal diagnosis is possible. Intrauterine transfusions are also appropriate for infants with severe alpha thalassemia. Clinical trials of prenatal and early postnatal bone marrow reconstitution with normal red cell progenitors are currently in progress.

Hemolysis may be prevented in infants with significant G6PD deficiency by avoiding drugs known to present an oxidative stress to the red cells.

Premature infants with low birth weight are at high risk for late-onset anemia because of low endogenous production of erythropoietin exacerbated by phlebotomy losses for laboratory surveillance. Inadequate nutrition and other factors may also play a significant role. **Recombinant human erythropoietin (r-HuEPO) has been successfully used to decrease the severity of anemia and lessen the use of blood transfusion in small premature infants. Long-term risks are unknown at present but appear to be minimal.** Benefits of therapy other than decreased exposure to blood transfusion are also unknown at present. Potential improvements in organ maturation or infant growth because of higher sustained levels of hemoglobin are speculative at present. The cost of a 6-week course of therapy with r-HuEPO is comparable in most institutions with that of conventional therapies with blood replacement.

Treatment with EPO should be considered in all infants of birth weight 800 to 1300 g. Infants <800 g may receive so many transfusions early in the hospital course that treating with r-HuEPO may confer no substantial additional benefit. Infants with birth weight >1300 g rarely require blood transfusion.

Treatment with r-HuEPO can begin when infants are stable and can tolerate iron supplementation, usually when tolerating approximately 60% of required enteral feedings. The recommended dose is 200 to 250 U/kg r-HuEPO IV or SC, three times weekly. The reticulocyte count should be monitored to document an adequate response. Oral iron supplementation should be initiated at the time of therapy, beginning with 2 mg/kg/day of elemental iron, and increasing to 6 mg/kg/day as tolerated. A baseline hematocrit and reticulocyte count should be obtained and followed weekly. Dosing should be adjusted to maintain a reticulocyte count >6%. Supplemental vitamin E, 15 to 25 IU/day, may be given at the start of therapy. Treatment is continued for 6 weeks or until 36 weeks' postconceptual age. Once treatment is discontinued, hematocrits should be monitored every other week until stable.[28,29]

The treatment of methemoglobinemia is oral methylene blue, except in the presence of G6PD deficiency in which treatment consists of ascorbic acid, 200 to 500 mg/kg/day.[17,37]

Polycythemia and Hyperviscosity

Physiology

Neonatal polycythemia is most commonly defined by a venous hematocrit greater than 65%.[14] Viscosity is related to but not identical to hematocrit. The viscosity of blood increases logarithmically in relation to the hematocrit.[23]

Although viscosity may be measured directly, hematocrit is often used as a indicator of viscosity. Blood sampling at 12 hours of postnatal age seems ideal to determine hematocrit and viscosity for diagnosis of polycythemic hyperviscosity.[45] Capillary hematocrit can be used as a screening test but should not be used alone for the diagnosis of polycythemia[20]; a venous sample should be analyzed to confirm an abnormally high capillary hematocrit.

Pathophysiology

Hyperviscosity is a syndrome of circulatory impairment secondary to increased resistance to blood flow. Complications of polycythemia and hyperviscosity include respiratory distress, congestive heart failure, hypoglycemia, hyperbilirubinemia, neurologic signs, and sequelae such as significant motor and mental retardation, cerebral infarcts, and cerebral palsy. Thromboemboli, cerebral artery thrombosis, NEC, and acute tubular necrosis are additional complications. Polycythemia can result from a large number of perinatal complications, as shown in Box 19-5.

In up to one third of monochorionic twins, there is a significant transfusion of blood from one twin into the other defined as a discrepancy in the infants' blood counts of greater than 5 g of hemoglobin. Usually, the recipient twin is larger and prone to cardiorespiratory symptoms, hyperviscosity, and hyperbilirubinemia, whereas the donor twin is smaller and at risk for congestive heart failure.[42]

Blood viscosity correlates better with symptoms than does hematocrit.[34] In addition, clinical signs and symptoms may be related to an underlying condition instead of polycythemia per se. In most nurseries, because instruments to measure viscosity are not readily available, neonatal hyperviscosity is diagnosed by a combination of symptoms and an abnormally high hematocrit.

Data Collection

History

In addition to a complete history of the pregnancy and delivery, questions should be directed to pertinent maternal medical conditions, including insulin-dependent diabetes mellitus, hypertension, and heart disease. Additional maternal risk factors include cigarette smoking and living at high altitude. Fetal risk factors include documentation of fetal growth restriction and delayed cord clamping.

Signs and Symptoms

Newborn infants with hematocrit values of greater than 65% to 70% may manifest symptoms because of increased viscosity.[45] Physical examination may be normal except for plethora and, occasionally, cyanosis. Neurologic findings may include lethargy, irritability, hypotonia, tremor, and poor suck. Tachypnea, tachycardia, and respiratory distress may be present. Poor gastrointestinal function is common with abdominal distension, decreased bowel sounds, and poor feeding.

Laboratory Data

The diagnosis of polycythemia is based upon hemoglobin and hematocrit in comparison with normal values for postconceptual and postnatal age. The diagnosis of hyperviscosity may be based upon direct viscosity measurement but usually is assigned based upon polycythemia in the presence of consistent clinical signs and symptoms. Affected infants often have thrombocytopenia, hyperbilirubinemia, and hypoglycemia. Tests of thyroid and adrenal function to rule out hyperthyroidism and adrenal hyperplasia should be performed with appropriate clinical indication. Chromosome analysis should be considered for babies with dysmorphic features.

Treatment

Therapy of polycythemia is generally based upon the presence of consistent signs and symptoms.

Box 19-5

Etiologies of Neonatal Polycythemia

A. Placental transfusion
　1. Delayed cord clamping (may increase the blood volume and red cell mass of the infant by as much as 55%)
　2. Twin-to-twin transfusion
B. Intrauterine hypoxia/placental vascular insufficiency
　1. Intrauterine growth restriction syndrome
　2. Maternal diabetes
　3. Maternal smoking
　4. Fetal risk factors
　5. Maternal hypertension syndromes
　6. Maternal cyanotic heart disease
C. Fetal factors
　1. Trisomy 13, 18, 21
　2. Hyperthyroidism
　3. Neonatal thyrotoxicosis
　4. Congenital adrenal hyperplasia
　5. Beckwith-Weidemann syndrome
D. High altitude
E. Idiopathic

Therapy, when indicated, is aimed at decreasing the hematocrit and includes removal of red cells by simple phlebotomy as well as partial exchange transfusion with replacement of removed red cell volume with volume expanders or plasma. Exchange transfusion often requires placement of a UVC. Risks of umbilical catheterization in polycythemic infants include portal vein thrombosis, phlebitis of the portal vein, and decreased plasma volume (if phlebotomy is used alone). In addition, infants with polycythemia and hyperviscosity are at increased risk of spontaneous large vessel thrombosis, especially renal vein thrombosis and stroke.

There is evidence that treating all infants with polycythemia may not improve outcome. In a study by Bada et al,[4] symptomatic infants received partial plasma exchange transfusion, which reduced blood viscosity, improved cerebral blood flow, and ameliorated symptoms. Infants who were asymptomatic before therapy showed little or no improvement in cerebral blood flow with partial exchange transfusion.

In a randomized controlled trial, Roithmaier et al[36] showed that partial exchange transfusion using crystalloid solution (Ringer's solution) was as effective as partial exchange transfusion using a colloid (plasma) in decreasing the hematocrit of polycythemic neonates. Crystalloid solutions are preferable to colloids because they are less expensive and infection-free.

Coagulation

Physiology

When a blood vessel is torn, blood will clot at the site of vessel injury through a series of carefully controlled enzymatic reactions. First, platelets that are small, platelike blood cells without nuclei adhere to the damaged endothelium both directly and by linkage via the von Willebrand protein to collagen, which is exposed beneath the blood vessel lining. The platelets release adenosine diphosphate (ADP) which recruits more platelets to the activation process. Activated platelets express a receptor for the blood protein fibrinogen, which binds to adjoining platelets and links them. Fibrinogen is a contractile protein that pulls platelets

together, forming a tightly woven net over the vessel tear. This is known as a platelet plug and is responsible for the initial cessation of bleeding, especially on mucous membranes of the nose, mouth, throat, and gastrointestinal and genitourinary tracts. At the same time, thromboxanes produced by the platelet prostaglandin pathway stimulate platelet aggregation, vasoconstriction, and decreased local blood flow.

Figure 19-2[27] shows a representation of the sequential reactions in activation of coagulation known as the "clotting cascade." The coagulation proteins in the blood are inert proenzymes until they are activated. The activation process involves exposure of a potent membrane glycoprotein receptor for clotting activation called tissue factor. Tissue factor is normally hidden in the subendothelium and becomes exposed by vascular injury or is presented on the intact blood vessel surface through the inflammatory process. Activated factor VII in the plasma binds to tissue factor and forms a complex that results in the sequential activation first of factor X and then of factor II (also called prothrombin). These biochemical reactions are similar in that they take place preferentially on procoagulant phospholipid surfaces of endothelial cells and platelets at the site of injury, involve calcium-dependent binding to the surface, and are accelerated by cofactors (factors VIII and V). This is known as the tissue factor pathway of coagulation activation.

The contact activation pathway is an alternative route to factor X activation. In this pathway, factor XII is activated by contact with negatively charged subendothelial collagen or by acidosis, cold, or heat injury. Activated factor XII subsequently activates factors XI and IX. Prekallikrein and high-molecular-weight kininogen serve as cofactors of activation. Contact activation initiates clot lysis and also many inflammatory pathways, including the complement system, which is important for host defense. The tissue factor and contact pathways activate each other and thus generally are not functioning completely independently.

Procoagulant factors II, VII, IX, and X and regulatory proteins; protein C and protein S are biochemically related. They are all produced in the liver and require vitamin K to become functional. Vitamin K catalyzes the transfer of carboxyl groups to glutamic acid residues of vitamin K-dependent

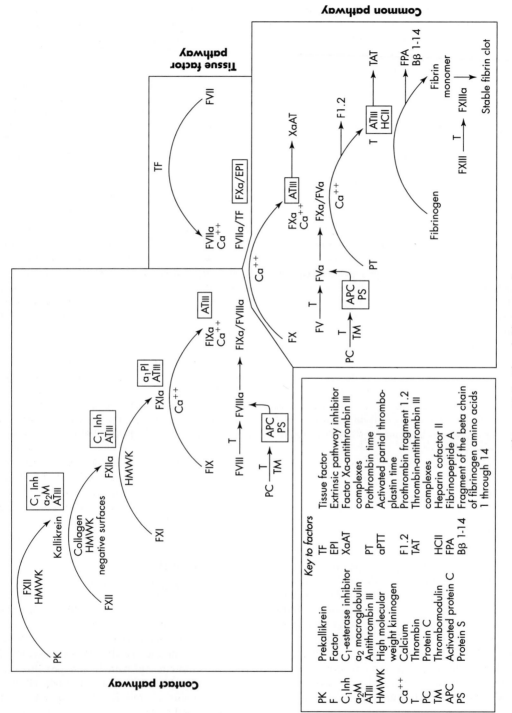

Figure 19-2 The clotting cascade.

proteins; only after carboxylation can these unique proteins then bind to surfaces via calcium.

Thrombin is the terminal coagulation enzyme and functions as an important regulator of coagulation. It is a potent platelet activator. Thrombin provides positive feedback activation of factors VIII and V and initiates the regulation of factors VIIIa and Va through activation of protein C. Thrombin cleaves fibrinogen to form a sticky fibrin strand. Factor XIII is activated by thrombin and cross-links the fibrin strand, greatly increasing its strength and stability. Fibrin then contracts and forms a tight dense clot. A fibrin clot holds opposed surfaces together for about a week as thrombin and other growth factors stimulate fibroblasts to grow. Ultimately, scar tissue bridges the original injury. When a blood clot is no longer needed, it is dissolved by an enzyme system called fibrinolysis. The blood zymogen plasminogen is activated by tissue plasminogen activator (TPA), which is released from endothelial cells. The active enzyme plasmin cleaves the fibrin clot into fragments of various sizes, called fibrin split products (FSPs). Split products that contain factor XIII mediated cross-linked fibrin are called the D-dimer fragments. Several proteins are responsible for regulating the coagulation process and ensuring that these powerful enzymes are not activated in the systemic circulation, causing uncontrolled blood clotting. The most important of these regulatory proteins are antithrombin III, protein C, and the protein C cofactor protein S. Heparin cofactor II, alpha$_2$-macroglobulin, and alpha$_1$-antitrypsin also function as coagulation regulatory proteins. Plasminogen activator inhibitor (PAI), histamine-rich glycoprotein, and fibrin binding of plasminogen regulate the activation of fibrinolysis.

Normal Values

Healthy term and preterm infants have platelet counts within the normal adult range. The coagulation system of the newborn infant is unique in that blood clotting proteins mature at different rates (Table 19-4).[16] Factors V, VIII, and XIII and fibrinogen are within the normal adult range by 20 weeks of fetal development. Low levels of these clotting proteins are never normal. The level of the von Willebrand protein is higher at birth than in the adult, and the von Willebrand protein subunits (called multimers) have an excess of the larger sized forms, which makes the protein more adherent to platelets and vessel walls. Fetal fibrinogen differs from the adult molecule in its content of sialic acid. This prolongs the thrombin time (TT) of the neonate. Vitamin K-dependent factors II, VII, IX, X, protein C, and protein S develop very slowly. Factor IX does not reach its full adult potential until 9 months of age; protein C may not reach adult levels until puberty. It is very difficult to determine if these proteins are genetically deficient during the neonatal period.

The clotting system is evaluated using a hemostasis screen, which includes a partial thromboplastin time (PTT), prothrombin time (PT), TT, fibrinogen concentration, and platelet count. The PTT may be within the adult range at term birth or may achieve the adult range by 2 months. The PTT of the stable preterm infant <1000 g is often extremely prolonged without signs of excessive bleeding. The PT is usually near normal at birth, may prolong slightly by day 3, and may reach adult normal values by day 5. The TT is slightly prolonged because of fetal fibrinogen until 3 weeks of age. The fibrinogen and platelet concentrations are within the normal adult range at birth in stable term and preterm infants. The bleeding time estimates platelet function. In this test a standard cut is made in the skin 0.5 to 1 cm long and 1 mm deep; the time necessary for this cut to stop bleeding is recorded. The bleeding time is rarely necessary in the evaluation of neonates. Platelet function is somewhat decreased in vitro at birth and for the first 3 weeks of age. In vivo the bleeding time is shorter in the neonate than in the adult, and clinically the neonate is hypercoagulable.

Pathophysiology

Thrombocytopenia

Thrombocytopenia is a general term that denotes a decreased number of platelets in the infant's blood. Thrombocytopenia is the most common coagulation disorder in the neonate. It is important to determine if the infant appears well or ill. The etiologies of thrombocytopenia in an otherwise well infant differ from those in an acutely ill neonate (Box 19-6).

Table 19-4
Coagulation Factor Values* for Fetus and Newborn Infant

Subjects	I (mg/dL)	II	V	VII	VIII:C	vWf:Ag	IX	X	XI
Fetus (~20 wk)	96	0.16	0.70	0.21	0.50	0.65	0.10	0.19	—
	(40)	(0.10)	(0.40)	(0.12)	(0.23)	(0.40)	(0.05)	(0.15)	—
Preterm newborn	250	0.32	0.80	0.37	0.75	1.50	0.22	0.38	0.20
(25-32 wk)	(100)	(0.18)	(0.43)	(0.24)	(0.40)	(0.90)	(0.17)	(0.20)	(0.12)
Preterm newborn	300	0.45	0.82	0.59	0.93	1.66	0.41	0.44	—
(33-36 wk)	(120)	(0.26)	(0.48)	(0.34)	(0.54)	(1.35)	(0.20)	(0.21)	—
Term newborn	240	0.52	1.00	0.57	1.50	1.60	0.35	0.45	0.42
(37-41 wk)	(150)	(0.25)	(0.54)	(0.35)	(0.55)	(0.84)	(0.15)	(0.30)	(0.20)
Older infant (age and level when adult value is approximated)	340 (21 days)	0.97 (45-60 days)	1.00 (1 day)	0.90 (21 days)	0.93 (1-2 days)	1.13 (1 wk)	0.7 (6 mo)	0.55 (6 wk)	0.52 (6 wk)

From Hathaway WE, Bonnar J: *Hemostatic disorders of the pregnant woman and newborn infant,* New York, 1987, Elsevier Science.
vWf, von Willebrand factor; *PK,* prekallikrein; *HMWK,* high-molecular-weight kininogen; *AT-III,* antithrombin III.
Values (data taken from references discussed in text) are expressed in units per milliliter as compared with normal adult subject reference plasma (100 percent = 1 U/ml); the mean and (lower limit of range or −2 SD) are shown.
*Clotting activity or chromogenic substrate methods (except protein C:Ag, protein S:Ag) in subjects in the first 24 hours of life.
†Cord. All other values are venous. All subjects received vitamin K at birth.

A well appearing infant is likely to suffer from immune thrombocytopenia, where the platelets are coated by circulating antibody and rapidly cleared from the circulation by the spleen and liver. Infants of mothers with idiopathic thrombocytopenic purpura (ITP) may have a low platelet count because the maternal antibody crosses the placenta to the infant but usually does not develop life-threatening hemorrhage. Alloimmune thrombocytopenia develops when the mother is negative for a platelet antigen, usually PLA-1, for which the father is positive. Fifty percent of recognized cases of alloimmune thrombocytopenia present in a mother's first infant. Subsequent infants can be more severely involved. Presentations of alloimmune thrombocytopenia range from asymptomatic infants in whom a low platelet count is detected coincidentally on a blood count to fatal cases of intracranial hemorrhage with onset in utero.

Constitutional thrombocytopenia is rare. Affected infants often manifest congenital skeletal malformations of the hands and arms. Thrombocytopenia absent radius (TAR) is a rare but well-characterized syndrome. A bone marrow examination is important to evaluate the megakaryocyte pool, which produces platelets. In Bernard-Soulier syndrome the platelet number is moderately decreased and giant platelets are seen on the peripheral smear. Infants with trisomy 21 (Down syndrome), 18, or 13 can manifest abnormal platelet counts without apparent illness. The bone marrow of infants with Down syndrome is highly reactive. Other features of trisomy 21 should be present.

Giant, cavernous hemangiomas often trap platelets in a syndrome known as Kasabach-Merritt, resulting in accelerated destruction. Clues to this syndrome include skin hemangiomas; bruits over the liver, spleen, or brain; or high output congestive heart failure with a structurally normal heart.

Thrombocytopenia develops in most infants with respiratory distress severe enough to require mechanical ventilation. The lowest platelet counts are usually found at about day 3 of life, and normal counts recover by 10 days if the infant's course is not complicated by infection or thrombosis. Infants less than 32 weeks' gestation with RDS and severe thrombocytopenia are at increased risk of intracranial hemorrhage.

Bacterial and viral infections must be excluded in any thrombocytopenic neonate. The infant of a

XII	PK	HMWK	XIII	Plasminogen	α_2-antiplasmin	AT-III	Protein C:Ag	Protein S:Ag
—	—	—	~0.30	—	—	0.23	0.10	—
—	—	—	—	—	—	(0.12)	(0.06)	—
0.22	0.26	0.28	0.11-0.40	0.35	74	0.35	0.29	—
(0.09)	(0.14)	(0.20)		(0.20)	(~50)	(0.20)	(0.21)	—
0.25	0.33	—	—	0.38	73	0.40	0.38	—
(0.09)	(0.23)			(0.26)	(~50)	(0.25)	(0.23)	—
0.44	0.35	0.64	0.61	0.49	83	0.56	0.50†	0.24†
(0.16)	(0.16)	(0.50)	(0.36)	(0.25)	(~65)	(0.32)	(0.30)	(0.10)
1.00	0.86	0.82	1.0	1.00	1.0	0.82	0.82	—
(14 days)	(6 mo)	(6 mo)	(1 mo)	(6 mo)	(1 wk)	(3-6 mo)	(24 mo)	—

mother with chorioamnionitis often demonstrates thrombocytopenia in the cord blood.

Thrombosis in a neonate often presents with an idiopathic falling platelet count. Thromboses are most commonly found at the tips of UACs and UVCs and can be diagnosed with ultrasound. An infected clot should be suspected in an infant with diagnosed catheter-related thrombosis and alterations in temperature, respiratory stability, or cardiovascular stability.

Thrombocytopenia in an ill infant is often part of the larger syndrome of DIC.[27] In DIC, activation of blood-clotting proteins is initiated by tissue factor from bacterial products (endotoxin) or inflammation, or through the contact system. The activation of clotting proteins leads to a hypercoagulable state, and thromboses occur, especially in the small vessels of the liver, spleen, brain, lungs, kidneys, and adrenals. The bone marrow and liver partially compensate by releasing platelets and clotting factors into the circulation. However, the regulatory system of coagulation is immature in the term and preterm neonate. The capacity to neutralize activated clotting proteins is quickly exhausted, and the resulting deficiencies of platelets and clotting factors is termed consumptive coagulopathy. DIC predisposes the preterm infant to intracranial hemorrhage. Venous thrombosis of the germinal matrix occurs as the initial lesion, fol-lowed by postthrombotic hemorrhage. Bleeding is also seen in the skin, around indwelling catheters, around endotracheal and chest tubes, and in the urine and stool.

Vitamin K Deficiency

The most important bleeding syndrome in the otherwise stable neonate is hemorrhagic disease of the newborn, caused by vitamin K deficiency.[19] There is a tenfold gradient in vitamin K concentration between the maternal and fetal plasma. Marginal fetal vitamin K levels are further compromised by maternal use of anticonvulsants or coumadin. Approximately 3% of cord blood samples from normal term pregnancies show biochemical evidence of noncarboxylated clotting proteins.[40] Early hemorrhagic disease of the newborn presents within the first 24 hours of life with massive cephalhematoma, gastrointestinal tract bleeding, or intracranial hemorrhage. Classic hemorrhagic disease of the newborn presents between 1 and 7 days of life; late vitamin K deficiency occurs between 1 week and 2 months of life. The recommendation of the American Academy of Pediatrics is to give every neonate 1 mg of vitamin K by intramuscular injection[5]; this is adequate to prevent bleeding in most infants. Vitamin K prophylaxis can be achieved using an oral vitamin K preparation. However, because oral therapy requires multiple doses over the first 6 weeks of life, it is difficult to ensure compliance and protect all infants using this formulation. Vitamin K concentrations are physiologically very low in human breast milk; cow's milk contains 10 times the amount of vitamin K (1.5 vs 15 mg/L respectively). Infants fed breast milk are at increased risk of vitamin K deficiency. In addition, infants with fat malabsorption secondary to cystic fibrosis, a_1-antitrypsin deficiency, or biliary atresia and infants treated with prolonged courses of antibiotics are at increased risk of vitamin K deficiency.

Hemophilia and Other Congenital Bleeding Disorders

The hemophilias are a group of life-long bleeding disorders caused by genetic deficiencies of one or more coagulation proteins. Factor VIII deficiency causes 80% of the hemophilias, and factor IX deficiency causes most of the remainder. Both factors VIII and IX are encoded on the X chromosome, and thus deficiency states are manifested in carrier mothers and affected sons. Deficiencies of other coagulation factors are inherited as autosomal traits with severe bleeding manifested with homozygous deficiency. Most infants with hemophilia appear to tolerate labor and a routine vaginal delivery with no undue problem. However, intracranial hemorrhage has been documented in many infants with hemophilia as a result of birth trauma.[7] Current recommendations call for vaginal delivery in the absence of complications; however, cesarean section should be elected if needed to avoid prolonged or difficult labor. Fifty percent of infants with severe hemophilia will hemorrhage from circumcision. The absence of procedure-related bleeding in the neonatal period does not exclude hemophilia owing to physiologically increased platelet function around birth. Prolonged bleeding from the umbilical cord stump is suggestive of factor XIII deficiency. Spontaneous intracranial hemorrhage also occurs in infants with homozygous factor XIII deficiency.

Data Collection

History

A history of maternal bleeding, medical and obstetric diagnoses, and medications should be elicited for every infant at birth. A careful family history for bleeding disorders in the parents, grandparents, siblings, aunts, uncles, and cousins of an infant should be taken as part of every admission evaluation. Specific questions must be asked about excessive bleeding with surgeries, menses, childbirth, traumas, and spontaneous bleeding events. Efforts should be made to obtain confirmatory medical records for any positive response. Procedures, including circumcision, should not be performed until the possibility of a bleeding disorder in the infant is excluded. The administration of vitamin K to the infant should be confirmed by review of the nursing notes.

Signs and Symptoms

Thrombocytopenia usually presents with small, flat hemorrhages into the skin called petechiae that do not blanch with pressure. Petechiae may be con-

---

Box 19-6

Etiology of Thrombocytopenia in the Newborn Infant

I. Well infant
  A. Immune
    1. Alloimmune thrombocytopenia
    2. Maternal idiopathic thrombocytopenia purpura
  B. Constitutional
    1. Thrombocytopenia absent radius
    2. Amegakaryocytic thrombocytopenia
    3. Wiskott-Aldrich syndrome
    4. Fanconi's anemia
    5. Bernard-Soulier syndrome
II. Sick Infant
  A. Respiratory distress syndrome
  B. Bacterial sepsis
  C. Viral infection
  D. Necrotizing enterocolitis
  E. Hyperviscosity
  F. Disseminated intravascular coagulation
III. May appear either well or sick
  A. Kasabach-Merritt (giant hemangioma)
  B. Trisomy 21, 18, 13
  C. Leukemia
  D. Thrombosis

centrated in skin creases of the neck and axilla and around the site of a tourniquet or may be scattered over the entire body. More severe thrombocytopenia results in large ecchymoses, which are flat bruises. Infants with severe thrombocytopenia may hemorrhage into the CNS or the gastrointestinal tract.

Bleeding with coagulation disorders causes palpable hematomas of the skin and scalp. Intracranial, retroperitoneal, and intraperitoneal, gastrointestinal and genitourinary bleeding may occur. Bleeding with surgeries or procedures may be immediate or delayed.

Laboratory Data

Any infant with bleeding signs should be evaluated with a hemostasis screen and a platelet count. The results of the hemostasis screen in the healthy infant and during many states of illness are shown in Table 19-5. The possibility of hemophilia should be excluded by specific factor assays. In addition, factors XIII, a_2-antiplasmin, and PAI-1 should be assayed in a term infant with unexplained significant hemorrhage, such as intracranial hemorrhage.

Treatment

Thrombocytopenia

Therapy for thrombocytopenia depends upon the overall health and stability of the neonate. The primary support of a thrombocytopenic infant is replacement transfusions of platelets, which are derived from CMV negative donors. A stable, otherwise healthy infant can tolerate a platelet count as low as 20,000/μl without undue risk of serious bleeding. However, an infant who is less than 30 weeks' gestation, mechanically ventilated, on ECMO, with indwelling UACs or UVCs and chest tubes, septic or otherwise unstable, will require a platelet count of 50,000/μl to prevent or treat bleeding.

Infants with alloimmune thrombocytopenia are likely to receive incompatible platelets from a random donor. Thrombocytopenia in this disorder responds well to intravenous gamma globulin (IVIG). Platelet transfusions, when needed, should be derived from the mother, if practical, or from a type-specific donor. Infants with Kasabach-Merritt may respond to steroids, antifibrinolytic agents, or interferon.

Transfusion of platelets into infants with thrombosis or DIC may aggravate the platelet consumption unless specific therapy of the underlying condition is also administered. The primary treatment of DIC is reversal of the trigger (Box 19-7). Adequate ventilation, support of circulation and perfusion, treatment of sepsis, and general supportive care usually interrupt the DIC process within 48 hours. Replacement of coagulation regulatory proteins in fresh frozen plasma or AT-III concentrate or inhibition of coagulation activation with low dose heparin is helpful in some cases.

Bleeding Disorders

Infants with vitamin K deficiency are treated with vitamin K, 1 mg by slow IV push. Fresh frozen plasma, 10 to 15 ml/kg may be given to control active bleeding.

Table 19-5
Coagulation Results in Normal Neonates and Neonates With Bleeding Syndromes

Description	PTT	PT	TT	FIB	D-Dimer	PLT CT
Healthy term	N-↑	N-↑	↑	NL	Neg	NL
Healthy preterm	↑↑	N-↑	↑	NL	Neg	NL
Vit K deficiency	↑↑	↑↑↑	↑	NL	Neg	NL
Liver disease	↑↑	↑↑↑	↑↑-↑↑↑	↓	Pos	↓
Hemophilia	↑↑↑	N-↑	↑	NL	Neg	NL
DIC	↑↑↑	↑↑	↑↑	↓	Pos	- ↓↓

PTT, Partial thromboplastin time; *PT,* prothrombin time; *TT,* thrombin time; *Fib,* fibrogen; *Plt Ct,* platelet count; *N,* normal; ↑, mildly prolonged; ↑↑, moderately prolonged; ↑↑↑, severely prolonged; ↓, decreased.

Treatment of congenital coagulation factor deficiencies is based upon the deficient factor. Factor VIII or IX should be replaced in a bleeding neonate (or for surgery) using only recombinant proteins because they have greater viral safety than human plasma-derived proteins. Factor XIII and fibrinogen may be replaced in cryoprecipitate. The von Willebrand protein is contained both in certain viral inactivated coagulation concentrates as well as in cryoprecipitate. Replacement of other clotting proteins usually requires fresh frozen plasma. DDAVP, a synthetic vasopressin that stimulates release of endothelial stores of factor VIII and the von Willebrand protein, is generally not used in the neonate because of the possibility of seizures related to hyponatremia in this age group. The hemophilia center should be involved in the diagnosis and management of all infants with congenital bleeding disorders.

Prevention and Parent Teaching

Mothers should be instructed during pregnancy regarding routine prevention of vitamin K deficiency with IM injection of vitamin K to the neonate. Primary care providers should be careful to document administration of vitamin K, especially for infants born at home.

Bleeding in an infant with a bleeding disorder can be minimized exerting care to prevent undue trauma. Intramuscular injections and other invasive procedures should be avoided if at all possible. The infant should be handled in as gentle a manner as possible. Pressure for tourniqueting and holding should be minimized. Extreme care should be taken with arterial puncture.

Replacement platelet or clotting factor infusions should be considered before any necessary invasive procedure. Parents should be educated about the nature of the bleeding disorder and its cause in their infant. They need to know whether this is a time-limited complication of the neonatal course or a long-term concern. Infants with constitutional thrombocytopenia or coagulopathy are at life-long risk of bleeding. The risk of platelet sensitization and the consequent aim to minimize platelet exposure must be conveyed to the parents. Any other family member at risk of a genetic cause of thrombocytopenia or bleeding should be identified, screened, and counseled.

Education of families about hemophilia or constitutional thrombocytopenia begins as soon as the diagnosis is established. Nurses should instruct parents about routine infant care and recognition of possible bleeding events in coordination with the hemophilia nurse coordinator.

Thrombosis

Pathophysiology

Thrombosis is an uncommon problem in pediatrics with increased incidence noted in both the neonatal period and after puberty. Physiologic correlates of the neonate's increased predisposition to thrombosis are shown in Boxes 19-8 and 19-9.

The most common sites of spontaneous thrombosis in the neonate are the renal veins, the CNS, and the aorta. Catheters placed for critical care support are associated with an increased risk of thrombosis.

Purpura Fulminans

Purpura fulminans is a syndrome of skin necrosis from venous thrombosis caused by severe deficiencies of protein C or protein S.[15,24] Most cases are caused by homozygous or double heterozygous genetic defects. Rarely, acquired deficiences from

---

Box 19-8

Prothrombotic Characteristics of Neonatal Blood

Increased hematocrit
Increased concentration and size of von Willebrand factor multimers
Low concentrations of physiologic anticoagulants, antithrombin III, protein C, and protein S
Low concentration of the fibrinolytic protein plasminogen
Small caliber blood vessels

Box 19-9

Pathologic Conditions Predisposing to Thrombosis in the Neonate

Hypotension
Hyperviscosity
Severe genetic and acquired deficiencies of antithrombin III, protein C, protein S, and plasminogen.[49,50]
Mechanical obstruction by catheters

---

maternal lupus anticoagulants can mimic the genetic syndromes. Consumption of protein C and protein S during bacterial sepsis usually presents at a later age and is less fulminant than the genetic syndromes.

Thrombocytosis

Thrombocytosis occurs with iron deficiency anemia. An iron-deficient neonate may have suffered from chronic blood loss in utero, either by hemorrhage into the placenta, to a twin, or with gastrointestinal bleeding. Neuroblastoma, a malignancy of neural crest cells, and Down syndrome may also be associated with thrombocytosis.

Data Collection

History

A history of thrombosis in the parents, grandparents, siblings, aunts, uncles, and cousins of the infant raises suspicion of genetic thrombophilia. Unfortunately, many family members affected with heterozygous deficiencies of protein C or protein S are asymptomatic until early to mid-adult life. A history of fetal or neonatal death with thrombosis is helpful.

Signs and Symptoms

Thrombosis.   Signs of decreased organ perfusion and subsequent dysfunction indicate the possibility of a thrombosis. The classic presentation of renal vein thrombosis includes hematuria, throm-

bocytopenia, and hypertension. Palpably enlarged kidneys may be noted on physical examination. The presence of unilateral or bilateral flank masses on the initial physical assessment indicates prenatal occurrence of renal vein thrombosis. Stroke usually presents with seizures during the first 24 hours of life. Aortic thromboses present with cool, pale extremities, decreased pulses and capillary refill, and upper extremity hypertension. Confirmation is made with ultrasound examination of the renal veins and aorta, renal scan, and computerized tomography (CT) or magnetic resonance imaging (MRI) of the brain.

Purpura Fulminans.   Purpura fulminans is a dramatic syndrome that usually presents within hours of birth. Infants develop patchy areas of skin thrombosis over the trunk and buttocks, usually in dependent areas. The lesions are palpable, initially dark red, and then quickly become dusky purple and then black; an eschar forms. The lesions are exquisitely painful. Most infants will manifest a white light reflex of the eyes from in utero thrombosis of the primary vitreal veins with subsequent retinal detachment, hemorrhage, and blindness. Imaging studies of the brain show evidence of CNS infarction in many infants. Renal vein thrombosis is not uncommon.

Thrombocytosis.   Infants rarely manifest signs of thrombocytosis. Occasionally, platelet counts of greater than 2,000,000/μl are associated with cerebral ischemia.

Treatment

Thrombosis.   The optimal therapy for neonatal thrombosis has not been determined. Two approaches include anticoagulation with unfractionated or low molecular weight heparin to prevent propagation of the clot or fibrinolytic therapy to dissolve the clot, as shown in Box 19-10. Fibrinolytic therapy may restore blood flow more rapidly. However, the risk of hemorrhage is greater with fibrinolytic therapy, especially CNS bleeding in an infant with brain ischemia from a previous episode of asphyxia or hypotension. Fibrinolytic therapy, if deemed acceptably safe, may be preferable for renal vein thrombosis and for life- or limb-threatening aortic thrombosis. Long-term anticoagulation with coumadin is necessary only in the small proportion of infants who have an ongoing trigger for thrombosis.

Purpura Fulminans.   The treatment of neonatal purpura fulminans is replacement of protein C or protein S. Fresh frozen plasma should be administered while confirmatory laboratory assays are being performed using 10 ml/kg every 8 to 12 hours. Concentrates of viral-inactivated, human plasma-derived protein C have been developed. The hemophilia center staff is the best resource regarding availability and safety of existing replacement proteins. Children with severe genetic deficiencies of protein C or protein S require life-long anticoagulation with coumadin at this time, because prophylactic replacement with the appropriate proteins is not currently available.

Infants with acquired deficiencies of protein C or protein S may respond to IVIG or steroids in addition to plasma replacement. Infants with sepsis will require fresh frozen plasma until antibiotics have successfully controlled their infection.

Box 19-10

Antithrombotic Therapy in the Neonate

Anticoagulant Therapy

Unfractionated heparin
  100 U/kg bolus
  25 U/kg/hr maintenance; adjusted to maintain anti-Xa level of 0.4-0.7 U/ml
Low-molecular-weight heparin
  1.7 mg/kg sc every 12 hr; adjusted to maintain anti-Xa level of 0.5-1.0 U/ml 6 hr after injection
Consider FFP 10 mL/kg or AT-III concentrate 50 U/kg q24 h to enhance heparin effect, if necessary

Fibrinolytic Therapy

Urokinase
  4400 U/kg bolus
  4400-50,000 U/kg/hr × 48 hr *or*
Tissue plasminogen activator
  0.1-0.5 mg/kg bolus
  0.1-0.5 mg/kg/hr × 48 hr *and*
Heparin 10 U/kg/hr (no bolus)
Consider fresh frozen plasma q24 h 10 ml/kg to replace plasminogen

---

Prevention and Parent Teaching

Parents of infants with severe genetic deficiencies of protein C or protein S will require intensive teaching regarding administration and monitoring of coumadin, observation for early lesions of purpura fulminans, as well as care and rehabilitation of early lesions, which lead to blindness, skin necrosis, and other lesions.

References

1. Alter BP: Fanconi's anemia: current concepts, *Amer J Pediatr Hematol Oncol* 14:170, 1992.
2. Apt L, Downey WS: "Melena" neonatorum: the swallowed blood syndrome: a simple test for the differentiation of adult and fetal hemoglobin in bloody stools, *J Pediatr* 47:6, 1955.
3. Ascari WQ, Levine P, Pollack W: Incidence of maternal Rh immunization by ABO compatible and incompatible pregnancies, *Br Med J* 1:399, 1969.
4. Bada HS et al: Asymptomatic syndrome of polycythemic hyperviscosity: effect of partial plasma exchange transfusion, *J Pediatr* 120:579, 1992.
5. Barness LA: *Vitamins in pediatric nutrition handbook,* Evanston, Ill, 1979, American Academy of Pediatrics.
6. Boussios T, Bertles JF, Goldwasser E: Erythropoietin: receptor characteristics during the ontogeny of hamster yolk sac erythroid cells, *J Biol Chem* 148:443, 1989.
7. Bray GL, Luban NLC: Hemophilia presenting with intracranial hemorrhage, *AJDC* 141:1215, 1987.

8. Chavez GF, Mulinare J, Edmonds LD: Epidemiology of Rh hemolytic disease of the newborn in the United States, *JAMA* 265:3270, 1991.
9. Clapp DW, Shannon KM: Embryonic and fetal erythropoiesis. In Feig SA, Freedman MH, editors: *Clinical disorders and experimental models of erythropoietin failure,* Boca Raton, Fla, 1993, CRC Press.
10. Cohen A, Manno C: Anemia. In Spitzer AR, editor: *Intensive care of the fetus and neonate* 90:1084, 1996.
11. Dallman PR: Anemia of prematurity, *Ann Rev Med* 32:143, 1981.
12. Finne PH, Halvorsen S: Regulation of erythropoiesis in the fetus and newborn, *Arch Dis Child* 47:683, 1972.
13. Gilmore JR: Normal hematopoiesis in intra-uterine and neonatal life, *J Pathol Bacteriol* 52:25, 1941.
14. Gross GP, Hathaway WE, McGaughey HR: Hyperviscosity in the neonate, *J Pediatr* 82:1004, 1973.
15. Hartman KP et al: Homozygous protein C deficiency: early treatment with warfarin, *Am J Pediatr Hematol Oncol* 11(4):395, 1989.
16. Hathaway WE, Bonnar J: *Hemostatic disorders of the pregnant woman and newborn infant,* 1987, New York, Elsevier Science Publishing Co.
17. Jaffe ER: The reduction of methemoglobin in erythrocytes of a patient with congenital methemoglobinemia, subjects with glucose-6-phosphate dehydrogenase deficiency, and normal individuals, *Blood* 21:561, 1963.
18. Kan YW, Forget BG, Nathan DG: Gamma-beta thalassemia: a cause of hemolytic disease of the newborn, *N Engl J Med* 286:129, 1972.
19. Lane PA, Hathaway WE: Vitamin K deficiency, *J Pediatr* 106:351, 1985.
20. Linderkamp O et al: Capillary-venous hematocrit differences in newborn infants, *Eur J Pediatr* 127:9, 1977.
21. Lipton JM, Alter BP: Blackfan-Diamond anemia. In Feig SA, Freedman MH, editors: *Clinical disorders and experimental models of erythropoietic failure,* Boca Raton, Fla, 1993, CRC Press.
22. Luchtman-Jones L, Schwartz A, Wilson D: Hematologic problems in the fetus and neonate. In Fanaroff A, editor: *Neonatal-Perinatal Medicine* 43(2):1201, 1997.
23. MackIntosh TF, Walker CHM: Blood viscosity in the newborn, *Arch Dis Child* 48:547, 1973.
24. Mahasandana C et al: Homozygous protein S deficiency in an infant with purpura fulminans, *J Pediatr* 117(5):750, 1990.
25. Manco-Johnson MJ: Neonatal antithrombin III deficiency, *Am J Med* 87(suppl):49, 1989.
26. Manco-Johnson MJ et al: Severe neonatal protein C deficiency: prevalence and thrombotic risk, *J Pediatr* 119(5):793, 1991.
27. Manco-Johnson MJ: Disseminated intravascular coagulation and other hypercoagulable syndromes, *Int J Pediatr Hematol Oncol* 1:1, 1994.
28. Mentzer WC Jr, Shannon KM, Phibbs RH: Recombinant human erythropoietin (Epoetin Alpha) in patients with the anemia of prematurity. In Eisley AJ et al, editors: *Erythropoietin, molecular cellular, and clinical biology* 20:374, 1991.
29. Meyer MP et al: Recombinant human erythropoietin in the treatment of the anemia of prematurity: results on a double blind, placebo controlled study, *Pediatrics* 93:918, 1994.
30. Oh W, Lind J: Venous and capillary hematocrit in newborn infants and placental transfusion, *Acta Paeditr* 55:38, 1966.
31. Oski FA: Iron deficiency anemia in infancy and childhood, *N Engl J Med* 329:190, 1993.
32. Paludetto R: Neonatal complications specific to twin (multiple) births (twin transfusion syndrome, intrauterine death of cotwins), *J Perinat Med* 19(1):246, 1964.
33. Pisciotto PT, editor: Pediatric transfusion practices. In *Blood transfusion therapy: a physician's handbook,* ed 3, Arlington, Va, 1989, American Association of Blood Banks.
34. Ramamurthy RD, Brans YW: Neonatal polycythemia. I. Criteria for diagnosis and treatment, *Pediatrics* 68:168, 1981.
35. Ramamurthy RS, Berlanga M: Postnatal alteration in hematocrit and viscosity in normal and polycythemic infants, *J Pediatr* 110:929, 1987.
36. Roithmaier A et al: Randomized controlled trial of Ringer solution versus serum for partial exchange transfusion in neonatal polycythemia, *Eur J Pediatr* 154:53, 1995.
37. Rosen PJ et al: Failure of methylene blue treatment in toxic methemoglobinemia associated with glucose-6-phosphate dehydrogenase deficiency, *Ann Intern Med* 75:83, 1971.
38. Shannon KM: Anemia of prematurity: progress and prospects, *Am J Pediatr Hematol Oncol* 12:14, 1990.
39. Shannon KM et al: Circulating erythroid progenitors in the anemia of prematurity: results on the double-blind, placebo-controlled study, *N Engl J Med* 317:728, 1987.
40. Shapiro AD et al: Vitamin K deficiency in the newborn infant: prevalence and perinatal risk factors, *J Pediatr* 109(4):675, 1986.
41. Shohat M, Reisner SH: Neonatal polycythemia. I. Early diagnosis and incidence relating to time of sampling, *Pediatrics* 73:7, 1984.
42. Tan KL et al: The twin tranfusion syndrome: clinical observation of 35 affected pairs, *Clin Pediatr* 18:111, 1979.
43. Todd D et al: The abnormal hemoglobin in homozygous alpha thalassemia, *Br J Hematology* 20:9, 1970.
44. Villalta IA et al: Diagnostic errors in neonatal polycythemia based on method of hematocrit determination, *J Pediatr* 115:460, 1989.
45. Woodrow JC, Donohue WTA: Rh-immunization by pregnancy: results of a survey and their relevance to prophylactic therapy, *Br Med J* 4:139, 1968.
46. Yaegashi N et al: Propagation of human parvovirus B19 in primary culture of erythroid lineage cells derived from fetal liver, *J Virol* 63:2422, 1989.
47. Zipursky A et al: Foetal erythrocytes in the maternal circulation, *Lancet* 1:451, 1959.
48. Zivny J et al: Regulation of erythropoiesis in fetus and mother during normal pregnancy, *Obstet Gynecol* 60:77, 1982.

Suggested Readings

Bifano EM, Ehrenkranz RA, editors: *Clinics in perinatology:perinatal hematology,* vol 22(3), Philadelphia, 1995, WB Saunders.

Bray GL, Luban NLC: Hemophilia presenting with intracranial hemorrhage: an approach to the infant with intracranial bleeding and coagulopathy, *Am J Dis Child* 141:1215, 1987.

Hathaway WE, Bonnar J: *Hemostatic disorders of the pregnant woman and newborn infant,* New York, 1987, Elsevier Science Publishing Co.

Manco-Johnson MJ et al: Severe protein C deficiency in newborn infants, *J Pediatr* 113(2):359, 1988.

Manco-Johnson MJ: Diagnosis and management of thromboses in the perinatal period, *Semin Perinatol* 14(5):393, 1990.

Manco-Johnson MJ: Disseminated intravascular coagulation and other hypercoagulable syndromes, *Int J Pediatr Hematol Oncol* 1:1, 1994.

Onwuzurike N, Warrier I, Lusher JM: Types of bleeding seen during the first 30 months of life in children with severe haemophilia A and B, *Haemophilia* 2:137, 1996.

Oski FA: The erythrocyte and its disorder. In Nathan DG, Oski FA, editors: *Hematology of infancy and childhood,* ed 4, Philadelphia, 1993, WB Saunders.

Polin RA, Fox WW: *Fetal and neonatal physiology,* vol 2, Philadelphia, 1992, WB Saunders.

Zipurski A et al: Isoimmune hemolytic disease. In Nathan DG et al: *Hematology of infancy and childhood,* ed 4, Philadelphia, 1992, WB Saunders.

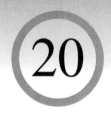

20 Jaundice

C. Gilbert Frank, Sharla C. Cooper, Gerald B. Merenstein

Jaundice, or hyperbilirubinemia, is an almost universal occurrence in the neonate although not usually of clinical significance. Past experiences have suggested the dangers of excessive levels of unconjugated bilirubin, but precise identification of what constitutes a "safe" level for the individual newborn remains elusive and is the subject of much ongoing investigation. This chapter provides the reader with a basic understanding of the multiple causes and contributing factors in the development of hyperbilirubinemia; the diagnosis, clinical significance, and complications of hyperbilirubinemia; and current treatment modalities and their complications.

Physiology

To understand the pathophysiology and clinical significance of hyperbilirubinemia, normal bilirubin metabolism in the newborn must be reviewed (Fig. 20-1). Most of the bilirubin (75% to 85%) produced by a newborn infant comes from the breakdown of the heme portion of erythrocyte hemoglobin. The remaining 15% to 25% of bilirubin is derived from nonerythroid heme proteins found principally in the liver and heme precursors in the marrow and extramedullary hemopoietic areas that do not go on to form red blood cells (early peak or shunt bilirubin).

Bilirubin metabolism is initiated in the reticuloendothelial system in principally the liver and spleen as old or abnormal red blood cells are removed from the circulation. The enzymes, microsomal heme oxygenase and biliverdin reductase, are responsible for the production of bilirubin and carbon monoxide. This bilirubin in its unconjugated or indirect-reacting form is released into the plasma.

At a normal plasma pH, bilirubin is very poorly soluble and binds tightly to circulating albumin that serves as a carrier protein. Albumin contains one high-affinity site for bilirubin and one or more sites of lower affinity. Bilirubin binds to albumin in a molar ratio of between 0.5 and 1 mole of bilirubin per mole of albumin. This ratio may be somewhat lower in the sick, VLBW infant. The ability of albumin to bind bilirubin is affected by a number of different factors, including plasma pH, free fatty acid levels, and certain drugs.

Bilirubin bound to albumin is carried to the liver and transported into the hepatocyte by carrier-mediated diffusion. Intracellularly, bilirubin is bound to ligandin (Y protein) and to a lesser extent to the Z protein. Conjugation occurs within the smooth endoplasmic reticulum of the cell. This reaction, catalyzed by the enzyme bilirubin UDP glucuronyl transferase, leads to the formation of bilirubin glucuronides that are water-soluble compounds. In addition to this enzyme, conjugation requires glucuronic acid synthesized from glucose. Conjugated bilirubin is then actively secreted into bile and passes into the small intestine.

Conjugated bilirubin is not reabsorbed from the intestine, but the bowel lumen of the newborn contains the enzyme beta-glucuronidase, which can convert conjugated bilirubin back into glucuronic acid and unconjugated bilirubin, which may be absorbed. This pathway constitutes the enterohepatic circulation of bilirubin and contributes significantly to the infant's bilirubin load.

The catabolism of 1 g of hemoglobin yields 35 mg of bilirubin. Because the red blood cell of the newborn has a shortened life span of 70 to 90 days (adult: 120 days), a significant bilirubin load is produced. The breakdown of bilirubin is the only chemical reaction in the body that results in formation of carbon monoxide, a marker sometimes used in studying bilirubin production.

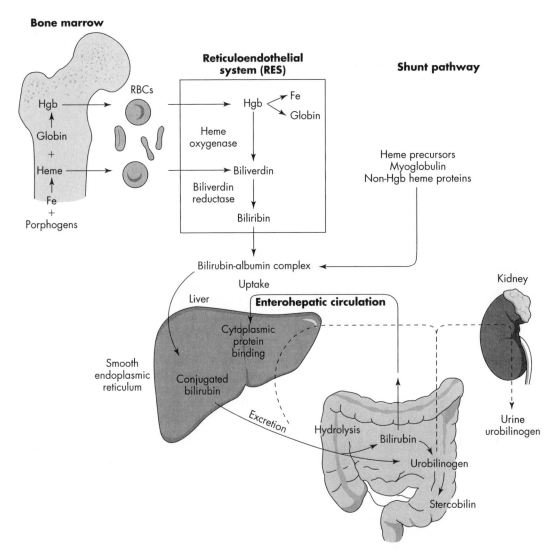

Figure 20-1 Pathways of bilirubin synthesis, transport, and metabolism. (From Gartner LM, Hollander M: Disorders of bilirubin metabolism. In Assali NS, editor: *Pathophysiology of gestation,* vol 3, New York, 1972, Academic Press.)

Albumin binding of unconjugated bilirubin may be important in the prevention of toxicity (kernicterus). Once the high-affinity site is saturated, there is a rapid increase in potentially toxic, free (nonbound) unconjugated bilirubin. A bilirubin/albumin molar ratio of 1 corresponds to approximately 8.5 mg bilirubin/g albumin. Although others have been suggested, the only drug demonstrated to carry an increased risk for kernicterus in the human is sulfisoxazole (Table 20-1).

In the hypoglycemic infant, glucuronide production may be limited, and thus conjugation is impaired. The presence of beta-glucuronidase in the bowel lumen during fetal life enables bilirubin to be reabsorbed and transported across the placenta for excretion by the maternal liver.

Table 20-1
Factors Affecting Bilirubin-Albumin Binding

Factors	Mechanism
pH (acidosis)	Decreases binding by decreasing affinity at the binding site and increasing tissue affinity
Hematin	Competitively inhibits binding at primary site
Free fatty acid (Intralipid)	Competitively inhibit binding at primary site
Infection	Mechanism not established
Drugs such as sulfa compounds, sodium salicylate, and phenylbutazone	Primarily competitive binding; principally at secondary site; best established for sulfisoxazole
Stabilizers for albumin preparations	Competitively inhibit binding at primary site
X-ray contrast media for cholangiography	Competitively inhibit binding at primary site

Etiology

Chemical hyperbilirubinemia occurs in virtually all newborns. The National Collaborative Perinatal Project[9] found that only about 6% of newborns weighing greater than 2500 g at birth would have serum bilirubin levels greater than 12.9 mg/dl. Pathologic (non-"physiologic") hyperbilirubinemia can be the result of increased production or decreased excretion of bilirubin or occasionally a combination of these two processes (Box 20-1).

Overproduction of Bilirubin

Hemolytic Disease of the Newborn

Hemolytic disease of the newborn may occur when blood group incompatibilities such as Rh, ABO, or in rare instances minor blood groups exist between a mother and her fetus. An Rh-negative mother can become sensitized to the Rh antigen in many ways. For example, sensitization can be caused by an improperly matched blood transfusion or the occurrence of fetal-maternal blood transfusion during pregnancy, delivery, abortion, or amniocentesis. The presence of the Rh antigen induces maternal

Box 20-1

Causes of Hyperbilirubinemia

A. Overproduction
1. Hemolytic disease of the newborn
2. Hereditary hemolytic anemias
   a) Membrane defects
   b) Hemoglobinopathies
   c) Enzyme defects
3. Polycythemia
4. Extravascular blood
   a) Swallowed
   b) Bruising/enclosed hemorrhage (e.g., cephalohematoma)
5. Increased enterohepatic circulation
B. Undersecretion
1. Decreased hepatic uptake
   a) Decreased sinusoidal perfusion
   b) Ligandin deficiency
2. Decreased conjugation
   a) Enzyme deficiency
   b) Enzyme inhibition and the Lucey-Driscoll syndrome[12]
3. Inadequate transport out of hepatocyte
4. Biliary obstruction
C. Combined
1. Bacterial infection
2. Congenital intrauterine infection
D. Breastfeeding
1. Breastfeeding jaundice
2. Breast milk jaundice
E. Miscellaneous
1. Hypothyroidism
2. Galactosemia
3. Infant of diabetic mother
F. Physiologic

antibody production, and IgG crosses the placenta into the fetal circulation. There it reacts with the Rh antigen on fetal erythrocytes. These antibody-coated cells are recognized as abnormal and are destroyed by the spleen. This results in increased amounts of hemoglobin, requiring metabolic degradation as discussed previously. As the destruction of erythrocytes and production of bilirubin progress, the ability of the fetus to compensate may be surpassed. The wide range of clinical features is discussed elsewhere.

With the widespread use of RhoGAM, the most

frequent cause of hemolytic disease of the newborn is ABO blood group incompatibility.

The classic example of hemolytic disease of the newborn has been erythroblastosis fetalis as a result of Rh incompatibility. Of the white population 15% is Rh negative. Fortunately the use of anti-D gamma globulin (RhoGAM), including antenatal administration at 26 to 28 weeks' gestation, has markedly decreased the incidence of this serious disease.

The IgG on the surface of the infant's red blood cells is the basis of the positive direct Coombs' test. Because prior sensitization with the Rh antigen is required for antibody production, the first Rh-positive infant is usually not affected.

ABO incompatibility is limited to mothers of blood group O and affects infants of blood group A or B. All group O individuals have naturally occurring anti-A and anti-B (IgG) antibodies, so previous sensitization is not necessary. Clinical disease is generally milder than that seen with Rh incompatibility.

Hereditary Hemolytic Anemias

Erythrocytes with abnormal membranes have abnormal osmotic fragility (generally increased) and an increased rate of splenic destruction. Hemoglobinopathies can be diagnosed by hemoglobin electrophoresis. Individuals with enzyme defects are unable to maintain the integrity of the red blood cells. A precipitating factor for the hemolysis is often not found in infants.

Examples of hemolytic anemias include hereditary spherocytosis and elliptocytosis. The family history may be positive in as many as 80% of cases.

G6PD deficiency is the most common enzyme defect. It is more common in certain ethnic groups, including Chinese, Greeks, and blacks. Deficiency of pyruvate kinase may also occur.

Polycythemia

Polycythemia (central venous hematocrit >65) is the condition in which an increased red blood cell mass, along with the shortened life span of these cells found in all newborns, results in an increased bilirubin load.

Polycythemia may be idiopathic or may occur as a result of a maternal-fetal transfusion, twin-to-twin transfusion, chronic in utero hypoxia, or delayed clamping of the umbilical cord at the time of delivery.

Extravascular Blood

Red blood cells trapped in the enclosed hemorrhages are broken down as resolution occurs.

Clinically, enclosed hemorrhage includes cephalhematoma, subgaleal hemorrhage, cerebral hemorrhage, intraabdominal bleeding, or any occult bleeding. Extensive bruising is associated with higher bilirubin loads as healing occurs. Swallowed maternal blood is another source of increased bilirubin load. Supernatant fluid of stool or gastric juices can be tested by the Apt test. Fetal hemoglobin will resist denaturation by alkali.

Increased Enterohepatic Circulation

The lumen of the newborn's bowel contains the enzyme beta-glucuronidase, which can convert conjugated bilirubin back into its unconjugated (absorbable) form and glucuronic acid.

Meconium contains a substantial amount of bilirubin. It is estimated that there is about 1 mg bilirubin/g meconium, or a total load of 100 to 200 mg. Any delay in the passage of meconium, such as can occur with Hirschsprung's disease (aganglionosis), intestinal atresia, intestinal stenosis, or the meconium plug and meconium ileus syndromes, will increase the bilirubin load that must be metabolized. Pathologic jaundice from these causes is rarely evident in the first 24 to 48 hours of life.

Undersecretion of Bilirubin

Infants with normal bilirubin production rates may be unable to remove this load for a variety of reasons.

Decreased Hepatic Uptake of Bilirubin

Diminished hepatic uptake of bilirubin may be a result of inadequate perfusion of hepatic sinusoids or deficient carrier proteins (Y and Z). Certain drugs and compounds such as steroid hormones, free fatty acids, and chloramphenicol may competitively bind to these proteins, creating a functional deficiency.

Inadequate perfusion of hepatic sinusoids occurs when there is a shunt through a persistent

ductus venosus or extrahepatic portal vein thrombosis, or with hyperviscosity and hypovolemia. This may occur in infants with severe congestive heart failure.

Although Y and Z protein are decreased in other primates, no actual deficiency has yet been demonstrated in the human newborn.

Decreased Bilirubin Conjugation

Decreased bilirubin conjugation may be a result of glucuronyl transferase deficiency, as in Crigler-Najjar syndromes I and II or Gilbert's syndrome. It may also be a result of enzyme inhibition, as in the Lucey-Driscoll syndrome.[12] The serums of some women and their infants contain an increased amount of an as yet unidentified factor that inhibits hepatic conjugation. Icteric infants with pyloric stenosis appear to have inhibition of glucuronyl transferase activity.[3]

Crigler-Najjar syndrome exists in two forms with either complete or partial absence of enzymatic activity. Type I, or complete absence, is an autosomal recessive disorder. Type II, or partial enzyme deficiency, is inherited as an autosomal dominant disorder and responds to enzyme induction with phenobarbital. Gilbert's syndrome is another autosomal dominant disorder with partial enzyme activity affecting individuals out of the newborn period with mild bilirubin elevation. Infants with Lucey-Driscoll syndrome may require exchange transfusion. Bilirubin levels rapidly decrease to normal after surgery for pyloric stenosis.

Inadequate Transport Out of the Hepatocyte

Dubin-Johnson and Rotor's syndromes are genetically inherited conditions (autosomal recessive and dominant, respectively) in which individuals are able to conjugate bilirubin normally but are unable to excrete it, resulting in direct hyperbilirubinemia.

Dubin-Johnson and Rotor's syndromes and generalized hepatocellular damage require specialized evaluation, including liver biopsy.

Biliary Obstruction

Biliary obstruction is often seen as a diagnostic dilemma between generalized hepatocellular damage and mechanical obstruction.

A variety of disorders can cause cellular damage, including infections such as hepatitis and metabolic disorders such as galactosemia. In the NICU the most common cause of cellular damage is the use of IV alimentation. The mechanism is not well established, but the damage takes at least 2 weeks to develop and is especially prominent in VLBW infants. Biliary atresia or, much less frequently, a choledochal cyst can cause mechanical obstruction to bile flow, resulting in a direct-reacting hyperbilirubinemia.

Combined Overproduction and Undersecretion

Bacterial infections (sepsis neonatorum) or the occurrence of intrauterine viral infections can result in increased bilirubin production and decreased hepatic clearance. Infants with NEC caused by a toxin-producing organism such as certain *Escherichia coli* may develop this form of hepatocellular damage.

Intrauterine infections, including congenital syphilis, toxoplasmosis, rubella, infection caused by CMV, herpes simplex, coxsackie B virus, and hepatitis virus, cause clinical jaundice. Infants with these infections will often have additional clinical stigmata of their infection.

Jaundice Associated with Breastfeeding

Breastfeeding Jaundice

In general, breastfed infants have higher bilirubin levels than bottle-fed infants, especially on the fifth day of life. It has been postulated that this early jaundice is related to decreased caloric and fluid intake from colostrum[5] and increased enterohepatic circulation resulting from low stool output and breast milk beta-glucuronidase.[8] In many studies there has been a relationship between the degree of hyperbilirubinemia and the amount of weight lost by the infant.

Breast Milk Jaundice

A small percentage (1% to 2%) of breastfed infants become jaundiced because of an inhibitor or inhibitory substance found in their mother's breast milk. Initially the inhibitory substance was considered a result of a progestational steroid, 3-alpha-20-beta pregnanediol,[7] but it has not been isolated consistently. It has been suggested that these milks contain elevated levels of beta glucuronidase or abnormally large amounts of unsaturated fatty acids inhibiting conjugation through an ill-defined mechanism such as unusually high lipoprotein lipase activity.[4,10,16] The rate of recurrance in families approaches 70%. It has also been suggested that enteric reabsorption of bilirubin is enhanced.[1]

Despite lack of supporting data that breastfed infants are underfed, it is common practice in some institutions to supplement with glucose water or electrolyte solutions after nursing. This is unnecessary, and supplemented infants have higher bilirubin levels. Optimal management includes early and frequent nursing (8 to 12 times/day).

Clinically, infants with breast milk jaundice have an unconjugated hyperbilirubinemia (greater than 12 mg/dl) that becomes exaggerated and persistent by about the fifth day of life. Levels may persist for 4 to 14 days, followed by very gradual declines. Interruption of breastfeeding for 24 to 48 hours results in a prompt fall in bilirubin levels, and resumption of nursing is not accompanied by "rebound" hyperbilirubinemia. This clinical pattern establishes the diagnosis of breast milk jaundice. It is essentially a diagnosis of exclusion in a healthy infant. As serum levels approach 20 mg/dl,

breastfeeding may be interrupted for 48 hours. It is important to support the mother during this period so as not to foster feelings of guilt or inadequacy. Early discharge of breastfed infants with inadequate follow-up may result in excessive levels of bilirubin and the possibility of kernicterus.

Physiologic or Developmental Jaundice

Physiologic or developmental jaundice is a diagnosis of exclusion. The newborn has a rate of bilirubin production of 8 to 10 mg/kg/24 hr, which is two to two and a half times the production rate in adults. Perfusion of the hepatic sinusoids may be somewhat compromised by incomplete closure of the ductus venosus or the presence of extramedullary hemopoietic tissue in the liver. Newborn monkeys have been shown to be deficient in the Y and Z proteins for the first few days of life, and this may also occur in the human newborn. Enterohepatic circulation contributes significantly to the bilirubin load.

The hormonal (estrogen) environment of the infant may inhibit liver function and bilirubin secretion. Although a level of 12.9 may define "pathologic" jaundice in the bottlefed infant, levels of up to 14.5 may be physiologic in the breastfed infant (Fig. 20-2).

Physiologic jaundice is partially attributable to a relative deficiency of glucuronyl transferase

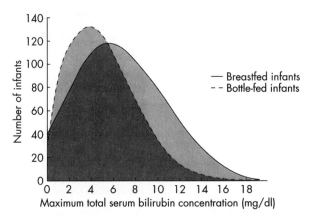

Figure 20-2   Distribution of maximum serum bilirubin concentration in white infants weighing more than 2500 g. Curves were computer-generated using exponential 1 knot spline regression. (From Maisell MJ, Gifford K: *Pediatrics* 78:837, 1986.)

activity. Enzyme activity increases rapidly after birth independent of the infant's gestational age. A major factor in physiologic jaundice remains the increased rate of bilirubin production (Box 20-2). Certain ethnic groups, including Eskimo, Oriental, and American Indian, have an increased incidence and severity of physiologic jaundice.

Miscellaneous Etiologies

Hypothyroidism

The mechanism of hyperbilirubinemia in hypothyroidism is not well understood, but in some animal studies thyroxin was needed for the hepatic clearance of bilirubin.

Hypothyroid infants have unconjugated hyperbilirubinemia that may be prolonged. They may fail to show any other signs or symptoms of hypothyroidism until later in their course. Therefore most states now routinely screen for hypothyroidism, galactosemia, and phenylketonuria.

Galactosemia

The mechanism in galactosemia may be related to a lack of substrate for glucuronidation and the accumulation of abnormal metabolic byproducts that are hepatotoxic.

Galactosemia is an autosomal recessive disorder characterized by increased jaundice in infants fed breast milk or lactose-containing formulas. The presence of nonglucose-reducing substances in the urine suggests galactosemia.

Infant of a Diabetic Mother

Hyperbilirubinemia in the IDM appears to be multifactorial. In addition to prematurity and a tendency to feed poorly, the IDM may have an increased bilirubin load secondary to an expanded red blood cell mass and hypovolemia.

Prevention

Anti-D gamma globulin (RhoGAM) antibody provides passive protection, allowing destruction of the fetal red blood cell and preventing maternal production of anti-Rh antibodies that might affect subsequent Rh-positive pregnancies.

Widespread use of RhoGAM has proved effective in preventing the sensitization of Rh-negative mothers after delivery or abortion of Rh-positive infants. Failures may occur if the amount of RhoGAM administered is insufficient compared with the load of fetal red blood cells received or if a significant fetal-maternal hemorrhage occurred before term. RhoGAM should be administered to Rh-negative women undergoing amniocentesis.

Early Feeding

The physiologic mechanism is not entirely known but may be caused by a decrease in intestinal transit time and decreased enterohepatic circulation.

When compared with infants not fed during the first 24 to 48 hours of life, infants fed earlier have lower peak bilirubin levels.

Phenobarbital

Phenobarbital acts as an inducer of microsomal enzymes, increasing the conjugation of bilirubin. It

---

Box 20-2

Criteria that Rule Out the Diagnosis of Physiologic Jaundice*

1. Clinical jaundice in the first 24 hours of life
2. Total serum bilirubin concentrations increasing by more than 5 mg/dl (85 μmol/L/day)
3. Total serum bilirubin concentration exceeding 12.9 mg/dl (221 μmol/L) in a full-term infant or 15 mg/dl (257 μmol/L) in a premature infant
4. Direct serum bilirubin concentration exceeding 1.5 to 2 mg/dl (26 to 34 μmol/L)
5. Clinical jaundice persisting for more than 1 week in a full-term infant or 2 weeks in a premature infant

*The absence of these criteria does not imply that the jaundice is physiologic. In the presence of any of these criteria, the jaundice must be investigated further.
From Maisels MJ: Neonatal jaundice. In Avery GB, editor: *Neonatology: pathophysiology and management of the newborn*, ed 2, Philadelphia, 1981, JB Lippincott Co.

also has a direct effect to stimulate bile secretion in infants with nonobstructive cholestasis. Phenobarbital also increases the concentration of ligandin. When used in conjunction with phototherapy, it does not increase the rate of decline.

Phenobarbital is effective when given to the mother before delivery. In infants with significant hemolytic disease of the newborn, it appears to slow the rate of rise of bilirubin and decrease the incidence of exchange transfusion. It is also indicated in infants with Crigler-Najjar syndrome type II. Its use is not indicated on a routine prophylactic basis, because such use would overtreat many infants, and other effects may be detrimental.

Tin Protoporphyrin and Tin Mesoporphyrin

Clinical trials have shown that administration of tin protoporphyrin (SnPP) or tin mesoporphyrin (SnMP) to preterm infants, term and near-term infants, or infants with ABO hemolytic disease of the newborn decrease bilirubin production. These compounds are potent competitive inhibitors of the enzyme heme oxygenase.[10,11,19] Heme is excreted directly into bile when bilrubin production is suppressed. Infants receiving a single dose of SnMP (6 μmol/kg body weight IM) have lower peak serum bilirubin levels and a decreased need for phototherapy. Side effects have been minimal and include a transient erythema in those infants requiring phototherapy after receiving SnMP. Additional studies to determine the role of these compounds in the management and prevention of neonatal jaundice are ongoing.

Data Collection

The history, physical examination, and laboratory data play an important role in the evaluation of the jaundiced newborn (Box 20-3).

History

The evaluation of the jaundiced infant begins with a good familial, perinatal, and neonatal history. The family history should include the occurrence of disorders associated with jaundice in other family members, especially siblings. The perinatal and obstetric history may provide clues or enable the clinician to anticipate possible hyperbilirubinemia. The infant's course since birth may be important.

Signs and Symptoms and Clinical Approach

A wide spectrum of signs and symptoms may occur in the jaundiced infant, often depending on the

---

Box 20-3

Evaluation of Unconjugated Hyperbilirubinemia in the Neonate

I. History
  A. Family
  B. Perinatal and obstetric
  C. Neonatal
II. Physical examination
  A. Pallor
  B. Hepatosplenomegaly
  C. Enclosed hemorrhage
  D. Petechiae
  E. Congenital anomalies
III. Laboratory data
  A. All jaundiced infants
    1. Maternal and infant blood type
    2. Coombs' test on cord blood
    3. Total/direct bilirubin (serial measurements)
    4. Complete blood count, including hematocrit, reticulocyte and platelet counts, white blood cell differential, and peripheral smear for red blood cell morphology
    5. Urinalysis, test for reducing substances
  B. Selected cases
    1. Protein, total and/or albumin
    2. Sepsis evaluation
    3. IgM
    4. Urine cytology for cytomegalovirus
    5. Viral cultures
  C. New techniques
    1. Transcutaneous bilirubinometry
    2. Bilirubin-binding tests

causes of the jaundice. In the absence of hemolysis, an infant may be asymptomatic with dermal icterus as the only clinical sign. The infant with hemolytic disease of the newborn may show signs of jaundice and pallor in association with severe anemia and hydrops fetalis or may appear entirely normal at birth. Hepatosplenomegaly resulting from congestion and extramedullary hemopoiesis may be present. Infants affected by hemolytic disease of the newborn also have pancreatic islet cell hyperplasia and are at increased risk for hypoglycemia. Careful physical examination may reveal the presence of a cephalhematoma or other enclosed hemorrhage. The occurrence of petechiae or purpura raises the possibility of intrauterine infection or sepsis. Congenital anomalies should be noted.

Laboratory Data

Knowledge of the mother's and infant's blood types and Rh will establish the potential for hemolytic disease. Direct Coombs' test on cord blood is positive in ABO disease. Later testing of the infant's blood in an ABO incompatibility may be Coombs' negative. In addition to hematocrit and reticulocyte determinations, a careful examination of the peripheral blood smear should be performed, looking for evidence of hemolysis such as increased numbers of nucleated red blood cells or the presence of fragmented cells, poikilocytosis, and anisocytosis.

Microspherocytosis is characteristic of ABO incompatibility and may at times be confused with hereditary spherocytosis. A knowledge of blood types and clinical course will help in differentiating these two. An abnormal white blood cell count or differential, or thrombocytopenia may suggest infection. In addition to jaundice and anemia in the first few days of life, infants with a hemolytic disease are at risk for development of a "late" anemia after discharge from the nursery. Fractionated (total/direct) bilirubin levels and serial levels help establish causes and enable the clinician to follow the rate of bilirubin rise. Protein and albumin determinations allow a gross assessment of adequacy of bilirubin binding. A great deal of clinical and laboratory research has been performed to determine the degree of and sites available for bilirubin albumin binding. This information may someday enable

the clinician to assess the risk for kernicterus and perform an exchange transfusion at the appropriate time, but these determinations are not presently recommended or available for routine use.

Items of interest include possible infection during the pregnancy or the use of oxytocin induction for delivery. Also of concern is the occurrence of an asphyxial episode during labor or delivery. Premature infants have higher mean bilirubin levels and a slightly later peak. A history of asphyxia and medication should be obtained. Also of interest is the infant's feeding and stool patterns. The time of onset or detection of jaundice may be important. Jaundice in the first 24 hours of life must always be considered abnormal.

Jaundice in the newborn can usually be detected clinically at a level of 6 to 7 mg/dl. Visible icterus appears first on the head and face and progresses in a cephalocaudal manner. The extremities are the last skin surface to be affected.

Immediate exchange transfusion with type O Rh-negative red blood cells may be necessary in Rh incompatibility with a severely affected infant. Hydrops fetalis is rare in hemolytic disease as a result of ABO incompatibility.

There is an increased incidence of jaundice in trisomic syndromes. Jaundice and umbilical hernia are associated with congenital hypothyroidism.

Minimal laboratory evaluation of the jaundiced newborn should include the mother's and infant's blood types, Rh status, and Coombs' test on cord blood. A CBC to include reticulocyte and platelet counts, white blood cell count and differential, peripheral smear for red blood cell morphology, and hematocrit should be performed. Infants suspected of bacterial sepsis should receive antibiotic treatment and a complete sepsis evaluation including cultures of blood urine, and cerebrospinal fluid. Bilirubin levels (total and direct) should be measured serially. Total protein and/or albumin levels may be helpful as the infant approaches exchange transfusion.

Urinalysis including evaluation for reducing substances may be helpful. Infants suspected of congenital infection should have additional tests, including IgM levels. Viral cultures and urine cytology for CMV may be performed. Newborn screening should be performed for hypothyroidism, galactosemia, and PKU.

Treatment

Treatment is aimed at preventing the complications of kernicterus and bilirubin encephalopathy. Phototherapy and exchange transfusion are widely used; however, decisions to utilize these therapies are complicated by an incomplete understanding of bilirubin toxicity, especially as applied to an individual infant. The American Academy of Pediatrics recently published a Practice Parameter: Management of Hyperbilirubinemia in the Healthy Term Newborn. These management guidelines are outlined in Table 20-2 and in the algorithm detailed in Figure 20-3. Extensive review of the literature dealing with full-term infants without hemolytic disease has found little evidence of adverse effects of bilirubin on IQ, neurologic examination, or hearing.[14] **Infants with hemolytic disease and premature (especially VLBW) infants should receive phototherapy and exchange transfusion at lower levels. A suggested guideline is to initiate phototherapy when the serum bilirubin is 5 mg/dl below the serum bilirubin concentration at which an exchange transfusion will be performed for that individual infant.[2] As more data become available, perhaps clearer guidelines can be established and more specific recommendations made for these infants.**

Phototherapy

Phototherapy is the most commonly employed means of treatment. The indication for phototherapy is to prevent the infant from requiring an exchange transfusion. It is estimated that 10% of newborns in the United States are treated with phototherapy.

Before the initiation of phototherapy in any infant, appropriate evaluation as to the cause of the jaundice must be performed. Indications for the initiation of phototherapy vary widely from nursery to nursery and depend on the individual infant's clinical status.

Phototherapy generally consists of a single tungston halogen lamp or a bank of four to eight cool white, daybright, or special blue fluorescent bulbs covered by a Plexiglass shield and placed 15 to 20 cm from the patient. Manufacturers' recommendations should be followed. Fiberoptic blankets delivering phototherapy from a high-intensity light source are also available either for use by themselves or in conjunction with other sources of phototherapy. The spectrum of light at 420 to 460 nm is the most effective. The energy output (irradiance) in this spectrum should be checked periodically to ensure maximum efficiency.

Phototherapy by photoisomerization and photooxidation results in the formation of more polar,

Table 20-2
Management of Hyperbilirubinemia in the Healthy Term Newborn*

Age (hr)	TSB* Level, mg/dl (µmol/L)			
	Consider Phototherapy†	**Phototherapy**	**Exchange Transfusion if Intensive Phototherapy Fails‡**	**Exchange Transfusion and Intensive Phototherapy**
≤24§	—	—	—	—
25-48	≥12 (170)	≥15 (260)	≥20 (340)	≥25 (430)
49-72	≥15 (260)	≥18 (310)	≥25 (430)	≥30 (510)
>72	≥17 (290)	≥20 (340)	≥25 (430)	≥30 (510)

From American Academy of Pediatrics: Practice parameter: management of hyperbilirubinemia in the healthy term infant, *Pediatrics* 94:558, 1994.
*TSB indicates total serum bilirubin.
†Phototherapy at these TSB levels is a clinical option, meaning that the intervention is available and may be used *on the basis of individual clinical judgment.*
‡Intensive phototherapy should produce a decline of TSB of 1 to 2 mg/dl within 4 to 6 hours and the TSB level should continue to fall and remain below the threshold level for exchange transfusion. If this does not occur, it is considered a failure of phototherapy.
§Term infants who are clinically jaundiced at ≤24 hours old are not considered healthy and require further evaluation

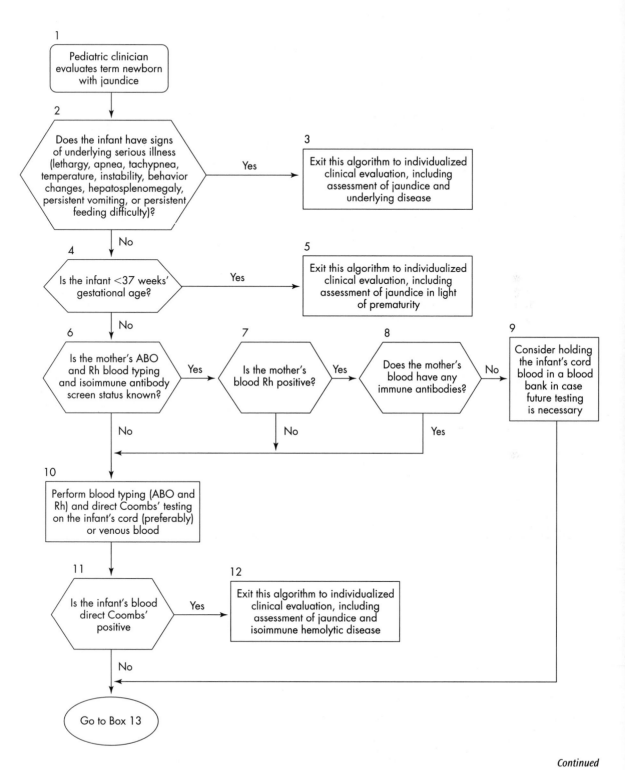

Continued

Figure 20-3 Algorithm. Management of hyperbilirubinemia in the healthy term infant.

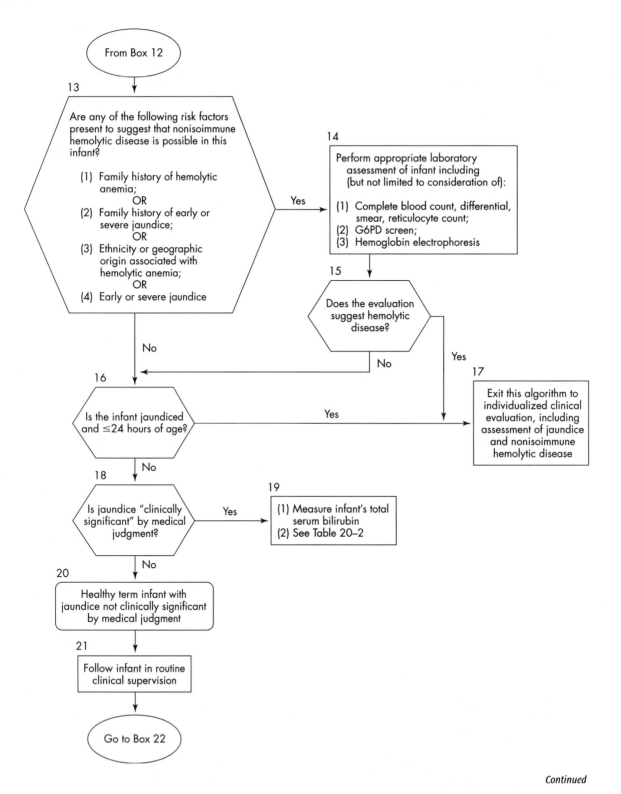

From Box 12

13

Are any of the following risk factors present to suggest that nonisoimmune hemolytic disease is possible in this infant?

(1) Family history of hemolytic anemia;
OR
(2) Family history of early or severe jaundice;
OR
(3) Ethnicity or geographic origin associated with hemolytic anemia;
OR
(4) Early or severe jaundice

Yes

14

Perform appropriate laboratory assessment of infant including (but not limited to consideration of):

(1) Complete blood count, differential, smear, reticulocyte count;
(2) G6PD screen;
(3) Hemoglobin electrophoresis

15

Does the evaluation suggest hemolytic disease?

No

Yes

17

Exit this algorithm to individualized clinical evaluation, including assessment of jaundice and nonisoimmune hemolytic disease

No

16

Is the infant jaundiced and ≤24 hours of age?

Yes

No

18

Is jaundice "clinically significant" by medical judgment?

Yes

19

(1) Measure infant's total serum bilirubin
(2) See Table 20–2

No

20

Healthy term infant with jaundice not clinically significant by medical judgment

21

Follow infant in routine clinical supervision

Go to Box 22

Continued

Figure 20-3, cont'd Algorithm. Management of hyperbilirubinemia in the healthy term infant.

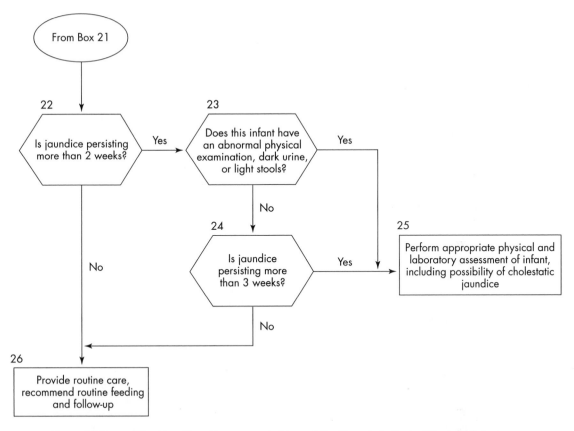

Figure 20-3, cont'd   Algorithm. Management of hyperbilirubinemia in the healthy term infant.

water-soluble bilirubin products. The most important of these reactions appears to be the formation of lumirubin,[13] a stable structural photoisomer. Lumirubin does not require conjugation and is rapidly excreted in bile and urine. The production of lumirubin is an irreversible reaction that appears to be dose related (Fig. 20-4).

The efficacy of phototherapy depends on energy output (irradiance) in the blue spectrum of the lights and on the surface area of the infant exposed to those lights.

Animal studies have demonstrated a potential retinal toxicity of light. It is not established that this occurs in the human newborn, but it remains a major concern.

Infants exposed to phototherapy, particularly the LBW infant and the infant under a radiant warmer, have significant increases in their IWL. These infants also have increased stool water losses and may develop a temporary lactose intolerance.

There are conflicting data in the literature on whether continuous or intermittent administration of phototherapy is most effective.

The concept behind phototherapy arose from the serendipitous observation that infants exposed to sunlight had less jaundice than infants positioned away from the windows.

Phototherapy is not a substitute for exchange transfusion when an exchange is indicated. The decision to treat with phototherapy must be made on an individual basis.

Special blue lights are the most effective but are not widely used, because they mask the clinical signs of cyanosis and color change in the infant.

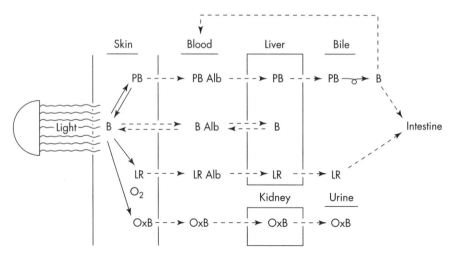

Figure 20-4   General mechanisms of phototherapy for neonatal jaundice. *Solid arrows* represent chemical reactions; *broken arrows* represent transport processes. Pigments may be bound to proteins in compartments other than blood. Some excretion of photoisomers, particularly lumirubin, in urine also occurs. *B,* Bilirubin (*Z,Z* isomer); *PB,* photobilirubin (*E,E* and *E,Z* isomers); *LR,* lumirubin (*E* and *Z* isomers); *O × B,* bilirubin oxidation products; *Alb,* albumin. (From McDonagh AF, Lightner DA: *Pediatrics* 75:443, 1985.)

Green light appears slightly less effective.[18] Many nurseries employ white fluorescent phototherapy bulbs. These are effective and permit better visual monitoring of the patient. The Plexiglas shield absorbs ultraviolet irradiation. Tungsten halogen lights are replacing fluorescent lights in many nurseries. Fiberoptic phototherapy blankets are now available. These systems (Wallaby Phototherapy System, Fiberoptic Medical Products, Inc., Allentown, Pennsylvania; and Biliblanket, Ohmeda, Columbia, Maryland) use a high-intensity halogen light source for transmission of light by fiberoptic bundles. Irradiance and efficacy appear comparable with standard phototherapy.[17] Purported advantages of these systems are elimination of the need for eye patches, exposure of greater surface area, and provision of phototherapy outside of the nursery with less interference in mother-infant bonding. These blankets are more convenient to use when phototherapy is required in an outpatient setting.

A photoreaction occurs in the very outer layers (top 2 mm) of the skin. Once phototherapy has been initiated, serum levels of bilirubin must be monitored frequently (every 4 to 12 hours), because

visual assessment of icterus is no longer valid. Hematocrit must also be monitored, especially in infants with hemolytic disease.

To increase exposure, most infants are placed naked under the lights with shielding over the eyes. In the small infant, diapers may cover a significant amount of surface area, and some clinicians have found that using a tie-on surgeon's mask as a "bikini bottom" is effective in containing stool and urine. The infant's position should be changed frequently. This permits maximum skin exposure to the lights.

Because of the potential for eye damage, the eyes should be covered while phototherapy is in use. Patches should completely cover the eyes without placing excessive pressure on the eyes and be carefully positioned to avoid occluding the nares. To permit evaluation of the infant's eyes, eye patches should be removed every 4 hours and changed every 8 hours. The patches should be left off during feedings and parental visits.

The infant's temperature should be monitored frequently. Infants in incubators or servocontrolled care centers may become overheated. The servocontrol probe should be shielded by an opaque covering. Infants treated in open cribs may become cold stressed. Fluid balance must be carefully monitored in the infant receiving phototherapy. Weights taken twice a day and close monitoring of intake and output such as urine volume and specific gravity may indicate a need for increased fluids, either orally or intravenously. The presence of reducing substances in the stool can be treated with a nonlactose-containing formula. With continuous phototherapy the infant will receive 18 to 20 hours of light per day with interruptions for feeding, blood drawing, and parental visits. In some studies, intermittent schedules such as 15 minutes on and 60 minutes off appear to be as effective as continuous schedules with much less irradiation, but the occurrence of in vitro complications may be greater. After phototherapy ceases, bilirubin levels should be followed for at least 24 hours to rule out the occurrence of significant rebound. Table 20-3 outlines some of the nursing assessments and management to be performed in infants undergoing phototherapy.

Exchange Transfusion

An exchange transfusion is indicated for correction of severe anemia, removal of antibody-coated red blood cells in hemolytic disease, or removal of excessive unconjugated bilirubin regardless of its cause. Phototherapy has significantly decreased the need for exchange transfusion. Again, the indications, especially in the VLBW infant, vary from nursery to nursery.

In the infant with severe hemolytic disease, a packed red blood cell exchange transfusion using type O Rh-negative blood may save the infant's life, correct anemia and hypoxemia, and permit successful transition.

Administration of 1 g/kg of salt-poor albumin 1 hour before the exchange transfusion has been shown in some studies to increase the efficiency of exchange by about 40%.[15] Aliquot size appears to have no significant effect on the efficiency of the exchange. Smaller aliquots are less stressful to the infant.

Citrate used as part of the anticoagulant solution binds divalent ions such as calcium and magnesium.

Immediately after the exchange, the bilirubin

level will be about 45% of the preexchange level. As plasma and tissue levels equilibrate, the bilirubin rises to about 60% of the preexchange level.

It must be stressed that the decision to perform an exchange transfusion must be individualized for each patient.

Central venous pressure must be carefully followed when performing an exchange transfusion with packed red blood cells. If necessary in the delivery room, a slow exchange is performed to reach a hematocrit of 45. Then the infant is transported to the NICU.

Exchange transfusion trays are commercially available and include a four-way stopcock, necessary tubing and syringes, 10% calcium gluconate, and a plastic bag for discarded blood.

Whole blood with a hematocrit of 50% to 55% is used for exchange transfusion. ABO type-specific Rh-negative blood should be used in cases with Rh incompatibility. Type O Rh-specific cells are indicated when ABO incompatibility exists. Citrate-phosphate-dextrose is the anticoagulant most widely used. Insist on fresh blood (<24 hours old). Albumin priming results in an expansion of plasma volume and should not be used in anemic or edematous infants.

For exchange transfusion the infant should be on a cardiac monitor and restrained in an incubator or on an infant care center with a radiant heater. Generally, 5 to 20 ml aliquots of blood are used, depending on the size and condition of the infant. The initial aliquot should be withdrawn and sent to the laboratory for bilirubin, hematocrit, calcium, and cultures. The rate of exchange is usually 2 to 4 ml/min. Blood used in the exchange should be warmed and mixed in the bag after every 50 to 100 ml. Central venous pressure measurements should be made about every 100 ml or every 50 ml in the hydropic infant.

The infant should be evaluated for hypocalcemia after each 100 ml of the exchange has been completed. Clinical signs and symptoms of hypocalcemia include irritability, tachycardia, or prolongation of the Q-oTc interval. If hypocalcemia is detected, 1 ml of a 10% calcium gluconate solution is slowly infused.

The final aliquot from an exchange should be sent for CBC, fractionated bilirubin, calcium ion, electrolytes, culture, and repeat type and cross-

Table 20-3
Nursing Management of Infants Undergoing Phototherapy

Nursing Assessment

Area	Parameter
Physical status	Intake and output
	Color
	Location of jaundice
	Skin integrity
	Stools (character, consistency)
	Vital signs
	Infant/environment temperature
	Hydration status
	Signs of phototherapy side effects
	Eye discharge and tearing
	Position
	Activity
Neurobehavioral status	Sleep-wake states
	Sensory threshold
	Behavioral responsiveness
	Feeding behaviors
	Consoling abilities
	Stress responses
	Interactive capabilities

Nursing Management

Nursing Diagnosis	Intervention
Fluid volume deficit (actual or potential)	Monitor intake and output.
	Monitor hydration status (weight, specific gravity, urine output).
	Monitor stooling pattern, character.
	Maintain adequate fluid intake (oral or parenteral).
Alteration in nutrition	Assess feeding behavior and activity.
	Monitor fluid and caloric intake, weight, abdominal girth.
	Remove eye shields during feeding.
	Hold during oral feedings as health and thermal status permit.
	Bring to alert state before feeding.
	Feed on demand if possible.
Impaired skin integrity	Observe color, rashes, excoriation.
	Clean skin with warm water.
	Clean perineal area after stooling.
	Turn frequently (also increases skin exposure to phototherapy).
	Ensure Plexiglas shield is in place between light source and infant to reduce exposure to UV light.

From Blackburn S: Hyperbilirubinema and neonatal jaundice, *Neonat Net* 14:15, 1995.

Table 20-3
Nursing Management of Infants Undergoing Phototherapy—cont'd

	Nursing Management	
Nursing Diagnosis	**Intervention**	
Potential for injury	Observe for side effects associated with phototherapy.	
	Observe for signs of sepsis.	
	Provide care to minimize side effects of phototherapy.	
	Shield eyes from lights with opaque patches.	
	Ensure eyelids are closed when shield is applied to prevent corneal injury.	
	Remove eye shield and observe eyes regularly.	
	Monitor position of eye shield to prevent occlusion of nose.	
	Avoid tight head band on eye shield to reduce risk of increased intracranial pressure, especially in preterm infants.	
	Observe for eye discharge, tearing.	
	Shield testes and possibly ovaries (data unclear about need to do this) with diaper.[17a]	
Alteration in thermal status	Place in warm, thermoneutral environment.	
	Monitor environmental and infant temperature.	
	Observe for hypothermia and hyperthermia.	
	Reduce heat losses from environmental sources.	
	Use servocontrol for infants in incubator or under radiant warmer.	
	Shield servocontrol thermistor from direct exposure to phototherapy lights.	

match for potential additional exchange transfusion. In addition to the individuals performing the exchange, one person must keep an accurate record of time, volumes withdrawn and infused, vital signs, and medications administered.

Complications

Hyperbilirubinemia

Hyperbilirubinemia is of clinical concern because of the complication of bilirubin encephalopathy (kernicterus). Kernicterus refers to yellowish staining in nuclear centers of the CNS, particularly in the basal ganglia, cerebellum, and hippocampus.

Development of toxicity may depend on albumin-bilirubin binding, although interruption of the blood-brain barrier may also play a role. Factors that interfere with albumin-bilirubin binding appear to predispose to the development of kernicterus and have been outlined earlier in this chapter (see Table 20-1). Free unconjugated bilirubin appears to be cytotoxic for CNS cells and uncouples oxidative phosphorylation and reduces protein synthesis in vitro at the mitochondrial level. Once toxicity has occurred, it appears to be irreversible.

Phototherapy

Despite its widespread use since 1958, questions about the safety and side effects of phototherapy remain. The potential for retinal damage, increase in IWLs, loose stools, lactose intolerance, temperature elevations, or cold stress have already been discussed. Infants who have an associated cholestatic jaundice and are exposed to phototherapy may develop the "bronze baby syndrome." This is presumably caused by retention of a bilirubin breakdown product produced by phototherapy. Increased platelet turnover and lower mean platelet counts may occur, although the mechanism is unknown. Transient skin rashes and tanning, particularly in black infants, have been reported. Tanning is a result of increased melanin production.

Cell culture studies have demonstrated DNA

damage when exposed to phototherapy, especially with intermittent administration. Other potential problems include interference with biologic (circadian) rhythms and with maternal-infant bonding. Although there may be some transient, short-term growth effects, long-term growth effects and development appear unaffected by phototherapy.

A list of complications of phototherapy follows:

- Potential retinal damage if eyes are exposed
- Increased IWL
- Loose bowel movements
- Temporary lactose intolerance
- Temperature maintenance (hyperthermia or hypothermia)
- Bronze baby syndrome
- Decreased platelet count
- Transient skin rashes and tanning
- Potential cellular damage
- Potential interference with biologic rhythm
- Potential interference with maternal-infant bonding

Exchange Transfusion

Exchange transfusion is a procedure with many potential complications and carries a mortality risk of about 0.5%. Some complications are shown in Table 20-4

Vascular complications are related to the use of umbilical catheters discussed in Chapter 7. NEC has been reported as a postexchange complication, probably as a result of bowel ischemia during the procedure.

Electrolyte and glucose disturbances are related to the blood preparation used during the exchange. Acid-citrate-dextrose and citrate-phosphate-dextrose blood have high levels of sodium and glucose and perhaps potassium. Initial hyperglycemia may be followed by reactive hypoglycemia as a result of an insulin response. Although acidic at the time of infusion, a postexchange alkalosis may occur as citrate is metabolized to bicarbonate in the liver.

Many of the electrolyte and acid-base disturbances may be avoided by the use of fresh, heparinized blood. Bleeding may occur in the overheparinized infant but is reversible with protamine sulfate. Thrombocytopenia may occur, especially

Table 20-4
Complications of Exchange Transfusion

System	Complications
Vascular	Embolization, thrombosis, and necrotizing enterocolitis
Cardiac	Dysrhythmias, volume overload, and arrest
Electrolyte	Hypernatremia, hyperkalemia, hypocalcemia, acidosis, and alkalosis after exchange
Clotting	Thrombocytopenia, overheparinization, and bleeding
Infection	Bacteremia and blood-borne, viral hepatitis
Others	Hemolysis from old donor blood or from mechanical or thermal injury, perforations of vessels and viscera, hypoglycemia from induced insulin release, and hypothermia from overexposure.

Modified from Odell GB: *Neonatal hyperbilirubinemia*, New York, 1980, Grune & Stratton.

in the infant requiring repeated exchange transfusions. Bacterial infection is rare, and routine antibiotic prophylaxis is not indicated. Most complications are avoidable if careful attention to technique is observed.

Clinical Complications

Hyperbilirubinemia

Early clinical signs of kernicterus include a poor Moro reflex with incomplete flexion of the extremities. Because of the infant's poor sucking ability, feeding may be difficult. In progressive cases the infant develops a high-pitched cry, is hypotonic, and may vomit. Opisthotonic posturing also may occur. In later life, severely affected survivors may manifest choreoathetosis, spastic cerebral palsy, mental retardation, sensory and perceptual deafness, and visual-motor incoordination. More subtle findings may occur in less severely affected infants and may not be apparent during the newborn period. There is speculation that some learning

disabilities may be related to hyperbilirubinemia even at what had been previously considered "safe" levels. Unfortunately, the critical level at which bilirubin toxicity occurs in either preterm or term infants has not been established.

Phototherapy

The infant with bronze baby syndrome develops a dark gray-brown discoloration of the skin, urine, and serum. There are generally no clinical symptoms with this syndrome, but there has been at least one reported death. After phototherapy ceases, the bronzing gradually resolves. In addition to shielding the eyes, it has been recommended that the gonads be shielded.

Exchange Transfusion

The use of freshly collected blood (<72 hours old) will help maintain acceptable potassium levels. Infants with hemolytic disease of the newborn are already at risk for hypoglycemia because of islet cell hyperplasia. Blood glucose levels must be followed closely in the first few hours after an exchange. Heparinized blood must be used within 24 hours of preparation of the unit. In addition to other forms of viral hepatitis, CMV and HIV may be transmitted to the infant, and one must screen for these.

Parent Teaching

Jaundice and its treatment can be very disturbing to parents. Parents often feel guilty that perhaps something they did or failed to do resulted in their infant's jaundice. Reassurance and support are vital, especially for the nursing mother, who may question her ability to adequately nourish her infant.

Phototherapy is especially distressing and should be explained to the parents before they see the infant under the lights. Parents may tend to believe that there may be problems with the infant's eyes despite reassurances to the contrary. The lights should be turned off and eye patches removed during visits so normal parent-infant interaction can occur. Side effects of phototherapy

such as loose or dark-green stools should be explained to parents.

Early discharge policies (<48 hours) have increased the need for outpatient evaluation and/or management of neonatal hyperbilirubinemia. Hyperbilirubinemia is the leading indication for hospital readmission in these infants.

As with many disorders in newborn infants, a little time spent in careful explanation with the parents can alleviate much fear, guilt, and occasionally anger and help establish a normal family relationship. Causes of jaundice should be explained to the parents, emphasizing that it is usually a transient problem and one to which all infants must adapt after birth. Giving the parents a pamphlet containing information on jaundice and its therapy may help reinforce the instructive efforts.

References

1. Alonzo EM et al: Enterohepatic circulation of nonconjugated bilirubin in rats fed with human milk, *J Pediatr* 118:425, 1991.
2. American Academy of Pediatrics/American College of Obstetrics and Gynecology: *Hyperbilirubinemia: guidelines for perinatal care,* ed 3, Elk Grove Village, Ill, 1992, American Academy of Pediatrics.
3. Bleicher MA et al: Extraordinary hyperbilirubinemia in a neonate with idiopathic hypertrophic pyloric stenosis, *J Pediatr Surg* 14:527, 1979.
4. Cole AP, Hargreaves T: Conjugation inhibitors in early neonatal hyperbilirubinemia, *Arch Dis Child* 47:415, 1972.
5. Cornwall R, Cornelius CE: Effect of fasting on bilirubin metabolism, *N Engl J Med* 283:204, 1970.
6. Gartner LM, Arias IM: Studies of prolonged neonatal jaundice in the breast-fed infant, *J Pediatr* 68:54, 1966.
7. Gourley G, Arend R: B-blucuronide and hyperbilirubinemia in breast fed and formula fed babies, *Lancet* 1:644, 1986.
8. Hardy JB et al: *The first year of life: the collaborative perinatal project of the National Institute of Neurological and Communicative Disorders and Stroke,* Baltimore, 1979, The Johns Hopkins University Press.
9. Hargreaves T: Effect of fatty acids on bilirubin conjugation, *Arch Dis Child* 48:446, 1973.
10. Kappas A et al: The use of tin protoporphyrin in the management of hyperbilirubinemia in newborn infants with direct Coombs positive ABO-incompatibility, *Pediatrics* 81:485, 1988.
11. Kappas A et al: Direct comparison of Sn-Mesoporphryin, an inhibitor of bilirubin production, and phototherapy in controlling hyperbilirubinemia in term and near term newborns, *Pediatrics* 95:468, 1995
12. Lucey JF, Arias I, McKay R: Transient familial hyperbilirubinemia, *Am J Dis Child* 100:787, 1960.

13. McDonagh A, Lightner D: "Like a shrivelled blood orange"—bilirubin, jaundice, and phototherapy, *Pediatrics* 75:443, 1985.

14. Newman TB, Maisels MJ: Does hyperbilirubinemia damage the brain of healthy full term infants? *Clin Perinatol* 17:331, 1990.

15. Odell GB, Cohen SN, Gordes EH: Administration of albumin in the management of hyperbilirubinemia by exchange transfusions, *Pediatrics* 30:613, 1962.

16. Poland RL, Schultz GE, Garg G: High milk lipase activity associated with breast milk jaundice, *Pediatr Res* 14:1328, 1980.

17. Rosenfeld W et al: A new device for phototherapy treatment of jaundiced infants, *J Perinatol* 10:243, 1990.

17a. Speck W: Effect on fertilization and embryonic development, *Pediatr Res* 10:506, 1979.

18. Tan KL: Efficiency of fluorescent daylight, blue and green lamps in the management of nonhemolytic hyperbilirubinemia, *J Pediatr* 90:448, 1989.

19. Valdes T et al: Control of jaundice in preterm newborns by an inhibitor of bilirubin production, *Pediatrics* 93:1, 1994.

Selected Readings

Allen FM, Diamond LK: *Erythroblastosis fetalis including exchange transfusion technique,* Boston, 1958, Little, Brown.

American Academy of Pediatrics: Practice parameter: management of hyperbilirubinemia in the healthy term infant, *Pediatrics* 94:558, 1994.

Auerbach K, Gartner L: Breastfeeding and human milk: their association with jaundice in the neonate, *Clin Perinatol* 14:89, 1987.

Blackburn S: Hyperbilirubinemia and neonatal jaundice, *Neonat Net* 14(7):15, 1995.

Broderson R: Free bilirubin in blood plasma of the newborn: effects of albumin, fatty acids, pH, displacing drugs and phototherapy. In Stern L, Oh W, Fris-Hansen B, editors: *Intensive care of the newborn,* ed 2, New York, 1978, Masson Publishing USA.

Brown AK, Johnson L: Loss of concern about jaundice and the reemergence of kernicterus in full-term infants in the era of managed care. In Fanaroff AA, Klaus MH, editors: *The yearbook of neonatal and perinatal medicine,* St Louis, 1996, Mosby.

Cashore WJ, Stein L: Neonatal hyperbilirubinemia, *Pediatr Clin North Am* 29:1191, 1982.

Catz C, Hanson JW et al: Summary of workshop: early discharge and neonatal hyperbilirubinemia, *Pediatrics* 96:743, 1995.

Gartner LM, Hollander M: Disorders of bilirubin metabolism. In Assali NS, editor: *Pathophysiology of gestation,* vol 3, New York, 1972, Academic Press.

Gartner LM, Lee KS: Jaundice and liver disease. In Fanaroff AA, Martin RJ, editors: *Neonatal-perinatal medicine: diseases of the fetus and infant,* ed 5, St Louis, 1992, Mosby.

Graziani LJ et al: Neurodevelopment of preterm infants: neonatal neurosonographic and serum bilirubin studies, *Pediatrics* 89:229, 1992.

Gross SJ: Vitamin E and neonatal bilirubinemia, *Pediatrics* 64:321, 1979.

Kopelman AE et al: The "bronze" baby syndrome: a complication of phototherapy, *J Pediatr* 8:466, 1972.

Levine R, Marsels M, editors: *Hyperbilirubinemia in the newborn, Report of the Eighty-fifth Boss Conference on Pediatric Research,* Columbus, Ohio, 1983.

Levine RL et al: Entry of bilirubin into the brain due to opening of the blood-brain barrier, *Pediatrics* 69:255, 1982.

Lucey JF: Neonatal jaundice and phototherapy, *Pediatr Clin North Am* 19:287, 1972.

Maisels MJ: Neonatal jaundice. In Avery GB, editor: *Neonatology: pathophysiology and management of the newborn,* ed 3, Philadelphia, 1987, JB Lippincott.

Maisels MJ, editor: Neonatal jaundice, *Clin Perinatol* 17:2, 1990 (14 articles).

Maisels MJ, Gifford K: Jaundice in full-term infants, *Am J Dis Child* 137:561, 1983.

Maisels MJ, Gifford K: Normal serum bilirubin levels in the newborn and the effect of breastfeeding, *Pediatrics* 78:837, 1986.

Maisels MJ: Phototherapy—25 years later. In Fanaroff AA, Klaus MH, editors: *The yearbook of neonatal and perinatal medicine,* St Louis, 1996, Mosby.

Odell GB: *Neonatal hyperbilirubinemia,* New York, 1980, Grune & Stratton.

Poland RL, Odell G: Physiologic jaundice: the enterohepatic circulation of bilirubin, *N Engl J Med* 284:1, 1971.

Poland RL, Ostrea EM Jr: Neonatal hyperbilirubinemia. In Klaus MII, Fanaroff AA, editors: *Care of the high risk neonate,* ed 3, Philadelphia, 1986, WB Saunders.

Robinson SH: The origins of bilirubin, *N Engl J Med* 279:143, 1968.

Scheidt PC et al: Phototherapy for neonatal hyperbilirubinemia: six year follow up of the National Institute of Child Health and Human Development Clinical Trial, *Pediatrics* 85:455, 1990.

Tan KL: Phototherapy for neonatal jaundice, *Clin Perinatol* 18:423, 1991.

Valaes T: Bilirubin metabolism: review and discussion of inborn errors, *Clin Perinatol* 3:177, 1976.

Yao TC, Stevenson DK: Advances in the diagnosis and treatment of neonatal hyperbilirubinemia. In Bifano EM, Ehrenkranz RA, editors: Perinatal hematology, *Clin Perinatol* 22:741, 1995.

Young CY et al: Phenobarbitone prophylaxis for neonatal hyperbilirubinemia, *Pediatrics* 48:372, 1971.

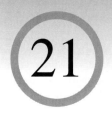

21 Infection in the Neonate

Gerald B. Merenstein, Karen Adams, Leonard E. Weisman

The newborn infant is uniquely susceptible to infectious diseases. Causes of infectious diseases with particular emphasis on prevention, history, presenting signs and symptoms, laboratory data, treatment, and parent teaching methods of prevention applicable to the care of the neonate are presented in this chapter. Abbreviations for this chapter are listed in Box 21-1.

Pathophysiology and Pathogenesis

Infections occur when a susceptible host comes in contact with a potentially pathogenic organism. When the encountered organism proliferates and overcomes the host defenses, infection results. Sources of infection in the newborn can be arbitrarily divided into three categories: (1) transplacental acquisition (intrauterine infection), (2) perinatal acquisition during labor and delivery (intrapartum infection), and (3) hospital acquisition in the neonatal period (postnatal infection) from the mother, hospital environment, or personnel.

In general, most infecting organisms can, under the proper circumstances, cross the placenta or ascend from the birth canal and invade the at risk neonate. These infections may result in abortion, stillbirth, and disease present at birth or in the neonatal period.

The main goal is to prevent infections in the fetus and newborn. Unfortunately, few proven measures exist for the prevention of transplacental or perinatal-acquired infections. These measures are important, because most nonbacterial infections (except syphilis and possibly toxoplasmosis, CMV, and herpes simplex) do not respond to current therapy.

Etiology

Thorough data collection for diagnosis of infectious diseases includes a review of the perinatal history, signs and symptoms, and laboratory data.

Intrauterine, intrapartum, or neonatal disease may be caused by a wide variety of organisms, many of which are discussed in this chapter.

Specific Infectious Diseases

The following specific infectious diseases are divided by their source of infection.

Transplacental (Intrauterine) Acquisition

Acquired Immunodeficiency Syndrome [3-6,19]

Prevention. The primary risk to infants for infection with HIV, the causative agent of acquired immunodeficiency syndrome (AIDS), is intrauterine, intrapartal, and postpartal exposure to a mother with HIV infection. HIV has been isolated from blood and many bodily fluids. Epidemiologic evidence has implicated only blood, semen, vaginal secretions, and breast milk in transmission. In countries such as the United States where safe alternatives exist, mothers with HIV infection should be discouraged from breastfeeding. HIV testing should be recommended and encouraged to all pregnant women.

Because the medical history and examination cannot reliably identify all patients infected with HIV (or other blood-borne pathogens) and because during delivery and initial care of the infant, perinatal care providers are exposed to large amounts of maternal blood, precautions (e.g., gloves) should be consistently used for *all* patients when handling the placenta or infant until all maternal blood has been washed away.

Box 21-1

Abbreviations

AIDS	Acquired immunodeficiency syndrome
CF	Complement fixation test
CIE	Counter immunoelectrophoresis
CSF	Cerebrospinal fluid
ELISA	Enzyme-linked immunosorbent assay
FA	Fluorescent antibody test
FAMA	Fluorescent antibody to membrane antigen
FTA-ABS	Fluorescent treponemal antibody absorption test
HbsAg	Hepatitis B surface antigen
HIV	Human immunodeficiency virus
IAHA	Immune adherence hemagglutination
IFA	Indirect fluorescent antibody test
IHA	Hemagglutination inhibition test
MHA-TP	Microhemagglutination test for *Treponema pallidum*
RPR	Rapid plasma reagin test
VDRL	Venereal Disease Research Laboratory test

Data Collection

History. Infection in the mother is primarily acquired sexually (bisexual partner, hemophiliac partner, prostitution, promiscuity) or via IV drug abuse. Infection may be asymptomatic. Transmission from infected mother to the fetus or infant occurs in 12.9% to 39% of births.

Signs and Symptoms. Infants with perinatally acquired HIV infection rarely have symptoms in the neonatal period, but the majority of these infants will present with clinical illness by 24 months of life. These may include failure to thrive, developmental disabilities, neurologic dysfunction, hepatosplenomegaly, generalized lymphadenopathy, parotitis, persistent oral candidiasis (thrush), and chronic or recurrent diarrhea. Lymphoid interstitial pneumonia is frequently seen in these infants. HIV-infected infants commonly have osteomyelitis, septic joints, pneumonia, sepsis, meningitis, and otitis media with common organisms (e.g., *Streptococcus pneumoniae, Haemophilus influenzae* type B), and these infections are frequently recurrent.

Laboratory Data. Although hypogammaglobinemia has been reported, hypergammaglobinemia is usually present.

The primary serologic laboratory test for HIV antibody is the enzyme-linked immunosorbent assay (ELISA). The Western blot test is used for confirmation of positive ELISA test results. Differentiation of the child with passively acquired antibody from the infant with active infection is critical but difficult. Acquired antibody is undetectable in 75% of infants by 12 months of age and in most infants by 15 to 18 months of age. Infants have also been described with negative serology but active infection. Early identification (3 to 6 months of age) may be possible using a combination of tests including viral cultures, polymerase chain reaction (PCR), and p24 antigen. It is not possible to exclude HIV unless two or more viral diagnostic tests (PCR or HIV culture) are negative at both greater than 1 month and greater than 4 months of age.

Treatment. Zidovudine (ZDV) reduces HIV transmission from infected mothers to their newborns.[23] ZDV should be given to infants of infected women immediately after birth but beginning no later than 24 hours of life and continued for 6 weeks. ZDV is administered orally at 2 mg/kg body weight/dose every 6 hours.[45] Infants who are perinatally infected with HIV are at high risk for developing *pneumocystis carinii* pneumonia (PCP) early in the first year of life. New guidelines recommend initiating prophylaxis for the prevention of PCP for all HIV-exposed infants at 4 to 6 weeks of age, regardless of their CD4+ cell count. For children on ZDV, PCP prophylaxis should begin after completion of the 6-week course of ZDV. PCP prophylaxis may be provided by 5 mg of trimethoprim (TMP) and 20 mg of sulfamethasoxazole (SMX)/kg body weight/day administered in 2 divided doses. TMP + SMX prophylaxis should be continued through the first year of life or until HIV is reasonably excluded.[35]

Parent Teaching. Care of the infant at risk for HIV requires close and long-term follow-up. Involvement of the parents is essential to this process. Education of the parents will maximize the success of such a care plan, and utilization of all available community resources should provide additional support. In addition to the rationale and importance for the medical management outlined above, the parents should be counseled concerning the need for immunizations following the American Academy of Pediatrics schedule (except IPV instead of OPV); rapid consultation with the child's physician if exposed to varicella (may need treatment with varicella zoster immune globulin [VZIG] within 96 hours of exposure) or measles (may need vaccination within 72 hours of exposure); or development of thrush, a diaper rash, or any other signs or symptoms of illness. Prevention of infections is important, and this requires good handwashing, regular bathing, appropriate food preparation skills (wash bottles, nipples, pacifiers), and good skin care (changing diapers, moisturizing skin in other areas to prevent drying and cracking).

Cytomegalovirus[12,55]

Prevention.   There are no practical methods for preventing CMV. Exposure avoidance is virtually impossible because of the ubiquitous and asymptomatic nature of the infections. Avoiding unnecessary blood transfusions or using CMV serum-negative blood donors has proved to be important in minimizing the occurrence of postnatally acquired CMV, particularly in premature infants.

The question frequently arises regarding assignment of staff to infants with the possible diagnosis of CMV. Staff members who may be pregnant have heightened concern regarding this issue. Staff members should be aware that many infants with CMV are often asymptomatic and therefore not identified while in the hospital. To avoid any problems, staff members should employ good handwashing technique with all infants. Wearing gloves when handling urine and other secretions is a strategy that can also be employed by staff members who are working in the NICU and are pregnant or attempting to become pregnant. The actual risk of an infected infant transmitting disease to a susceptible health care worker is unknown but probably small.

Data Collection

History.   Congenital infections are represented by a wide spectrum of disease from asymptomatic disease to profoundly symptomatic disease. Infection in the mother is usually asymptomatic.

Signs and Symptoms.   An infant with CMV is usually asymptomatic. Congenital manifestations include IUGR, neonatal jaundice (increased direct fraction), purpura, hepatosplenomegaly, microcephaly, seizures, intracerebral calcification, chorioretinitis, and progressive sensorineural hearing loss.

Laboratory Data.   CMV may be cultured from urine, pharyngeal secretions, and peripheral leukocytes. Isolation of the virus within 2 weeks of birth indicates transplacental acquisition. A paired sera demonstration of a fourfold titer rise or histopathologic demonstration of characteristic nuclear inclusions in certain tissues can confirm infection. Examining the urine for intranuclear inclusions is not helpful.

Treatment.   Currently, ganciclovir, forscarnet, and cidofovir are the only licensed antiviral agents effective against CMV. These drugs are only approved for treatment of life- and sight-saving disease. A multicenter controlled study is currently underway to evaluate ganciclovir in the treatment of infants with symptomatic CMV and CNS involvement.

Parent Teaching.   The need for good handwashing technique by parents and care givers of infants with suspected CMV should be included in discharge instructions.

Rubella[2,3,20]

Prevention.   Medical personnel should ensure that all mothers have a protective hemagglutination titer before conception. If the woman is susceptible, vaccinate her with rubella vaccine before conception. If a woman is found to be rubella nonimmune during pregnancy, she should receive rubella immunization in the postpartum period.

All perinatal health care workers should have rubella titers drawn to identify immunity status and should be reimmunized if this is not adequate.

Women of childbearing age who do not have immune titers should be encouraged to have rubella immunization.

Data Collection

History.   Rubella in the first 4 to 5 months of pregnancy has a high incidence of sequelae in the infant. A mother with rubella may be relatively asymptomatic or mildly ill with respiratory symptoms with or without a rash.

Signs and Symptoms.   Congenital manifestations of rubella include IUGR, sensorineural deafness, cataracts, neonatal jaundice (increased direct fraction), purpura, hepatosplenomegaly, microcephaly, chronic encephalitis, chorioretinitis, and cardiac defects (especially PDA and peripheral pulmonic stenosis). Less frequent manifestations include bone lesions and pneumonitis.

Laboratory Data.   The virus may be isolated from the throat, blood, urine, and cerebrospinal fluid (CSF). A paired sera demonstration of a fourfold titer rise such as a hemagglutination inhibition test (IHA) or a fluorescent antibody test (FA) is diagnostic.

Parent Teaching.   Infants with congenital rubella may secrete the virus for many years. This requires that discharge instructions include preventive strategies that need to be employed to decrease the chance of contact of susceptible pregnant women with the infant. Parents need to be informed of their responsibility to ensure that potentially seronegative women of childbearing age avoid direct contact with the infant. The challenge arises to impress this on the family and at the same time avoid ostracizing the infant or negatively affecting the parent-infant attachment process. In discharge planning with these families, a collaborative approach should be employed using community health, medical, nursing, and social work input and support.

Syphilis [2,3,40,56]

Prevention.   Avoid exposing the mother to syphilis. Monitor the serum early and late in pregnancy, and treat the mother for the appropriate stage of disease. Erythromycin, previously used in penicillin-sensitive women, is not considered adequate treatment during gestation because of (1) 30% treatment failure rates in adults and (2) failure to establish a cure in the newborn because of poor transplacental passage of erythromycin. Infants born to women treated with erythromycin should be considered high risk for infection and appropriately evaluated and treated.[56] If penicillin allergy is confirmed in the pregnant woman, then acute desensitization is necessary. Desensitization can be accomplished using increasing doses of oral penicillin over 4 to 6 hours.

Data Collection

History.   A congenital infection may be manifested by a multisystem disease. A primary syphilitic chancre on the cervix or rectal mucosa in a mother may be unnoticed.

Signs and Symptoms.   An infant exposed to syphilis may be asymptomatic at birth or involve virtually all organ systems. Clinical findings may include hepatitis, pneumonitis, bone marrow failure, myocarditis, meningitis, nephrotic syndrome, rhinitis (snuffles), and a rash involving the palms and soles.

Laboratory Data.   The microscopic darkfield examination identifies spirochetes from nonoral lesions. Nonspecific, nontreponemal, reaginic tests, such as Venereal Disease Research Laboratory (VDRL) tests and rapid plasma reagin (RPR) tests, followed serially with a rise or absence of fall after birth, are diagnostic. Specific treponemal antibody serologic tests such as a fluorescent treponemal antibody absorption test (FTA-ABS) and a microhemagglutination test for *Treponema pallidum* (MHA-TP) may also be diagnostic, but an FTA-ABS IgM test is unreliable. A long-bone x-ray examination showing metaphysitis or periostitis may help in diagnosing syphilis. VDRL tests on CSF are mandatory in all infants suspected of having congenital syphilis. When the diagnosis of active congenital syphilis is equivocal, it is often best to treat and ascertain the diagnosis by serial serologic determinations.

Treatment.   See Table 21-1.

Parent Teaching.   Adequate follow-up of both symptomatic and asymptomatic neonates is very important. A physical evaluation should be conducted at 1, 2, 3, 6, and 12 months. Serologic testing

Table 21-1
Recommended Therapy for Indicated Conditions

Condition	Treatment*
Sepsis and/or Meningitis	
Initial therapy	
Early-onset	IV ampicillin and gentamicin or IV amikacin (if gentamicin-resistant organisms are present in nursery, ampicillin plus cefotaxime is a suitable alternative, particularly if meningitis is present)
Late-onset	IV vancomycin plus cefotaxime or IV aminoglycoside (See Early Onset.)
Once specific organisms are identified	
Group B streptococci	IV ampicillin and gentimicin for 10-14 days (gentamicin may be discontinued if strain is not tolerant)
Coliform species	IV ampicillin and gentimicin for 10-14 days (cefotaxime may replace gentamicin)
Listeria monocytogenes	IV ampicillin and IV gentamicin for 14-21 days
Enterococci	Same as for *Listeria monocytogenes*
Group A streptococci	IV penicillin G for 10-14 days
Group D streptococci (non-enterococcal)	Same as for group A streptococci
Staphylococcus aureus	IV nafcillin for 10-14 days; IV vancomycin for methicillin-resistant strains
Staphylococcus epidermidis	IV vancomycin for 10-14 days
Pseudomonas aeruginosa	IV mezlocillin and IV gentamicin for 10-14 days
Anaerobes	IV chloramphenicol if levels can be monitored (levels should be in 20-25 µg/ml range) or IV clindamycin
Pneumonia	
Group B streptococci	Same as for sepsis (respiratory distress syndrome may mimic pneumonitis and vice versa)
Staphylococcus aureus	Same as for sepsis
Chlamydia trachomatis	PO erythromycin for 14 days
Pneumocystitis carinii	PO or IV trimethoprim and sulfamethoxazole or IV pentamidine isethionate
Pertussis	PO erythromycin for 14 days (clinical course is unchanged but shedding of organism is diminished significantly)
Other organisms	Same as for sepsis
Skin and Soft-tissue Infections	
Impetigo	IV nafcillin or PO dicloxacillin for 7 days (depending on clinical severity)
Group A streptococcal infections	IV penicillin G for 7 days
Breast abscess	IV nafcillin and gentamicin for 7 days pending identification of etiologic agent (change to IV penicillin if streptococcus is etiologic) (IV ampicillin and/or gentamicin should be used for coliform species pending sensitivities); value of surgical drainage is individualized
Omphalitis and/or funisitis	IV nafcillin for 7 days (penicillin may be used if infection is caused by group A or B streptococci)
Gastrointestinal Infections	
Salmonella species	IV ampicillin for 7-10 days, IV chloramphenicol for 7-10 days, or IV gentamicin for 7-10 days depending on sensitivities (focal complications of meningitis and arthritis should be monitored closely)

*See Table 21-6 for dosages.
Modified from Nelson JD: *Pocketbook of pediatric antimicrobial therapy,* ed 5, Dallas, 1983, Jodone Publishing.

Continued

Table 21-1
Recommended Therapy for Indicated Conditions—cont'd

Condition	Treatment*
Gastrointestinal Infections—cont'd	
Shigella species	PO trimethoprim/sulfamethoxazole or PO or IV ampicillin depending on sensitivities
Enteropathogenic *E. coli*	PO colistin, 10-15 mg/kg/day divided q8h, for 5-7 days
Necrotizing enterocolitis	IV ampicillin and IV gentamicin for 2-3 weeks (if *Pseudomonas* is isolated, IV mezlocillin may be substituted for ampicillin); supportive measures (gastrointestinal suction) are appropriate
Osteomyelitis or Septic Arthritis	
Group B streptococci	IV penicillin G for 21 days minimum
Staphylococcus aureus	IV nafcillin for 21 days minimum
Coliform species	IV gentamicin for 21 days minimum (IV ampicillin for 21 days minimum if organism is sensitive)
Gonococcus species	IV penicillin G for 10 days
Unknown	IV nafcillin and gentamicin for 21 days minimum
Urinary Tract Infections	Suspect predisposing anatomic defect if urinary tract infection; individualize workup and follow-up
Coliform species	Gentamicin, 3 mg/kg/day divided q8h, for 10 days
Enterococcus species	Ampicillin, 30 mg/kg/day divided q8h, for 10 days
Miscellaneous Conditions	
Congenital syphilis	
Without CNS involvement	IM procaine penicillin G (50,000 units/kg) daily for 10-14 days (follow-up VDRL tests should revert to negative if treatment is adequate by 1 year)
With CNS involvement	IV aqueous crystalline penicillin 100,000 to 150,000 units/kg/day divided q8-12h for 10-14 days.
Toxoplasmosis	PO sulfadiazine, 100-120 mg/kg/day divided q12h and PO pyrimethamine, 1 mg/kg/day divided q12h (duration of treatment is debatable but should be long [i.e., months], supplemental folic acid, 1 mg/day, should be added)
Herpes simplex infections	IV acyclovir, 30 mg/kg/day as 1 hr infusion divided q8h, for 10 days
Conjunctivitis	
Chlamydia species	PO erythromycin for 10 days (topical may be ineffective)
Gonococcus species	IV penicillin G for 10 days; cefoxitin for penicillin-resistant strains
Otitis media	
In otherwise normal neonate	PO amoxicillin/clavulinic acid (Augmentin), 40 mg/kg
In neonate with nosocomial infection	PO or IV ampicillin and IV gentamicin (if there is no response to treatment, consider diagnostic tympanocentesis; *S. aureus* and coliform species may be present)

*See Table 21-6 for dosages.

should be performed at 3 months, and if still reactive, at 6 and 12 months. If titers fail to decline, increase, or are still present after 12 months, the infant should be reevaluated and retreated. Infants with neurosyphilis should have repeat CSF examinations every 6 months until it is normal and VDRL nonreactive. If CSF VDRL is still reactive at 6 months or CSF is abnormal at 24 months, reevaluation and retreatment is indicated.

Toxoplasmosis[2]

Prevention.   Women should avoid unnecessary exposure to raw meat and cat feces. Using a pair of gloves when emptying the litter box may provide protection if the pregnant woman (or women attempting to become pregnant) must empty the litter box.

Data Collection

History.   Congenital infections are represented by a wide range of disease from asymptomatic disease to profound symptomatic disease. Mothers may have noted an influenza-like illness, posterior cervical adenitis, or chorioretinitis but usually lack accompanying signs or symptoms. A history of exposure to cat feces or ingestion of raw meat may occasionally be obtained.

Signs and Symptoms.   Manifestations in the newborn may be prematurity, IUGR, hydrocephalus, chorioretinitis, seizures, cerebral calcifications, hepatosplenomegaly, thrombocytopenia, jaundice, generalized lymphadenopathy, and a rash.

Laboratory Data.   Isolating *Toxoplasma gondii* from blood or body fluids is difficult and tedious. Cysts may be found in the placenta or tissues of a fetus or newborn. Most congenitally infected infants will have a Sabin-Feldman dye test titer greater than 1:1000 at birth.

Treatment.   See Table 21-1.

Perinatal Acquisition During Labor and Delivery

Chlamydia Trachomatis[3,23]

Prevention.   Eye prophylaxis with erythromycin (preferred) or tetracycline ophthalmic ointment minimizes the development of conjunctivitis but has no effect on the subsequent development of pneumonitis.

Data Collection

History.   A mother with *Chlamydia trachomatis* is usually asymptomatic during her pregnancy.

Signs and Symptoms.   Conjunctivitis may be manifested as congestion and edema of the conjunctiva with minimal discharge developing 1 to 2 weeks after birth and lasting several weeks with recurrences, particularly after topical therapy. Infants with pneumonitis usually do not have a fever but have a prolonged staccato cough, tachypnea, mild hypoxemia, and eosinophilia. Otitis media and bronchiolitis may also occur.

Laboratory Data.   Definitive diagnosis is made by isolating the organism in tissue culture. Demonstrating chlamydial antigen in clinical specimens by the direct fluorescent antibody method or enzyme immunoassay is very reliable. To enhance the likelihood of obtaining an adequate sample, it is important to scrape the lower conjuctiva (for conjunctivitis) or obtain deep tracheal secretions or a nasopharyngeal aspirate (for pneumonia). Scraping conjunctival epithelial cells and demonstrating characteristic intracytoplasmic inclusion bodies by a Giemsa stain is diagnostic. Although serologic tests for conjuctivitis are unreliable, a significant titer rise in IgM specific antibody may be reliable in cases of pneumonia. Eosinophilia (>300 to 400/mm^3), may be suggestive of pneumonia.

Enterovirus (Coxsackievirus A and B, Echovirus, and Poliomyelitis)

Prevention.   To prevent poliomyelitis, maintain poliomyelitis immunity with active immunization before conception. Passive protection with pooled human serum globulin may help in selected exposures (0.2 ml/kg body weight, given IM). Routine nursery infection control procedures must be observed. It is recommended that only inactivated polio virus (IPV) vaccine, and not oral polio virus (OPV) vaccine, be utilized in the nursery. The IPV is administered intramuscularly and contains no live virus, whereas OPV is administered orally and contains live but attenuated virus that has been reported to cause infection in immunocompromised patients.

Data Collection

History.   Infection may occur year-round but is more prevalent from June to December in temperate climates. Most *Enterovirus* infections are asymptomatic. Poliomyelitis is rare because of a high vaccine-induced immunity in the United States.

Signs and Symptoms.   Mothers with entero viral infections are usually mildly ill with fever or diarrhea. Infants may be asymptomatic or have fever or diarrhea. Fulminating encephalomyocarditis or acute hepatic necrosis may occur within several days of birth, but their occurrence is rare.

Laboratory Data. The virus may be isolated from the throat, rectum, or CSF. Isolating coxsackievirus A may require suckling mouse inoculation. Serologic screening is impractical because of the large number of serotypes.

Group B Streptococcus[13,37,57]

Prevention. Intrapartum (during labor) treatment of the mother with penicillin appears to prevent group B streptococcus (GBS) disease in the neonate and decrease maternal postpartum endometritis.[13] Neonatal sepsis has been reported with less than 4 hours of maternal antibiotics at term and with up to 48 hours in preterm infants.[57]

Data Collection. See section on bacterial infections and bacterial sepsis.

Treatment. See Table 21-1.

Hepatitis B[3,7-9,21,62]

Prevention. Prenatal screening of women for hepatitis B surface antigen (HBsAg) is indicated and cost-effective. Use of active and passive immunization in infants born of HBsAg-positive mothers is indicated (Tables 21-2 and 21-3). Use of active immunization for infants born to HBsAg-negative women is all recommended.

Data Collection

History. Mothers who are HBsAg positive because of the chronic carrier state or acute disease before delivery may pass the infection to their infants at delivery.

Women at high risk include women of Asian, Pacific Island, or Alaskan Eskimo descent; women born in Haiti or sub-Saharan Africa; or women with a history of liver disease, IV drug abuse, or frequent exposure to blood in a medical-dental setting.

Signs and Symptoms. The neonate with hepatitis B is usually asymptomatic. Occasionally, infected infants demonstrate elevated liver enzymes or acute fulminating hepatitis. Neonatal infection with subsequent chronic carriage has been implicated in the development of primary hepatocellular carcinoma later in life.

Laboratory Data. Virtually all infants at risk of acquiring hepatitis from their mother are HBsAg negative at birth. Many untreated infants become HBsAg positive 4 to 12 weeks postnatally and become lifelong asymptomatic carriers or develop hepatitis B.

Table 21-2
Acceptable Methods of Passive Immunization in Newborns

Disease	Indications for Use in Newborns	When to Use	Product*	Dose
Hepatitis A	Active infection in mother or close family contacts	As soon as possible	HISG	0.02-0.04 ml/kg body weight given intramuscularly (IM)
Hepatitis B	Mothers with acute type B infection or mothers who are antigen positive	As soon as possible (within 12 hr)	HBIG†	0.5 ml/kg body weight given IM
Tetanus	Inadequately immunized mothers with contaminated infant (e.g., dirty cord)	As soon as possible	TIG	250 units given IM (optimal dose not established)
Varicella	Infant born to a mother who develops lesions less than 5 days before delivery or within 2 days after delivery	Within 72 hr of birth	ZIG	2 ml given IM

*HSIG, Human immune serum globulin; HBIG, hepatitis B immune globulin; TIG, tetanus globulin (human); ZIG, zoster immune globulin.
†Should be used in conjunction with active immunization with HBV vaccine (Table 21-3).
Modified from Remington JS, Klein JO, editors: *Infectious diseases of the fetus and newborn infant,* ed 2, Philadelphia, 1983, WB Saunders.

Herpes Simplex (Types 1 and 2)*

Prevention. The key to preventing herpes simplex is avoiding exposure. Mothers with active lesions or prodrome should have cesarean section preferably within 4 to 6 hours of membrane rupture. Treatment with acyclovir should begin at the first sign of neonatal disease or when infants have been exposed to an active lesion.

Communication is required between obstetric and neonatal staff to determine the status of a family with a history of herpes. Unnecessary restrictions should not be placed on postpartum mothers who are not actively infected. Health professionals need to employ all family-centered strategies used in their institutions with these families unless these are precluded by the need for the infant's treatment.

Data Collection

History. Disease caused by type 1 herpes simplex is usually spread via the respiratory route, whereas disease caused by type 2 herpes simplex is usually spread via the genital route.

Many mothers who transmit herpes simplex to their newborn infants are asymptomatic. The risk to the infant from recurrent lesions is minimal.

Signs and Symptoms. Infants with herpes simplex have a spectrum of illnesses ranging from

localized skin lesions to generalized infections involving the liver, lungs, and CNS. This disseminated disease has a high morbidity and mortality.

Laboratory Data. A cytologic examination of the base of skin vesicles with a Giemsa stain (Tzanck test) may reveal characteristic but nonspecific giant cells and eosinophilic intranuclear inclusions. The virus may be readily identified on a tissue culture within 24 to 48 hours from the respiratory and genital tracts, blood, urine, and CSF. Rapid viral diagnosis by fluorescent tests is widely available. Although tests of paired serology such as complement fixation test (CF), ELISA, and neutralization are available, they are of little value in the acute clinical situation.

Treatment. See Table 21-1.

Parent Teaching. Families with herpes simplex require consistent and detailed teaching regarding prevention of transmission of herpes to the infant. Breastfeeding mothers can be reassured that they may continue to breastfeed as long as there are no lesions on their breasts. Emphasis should be placed on the need for breastfeeding mothers to check their breasts for lesions.

Parents with active herpes simplex need to employ good handwashing technique while caring for their infants. Parents with oral herpes should avoid kissing their infants while lesions are open and draining.

* References 3, 14, 15, 39, 50, 59, 61.

Table 21-3
Acceptable Methods of Active Immunization in Newborns

Disease	Indications for Use in Newborns	When to Use	Product	Dose
Hepatitis B	HBsAg-positive*	3 separate doses at birth,† 1 month, and 6 months	Recombivax Engerix-B	0.5 ml IM 0.5 ml IM
	HBsAg-negative*		Recombivax Engerix-B	0.25 ml IM 0.5 ml IM
Pertussis	To control rare outbreak in nursery	As soon as possible	Pertussis	0.25-0.5 ml administered subcutaneously
Tuberculosis	Selected infants at risk of contracting tuberculosis	As soon as possible	BCG*	0.1 ml given intradermally and divided into two sites over deltoid muscle

*HBsAg, Hepatitis B surface antigen; BCG, Calmette-Guérin bacillus.
†As soon as possible.

Listeria Monocytogenes[3,26]

Prevention. Pregnant women should avoid drinking unpasteurized milk to prevent *Listeria monocytogenes* infection.

Data Collection. See section on bacterial infections and bacterial sepsis.

Treatment. See Table 21-1.

Mycobacterium Tuberculosis[2]

Prevention. Mothers at risk for *Mycobacterium tuberculosis* infection may be identified with a tuberculin test during pregnancy. If the mother is a tuberculin converter (a positive skin test within the past 2 years), a chest x-ray examination should be obtained. If the mother has active tuberculosis, she should be treated with isoniazid and rifampin with the addition of ethambutol initially until sensitivity testing is available. Pyridoxine should always be given with isoniazid during pregnancy because of the increased requirements for this vitamin in pregnant women. If the mother does not have active tuberculosis, household contacts should be screened. If disease is identified in the mother or household contacts, the infant is at high risk for developing tuberculosis.

Separate infants of mothers with active disease from the mother until the mother is not contagious (usually negative sputum). Treat high-risk infants with isoniazid (10 mg/kg/day) or a tuberculosis vaccine (*Calmette-Guérin* bacillus) (see Table 21-3).

Data Collection

History. A strong history of maternal contact with tuberculosis favors the diagnosis. This is especially true in high-risk populations (Southeast Asian, American Indians, and families with a known cavitary disease). Mothers with HIV infection are at an increased risk for developing active tuberculosis.

Signs and Symptoms. Mothers may be relatively asymptomatic or have signs and symptoms that are generalized (fever and weight loss) or localized to the respiratory tract. A congenital infection is extremely rare. Nonspecific signs and symptoms such as failure to thrive and unexplained hypothermia or hyperthermia are the most common manifestations in the neonatal period.

Laboratory Data. Acid-fast organisms found on smears of gastric aspirates, sputum, CSF, or infected tissues strongly suggest tuberculosis in the neonate. Isolating *Mycobacterium tuberculosis* by culture is diagnostic and should be aggressively sought. The tuberculin test is usually positive (>10 mm induration) in active tuberculosis. However, a positive skin test requires 3 to 12 weeks after infection to manifest itself and is usually negative in the neonate. A chest x-ray examination also is usually negative in the neonate.

Treatment. Since congenital tuberculosis is such a rare condition, optimal therapy has not been established. However, most recommendations suggest four-drug therapy (isoniazid, rifampin, pyrazinamide, plus either ethambutol or streptomycin).

Parent Teaching. Infants who are treated with isoniazid or breastfed infants whose mothers are treated with isoniazid should receive pyridoxine supplementation.

Neisseria Gonorrhea

Prevention. Screening high-risk mothers before delivery may identify asymptomatic gonorrhea. Treating positive mothers before delivery or exposed infants at delivery is necessary.

Administering silver nitrate, erythromycin, or tetracycline in the eyes is mandatory in all vaginal deliveries.

Data Collection

History. Mothers with previous venereal disease are a high-risk group, because 80% of the infected women may be asymptomatic.

Signs and Symptoms. The predominant manifestation of gonorrhea is ophthalmia neonatorum, although a systemic, blood-borne infection may rarely occur involving the joints, lungs, endocardium, and CNS. Conjunctivitis usually begins 2 to 5 days after birth. Eye prophylaxis minimizes but does not guarantee freedom from infection. Scalp abscess resulting from fetal monitoring has been reported.

Laboratory Data. A gram stain of purulent eye discharge revealing gram-negative intracellular diplococci is diagnostic. Culture confirmation using fermentation or fluorescence establishes the diagnosis of gonorrhea. The organism is labile, so cultures should be taken to the laboratory and plated immediately. When gonorrhea is diagnosed, other sexually transmitted diseases may be present concomitantly (especially chlamydia).

Treatment.   See Table 21-1.

Varicella[3]

Prevention.   See Table 21-2.

Data Collection
History.   The history of varicella in the mother before conception virtually excludes the diagnosis. Varicella presents in the mother with a fever, respiratory symptoms, and characteristic vesicular rash primarily on the trunk. If this occurs within 5 days of delivery, it threatens a newborn. Preventive measures should be instituted as soon as possible. Acute perinatal varicella is frequently a devastating systemic disease. Nosocomially acquired transmission of varicella is a potentially significant problem for high-risk infants: premature infants born to susceptible mothers, infants who are severely premature regardless of maternal status, and immunocompromised patients of all ages (Table 21-4).

Signs and Symptoms.   Congenital varicella is rare but has followed maternal varicella in the first trimester of pregnancy. Congenital manifestations include limb atrophy, skin scars, and CNS and eye abnormalities.

Laboratory Data.   The demonstration of multinucleated giant cells containing intranuclear inclusions in skin scrapings on Giemsa stain is non-specific but helpful. Isolating the virus from the skin lesions or respiratory tract is difficult. A number of serologic tests such as the fluorescent antibody to membrane antigen test (FAMA), immune adherence hemagglutination test (IAHA), ELISA, and neutralization test are available but are not helpful in the acute clinical situation. Complement fixation (CF) serologic tests are relatively insensitive.

Early-Onset Bacterial Disease[31,32,46,52,60]

Prevention.   For GBS only see page 420.

Data Collection
History.   Early-onset disease is almost always acquired perinatally and is discussed here. Late-onset disease is discussed in the section on postnatally acquired disease. Early-onset disease presents as a fulminate multisystem illness during the first days of life. Many of these infants are premature and have a history of one or more significant obstetric complications, including premature rupture of maternal membranes, premature onset of labor, chorioamnionitis, or peripartum maternal fever, prolonged membrane rupture (>18 hours), maternal genitourinary tract infection, fetal distress, or aspiration by the neonate.[31] Bacteria responsible for early-onset disease are acquired from the birth canal before or during delivery and are shown in Box 21-2. Early-onset bacterial disease has a high mortality.

Signs and Symptoms.   Neonatal bacterial sepsis is characterized by systemic signs of infection associated with bacteremia. Meningitis in the neonate can be a sequelae of bacteremia. In addition, blood-borne bacteria may localize in other tissues, causing focal disease. Both patterns of bacterial disease, early-and late-onset, have been associated with systemic infections during the neonatal period.

In general, signs, particularly of early-onset disease, are nonspecific and nonlocalizing. Symptoms include temperature instability (hypothermia and/or hyperthermia), respiratory distress (apnea, cyanosis, and tachypnea), lethargy, feeding abnormalities (vomiting, increased residuals, and abdominal distention), jaundice (particularly increased direct fraction), seizures, or purpura (Fig. 21-1).

Laboratory Data.   Isolating bacteria from a nonpermissive site (blood, CSF, urine, closed body space) is the most valid method of establishing the diagnosis of bacterial sepsis. Surface cultures (including ear and gastric aspirates) do not establish the presence of active systemic infection but merely indicate colonization. Bacterial antigens or endotoxins may be demonstrated in sera, CSF, urine, or body fluids by a variety of methods (counter immunoelectrophoresis [CIE], latex agglutination [LA], and limulus lysate test). Such a demonstration is not totally definitive, nor does it allow the determination of the antibiotic sensitivity of the offending organism. False-positive reactions may be caused by skin surface contamination or gastrointestinal absorption of antigen.[9] The CSF is examined in most infants suspected of sepsis,

Table 21-4
Infection Control Measures and Isolation Techniques for Specific Diseases

Disease/Organism	Recommended Precautions					Infective Material	Duration of Isolation/ Precaution	Comments
	Hand Washing	Private Room or Cohort	Mask	Gown	Gloves			
AIDS/HIV	X	D	No	(X)	(X)	Blood and body fluids	Duration of illness	Utmost care needed to avoid needle sticks
Adenovirus	X	X	No	(X)	No	Respiratory secretions and feces	Duration of hospitalization	During outbreaks cohort patients suspected of having adenovirus infection
Conjunctivitis Gonococcal (Ophthalmia neonatorum)	X	X	No	No	(X)	Purulent exudate	Until 24 hours after initiation of effective therapy	
Chlamydia	X	No	No	No	(X)	Purulent exudate	Duration of illness	
Coxsackievirus	X	D	No	(X)	(X)	Feces and respiratory secretions	7 days after onset	
Cytomegalovirus	X	No	No	No	(X)	Urine and respiratory secretions		Counsel pregnant personnel
Diarrhea	X	D	No	(X)	(X)	Feces	Duration of illness	Identify colonized or infected infants by culture; institute cohorting
Echovirus	X	D	No	(X)	(X)	Feces and respiratory secretions	For 7 days after onset of illness	
Gastroenteritis	X	X	No	(X)	(X)	Feces	Duration of illness	
Hepatitis Type A	X	D	No	(X)	(X)	Feces	For 7 days after onset of illness	Most contagious before symptoms
Type B	X	No	No	(X)	(X)	Blood and body fluids	Duration of positivity	Avoid needle sticks

Infection						Infective material	Duration of precautions	Comments
Herpes simplex	X	X	No	(X)	(X)	Lesions, secretions, urine, and stool	Duration of illness	
Influenza A or B	X	X	No	(X)	(X)	Respiratory secretions	Duration of illness	Cohort patients suspected of having influenza during outbreak; staff should receive yearly influenza vaccine
Meningitis								
Aseptic	X	D	No	(X)	(X)	Feces	Duration of illness	Cohort colonized or infected infants during a nursery outbreak
Bacterial	X	No	No	No	No			
Necrotizing enterocolitis	X	No	No	(X)	(X)	(?) Feces	Duration of illness	Cohort ill infants
Respiratory syncytial virus	X	X	X	(X)	(X)	Respiratory secretions	Duration of illness	Cohort suspect infants, especially premature infants, during outbreaks
Rubella	X	X	X	No	No	Respiratory secretions	Duration of hospitalization	Infants may shed virus for as long as 2 years; seronegative women should avoid contact

X, Recommended at all times; (X), recommended if soiling is likely, or if touching infective materials; D, desirable but optional.

Continued

Table 21-4
Infection Control Measures and Isolation Techniques for Specific Diseases—cont'd

Disease/Organism	Recommended Precautions					Infective Material	Duration of Isolation/ Precaution	Comments
	Hand Washing	Private Room or Cohort	Mask	Gown	Gloves			
Staphylococcal disease (S. aureus)	X	D	No	(X)	(X)	Purulent exudate	Duration of illness	
Streptococcal disease Group A	X	D	No	(X)	(X)	Respiratory secretions	24 hours after initiation of effective therapy	
Group B	X	D	No	(X)	(X)	Respiratory and genital secretions		Cohort ill and colonized infants during a nursery outbreak
Syphilis	X	No	No	No	(X)	Lesion secretions and blood	24 hours after start of effective therapy	
Toxoplasmosis	X	No	No	No	No		None	
Varicella	X	X	X	X	X	Respiratory and lesion secretions	Until lesions are crusted	Neonates born to mothers with active chickenpox should be placed on isolation precautions at birth; persons who are not susceptible do not need to mask
Vancomycin-resistant organisms	X	X	No	X	X	Secretions	Duration of illness	

because meningitis is a frequent manifestation of sepsis in the neonate, especially in symptomatic infants, and infants with GBS sepsis and with late-onset disease[53,57] (Table 21-5). It has been suggested that, because of the low yield and potential adverse effects from lumbar puncture, examination of CSF be deferred in asymptomatic infants being evaluated for maternal risk factors or respiratory distress.[27,53,58] The CSF is examined in most infants suspected of sepsis, because meningitis is difficult to exclude without a lumbar puncture and its diagnosis affects therapy and follow-up in the neonate.

Several laboratory aids are used in assessing neonatal sepsis, but it must be realized that these tests are nonspecific and occasionally may be misleading.[22] They include the CBC, band neutrophil ratio, and platelet count, all of which may be associated with bacterial sepsis[24,40] (Figs. 21-2 to 21-5). The usefulness of these tests is improved if a second CBC is obtained in 12 to 24 hours.[32] Acute phase reactants, including C-reactive protein, fibrinogen, haptoglobin, and erythrocyte sedimentation rates, are occasionally useful adjunctive tests clinically, and chest x-ray examination and x-ray evaluation of specific indicated areas may also help. Several other nonspecific laboratory abnormalities may accompany neonatal sepsis, including hyperglycemia, hypoglycemia, and unexplained metabolic acidosis.

Treatment. Antibiotics are the cornerstone of the treatment for presumed or confirmed infections in neonates. The indiscriminate or inappropriate use of systemic antibiotics may cause undesirable side effects, favor the emergence of resistant strains of bacteria, and alter the normal flora of the newborn. Adequate and appropriate specimens for culture should be obtained before antibiotic therapy is initiated. Broad-spectrum antibiotic coverage, usually with ampicillin and an aminoglycoside for early-onset sepsis, is commonly initiated pending culture and sensitivity results. Once causative organisms are identified and antibiotic sensitivities established, the most appropriate and least toxic antibiotic or antibiotic combination should be continued for an appropriate period by a suitable route. If adequate cultures are negative after a reasonable period

---

Box 21-2

Organisms Causing Early-Onset Bacterial Sepsis

Common Organisms

Group B streptococcus
Escherichia coli
Haemophilus influenzae (type B and nontypable)
Coagulase-negative staphylococcus

Unusual Organisms

Staphylococcus aureus
Neisseria meningitidis
Streptococcus pneumoniae
Listeria monocytogenes

Rare Organisms

Klebsiella pneumoniae
Pseudomonas aeruginosa
Enterobacter species
Serratia marcescens
Group A streptococcus
Anaerobic species

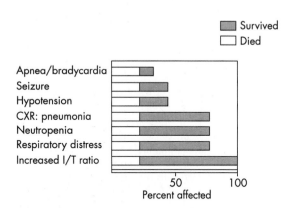

Figure 21-1 Clinical and laboratory findings in nine infants with signs and symptoms of early-onset group B streptococcal disease. (From Nelson SN, Merenstein GB, Pierce JR: *J Perinatol* 6:234, 1986.)

(48 to 72 hours), antibiotic therapy may be discontinued in most situations. It is important to realize that antibiotics are not the entire solution to treating the infected newborn. Meticulous attention to the treatment of associated conditions,

Table 21-5
Normal Cerebrospinal Fluid Values in Neonates

	White Blood Cells	Polymorphonuclear Neutrophilic (Leukocytes)	Protein (mg/dl)	Glucose (mg/dl)
Premature Infants				
Reported means	2-27		75-150	79-83
Reported ranges	0-112		31-292	64-106
Term Infants				
Reported means	3-5	2-3	47-67	51-55
Reported ranges	0-90	0-70	17-240	32-78

Modified from Remington JS, Klein JO, editors: *Infectious diseases of the fetus and newborn infant,* ed 2, Philadelphia, 1983, WB Saunders.

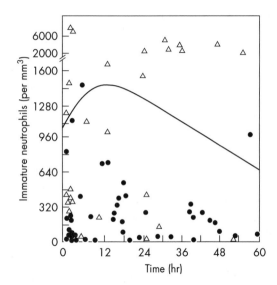

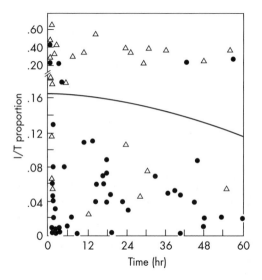

Figure 21-2   Total immature neutrophil counts during first 60 hours of life in infants with sepsis (△) and those delivered of women with pregnancy-induced hypertension (•). (From Engle WD, Rosenfeld CR: *J Pediatr* 105: 982, 1984.)

Figure 21-3   Immature-to-total neutrophil proportion during first 60 hours of life in infants with sepsis (△) and those delivered of women with pregnancy-induced hypertension (•). (From Engle WD, Rosenfeld CR: *J Pediatr* 105:982, 1984.)

such as shock, hypoxemia, thermal abnormalitites, electrolyte or acid-base imbalance, adequate nutrition, anemia, drainage of pus, and removal of foreign bodies, may be as important as choosing the proper antibiotic. Further investigation is required before newer adjunctive therapies such as IV immunoglobin and cytokin can be recommended. Table 21-1 provides guidelines for choosing the proper antibiotic for indicated conditions;

Table 21-6 gives the proper dose, route, and frequency of administration of commonly used antibiotics in the newborn nursery. Table 21-7 describes the passage of antibiotics across the placenta, and Table 21-8 describes their passage into breast milk.

Parent Teaching.   Transplacental infection often results in fetal abnormality and/or death. New-

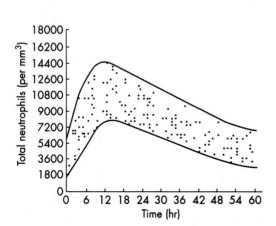

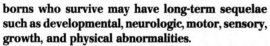

Figure 21-4 Total neutrophil count reference range in first 60 hours of life. *Heavy line* represents envelope bounding these data. (From Manroe BL, Weinberg AG, Rosenfeld CR: *J Pediatr* 95:89, 1979.)

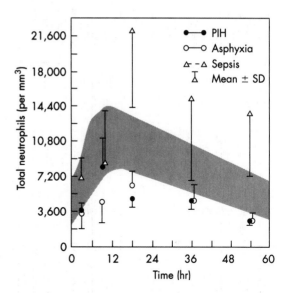

Figure 21-5 Distribution of absolute total neutrophil counts in first 60 hours of life in infants with sepsis (n = 13), asphyxia neonatorum (n = 12), and those delivered of women with pregnancy-induced hypertension (PIH) (n = 20). (From Engle WD, Rosenfeld CR: *J Pediatr* 105:982, 1984.)

borns who survive may have long-term sequelae such as developmental, neurologic, motor, sensory, growth, and physical abnormalities.

Before antibiotic use, the mortality from bacterial sepsis was 95% to 100%, but antibiotics and supportive care have reduced the mortality to less than 50%. Debilitated infants (preterm and sick neonates) are at greater risk and have a higher incidence of morbidity and mortality than term healthy neonates. The most common complications of bacterial sepsis are meningitis and septic shock. The outcome is influenced by early recognition and vigorous treatment with appropriate antibiotics and supportive care.

Postnatal Acquisition Late-Onset Bacterial Disease[11,28,37,42,48,54,56]

Prevention. The Centers for Disease Control (CDC) defines all neonatal infections acquired intrapartum or during hospitalization as nosocomial. Infants requiring the specialized care of NICUs are highly susceptible to infections. Prematurity, stress, immature immune systems, and complicated medical and surgical problems con-

tribute to their increased susceptibility. In addition, most infants in the NICU require a variety of invasive diagnostic, therapeutic, and monitoring procedures; many of these procedures bypass natural physical barriers that may allow colonization to occur and a nosocomial (late-onset) infection to develop.

Infection control principles and practices for the prevention of these nosocomial infections are outlined in Table 21-9.[2,3,16,29,38] Table 21-4 outlines infection control measures and isolation techniques for specific diseases.[2,18,30]

Data Collection

History. Late-onset disease may occur as early as 5 days of age but is more common after the first week of life. These infants may have a history of obstetric complications, but they are less common than obstetric complications in early-onset disease. Bacteria responsible for late-onset sepsis and meningitis include those acquired from the maternal genital tract and organisms acquired after birth from human contact or from contaminated equipment or material (Box 21-3, p. 434).

Table 21-6
Antibiotic Dosages for Neonates

Antibiotic	Route	Daily Dosage and Intervals	
		<7 Days of Age	>7 Days of Age
Amikacin sulfate	IV, IM	15 mg/kg/day divided q12h	15-20 mg/kg/day divided q8-12h
Amoxicillin	PO	50 mg/kg/day divided q12h	50 mg/kg/day divided q8h
Amoxicillin/clavulinic acid	PO	Not recommended	40 mg/kg/day divided q8h
Amphotericin B*	IV	0.1 mg/kg over 6 hr infusion initially, increase to 1 mg/kg/day in small increments	Same
Ampicillin			
Meningitis	IV	100 mg/kg/day divided q12h	150-200 mg/kg/day divided q6-8h
Other indications	IV, IM, PO	50 mg/kg/day divided q12h	75 mg/kg/day divided q8h
Carbenicillin	IV, IM	200 mg/kg/day divided q12h	300-400 mg/kg/day divided q6-8h
Cefazolin*	IV, IM	40 mg/kg/day divided q12h	40 mg/kg/day divided q12h
Cefotaxime	IV, IM	100 mg/kg/day divided q12h	150 mg/kg/day divided q8h
Cefoxitin	IV	15 mg/kg/day divided q8h	30 mg/kg/day divided q6h
Chloramphenicol succinate (not recommended unless serum concentrations are monitored)	IV, PO	25 mg/kg once daily	25-50 mg/kg/day divided q12-24h
Clindamycin*	IV, PO	25 mg/kg/day divided q8h	25-40 mg/kg/day divided q6h
Colistin	PO	4 mg/kg divided q6h	Same
Dicloxacillin*	PO	25 mg/kg twice daily	25 mg/kg divided q8h
Erythromycin estolate	PO	20 mg/kg/day divided q12h	20-30 mg/kg/day divided q8-12h
Gentamicin	IV, IM	5 mg/kg/day divided q12h	7.5 mg/kg/day divided q8h
Kanamycin	IV, IM	15-20 mg/kg/day divided q12h	20-30 mg/kg/day divided q8-12h
Methicillin	IV, IM	50-75 mg/kg/day divided q8-12h	100-150 mg/kg/day divided q6-8h
Metronidazole	IV, PO	15 mg/kg loading dose; then 15 mg/kg/day divided q12h	Same
Moxalactam	IV, IM	100 mg/kg/day divided q12h	150 mg/kg/day divided q8h
Nafcillin	IV	40 mg/kg/day divided q12h	60-80 mg/kg/day divided q6-8h
Neomycin	PO	25 mg/kg divided q6h	Same
Nystatin	PO	400,000 units/day divided q6h	Same
Mezlocillin	IVM, IM	150-225 mg/kg/day divided q8-12h	225-300 mg/kg/day divided q6-8h
Penicillin G			
Meningitis	IV	100,000-150,000 units/kg/day divided q8-12h	150,000-250,000 units/kg/day divided q6-8h
Other indications	IV	50,000 units/kg/day divided q12h	75,000 units/kg/day divided q6-8h
Penicillin G, benzathine	IM	50,000 units/kg (1 dose only)	Same
Penicillin G, procaine	IM	50,000 units/kg/day once daily	Same
Pentamidine isethionate*	IV	4 mg/kg/day for 14 days (Available from CDC, Atlanta, Ga)	Same
Ticarcillin	IV, IM	150-225 mg/kg/day divided q8-12h	225-300 mg/kg/day divided q6-8h
Tobramycin	IV, IM	4 mg/kg/day divided q12h	6 mg/kg/day divided q8h
Trimethorpim/sulfamethoxazole (TMP/SMX)	IV, PO	10-20 mg/kg/day TMP or 50-100 kg/day SMX	Same
Vancomycin	IV	30 mg/kg/day divided q12h	45 mg/kg/day divided q8h

*Pharmacokinetics in newborns are not well characterized. These drugs should be used with extra caution in neonates (pediatric infectious disease consultation recommended).

Although prematurity remains the most significant factor, invasive procedures performed on the neonate, such as intubation, catheterization, and surgery, also increase the risk for bacterial infection.

Signs and Symptoms.   Similar to early-onset sepsis, they are nonspecific (see page 423).

Laboratory Data.   A complete set of cultures should be obtained but have similar limitations as in early-onset infection.

Treatment.   Broad-spectrum antibiotic coverage, usually vancomycin and an aminoglycoside or a third generation cephalosporin, is commonly initiated pending culture and sensitivity results (see pages 427 to 428). Vancomycin resistance is, however, emerging as a potential problem in the care of sick neonates.[51] To minimize the development of these resistant organisms, the CDC has recommended prudent vancomycin use, education of medical personnel about the problem of vancomycin resistance, early detection and prompt reporting of organisms, and immediate implementation of appropriate infection control measures (see Table 21-4).

Fungal Infection[10,11,43,48]

Fungal infections in neonates can cause significant morbidity and mortality. They are usually seen in VLBW infants, infants with congenital anomalies requiring surgery, and/or infants who require multiple or prolonged vascular catheters.

Prevention.   Because these infants are often colonized at birth, strict adherence to aseptic technique when dealing with central catheters is essential. Antibiotic use should be minimized and limited to treatment of specific illnesses.

Data Collection

History.   VLBW infants, infants requiring surgery, and/or infants requiring invasive procedures such as arterial or venous catheters are at increased risk for fungal infection. The use of lipids increases the risk for infection with lipophilic organisms.

Signs and Symptoms.   These may be nonspecific, nonlocalizing, and difficult to differentiate from infants with bacterial sepsis.

Table 21-7
Passage of Antibiotics Across the Placenta*

% Antibiotic in Indicated Category	Antibiotic
Equal to serum concentration	Amoxicillin
	Ampicillin
	Carbenicillin
	Chloramphenicol
	Methicillin
	Nitrofurantoin
	Penicillin G
	Sulfonamides
	Tetracyclines
	Trimethoprim
50% of serum concentration	Aminoglycosides
10%-15% of serum concentration	Amikacin
	Cephalosporins
	Clindamycin
	Nafcillin
	Tobramycin
Negligible (less than 10% of serum concentration)	Dicloxacillin
	Erythromycin

*Several factors determine the degree of transfer of antibiotics across the placenta, including lipid solubility, degree of ionization, molecular weight, protein binding, placental maturation, and placental and fetal blood flow.

Table 21-8
Passage of Antibiotics into Breast Milk*

% Antibiotic in Indicated Category	Antibiotic
Equal to serum concentration	Isoniazid
	Metronidazole
	Sulfonamides
	Trimethoprim
50% of serum concentration	Chloramphenicol
	Erythromycin
	Tetracyclines
Less than 25% of serum concentration	Cefazolin
	Kanamycin
	Nitrofurantoin
	Oxacillin
	Penicillin G
	Penicillin V

*Data on concentrations of antibiotics in human breast milk are sparse. Because most antibiotics are present in breast milk in microgram amounts, they are normally not ingested by the infant in therapeutic amounts.

Table 21-9

Infection Control Principles and Practices to Prevent Nosocomial Infection

Principle	Practice
Hand Washing	
Hand washing is the most important procedure for controlling infection in the NICU.	1. Before each shift, wash hands, wrists, forearms, and elbows with an antiseptic. Scrub hands with a brush or pad for 2-3 minutes and rinse thoroughly. Chlorhexidine, hexachlorophene, and iodophors are the preferred products.
	2. Wash hands for 10-15 seconds between infant contacts. Soap and water are adequate unless the infant is infected or contaminated objects have been handled.
	3. Use an antiseptic for hand washing before surgical or similar invasive procedures.
Patient Placement	
Overcrowding in the NICU increases risk of cross-contamination.	1. Provide 4-6 feet intervals between infants.
Skin and Cord Care	
The skin, its secretions, and normal flora are natural defense mechanisms that protect against invading pathogens. Manipulating an infant's skin must be minimized.	1. The American Academy of Pediatrics suggests using a dry technique: a. Delay initial cleansing until temperature is stable. b. Use sterile cotton sponges and sterile water or a mild soap to remove blood from face and head and meconium from perineal area. c. *Do not* touch other areas unless grossly soiled.
No single method of cord care has proved to prevent colonization or limit disease.	2. Local application of alcohol, triple dye, and various antimicrobial agents is currently used.
Medical Devices	
Medical devices facilitate infections by the following: 1. Bypassing normal defense mechanisms, providing direct access to blood and deep tissues 2. Supporting growth of microorganisms and becoming reservoirs from which bacteria can be transmitted with the device to another patient 3. Providing a "protected site" when placed in deeper tissue, so phagocytosis or defense mechanisms cannot eradiate the organisms 4. Using sterile medical devices that are occasionally contaminated from the manufacturer or central supply	1. IV infusion devices predispose infants to phlebitis and bacteremia. Preventive measures include preparing the site with tincture of iodine (2% iodine in 70% alcohol), an iodophor, or 70% alcohol; anchoring the IV securely; performing site assessment and care every 24 hr (routine site care is not necessary with polyurethane dressings); rotating the IV site every 48-72 hr; changing the IV tubing every 24-48 hr on regular IVs; and discontinuing the IV at the first sign of complication. 2. Arterial lines predispose infants to bacteremia. Preventive measures include aseptically inserting the catheter using gloves, inspecting the site and performing site care every 24 hr, treating the catheter and stopcocks as sterile fields, and minimizing manipulation by drawing all blood specimens at the same time. 3. Intravascular pressure—monitoring systems predispose infants to septicemia. Preventive measures include replacing the flush solution every 24 hr, replacing the chamber dome, and replacing the tubing and continuous flow device (if used) at 48 hr intervals and between each patient. 4. Respiratory therapy devices increase the risk of contamination. Preventive measures include using aseptic technique during suctioning; dating opened solution for irrigation, humidification, and nebulization, and discarding after 24 hr; ensuring routine replacement and cleaning of all respiratory equipment, including Ambu bags, cascade nebulizers, endotracheal tube adaptors and tubing; and checking sputum cultures and gram stains every several days to assess the degree of colonization or infection in the intubated patient.

Table 21-9
Infection Control Principles and Practices to Prevent Nosocomial Infection—cont'd

Principle	Practice
Specimen Collection Improperly collected specimens cause infection at the site of collection or erroneous diagnosis leading to the administration of the wrong antibiotic or delayed administration of the appropriate antibiotic.	1. Wash hands before collecting specimen. 2. Observe aseptic technique to reduce risk of infection and to avoid contamination of specimen. 3. Deliver specimens to the laboratory immediately. 4. *Do not use femoral sticks.*
Nursery Attire Personal clothing and unscrubbed skin area of personnel should not touch infants.	1. Short-sleeved scrub gowns accommodate washing to elbows. 2. Long-sleeved gowns should be worn and changed between handling of infected or potentially infected infants. 3. Sterile gowns are necessary for sterile procedures.

Employee Health
Transmission of disease among patients and employees can occur bidirectionally. Each NICU must establish reasonable guidelines for restriction of assignments based on the employee's potential to transmit disease and the potential risk of acquiring disease.
	1. Conditions that commonly restrict personnel from patient care in the NICU are skin lesions and draining wounds, acute respiratory infections, fever, gastroenteritis, active herpes simplex (oral, genital, or paronychial), and herpes zoster.
	2. Conditions that are transmitted from infants to personnel are
	  a. Rubella—Obtain rubella titers from women of childbearing age; if a protective level is not present, they should be vaccinated.
	  b. Cytomegalovirus—CMV is a potential threat to pregnant women. Adherence to good infection control practices may reduce this threat.
	  c. Hepatitis B is usually not a major problem in the NICU, because host infants are not infectious in the early neonatal period. An effective vaccine is available and may be considered for high-risk individuals (see Tables 21-2 and 21-3).
	  d. Use of gloves with body fluid contact will decrease the risk of transmission of HBV and HIV.

Cohorting Cohorting is an important infection control measure used primarily during outbreaks or epidemics in the NICU. The object of cohorting is to limit the number of contacts of one infant with other infants and personnel.	1. Group together infants born within the same time frame (usually 24-48 hr) or who are colonized or infected with the same pathogen. These infants should remain together until discharged. 2. Provide nursing care by personnel who do not care for other infants. 3. After all infants in cohort are discharged, clean room before admittance of a new group of infants.

Laboratory Data. Routine laboratory data, such as clinical signs and symptoms, are rarely helpful in differentiating fungal from bacterial infection. Positive cultures from urine or blood indicate systemic infection. Tracheal cultures may be helpful in infants with acquired pneumonia. Urine and buffy coat smear of blood from central catheters should be examined for evidence of budding yeast.

Treatment. The treatment of fungal infection will vary from infant to infant. Very few infants will

Table 21-10
Antifungal Therapy

Drug	Dosage	Comments
Amphotericin B	0.1 to 1 mg/kg/day IV; begin at 0.1 mg/kg and increase daily as tolerated	Nephrotoxic
5-Fluorocytosine (5-FC)	50 to 100 mg/kg/day PO, q6h	Hepatotoxic; bone marrow suppression

Box 21-3

Organisms Causing Late-Onset Sepsis

Coagulase-negative staphylococcus
Escherichia coli
Klebsiella species
Enterobacter species
Candida species
Malassezzia furfur
Other enteric organisms
Group B streptococcus
Methicillin-resistant *Staphylococcus aureus*

respond to simple interventions such as stopping broad-spectrum antibiotics, stopping lipid infusions, or removing central catheters. Almost all will require treatment with antifungal agents such as amphotericin B and/or 5 fluorocytosine (5-FC) (Table 21-10).

Parent Teaching

Parents who have infants with viral or bacterial infection require support and information regarding their infant's condition. Questions arise regarding treatment and prognosis, as well as possible long-range effects of the infection. Parents experience significant guilt feelings based on misperceptions regarding what role they had in causing the infection. Health care professionals need to remain sensitive to the crisis that parents are experiencing and address the issues of etiology as well as treatment and prognosis. Valid and factual data as well as information regarding complications and

long-term effects should be shared with parents in a timely manner.

Controlling infection in the nursery is of prime importance but does not include excluding the parents from caring for their sick infant. Everyone must adhere to proper hand washing, gowning, and isolation techniques. Educating the parents and siblings about the importance of these procedures, along with appropriate reminders, ensures cooperation. With proper precautions, there is no evidence of increased incidence of infection with parent and sibling visits.

All those entering the nursery must be screened for the presence of illness. Anyone with a fever, respiratory symptoms (cough, runny nose, sore throat), gastrointestinal symptoms (nausea, vomiting, diarrhea), or skin lesions should not come in contact with the infant. People with communicable disease (e.g., varicella) or recent exposure to a communicable disease also should not come in contact with the sick neonate.

Daily cord care should be demonstrated, and a return demonstration by the parents should be observed before discharging the infant. Every parent should be taught the signs and symptoms of neonatal illness, because early recognition of signs and symptoms expedites prompt treatment. Parents must be taught to take axillary temperatures and to read a thermometer. They need to be aware that both hypothermia and hyperthermia may be signs of neonatal illness.

References

1. Abzug MJ et al: Evolution of the placental barrier to fetal infection by murine enterovirus, *J Infect Dis* 163:1336, 1991.
2. American Academy of Pediatrics: *Report of the committee on infectious disease,* ed 23, Oak Grove Village, III, 1994, American Academy of Pediatrics.

3. American Academy of Pediatrics and American College of Obstetricians and Gynecologists: *Guidelines for perinatal care,* ed 3, Oak Grove Village, Ill, 1992, American Academy of Pediatrics.

4. American Academy of Pediatrics Task Force on Pediatric AIDS: Perinatal HIV infection (AIDS), *Pediatrics* 82:941, 1988.

5. American Academy of Pediatrics Task Force on Pediatric AIDS: Pediatric guidelines for infection control of HIV (AIDS virus) in hospitals, medical offices, schools and other settings, *Pediatrics* 82:801, 1988.

6. American Academy of Pediatrics Task Force on Pediatric AIDS: Perinatal human immunodeficiency virus (HIV) testing, *Pediatrics* 95:303, 1995.

7. American Academy of Pediatrics Committee on Infectious Disease: Universal hepatitis B immunization, *Pediatrics* 89:795, 1992.

8. Arevalo JA, Washington AE: Cost-effectiveness of prenatal screening and immunization for hepatitis B virus, *JAMA* 259:365, 1988.

9. Ascher DP et al: Group B streptococcal latex agglutination testing in the neonate, *J Pediatr* 119:458, 1991.

10. Ascuitto RJ et al: Buffy coat smears of blood drawn through central venous catheters as an aid to rapid diagnosis of systemic fungal infection, *J Pediatr* 106:445, 1985.

11. Bailey JE: Neonatal candidiasis: the current challenge, *Clin Perinatol* 18:303, 1991.

12. Boppanna SB et al: Symptomatic congenital cytomegalovirus infection: neonatal morbidity and mortality, *Pediatr Infect Dis J* 11:93, 1992.

13. Boyer SM, Gotoff SP: Prevention of early-onset group B stretococcal disease with selected intrapartum chemoprophylaxis, *N Engl J Med* 31:16655, 1986.

14. Brown ZA et al: Effects on infants of a first episode of genital herpes during pregnancy, *N Engl J Med* 317:1246, 1987.

15. Brown ZA et al: Neonatal herpes simplex virus infection in relation to asymptomatic maternal infection at the time of labor, *N Engl J Med* 324:1247, 1991.

16. Burch SM, Chadwick JV: Use of a retroset in the delivery of intravenous medications in the neonate, *Neonat Ne* 6:51, 1987.

17. Cairo MS: Cytokines: a new immunotherapy, *Clin Perinatol* 18:343, 1991.

18. Centers for Disease Control: *Guidelines of isolation precautions,* ed 4, Washington DC, 1983, US Government Printing Office.

19. Centers for Disease Control: Guidelines for prevention of transmission of human immunodeficiency virus and hepatitis B virus to health care and public safety workers, *MMWR* 38(S-6):1-37, 1989.

20. Centers for Disease Control: Increase in rubella and congential rubella syndrome—United States 1988-90, *MMWR* 40:93, 1991.

21. Centers for Disease Control: Hepatitis B virus, a comprehensive strategy for eliminating transmission in the United States through universal childhood vaccination, *MMWR* 40(RR-13):1-25, 1991.

22. Christensen RD et al: Fatal early onset group B streptococcal sepsis with normal leukocyte counts, *Pediatr Infect Dis J* 4:242, 1985.

23. Connor EM et al: Reduction of maternal-infant transmission of HIV-1 with zidovudine treatment, *N Engl J Med* 331:1173, 1994.

24. Cromblehome W: Neonatal chlamydial infections, *Contemp Ob-Gyn* p. 57, 1991.

25. Engle WD, Rosenfeld CR: Neutropenia in high risk neonates, *J Pediatr* 105:982, 1984.

26. Enocksson E et al: Listeriosis during pregnancy and in neonates, *Scand J Infect Dis* 71(suppl):89, 1990.

27. Fielkow S, Reuter S, Gotoff SP: Cerebrospinal fluid examination in symptom free infants with risk factors for infection, *J Pediatr* 119:971, 1991.

28. Freeman J et al: Birth weight and length of stay as determinants of nosocomial coagulase negative Staphylococcal bacteremia in neonatal intensive care unit populations: potential for confounding, *Am J Epidemiol* 132:1130, 1991.

29. Fryklund B, Tullu K, Burman LG: Epidemiology of enteric bacteria in neonatal units—influence of procedures and patient variables, *J Hosp Infect* 18:15, 1991.

30. Garner JS, Simmons BP: Guidelines for isolation precautions in hospitals, *Infect Control* 4(suppl):245, 1983.

31. Gerdes JS: Clinicopathologic approach to the diagnosis of sepsis, *Clin Perinatol* 18:361, 1991.

32. Gibbs R, Duff P: Progress in pathogenesis and management of clinical intraamniotic infection, *Am J Obstet Gynecol* 164:1317, 1991.

33. Gray JG: Lues-lues: maternal and fetal considerations of syphilis, *Obstet Gynecol Surv* 50:845, 1995.

34. Greenberg DN, Yoder BA: Changes in the differential white blood count in screening for group B streptococcal sepsis, *Pediatr Infect Dis J* 9:886, 1990.

35. Grubman S, Simonds RJ: Preventing *pneumocystis carnii* pneumonia in human immunodeficiency virus-infected children: new guidelines for prophylaxis, *Pediatr Infect Dis J* 15:165, 1996.

36. Hall SL: Coagulase negative staphylococcal infections in neonates, *Pediatr Infect Dis J* 10:57, 1991.

37. Guidelines for preventing perinatal GBS infection, *Contemp Obstet Gynecol* 84, 1996.

38. Hargrove C: Administration of intravenous medications in the NICU: the development of a procedure, *Neonat Net* 6:51, 1987.

39. Hutto C et al: Intrauterine herpes simplex infections, *J Pediatr* 110:97, 1987.

40. Ikeda MK, Jensen HB: Evaluation and treatment of congenital syphilis, *J Pediatr* 117:843, 1990.

41. Kliegman RM, Clapp DW: Rational principles for immunoglobulin prophylaxis and therapy for neonatal infections, *Clin Perinatol* 18:303, 1991.

42. Landers S et al: Factors associated with umbilical catheter related sepsis in neonates, *Am J Dis Child* 145:675, 1991.

43. Long JG, Keyserling HL: Catheter-related infections in infants due to an unusual lipophilic yeast—*Malassezzia furfur, Pediatrics* 76:8896, 1985.

44. Manroe BL et al: The neonatal blood count in health and disease. I. Reference values for neutropenic cells, *J Pediatr* 95:89, 1979.

45. Mofenson LM: The role of antiretroviral therapy in the management of HIV infection in women, *Clin Obstet Gynecol* 39:361, 1996.

46. Nelson SN, Merenstein GB, Pierce JR: Early onset group B Streptococcal disease, *J Perinatol* 6:234, 1986.

47. Noel GJ et al: Multiple methicillin-resistant staphylococcus aureus strains as a cause for a single outbreak of severe disease in hospitalized neonates, *Pediatr Infect Dis J* 11:184, 1992.

48. Phillips G, Golledge C: Fungal infection in neonates, *J Antimicrob Chemother* 28:159, 1991.

49. Pierce JR, Merenstein GB, Stocker JT: Immediate postpartum cultures in an intensive care nursery, *Pediatr Infect Dis J* 3:510, 1984.

50. Prober CG et al: Low risk of herpes simplex virus in neonates exposed to the virus at the time of vaginal delivery to mothers with recurrent genital herpes simplex infection, *N Engl J Med* 316:240, 1987.

51. Recommendations for preventing the spread of vancomycin disease, *MMWR* 44:1, 1994.

52. Rusi P et al: *Haemophilus influenzae:* an important cause of maternal and neonatal infections, *Obstet Gynecol* 77:92, 1991.

53. Schwerenski J, McIntyre L, Bauer CR: Lumbar puncture frequency and cerebrospinal fluid analysis in the neonate, *Am J Dis Child* 145:54, 1991.

54. St Geme JW, Harris MC: Coagulase negative staphylococcus infection in the neonate, *Clin Perinatol* 18:281, 1991.

55. Stagno S et al: Congenital cytomegalovirus infection: the relative importance of primary and recurrent maternal infection, *N Engl J Med* 306:945, 1982.

56. Stoll BJ: Congenital syphilis: evaluation and management of neonates born with reactive serologic tests for syphilis, *Pediatr Infect Dis J* 13:845, 1994.

57. Weisman LE et al: Early onset group B streptococcal sepsis: a current assessment, *J Pediatr* 121:428, 1992.

58. Weiss MG, Ionides SP, Anderson CL: Meningitis in premature infants with respiratory distress: role of admission lumbar puncture, *J Pediatr* 119:973, 1991.

59. Whitley R et al: A controlled trial comparing vidarbine with acyclovir in neonatal herpes simplex virus infection, *N Engl J Med* 324:444, 1991.

60. Wiswell TE, Hachey WE: Multiple site blood cultures in the evaluation for neonatal sepsis during the first week of life, *Pediatr Infect Dis J* 10:365, 1991.

61. Wittek AE et al: Asymptomatic shedding of herpes simplex virus from the cervix and lesion site during pregnancy: correlation of antepartum shedding with shedding at delivery, *Am J Dis Child* 138:439, 1984.

62. Wong VCW et al: Prevention of HBsAg carrier state in the newborn infants of mothers who are chronic carriers of HBsAg and HBeAg by administration of hepatitis-B vaccine and hepatitis-B immunoglobin, *Lancet* 1:921, 1984.

63. Yamauchi T: Nosocomial infections in the newborn, *Curr Opin Infect Dis* 4:474, 1991.

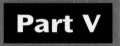

Part V *Common Systemic Diseases of the Neonate*

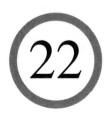

22 Respiratory Diseases

Mary I. Enzman Hagedorn, Sandra L. Gardner, Steven H. Abman

Despite the marked improvement in the outcome of premature newborns with respiratory distress over the past decade, significant mortality and high morbidity persist. Much of the improvement in neonatal mortality has been the result of successful treatment and management of respiratory diseases in the neonate. An overview of some of the common respiratory diseases, their treatments, and outcomes are presented in this chapter. General principles and concepts related to respiratory physiology, etiology, and symptomatology are presented, followed by specific disease processes and their management. In addition, recent developments in novel therapies such as nitric oxide and partial liquid ventilation are presented.

General Physiology

Any discussion of general respiratory physiology must include some elements of anatomy and embryology and their significance to the clinician (Table 22-1).

Surface-active compounds such as phosphatidylcholine and phosphatidylglycerol stabilize the alveoli. Surface tension forces act on air-fluid interfaces, causing a water droplet to "bead up." The surface-active compound (e.g., soap added to a water droplet) reduces the surface tension and allows the droplet to spread out in a thin film. In the lung, surface tension forces tend to cause alveoli to collapse. A compound such as surfactant reduces surface tension and allows the alveoli to remain open.

The situation, however, is more complicated than just described. LaPlace detailed the magnitude of the pressure (P) exerted at the surface of an air-liquid interface as equaling twice the surface tension (st) divided by the radius (r) of curvature of the surface (P = 2 st ÷ r). In the absence of surfactant an alveolus with a small radius of curvature has a greater magnitude of pressure at its surface (tending to collapse it) than does an alveolus with a larger radius of curvature. Therefore smaller alveoli would tend to collapse and empty contained gas into larger alveoli.

Surfactant modifies surface tension by decreasing surface tension when the radius of curvature is small and increasing surface tension when the radius of curvature is greater. An alveolus with a larger radius of curvature has a greater than expected pressure (tending to reduce its volume), and an alveolus with a smaller radius of curvature has less than expected pressure. Therefore the alveoli are stabilized at a uniform radius of curvature (uniform volume).

Surfactant provides a number of useful properties in addition to reducing surface tension, which increases lung compliance, provides alveolar stability, and decreases opening pressure. It also enhances alveolar fluid clearance, decreases precapillary tone, and plays a protective role for the epithelial cell surface. Surfactant is constantly

Table 22-1
Lung Development

Stage and Major Events	Significance
Embryonic (up to 5 Weeks)	
Single ventral outpocketing quickly divides into two lung buds	Airways begin to differentiate
Mesenchyme surrounds endodermal lung buds, which continue to divide and extend into the mesenchyme	
Branching of the airways begins	Branching anomalies (e.g., pulmonary agenesis and sequestered lobe) occur early in fetal life
Pulmonary arteries invade lung tissue, following the airways, and divide as the airways divide	
Pulmonary veins arise independently from the lung parenchyma and return to the left atrium, thus completing the pulmonary circuit	
Pseudoglandular (5-16 Weeks)	
Progressive airway branching begins; bronchi and terminal bronchioles form	All subdivisions that will form airways are complete by the sixteenth week
Muscle fibers, elastic tissue, and early cartilage formation can be seen along the tracheobronchial tree	
Mucous glands are found at 12 weeks and increase in number until 25-26 weeks, when cilia begin to develop	
Diaphragm develops	Herniation of the diaphragm occurs
Cannicular (13-25 Weeks)	
Airway changes from glandular to tubular and increases in length and diameter	Air conducting portion (bronchi and terminal bronchioli) continues luminal development
20 Weeks	
Fetal airways end in blind pouches lined with cuboid epithelium; a relatively large amount of interstitial mesenchyme is present; few pulmonary capillaries are present, and they are not closely associated with the respiratory epithelium	

being formed, stored, secreted, and recycled. Conditions that interfere with surfactant metabolism include acidemia, hypoxia, shock, over-inflation, underinflation, pulmonary edema, mechanical ventilation, and hypercapnia. Surfactant production is delayed in IDMs in classes of A, B, and C; infants with erythroblastosis fetalis; and infants who are the smaller of twins. Surfactant production is accelerated in the following:

- IDMs of classes D, F, and R
- Infants of heroin-addicted mothers

- Premature rupture of membranes of greater than 48 hours' duration
- Infants of mothers with hypertension
- Infants subjected to maternal infection
- Infants suffering from placental insufficiency
- Infants affected by administration of betamethasone or thyroid hormone to the mother
- Infants affected by abruptio placentae

The fetal lung is filled with a volume of liquid (20 to 30 ml/kg) equal to the functional residual capacity. This fluid is not amniotic fluid but rather

Table 22-1
Lung Development—cont'd

Stage and Major Events	Significance
22-24 Weeks	
Rapid proliferation of the pulmonary capillary bed, an increase of the surface area of the respiratory epithelium, and formation of alveolar ducts and sacculi occur	Development of the gas exchange portion (the respiratory bronchi and alveolar ducts) begins; pulmonary vasculature develops most rapidly
Respiratory epithelium contains cells that become differentiated into type I and type II pneumocytes	
Type I pneumocytes produce an extremely thin squamous epithelial layer that lines the alveoli and fuses to the underlying capillary endothelial cells	By the late fetal period the resulting membrane between the alveoli and capillaries allows sufficient gas exchange to support independent life
Type II pneumocytes (cuboid cells) are the site of surfactant synthesis and storage	At 22 weeks, surface-active phospholipid (lecithin) can first be detected
Terminal (24-40 Weeks)	
Lung differentiation: proliferation of the pulmonary vascular bed, creation of new respiratory units (alveolar ducts and alveoli), decrease in amount of interstitial mesenchyme, and fusion of the gas exchange epithelium to the pulmonary capillary epithelium occur	Before this time the fetal lungs are incapable of supporting adequate gas exchange because of insufficient alveolar surface area and inadequate pulmonary vasculature
34-36 Weeks	
Phosphatidylglycerol appears, and a dramatic increase in the principal surfactant compound phosphatidylchoine occurs	Adequate amounts of surface-active material protects against the development of respiratory distress syndrome
Alveolar (Postnatal Lung Development) (Late Fetal Life to 8-10 Years of Age)	
At term the number of airways is complete; there is sufficient respiratory surface for gaseous exchange, and the pulmonary capillary bed is sufficient to carry the gases that have been exchanged	Although the infant is capable of sustaining respiratory effort and the lung is able to provide oxygenation and ventilation at birth, lung development is still incomplete
Alveoli continue to increase in number, size, and shape; they enlarge and become deeper to maximize the exposed surface area for gas exchange	Ongoing lung development implies that infants who have suffered severe lung disease at birth need not become life-long pulmonary cripples

a liquid that has been produced in the lung and discharged through the larynx and mouth into the amniotic fluid. Lung fluid is continuously produced at a rate of approximately 2 to 4 ml/kg/hr.

Because of the movement of lung fluid and its components (notably lecithin) into amniotic fluid, the lecithin/sphingomyelin (L/S) ratio has become a notable clinical tool. Noting a sharp increase in the L/S ratio, Gluck and Kulovich[61] found they could predict infants at risk for RDS. In general,

L/S ratios of more than 2:1 are not associated with RDS, whereas ratios of less than 2:1 are associated with it. Phosphatidyglycerol (PG), the second most common phospholipid in surfactant, appears at about 36 weeks' gestation and increases until term. The presence of PG is associated with a very low risk of RDS, whereas its absence is associated with the development of RDS. Unlike the L/S ratio, PG determination is valid in the presence of blood-contaminated amniotic fluid.

During vaginal delivery, approximately one third of the lung fluid may be removed during the thoracic "squeeze" as the infant passes through the birth canal; the remainder of the fluid is removed mainly by the pulmonary lymphatics, although pulmonary capillaries may play a role. After a cesarean section, all of the lung fluid will be removed by the pulmonary lymphatics and capillaries.

The first breath of life, a response to tactile, thermal, chemical, and mechanical stimuli, initiates respiratory effort. The fluid-filled lungs, surface forces, and tissue-sensitive forces are obstacles to the first breath. At birth, gas is substituted for liquid to expand the alveoli. After the alveoli are "opened" during the first few breaths, a film of surface-active material stabilizes the alveoli.

The first breath of life is certainly the most difficult one. During the first breath, a pressure of 60 to 80 cm of water may be required to overcome the effects of the surface tension of the air-liquid interface, particularly the small airways and alveoli. Thus on each subsequent breath, less pressure is required to allow for a similar increase in air volume in the lung. The effort of breathing is lessened with subsequent breaths.

General Etiology

Respiratory disease may be defined as a progressive impairment of the lungs to exchange gas at the alveolar level. Although the pathologic process causing respiratory disease in the neonate may occur in any portion of the respiratory system (or in other organ systems), the final common pathway in respiratory disease is impairment of gas exchange.

Prematurity is the single most common factor in the occurrence of RDS. Its incidence is inversely proportional to gestational age and occurs most frequently in infants of less than 1200 g and 30 weeks' gestation. Male infants outnumber female infants 2:1.

The principal factor operating in the development of RDS in very premature infants is surfactant deficiency.

Multiple gestations increase the risk of respiratory disease related to lung maturity in the second, third, or more siblings. There is a tendency for the second and subsequent infants to be smaller and suffer perinatal asphyxia. Grand multiparity is associated with increased risk of respiratory disease, particularly when other siblings have had RDS.

Prenatal maternal complications increase the risk for respiratory disease in the infant. Maternal illnesses such as cardiorespiratory disease, hypoxia, hemorrhage, shock, hypotension, or hypertension result in decreased uterine blood flow with subsequent hypoxia or ischemia at the placental level. Severe maternal anemia causes fetal cardiac depression and respiratory depression. Maternal diabetes may result in preterm delivery because of fetal and maternal indications. There is also a greater incidence of false-positive L/S ratios in diabetic populations. There has been a propensity of IDMs to develop RDS despite documentation of L/S ratios greater than 2:1. (A combination of L/S ratios $\geq 2:1$ and the presence of PG confirms fetal lung maturity.) Abnormal placental conditions (compressed umbilical cord caused by prolapse or breech delivery, placental disease such as infarcts or syphilis, or hemorrhage as a result of placenta previa or abruptio) affect oxygen transfer from mother to fetus and result in an asphyxial insult to the developing fetal lung. Premature rupture of the membranes predisposes the fetus or newborn to the development of infections such as pneumonia, sepsis, or meningitis. Premature or prolonged rupture of the membranes not associated with neonatal infection accelerates fetal lung development and thereby lessens the incidence of RDS. Prenatal administration of glucocorticoids,[125] maternal toxemia, and maternal heroin addiction also hasten fetal lung maturation.

Factors affecting the fetus during the birthing process may lead to respiratory distress. Depression of the respiratory center can be a result of maternal medications that cross the placenta. An infant delivered shortly after administration of maternal analgesia or anesthesia may have only minimal respiratory efforts at birth. Excessive uterine activity, usually as a result of oxytocin induction or augmentation of labor, results in decreased uterine blood flow, late fetal heart deceleration, and respiratory depression in the infant at birth.

Respiratory disease may be the result of direct trauma to the respiratory center or a cerebral hemorrhage in close proximity to it. Fetal shock caused by difficult labor or dystocia, tight nuchal cord, cerebral hemorrhage, or hemorrhage from the fetal side of the placenta results in CNS depression and hypoxia. Bleeding results in a generalized hypovolemic condition characterized by decreased oxygen-carrying capacity. Fetal or neonatal asphyxia and blood loss lead to progressive respiratory distress. Delivery by cesarean section prevents one third of the lung fluid from being expelled by the thoracic squeeze of vaginal birth. Thus after cesarean birth, all lung fluid must be absorbed through circulatory and lymphatic channels; therefore a greater incidence of transient tachypnea of the newborn may occur as the increased volume of retained fluid is absorbed.

The role of cesarean section in the development of RDS is still controversial. However, the general consensus is that cesarean section delivery in the absence of fetal distress is not associated with an increased incidence of RDS. Yet a correlation appears between absence of labor and increased risk of developing RDS, but the amount of retained lung fluid may be the significant factor.

Obstruction of the airway caused by aspiration of meconium or amniotic fluid occurs either spontaneously at birth or during resuscitative efforts. Although the lungs initially fill with air, subsequent atelectasis occurs as complete airway obstruction prevents further entrance of air. Conversely, a "ball valve" effect or "air-trapping" effect may occur as air is allowed in but is unable to escape because of intermittent obstruction. The presence of amniotic debris, vernix, lanugo, and meconium in the respiratory tract increases the incidence and severity of pulmonary infection. Diaphragmatic paralysis occurs after phrenic nerve injury during birth (usually of an LGA infant) and is often associated with Erb's palsy. The paradoxic movement of the paralyzed diaphragm during inspiration and expiration results in inadequate tidal volume and impaired gaseous exchange.

Existing neonatal conditions increase the risk of respiratory disease. Congenital defects that prevent transmission of the stimulus to or from the respiratory center, prevent normal respiratory effort, reduce gas exchange surface area, or hamper the delivery of oxygen to the site of exchange will predispose the infant to respiratory embarrassment. Such defects include heart or great vessel anomalies, diaphragmatic hernia and hypoplastic lung, respiratory tract anomalies (e.g., choanal atresia or tracheoesophageal fistula), chest wall deformities, and CNS defects.

Diseases of the infant can also lead to respiratory disease. Hemolytic disease such as ABO and Rh incompatibility results in anemia and, if severe, in hypovolemic shock. Blood incompatibilities increase respiratory distress by decreasing the oxygen-carrying capacity of the blood. Infections stress the body's systems, increase oxygen requirements, and contribute to an impairment of surfactant production. Chronic lung disease in the form of BPD occurs in 35% to 40% of 750 to 1500 g infants with or without surfactant therapy.[38] Prolonged treatment of RDS may be necessitated by the severity of the disease but may increase the risk of developing chronic lung disease.

General Prevention

Antepartum

Prevention of respiratory disease begins with prevention of conditions that predispose to respiratory distress. These conditions that constitute "reproductive risks" have been identified and can be categorized as psychosocial, genetic, biophysical, or economic in nature. Once an individual is identified among a high-risk category, comprehensive prenatal care with immediate attention given to maternal complications that arise is crucial (see Chapters 2 and 3).

Intrapartum

Fetal well-being is assessed by using electronic monitoring of uterine activity and fetal heart rate and fetal scalp blood sampling. Electronic fetal heart rate monitoring enables instantaneous fetal heart rate tracings as opposed to the previous method of intermittent evaluation by stethoscope. Fetal heart rate monitoring allows for coincident correlation between uterine contractions and fetal response. These tools enable the practitioner to evaluate how well the fetus withstands the stresses of labor and to make decisions regarding the laboring course.

Fetal cardiac response to stress is unlike the older child or adult's response to hypoxia, hypercapnia, and acidosis with tachycardia from sympathetic nervous system discharge. The fetus responds to these same stresses with an initial increase in heart rate. This is quickly followed by bradycardia from parasympathetic stimulation when the hypoxia, hypercapnia, and acidosis persist (see Chapter 2).

Postpartum

After delivery the infant should be maintained in an environment that minimizes stress and thereby minimizes the oxygen requirement. All infants, but particularly at-risk infants, should be maintained within the narrow parameter of physiologic homeostasis (see Part II).

General Data Collection

Because the clinical manifestations of many neonatal illnesses include respiratory symptoms (cardiac, metabolic, neurologic, and hematologic), a systematic and thorough approach to data collection is essential in evaluating an infant in respiratory distress.

History

The perinatal history (antepartum, intrapartum, and postpartum) should be reviewed for risk factors (see Chapter 2).

Signs and Symptoms

Vital signs such as temperature, pulse, respiration, and blood pressure should be evaluated. Hypothermia and hyperthermia increase oxygen requirements by altering the basal metabolic rate. Hypotension is often associated with respiratory disease.

Respiratory Examination

Respiratory effort is normally irregular in rate and depth, and is chiefly abdominal, rather than thoracic, with a rate of 30 to 60 breaths/min. Bradypnea is characterized by a rate below 30 breaths/min that is regular (as opposed to periodic or apneic) and may be caused by an insult to the respiratory center of the CNS. Tachypnea, a rate above 60 breaths/min after the first hour of life, is the earliest symptom of respiratory (and often other) diseases. As a compensatory mechanism, tachypnea attempts to maintain alveolar ventilation and gaseous exchange. As a decompensatory mechanism, tachypnea increases oxygen demand, energy output, and the "work" of breathing.

Periodic respirations are cyclic respirations of apnea (5 to 10 seconds) and ventilation (10 to 15 seconds). The average respiratory rate is 30 to 40 breaths/min. Periodic breathing is a common occurrence in small preterm infants as a result of an immature CNS. Apnea is a nonbreathing episode lasting longer than 20 seconds and accompanied by physiologic alterations. The syndrome of apnea is discussed later in this chapter.

Use of accessory muscles of respiration is indicative of a marked increase in the work of breathing. Retractions reflect the inward pull of the thin chest wall on inspiration. Retracting is best observed in relation to the sternum (substernal and suprasternal) and the intercostal, supracostal, and subcostal spaces. The increased negative intrathoracic pressure necessary to ventilate the stiff, noncompliant lung causes the chest wall to retract. This further compromises the lung's expansion. The degree of retraction is directly proportional to the severity of the disease.

Nasal flaring is a compensatory mechanism that attempts to take in more oxygen by increasing the size of the nares and thus decreasing the resistance (by as much as 40%) of the narrow airways. Grunting is forced expiration through a partially closed glottis. The audible grunt may be heard with or without the aid of a stethoscope. As a compensatory mechanism, grunting stabilizes the alveoli by increasing transpulmonary pressure and increases gaseous exchange by delaying expiration.[74]

Color is normally pink after the first breaths of

life. Acrocyanosis, peripheral cyanosis of the hands and feet in the first 24 hours of life, is normal. Pallor with poor peripheral circulation may indicate systemic hypotension. Ruddy, plethoric skin color may indicate hyperviscosity or polycythemia, or both, as causes of respiratory symptoms. However, the lack of a deep-red coloring does not rule out polycythemia or hyperviscosity.

Cyanosis, a late and serious sign, is a blue discoloration of the skin, nail beds, and mucous membranes. Differentiation between peripheral cyanosis (of hands and feet) and central cyanosis (of mucous membranes of mouth and generalized body cyanosis) is essential. Because a large decrease in Pao_2 may be tolerated without detectable cyanosis, the lack of cyanosis does not ensure a healthy infant. When hypoxemia reaches a level that produces frank cyanosis, the insufficiency is usually in advanced stages (see Chapter 10). Therefore cyanosis or its lack is not a reliable sign in the neonate.

Symmetry of the newborn chest is characterized by a relatively round or barrel shape, because the anteroposterior diameter equals the transverse diameter. With prolonged respiratory distress, there is an increase in the anteroposterior diameter, so that the neonate becomes pigeon-chested.

Auscultation of the newborn chest includes comparing and contrasting one side with the other and noting the quality of breath sounds and the presence or absence of rales, rhonchi, or other abnormal sounds. Because of the relatively small size of the newborn's chest, it is hyperresonant, so that breath sounds are widely transmitted. Therefore one cannot always rely on auscultation to detect pathologic conditions (e.g., pneumothorax). Percussion of the chest to determine the presence of air, fluid, or solids may not be useful in the neonate because of small chest size and hyperresonance. Palpation of the neonatal chest wall while the infant is crying may detect gross changes in sound transmission through the chest. Palpation of crepitus in the neck, around the clavicles, or on the chest wall suggests the complication of air leak.

Nonrespiratory Examination

Hypotonia is characterized by a froglike positioning and a lax, open mouth. Progressing from flexion to flaccidity indicates progression of hypoxia and exhaustion from the work of breathing. Cardiac findings such as a murmur, absence of pulses, bounding pulses, palmar or calf pulses, weight gain, hepatosplenomegaly, cyanosis, edema, bradycardia, or tachycardia indicate congestive heart failure or congenital heart defects. A scaphoid abdomen indicates a diaphragmatic hernia.

Laboratory Data

Because the clinical presentation of many respiratory and nonrespiratory diseases is the same, a chest x-ray examination may be the only way to differentiate cause and establish the proper diagnosis. X-ray evaluation helps eliminate congenital anomalies (e.g., diaphragmatic hernia with lung hypoplasia, masses, and obstruction) as the cause when acquired respiratory disease (e.g., RDS, transient tachypnea of the newborn, and pneumonia) is the cause of the distress. X-ray films confirm the presence of pneumothorax or other pulmonary air leaks.

Arterial blood gases are used to demonstrate derangements of oxygenation and acid-base balance, and to differentiate between respiratory and metabolic components. Initial baseline values are followed by serial observations at least every 15 to 30 minutes after any change in therapy. This may be modified with pulse oximetry or transcutaneous monitoring. Shunt study may differentiate between lung origin and cardiac origin of respiratory distress. The symptoms of pulmonary disease (cyanosis and low Pao_2) are often alleviated with crying, increased Fio_2, and/or continuous positive airway pressure. If the same symptoms are cardiac in origin, they remain unchanged or worsen with these interventions. Administration of 100% Fio_2 for 10 minutes or longer may result in an increased Pao_2 (>100 mm Hg), whereas in cardiac disease caused by right-to-left shunting there is no change in Pao_2 after 100% Fio_2 administration. CAUTION: In the presence of severe lung disease with significant right-to-left shunting, cyanosis and Pao_2 may not be changed with 100% Fio_2.

The hematocrit is used to rule out anemia or polycythemia as the cause of the respiratory distress. In anemia, inadequate oxygen content promotes tissue hypoxia. In polycythemia, increased viscosity and sludging of blood flow adversely affect tissue oxygenation.

The white blood cell count and differential aid in diagnosing sepsis as the cause of distress. A blood culture is invaluable in suspected infection and should be obtained before antibiotic therapy. Blood glucose determination to rule out hypoglycemia as a cause is particularly important in IDMs, SGA infants, LGA infants, and preterm AGA infants. An electrocardiogram, ECG, and cardiac catheterization are used to rule out cardiac abnormalities.

An EEG and ultrasound examination of the brain help to rule out CNS abnormalities. Serum electrolytes (calcium, sodium, and potassium) aid in eliminating metabolic aberration as the cause of the distress.

General Treatment Strategies

Treatment of any condition should be directed at correction of its underlying cause. Unfortunately, present technology does not always permit therapeutic maneuvers directed at the underlying cause of many neonatal respiratory diseases. In meconium aspiration syndrome, if prevention of the aspiration through thorough suction is to no avail, damage to the neonatal lung results. No therapeutic measure is available at present to augment the healing process. Therapy is thus directed at preventing or alleviating the consequences of neonatal lung diseases such as hypoxemia and acidemia, allowing healing to take place and reducing iatrogenic complications.

Respiratory support is the hallmark of treatment of neonatal respiratory disease. Respiratory support involves increasing inspired oxygen tensions and providing ventilation if required.

Supplemental Oxygen

When the neonate is unable to maintain adequate oxygenation, supplemental oxygen must be provided. Because oxygen is a drug, it must be treated as such and given only for medical indications. Biochemical criteria ($Pao_2 < 60$ mm Hg) and clinical criteria such as respiratory distress, central cyanosis, apnea, asphyxia, and hypotonia are indications to prescribe oxygen.

Regardless of the mode of delivery (hood, ventilator, bag, or mask), safe and effective oxygen administration follows certain principles:

- No concentration of oxygen has been proved to be "safe." A concentration (e.g., 30%, 40%, 80%, 100%) that is therapeutic for one infant may be toxic for another.
- To titrate inspired oxygen concentrations to the individual infant's need, arterial PO_2 must be measured and maintained between 60 and 80 mm Hg.
- Oxygen administration without some form of continuous monitoring of the infant's oxygenation (e.g., arterial blood gases, pulse oximetry and/or transcutaneous monitoring) is dangerous and not recommended.[5]
- Delivered oxygen should be humidified (30% to 40%), because dry gases are irritating to the airways and humidity decreases insensible water losses. To prevent respiratory therapy equipment from becoming a source of infection, humidifiers and tubing should be replaced at least every 48 hours.
- Oxygen should be warmed (31° to 34° C [88° to 94° F]) so temperature at the delivery site is the same as the incubator temperature. Oxygen delivered by endotracheal tube should be warmed to core temperature (i.e., 36.5° to 37° C). This prevents cold stress and increased oxygen consumption from blowing cold air in the infant's face.[151]
- Oxygen concentration must be monitored by continuous or intermittent sampling (at least every hour) and recorded. Oxygen monitors and analyzers should be calibrated every 8 hours.
- A stable concentration of oxygen is necessary to maintain Pao_2 within normal limits. A sudden increase or decrease in oxygen concentration may result in a disproportionate increase or decrease in Pao_2 caused by vasodilation or vasoconstriction in response to oxygen.[151] Adjustment of supplemental oxygen (particularly lowering Fio_2) must be done slowly to avoid the "flip-flop phenomenon." Hypoxic insult initiates pulmonary

vasoconstriction, which causes hypoperfusion and increased pulmonary vascular resistance. The infant should be weaned from supplemental oxygen cautiously[151] (see "rule of seven," Chapter 10, p. 166).

- Observing color, respiratory effort, activity, and circulatory response and monitoring arterial oxygen concentration aid in determining the need for oxygen therapy and for adjustments to it.
- Clinical observations, Fio_2 concentrations, and time of adjustments must be described, recorded, and reported.
- Oxygen concentration should be returned to previous levels if clinical observations of distress and inability to tolerate decreased levels of oxygen occur.

Delivery Methods

For instructions on the bag and mask resuscitation method see Chapter 4.

An oxygen hood is a clear plastic hood that fits over the infant's head to deliver a constant concentration of oxygen. If the infant has sufficient ventilation to maintain a normal arterial carbon dioxide tension, oxygenation by increased inspired oxygen tensions through an oxygen hood may be all the respiratory support that is required. This degree of support is particularly applicable in cases of mild RDS, transient tachypnea of the newborn (TTN), meconium aspiration, or neonatal pneumonia.

A blender system is the most reliable way to administer a fixed oxygen concentration via a hood. An appropriately sized hood should be used. If it is too large, the infant may slip out of the hood and Fio_2 may be diluted by leaks; if it is too small, pressure points may develop, especially around the neck. Another source of oxygen must be provided when the infant's head is removed from the hood because of feeding, being held, or suctioning. This secondary source may be set up from the blender source so that the infant's Pao_2 remains constant during suctioning or feedings. The infant may need increased Fio_2 from the secondary source, and this can be easily adjusted according to assessments made with pulse oximetry or a transcutaneous monitor (TCM); these changes should be recorded.

For both home and hospital use, the nasal cannula provides an acceptable way to administer oxygen to the dependent infant who is developing social and motor skills.[162] Oxygen cannulas for neonatal and infant use are now commercially available.

- Choose the appropriately sized cannula for the infant.
- Position the cannula across the infant's upper lip. Secure it to the infant's face by first applying Stomahesive or Tegaderm (Op-site) directly to the infant's cheeks and taping the cannula to it to prevent skin irritation.

CAUTION: Neonates are obligatory nasal breathers, so that nasal obstruction (mucus or milk) will decrease the amount of oxygen actually received. Therefore nares should be suctioned as needed. The exact concentrations of oxygen delivered by cannula cannot be measured.[166] Flow rates are titrated by monitoring Pao_2, pulse oximetry levels, or $TcPo_2$ and by evaluating the clinical course. Use of nasal cannulas with oxygen rates >0.5 liters/min may result in inadvertent administration of continuous distending (positive) pressure and result in increased respiratory effort (i.e., tachypnea, retractions, exaggerated periodic breathing).[109,166] Oxygen tubing should be long enough to provide opportunities for social and gross motor skill development.

Continuous Distending Pressure

Application of a continuous distending pressure (CDP) to the lungs increases functional residual capacity and Pao_2. It improves oxygenation by decreasing intrapulmonary shunting and by improving the match of ventilation and perfusion. The application of CDP improves compliance of the lung and lessens the work of breathing.[64]

In RDS, where the functional residual capacity is reduced, increased respiratory oxygen tensions via an Oxyhood may not be sufficient to maintain an adequate arterial oxygen tension. More invasive techniques may be required.

CPAP or continuous negative pressure (CNP) are two methods of delivery of CDP. If the infant cannot maintain a Pao_2 of 60 mm Hg in 0.6 Fio_2, a trial of CPAP, either by the nasal route or through an endotracheal tube, is indicated. Initial levels of CPAP should be in the range of 4 to 5 cm of water. CPAP should be increased to 8 to 10 cm of water by 2 cm increments if required to raise the infant's Pao_2 (as measured by arterial blood gas determinations, noninvasive monitoring, or both). Arterial blood gas determinations are performed 15 to 30 minutes after initiating CDP and with each adjustment.

Indications and complications in the use of CPAP are listed in Table 22-2. If the infant is able to maintain ventilation as indicated by normal arterial carbon dioxide tension, no further respiratory support may be required. Early institution of CDP reduces the need for mechanical ventilation.

Although negative pressure devices, head chambers, and face masks have been used to deliver CDP, using nasal prongs placed in the infant's nares or endotracheal intubation is preferred. A variety of nasal prongs are available. An orogastric tube (feeding tube) should be used for gastric decompression when implementing nasal prongs.

When the infant's Pao_2 is consistently over 70 mm Hg, inspired oxygen concentration and/or CDP may be lowered. Oxygen concentration is usually lowered in 5% to 10% increments to a level of 40% to 60%. CDP is lowered in increments of 1 cm of water to a level of 2 cm of water before discontinuing either prongs or an endotracheal tube. The infant may then be placed into an oxygen hood with the same Fio_2. Pao_2 (or $TcPo_2$) should be checked 15 to 30 minutes after each change.

Pulmonary Hygiene

Pulmonary hygiene is normally maintained by ciliary activity, a covering of mucus, and narrowing and dilation of the bronchi with respiration and coughing. Anatomic and physiologic variations in the neonate alter these normal pulmonary mechanisms. The small airway of the neonate has a diameter that is four times smaller than that of the normal adult. Debris that causes only a moderate obstruction for the adult airway causes a disproportionately greater obstruction of the smaller airway of the neonate. Also, the neonate normally has an underdeveloped cough reflex. The sick neonate with insufficient respiratory effort and a weak or nonexistent cry has underventilated lungs. Often the neonate that is attached to multiple life-support system is cared for in the same position. This localizes secretions in the dependent pulmonary tree and sets the stage for hypostatic pneumonia.

Combined chest physiotherapy and suctioning has become increasingly popular as a treatment modality for infants suffering from RDS. There is, however, a paucity of literature to substantiate this treatment.

Whenever the normal mechanisms for mobilizing and removing pulmonary secretions are inefficient or inactive, pulmonary hygiene is indicated. Pulmonary hygiene consists of two major components: chest physiotherapy and suctioning. The goals of pulmonary hygiene are as follows:

- To facilitate removal of pulmonary debris by loosening and mobilizing secretions into the mainstem bronchi for suctioning
- To maintain a patent airway
- To promote optimal pulmonary ventilation
- To prevent pulmonary infection from accumulated secretions

In the neonatal period, pulmonary hygiene is indi-

Table 22-2 Continuous Positive Airway Pressure	
Indications	**Complications**
Infant who breathes spontaneously yet has mild to moderate respiratory distress syndrome	Respiratory difficulty secondary to narrowing of the nasal passage with prongs or trachea with the presence of an endotracheal tube
Very-low-birth-weight infant with secondary apnea	Pneumothorax
During the weaning process for ventilatory support	Air Leaks
	Nasal irritation, trauma, infection

cated for intubated patients with conditions associated with atelectasis, increased secretions, and pulmonary debris (pneumonia, meconium aspiration, RDS, and BPD).

CAUTION: The following are guidelines for pulmonary hygiene. These procedures must be individualized.

- Any manipulation of the sick neonate has the potential for decreasing oxygenation and precipitating hypoxia.[45] Pulse oximetry and transcutaneous Po_2 readings show that pulmonary hygiene and other procedures (i.e., feeding, peripheral blood drawing, and turning) may cause lowering of oxygen tensions.[45,110] Therefore increased inspired oxygen tensions may need to be provided during these procedures.
- Pulmonary hygiene with a subsequent rest period (until vital signs and oxygenation return to baseline) should be done before feeding.
- Percussion should be performed over the chest wall but not over the liver, kidneys, sternum, vertebrae, or stomach.
- Infants receiving chest physiotherapy may appear stressed. Bradycardia, cyanosis, hypotonia, fighting, struggling, and alterations in oxygenation are signs of stress that should be observed during pulmonary hygiene. The procedure should be altered by the care provider to decrease stress and subsequent physiologic alterations.
- Position modifications or deletions may be necessary based on clinical manifestations of stress.
- The length of time for certain segments and for the procedure as a whole must be kept to a minimum to conserve the neonate's energy and prevent hypoxia.
- The affected areas are the prime consideration; prophylactic pulmonary hygiene is secondary. The right upper and middle lobes of the lung are the most common sites for the development of secondary pneumonia and atelectasis.[42]
- Physical assessment and estimates of secretions gauge the effectiveness and frequency of therapy.
- Communication among care providers main-

tains continuity in setting priorities, providing adequate pulmonary hygiene, and recognizing what stresses the individual infant.

Chest Physiotherapy

Chest physiotherapy consists of positioning, percussion, and vibration.

Positioning. Postural changes use gravity to facilitate the movement of pulmonary debris from smaller to larger bronchi. Specific lung segments must be uppermost and angled so that they drain into their major bronchi (Box 22-1). To facilitate maximum drainage, the infant is positioned 5 to 10 minutes before the onset of percussion and vibration. In the usual course of care, position changes every 1 to 2 hours are a continuum of intermittent postural drainage. Prone positioning promotes ventilation by increasing lung expansion, increasing Pao_2, and draining the usually dependent posteriorly directed airways.[42,163] If a position is stressful, it should be modified, the amount of time spent in it should be decreased, or it should be deleted according to the infant's tolerance.

Percussion. Percussion of the chest wall with a nontraumatic, commercial device creates a suction action that loosens secretions. The chest wall is gently tapped (for 30 seconds to 1 minute) over the affected area and then prophylactically over other frequently involved segments. Based on the infant's condition and tolerance, 1- to 2-inch segments are percussed. For very small or unstable infants, only one segment may be percussed with each treatment. Notation of the treated area must be exact, so that rotation and treatment of all areas occurs. Frequency varies from 1 to 4 hours depending on the disease process, amount of congestion, and tolerance.

Fractures have been documented in infants with BPD that apparently are the result of vigorous percussion.[43]

Vibration. Vibration of the neonatal chest with fingertips, a padded electric toothbrush, or mechanical vibrator may follow percussion or be performed in lieu of percussion. When done on expiration, vibration of specific lung segments mobilizes secretions. As with percussion, priority is

Box 22-1

Postural Changes to Facilitate Drainage

Upper Lobes

Position 1: An upright position drains apical segments of the upper lobes.

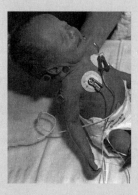

Position 2: A supine position 30-degree upright angle drains the anterior segments of the upper lobes.

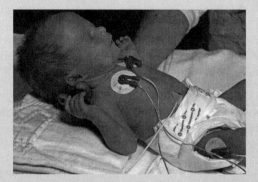

Position 1: A 30-degree upright angle drains the lateral bronchi of the apical segment of the right lung when infant is on left side and the apical posterior segment of the left lobe when infant is on right side.

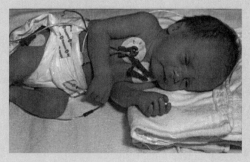

Modified from Dunn D, Lewis AT: *Pediatr Clin North Am* 20:490, 1973.

Box 22-1

Postural Changes to Facilitate Drainage—cont'd

Upper Lobes   Position 2: A rotation forward 45 degrees drains posterior bronchi of the upper lobe and apical segments. In addition, rotation to the right also drains the left posterior segment of the left upper lobe.

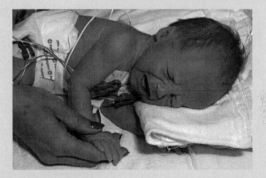

With the right side elevated 45 degrees in the prone position, the posterior segment of the right upper lobe is drained.

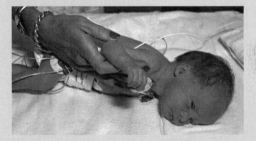

In a supine position the anterior segment of the upper lobes is drained.

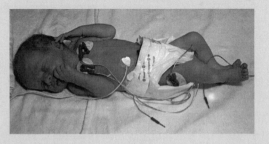

Continued

Box 22-1

Postural Changes to Facilitate
Drainage—cont'd

**Middle Lobe
and Lingula**

With the head tilted downward 15 degrees and a 45-degree rotation to the left, the right middle lobe is drained. With the head tilted downward 15 degrees and a 45-degree rotation to the right, the lingula of the left upper lobe is drained.

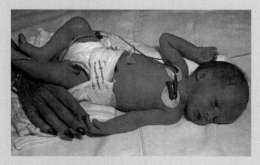

Lower Lobes

In a prone position the superior segments of the lower lobes drain.

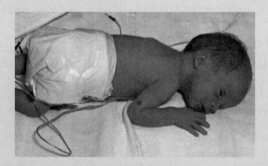

In the supine position with the head tilted downward 30 degrees, the anterior segments of the lower lobes drain.

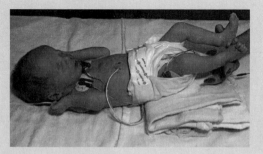

Box 22-1

Postural Changes to Facilitate Drainage—cont'd

Lower Lobes—cont'd In side-lying position with the head tilted downward 30 degrees, the lateral basal segments are drained. While lying on the right side, the medial basal segment of the right side drains.

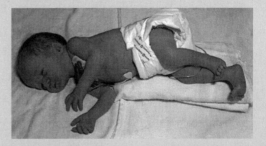

In a prone position the superior segments of the lower lobes drain.

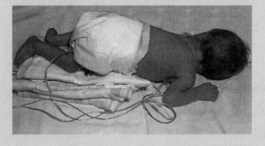

given to involved areas, with prophylactic therapy rotated among the other segments.

The use of positioning, percussion, and vibration increases recovery of the infant's secretions more than the use of gravity alone. Recent studies have shown vibration to be as efficacious for mobilizing secretions as percussion and may be less traumatic and stressful for the infant.[33]

Suctioning

Once secretions are loosened and mobilized, they must be removed through the nose and mouth or by tracheal suctioning.

Nasooropharyngeal Suctioning. When the infant has no artificial airway, suctioning the nasooropharynx serves two purposes: removing secretions and initiating a cough reflex that mobilizes secretions. With either a suction bulb or catheter, the infant is suctioned immediately after chest physiotherapy. Providing an oxygen source during the procedure is important. Because stimulation of the nares causes reflex inspiration with possible inhalation of oropharyngeal contents, first the mouth and then the nose should be suctioned. The results should be recorded.

CAUTION: Suctioning should be avoided for 30 minutes to 1 hour after feeding unless it is necessary to establish a patent airway. The catheter should be gently inserted upward and back into the nares, never forced. If the catheter is hard to pass or the nares seem blocked, this procedure should be abandoned to prevent swelling and/or trauma. The catheter may initiate vasovagal stimulation with resultant bradycardia.

Endotracheal suctioning (Oral Tube or Nasotracheal Tube). An artificial airway prevents normal warming, humidifying, and cleansing of the air by the upper airway. The presence of the foreign body (the tube) also increases pulmonary secretions. To maintain a patent airway, sterile endotracheal suction should be performed as assessment indicates (i.e., changes in breath sounds, increased irritability, agitation, or labile oxygenation). The following equipment is used for conventional suction procedure:

- Sterile suction catheter (of appropriate size; measurement of the length to be passed is essential)
- Sterile gloves
- Sterile normal saline (without preservative)
- Stethoscope
- Suction machine (80 to 100 mm Hg negative pressure)

The sterile catheter and glove package are opened. Sterile normal saline (0.25 to 0.5 ml) is drawn up in a 1 ml syringe. The resuscitation bag is connected to oxygen, and the patency is checked so that, if the neonate becomes apneic or bradycardic during the procedure, resuscitation equipment is immediately available. If the infant is on a ventilator equipped with a bag, this may be used for resuscitation if necessary.

Wall suction is adjusted to minimum pressure for effective suctioning. Hands are washed before and after every contact with the neonate. Assessment of the neonate's condition is made before initiating a suction procedure by observing vital signs (pulse and respirations), color, and pulse oximeter reading. Auscultation of the chest for adventitious sounds (rales, rhonchi, or wheezing) helps to evaluate the condition and indicate a need for suction. Because suctioning is one of the most stressful procedures performed in infants, suctioning should not be routine but instead should be based on assessment criteria of breath sounds, oxygenation, etc.

Procedure for Conventional Suction

- Disconnect and instill 0.25 to 0.5 ml of normal saline into tracheal tube and reconnect infant to ventilator. Saline (without preservative) thins secretions and facilitates their removal from the major bronchi. The amount of saline depends on the size of the infant (<2000 g—0.25 ml; >2000 g—0.5 ml) and the viscosity of secretions.
- Ventilate with deep inflating breaths. Use six to eight extra breaths at the same oxygen concentration (Fio_2), matching pressure to the ventilator settings. Increase Fio_2 if clinically indicated, using oximetry or a TCM. Hyperoxygenation, increasing the Fio_2 to 100% for ventilation, raises Pao_2 and has been associated with hyperoxia and its attendant consequences (i.e., retinopathy of prematurity). Hyperinflating the lungs helps to minimize hypoxia during suction without the danger of exposure to dangerously elevated Pao_2. Hyperinflation between each suction maneuver and at completion of suctioning restores functional residual capacity and prevents atelectasis. The response to hyperinflation depends on the infant's behavior during the procedure. If the infant is relaxed and at rest, the therapeutic effect of increased Pao_2 occurs; if the infant is fighting and struggling against the bag, the Pao_2 may fall precipitously.[130] Coordinating bag inflation with the infant's normal inspiration will tend to minimize struggling and the fall in Pao_2.
- Put gloves on and attach sterile catheter to suction tubing. Some systems provide sterile catheters "in line" and obviate the need for gloving.
- With nondominant hand, disconnect from ventilator.
- Gently pass catheter down endotracheal tube to measured length (this will prevent damage to bronchial mucosa that can occur using method of passing suction catheter until meeting resistance).
- Occlude suction hole in catheter and withdraw. Use continuous suction so that secre-

tions are not "released" with intermittent suction. Do not use an up-and-down motion while removing the catheter, because this will decrease oxygenation and promote hypoxia. Occlude tracheal tube with catheter for no longer than 5 to 10 seconds because of the danger of prolonged hypoxia. Only one suction attempt should be made before the infant is again ventilated. Assess tolerance of procedure by observing pulse oximeter and infant's color, heart rate, tone, and activity.
- Replace on ventilator and hyperinflate with appropriate Fio_2 for six to eight breaths or until adequate oxygenation has been established.

Procedure for Closed System Suction
Equipment to be Prepared
- Inline suction catheter (changed daily; measurement of the length to be passed is essential)
- Sterile normal saline (without preservative)
- Suction canister (80 to 100 mm HB negative pressure)

Procedure
- Unlock the inline suction catheter. Press suction control valve and check suction pressure.
- Place saline syringe on the proximal port of the adapter and instill 0.25 to 0.5 ml before suctioning.
- Slide the catheter through the plastic cover down the endotracheal tube to the predetermined distance.
- Apply suction while withdrawing the catheter tip to the catheter window (the plastic cover will inflate from ventilation if the catheter is pulled back too far; the catheter will completely or partially occlude the ventilatory circuit if not pulled back far enough).
- To irrigate the catheter after suction: place normal saline syringe at the distal port adapter and squeeze saline into the port while simultaneously applying suction. Remove the saline and close the port when the catheter has been thoroughly rinsed.
- Rotate and lock the suction control cap to discontinue suction.
- Repeat procedure as indicated by results

obtained. All suctioning should take place with the head midline, because the catheter is only being passed the length of the endotracheal tube and not to the carina.
- Suction the nasopharynx and oropharynx prn.
- To facilitate pulmonary drainage, improve ventilation, and preserve skin integrity, change infant's position after suctioning. Adequate hydration thins secretions and thus facilitates their removal.
- Check respirator settings, including alarm system in "on" position. Check tube position to be sure the tracheal tube is not strained or bent.
- Reassess infant's condition after procedure by observing vital signs, color, and pulse oximeter, and auscultating chest to evaluate effectiveness of therapy. Ensure proper tube placement and adequate bilateral ventilation. Note tolerance of procedure on record, as well as need for increased oxygen or rate during suctioning.
- Note amount and type of secretions obtained.

NOTE: When two persons are available for suctioning, one remains "sterile" and does the suctioning while the other detaches the tracheal tube from the ventilator and hyperventilates the infant between suctionings.

Endotracheal suctioning is associated with physiologic alterations such as hypoxia, bradycardia, cardiac dysrhythmias, increased intracranial pressure, and atelectasis.[45,46] Pulse oximetry is a valuable tool in assessing oxygenation status during pulmonary hygiene. If oxygen saturation falls during suction, hyperventilate with a bag and/or increase Fio_2 10% to 15% above baseline concentration until recovery occurs. Muscle relaxation or paralysis with medications may be used to decrease periods of hypoxia or hyperoxia and increased intracranial pressure.[46]

Use of a closed suction system (i.e., an adapter to suction without disconnection from the ventilatory) reduces associated hypoxemia and bradycardia by enabling oxygenation and ventilation to continue during suction.[63,66,67] Advantages of the closed system include (1) enclosure of catheter in clear sheath that keeps it clean and enables visualization of secretions, (2) use of less suction pressure, (3) decreased need for two-person technique, and (4) cost-effectiveness. Despite less hypoxemia and bradycardia, a national survey of NICUs showed <5% using a closed suction system.[156]

Other aspects of therapy for the neonate with respiratory disease include the following:

- Supportive care and monitoring (see Chapters 2 through 12)
- Nutritional and metabolic care (see Chapters 13 through 18)
- Infection control and care of hematologic diseases (see Chapters 19 through 21)
- Care of family—parents and siblings (see Chapters 28 through 30)

Endotracheal Intubation

Endotracheal intubation may be accomplished by the orotracheal route or the nasotracheal route. Nasotracheal intubation is more difficult to perform, but it is easier to anchor the tube to prevent accidental extubation. It may be more appropriate for the larger, more vigorous infant. Smaller infants under 1250 g seem to do well with orotracheal tubes.

An endotracheal tube diameter that approximates the diameter of the infant's fifth digit generally fits snugly into the trachea. To measure for an endotracheal tube, the distance from the oral (or nasal) orifice to midway between the glottis and carina may be calculated by multiplying the crown-heel length by 0.2. In an emergency the distance from the lips to midway between the glottis and carina may be approximated by the 7-8-9-10 rule. The distance is 7 cm in an 1 kg infant, 8 cm in a 2 kg infant, 9 cm in a 3 kg infant, and 10 cm in a 4 kg infant.

Intubation Procedure

For long-term stability, commercially available endotracheal tube anchors prevent accidental extubation. Some nurseries still prefer fixing tubes with tape or sutures (see Chapter 4).

Extubation Procedure

Assess the infant's condition by observing the heart rate, color, and respiratory rate and effort, and by auscultating the chest. If the infant's condition is stable, proceed with extubation. Extubate before feeding, or empty the stomach to prevent vomiting. Because neonates are obligatory nasal breathers, the nasopharynx must also be suctioned and patent for extubation.

Hyperinflate with deep breaths with the infant's head in the midline and remove the tube on inflation[99] (to provide adequate lung expansion and prevent atelectasis), on expiration[64] (so that secretions that have accumulated around the tracheal tube are "blown away" on exhalation and tube removal), or while suctioning (to remove secretions that have accumulated around the tube). Place in a warm, humidified oxygen hood at Fio_2 to keep pulse oximeter at 92% to 94%.

Reassess the infant's condition, especially for signs of increased work of breathing and distress. Document tube removal and the infant's tolerance. Check arterial blood gases 15 to 20 minutes after extubation to assess oxygenation and ventilation status. Perform a chest x-ray examination to document atelectasis or fully expanded lungs. Continue pulmonary hygiene as long as the infant has secretions. Observe for complications of intubation (Table 22-3).

Mechanical Ventilation

Mechanical ventilation is used in neonates to correct abnormalities in oxygenation ($\downarrow Pao_2$), alveolar ventilation ($\uparrow Paco_2$), or respiratory effort (apnea or ineffectual respirations). It is not used to treat the primary disease, but frequently it is used to support the infant until the disease is treated or resolved. **Those newborns who meet the criteria in (Box 22-2) are candidates for assisted ventilation.**

Ventilator Settings

To individualize assisted ventilation, knowledge of the ventilator capabilities is essential.

Intermittent Mandatory Ventilation.   Most mechanical ventilators in common use today allow for intermittent mandatory ventilation (IMV). IMV provides a continuous flow of gas that is available to the infant during spontaneous respirations. Periodic occlusion of the system diverts gas under pressure to the infant. Because IMV provides for spontaneous and mechanical ventilation, only thea-

Table 22-3
Complications of Endotracheal Intubation

Complication	Comments
Immediate	
Malposition	
Too low	Usually in right mainstem bronchus; no or diminished breath sounds in left chest or upper right lobe; asymmetrical chest movement; atelectasis (withdraw tube until breath sounds are heard bilaterally and equally)
Too high	Inadequate ventilation bilaterally, especially at lung bases
Esophagus	Air movement auscultated in stomach with no or inadequate breath sounds
Obstruction	
Plug	Partial—no change or diminished breath sounds audible
	Complete—distant or no breath sounds audible
Kinking of the tube	
Head position	Flexion or extension of the head results in diminished or blocked air flow
Perforation	
Vocal cords	
Trachea	
Pharynx	
Esophagus	
Pulmonary Hemorrhage	
Infection	
Air Leak	
Increased Intracranial Pressure	
Postextubation	
Migratory lobar collapse	Prevent and treat with pulmonary hygiene
Diffuse microatelectasis	In very-low-birth-weight infants may be associated with apnea; treatable by pulmonary hygiene or nasal CPAP, or both
Long Term	
General	Vocal cord inflammation, stenosis, and eventual dysfunction; tracheoesophageal fistula; subglottic stenosis; tracheal inflammation and stenosis; necrotizing tracheobronchitis contributes to bronchopulmonary dysplasia
Specific to the Type of Tube	
Orotracheal	Abnormal dentition; gingival and palatal erosion; palatal grooves
Nasotracheal	Otitis media; erosion of alae nasae and nasal septum; nasal stenosis

mount of ventilatory assistance that is needed by the individual infant is provided.

Synchronized Intermittent Mandatory Ventilation (SIMV). SIMV enables synchronization of ventilation breaths by sensing (through an airway or diaphragmatic sensor) the neonate's initiation of respiration, then triggering of a mechanical breath. Synchronized ventilation prevents the generation of excessive pressure within the respiratory tract when infant exhalation coincides with mechanical ventilation. Use of SIMV is associated with a decrease in (1) oxygen need, (2) duration of ventilator therapy, (3) incidence of BPD, and (4) severity of IVH.[16,79,122,161]

Continuous Distending Pressure. CDP is expressed in centimeters of water. CDP may be given without IMV (CPAP) or with it (positive end expiratory pressure [PEEP])

The effects of CDP include increased alveolar stability, increased functional residual capacity, decreased risk of atelectasis, increased intrathoracic pressure, and impeded passage of fluid from lung capillaries to alveolar spaces, aiding in the prevention or treatment of pulmonary edema. Effects of changes in PEEP are dependent upon severity of lung disease and degree of lung inflation. High PEEP in the presence of relatively compliant lungs will cause overdistention, worsen Pao_2, and in-

---

Box 22-2

Criteria that Qualify Newborns for Assisted Ventilation

I. Blood gases
   A. Severe hypoxemia (Pao_2 <50 to 60 mm Hg with Fio_2 of 0.7 to 1.0,[15] or Pao_2 <60 mm Hg with Fio_2 >0.4 in infant <1250 g)[45]
   B. Severe hypercapnia ($Paco_2$ >55 to 65 mm Hg with pH <7.20 to 7.25)[23]
II. Clinical
   A. Apnea and bradycardia requiring resuscitation in infants with lung disease or unresponsive to CPAP, or theophylline therapy in preterm infants with normal lungs
   B. Inefficient respiratory effort such as gasping respirations from asphyxia, narcosis, or primary cardiopulmonary disease
   C. Shock and asphyxia with hypoperfusion and hypotension
   D. RDS in infants weighing <1000 g, frequently making them incapable of maintaining ventilation (in these infants it has been suggested that mechanical ventilation without a trial of CPAP is appropriate)[49]

CPAP, Continuous positive airway pressure; *RDS,* respiratory distress syndrome.

---

crease pulmonary vascular resistance. In addition, overdistention may increase the risk of barotrauma. However, the use of levels of PEEP that are too low contributes to hypoxia and pulmonary hypertension because of low lung volumes. Experimentally, acute lung injury is actually worsened by the failure to recruit adequate lung volume by using insufficient PEEP.

Peak Inspiratory Pressure (PIP). PIP is the maximum pressure measured during the delivery of gas (inspiration) during conventional mechanical ventilation. PIP reflects the effects of the amount of gas delivered to the lungs in a given breath (tidal volume) and the underlying mechanical properties of the lungs. For example, if the same PIP is used in neonates with severe RDS (with stiff, noncompliant lungs) as in neonates ventilated for apnea with minimal lung disease, the tidal volume will be much greater in the later group. Recent studies suggest that overdistention of the lungs caused by excessive tidal volumes, and not pressure itself, worsens acute lung injury (so called "volutrauma"). Thus adverse effects of high PIP are dependent upon the degree of lung disease.

Rate. The rate reflects how often a volume of gas in the system is delivered to the infant. It is expressed as breaths per minute. Too rapid a rate, especially with a poorly inflated lung, can cause lung injury caused by gas trapping ("inadvertent PEEP").

Inspiration/Expiration Ratio. The inspiration/expiration ratio (I/E ratio) reflects the relationship between time spent in inspiration and time spent in expiration. When the rate is 60 breaths/min and the total respiratory cycle is 1 second, an I/E ratio of 1:1 means 0.5 second is inspiration and 0.5 second is expiration. If the I/E ratio is 1:2 with a rate of 60 and the total respiratory cycle is 1 second, inspiration is 0.33 second and expiration is 0.66 second.

Prolonged inspiration may be associated with more efficient ventilation, optimal arterial oxygenation, a higher risk of air leak, and impeding of venous return.[23] Prolonged expiration also improves oxygenation, especially in air-trapping conditions (such as rapid rate ventilation or airway disease).[17]

Mean Airway Pressure. Mean airway pressure (MAP) is the amount of pressure transmitted to the airway throughout an entire respiratory cycle.[17] Any change in ventilator settings affects the MAP. MAP is most affected by changes in PEEP, inspiratory time, or I/E ratio.[9] MAP is associated with optimal oxygenation ($\uparrow$ Pao_2) and ventilation ($\downarrow$ $Paco_2$) when pressures range between 6 and 14 cm of water.[17] When MAP exceeds 14 cm of water, there is a progressive deterioration of the blood gases ($\downarrow$ Pao_2, $\uparrow$ $Paco_2$).[17] The effects of any given level of MAP are dependent upon the changes in mechanical properties of the lung caused by the primary disease. For example, high MAP may be needed to improve oxygenation in severe RDS or meconium aspiration syndrome, especially in term neonates. Low MAP in this setting will cause sustained hypoxemia and atelectasis. In contrast, use of high MAP in neonates in the presence of minimal lung disease will cause overdistention and deterioration of arterial blood gas tensions. In general, the goal of increasing MAP is to improve Pao_2 and is usually achieved by small increases in PEEP or prolongation of inspiratory time. Repeat chest x-ray examination and continuous monitoring of blood pressure and oxygenation (by pulse oximeter) will help determine the optimal level of MAP.

Usual starting pressures for beginning ventilatory support are listed in Table 22-4.

The inspired oxygen tension is adjusted to provide an adequate arterial oxygen tension. If the infant still has difficulty maintaining an adequate carbon dioxide tension, a faster rate and/or greater inspiratory pressure would be indicated.

Table 22-5 lists the usual effects to be expected from changing specific ventilator settings.

To evaluate the efficacy of mechanical ventilation and any adjustments made with the system, continuous monitoring with pulse oximeters or transcutaneous monitors (see Chapter 7) must be maintained and/or blood gases obtained. Blood gases should be obtained 15 to 30 minutes after beginning ventilatory support or after any change in settings, every 4 to 6 hours if no change is made in ventilator settings, and as needed based on the clinical condition of the infant.

Arterial blood gases should be maintained in the following range, although some advocate accepting high $Paco_2$ and lower Pao_2 in some infants (see Chapter 10):

Pao_2	**60 to 80 mm Hg**
$Paco_2$	**35 to 45 mm Hg**
pH	**7.35 to 7.45**

Optimal arterial blood gas tensions are somewhat controversial. To decrease the risk of acute lung injury by minimizing lung overdistention and barotrauma, some neonatologists advocate strategies that target lower Pao_2 and higher $Paco_2$ ("permissive hypercapnia"). The risks and benefits of such strategies depend on the specific clinical setting. If excessive ventilator settings are required to lower $Paco_2$, allowing $Paco_2$ to rise (as long as the pH is greater than 7.25) is often accepted in an attempt to avoid lung injury. Whether high $Paco_2$ will increase cerebral blood flow, thus worsening the neonate's neurologic outcome is uncertain. However, hyperventilation (low $Paco_2$) can decrease cerebral blood flow and oxygen delivery to the brain and may contribute to adverse long-term neurologic sequelae. In addition, since the goal of respiratory care is to optimize oxygen delivery to tissues, the effect of a given Pao_2 is partly dependent on cardiac function (see Chapter 23) and hemoglobin level (see Chapter 19). Accepting lower Pao_2 and O_2 saturation may lead to worse outcomes in the setting of systemic hypotension and poor cardiac function (e.g., sepsis).

Several therapeutic interventions, including surfactant, high-frequency ventilation (HFV), steroids, and ECMO, have been shown to be effective in special clinical settings. In addition, more

---

Table 22-4
Starting Pressures for Beginning Ventilatory Support

Parameter	Range
Fio_2	At previous level or 10% higher than previously required concentration
PEEP	4 to 6 cm water
PIP	16 to 20 cm water
Rate	40 to 60
I/E ratio	1:1 to 1:2

PEEP, Positive end expiratory pressure; *PIP,* peak inspiratory pressure.

Table 22-5
Usual Effects of Changing Mechanical (Traditional) Ventilator Settings

Increasing	Causes			Complications
	Pa_{O_2}	Pa_{CO_2}	pH	
Fi_{O_2}	↑	0	0	Oxygen toxicity (bronchopulmonary dysplasia, retrolental fibroplasia); absorption atelectasis; Fi_{O_2} may have no effect on oxygenation in the presence of severe R → L (right to left) shunt (PPHN), congenital heart disease, or marked intrapulmonary shunting due to severe parenchymal lung disease
CPAP/PEEP	↑	0/↑	0/↓	Hypoventilation with respiratory acidosis; decreased cardiac output with metabolic acidosis; air leaks
PIP	↑	↓	↑	Barotrauma with air leaks and bronchopulmonary dysplasia; respiratory alkalosis
Rate	↓	↓	↑	Respiratory alkalosis
I/E ratio (1:1 to 1:2)	↑	0	0	Increased intrapleural pressure; decreased venous return

CPAP, Continuous positive airway pressure; *PEEP,* positive end expiratory pressure; *PIP,* peak inspiratory pressure.

recently, novel therapies, including inhaled NO and partial liquid ventilation (PLV) are currently under study.

High-Frequency Ventilation

Barotrauma is a major contributing factor to the development of chronic lung disease or death from progressive lung injury in newborns treated with conventional mechanical ventilation. The goal of new ventilatory strategies such as HFV is to reduce barotrauma by its application early in the course of RDS, or to reduce the progression of injury in infants already having advanced pulmonary interstitial emphysema, recurrent pneumothoraxes, or bronchopleural fistula. In addition to minimizing lung injury, the goal of HFV is to enhance oxygenation more effectively than conventional ventilation in some clinical settings. For example, the use of high-frequency oscillating ventilators (HFOV) has been shown to reduce the need for ECMO in term neonates.[26]

HFV differs from conventional modes of ventilator support in that it uses smaller tidal volumes at supraphysiologic frequencies, allowing for generation of lower intrathoracic pressure. At high frequencies the calculated tidal volume is less than dead space. Thus the physics of gas flow and exchange are different from the traditional teaching of lung mechanics and are thought to be related to augmented diffusion. Reduction in barotrauma occurs by allowing for ventilation with a very small pressure amplitude around the mean airway pressure in the distal airway. Therefore at high frequencies (commonly 10 to 15 Hertz), the peak inspiratory and expiratory pressures approach MAP (i.e., lower downstream pressures). Because of this effect, higher MAP can be used to improve oxygenation without worsening lung injury. As observed with overdistention with conventional ventilation, excessive MAP to achieve optimal lung inflation and oxygenation may account for the marked center-to-center differences in HFOV use.[77]

HFV can be achieved by jet ventilators or by oscillators. Jet ventilators deliver short bursts of high-flow gases directly into the proximal airway via a small cannula and have a passive exhalation cycle. Oscillators vibrate columns of air and have active exhalation cycles. Although clinical comparisons of these two methods are still pending, a high incidence of necrotizing tracheitis has been reported with high-frequency jet ventilation. This problem, however, appears to be related more to insufficient humidification during jet ventilation.[28] Hypotension caused by reduced cardiac output is prevented by avoiding hyperinflation.[28]

Animal studies of preterm baboons have demonstrated dramatic effects of homogeneity of ventilation applied shortly after birth in comparison with conventional methods, and the potential application of this method in early RDS to lessen the incidence of BPD has been suggested.[120] Clinical studies have demonstrated that with HFV it is possible to ventilate infants with severe BPD and pulmonary interstitial emphysema at lower levels than with conventional methods and improve gas exchange in severely ill neonates. However, early application of HFV, using either oscillators or jet ventilators, has failed to reduce morbidity and mortality of RDS.[22,76] The role of HFV in the treatment of newborns needs further delineation with RCTs. HFOV in combination with other therapies, especially inhaled NO, may contribute more to improved clinical outcome than either therapy used alone.[2]

Extracorporeal Membrane Oxygenation

ECMO is a modification of cardiopulmonary bypass that allows for more prolonged therapy than is traditionally performed in the operating room for cardiac surgery. ECMO establishes a pulmonary bypass circuit, allowing gas exchange to occur outside of the lung by perfusion of blood through a membrane oxygenator. Blood is drawn from a catheter in the right internal jugular vein or right atrium, oxygenated as it crosses the membrane, and then returned to the patient via the right common carotid artery (venoarterial ECMO) or the femoral vein (venovenous ECMO). The pump produces a continuous, nonpulsatile flow through the membrane oxygenator as the patient is kept heparinized and continues to be ventilated at low pressures, rates, and oxygen tensions. The goal of this therapy is to "buy time" for the severely injured lung to heal while attenuating ongoing lung injury by decreasing exposure to hyperoxia and barotrauma. Therapy can be continued for several days, until lung recovery appears sufficient to maintain adequate gas tension without ECMO. Early clinical success has been reported in such disorders as severe RDS, meconium aspiration syndrome, and PPHN.

A multicenter randomized trial of ECMO therapy in the United Kingdom has demonstrated improved survival in term neonates with severe hypoxemic respiratory failure and PPHN.[159] Controversy persists, however, regarding the optimal timing of ECMO therapy for hypoxemic neonates. Delays in applying ECMO therapy may potentially worsen outcome; however, ECMO therapy is invasive, costly, and is associated with adverse outcomes, including intracranial hemorrhage. In addition, the use of alternative therapies such as surfactant, inhaled NO, and HFOV have reduced the need for ECMO in many hypoxemic term neonates. Considerable variability exists between centers, however, suggesting that the use of these techniques is partly dependent upon the clinical strategy and other issues in patient management. Ongoing clinical studies are evaluating the relative roles for these interventions in reducing the need for ECMO without worsening the risks for mortality or long-term sequelae, such as chronic lung disease and neurodevelopmental outcome.[91]

Inhaled Nitric Oxide. Inhaled NO is one of the exciting new developments in the treatment of hypoxemic newborns. Based on the initial discovery that vascular endothelial cells produce a potent vasodilator substance ("endothelium-derived relaxing factor"), which was later identified as NO,[84] clinical research into the use of NO began. Since NO could be delivered as a gas, its potential role for clinical treatment of pulmonary hypertension and hypoxemia was quickly recognized and tested in adults with primary pulmonary hypertension.[131] Experimental studies demonstrated that low doses of inhaled NO cause potent, selective, and sustained pulmonary vasodilation in the perinatal pulmonary circulation.[94] The vasodilator response is due to NO stimulation of soluble guanylate cyclase activity, increasing cyclic guanosine monophosphate (GMP) in vascular smooth muscle and causing vasorelaxation. Selectivity of inhaled NO for the pulmonary circulation is based on direct delivery of NO into the lung; since NO is avidly bound by hemoglobin in red blood cells and inactivated after metabolism to nitrite and nitrate, there are no direct effects on systemic arterial pressure. Since hypoxia in PPHN is mostly due to right-to-left shunting across the ductus arteriosus and foramen ovalae, selective pulmonary vasodilation is essential for improving oxygenation. Early clinical studies of inhaled NO demonstrated brief exposure to inhaled NO, acutely improved oxygenation, and lowered pulmonary artery pressure.[95,140] With prolonged low-dose inhaled NO treatment (6 ppm), sustained responsiveness to inhaled NO led to complete clinical recovery without the need for ECMO therapy. The effectiveness of this low-dose clinical strategy was confirmed in a subsequent study.[94] Preliminary data from a randomized multicenter study has demonstrated decreased need for ECMO in severe PPHN. Clinical studies have further demonstrated that combined therapy of inhaled NO with HFOV may be more effective than either therapy alone in select cases.[95] Inhaled NO also improves oxygenation in premature neonates with severe RDS, but there are concerns regarding potential toxicities, including pulmonary edema or hemorrhage, chronic lung disease, and increased severity of intracranial hemorrhage. Whether these toxicities occur in preterm or term neonates is uncertain, and randomized controlled studies examining relative risks and benefits are needed. At this time, the use of inhaled NO remains experimental and has not been approved by the Food and Drug Administration (FDA).

Partial Liquid Ventilation.[30]   Although prenatal steroids, surfactant, and HFOV therapies have improved the clinical course of sick preterm newborns with respiratory failure, the morbidity of severe RDS persists. Based on experimental studies from over the past 40 years, it has been recognized that perfluorocarbon liquids can improve oxygenation (in animal models) in various respiratory disorders.[146] Experimental studies of liquid ventilation have demonstrated its high oxygen solubility and striking surface tension-lowering properties, suggesting its potential efficacy in clinical disease. Early clinical use of ventilation with perfluorocarbons suggests improved oxygenation in selected patients.[107] Ongoing clinical trials are evaluating its potential role in neonatal respiratory failure.

Weaning from the Ventilator

When the infant's condition improves, ventilatory support is slowly removed. Evidence of improvement includes biochemical parameters and clinical parameters:

- Arterial blood gases are stable and physiologic.

- There are spontaneous respiratory efforts against the ventilator when it is connected or against suctioning.
- There is increased activity and muscle tone and progressively decreasing Fio_2 requirement.

With IMV there is a gradual decrease in mechanical ventilation with a corresponding increase in spontaneous respiration. One ventilator setting at a time is changed, and arterial blood gases and pulse oximetry values are evaluated to determine the infant's response before another adjustment is made. Because each ventilator parameter has risks and benefits, each parameter must be evaluated before the decision is made as to which one will be lowered. Because high concentrations of oxygen may be toxic to the lungs and hyperoxia may damage the eyes, oxygen is usually lowered first to a level below 80% in 5% to 10% increments. PIP is lowered in 1 to 2 cm increments to a level of 16 cm of water, and respiratory rate is lower in 1 to 5 breaths/min increments until the infant is on CPAP alone or has a rate of 5 breaths/min or less. Once adequate oxygenation and ventilation on CPAP alone have been maintained, the infant may be extubated and placed in an oxygen hood. Oxygen should be adjusted with the use of pulse oximetry.

During the recovery phase of RDS (approximately 72 hours), changes in lung compliance occur rapidly. Hyperoxia, air leaks, increased intracranial pressure, and decreased cardiac output easily occur if high pressures and high oxygen concentrations are not decreased as rapidly as the lung is recovering.

Infants who are difficult or impossible to wean from the ventilator may have BPD, PDA, or CNS damage that affects the respiratory control center.

General Complications

Acute Complications

Acute and chronic complications are the result of the disease process, treatment, or both. Beginning with the least invasive therapy and progressing to more complicated ones only as needed accomplishes two goals. It individualizes therapy and minimizes risk of complications. Continuous monitoring of the individual infant's progress is vital in decreasing complications from the disease and from the interventions used to support the infant or to treat the primary condition. Complications of respiratory diseases are listed in Box 22-3.

Sudden deterioration of the infant's condition is an emergency, and the cause must be found and corrected as soon as possible to minimize further damage. Causes of sudden deterioration are listed in Box 22-4.

Respiratory

Management of the infant who has suddenly deteriorated begins with a visual inspection. The oxygen hood, CPAP, or ventilator must be properly connected and free of water. If all connections are intact, the infant must be disconnected from assisted ventilation and connected to a resuscitation bag (that is connected to an oxygen source and kept at the bedside). Manual ventilation matching pressure, rates, and Fio_2 to ventilator settings must be maintained. If the infant improves with these inter-

ventions, mechanical failure of the ventilator should be suspected. Assistance should be summoned to find the mechanical problem or replace the system. The infant's respiratory effort must be manually assisted until the problem is solved.

If the infant does not improve with manual ventilation, there is probably a problem with the tube. The infant's condition can be assessed by auscultating the chest for quality of breath sounds. Findings and what they suggest are listed in Table 22-6.

The endotracheal tube should be suctioned quickly. If there is no improvement in clinical condition or air entry, the tube should be replaced while supporting the infant with bag and mask ventilation. If the tube is too low, it can be repositioned by pulling it back 0.5 to 1 cm. If air entry and clinical condition improve with auscultation, the tube must be secured in the new position and an x-ray examination made for tube placement. If assessment of the chest leads to suspicion of accidental extubation, the tube must be removed, ventilation with bag and mask administered, and reintubation performed. If the infant does not improve with manual ventilation and the tube is in place, an air leak or IVH could be the cause.

Monitors and ventilators are equipped with alarm systems to warn care providers of sudden

---

Box 22-3

Complications of Respiratory Disease

I. Acute
  A. Sudden deterioration of condition
  B. Air leaks
  C. Central nervous system
    1. Hypoxic-ischemic injury
    2. Increased intracranial pressure
    3. Hemorrhage
  D. Cardiac
    1. Patent ductus arteriosus
    2. Decreased cardiac output
  E. Infection
  F. Bleeding diathesis
  G. Tube
  H. Pulmonary hemorrhage
II. Chronic
  A. Oxygen toxicity and barotrauma (BPD)
  B. Hyperoxia (retinopathy of prematurity)
  C. Hypoxia
  D. Tube

Box 22-4

Causes of Sudden Deterioration

I. Tube
  A. Accidental extubation
  B. Accidental disconnection
  C. Plug
II. Machine malfunction
  A. Ventilator or CPAP device
  B. Oxygen blender
  C. Tubing and connections
III. Alarm system "off"
IV. Severe hypoxia
V. Metabolic factors
VI. Air leak
VII. Intraventricular hemmorhage

CPAP, Continuous positive airway pressure.

Table 22-6
Findings and Cause of Infant's Condition with Chest Auscultation

Finding	Possible Cause
No air entry bilaterally	Air leak
	Plugged endotracheal tube
Diminished air entry	Air leak
	Endotracheal tube too high
Air entry over stomach	Accidental extubation
Air entry unequal	Air leak
	Endotracheal tube too low
Cardiac point of maximum intensity shifted	Air leak with tension

changes in the infant's condition or in supportive systems. It is imperative that all alarm systems be maintained in the "on" position. Turning the alarms "off" during care for such procedures as suctioning and weighing creates the risk of forgetting to turn them "on" again. In a busy NICU the compromised infant may not be visually noticed until the hypoxia is so severe that resuscitation is more difficult or impossible. Monitor parameters (both high and low alarm settings) must be individualized for each infant and recorded (see Chapter 7).

The sick neonate may experience a severe hypoxic insult when oxygen is too rapidly altered during caregiving procedures. Feeding, weighing, or turning without an alternative oxygen source may cause a sudden decrease in Pa_{O_2}, pulmonary vasoconstriction, hypoperfusion, and an iatrogenic worsening of the condition. Prolonged endotracheal tube suctioning (15 to 20 seconds) causes hypoxia and atelectasis. Care must be organized to conserve energy, minimize hypoxic insults, and maintain the infant in physiologic homeostasis.[34,45,110] Alternative oxygen sources must be provided when the usual method of oxygen delivery is disrupted for giving care. Small alterations in Fi_{O_2} prevent rapid increases or decreases in oxygen tension.

Metabolic Factors

Hypoglycemia must never be overlooked as the cause of sudden collapse. Undetected infiltration or disconnection of IV fluids may cause a precipitous drop in blood glucose, with respiratory irregularity, apnea, or seizures. Quickly checking the blood glucose with a reagent strip is always warranted. If low blood glucose is not the cause of the sudden deterioration, it may be a complication of the asphyxial episode. After the infant is stabilized, screening for hypoglycemia and providing adequate fluids and glucose are appropriate (see Chapter 14).

Hypothermia and overwhelming sepsis with their associated metabolic derangements may be the cause of sudden deterioration. Muted response to cold stress is a sequela of asphyxial insult, and cold stress must be avoided after the acute episode. A high level of suspicion for infection should accompany sudden deterioration (see Chapters 6 and 21).

Air Leaks

Physiology. When air dissects from an alveolus, it follows the tracheobronchial tree and may accumulate in the mediastinum (pneumomediastinum), in the pleural space (pneumothorax), in the space surrounding the heart (pneumopericardium), or in the peritoneal cavity (pneumoperitoneum). Air leaks are complications of respiratory diseases and treatment strategies.

The free air released from ruptured alveoli may lead to pulmonary interstitial emphysema (PIE) (Fig. 22-1). This free air intravasates into interstitial tissue and can compromise pulmonary vascular circulation and decrease ventilation of the lungs. Localized pulmonary interstitial emphysema sometimes resolves spontaneously. Frequently it can continue for weeks or even months. Use of HFV has improved the outcome of these infants.

Etiologies. Those infants at increased risk for the development of air leaks fall into three specific categories: healthy term neonates, those with pulmonary diseases, and those receiving positive pressure support (CPAP and IMV).

Healthy term neonates generate pressures of 40 to 80 cm of water for their first breath of life. Therefore a spontaneous air leak is more common in the neonatal period (2% to 10%) than at any other time of life.

Pulmonary diseases such as RDS as a result of stiff, noncompliant lungs require higher pressures for alveolar ventilation. Aspiration syndromes

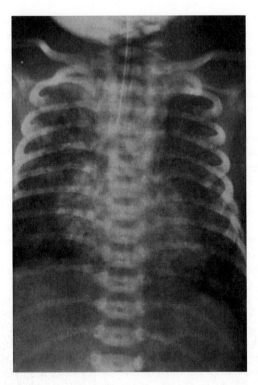

Figure 22-1 Pulmonary interstitial emphysema (PIE).

cause a ball-valve obstruction of debris with distal air trapping (meconium, milk, amniotic fluid, blood, and mucus). Hypoplastic lungs create a risk for air leaks because lung growth and development are abnormal and the lungs are stiff and noncompliant (diaphragmatic hernia and oligohydramnios syndrome). In either congenital lobar or pulmonary interstitial emphysema, alveolar rupture is associated with positive-pressure ventilation.

Positive-pressure ventilation, especially with excessive pressure, results in overdistention with alveolar rupture and air dissection. It occurs in 16% to 36% of infants who are ventilated by CPAP or IMV, or resuscitated with a bag and mask or with an endotracheal tube and bag.

Prevention. Using the least amount of positive pressure to obtain physiologic results decreases the chances of air leaks. The incidence of pneumothorax is reduced in surfactant-treated prematures and with the use of HFV.[28,74] Scrupulously clearing the airway before auscultation and using pressure gauges on resuscitation equipment may prevent aspiration and the possibility of inadvertently using pressure that is too high. Rapid recognition of at-risk infants, recognition of clinical manifestations and diagnosis, and rapid emergency treatment improve survival and decrease the long-term sequelae of hypoxia and ischemia.

Data Collection

History. Pneumothorax or other air leaks should be suspected when any one of the following infants takes a sudden turn for the worse:

- A preterm infant with RDS either with or without positive-pressure support
- A term or postterm infant with meconium-stained amniotic fluid
- An infant with an x-ray picture of interstitial or lobar emphysema
- An infant requiring resuscitation at birth
- An infant receiving CPAP or positive-pressure ventilation

Signs and Symptoms. Asymptomatic air leaks occur in term neonates, frequently require no treatment, and resolve spontaneously in 24 to 48 hours. Gradual onset of symptoms is characterized by increasing difficulty in ventilation, oxygenation, and perfusion. Early clinical manifestations may include restlessness and irritability; lethargy; tachypnea; and use of accessory muscles including grunting, flaring, and retractions. These subtle clinical changes may be unnoticed until the infant progresses to a sudden, profound collapse.

Sudden and severe deterioration in clinical course is characterized by:

- Profound generalized cyanosis
- Bradycardia
- Decrease in height of QRS complex on monitor
- Air hunger including gasping and anxious facies
- Diminished or shifted breath sounds
- Chest asymmetry
- Diminished, shifted, or muffled cardiac sounds and point of maximal intensity
- Severe hypotension and poor peripheral perfusion

- Easily palpable liver and spleen
- Subcutaneous emphysema
- Cardiorespiratory arrest

Laboratory Data. Arterial blood gas determinations reveal increasing hypoxemia ($\downarrow$ Pa$_{O_2}$), increasing hypercapnia ($\uparrow$ Pa$_{CO_2}$), and a persistent metabolic acidosis with gradual onset of symptoms. Transillumination of the chest with a fiberoptic probe may reveal hyperlucency of the affected side when compared with the other side.[104] A chest x-ray examination is the definitive diagnostic technique in air leaks. Because clinical manifestations of many other diseases may be similar to air leaks, the only way to be sure of the diagnosis is to take a chest x-ray examination. Anteroposterior and lateral films must be obtained. Occasionally a decubitus lateral x-ray film may be of value.

Treatment. An air leak is a surgical emergency of the chest. Tension within the chest cavity compromises lung excursion and cardiac output; without prompt treatment the infant will not survive. Trained care providers must be immediately available to provide emergency management in any institution that provides positive-pressure ventilatory support.

Evacuation of trapped air to decrease tension and allow proper organ function is the goal of treatment. Pneumomediastinum rarely needs to be treated, but pneumopericardium may result in cardiac tamponade and need needle aspiration and/or tube drainage. Pneumoperitoneum must be differentiated from a perforated viscus.

A suggested conservative treatment is endotracheal intubation of the unaffected lung. The tube is advanced 1 to 2 cm beyond the carina to occlude the involved lung. This procedure is difficult to perform if the left lung is involved. If the pulmonary interstitial emphysema is localized to one lung or lobe of the lung, differential ventilation or surgical removal of the lobe may be curative. Pneumothorax may be treated with needle aspiration of air. Tube thoracotomy with suction drainage is frequently required.

Immediate Supportive Care. The head of the bed is elevated 30 to 40 degrees. This decreases the work of breathing by using gravity to localize the air in the upper chest and to push the abdominal organs downward away from the diaphragm.

Oxygen at 100% concentration is administered. The two goals for using 100% oxygen for immediate care are to attempt to improve oxygenation in a severely compromised infant and to use a nitrogen washout technique to increase by as much as sixfold the rate of absorption of the trapped air.[100]

CAUTION. Prolonged administration of 100% oxygen to treat an air leak in term infants has been used. However, exclusive use of 100% oxygen to treat trapped air is not recommended in the preterm infant because of the risk of developing retinopathy of prematurity and the length of time necessary to obtain complete resolution.

The severely compromised infant requires immediate emergency procedures. A diagnostic and therapeutic thoracentesis may be necessary in life threatening situations where there is not time to wait for x-ray examination.

Needle Aspiration. A scalp vein needle (23 to 25 gauge), a three-way stopcock, and a 10 to 20 ml syringe may be used for needle aspiration. The equipment is connected (syringe-stopcock-needle), the chest is prepared for asepsis, and the needle is inserted in the third intercostal space in the anterior axillary line. A slight pop may be felt when the pleura is entered. Air is withdrawn into the syringe and evacuated into the room by turning the stopcock. This procedure is repeated until no more air can be aspirated or until a chest tube can be placed.

Chest Tube. Tube thoracotomy is the definitive treatment for pneumothorax. The insertion of a chest tube is an invasive procedure that requires strict surgical technique, with each operator wearing a gown, gloves, mask, and cap. The infant should be appropriately positioned, restrained, and monitored before the chest is prepared for asepsis. Ideally, the anterior chest wall should be prepped a minimum of 3 minutes. If a special tray is not available, a minor suture tray will usually contain the necessary instruments. Necessary equipment is as follows:

- Chest tube (no. 8 to 12 Fr Argyle)
- Iodine or Betadine scrub solution
- Gloves, gown, mask, hat
- Sterile drapes
- Syringes
- Sterile sponges (gauze)

- Medicine cups
- Lidocaine 1% without epinephrine
- Scalpel blades (no. 11 or 15)
- Hemostat (mosquito and Kelly)
- Scissors
- Needle holder
- Sterile suture
- Sterile connectors (straight)
- Tubing
- Infant disposable underwater seal drainage system (two- or three-bottle or Pleurevac system)
- Suction
- Sterile saline
- Tape

The insertion site depends on the clinician's preference. In the lateral approach, the site is the fourth to sixth intercostal space on or lateral to the anterior axillary line. In the superior approach, the site is the second or third intercostal space on or just lateral to the midclavicular line (Fig. 22-2). Some researchers have documented that the superior approach is more effective for aspiration of pneumothoraxes.[120]

After infiltration of the area with 1% lidocaine, a small incision is made. A purse-string suture should be placed around the incision with ends left loose. A curved hemostat is inserted into the incision and opened. The catheter is advanced through the interspace and into the pleural space. The most frequent error on the part of the inexperienced operator is applying too little force to enter the pleural cavity. The purse-string is tightened and tied, and then tied to the chest tube. The tube is connected to the underwater drainage system, which may then be connected to a continuous suction (10 to 20 cm of water is most commonly recommended). The tube should be secured with tape. An x-ray examination is used to confirm

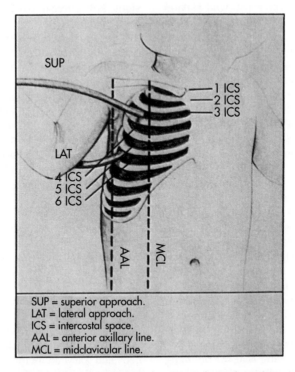

Figure 22-2 Chest tube insertion site. *SUP,* Superior approach; *LAT,* lateral approach; *ICS,* Intercostal space; *AAL,* anterior axillary line *MCL,* midclavicular line. (From Oellrich RG: Pneumothorax; chest tubes and the neonate, *MCN,* 10:31, 1985.)

placement of the tube and to evaluate the effectiveness of the therapy.

Complications.   In some instances complications have arisen from the placement of chest tubes in neonates. These include hemorrhage, lung perforation, infarction, and phrenic nerve injury with eventration of the diaphragm. Clinical signs of eventration (elevation of the diaphragm into the thoracic cavity) include a shift of the umbilicus upward and toward the affected side.[115]

Care of Chest Tube and Drainage System.   The chest tube drainage system removes air and fluid material from the pleural space to restore negative pressure and expand the lung. Care providers must be familiar with the operation of the drainage system used in the nursery. The single-bottle water seal system drains air and fluid by gravity and blocks atmospheric air from being drawn into the pleural space. In addition to the water seal, the multiple-bottle systems allow suction to be applied to facilitate drainage and expansion. The Pleurevac system is a single plastic unit divided into three chambers: the collection, water seal, and suction chambers.

Oscillation of fluid in the tube demonstrates effective communication between the pleural space and the drainage bottle. In the small, sick infant, intrapleural pressure may only cause fluctuation in the tube at the chest wall. Fluctuation in either the tube or bottle should be observed. Fluctuation may cease as a result of fibrin or blood clots obstructing the tube, kinked or compressed tubing, or the suction apparatus not working properly. Milking and stripping the chest tube is generally unnecessary if only air is being removed. Presence of clots or debris may require gentle kneading of the tube.[25] Milking and stripping generate tremendously high pressures that may entrap and damage the lung in the chest tube eyelets.[41]

Bubbling in the drainage bottle indicates that air is being removed from the pleural space. Continuous bubbling may indicate an air leak in the system. To locate the source of the leak, the tube is momentarily clamped (beginning close to the chest and working toward the bottle) with a rubber-tipped hemostat. When the clamp is placed between the air leak and the water seal, the bubbling will stop. Patency of the tube, fluctuation, and bubbling should be observed and charted hourly.

Excessive or insufficient fluid in the drainage bottles may interfere with proper function of the drainage system. The bottle may need to be changed, or sterile saline may need to be added.

Frequent turning is important for maximum drainage and lung expansion. Proper stabilizing and positioning of the chest tube is necessary for function, comfort, and prevention of accidental removal. The tubing may be secured by encircling it with an adhesive tab, placing a safety pin through the tape (not the tube), and securing it to the bed. If the tube becomes dislodged, the opening should be covered with sterile gauze and pressure applied until the tube can be replaced.

When the infant is moved for such procedures as x-ray examination and weighing, the tube must be stabilized by holding it close to the chest. If the closed system is disturbed (e.g., broken bottle), the tube should be clamped with a rubber-tipped hemostat that should always be kept at the bedside. The chest tube should be clamped for as short a time as possible. After necessary clamping, vital signs and clinical conditions should be closely monitored.

Bottles should be stabilized by being taped to an incubator or warmer so that they are not accidentally broken or picked up. The bottles must always be below the level of the infant's chest to prevent water from being pulled into the pleural space.

Removal of Chest Tubes.   When bubbling has ceased for at least 24 hours, and the chest x-ray films show no free air for 12 to 24 hours, the chest tube may be removed. Rapid, sterile removal of the tube is followed by application of a petrolatum gauze pressure dressing.

CNS Insult

Acute insult to the CNS may result in increased intracranial pressure, hemorrhage, or hypoxic ischemic brain injury (see Chapter 25).

Cardiac Complications

CDP or IMV may exert sufficient pressure on the pulmonary capillary bed to raise pulmonary artery pressure and interfere with cardiac output.[82] The effect of CDP or IMV on the pulmonary vascular bed and cardiac output may be alleviated by lowering the PIP, or PEEP, or both. At times a fluid infusion to increase the intravascular volume may overcome the resistance to the pulmonary blood flow. The effect of MAP on cardiac output is difficult to monitor in most NICUs, because pulmonary artery or pulmonary wedge pressures are not routinely obtained. Until such time as these measurements are routinely obtained, the best CPAP is determined only on clinical grounds.

PDA is the most common cardiac complication in neonates with respiratory disease. Most often it is manifested by an increasing oxygen requirement or increased dependency on ventilatory support (see Chapter 23).

Infection and Bleeding

Procedures such as intubation expose the neonate to the risk of acquired infection. Scrupulous attention to technique when caring for respiratory equipment and performing procedures such as suctioning the endotracheal tube minimizes the risks of infection. Hand washing before and after every contact with the neonate is the best method of preventing hospital-acquired infection in an already compromised, sick neonate. Neonates who are severely ill with respiratory disease may exhibit bleeding diathesis at birth or during the acute phase of their disease. Early recognition and treatment is important (see Part IV).

Chronic Complications

Bronchopulmonary Dysplasia

BPD was first described by Northway and Rosan[129] as serial roentgenographic changes occurring in the lungs of premature infants who survived hyaline membrane disease. BPD also occurs in a variety of conditions, including esophageal atresia, aspiration pneumonia, congenital heart disease, PDA, and meconium aspiration.[81,87,89]

Recent changes in neonatal care have modified the classic stages of BPD as first described by Northway et al.[129] In comparison with earlier studies, current neonates with chronic lung disease are far more premature and have lower birthweights, and generally lack many of the radiographic changes of cystic lung disease. Despite these changes the incidence of chronic lung disease after NICU care remains a significant clinical problem with an incidence approaching 35% to 40% in 750

to 1500 g infants with or without surfactant therapy.[38]

Pathophysiology. The pathogenesis of BPD is one of constant and recurring lung injury with ongoing repair and healing of the injury. Chronic injury and repair may in itself prolong the need for the very factors that contribute to the development of BPD: oxygen therapy and mechanical ventilation. In RDS there is injury to the alveolar mucosa, airway mucosa, serum exudation membranes, and fibrin coagulation-forming hyaline membranes. If sufficient hypoxia occurs with resultant damage, the alveolar and airway epithelium and its basement membrane will hemorrhage, and round cell infiltration will begin. Cellular and noncellular debris fill the alveoli and small airways. The obstruction causes microatelectasis, and nonobstructed airways become hyperexpanded and emphysematous.

In the healing and repair process, type II alveolar cells or their precursors multiply and differentiate into type I pneumocytes, which provide alveolar epithelium. Cells of the basal layer of the pseudostratified, ciliated, columnar epithelium lining the airways multiply and migrate to cover the injured airway and rejuvenate the epithelium. During this healing phase the rapidly multiplying and differentiating transitional cells are squamous or cuboidal and therefore appear "metaplastic." Epithelial metaplasia is one of the characteristics of BPD.

As healing occurs, increased inspired oxygen tensions, barotrauma, and infection continue to injure the cells that are taking part in the healing process.

Etiology.   BPD is an iatrogenic disease caused by oxygen toxicity and barotrauma resulting from pressure ventilation. In addition, there is evidence to suggest that lung immaturity, fluid overload, infection, ligation of the PDA, and familial predisposition to asthma also contribute to the development of BPD.[127,128,158]

Oxygen Toxicity.   BPD has been documented in both long- and short-term exposure to oxygen at both low and high levels (greater than 80%), as well as in infants treated with mechanical ventilation without supplemental oxygen.[126] As a result of these findings, many units have instituted guidelines for oxygen use and monitoring of levels with pulse oximetry. In addition, peak pressures should be monitored closely and reduced whenever possible to prevent barotrauma.

Barotrauma. BPD has also been related to barotrauma. BPD has been described in infants who have received peak inspiratory pressures of greater than 35 cm of water[153] and in those with pneumothorax and PIE.[123] A decrease in the incidence of BPD has been noted when lower peak inspiratory pressures were used.[138] Although peak inspiratory pressures should be limited whenever possible, some infants with very noncompliant lungs require the use of high pressure for survival. Use of surfactant therapy and newer ventilatory techniques have decreased the pressures necessary to adequately oxygenate and ventilate the neonate as well as resultant airleaks. Preliminary studies in the use of high-frequency ventilation suggest that this type of ventilation may cause yet another form of barotrauma.

Patent Ductus Arteriosus. There is a high incidence of BPD among infants with PDA[58] and congestive heart failure.[18,58,85,158] The amount of oxygen and peak inspiratory pressure required to support the neonate through the pulmonary complications of PDA may result in damage from oxygen toxicity and barotrauma. The increased pulmonary blood flow that occurs may also contribute to pulmonary damage. Because of these findings, medical closure of the ductus with indomethacin or surgical ligation is advocated (see Chapter 23) but has not affected the incidence of BPD.[15]

Nutrition. Inadequate nutrition caused by poor intake and/or increased nutritional requirements resulting in catabolism may potentiate the effects of oxygen and barotrauma on the neonatal lung.[53] Inadequate intake of antioxidants, trace elements, vitamins, and polyunsaturated fatty acids may also predispose the lung to injury.[38]

Fluids. BPD has also been detected in infants who have developed symptoms of fluid overload within the first few days of life.[18] Fluid balance in the VLBW infant is complicated by huge IWLs and often an intolerance to enteral feedings. Intake, output, and changes in weight must be closely monitored to calculate the fluid needs.

Family History of Asthma. Infants who develop BPD may have relatives with asthma who require hospitalization.[128] The lungs of these infants may be less tolerant of the insults of pulmonary disease, oxygen, pressure, and fluids.

Prematurity. Premature births alone may have a significant effect on pulmonary development, because prematurity results in differences in the development of small airways.[158] As a result, premature infants could be more susceptible to additional damage to the small airways from oxygen, ventilator pressure, fluids, and circulatory overload. As the survival rate of premature infants of less than 28 weeks' gestation increases, the occurrence of BPD is increasing.

Despite management of risk factors and the use of surfactant and other technologies, BPD is increasing especially in the VLBW, early gestational age preterm infant. However, the current form of BPD is less severe with fewer infants requiring tracheostomies and chronic ($\geq$6 months) ventilation.[38]

Oxygen and Antioxidants.[38]   Oxygen accepts free electrons generated by oxidative metabolism within the cell and produces free radicals, molecules that are toxic to living cells and/or tissues. Normally, antioxidants protect cells against free radicals, but this balance may be upset by (1) increased free radical production or (2) decreased antioxidant defense. The preterm neonate may be deficient in antioxidants and thus more susceptible to lung damage from free radicals.

Inflammation.   Oxygen radicals, barotrauma, infection, etc. initiate the inflammatory process, resulting in the infiltration of leukocytes, with release of other inflammatory mediators, resulting in pulmonary damage (i.e., decrease in capillary endothelial integrity, albumin leakage in the alveoli resulting in pulmonary edema). Activated neutrophils release enzymes that directly destroy the elastin and collagen of the lung. This inflammatory cycle produces significant pulmonary injury during a critical period of rapid lung growth and development (24 to 40 weeks) (see Table 22-1).

Prevention.   Premature infants treated with surfactant replacement show a lower incidence of BPD.[111] Steroids used antenatally[125] and early in the course of RDS[32,154] decrease the incidence and severity of BPD. Premature and full term infants (with pneumonia, MAS) treated with surfactant replacement have a lower incidence of BPD because of (1) better ventilation and pressure distri-

bution in the alveoli, (2) stabilization of the alveoli, and (3) prevention of overdistention.[9,111-113] Use of nasal CPAP may reduce or eliminate the need for intubation and mechanical ventilation, as well as assist in successful extubation.[80] In an attempt to prevent reinjury and allow healing, inspired oxygen tensions should be kept as low as is reasonable to provide adequate arterial oxygen tension. Pressures on the ventilator should be reduced when possible to prevent barotrauma. Although the collaborative HFV trial did not demonstrate a difference in the incidence of BPD between HFV and conventional ventilation,[77,60] early use of HFV and/or use of HFV with surfactant may decrease lung damage and resultant BPD.[37,38] For infants >36 weeks' gestational age who are unresponsive to conventional ventilation, ECMO is utilized in selected cases. Infections should be treated with appropriate antibiotic agents and PDA vigorously treated medically and/or surgically. Use of human recombinant antioxidant enzymes to prevent BPD is being studied.[38]

Data Collection

History.   A history of prematurity, moderate to severe RDS, intubation with oxygen and positive-pressure ventilation in the first week of life, inability to be weaned from the ventilator, and increasing oxygen requirement at the end of the first week of life are associated with BPD. Long-term features include tachypnea, rales, retractions, abnormal chest x-ray examination results, and the need for supplemental oxygen for more than 28 days[14] or to the expected date of delivery.[155]

Signs and Symptoms.   Tachypnea, exercise intolerance (feeding and handling), oxygen dependence, and respiratory distress (retractions, nasal flaring, fine rales at the bases or throughout the lung fields) may all be associated with BPD.

Laboratory Data.   X-ray findings (Fig. 22-3) correlate with the stage of disease; however, the pathologic changes are often more severe than the chest x-ray findings indicate.[43,129]

Stage I	Reticulogranular pattern and air bronchogram or RDS (first 3 days of life)
Stage II	Coarse granular infiltrates that are dense enough to obscure the cardiac markings (first 3 to 10 days of life)
Stage III	Multiple small cyst formation within

the opaque lungs and visible cardiac borders (first 10 to 20 days of life)

Stage IV	Irregular larger cyst formation that alternates with areas of increased density (after 28 days of life)

Cardiovascular changes include (1) right ventricular hypertrophy on ECG, (2) elevated right ventricular systolic time intervals or left ventricular and septal wall thickening on echocardiogram, or (3) elevated pulmonary vascular pressures and resistance at cardiac catheterization.[38]

Treatment.   The therapeutic goal is to reduce those factors that produce reinjury and to allow the lung to heal so that normal function can be resumed. This process may take weeks, months, or even years in severe lung injuries or in small infants under 1000 g.

Concurrent supportive therapies include (1) maintenance of adequate oxygenation and ventilation, (2) adequate nutrition and fluid restriction, (3) early PDA closure, and (4) pharmacologic management. Sufficient PIP should be used to prevent atelectasis while maintaining the lowest Fio_2 (if possible ≤.5)[38] to maintain adequate oxygenation (i.e., Pao_2 60-80 mm Hg; O_2sat 90% to 95%). Weaning from mechanical ventilation is done slowly and may be facilitated by (1) use of SIMV that reduces the work of breathing, (2) use of methylxanthines before extubation, and (3) use of nasal CPAP after extubation.[80,160] Usually in BPD the infant's ability to maintain ventilation develops before the ability to maintain adequate oxygenation. Often infants are discharged from the NICU on home oxygen therapy. Neonates with BPD have an increased resting metabolic expenditure as the major reason for growth failure, especially in the smallest, sickest infants.[105] These infants may require 150 to 200 kcal/kg/day to support adequate growth (i.e., 10 to 30 g/day weight gain).[57,167] Without adequate protein and/or caloric intake, damaged pulmonary tissue cannot heal[53] and provision of appropriate nutrition to the neonate with BPD is essential (see Chapters 13 to 16).

Pharmacologic management of BPD includes the use of bronchodilators, steroids, and diuretics (Table 22-7).[1] Inhaled and systemic bronchodilators improve lung mechanics and gaseous ex-

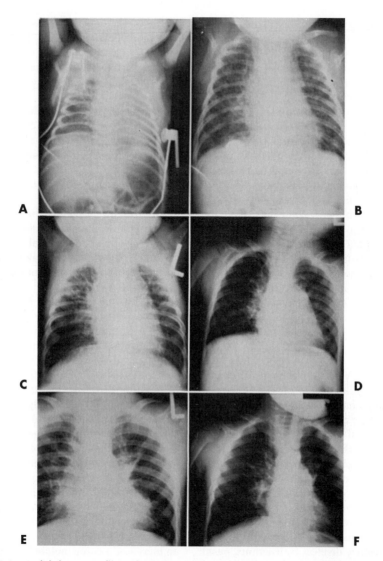

Figure 22-3   Serial chest x-ray films of premature infant with BPD over 2½ year period. **A,** Newborn. **B,** 2 months. **C,** 3 months. **D,** 1 year. **E,** 2 years. Infant's disease process was characterized by multiple hospitalizations for reactive airway disease and pulmonary hypertension. Note progressive lung disease characterized by hyperinflation and eventual clearing of infiltrate by 2½ years of age (**F**).

change by relaxation of bronchial smooth muscle.[35,36,54,90] However, bronchodilators may fail to relieve airway obstruction because of relatively poor development of bronchial smooth muscle in preterm infants.

Methylxanthine therapy promotes weaning of infants with RDS from low rates of ventilatory support.[73] Diuretics and diuretics combined with methylxanthines improve lung mechanics, clinical respiratory status, and ability to wean from mechanical ventilation.[36,90]

In addition to the efficacy of prenatal steroids

Table 22-7
Pharmacologic Agents Used in Treatment of BPD

Drug	Dosage	Comments
I. Bronchodilators		
A. Inhaled		
1. Beta₂-agonists		
a. Albuterol (Proventil, Ventolin)	0.1 mg/kg up to 5 mg in 2 ml of normal saline q4-6h Max dose-0.5 ml or 2.5 mg/ treatment; up to 6 treatments/ 24 hr	Drug of choice for bronchospasm—improves pulmonary resistance and lung compliance by bronchial smooth muscle relaxation; tachycardia, tremors, nausea and vomiting; can cause paradoxical bronchoconstriction; irritability; onset 5-15 min; peak action in 30 min to 2 hr; duration 3-4 hr
b. Terbutaline (Brethine)	0.03-0.3 mg/kg/day	Same as for Albuterol above; onset 5-30 min; duration 3-4 hr
2. Histamine inhibitor (Cromolyn: 20 mg/2 ml solution for nebulizer)	10-20 mg tid	Prevents release of inflammatory mediators and reduces airway hypersensitivity; urticaria, rash, and throat irritation; dosage may need adjusting in patients with hepatic and/or renal dysfunction
B. Systemic		
1. Methylxanthines		
a. Caffeine citrate	Loading: 20 mg/kg Maintenance: 5 mg/kg/day IV or PO	Promotes weaning from low rates of ventilatory support[48] by reduction of pulmonary resistance, improved lung compliance, and improved skeletal muscle and diaphragmatic contractility; has diuretic effect; half-life as long as 100 hr, excreted unchanged in urine; safer drug with fewer side effects than theophylline; side effects rare but include tachycardia, diuresis, dysrhythmias, glucosuria, seizures, ketonuria, vomiting, hyperglycemia, jitteriness, hemorrhagic gastritis
b. Theophylline (PO)	4-6 mg/kg of active theophylline, which should produce a serum level of 10-20 µg/ml; maintenance calculated by rate of plasma clearance, usually 3-7 mg/kg/day q12h	Half-life is 30-40 hr, metabolized to caffeine in the liver and excreted in urine; multisystem effect: CNS stimulant; increases respiratory rate, inspiratory drive, and surfactant production; increases GFR; increases heart rate, contractility, and output; decreases GI motility and increases GI secretions; increases glucose levels, ketonuria, and glycosuria; increases muscle contractility; increases catecholamine and insulin levels; side effects: same as for caffeine citrate
2. Beta₂-agonists		
a. Terbutaline	5 µg/kg SC q4-6h	Improves pulmonary mechanics; side effects same as for Albuterol above; adjunct to methylxanthines
b. Albuterol	0.15 mg/kg/dose PO q8h	Reduces pulmonary resistance; adjunct to methylxanthines; side effects same as for Albuterol above

tid, Three times a day; *GFR*, glomerular filtration rate; *GI*, gastrointestinal; *BUN*, blood urea nitrogen; *BPD*, bronchopulmonary dysplasia; *KCL*, potassium chloride; *bid*, twice a day.

Continued

Table 22-7
Pharmacologic Agents Used in Treatment of BPD—cont'd

Drug	Dosage	Comments

II. Steroids
A. Inhaled
  1. Corticosteroids (Dexa-
  methasone [Decadron])
	100 µg/inhalation from metered
	dose inhaler (MDI)
		30%-60% systemic bioavailability vs 53%-78% from oral intake; majority removed from lung within 20 min after administration; difficult to administer with MDI; amount of drug delivered is unpredictable; MDIs should not be used in ventilated infants with tidal volume <100 ml because of the potential hypoxic mixture resulting from the volume of chlorofluorocarbon gas released by the MDI[8]; side effects: oral candidiasis, bronchospasm, and adrenal suppression

2. Glucocorticosteroids
  a. Flunisolide (Na-
  salide)
	250 µg/inhalation	Unknown stability—do not mix with other drugs; bronchospasm may result from buffers and/or preservatives; side effects: same as for dexamethasone above

b. Beclomethasone
  (Beconase;
  Vancenase)
	42 µg/inhalation	

B. Systemic (Cortico- steroids—Dexameth- asone [Decadron])	0.5 mg/kg/day IV or PO q12h for 3 days; decrease to 0.3 mg/kg/ day for 3 days Taper 10%-20% q3days	Hyperglycemia; hypothalamic-pituitary-adrenal axis suppression; protein depletion and/or tissue catabolism (increase BUN; failure to gain weight); gastric irritation, perforation, bleeding; restlessness and/or irritability; myocardial hypertrophy; hypertension; (?) increased risk for infection

III. Diuretics

A. Furosemide (Lasix)	1-2 mg/kg/dose IV bid or 2-4 mg/kg/dose PO bid	Treatment of choice for fluid overload in BPD—decrease interstitial edema and pulmonary vascular resistance; daily or alternate day administration improves pulmonary mechanics and facilitates weaning from ventilator; side effects: metabolic alkalosis, hypokalemia, hypocalcemia, hypochloremia, hyponatremia, renal calcifications, gallstones, ototoxicity; KCL supplementation; onset 5 min IV; 1 hr, PO; duration 2-4 hr
B. Thiazides		
1. Chlorthiazide (Diuril)	5-20 mg/kg/dose IV or PO bid	Less potent than furosemide; promotes potassium and bicarbonate excretion with sodium and chloride; spares calcium; given with spironolactone; combination of thiazide and spironolactone results in improved lung mechanics and increased urine output; side effects: electrolyte imbalance, hypercalcemia, hyperglycemia, decreased magnesium level, hypersensitivity, GI upset, glycosuria
2. Hydrochlorthiazide (Hydro Diuril)	1-2 mg/kg/dose PO bid	Side effects: electrolyte imbalance, hypercalcemia, hyperglycemia, metabolic alkalosis; increased urinary losses of sodium, potassium, magnesium, chloride, phosphorus, and bicarbonate; spares calcium; onset 1-2 hr; duration 6-12 hr
3. Spironolactone (Aldactone)	1.5 mg/kg/dose PO bid	Weak diuretic; causes increased sodium chloride and water loss; spares potassium; side effects: irritability, lethargy, GI upset, rash; onset 3-5 days
4. Bumetanide (Bumax)	0.015 mg/kg/day up to 0.1 mg/kg/day PO	40 times the potency of Lasix; used in neonates and infants who are refractory to Lasix therapy; side effects same as for Furosemide above, plus hypophosphatemia

in reducing the severity of RDS in premature neonates,[125] postnatal use of steroids appears to decrease the incidence of BPD. Several clinical studies have demonstrated more rapid ventilator weaning and decreased need for supplemental oxygen in at-risk neonates.[72,92,169,170] In addition, steroids reduce lung inflammation and improve pulmonary function in severe RDS.[102] Steroid use has been associated with multiple side effects, including poor growth, hypertension, hyperglycemia, sepsis, azotemia, and myocardial hypertrophy.* Current studies are examining whether inhaled steroids[10,149] will be effective while decreasing the incidence and severity of these side effects.

Complications. Complications of BPD are most common in the smallest, sickest infants (Box 22-5).

---

* References 19, 32, 48, 102, 142, 154, 164.

Retinopathy of Prematurity (Retrolental Fibroplasia)

The association between oxygen administration, prematurity, and subsequent retinal changes often resulting in blindness has been recognized since the 1950s.[98] Severe restriction in the use of oxygen with the premature infant resulted in less ROP, but also in an increased morbidity and mortality.[11,119] With increased survival of the very preterm infant, liberalization of the use of oxygen, and improved technology for support and assisted ventilation, there is a resurgence of ROP.

Physiology. The pathophysiologic process in the development of ROP is not completely understood. Many factors play a role in the pathogenesis. When hyperoxia is involved, it is the pressure in arterial blood (Pao_2) rather than the concentration administered (Fio_2) that is important.

In response to hyperoxia, the retinal vessels constrict. They may permanently constrict and become necrotic (vasoobliteration). The vessels that have not been obliterated may proliferate in an attempt to reestablish retinal circulation. Proliferating vessels may extend into the vitreous, causing fluid leakage and/or hemorrhage, with retinal scar formation, traction on the retina, detachment, and blindness.

The degree of nasal retinal vascularization at birth determines the susceptibility to the insult of hyperoxia. The majority of retinal vascularization is complete by 32 weeks' gestation. However, even at 40 weeks the temporal periphery of the retina may still not be completely vascularized.

Early changes may first be evident at the temporal periphery, because this area is the last to be completely vascularized. Proliferation of new vessels may remain localized and spontaneously resolve or may progress to cause total retinal detachment.

ROP is classified by location of disease in the retina (zone), by degree (stage) of vascular abnormality, and by extent of developing vasculature (clock hour)[4,7] (Fig. 22-4 and Table 22-8). Changes are first readily seen between 6 and 8 weeks of life. Seventy-five percent of mild forms of ROP spontaneously resolve.

Etiology. ROP is considered primarily a disease of prematurity. The incidence is inversely propor-

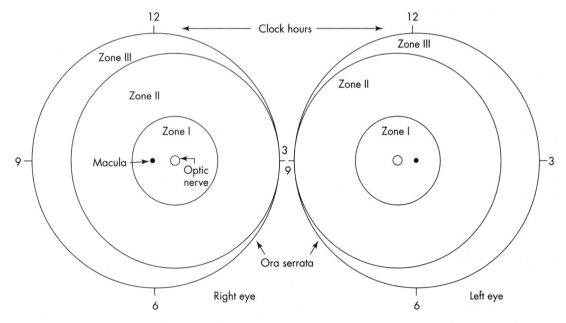

Figure 22-4 International classification of retinopathy of prematurity (ROP). (From AMA: *Arch Ophthamol* 102:1131, 1984. Courtesy Ross Laboratories, Columbus, Ohio.)

Table 22-8
Stages of Retinopathy of Prematurity (ROP)

Stages	Description
Stage 1: Demarcation line	A thin white line separates the avascular retina anteriorly from the vascularized retina posteriorly. Abnormal branching vessels lead to the demarcation line, which is flat and lies in the plane of the retina.
Stage 2: Ridge	The ridge has a definite height and width, occupies a volume, and extends up out of the plane of the retina. Its color may change from white to pink. Small, isolated tufts of new vessels may appear posterior to the structure.
Stage 3: Ridge with extraretinal fibrovascular proliferations	To the ridge of stage 2 is added the presence of extraretinal fibrovascular proliferative tissue. Characteristic locations: 1. Continuous with the posterior aspect of the ridge (ragged ridge) 2. Immediately posterior to the ridge but not always appearing to be connected to it 3. Into the vitreous perpendicular to the retinal plane
Stae 4: Retinal detachment	To stage 3 is added unequivocal detachment of the retina caused by exudative effusion of fluid, traction, or both.
"PLUS" disease	Progressive vascular incompetence is noted primarily by increasing dilation and tortuosity of peripheral retinal vessels. Only when posterior veins are enlarged and arterioles are tortuous is the designation "+" added to the ROP stage number (e.g., stage 3 + ROP).

From American Medical Association: *Arch Ophthalmol* 102:1130, 1984. Courtesy Ross Laboratories, Columbus, Ohio.

tional to birth weight and gestational age. Damage may occur in any preterm infant and has its highest incidence in the infant younger than 28 weeks' gestation. Infants weighing less than 1500 g (appropriate weight for gestational age) have the highest incidence of disease (16% to 34%)[67] and the highest incidence of blindness (5% to 11%)[67,134]

Prevention. Adherence to the principles of oxygen therapy is essential as the first line of defense against developing ROP. Because an infant who is very hyperoxic (Pao_2 > 200 mm Hg) will clinically look no different from an infant whose Pao_2 is normal (approximately 80 torr), monitoring of arterial blood gases or transcutaneous oxygen is mandatory whenever oxygen is administered. Oxygen tension should be measured 15 to 30 minutes after initiating, altering, or discontinuing therapy.

The usefulness and safety of vitamin E is still unclear. Its use is considered experimental, and its routine administration for the prevention of ROP is not recommended. Vitamin E supplementation to achieve serum levels as high as 4 to 5 mg/dl may be used in combination with cryotherapy to decrease the sequalae of ROP.[88]

Data Collection. Visualization of the retina is difficult and not predictive of occurring vasoconstriction and retinal changes as a result of hyperoxia. Indirect funduscopic examination by a neonatal ophthalmologist at 4 to 6 weeks may document retinal changes. Contributing factors to the development of ROP include the following:

- Prematurity—very low birth weight (<1500 g)
- Hyperoxia/hypoxia
- Blood transfusions
- Pregnancy complications (hypertension, preeclampsia, diabetes, bleeding, smoking)
- Apnea/bradycardia
- Asphyxia/acidosis
- Sepsis
- Hypercapnia/hypocapnia
- IVH
- BPD
- PDA
- Ventilatory support (prolonged and with episodes of hypercapnia, hypoxia, or both)
- Multiple gestation

- Nutritional deficiency (i.e., antioxidants)
- Exposure to bright lights

Treatment. The best treatment is prevention. NOTE: Even strict adherence to all principles of good care may still not prevent ROP in VLBW infants.

Noninvasive continuous monitoring (pulse oximetry) enables trending of an infant's fluctuations (hypoxia or hyperoxia) with ventilatory changes, handling, and activity (see Chapter 7). Cryotherapy performed by a qualified, experienced pediatric ophthalmologist shows a 50% reduction in severe vision loss in treated infants.[31] Laser surgery is less invasive, requires no anesthesia, and enables deeper tissue penetration and more predictable tissue interaction. In addition, it is less painful postoperatively than cryosurgery.[83,136,145]

Complications. Complications of cryotherapy include infection, periorbital edema, retinal scarring, and detachment. Complications of laser surgery include choroidal hemorrhage, scarring, and (rarely) pain. When the eyes are not used, microphthalmia (small sunken eyes) results. Glaucoma, strabismus, amblyopia, and late retinal detachment (in teens or early twenties) may develop. Severe myopia may develop as early as 6 months of age. Early detection and correction with lenses is essential to save the child's remaining sight.

Parent Teaching. Blindness is defined by most of our society as one of the worst handicaps. Parents will experience grief over this devastating loss and will need help to cope before they will be able to bond to their blind child.

Blind infants are unable to communicate with care providers through the signs and signals of facial expressions.[52] Because of the absence of eye language, no cues to infant needs and no feedback of preference, recognition, and delight can be given. Absence of a smile from the blind infant connotes a negative response to the care provider. When care providers understand these behavioral differences, they can assist parents to understand the lack of facial expression. Instead of facial expression, parents are taught to read the special hand language of their infants as an expression of emotions, intentions, preference, and recognition.[52] **Appropriate referrals to occupational therapy, physical therapy, and community resources for extrasensory stimulation for the infant may help avoid developmental delays from insufficient or inappropriate stimulation.**

Chronic CNS Sequelae

For large infants (>1500 g) with mild-to-moderate RDS, the current developmental outcome is probably comparable with that of infants without RDS.[23] The highest incidence of abnormal findings occurs in infants with intracranial hemorrhage, the lowest birth weights (<1500 g), and BPD.*

Transient neurologic abnormalities such as hypotonia and/or hypertonia and persistence of primitive reflexes occur in 70% to 80% of high-risk infants.[69] In 10% to 26% of these infants major neurologic defects such as cerebral palsy, hydrocephalus, seizures, and mental retardation are diagnosed in the first 2 years of life.[69,126,152] However, minor defects that are not severely handicapping, such as learning disorders, hyperactivity, minor retardation, altered muscle tone, and fine and gross motor incoordination may not be diagnosed as early. Subtle perceptual problems may be diagnosed in the preschool child or even in the school age child with inadequate school performance.[69,101,118,143] By preschool, severe neurodevelopmental problems may exist in 50% of survivors.[87,93,108] Cerebral palsy remains the most common neurologic defect in survivors (3% to 26%).†

Respiratory Distress Syndrome

Pathophysiology

RDS is a disease of immature lung anatomy and physiology. Anatomically the preterm lung is unable to support oxygenation and ventilation, because alveolar saccules are insufficiently developed, causing a deficient surface area for gas

exchange. Also, the pulmonary capillary bed is deficient and the interstitial mesenchyme is present to a greater extent, increasing the distance between the alveolar and the endothelial cell membranes.

Physiologically the volume of surfactant is insufficient to prevent collapse of unstable alveoli. Because the alveoli collapse with each breath, normal functional residual capacity is not established. Because of alveolar collapse, oxygenation and ventilation are insufficient, and each breath requires increased energy output.

Compliance is related to the volume achieved during a given application of pressure. Compliance of the lung is equal to the ratio of the change in volume to the change in pressure. The lung in RDS has low compliance (i.e., little change in volume is achieved with a relatively great application of pressure), thereby contributing to increased work of breathing. However, the chest wall of the neonate is unfortunately very compliant; a slight application of pressure results in a large change in volume. The infant may not be able to create enough inspiratory pressure to open the alveoli as the chest wall retracts and collapses about the relatively stiff lung. Thus in RDS the diaphragm contracts, creating an inspiratory pressure that moves less volume into the lung than expected and simultaneously causes large sternal and intercostal retractions of the chest wall.

The increased effort of these opposing forces usually results in hypoxemia and acidemia that cause constriction of the pulmonary vascular (arterial) musculature, severely limiting pulmonary capillary blood flow. The integrity of pulmonary capillary blood flow is critical for the integrity of the alveolar epithelial membrane and the production of surfactant. Without adequate pulmonary capillary blood flow, the type II pneumocytes become deficient in precursor material required for production of surfactant. Lack of surfactant production compounds the deficiency and leads to low compliance. These physiologic factors promote increased work of breathing and aggravate the ongoing ventilatory problems.

In the fetus, pulmonary vascular resistance is high, and pulmonary artery blood pressure is greater than systemic blood pressure, causing blood flow from the main pulmonary artery to travel through the open ductus arteriosus to the descending aorta. A second right-to-left shunt occurs across

---

* References 3, 62, 68, 69, 87, 89, 144, 148, 152, 165.

† References 62, 69, 70, 87, 89, 93, 108, 143, 152.

the foramen ovale in the fetus. The high pulmonary vascular resistance is "reactive" to the normal fetal "hypoxemia," because the pulmonary vascular resistance and the pulmonary artery blood pressure decrease as the Pao_2 of the neonate increases. At birth the ductus arteriosus actively constricts in response to the increase in Pao_2 (Pao_2 >50 mm Hg), eliminating blood flow across the ductus and completing the transition to neonatal circulation. The fetal circulatory pattern may persist from birth or be initiated by a transient hypoxemic episode. In the instance of neonatal hypoxemia, the pulmonary vasculature "reacts" by vasoconstriction, raising pulmonary vascular resistance, and the ductus arteriosus "reacts" by relaxing, once again allowing blood flow from the pulmonary artery to the descending aorta, as normally occurs in the fetus. Pulmonary vascular resistance is increased with shunting through the ductus arteriosus. Fetal circulatory patterns are perpetuated by hypoxemia and acidemia and produce systemic hypoxemia that aggravates and perpetuates the condition.

Endothelial damage and alveolar necrosis aggravate the already existing surfactant deficiency. A cyclic deterioration is established, and hypoxia and acidosis persist unless treatment is initiated.

Microscopically, the events that occur in the lung include injury to and death of the alveolar epithelial cells and airway epithelial cells. This injury and death are followed by sloughing of the cells from the respiratory basement membrane, leaving the basement membrane denuded followed by exudation of serum. Fibrin in the serum clots, and hyaline membranes are formed, covering the denuded basement membranes in the airways and alveolar spaces. If there is sufficient hypoxic damage to the cells and basement membranes, frank hemorrhage may fill the alveolar spaces. These factors serve to decrease the total surface area of the gas exchange membrane. The end result is hypoxemia, acidemia, and increasing respiratory distress.

The entire sequence of events in RDS is related to the inability to maintain lung expansion and alveolar stability as a result of surfactant deficiency. RDS evolves from two interrelated problems: atelectasis and persistence of or reversion to the fetal levels of pulmonary hypertension[135] (Figs. 22-5 and 22-6).

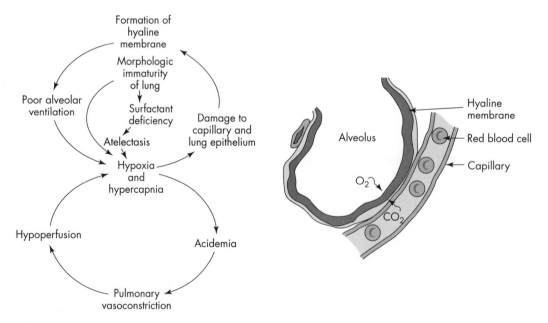

Figure 22-5 Interdependent relationship of factors involved in pathology of RDS. (From Pierog SH, Ferrara A: *Medical care of the sick newborn,* ed 2, St Louis, 1976, Mosby.)

Etiology

RDS occurs in infants born prematurely and is a consequence of immature lung anatomy and physiology. In the premature infant or stressed infant, atelectasis from the collapse of the terminal alveoli because of lack of surfactant appears after the first few hours of life. In the premature infant, surfactant production is limited, and stores are quickly depleted. Surfactant production may be further diminished by other unfavorable conditions such as high oxygen concentration, poor pulmonary drainage, excessive pulmonary hygiene, or effects of respirator management.

Data Collection

History

A history of prematurity, cesarean section, and/or asphyxial episodes may be seen in infants with RDS.

Physical Examination

Infants with RDS often show signs of tachypnea, grunting, flaring, and retractions within the first few minutes to hours of life. Pallor or cyanosis may also be present. The trachea is midline, and there is a normal apical pulse. Auscultation of the chest reveals decreased breath sounds and often rales. Many of these infants may be hypotensive with prolonged capillary refill.

Laboratory Data

A chest x-ray examination reveals a ground-glass appearance that represents areas of atelectatic respiratory alveoli adjacent to expanded or even hyperexpanded respiratory units. This can also be described as a bilateral reticulogranular pattern with air bronchograms (Fig 22-7 and 22-8).

Arterial blood gases reveal hypoxemia and often acidemia that may be metabolic, respiratory, or a combination of both (see Chapter 10).

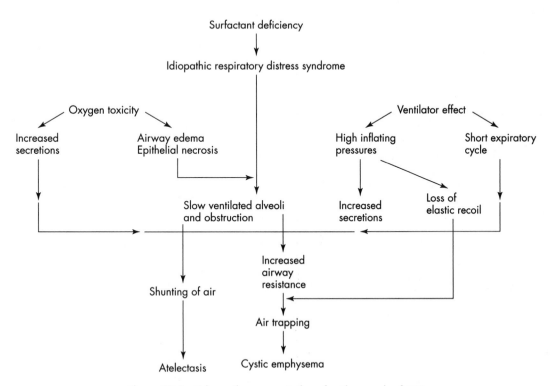

Figure 22-6 Schematic representation of pathogenesis of RDS.

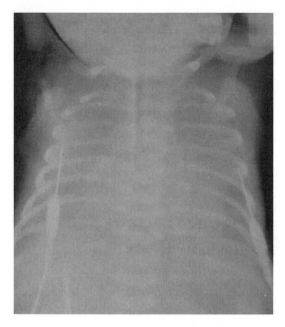

Figure 22-7 Chest x-ray film of 28-week preterm infant with severe RDS. Note "white-out" appearance.

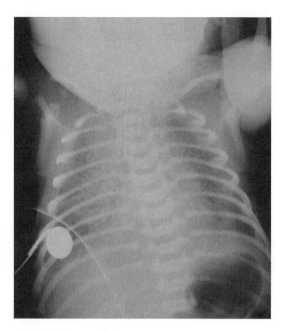

Figure 22-8 Chest x-ray film of 27-week premature infant with RDS. Note characteristic infiltrate pattern with air bronchograms.

Treatment

Surfactant Replacement Therapy

Because surfactant deficiency is the primary abnormality of RDS, the development of an effective clinical strategy for administering exogenous surface-active material to premature infants has been the focus of research efforts for many years. Animal studies have found the administration of surfactant into the airway of premature fetal animals before ventilation markedly improved gaseous exchange and survival.[44,86] Administration of surfactant harvested from mature bovine lung or human amniotic fluid from normal term pregnancies has led to dramatic and rapid improvement in gas exchange, decreased the need for high levels of supplemental oxygen and ventilator therapy, caused less barotrauma, and improved chest x-ray findings in infants treated shortly after birth.[55] The effects of synthetic surfactant administered at birth and at 12 hours of age show that the surfactant group had fewer deaths, a lower incidence of BPD, and less barotrauma and related complications.[29,111,113,117] Current concerns about possible immunogenicity, negative interactions with endogenous surfactant production, and the optimal clinical strategies (such as how much surfactant to administer, how many doses, and the optimal method of delivery), are under study. Surfactant therapy in premature infants with RDS constitutes a major historical milestone in neonatal care (see Chapter 1). **Surfactant preparations are commercially available as (1) organic solvent extract of minced bovine lung, and (2) artificial or synthetic surfactant. Table 22-9 summarizes the commercially available products for surfactant replacement.**

Prophylactic or rescue therapy with exogenous surfactant has markedly improved the outcome of infants with RDS (see Table 22-9). Otherwise, treatment is directed toward the indications in Box 22-6.

Table 22-9
Surfactant Replacement Therapy

Drug/Source	Indications	Administration and Dosage	Adverse Effects
Beractant (Survanta) exogenous surfactant from bovine lung extract	Prevention and treatment ("rescue") of RDS in premature infants; significantly reduces the incidence of RDS, mortality caused by RDS, and air leak complications **Prevention:** In premature infants <1250 g birth weight or with evidence of surfactant deficiency, give as soon as possible, preferably within 15 minutes of birth **Rescue:** To treat infants with RDS confirmed by x-ray examination and requiring mechanical ventilation, give as soon as possible, preferably by 8 hours of age	**Administration:** For *intratracheal* administration only (instillation through a 5 Fr end-hole catheter inserted into the infant's endotracheal tube with the tip of the catheter just beyond the end of the endotracheal tube and above the infant's carina); each dose is 100 mg of phospholipids/kg birth weight (4 ml/kg); four doses can be administerd in the first 48 hours of life; give doses no more frequently than every 6 hours; repeat doses are based on the infant's birth weight	The most commonly reported adverse experiences are associated with the dosage procedure: transient bradycardia and oxygen desaturation
Colfosceril (Exosurf) artificial surfactant	Prevention and treatment ("rescue") of RDS in premature infants	**Administration:** Suction the infant before administration, but do not suction for 2 hours after administration, except when clinically necessary; administer via the sideport on the special endotracheal tube adapter without interrupting mechanical ventilation **Dosage:** Each dose is administered in two 2.5 ml/kg half-doses; each half-dose is instilled slowly over 1 to 2 minutes in small bursts	See above

RDS, Respiratory distress syndrome.
From Yeh TF: *Neonatal therapeutics,* St Louis, 1991, Mosby; Olin B, Hebel S, Dombek C: *Drug facts and comparisons,* St Louis, 1992, Wolters Kluwer.

Box 22-6

Treatment for RDS

I. Reducing hypoxemia (see section on general treatment strategies in this chapter and in Chapter 10)
  A. Maintain in neutral thermal environment (see Chapter 6)
  B. Maintain blood pressure and hematocrit (see Chapters 5 and 19)
  C. Decrease stimuli from the NICU environment (see Chapter 12)
  D. Recognize and relieve pain and/or agitation (see Chapter 11)
II. Correcting acidemia (see Chapter 10)
III. Increasing the functional residual capacity (see section on general treatment strategies)
  A. Maintaining appropriate temperature (see Chapter 6)
  B. Monitoring vital signs and arterial blood gases (see Chapters 7 and 10)
  C. Providing appropriate fluid, electrolytes, glucose, and calories (see Part III)
  D. Observing for complications of disease and treatments (see section on general complications)
IV. Monitor for complications (see section on general complications, acute and chronic)

RDS, Respiratory distress syndrome; *NICU,* neonatal intensive care unit.

Transient Tachypnea of the Newborn

Pathophysiology

Transient tachypnea of the newborn (TTN) is the result of delayed reabsorption of normal lung fluid, and thus an alternative name is "wet lung." Lung fluid accumulates in the peribronchiolar lymphatics and the bronchovascular spaces. Thus TTN is an "obstructive" lung disease, whereas RDS is a "restrictive" lung disease.

Etiology

TTN generally occurs in term or near-term infants with a history of cesarean section or precipitous delivery. In these situations there is a lack of the gradual compression of the chest that perhaps would eliminate some fluid during a normal vaginal delivery. This accumulation of interstitial fluid interferes with the forces that tend to hold the bronchioli open. This interference causes the bronchioli to collapse. The result is air trapping.

Data Collection

History

As previously stated, term or near-term infants with a history of cesarean section or precipitous delivery are predisposed to TTN. Onset is usually 2 to 6 hours after birth.

Physical Examination

Respiratory distress including tachypnea, retractions, grunting, and flaring may be seen. Cyanosis in room air may also be present.

Laboratory Data

Mild hypoxemia (requiring <40% oxygen) and mild acidemia are usually present. A significant degree of hypoxemia or acidemia will tend to constrict the pulmonary vasculature and aggravate the problem. Chest x-ray examination reveals hyperexpansion with streaky infiltrates radiating from the hilum. These infiltrates are thought to represent interstitial fluid along the bronchovascular spaces. The air trapping causes the appearance of hyperexpansion on the chest x-ray film.

Treatment

In general, support of the patient with TTN requires only the provision of sufficient supplemental oxygen to maintain an arterial oxygen tension of more than 70 to 80 mm Hg and maintenance of usual supportive neonatal care. Although diuretic agents have been advocated, usually little more than general support is necessary while the normal absorption of lung fluid through the lymphatics takes place.

Meconium Aspiration Syndrome

Pathophysiology

Before meconium aspiration can occur, meconium must find its way into the amniotic fluid. This condition occurs more often in term or postterm infants when a hypoxic episode is experienced in utero. With fetal asphyxia the anal sphincter relaxes and colonic peristalsis ensues, expelling meconium into the amniotic fluid. Subsequently a second episode of asphyxia occurs during which the infant makes gasping respiratory movements. These movements open the glottis so that meconium flows into the oropharynx and on into the lung. Thus the pathophysiology of lung disease in MAS is in part related to the mechanisms causing fetal stress as well as the direct adverse effects of meconium in the lung.

Etiology

Meconium aspiration produces disease by several mechanisms: meconium may physically obstruct the glottis, trachea, or any number of smaller airways; it promotes development of infection seemingly by increasing the virulence of infecting organisms; and the increase in pulmonary vascular resistance caused by asphyxial episodes results in increased right-to-left shunting (Fig 22-9).

Prevention

Before birth, meconium aspiration may be prevented by early recognition of the compromised fetus and appropriate intervention.

At birth, suction of the infant's oropharynx on the perineum before the first breath may be preventive. On delivery of the head and before delivery

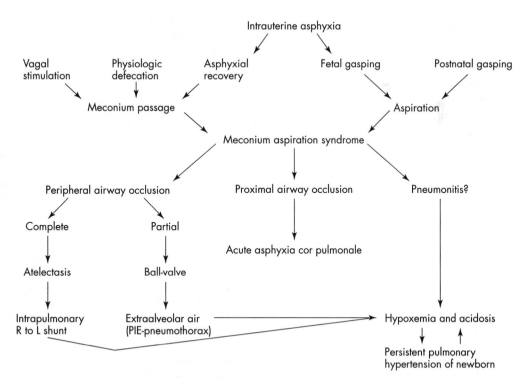

Figure 22-9 Schematic representation of pathogenesis of meconium aspiration syndrome. (Modified from Basick R: *Pediatr Clin North Am* 24:467, 1977.)

of the rest of the body of an infant with meconium-stained fluid, removing meconium, blood, and mucus from the infant's nose, mouth, and pharynx with a wall suction apparatus is essential. This prevents aspiration of the contents into the bronchi with the first gasp of respiration[24] NOTE: Aspiration of amniotic contents into upper large airways before the first respiratory efforts may occur with the onset of gasping in utero.

After birth, intubation and suction of the trachea may be useful. Pulmonary lavage is not effective and is not recommended.

Data Collection

History

History of asphyxia, IUGR, postterm delivery, and meconium-stained amniotic fluid may be present.

Physical Examination

Tachypnea, rales, and cyanosis are seen in mild cases. In moderately severe cases, grunting, retractions, and nasal flaring may also be seen. In severe cases the infant is asphyxiated and severely depressed at birth. There is profound cyanosis and pallor, irregular gasping respirations, and an increased anteroposterior diameter of the chest.

Laboratory Data

The chest x-ray examination shows marked air trapping and hyperexpansion. There are bilateral, coarse, patchy infiltrates (Fig. 22-10). Air leaks are frequently seen. Pleural effusion may occur as a result of the inflammatory process in the lung.

Severe hypoxemia as a result of ventilation perfusion inequality and right-to-left shunting caused by pulmonary hypertension is usually present. Severe hypercapnia is usually present. Severe acidosis is usually a combined respiratory and metabolic acidosis.

Treatment

Because the major problem in meconium aspiration is hypoxemia, treatment should be directed at improving oxygenation. Mildly affected infants will frequently require only warmed, humidified oxygen by hood. Increasing severity of meconium

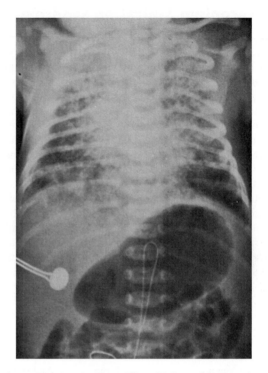

Figure 22-10 Chest x-ray film of infant with meconium aspiration. Note diffuse infiltrates.

aspiration will require increased levels of intervention. Some infants will respond to CPAP (4 to 6 cm of water), but others will require full ventilator support. Because these infants are usually term or postterm, they may fight assisted ventilation and require paralyzation to ventilate and oxygenate the lungs adequately. A 0.03 to 0.06 mg/kg/dose of pancuronium bromide (Pavulon) will paralyze the infant. Repeat doses are given as needed. With paralysis, these infants require rapid rates (60 to 80 breaths/min) and high pressure (>30 cm of water). PEEP of 4 to 6 cm of water may also be used. Recent studies suggest that surfactant replacement therapy can improve oxygenation in some patients with severe respiratory failure and meconium aspiration.[9,114] In addition, HFOV decreased the need for ECMO in one study, but responsiveness to HFOV after failing conventional ventilation is variable.[28]

Mucosal irritation and increased mucosal secretion hamper respiratory and mucociliary clearance efforts. Frequent pulmonary hygiene every 2 to 3 hours will help alleviate this problem.

As with any sick infant, close attention must be given to physiologic support and homeostasis (see also section on general treatment strategies, Chapters, 6, 7, and 10, and Part III).

Complications

Persistent pulmonary hypertension is a frequent complication of meconium aspiration, and it compounds the difficulties in oxygenating the infant.[5] An air leak is a complication of both the disease (ball-valve obstruction causing air trapping) and the treatment (CPAP or ventilator support). The underlying asphyxia can be viewed as either a cause or a complication (see Chapter 4).

Persistent Pulmonary Hypertension of the Newborn (Persistent Fetal Circulation)

PPHN presents as severe pulmonary hypertension with pulmonary artery pressure elevation to levels equal to or higher than systemic pressure and large right-to-left shunts through both the foramen ovale and the ductus arteriosus. Despite improved identification and aggressive treatment, mortality and morbidity remain high. Resultant morbidity in surviving infants includes chronic lung disease, neurologic sequelae, neurosensory hearing loss, and pneumothorax.[13,47,124]

Physiology

Once the placental blood source is severed, adequate oxygenation of the newborn depends on inflation of the lungs, closure of the fetal shunts, a decrease in pulmonary vascular resistance, and an increase in pulmonary blood flow. Normally, pulmonary vascular resistance decreases with the first breath of life. When it remains high, successful transition from fetal to neonatal circulation does not occur. In the infant manifesting PPHN, high pulmonary vascular resistance and pulmonary hypertension impede pulmonary blood flow. This leads to hypoxemia, acidemia, and eventually lactic

acidosis. The pulmonary arterioles respond to this process with further constriction, promoting an additional decrease in blood flow; thus a cyclic pattern is set up. Pulmonary vascular resistance also maintains higher right-sided pressures in the heart that equal or exceed systemic pressures. This promotes the right-to-left shunting that is characteristic of this disease.[40] PPHN also produces direct and indirect effects on myocardial function. A combination of pressure alterations, hypoxia, and acidemia leads to a cyclic pattern of decreased cardiac output, decreased pulmonary blood flow, and further vasoconstriction (Figs. 22-11 to 22-14).

Etiology

PPHN occurs as an idiopathic or unexplained condition. Because full development of the pulmonary arterial musculature occurs late in gestation, persistent PPHN is primarily a condition of the term and postterm infant. In utero, development of increased vascular smooth muscle or perinatal factors that cause or contribute to vasospasm are thought to be prime mechanisms of PPHN.

Prevention

Prevention of PPHN includes minimizing intrauterine and perinatal risk factors when possible, maintaining postnatal physiologic homeostasis, and detecting and correcting any underlying abnormality.

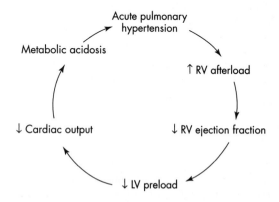

Figure 22-11   Effect of pulmonary hypertension on cardiac output. *RV,* Right ventricle; *LV,* left ventricle. (From Perkin RM, Anas NG: *J Pediatr* 105:511, 1984.)

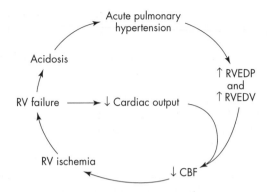

Figure 22-12   Effect of pulmonary hypertension on right ventricular function. *RV,* Right ventricle; *RVEDP,* right ventricular end-diastolic pressure; *RVEDV,* right ventricular end-diastolic volume; *CBF,* coronary blood flow. (From Perkin RM, Anas NG: *J Pediatr* 105:511, 1984.)

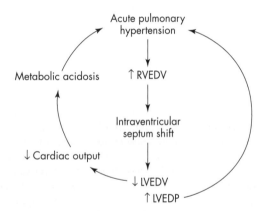

Figure 22-13   Effect of pulmonary hypertension on left ventricular function. *RVEDV,* Right ventricle end-diastolic volume; *LVEDV,* left ventricular end-diastolic volume; *LVEDP,* left ventricular end-diastolic pressure. (From Perkin RM, Anas NG: *J Pediatr* 105:511, 1984.)

Data Collection

History

Risk factors of PPHN are listed in Box 22-7.

There are two major considerations in the history of these infants: (1) the recognition of major disease processes or syndromes that are highly associated with pulmonary hypertension and (2) the timing of the onset of cyanosis and the deterioration of the infant.

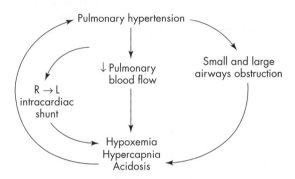

Figure 22-14   Effect of pulmonary hypertension on gas exchange. *R → L,* right to left. (From Perkin RM, Anas NG: *J Pediatr* 105:511, 1984.)

Physical Examination

The initial clinical presentation is usually a full-term or postterm infant with worsening cyanosis. Tachypnea is a common finding and when accompanied by retractions is indicative of decreased pulmonary compliance. Cyanosis may either be intense at birth or progressively worsen in association with increased right-to-left shunting. The milder cases of PPHN have minimal tachypnea and cyanosis, frequently associated with stress from crying or feeding. The severe cases are characterized by marked cyanosis, tachypnea, and decreased peripheral perfusion.

Increased pulmonary artery pressure results in the following symptoms[76]:

- Pulmonic systolic ejection clicks
- Second heart sound that is single, loud, or narrowly split with a loud pulmonary component
- Prominent right ventricular impulse that is visible or palpable at the lower left sternal border
- Soft systolic murmur in the pulmonary area

Laboratory Data

The laboratory evaluation of the infant with potential PPHN should include a CBC with differential, platelet count, chest x-ray examination, and serum glucose, calcium, and arterial blood gas determinations. The CBC is used to detect anemia that could contribute to systemic hypertension, to de-

---

Box 22-7

Risk factors of PPHN

I. Intrauterine factors
   A. Fetal hypertension
   B. Chronic in utero hypoxia
   C. Pulmonary hypoplasia (diaphragmatic hernia or oligohydramnios)[137]
   D. In utero ductus arteriosus closure (maternal drugs, i.e., indomethacin or salicylic agents)
   E. Asphyxia
   F. Maternal ingestion of prostaglandin inhibitors, dilantin, or lithium[50,133,157]
II. Premature factors
   A. Surfactant deficiency
III. Postnatal factors
   A. Polycythemia[59]
   B. Hypothermia
   C. Hypoglycemia or hypocalcemia[59]
   D. Acidosis
   E. Meconium aspiration syndrome[12]
   F. Parenchymal pulmonary disease
   G. Pneumonia (beta strep)
   H. Transient tachypnea of the newborn[21]
   I. Alveolar hypoventilation[141]
   J. Myocardial dysfunction and ischemia[59]
   K. Sepsis[147]
   L. Acquired surfactant deficiency (i.e., chemical meconium aspiration syndrome, pneumonia, and aspiration)

PPHN, Persistent pulmonary hypertension of the newborn.

---

tect plethora that could lead to increased pulmonary vascular resistance, and to detect an infectious process such as group B streptococcal sepsis or pneumonia.

Arterial blood gases demonstrate acidosis, hypoxia, and increased Pa_{CO_2}. If a blood gas is obtained simultaneously in the right radial artery (preductal) and in the descending aorta (postductal), the right-to-left shunt can be documented (preductal Pa_{O_2} > postductal). Simultaneous preductal and postductal pulse oximetry and/or transcutaneous oxygen measurements may also be useful in the diagnosis.

The most common radiographic findings associated with PPHN include the following[76]:

- Prominent main pulmonary artery segment
- Mild-to-moderate cardiomegaly
- Variable pulmonary vasculature (increased, decreased, or normal)
- Signs of left ventricular dysfunction that include pulmonary venous congestion and cardiomegaly

The electrocardiogram is usually normal but may demonstrate right ventricular hypertrophy and signs of myocardial ischemia. Echocardiography is helpful in evaluating cardiac structures and ruling out cyanotic lesions. It is often helpful in the evaluation of pulmonary valve pattern for evidence of pulmonary hypertension.

Other diagnostic tests are outlined in Table 22-10.

Treatment

Treatment of PPHN focuses on intervening in or preventing the development of the cyclic pattern previously described.[150] Infants presenting with low systemic blood pressure and cyanosis should have immediate supportive treatment. Intervention is aimed at using various maneuvers to increase pulmonary blood flow.[39,51,132] Pulmonary blood flow should increase if the pulmonary vascular resistance is decreased or if systemic vascular resistance is increased. In both instances right-to-left shunting is impeded. Conventional treatment modalities include direct dilation of pulmonary vasculature through intubation and mechanical ventilation using hyperoxia and hyperventilation, which produce alkalosis. The infant should be ventilated with whatever combination of rate, pressure, and oxygen is needed to lower Pa_{CO_2} and raise pH (Tables 22-11 and 22-12). Although the exact mechanism is unknown, alkalosis and/or hypocarbia produce a direct vasodilatory effect on pulmonary vasculature, decreasing pulmonary vascular resistance and thereby improving oxygenation.[51] Large, vigorous infants may require sedation with fentanyl (2 to 4 µg/kg),[71] or muscle paralysis with pancuronium bromide (0.03 to 0.06 mg/kg/dose) to promote effective ventilation.

In addition to mechanical ventilation, the use of

Table 22-10
Diagnostic Tests for PPHN

Test	Use
Hyperoxia test	If P_{O_2} does not increase in 100% oxygen, a right-to-left shunt is demonstrated (may be secondary to either PPHN or congenital heart disease)
Comparison of preductal and postductal arterial P_{O_2}	Demonstrates ductal shunting; if negative, it does not rule out PPHN; most congenital heart disease has no ductal shunting
Contrast echocardiography "bubble echo"	Demonstrates foramen ovale shunting but should be present in most PPHN
Hyperoxia-hyperventilation	Most definitive test; if P_{O_2} <50 mm Hg prehyperventilation and rises to above 100 mm Hg, is almost always PPHN

PPHN, Persistent pulmonary hypertension of the newborn.
From Duara S, Gewitz MH, Fox WW: *Clin Perinatol* 11:641, 1984.

Table 22-11
pH and P_{CO_2} Control in PPHN

Steps	Control in PPHN
1	Object is to reduce right-to-left shunt by hyperventilation → increase pH and reduce P_{CO_2} → reduce pulmonary artery pressure → reduce right-to-left shunt.
2	Each patient seems to have a *critical* level of P_{CO_2} below which P_{O_2} begins to rise. The clinician must determine the necessary level of P_{CO_2} early during treatment.
3	Use P_{CO_2} levels as low as 16 torr, if necessary, to control P_{O_2}. If P_{O_2} is not controlled, the prognosis is poor.
4	In the acute, critical stages of the disease, use high ventilator rates and whatever inflating pressure is necessary to decrease P_{CO_2} to the critical level.
5	Ventilator rates of 100 to 150 breaths/min are recommended during initial therapy to lower the inflating pressure and maintain a low P_{CO_2}.

PPHN, Persistent pulmonary hypertension of the newborn.
Modified from Fox WW, Duara S: *J Pediatr* 103:505, 1983.

pharmacologic vasodilators, such as tolazoline, sodium nitroprusside, prostaglandin E1, and others, have been recommended to decrease pulmonary vascular resistance.[104] Tolazoline is a potent vasodilator of the pulmonary and systemic circulation that may be used in the treatment of PPHN. The pulmonary vascular response should be assessed by rapidly (10 to 15 minutes) infusing 1 to 2 mg/kg of tolazoline through a peripheral scalp vein that drains into the superior vena caval system. If the response is favorable (improved Pa_{O_2}), a continuous infusion of 0.5 to 1 mg/kg/hr may be instituted. When tolazoline is being used, another IV line is needed to administer fluids and medications to support the systemic blood pressure. The infant must also be observed for gastrointestinal bleeding, pulmonary hemorrhage, and/or systemic hypotension. In the presence of systemic hypotension, volume expansion with albumin, plasma, or blood should be instituted. In the event of hypotension refractory to volume expansion, isoproterenol or dopamine should be considered.

Because of tolazoline's side effects, many clinicians use sodium nitroprusside, PgE1, or other agents (Table 22-13). Infusion of vasopressors (dopamine, dobutamine, and isoproterenol) and/or afterload reducers (nitroprusside) has been advocated to increase cardiac output and perfusion.[39] Vasopressors decrease the ratio of pulmonary systemic vascular resistance, thereby decreasing the amount of right-to-left shunting and increasing cardiac output. Continuous infusions of systemic vasopressors are primarily used as an adjunct to or to counterbalance the hypotension caused by systemic vasodilators.

As previously discussed, inhaled NO (1 to 10 ppm) has been shown to be effective in many neonates with PPHN.[121] Its advantages over pharmacologic agents is due to the selective and potent vasodilatory effects without causing systemic hy-

Table 22-12
Guidelines for Operation of Mechanical Ventilator in PPHN

Factor	Goal	Common error
Inspiratory pressure	Level necessary to $\downarrow$ P_{CO_2}	Inadequate inspiratory pressure (no movement of chest wall, or decreasing P_{CO_2}); reading on hand manometer may differ from that on ventilator
Ventilator rate	Rapid rates (up to 150 breaths/min) to $\downarrow$ P_{CO_2}, with lowest inspiratory pressure possible	Use of ventilator with maximum rate below level needed to $\downarrow$ P_{CO_2}; may require hand ventilation to achieve high rates
Positive end-expiratory pressure	Low values unless pulmonary parenchymal disease exists	Failure to try different levels as patient condition changes
Inspired O_2 concentration	P_{O_2} >100 to 120 torr	Weaning too rapidly
Inspiratory/expiratory ratio	Short inspiratory time to prevent air trapping at rapid rates	Inadequate flow rates to achieve short inspiratory time

PPHN, Persistent pulmonary hypertension of the newborn.
Modified from Fox WW, Duara S: *J Pediatr* 103:511, 1983.

potension. Responsiveness to inhaled NO is partly dependent upon the disease associated with pulmonary hypertension. For example, neonates with idiopathic PPHN without parenchymal lung disease respond more often to an inhaled NO than neonates with MAS and pulmonary hypertension. Similarly, the use of HFOV is more often effective in PPHN neonates with lung disease. Finally, many neonates who fail to respond to inhaled NO or HFOV alone respond well to the combination of these therapies.[97]

Because maintaining adequate oxygenation is a prime goal of care of infants with PPHN, alterations in "routine" care and handling are essential. Because handling a sick newborn for any reason causes a fall in Pa_{O_2}, the benefits of handling for routine care such as changing linens, weighing, suctioning, and taking vital signs must be balanced against the risk of iatrogenic hypoxia. Pa_{O_2} variations in the newborn are as follows[34,45]:

At rest	±15 mm Hg variation
While crying	$\downarrow Pa_{O_2}$ by as much as 50 mm Hg
With routine care	$\downarrow Pa_{O_2}$ by as much as 30 mm Hg

Organized, coordinated care and minimized disturbances are therefore very important. If the infant is not sedated or paralyzed, keeping the infant calm is very important because severe hypoxia will accompany crying. Using pacifiers and decreasing noxious stimuli (e.g., invasive procedures) keeps struggling and crying to a minimum. Continuously monitoring vital signs, blood pressure, and transcutaneous blood gases or pulse oximetry decreases the need for physical manipulation and disturbance.

Complications

Complications are usually associated with treatment and underlying causes and not primarily with PPHN. Risks of conventional ventilation include air leaks, oxygen toxicity, and barotrauma, which can lead to the development of chronic lung disease. Hypocarbia has been known to decrease cerebral blood flow.[20] There has been concern that the prolonged profound hypocarbia produced by hyperventilation could cause severe ischemic damage to the rapidly growing newborn brain.

Apnea

Physiology

The two major control mechanisms that regulate pulmonary ventilation are the neural and chemical systems. The cerebral cortex and brainstem are the governing agents for the neural control system,

Table 22-13
Vasopressor Response in the Neonate

Drug Dose	Disadvantages
Dopamine	
<4 µg/kg/min: renal vasodilation, mesenteric and cerebral vasodilation (effects unknown) plus increase in cardiac output	May decrease systemic arterial pressure
5-20 µg/kg/min: increase in cardiac output depending on myocardial norepinephrine	Loss of renal and mesenteric perfusion
>20 µg/kg/min: systemic arterial pressure increases more than pulmonary artery pressure	Cardiac output may decrease Myocardial oxygen consumption increases Marked increase in left ventricular afterload Dysrhythmias noted
Dobutamine	
10 µg/kg/min: increases cardiac contractility directly; cardiac output increases depending on myocardial catecholamine stores	No selective renal or mesenteric vasodilation Tends to increase skeletal blood flow at the expense of viscera Increase in pulmonary artery pressure
Isoproterenol	
0.05-1.0 µg/kg/min: lowers pulmonary vascular resistance in pulmonary hypertensive and vascular disease in child and adult; lowers hypoxemia-induced pulmonary vascular resistance in animal models	Dysrhythmias No specific vasodilation effects
Nitroprusside	
0.4-5.0 µg/kg/min: cardiac output increases because of decreased left ventricular afterload; systemic vascular resistance (indicated by blood pressure) decreases because of decrease in left ventricular afterload	Systemic vascular resistance remains constant if CO_2 increases

Modified form Drummond W: *Clin Perinatol* 11:715, 1984.

which regulates respiratory rate and rhythm. The peripheral components of this system are found in the upper airway and lung. The chemical control center is found in the medulla and is sensitive to changes in $Paco_2$. The peripheral portion of the chemical system lies in the carotid and aortic vessels and is sensitive to changes in $Paco_2$.[116] Alveolar ventilation is controlled by the chemical system, and this system is the principal defense against hypoxia. Neonates have a unique response to hypoxemia and carbon dioxide retention. Unlike adults, who have sustained increase in ventilation, infants have a brief period of increased ventilation followed by respiratory depression.

Carbon dioxide responsiveness is less devel-oped in the preterm infant and may be the result of decreased sensitivity in the chemical center or mechanical factors that prevent an increase in ventilation.[116] Apnea of prematurity or primary apnea is not associated with other specific disease entities. The younger the gestational age, the greater the incidence of apnea. Apnea may be associated with hypoxemia, neuronal immaturity, sleep, catecholamine deficiency, and respiratory muscle fatigue.

Etiology

Clinically, various conditions may cause apnea in the premature infant by producing hypoxia and/or

Table 22-14
Causes of Apnea in the Premature Infant

Causes	Specifics
Infection	Pneumonia, sepsis, meningitis
Respiratory distress	RDS, airway obstruction, CPAP application, postextubation, congenital anomalies of the upper airways
Cardiovascular disorders	Patent ductus arteriosus, congestive heart failure
Gastrointestinal disorders	Gastroesophageal reflux, necrotizing enterocolitis
CNS disorders	Depressant drugs, intraventricular hemorrhage, seizure, kernicterus, infection, tumors
Metabolic disorders	Hypoglycemia, hypocalcemia, hyponatremia
Environmental	Rapid increase of environmental temperature, hypothermia, vigorous suctioning, feeding, stooling, stretching
Hematopoeitic	Polycythemia, anemia

RDS, Respiratory distress syndrome; *CPAP,* continuous positive airway pressure.

altering the sensitivity of peripheral or central chemoreceptors[116] (Table 22-14). Neuronal immaturity seems a plausible cause for apnea. Respiratory efforts are more unstable at a younger gestational age. The decreased response appears to be the result of a general lack of dendritic formation and limited synaptic connections, therefore decreasing the excitatory drive. Another postulation is that apneic episodes are manifestations of synaptic disorders that occur without a motor component. Such phenomena have been confirmed on electroencephalogram. Infants depend on alternating excitation and inhibition to establish rhythmic breathing, and therefore imbalances (e.g., hypoxia, hypoglycemia, or hypocalcemia) may cause respiratory arrest.

Apnea has been noted to appear with greater frequency during sleep and especially during REM or active sleep in both term and preterm infants. Apnea is uncommon in non-REM sleep, but periodic breathing may be observed. The effects of REM sleep are inhibition of spinal motor neurons,

increase in brain activity causing increasing eye movements and muscular twitching, and changes in brain temperature and cerebral blood flow and CNS arousal shown by electroencephalogram changes.

Decreased amounts of peripheral catecholamines in the premature infant have also been postulated as a cause of apnea. This would become critical if hemorrhage or infection was also present in the premature infant and stores were depleted.

The premature infant has a more compliant chest cage and less compliant lungs; this situation results in a greater workload. Respiratory muscle fatigue occurs easily in the absence of fatigue-resistant fibers.

Apnea associated with the sleep state becomes more significant in that premature infants, particularly those less than 32 weeks of gestation, spend 80% of their time asleep. Equally significant is the time spent in REM sleep, the predominant sleep state of premature infants. The percentage of quiet sleep or non-REM sleep will increase from 20% to 60% of the total sleep period by the time an infant is 3 months old.

Secondary apnea may be associated with a particular disease entity or in response to special procedures. Many disorders leading to secondary apnea may exert their influence through hypoxemia and subsequent respiratory center depression.

The majority of cases of secondary apnea arise from four conditions. In RDS, apnea is related to the degree of parenchymal disease and may result from muscle fatigue. With CNS hemorrhage and seizures, apnea arises from asphyxia with subsequent hypoxemia and respiratory center depression or actual brain injury. Apnea is related to central depression in sepsis. In addition, carbon dioxide retention and hypoxemia associated with the left-to-right shunting of a PDA may cause apnea.

Iatrogenic causes of apnea include increased environmental temperature, sudden increases in environmental temperature, vagal response to suctioning of the nasopharynx or to a gavage tube, gastrointestinal reflux, and obstruction of the airway. Reflex apnea occurs when foreign material (milk) is present in the oropharynx. The reflex is protective in that it prevents inhalation of the substance into the airway. Obstruction may occur from improper neck positioning or aspiration.

Prevention

All infants assessed as high risk for apneic spells should be carefully monitored for a period of at least 10 to 12 days. Impedance apnea monitors do not distinguish normal respiratory efforts from gasping movements associated with obstruction. Both heart rate and respiratory rates should be monitored. Alarm systems should be used at all times. A qualified observer is essential.

Pulse oximetry monitors may detect hypoxemic conditions that may lead to apneic spells. In the premature infant younger than 32 weeks gestation this type of apnea is common. Care should be organized to decrease stressful, hypoxic episodes.

Apneic episodes may be prevented or decreased by several means. Gentle tactile stimulation alone has been shown to be effective in decreasing and preventing apneic spells in most premature infants. Noxious stimuli such as vigorous shaking or banging on the incubator should be avoided. If tactile stimulus is ineffective and temporary bag and mask ventilation is required, attention should be paid to preventing undue pressure on the lower chin and neck so that the airway remains clear. Bagging that is too vigorous may also stimulate pulmonary stretch receptors and induce apnea; therefore it should be avoided. Waterbed flotation may decrease the frequency of apnea but generally does not completely eliminate it.

Because increased environmental temperature and sudden changes in temperature have resulted in apneic episodes, prevention includes maintaining the environmental temperature at the lower end of the normal spectrum, particularly if an apneic episode has already occurred. Incubator temperature may require a 0.5° to 1.0° C (1° to 2° F) decrease to counter the problem. Phototherapy may provide sufficient radiant energy to increase the infant's temperature and contribute to the incidence of apnea. Care should be taken to avoid sudden changes in temperature. An infant should not be placed on a cold scale; the infant should be placed in a prewarmed incubator or bed. Oxygen should be warmed and humidified before administration.

Careful attention must be paid to prevent airway obstruction. Small neck rolls under the neck and shoulders have been used to decrease neck flexion and prevent airway obstruction when in the supine position. Close monitoring should be done during procedures such as lumbar puncture where accidental airway obstruction may occur.

Data Collection

Evaluation of apnea should include studies to rule out treatable causes.

History

Evaluation of the prenatal and birth history may give a clue to the causes and also provide a basis for further study.

Physical Examination

A thorough physical and neurologic examination rules out grossly apparent abnormalities. Observation and documentation of apneic and bradycardia episodes and any relationship to precipitating factors help differentiate primary from secondary apnea.

Laboratory Data

A CBC helps assess infection and anemia as causes of apnea. Serum glucose, calcium, phosphate, magnesium, sodium, potassium, and chloride levels help assess metabolic causes. Arterial blood gas measurements help assess hypoxemia and metabolic and respiratory contributions to apnea. Blood, urine, and CSF culture help rule out sepsis as the cause of apnea. The CSF culture is usually done only when other signs and symptoms of infection are present. Chest x-ray examinations help in assessing cardiac and respiratory causes. The examinations may also rule out aspiration of abdominal contents caused by gastroesophageal reflux. Ultrasound examination of the head and electroencephalogram may be used to rule out IVH or other neurologic causes of apnea.

Treatment

Treatment of secondary apnea is aimed at the diagnosis and management of the specific causes. In the treatment of primary apnea (apnea of prematurity), initial efforts should begin with the least invasive intervention possible. Gentle tactile stimulation is frequently successful, especially with early recognition and intervention. When infants do not immediately respond to external stimuli, bag and mask ventilation must be initiated. Gener-

ally, an Fio_2 approximating that used before the spell but not exceeding a 10% increase will alleviate hypoxemia and avoid marked elevations in the arterial Pao_2. The use of pulse oximetry or a $TcPo_2$ monitor will allow closer following of Pao_2 fluctuation and help prevent complications of oxygen toxicity. Elevation in ambient oxygen concentrations, although decreasing the frequency of apnea, causes prolongation of apnea spells.

Apnea will respond to low pressure (3 to 5 cm of water) nasal CPAP. Mechanical ventilation may be required if the infant fails to respond to lesser measures and continues to have repeated and prolonged apneic episodes. It may also be required in extremely immature, unstable, or debilitated infants.

Methylxanthines (caffeine, theophylline, and aminophylline) are used to treat apnea of prematurity (Table 22-15). They are used only in primary apnea (i.e., when pathologic causes have been eliminated). Treatment should follow a strict protocol, and serum levels must be checked. Methylxanthines are potent cardiac, respiratory, and CNS stimulants and smooth muscle relaxers. Their effect on decreasing the frequency of apnea is related to central stimulation rather than to changes in pulmonary function.

Complications

Side effects of xanthines include gastric irritation, hyperactivity (restlessness, irritability, and wakefulness), myocardial stimulation (tachycardia and hypotension), and increased urinary output.

Prognosis for apnea arising from an underlying cause depends on the outcome of the disease process itself. The prognosis for apnea is generally good in infants who are otherwise well and healthy and for whom the apnea is not prolonged. The prognosis becomes increasingly less favorable with an increased frequency and duration of episodes. Prompt recognition and intervention decrease the possibility of severe complications from hypoxia.

Parent Teaching

Parental attachment to the infant with respiratory disease is especially difficult. It is made more difficult if the infant is also premature. Normal interaction is curtailed by the infant's condition and appearance, the environment, and the parent's reaction to these factors. The infant who is in an oxygen hood or being ventilated may give inadequate cues to arouse parental attachment and instead may, arouse feelings of grief and loss (see Part VI).

The goal of discharge planning is the best possible outcome with the least family disruption. Evaluation of parental readiness to care for their infant is essential to effective teaching and learning. Physical surroundings and preparations for the infant are assessed when possible by a home visit. Parental concerns at bringing home an infant

Table 22-15
Methylxanthines Used to Treat Apnea of Prematurity

Drug	Dosage	Therapeutic Levels	Side Effects
Caffeine citrate	Loading: 20 mg/kg Maintenance: 2.5 mg/kg/day	Afterload: 8-14 µg/ml Maintenance: 7-20 µg/ml	Tachycardia, dysrhythmias, diuresis, glucosuria, keto-nuria, hyperglycemia, jit-teriness, seizures, vomit-ing, nausea, hemorrhagic gastritis
Theophylline	Loading: 5-6 mg/kg Maintenance: 1 mg/kg q8h to 3 mg/kg q12h	5-15 µg/ml, although levels of 3-4 µg/ml have been shown to be effective in decreasing apnea	See above

with special care needs must be assessed and discussed. The parents learn to be comfortable in handling and caring for their infant gradually throughout hospitalization. A specially designated or decorated room is used for family visiting and caretaking. Before discharge, the mother and/or father spend the night caring for the infant. Positive reinforcement and praise from the professional staff should be freely given to parents who attend classes and successfully master the tasks of caregiving for their infant.

Special equipment such as oxygen tanks, nasal cannulas, a respirator, and suction equipment for home use must be acquired before discharge. Sources, mode of delivery, and use of equipment must all be taught to parents before discharge. Pulmonary hygiene for infants with prolonged difficulty in handling secretions must also be taught. Written protocols and instructions should be provided to parents whenever possible. Parents must be informed of dosage, route of administration, side effects, and planned duration of use of all medications.

Because fluid and nutritional status is so important to any infant with a chronic condition, nutritional information for parents is required. Infants with tachypnea (BPD) often have difficulty with coordinating suck and swallow. Often smaller, more frequent feedings are necessary when using supplemental oxygen. Alternative feeding methods such as gavage feeding may be necessary to safely provide enough calories with a minimum of work.

Apnea is especially distressing to parents because of their fears of recurrence once the child goes home. If apnea is related to an underlying disease, treatment of the cause should result in resolution of the apneic episodes. Parents can be reliably assured that recurrence is unlikely unless the disease recurs. With apnea of prematurity, such assurances cannot be offered. However, the assurance can be offered that infants do grow into a regular ventilatory pattern as their respiratory center matures and that all means to protect the infant will be used until that time. Also, the parents can be assured that the infant will not go home until he or she is ready and the parents are adequately prepared to handle situations that may arise.

Before an infant needing a home monitoring system is discharged from the hospital, the parents must be given adequate support and instruction. Classes on the use of the apnea monitors must include demonstration of the equipment and return demonstrations. Minor equipment checks and repairs should be mastered before discharge.

Support by the primary care providers after discharge is essential. Parents must have telephone numbers of the medical facility and personnel they can call 24 hours a day in case of problems or equipment failure.

Anticipatory support includes discussion of potential stress factors related to having an infant on a monitor at home: sibling rivalries, marital stresses, scheduling problems, potential problems with babysitters, and the parent's own fears of the situation. An apnea monitor in the home may provoke anxiety in spite of discussion and instruction.

The parents of every infant who has apneic episodes or serious respiratory disease must be taught CPR. This is a skill that is learned over the course of time by reading written materials and seeing and returning the demonstration. Learning CPR cannot be done on the day of discharge but must be a staged process of individual and class instruction. Supplying instructional pamphlets written just for parents aids in initial learning and provides a quick reference. If other family members or babysitters will provide child care during work or evening hours, they too must be able to resuscitate the infant.

Other emergency actions for which parents must be prepared include clearing the infant's airway, calling for help (having emergency phone numbers easily accessible), planning for an alternate communication source (i.e., neighbor's phone), and notifying the community rescue squad of the infant's presence in the home.

Parents must be taught how to recognize signs of illness or significant deterioration in the condition of their infant. In addition to information about special care needs, parents need information about normal newborn care. Developing realistic expectations and positive parenting skills is as important to these parents as to all new parents.

For the parents of an infant with special respiratory problems, the importance of continuous follow-up care must be emphasized. Follow-up visits should coincide with developmental stages, the natural course of the disease, and expected complications of the disease.

The parents whose child has special respiratory needs must learn a myriad of involved technical information. The primary care provider (frequently the primary nurse) is responsible for organizing, teaching, coordinating, and documenting the information. This nurse is also responsible for ensuring that the parents have not only been taught but in fact understand.

References

1. Abman S, Groothuis J: Pathophysiology and treatment of BPD, *Pediatr Clin North Am* 41:277, 1994.
2. Abman S, Kinsella J: Inhaled nitric oxide therapy of pulmonary hypertension and respiratory failure in premature and term neonates, *Adv Pharmacol* 34:457, 1995.
3. Allen M et al: The limit of viability: neonatal outcome of infants born at 22-25 weeks gestation, *N Engl J Med* 329:1597, 1993.
4. American Academy of Pediatrics: An international classification of retinopathy of prematurity, *Pediatrics* 74:127, 1984.
5. American Academy of Pediatrics and American College of Obstetricians and Gynecologists: *Guidelines for perinatal care,* ed 3, Evanston, Ill, 1992, American Academy of Pediatrics.
6. American Academy of Pediatrics, Committee on Fetus and Newborn: Vitamin E and the prevention of retinopathy of prematurity, *Pediatrics* 76:315, 1985.
7. American Medical Association: International classification of retinopathy of prematurity, *Arch Ophthalmol* 102:1130, 1984.
8. American Respiratory Care Foundation and American Association for Respiratory Care: aerosol consensus statement, *Chest* 100:1106, 1991.
9. Auten R et al: Surfactant treatment of full-term newborns with respiratory failure, *Pediatrics* 87:101, 1991.
10. Avent M, Gal P, Ransom J: The role of inhaled steroids in the treatment of BPD, *Neonat Net* 13:63, 1994.
11. Avery ME, Oppenheimer EH: Recent increases in mortality from hyaline membrane disease, *J Pediatr* 57:553, 1960.
12. Bacsik R: Meconium aspiration syndrome, *Pediatr Clin North Am* 24:463, 1977.
13. Ballard R, Leonard C: Developmental follow-up of infants with persistent pulmonary hypertension of the newborn, *Clin Perinatol* 11:737, 1984.
14. Bancalari E, Gerhardt T: Broncho-pulmonary dysplasia, *Pediatr Clin North Am* 33:1, 1986.
15. Bancalari E, Sosenko J: Pathogenesis and prevention of chronic lung disease: recent developments, *Pediatr Pulmonol* 8:109, 1990.
16. Bernstein G et al: Prospective randomized multicenter trial comparing synchronized and conventional intermittent mandatory ventilation (SIMV vs. IMV) in neonates, *Soc Pediatr Res Abstract* 35(4):part 2, 1994.
17. Boros SJ et al: The effect of independent variations in I:E ratio and end expiratory pressure during mechanical ventilation in hyaline membrane disease: the significance of mean airway pressure, *J Pediatr* 91:114, 1977.
18. Brown E et al: BPD: possible relationship to pulmonary edema, *J Pediatr* 92:982, 1978.
19. Brownlee K et al: Catabolic effect of dexamethasone in the preterm baby, *Arch Dis Child* 67:471, 1992.
20. Bruce D: Effects of hyperventilation on cerebral blood flow and metabolism, *Clin Perinatol* 11:737, 1984.
21. Bucciarelli R et al: Persistence of fetal cardiopulmonary circulation: one manifestation of transient tachypnea of the newborn, *Pediatrics* 58:192, 1976.
22. Carlo WA et al: Early randomized intervention with high frequency jet ventilation in RDS, *Pediatrics* 117:765, 1990.
23. Carlo WA et al: Assisted ventilation and the complications of respiratory distress. In Fanaroff AA, Martin RJ, editors: *Neonatal-perinatal medicine,* ed 5, St Louis, 1992, Mosby.
24. Carson B et al: Combined obstetric and pediatric approach to prevention of meconium aspiration syndrome, *Am J Obstet Gynecol* 126:712, 1976.
25. Carroll P: Pneumothorax in the newborn, *Neonat Net* 10:27, 1991.
26. Carter J, Gertmann D, Clarck R et al: HFOV and ECMO for the treatment of acute neonatal respiratory failure, *Pediatrics* 124:661, 1994.
27. Chang H: Mechanisms of gas transport during ventilation with high frequency oscillation, *J Appl Physiol* 56:533, 1984.
28. Clark R: High frequency ventilation, *J Pediatr* 124:661, 1994.
29. Courtney S et al: Double blind one year follow-up of 1540 infants with RDS randomized to rescue treatment with two doses of synthetic surfactant or air in four clinical trials, *J Pediatr* 126:543, 1995.
30. Cox C, Wolfson M, Shafer T: Liquid ventilation: a comprehensive overview, *Neonat Net* 15:31, 1996.
31. CRYO-ROP Cooperative Group: Multicenter trial of cryotherapy for ROP, *Arch Ophthalmol* 106:471, 1988.
32. Cumming J, D'Eugenio D, Gross S: A controlled trial of dexamethasone in preterm infants at high risk for BPD, *N Engl J Med* 320(23):1505, 1989.
33. Curran C, Kachoyeanos M: The effects on neonates of two methods of chest physical therapy, *Matern Child Nurs J* 4:312, 1979.
34. Dangeman BC et al: The variability of Pao2 in newborn infants in response to routine care, *Pediatr Res* 10:149, 1976.
35. Davis J et al: Changes in pulmonary mechanics after caffeine administration in infants with BPD, *Pediatr Pulmonol* 6:49, 1989.
36. Davis J, Sinkin R, Aranda J: Drug therapy for BPD, *Pediatr Pulmonol* 8:117, 1990.
37. Davis J et al: High frequency jet ventilation and surfactant treatment of newborns in severe respiratory failure, *Pediatr Pulmonol* 13:108, 1992.

38. Davis J, Rosenfeld W: Chronic lung disease. In Avery G, Fletcher M, MacDonald M, editors: *Neonatology: pathophysiology and management of the newborn,* ed 4, Philadelphia, 1994, JB Lippincott.

39. Drummond W: Use of cardiotonic therapy in the management of infants with persistent pulmonary hypertension of the newborn, *Clin Perinatol* 11:715, 1984.

40. Duara S, Gewitz MH, Fox WW: Use of mechanical ventilation for clinical management of persistent pulmonary hypertension of the newborn, *Clin Perinatol* 11:641, 1984.

41. Duncan C, Erikson R: Pressures associated with chest tube stripping, *Heart Lung* 11:166, 1982.

42. Dunn D, Lewis A: Some important aspects of neonatal nursing related to pulmonary disease and family involvement, *Pediatr Clin North Am* 20:481, 1973.

43. Edwards DK, Colby TV, Northway WH: Radiologic pathologic correlations in bronchopulmonary dysplasia, *J Pediatr* 85:834, 1979.

44. Enhorning G, Robertson B: Lung expansion in the premature rabbit fetus after tracheal deposition of surfactant, *Pediatrics* 50:58, 1972.

45. Evans J: Incidence of hypoxia associated with caregiving in premature infants, *Neonat Net* 10:17, 1991.

46. Fanconi S, Duc G: Intratracheal suction in the sick preterm infant: prevention of intracranial hypertension and cerebral hypoperfusion by muscle paralysis, *Pediatrics* 79:538, 1987.

47. Ferrera B et al: Efficacy and neurological outcome of profound hypocapneic alkalosis for the treatment of persistent pulmonary hypertension in infancy, *J Pediatr* 105:457, 1984.

48. Ferrara T, Couser R, Hoekstra R: Side effects and long-term follow-up of corticosteroid therapy in VLBW infants with BPD, *J Perinatol* 10:137, 1990.

49. Finer NN, Kelly MA: Optimal ventilation for the neonate. II. Mechanical ventilation, *Perinatol Neonatol* 7:63, 1983.

50. Fittenberg J: Persistent pulmonary hypertension after lithium intoxication in the newborn, *Eur J Pediatr* 138:321, 1982.

51. Fox WW, Duara S: Persistent pulmonary hypertension in the neonate: diagnosis and treatment, *J Pediatr* 103:505, 1983.

52. Fraiberg S: Blind infants and their mothers: an examination of the sign system. In Lewis M, Rosenblum L, editors: *The effect of the infant on its caregiver,* New York, 1974, John Wiley & Sons.

53. Frank L, Sosenko I: Undernutrition as a major contributing factor in the pathogenesis of BPD, *Am Rev Respir Dis* 138:724, 1988.

54. Frank M: Theophylline: a closer look, *Neonat Net* 6:7, 1987.

55. Fujiwara T et al: Artificial surfactant therapy in HMD, *Lancet* 1:55, 1980.

56. Gal P et al: Beclomethasone for treating premature infants with BPD: guidelines for patient selection (letter), *J Pediatr* 5:122, 1991.

57. Gardner S, Hagedorn M: Physiologic sequelae of prematurity: the nurse practitioner's role. Part V. Feeding difficulties and growth failure (pathophysiology, cause and data collection), *J Pediatr Health Care* 5:122, 1991.

58. Gay J, Daily W, Meyer B: Ligation of the PDA in premature infants: report of 45 cases, *J Pediatr Surg* 8:677, 1973.

59. Gersony W: Neonatal pulmonary hypertension: pathophysiology, classification, etiology, *Clin Perinatol* 11:517, 1984.

60. Gerstman DR et al: The Provo multicenter early high frequency oscillatory ventilation trial: improved pulmonary and clinical outcomes in respiratory distress syndrome, *Pediatrics* 98:1044, 1996.

61. Gluck L, Kulovich M: Fetal lung development, *Pediatr Clin North Am* 20:367, 1973.

62. Goldson E: The micropremie: infants with birth weight less than 800 gms, *Infants and Young Children* 8:1, 1996.

63. Graff M et al: Prevention of hypoxia and hyperoxia during endotracheal suctioning, *Crit Care Med* 15:1133, 1987.

64. Gregory G: Respiratory care of newborn infants, *Pediatr Clin North Am* 19:311, 1972.

65. Groothuis J, Rosenberg A: Home oxygen promotes weight gain in infants with BPD, *Am J Dis Child* 141:992, 1987.

66. Gunderson L, McPhee A, Donovan E: Partially ventilated endotracheal suction, *Am J Dis Child* 140(5):462, 1986.

67. Gunn T: Risk factors in retrolental fibroplasia, *Pediatrics* 65:1096, 1980.

68. Hack M, Fanaroff A: Outcomes of extremely low birth weight infants between 1982 and 1988, *N Engl J Med* 321:1642, 1989.

69. Hack M: Follow-up of high risk neonates. In Fanaroff AA, Martin RJ, editors: *Neonatal-perinatal medicine,* ed 5, St Louis, 1992, Mosby.

70. Hack M et al: School age outcomes in children with birth weights <750 gm, *N Engl J Med* 331:753, 1994.

71. Hansen D, Hickey P: Anesthesia for hypoplastic left heart syndrome: use of high dose fentanyl in 30 neonates, *Anesth Analg* 65:127, 1986.

72. Harka K et al: Dexamethasone therapy for chronic lung disease in ventilator-and-oxygen-dependent infants: a controlled trial, *J Pediatr* 115(6):979, 1989.

73. Harris M et al: Successful extubation of infants with respiratory distress syndrome using aminophylline, *J Pediatr* 103:303, 1983.

74. Harrison VC, Heese H, Klein M: The significance of grunting in hyaline membrane disease, *Pediatrics* 41:549, 1968.

75. Harbar JD et al: A multicenter randomized placebo controlled trial of surfactant therapy for RDS, *N Engl J Med* 302:959, 1989.

76. Henry G: Noninvasive assessment of cardiac function and pulmonary hypertension in persistent pulmonary hypertension, *Clin Perinatal* 11:626, 1984.

77. HiFi Study Group: HFOV compared with conventional mechanical ventilation in the treatment of respiratory failure in preterm infants, *N Engl J Med* 320:88, 1989.

78. HiFi Study Group: HFO ventilation compared with conventional mechanical ventilation in the treatment of respiratory failure in preterm infants: assessment of pulmonary function at 9 months of corrected age, *J Pediatr* 116:933, 1990.

79. Hird M et al: Patient triggered ventilation using a flow triggered system, *Arch Dis Child* 66:1140, 1991.

80. Higgins R, Richter S, Davis J: Nasal continuous positive airway pressure facilitates extubation of VLBW neonates, *Pediatrics* 88:999, 1991.

81. Hodson W et al: BPD: the need for epidemiological studies, *J Pediatr* 95:848, 1979.

82. Holzman BH, Scarpelli EM: Cardiopulmonary consequences of positive end expiratory pressure, *Pediatr Res* 13:1112, 1979.

83. Hunsucker K et al: Laser surgery for ROP, *Neonat Net* 14:21, 1995.

84. Ignarro L et al: Endothelium-derived relaxing factor produced and released from artery and vein is nitric oxide, *Proc Natl Acad Sci USA* 84:9265, 1987.

85. Jacob J et al: The contribution of PDA in the neonate with severe RDS, *J Pediatr* 96:79, 1979.

86. Jobe A et al: Duration and characteristics of treatment of premature lambs with natural surfactant, *J Clin Invest* 67:370, 1981.

87. Johnson A et al: Functional abilities at age 4 years of children born before 29 weeks of gestation, *Br Med J* 306:1715, 1993.

88. Johnson L et al: Severe retinopathy of prematurity in infants with birth weights less than 1250 grams: incidence and outcome treatment with pharmacologic serum levels of vitamin E in addition to cryotherapy from 1985 to 1991, *J Pediatr* 127:632, 1995.

89. Jones R et al: Controlled trial of dexamethasone in neonatal chronic lung disease: a three-year follow-up, *Pediatrics* 96:897, 1995.

90. Kao LC et al: Oral theophylline and diuretics improve pulmonary mechanics in infants with bronchopulmonary dysplasia, *J Pediatr* 111(3):439, 1987.

91. Kanto W: A decade of experience with neonatal extracorporeal membrane oxygenation, *J Pediatr* 124: 335, 1994.

92. Kazzi N, Brans Y, Poland R: Dexamethasone effects on the hospital course of infants with BPD who are dependent on artificial ventilation, *Pediatrics* 86(5):722, 1990.

93. Kilbride H et al: Neurodevelopmental follow-up of infants with BW <801 gms with intracranial hemorrhage, *J Perinatol* 9:376, 1989.

94. Kinsella J et al: Hemodynamic effects of exgenous NO in ovine transitional pulmonary circulation, *Am J Physiol* 263:H875, 1992.

95. Kinsella J et al: Low dose inhaled NO in PPHN, *Lancet* 340:819, 1992.

96. Kinsella J et al: Clinical responses to prolonged treatment of PPHN with low doses of nitric oxide, *J Pediatr* 123:103, 1993.

97. Kinsella J, Alman S: Recent development in the pathophysiology and treatment of PPHN, *J Pediatr* 126:853, 1995.

98. Kinsey VE: RLF: Cooperative study of retrolental fibroplasia and use of oxygen, *Arch Ophthalmol* 56:481, 1956.

99. Klaus M, Fanaroff A: *Care of the high-risk neonate,* ed 3, Philadelphia, 1986, WB Saunders.

100. Klaus M, Meyer BP: Oxygen therapy for the newborn, *Pediatr Clin North Am* 13:725, 1966.

101. Klein N et al: Children who were very low birth weight: development and academic achievement at 9 years of age, *J Dev Behav Pediatr* 10:32, 1989.

102. Knoppert D, Mackanjee H: Current strategies in the management of BPD: the role of corticosteroids, *Neonat Net* 13:53, 1994.

103. Kuhns LR et al: Diagnosis of pneumothorax and pneumomediastinum in the neonate by transillumination, *Pediatrics* 56:355, 1975.

104. Kulik T, Lock J: Pulmonary vasodilator therapy in persistent pulmonary hypertension of the newborn, *Clin Perinatol* 11:694, 1984.

105. Kurzner S et al: Growth failure in infants with BPD: nutrition and increased resting metabolic expenditure, *Pediatrics* 8:379, 1988.

106. Laforce W, Bruno D: Controlled trial of beclomethasone dipropionate by the nebulization in oxygen and ventilator-dependent infants, *J Pediatr* 122:285, 1993.

107. Leach C et al: Partial liquid ventilation with perflubron in premature infants with severe RDS, *N Engl J Med* 335:761, 1996.

108. Lipper E et al: Survival and outcome of infants weighing 800 gm at birth, *Am J Obstet Gynecol* 163:146, 1990.

109. Locke R et al: Inadvertent administration of positive end-distending pressure during nasal cannula flow, *Pediatrics* 91(1):135, 1993.

110. Long JG, Phillip AGS, Lucey JF, Excessive handling as a cause of hypoxemia, *Pediatrics* 65:203, 1980.

111. Long W et al: Controlled trial of synthetic surfactant in infants weighing 1250 gms or more with respiratory distress syndrome, *N Engl J Med* 325:1696, 1991.

112. Long W et al: Effects of two rescue doses of a synthetic surfactant on mortality rate without bronchopulmonary dysplasia in 700-1350 gm infants with RDS: the American Exosurf neonatal study group I, *J Pediatr* 118:595, 1991.

113. Long W et al: Symposium on synthetic surfactant II: health and developmental outcomes at one year, *J Pediatr Suppl* 126:51, 1995.

114. Lotze A et al: Improved pulmonary outcome after exogenous surfactant therapy for respiratory failure in term infants requiring ECMO, *J Pediatr* 122:261, 1993.

115. Marinelli P et al: Acquired eventration of the diaphragm: a complication of chest tube placement in neonatal pneumothorax, *Pediatrics* 67:552, 1981.

116. Martin RJ, Miller MB, Carlo WA: Pathogenesis of apnea in preterm infants, *J Pediatr* 109:733, 1986.

117. Mauskopf J et al: Synthetic surfactant for rescue treatment of RDS in premature infants weighing from 700-1350 gms: impact on hospital resource use and charges, *J Pediatr* 125:94, 1995.

118. McCormick M et al: Very low birth weight children: behavior problems and school difficulty in a national sample, *J Pediatr* 117:687, 1990.

119. McDonald AD: Cerebral palsy in children of very low birth weight, *Arch Dis Child* 38:579, 1963.

120. Meredith R et al: Role of lung injury in the pathogenesis of HMD in premature baboons, *J Appl Physiol* 66:2150, 1989.

121. Miller C: Nitric oxide therapy for PPHN, *Neonat Net* 14:9, 1995.

122. Mitchell A et al: Limitations of patient triggered ventilation in neonates, *Arch Dis Child* 64:924, 1989.

123. Moylan F et al: The relationship of BPD to the occurrence of alveolar rupture during positive pressure ventilation, *Crit Care Med* 6:140, 1978.

124. Munoz K, Walton J: Hearing loss in infants with persistent pulmonary hypertension of the newborn, *Pediatrics* 81:650, 1988.

125. National Institutes of Health: Effect of corticosteroids for fetal maturation in perinatal outcomes, *NJH* 12(2):1, 1994.

126. Neonatal care for low birth weight infants: costs and effectiveness, Washington, DC, 1987, Office of Technology Assessment. (Health Technology Case Study 38, publication OTM-HCS-38).

127. Nickerson B: BPD chronic pulmonary disease following neonatal respiratory failure, *Chest* 87:528, 1985.

128. Nickerson B, Taussig L: Family history of asthma in infants with BPD, *Pediatrics* 65:1140, 1980.

129. Northway WH, Rosan RC: Radiographic features of pulmonary oxygen toxicity in the newborn: bronchopulmonary dysplasia, *Radiology* 91:49, 1968.

130. Okken A, Rubin IL, Martin RJ: Intermittent bag ventilation of preterm infants on CPAP: the effect on transcutaneous Po$_2$, *Pediatrics* 93:279, 1978.

131. Pepke-Zaba J et al: Inhaled NO as a cause of selective pulmonary vasodilation in pulmonary hypertension, *Lancet* 338:1173, 1991.

132. Perkin RM, Anas N: Pulmonary hypertension in pediatric patients, *J Pediatr* 105:511, 1984.

133. Perkin RM, Levin D, Clark R: Serum salicylate levels and right to left ductus shunts in newborn infants with persistent pulmonary hypertension of the newborn, *J Pediatr* 96:721, 1980.

134. Phelps D: Retinopathy of prematurity: an estimate of vision loss in the United States, *Pediatrics* 67:924, 1981.

135. Pierog SH, Ferrara A: *Approach to medical care of the sick newborn,* ed 2, St Louis, 1976, Mosby.

136. Preslan M: Laser therapy for ROP, *J Pediatr Opthalmol Strabis* 30:80, 1993.

137. Reale F, Esterly J: Pulmonary hypoplasia: a morphometric study of the lungs of infants with diaphragmatic hernia, ancephaly, renal malformations, *Pediatrics* 51:91, 1973.

138. Rhodes P, Hall R, Leonides J: Chronic pulmonary disease in neonates with assisted ventilation, *Pediatrics* 55:788, 1975.

139. Rhodes P et al: Minimizing pneumothorax and BPD in ventilated infants with hyaline membrane disease, *J Pediatr* 103:634, 1983.

140. Roberts J et al: Inhaled NO in PPHN, *Lancet* 340:818, 1992.

141. Rudolph A: High pulmonary vascular resistance after birth, *Clin Pediatr* 19:585, 1980.

142. Rush M, Hazinski T: Current therapy of BPD. In Holtzman R, Frank L, editors: *Clinics in perinatology,* Philadelphia, 1992, WB Saunders.

143. Saigal S et al: Cognitive abilities and school performance of extremely low birth weight children and matched term control children at age 8 years, a regional study, *J Pediatr* 118:751, 1991.

144. Saigal S et al: Comprehensive assessment of the health status in ELBW children at 8 years of age: comparison with a reference group, *J Pediatr* 125:411, 1993.

145. Schecter R: Laser treatment of ROP, *Arch Ophthalmol* 111:730, 1993.

146. Shaffer T, Greenspan J, Wolffson M: Liquid ventilation. In Boynton B, Carlo W, Jobe A, editors: *New therapies for neonatal respiratory failure,* New York, 1994, Cambridge University Press.

147. Shankaran S, Farooki Z, Desai R: Beta hemolytic streptococcal infection appearing as persistent fetal circulation, *Am J Dis Child* 136:725, 1982.

148. Skidmore M et al: Increased risk of cerebral palsy among very low birth weight infants with chronic lung disease, *Dev Med Child Neurol* 32:325, 1990.

149. Southgate W: Aerosolized pharmacotherapy in the neonate, *Neonat Net* 14:29, 1995.

150. Southwell S: Update on the treatment of persistent pulmonary hypertension of the newborn, *Neonat Net* 4:19, 1986.

151. Stern L: Therapy of the respiratory distress syndrome, *Pediatr Clin North Am* 19:221, 1972.

152. Synnes A et al: Perinatal outcomes of a large cohort of extremely low gestational age infants (23-28 wks), *J Pediatr* 125:952, 1994.

153. Taghizadih A, Reynold E: Pathogenesis of bronchopulmonary dysplasia following hyaline membrane disease, *Am J Pathol* 82:241, 1976.

154. The Collaborative Dexamethasone Trial Group: Dexamethasone therapy in neonatal chronic lung disease: an international placebo-controlled trial, *Pediatrics* 88(3):421, 1991.

155. The OSIRIS Collaborative Group: Early vs. delayed neonatal administration of a synthetic surfactant: the judgment of OSIRIS, *Lancet* 340 (8832):1363, 1993.

156. Tolles C, Stone K: National survey of neonatal endotracheal suctioning practices, *Neonat Net* 9:7, 1990.

157. Truog W, Feusner J, Baker D: Association of hemorrhagic disease and the syndrome of persistent fetal circulation with definitive diagnosis by two dimensional echocardiography, *Am Heart J* 102:936, 1981.

158. Truog W et al: BPD and pulmonary insufficiency of prematurity, *Am J Dis Child* 139:351, 1985.

159. United Kingdom Collaborative ECMO Trial Group: UK collaborative randomized trial of neonatal ECMO, *Lancet* 348:75, 1996.

160. Viscarde R et al: Efficacy of theophylline for prevention of post-extubation respiratory failure in VLBW infants, *J Pediatr* 107:469, 1985.

161. Visveschwara N et al: Patient triggered synchronized assisted ventilation of newborns: report of a preliminary study and three years experience, *J Perinatol* XI(4):347, 1991.

162. Voyles JB: BPD, *Am J Nurs* 81:51, 1981.

163. Wagaman M et al: Improved oxygenation and lung compliance with prone positioning of neonates, *J Pediatr* 94:787, 1979.

164. Werner J et al: Hypertrophic cardiomyopathy associated with dexamethasone therapy for BPD, *J Pediatr* 120:286, 1992.

165. Whyte H et al: Extreme immaturity: outcome of 568 pregnancies of 23-26 wks gestation, *Obstet Gynecol* 82:1, 1993.

166. Wilson J et al: Evaluation of oxygen delivery with use of nasopharyngeal catheters and nasal cannulas, *Neonat Net* 15(4):15, 1996.

167. Winters R: *Principles of pediatric fluid therapy,* Boston, 1982, Little, Brown.

168. Wright J: Closed-suctioning procedure in neonates, *Neonat Net* 15:87, 1996.

169. Yeh T et al: Early postnatal dexamethasone therapy in premature infants with severe RDS: a double-blind controlled study, *J Pediatr* 117:273, 1990.

170. Yoder M, Chua R, Tepper R: Effects of dexamethasone on pulmonary inflammation and pulmonary function of ventilator-dependent infants with BPD, *Am Rev Respirator Dis* 143:1044, 1991.

171. Yuskel B, Greenough A: Randomized trial of inhaled steroids in preterm infants with respiratory symptoms at follow-up, *Thorax* 47:910, 1992.

Resources for Parents

Videotapes

Cardiopulmonary resuscitation and emergency procedures for choking for infants and young children, University of Colorado Health Sciences Center School of Nursing, 1988. Distributed by Learner Managed Designs, Lawrence, Kansas.

Home oxygen for infants and young children, University of Colorado Health Sciences Center School of Nursing. Distributed by Learner Managed Designs, Lawrence, Kansas.

Booklet

Srokosz CL, editor: *A home oxygen programme for infants,* distributed by Hospital Education Services, PO Box 5777, London, Ontario, Canada NGA 416.

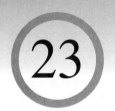

Cardiovascular Diseases and Surgical Interventions

Elaine Daberkow-Carson, Reginald L. Washington

Approximately 1 of every 100 infants has a congenital heart defect. Some infants have life-threatening defects requiring immediate action within the first few hours or days of life.[6] Others require no intervention until later in life or possibly not at all. It is important for the practitioner to recognize the presence of congenital heart disease, differentiate it from other conditions, and institute appropriate treatment. This chapter is designed to give the reader a clear understanding of neonatal circulation, signs and symptoms of congenital heart disease, and current management practices.

Congenital Heart Disease Overview

Physiology

Profound hemodynamic changes occur with the delivery of the newborn. Rudolph[14] provides an excellent detailed review of this topic. However, because a basic understanding of these physiologic principles is mandatory in understanding congenital heart disease, they are briefly presented here.

Fetal Circulation

Three shunts affect fetal circulation: the ductus venosus, the ductus arteriosus, and the foramen ovale. These three shunts allow mixing of the fetal blood and are important in the development of a normal heart.

The blood with the highest oxygen saturation in the fetus is in the umbilical veins and is shunted directly to the heart, bypassing the liver through the ductus venosus. Once in the heart, most of this highly saturated blood is shunted directly through the foramen ovale to the left atrium, left ventricle, aorta, and the coronary, carotid, and subclavian arteries. Therefore the blood with the highest oxygen saturation is directed to the tissues with the highest oxygen demand—the myocardium and the brain. The desaturated blood returning to the superior vena cava is primarily directed into the right ventricle, main pulmonary artery, ductus arteriosus, and descending aorta where it ultimately enters the placental circulation and is resaturated. Only a small percentage of blood flow is directed to the fetal lungs, where oxygen is delivered to the lung tissue rather than extracted from it.

Changes that Occur in the Fetal Circulation with Birth. In utero, the systemic vascular resistance is low primarily because of the low resistance in the placenta. The pulmonary arterioles, which are constricted and hypertrophied, are relatively resistant to blood flow. At birth the placenta is removed from the circulation, thereby greatly increasing the systemic vascular resistance. Initiation of respirations produces increased oxygen tension, which decreases pulmonary vascular resistance and increases pulmonary blood flow. In addition, the left atrial pressure increases, closing the foramen ovale and eliminating the right-to-left shunt through the foramen ovale (see Fig. 4-1).

The ductus arteriosus is extremely sensitive to the oxygen content of the blood, and the neonatal Pao_2 increases after birth. This increase in oxygen content initiates the constriction of the ductus arteriosus.

Once these changes take place, the newborn's circulation resembles that of an adult. Desaturated blood returns to the heart by the inferior and superior venae cavae, and enters the right atrium, right ventricle, pulmonary artery, and pulmonary circulation where oxygen and carbon dioxide are exchanged. The saturated blood then returns to the heart through the pulmonary venous system and enters the left atrium, left ventricle, and ultimately the aorta and systemic arterial system. However, pulmonary vascular resistance and pressures in the right ventricle and pulmonary system remain elevated in the neonate because of the hypertrophy of the pulmonary vessels. This hypertrophy slowly resolves, and the pulmonary vascular resistance and right heart pressures decrease to normal low levels between 1 and 2 months of age.

Etiology

Traditionally, the etiology of congenital heart defects has been viewed as multifactorial, involving a complex interaction between genetic and environmental factors.[13] Recent population-based studies have revealed data challenging these views. One study, the Baltimore-Washington Infant Study, identified all liveborn infants with a heart defect in the Midatlantic region and compared environmental and genetic characteristics.[12] The single greatest risk factor was genetic, defined as a history of congenital cardiovascular disease in the family. Additionally, familial congenital heart defects were often concordant by phenotype and developmental mechanism (see Table 23-1 for the most common environmental risk factors and Box 23-1 for other risk factors associated with an increased likelihood of congenital heart defects).[12] These studies, plus the recent advances toward identification of specific genes responsible for certain cardiovascular defects, suggest that genetic factors play a far more prevalent role than previously thought.

About 8% of congenital heart defects are associated with specific syndromes (e.g., trisomy 21 syndrome and Turner's syndrome) (Table 23-2). An additional 2% of congenital heart defects predominantly originate because of known environ-

Table 23-1
Most Common Environmental Triggers and Specific Defects Associated with Each

Potential Teratogens	Frequency of Cardiovascular Disease (%)	Most Common Malformations
Drugs		
Alcohol	25-30	Ventricular septal defect, patent ductus arteriosus, atrial septal defect
Amphetamines	5-10	Ventricular septal defect, patent ductus arteriosus, atrial septal defect, transposition of great arteries
Anticonvulsants	2-3	Pulmonary stenosis, aortic stenosis, coarctation of aorta, patent ductus arteriosus
Trimethadione	15-30	Transposition of great arteries, tetralogy of Fallot, hypoplastic left heart syndrome
Lithium	10	Ebstein's anomaly, tricuspid atresia, atrial septal defect
Sex hormones	2-4	Ventricular septal defect, transposition of great arteries, tetralogy of Fallot
Infections		
Rubella	35	Peripheral pulmonary artery stenosis, ventricular septal defect, patent ductus arteriosus, atrial septal defect
Maternal Conditions		
Diabetes	3-5	Transposition of great arteries, ventricular septal defect, coarctation of aorta
	30-50	Cardiomegaly, myopathy
Lupus erythematosus	?	Heart block

Box 23-1

Other Risk Factors Associated with Congenital Heart Defects

Exposure to Environmental Agents During Work and/or Hobby

- Paternal exposure to cold temperature
- Maternal exposure to various solvents, hairdyes, autobody repair work

Drug Exposure

- Diazepam, phenothiazines
- Corticosteroids
- Gastrointestinal drugs
- Paternal exposure to cocaine

Maternal Reproductive History

- Genetic risk factor (family history of congenital heart disease), >3 prior pregnancies and an increased number of miscarriages
- Without genetic risk but with premature births and previous induced abortion

Syndromic Associations

- 27.7% of all cases had either chromosomal anomalies, heritable syndromes, or an additional major organ system defect (see Table 23-2)

---

mental factors (rubella, maternal anti-convulsant therapy, or maternal alcohol consumption). Approximately 1% of infants in North America have congenital heart disease. Approximately 50% of these have a ventricular septal defect (VSD) alone or in combination with other cardiac abnormalities. Table 23-3 shows the most common congenital heart defects and their time of presentation.

Data Collection

History

A family history of congenital heart disease, a prenatal history of maternal viral infections (rubella and CMV) or drug or toxic substance ingestion, asphyxia or dysrhythmias before or at birth, a history of hydrops fetalis, or Rh incompatibility give clues about the possible presence of congeni-

tal heart disease.[3] The timing of the onset of symptoms may indicate the type of anomaly (see Table 23-3).

Clinical Presentation of Infants with Severe Cardiac Disease

Newborns with severe congenital heart disease usually have one or more of the following signs or symptoms: (1) cyanosis, (2) respiratory distress, (3) congestive heart failure and diminished cardiac output, (4) abnormal cardiac rhythm, and (5) cardiac murmurs. Although cardiac murmurs in the neonatal period do not necessarily indicate severe cardiac disease, they must be carefully evaluated. Absence of a murmur does not exclude cardiac disease. Infants with severe, life-threatening congenital anomalies of the cardiovascular system may not have a murmur.

Each of these previously mentioned categories is considered on an individual basis. The reader is reminded that the differential diagnosis of any individual sign or symptom is important, especially in the neonatal period when there is considerable overlap and several disease entities have identical symptoms. This section discusses each sign or symptom and briefly discusses the laboratory evaluation of each.

Cyanosis. Cyanosis is a bluish discoloration of the skin, nail beds, and mucous membranes resulting from the presence of 3 mg/dl or more of reduced hemoglobin in the arterial blood or 4 to 5 mg/dl or more of reduced hemoglobin in the peripheral capillary blood. Cyanosis therefore depends on the total hemoglobin concentration and the arterial oxygen saturation and requires immediate assessment.

When the causes of cyanosis are being considered, the six components of oxygen delivery must be considered individually. These are made up of the CNS, musculoskeletal system, airways, gas exchange interface in the lungs, hemoglobin, and cardiovascular system. Each of these is briefly reviewed here. The reader is referred to other sections of this book for a more complete discussion of the individual lesions.

Several disorders of the CNS and neuromuscular system cause poor oxygenation as a result of the abnormal rate or rhythm of respiration. Iatrogenic depression of the cardiovascular system may result

Table 23-2
Chromosomal Aberrations Evident in Neonatal Period that Are Associated with Congenital Heart Disease

Population	Incidence of Congenital Heart Disease (%)	Most Common Lesions		
		1	2	3
Trisomy 21 syndrome	50	Ventricular septal defect, endocardial cushion defect	Atrial septal defect	Patent ductus arteriosus
Trisomy 18 syndrome	99+	Ventricular septal defect	Patent ductus arteriosus	Pulmonary stenosis
Trisomy 13 syndrome	90	Ventricular septal defect	Patent ductus arteriosus	Dextrocardia
Turner's syndrome	35	Coarctation of aorta	Aortic stenosis	Atrial septal defect

Table 23-3
Diagnosis of Infants at Selected Ages*

0-6 Days (%)		7-13 Days (%)		13-20 Days (%)	
Transposition of great arteries	(17)	Coarctation of aorta	(19)	Ventricular septal defect	(20)
Hypoplastic left ventricle	(12)	Ventricular septal defect	(15)	Transposition of great arteries	(17)
Lung disease	(10)	Hypoplastic left ventricle	(11)	Coarctation of aorta	(16)
Tetralogy of Fallot	(9)	Transpostion of great arteries	(9)	Tetralogy of Fallot	(8)
Coarctation of aorta	(7)	Tetralogy of Fallot	(6)	Endocardial cushion defect	(6)
Ventricular septal defect	(7)	Heterotaxia	(4)	Heterotaxia	(6)
Pulmonary atresia (with intact ventricular septum)	(7)	Truncus arteriosus	(4)	Patent ductus arteriosus	(4)
Heterotaxia	(6)	Single ventricle	(4)	Total anomalous pulmonary venous return	(3)
Other	(25)	Other	(28)	Other	(20)
Total 896	(100)	Total 210	(100)	Total 116	(100)

*These numbers are intended as a rough guideline because there is considerable overlap. Infants with congenital heart disease are often active initially and appear well for several hours or days after birth. In contrast, infants with respiratory distress often have characteristic symptoms within the first several hours after birth.
From Fyler D et al: *Pediatrics* 65:391, 1980.

from the anesthetic administered to the mother before delivery. Birth trauma can cause either asphyxia or diaphragmatic paralysis and result in generalized cyanosis. Metabolic abnormalities that cause neuroencephalopathy and resultant cyanosis are hypoglycemia and hypocalcemia.

Several disorders of the lung result in poor oxygenation from alveolar hypoventilation. These include hypoplastic lung, bronchiogenic cysts, pulmonary arteriovenous malformation, atelectasis with resultant lobar emphysema, pneumothorax,

aspiration pneumonia, RDS, and shock lung. Differentiating between these disorders and primary cardiac disease is often difficult.

Because the cyanosis depends on the amount of reduced hemoglobin present, any abnormality of the blood that alters either the hemoglobin structure or content may result in cyanosis. Disorders such as polycythemia, hypovolemia, methemoglobinemia, and other hemoglobinopathies may account for cyanosis and must always be considered.

Finally, several disorders of the cardiovascular-pulmonary system may cause cyanosis, even though they do not involve actual structural defects. These include persistent pulmonary hypertension, pulmonary edema, dysrhythmias, and low cardiac output from any cause.

Respiratory Distress.   Respiratory distress may occur from pulmonary venous congestion as a result of a defect in the cardiovascular system, pulmonary disease, or both. This differentiation is often difficult, and newborns may have both primary pulmonary disease and cardiac defects.

Most infants with cyanosis from congenital heart disease do not have respiratory distress. When respiratory distress is present, the cyanosis is not proportional to the amount of respiratory distress evaluated from the physical and chest x-ray examinations. If cyanosis is present and is caused by a fixed right-to-left shunt (cardiac lesion) increasing inspired oxygen will have little effect on the arterial blood gases. However, if the cyanosis is caused by a diffusion defect in the lungs (pulmonary disorder), the degree of cyanosis often decreases with increasing inspired oxygen.

The shunt study is beneficial in differentiating respiratory disease from cyanotic heart disease. Shunt studies are performed by obtaining arterial blood gases (preferably from the right radial artery) when the infant is in room air and then after the infant has been in 100% oxygen for 5 to 10 minutes. If the Pao_2 is greater than 150 torr, the presence of a right-to-left shunt and cyanotic congenital heart disease as the cause of cyanosis is unlikely.

Congestive Heart Failure.   Congestive heart failure is a clinical syndrome reflecting the inability of the myocardium to meet the metabolic requirements of the body. Therefore the signs and symptoms of congestive heart failure reflect the decreased cardiac output and decreased tissue perfusion.

Congestive heart failure may be caused by (1) volume overload, (2) pressure overload, (3) cardiomyopathy, or (4) dysrhythmias. However, in the newborn, asphyxia and anemia must also be considered as causes of congestive heart failure.

The common symptoms associated with congestive heart failure can be explained using the physiologic principles previously outlined.

Tachycardia.   The heart attempts to compensate for the decrease in cardiac output by increasing either the heart rate or the stroke volume ($CO = HR \times SV$). The newborn has a reduced capacity to increase stroke volume, primarily because the fetal myocardium has relatively few contractile elements and is poorly innervated by the sympathetic nervous system. Therefore the newborn increases cardiac output mainly by increasing the heart rate, resulting in tachycardia.

Cardiac Enlargement.   Dilation and/or hypertrophy of the heart occurs in response to the volume or pressure overload, or the dysfunction associated with cardiomyopathies and dysrhythmias. Dilation of the cardiac chambers is evident on chest x-ray examination, with enlargement of the cardiac silhouette.

Tachypnea.   Inefficient emptying or overloading of the lungs results in interstitial pulmonary edema. Tachypnea is the first clinical manifestation of pulmonary edema. As pulmonary edema progresses, however, alveolar and bronchiolar edema occur, resulting in intercostal retractions, grunting, nasal flaring, dyspnea, rales, and possibly cyanosis.

Gallop Rhythm.   The gallop rhythm is an abnormal filling sound caused by the dilation of the ventricles. It is heard as a triple rhythm on auscultation.

Decreased Peripheral Pulses and Mottling of the Extremities.   Decreased cardiac output results in a compensatory redistribuiton of blood flow to vital tissues. Peripheral tissue perfusion is therefore decreased, resulting in mottling of the skin and a grayish or pale skin color, as well as decreased pulses.

Decreased Urine Output and Edema.   Decreased renal perfusion results in decreased glomerular filtration. This is interpreted by the body as a decrease in intravascular volume, initiating compensatory mechanisms such as vasoconstriction and fluid and sodium retention. Infants normally manifest this as weight gain or may have periorbital edema.

Diaphoresis.   Diaphoresis represents the increased metabolic rate with congestive heart failure and most likely increased activity of the autonomic nervous system. The increased metabolic rate is in response to the increased workload of the heart in failure.

Hepatomegaly.   The right ventricle in congestive heart failure is less compliant and may not adequately empty, leading to elevated pressures in the right atrium, central venous system, and hepatic system. Hepatomegaly results from hepatic congestion caused by the elevated central venous pressure.

Decreased Exercise Tolerance.   The decreased perfusion to peripheral tissues and the increased energy required by the heart in failure leave little energy reserve for activities such as feeding and crying. The infant may sleep a majority of the time, fall asleep during feedings, and have a weak cry.

Failure to Thrive and Feeding Problems.   Multiple factors contribute to the infant's failure to thrive and feeding difficulties. Tachypnea compromises the infant's ability to feed. The basal metabolic rate increases in infants with congestive heart failure, necessitating a higher caloric intake (150 cal/kg/day or more). The infant must expend more energy to consume the calories but lacks the energy to do so.

Diminished Cardiac Output.   An infant with poor peripheral pulses and skin mottling often has a profound decrease in cardiac output. This is commonly found in infants with coarctation of the aorta or hypoplastic left heart syndrome but may also be noted in asphyxia, metabolic disease, and sepsis.

The "E" class of prostaglandins, such as PGE, prolongs the patency of ductal tissue and is useful in certain "ductal-dependent" lesions (coarctation of the aorta, transposition of the great arteries, tricuspid atresia, pulmonary atresia or hypoplastic left heart syndrome) (Table 23-4).

Abnormalities of the cardiac rhythm and murmurs are discussed individually later.

Cardiac Examination

See section on specific cardiac lesions.

Laboratory Data

Arterial Blood Gases.   The $Paco_2$ in cardiac disease is often normal or increased if a primary pulmonary disease is present. Frequent monitoring of blood gases is unnecessary, but the acid-base balance should be monitored closely. The $Paco_2$ may be normal or decreased, depending on the cardiac lesion and pulmonary status of the infant.

Chest X-ray Examination.   The chest x-ray examination may be normal even if life-threatening congenital heart disease is present. However, the degree of pulmonary vascularity helps define the type of congenital heart disease present and is characterized as being increased, normal, or decreased. Likewise, the heart size should be evaluated and is described as being increased, normal, or decreased.

Electrocardiogram.   See the section on specific cardiac lesions.

Echocardiogram.   Echocardiograms are used to define cardiac anatomy, assess pressures, measure gradients, and evaluate cardiac function. The transthoracic echocardiogram is the most commonly used approach. It is noninvasive and performed with the transducer on the infant's chest. The transesophageal echocardiogram (TEE) is used for intraoperative and postoperative evaluations, as well as in patients in whom it is not possible to obtain adequate views of the cardiac anatomy or evaluation of function by transthoracic echo. TEE requires general anesthesia for control of the airway and patient comfort. TEE can be performed on infants as small as 2500 grams.

MRI offers three-dimensional reconstruction and high-resolution images of the heart and great vessels. The MRI is of particular use in evaluation of extracardiac vascularity, such as arch anomalies, vascular rings, and pulmonary arterial venous anomalies. The MRI provides high spatial resolution, excellent soft-tissue definition, a large field of view, and unrestricted demonstration of cardiovascular morphology. It does require sedation and a stable patient, and it is expensive.

General Treatment Strategy

Optimal management of infants with heart disease requires specialized expertise. Infants are monitored closely for hypoxia, hypoglycemia, acidosis, and congestive heart failure.

The infant must be kept in an incubator or warmer in which body temperature is maintained while color changes (pallor and increased cyanosis) may be observed. A cardiorespiratory monitor for continuous cardiac monitoring detects bradycardia, tachycardia, and dysrhythmias. Monitoring of oxygen saturations is helpful in determining

Table 23-4
Cardiac Drugs

Drug	Route	Dose	Onset of Action	Comments
Atropine	IV	0.01-0.03 mg/kg/dose prn (max 0.4 mg)	Seconds	May cause tachycardia, urinary retention, or hyperthermia
	PO	0.01-0.03 mg/kg/dose q4-6h (max 0.4 mg)	Minutes	May cause tachycardia
Calcium chloride (10% solution)	IV	0.2-0.3 ml (20-30 mg)/kg/dose q10min prn (max 500 mg)	Minutes	Slow infusion; *must* be IV; potentiates digoxin; bradycardia
Diazoxide (Hyperstat)*	IV	5 mg/kg/dose q30min prn	1-2 min	May cause hypotension or hyperglycemia
Dobutamine (Dobutrex)†	IV	2-10 µg/kg/min	Minutes	Do not use in IHSS or tetralogy of Fallot; may cause ventricular ectopy, tachycardia, or hypertension Incompatible with alkaline solutions
Dopamine (Intropin)*	IV	5-30 µg/kg/min	Minutes	Often combined with a vasodilator when used at higher doses to counteract alpha vessel constriction; inactivated in alkaline solution
Epinephrine (1:10,000)	IV	0.1 ml/kg/dose (max 5 ml/dose) q3-5min prn (0.01 mg/kg/dose)	Seconds	May cause tachycardia, dysrhythmias, or hypertension; not effective if acidosis is present
Furosemide (Lasix)	IV	1-2 mg/kg/dose	5-15 min	May cause metabolic alkalosis + hypokalemia
	PO	1-4 mg/kg/dose	30-60 min	Follow electrolytes; may need KCl supplementation; renal calcification
Hydralazine (Apresoline)	IV	0.1-0.5 mg/kg/dose q3-6h	15-30 min	May cause lupuslike syndrome, tachycardia, or hypotension
	PO	0.1-0.5 mg/kg q6h; may increase to max of 2 mg/kg q6h	Often days until titrated effect achieved	Same as above
Hydrochlorothiazide (HydroDiuril)	PO	1-2 mg/kg q12h	1-2 hr	May cause electrolyte imbalance; may need KCl supplementation
Indomethacin	IV	0.1-0.2 µg/kg/dose; may be repeated q8h for total of 3 doses		Less effective if administered after 7 days of age; probably will have no effect after 14 days of age
Isoproterenol (Isuprel)‡	IV	0.1-0.4 µg/kg/min	30-60 sec	May cause tachycardia/ventricular tachydysrhythmias; may also cause subendocardial ischemia
Lidocaine (Xylocaine)	IV	IV bolus 1-3 mg/kg; IV drip 30-50 µg/kg/min		May cause dysrhythmia, CNS agitation, or depression

*Safety and efficacy of these agents in children have not been established.
†Mix: 6 × weight (kg) = milligrams to be added to 100 ml D₅W. Yields: 1 ml/hr = 1 µg/kg/min.
  Example: 6 × 3 kg = 18 mg (dopamine, dobutamine, or Nipride) to be added to 100 ml D₅W.
‡Mix: 0.6 × weight (kg) = milligrams to be added to 100 ml D₅W. Yields: 1 ml/hr = 0.1 µg/kg/min.
  Example: 0.6 × 3 kg = 1.8 mg (Isuprel) to be added to 100 ml D₅W.
†,‡From Pediatric Life Support, Children's Hospital and Medical Center, Seattle, Washington, 1987.

Table 23-4
Cardiac Drugs—cont'd

Drug	Route	Dose	Onset of Action	Comments
Nitroprusside (Nipride)†	IV	1-10 µg/kg/min over 10 min to control blood pressure; chronic infusion—2 µg/kg/min (protect from light; change solution q4h)	Seconds	May cause hypotension and reflex tachycardia; may cause thiocyanate toxicity, especially if decreased renal function is present
Phentolamine (Regitine)	IV	1-20 µg/kg/min	5-10 min	May cause hypotension; commonly used with an inotropic agent
Phenytoin (Dilantin)	PO	5 mg/kg/day qid	N/A	May cause hypotension
	IV	Load: 10-15 mg/kg over 5 min slow infusion Maintenance: 3-5 mg/kg/day bid	5-10 min	May cause cardiac depression
	PO	3-5 mg/kg/day bid	2-4 hr	Therapeutic blood levels (5-20 µg/ml)
Procainamide (Pronestyl)	IV	Load: 10-15 mg/kg/dose (max 1000 mg) over 5 min Maintenance: IV 30-80 µg/kg/min	1-5 min	May cause hypotension or lupus-like syndrome
	IM	5-8 mg/kg q6h	15-30 min	Same as above
Propranolol (Inderal)	IV	Dysrhythmias: 0.01-0.15 mg/kg/dose slow IV q6-8h prn (max single dose, 10 mg); hypercyanotic spell: 0.15-0.25 mg/kg/dose slow IV push q 15 min (max dose 10 mg)	2-5 min	May severely decrease cardiac output
	PO	Dysrhythmias: 0.5-1.0 mg/kg/dose tid-qid (max daily dose 60 mg); hypercyanotic spells: 1-2 mg/kg/dose qid	30-60 min	Same as above
Prostaglandin E₁ (Prostin VR)	IV	0.01-0.1 µg/kg/min	Minutes	May cause apnea, fever, or hypotension
Quinidine gluconate (Duraquin)	PO	5-10 mg/kg q6h	4-8 hr	May cause gastrointestinal symptoms, hypotension, or blood dyscrasia
Spironolactone (Aldactone)	PO	1-2 mg/kg/day	3-5 days	Hyperkalemia, gastrointestinal upset, drowsiness
Tolazoline	IV	Test: 1-2 mg/kg slow IV push Maintenance: 1-2 mg/kg/hr	Minutes	May cause hypotension; gastrointestinal or pulmonary hemorrhage
Adenosine	IV	30-250 µg/kg		Slows the spontaneous heart rate and prolongs the PR interval, may cause transient complete heart block and hypotension, half-life is only 9.3 seconds so its effects quickly dissipate

adequacy of pulmonary blood flow and/or increased need for oxygen. The respiratory effort is assessed for tachypnea, shallow breathing, apnea, retractions, grunting, and nasal flaring. Observe and document activity level such as muscle tone, spontaneous movement, and seizure activity.

Management of Congestive Heart Failure

The medical management of congestive heart failure attempts to reverse the process outlined previously and helps the heart compensate with increased cardiac output.

Digoxin acts primarily as a positive inotropic (improves contractility) agent but decreases the heart rate and increases urine output (Box 23-2). This drug should be used with caution if acidosis, myocarditis, or obstructive lesions (e.g., tetralogy of Fallot, subvalvular pulmonary stenosis, and asymmetric septal hypertrophy) are present.

Diuretics such as furosemide (see Table 23-4) help decrease total body water (which is increased as a result of congestive heart failure). In general, chronic fluid restriction and low-salt diets are not commonly used in newborns or infants with congestive heart failure.

Infants with congestive heart failure may be difficult to feed, and the process is often frustrating. They may have trouble sucking, swallowing, and breathing simultaneously. They may need to rest frequently during a feeding, thus prolonging feeding times, and they may fall asleep exhausted before adequate caloric intake is achieved. Because caloric requirements are higher in infants with congenital heart disease, adequate nutrition must be assured by (1) observing the infant's ability to nipple feed (a soft free-flowing [premature] nipple offers the least resistance to sucking and helps the infant conserve energy), (2) providing adequate calories for growth and if necessary using alternative feeding methods (i.e., gavage or continuous nasogastric drip) if the infant is sucking poorly, (3) anticipating the infant's hunger and offering feedings before the infant uses energy by crying, (4) positioning the infant in a semi-erect position for feeding, (5) burping the infant after every half ounce to help minimize vomiting, and (6) weighing the infant daily and checking for appropriate weight gain. Before discharge from the nursery, the infant should be in stable condition (e.g., feeding well and gaining weight appropriately).

An important fact for families to understand is that many infants will gain weight very slowly because of their cardiac defects, regardless of the method of feeding that is used. The family of an infant in congestive heart failure needs support

---

Box 23-2

Digoxin Dosages and Common Side Effects

Digitalizing Schedule

Preterm infant
   PO route: 20 μg/kg total dose*
Term infant
   PO route: 30 μg/kg total dose*

Total dose is usually divided into three doses giving one half, then one fourth, then one fourth of the total dose q8h. Check ECG rhythm strip for rate, PR interval, and dysrhythmias before each dose.

Maintenance Schedule

Preterm infant
   PO route: 5-10 μg/kg/day*
Term infant
   PO route: 5-10 μg/kg/day*

Total dose should be divided bid. Allow 12-24 hr between last digitalizing and first maintenance doses. It takes about 6 days to "digitalize" a patient with maintenance doses alone. The sign of digitalis effect is usually prolongation of the PR interval. The first sign of digitalis toxicity is usually vomiting, dysrhythmias, or bradycardia.

Drugs such as quinidine, amiodarone, and diuretics predispose to digoxin toxicity. The clearance of digoxin is directly related to renal function. Dosage must be reduced in patients with impaired renal function.

* IV dose is 75% PO dose.

and teaching. Explanation of the term *congestive heart failure* should be given early, because it is a frightening term for parents. The words "heart failure" are often interpreted as "heart attack." It is important that parents understand that saying an infant is in heart failure does not imply that the infant's heart will stop. A simple explanation describing heart failure as a condition in which the heart shows signs of being less able to pump sufficient blood to meet all the needs of the body is helpful in decreasing anxiety for the family.

Specific Conditions[5,8,11]

Patent Ductus Arteriosus

Physiology

The ductus arteriosus is a normal pathway in the fetal circulatory system and allows blood from the right ventricle and pulmonary arterial system to flow into the descending aorta for ultimate delivery to the placenta (Fig. 23-1). Functionally, the PDA closes within a few hours to several days after birth, but this closure is often delayed in premature infants. After birth, as a result of a decrease in the pressure of the pulmonary circulation and an increase in the pressure of the aorta, the blood flow

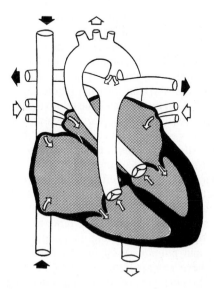

Figure 23-1   Patent ductus arteriosus. (Courtesy Ross Laboratories, Columbus, Ohio.)

through a PDA is predominantly from the aorta to the pulmonary artery (left-to-right shunt). The hemodynamic changes and the resultant clinical manifestations of a PDA depend on the magnitude of the pulmonary vascular resistance and the size of the ductal lumen.

Approximately 15% of infants with PDAs have additional cardiac defects, (VSD, coarctation of the aorta, aortic stenosis, or pulmonary stenosis). PDA can be associated with known syndromes, most commonly rubella.

Data Collection

History.   Asphyxial insult or RDS, inability to wean from a respirator, and an increasing Fio_2 demand usually accompany PDA.

Physical Findings.   Increased flow to the pulmonary circulation and volume overload of the left ventricle are the two major physiologic abnormalities in a PDA.

  Cyanosis.   Generally, cyanosis is not present in an isolated PDA, because the predominant shunt is from left to right.

  Heart Sounds.   Infants with a PDA may have audible murmurs as a result of the left-to-right shunting through the ductus during systole. A grade I through III systolic murmur is best heard at the upper left sternal border with radiation to the left axilla and faintly to the back. Although this murmur may occasionally flow into diastole, the classical continuous machinery-like murmur is an unusual occurrence in the newborn period. It is often helpful to briefly disconnect the newborn from the ventilator before auscultating. There are cases of large PDAs in which no murmur is audible.

  Pulses.   Because of the rapid upstroke and wide pulse pressure, the peripheral pulses are bounding. Pulses are hyperdynamic and easily palpated. Assessment of the pulses should include palpation of palmar, plantar, and calf pulses. The calf pulses are not usually palpable in infants. The presence of an easily palpated pulse in these areas suggests the presence of an aortic run-off lesion, which is most commonly a PDA.

  Congestive Heart Failure.   Because of the volume overload of the left ventricle, the infant may show signs of congestive heart failure and pulmonary edema (see section on congestive heart failure).

Laboratory Data

Arterial Blood Gases.   The arterial blood gases are normal.

Chest X-ray Examination.   Chest x-ray examination is normal in small shunts. Cardiomegaly is present with increased pulmonary vascularity in large shunts.

Electrocardiogram.   The ECG may be normal, demonstrate left ventricular hypertrophy, or demonstrate combined ventricular hypertrophy. Ischemia is rarely seen.

Echocardiogram.   An increased left atrial/ aortic ratio suggests a moderate to large left-to-right shunt (i.e., PDA, VSD). An echocardiogram should be performed before medical or surgical closure of the PDA to rule out a ductal-dependent lesion or other associated anomalies. Color flow mapping allows for visualization of the PDA, as well as determination of the direction of blood flow across the PDA (i.e., left to right, right to left, or bidirectional).

Cardiac Catheterization.   If the echocardiogram has eliminated a ductal-dependent lesion, cardiac catheterization is usually not required before treatment.

Treatment

Medical Management. Asymptomatic infants with PDAs generally do not require medical management or surgical ligation. These infants should be monitored for evidence of congestive heart failure, failure to thrive, increasing oxygen requirement, or other complications.

Symptomatic infants require ductal closure by either ductal ligation or indomethacin therapy. Medical management such as fluid restriction is rarely successful. Indomethacin is administered orally (PO) or intravenously (IV) at a dose of 0.1 to 0.2 mg/kg/dose and may be repeated every 8 hours for a total of three doses. It is much less effective if administered after 7 days of age and probably will have no effect after 14 days of age. Urine output should be continuously monitored, and if there is a dramatic decrease, the drug should be discontinued.

Surgical Treatment.   Surgical ligation or clipping the ductus arteriosus through a lateral thoracotomy incision is a low-risk procedure when performed by an experienced surgical team. Coil closure of a PDA in the cardiac catheterization laboratory or video-assisted transthoracic endoscopic closure of a PDA is usually not done in infants less than 3 to 6 months of age.

Complications and Residual Effects

Complications and residual effects, although rare, include (1) recannulization, (2) recurrent laryngeal or phrenic nerve palsies, or (3) false aneurysms. The surgical mortality in the neonatal period is generally less than 1%.

Prognosis and Follow-Up

Asymptomatic infants have an excellent prognosis, although close follow-up is necessary because if the ductus remains patent until 9 to 12 months of age, ligation is recommended.

Symptomatic infants with a persistent ductus arteriosus generally experience failure to thrive, continued congestive heart failure, increased oxygen requirements with resultant BPD, or pulmonary infections.

Ventricular Septal Defect

Physiology

VSDs may involve various portions of the ventricular septum and are classified according to the anatomic position that they occupy when viewed from the right ventricle (Fig. 23-2).

A VSD may occur as an isolated anomaly or may be part of a more complex cardiac lesion. Only isolated VSDs are discussed in this section. The effect of the VSD on the circulation depends on both the size of the VSD and the relative pulmonary vascular resistance. Pulmonary vascular resistance is nearly systemic immediately after birth but rapidly falls to one-fourth to one-third systemic in the first several days of life.

In a small VSD the left-to-right shunting at the ventricular level is minimal and the infants are asymptomatic.

Larger VSDs may have a mild to moderate left-to-right shunt, resulting in congestive heart failure and pulmonary edema. Premature infants tend to have lower pulmonary vascular resistance at birth, allowing greater left-to-right shunting, and therefore may be symptomatic. Infants with severe lung disease (RDS, BPD, or pneumonia) may have

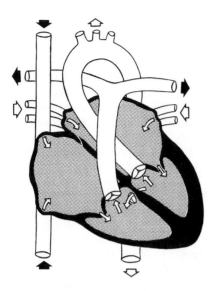

Figure 23-2 Ventricular septal defects. (Courtesy Ross Laboratories, Columbus, Ohio.)

elevated pulmonary vascular resistance and therefore minimal left-to-right shunting.

Data Collection

See Table 23-1 for infants at increased risk.

Physical Findings

Cyanosis. Infants with isolated VSDs are rarely cyanotic in the neonatal period.

Heart Sounds. Most infants with VSDs have a heart murmur. The time when this murmur is first audible depends on the pulmonary vascular resistance and the size of the defect. The murmur is typically a grade II to III/VI systolic murmur heard best at the lower left sternal border. A diastolic flow rumble at the apex indicates a large left-to-right shunt.

Congestive Heart Failure. Congestive heart failure is unusual in the newborn with an isolated VSD. When it occurs, however, it is a result of the volume overload of the left ventricle (see section on congestive heart failure).

Laboratory Data

Arterial Blood Gases. Arterial blood gases are normal.

Chest X-ray Examination. A chest x-ray examination shows a normal to increased heart size with an increased pulmonary vascular flow.

Electrocardiogram. The ECG in an infant with a VSD is usually normal but may demonstrate ventricular hypertrophy.

Echocardiogram. A two-dimensional echocardiogram is able to demonstrate the VSD in 90% of the cases. Doppler interrogation of the ventricular septum and/or color flow mapping have greatly increased the accuracy of diagnosing a VSD noninvasively. The use of color flow is particularly advantageous in identifying the presence of multiple VSDs and the direction of blood flow across the VSD.

Cardiac Catheterization. A cardiac catheterization is diagnostic but not required in the neonatal period unless there is some question regarding the diagnosis or if surgery is being considered.

Treatment

Medical Management. If the patient demonstrates failure to thrive or intractable congestive heart failure with maximum medical management, surgical intervention at any age is necessary (see section on general treatment strategy).

Surgical Treatment. Surgical treatment of a VSD consists of either suture closure or patching (using most commonly a synthetic material such as Dacron). In general, a VSD may be approached through a median sternotomy incision, then through the right atrium and tricuspid valve, thereby avoiding a right or left ventriculotomy.

If the infant is small (<2 kg) or single or multiple muscular VSDs are present, it may be necessary to perform a palliative procedure of pulmonary artery banding to decrease pulmonary blood flow until the infant is older and can undergo debanding and closure of the VSDs.

Complications and Residual Effects

Complications and/or residual effects may include (1) a persistent shunt (residual VSD), (2) conduction abnormalities (right bundle-branch block and third-degree heart block), and (3) aortic or tricuspid insufficiency (<1%).

The mortality in infants is less than 10%, with higher mortality found in the neonatal period. Contraindications to primary VSD closure include the diagnosis of double-outlet right ventricle and multiple muscular VSDs. The combined risk of pulmonary banding plus later debanding and VSD closure is about 10%.

Prognosis and Follow-Up

Approximately 50% to 75% of small VSDs will spontaneously close.

If a large left-to-right shunt is persistent after 9 to 24 months of age, the infant is susceptible to pulmonary vascular disease.

Coarctation of the Aorta

Physiology

Coarctation of the aorta is a localized constriction of the aorta that usually occurs at the junction of the transverse aortic arch and the descending aorta in the vicinity of the ductus arteriosus (Fig. 23-3). However, coarctation can occur anywhere in the aorta from above the aortic valve to the abdominal aorta. The precise location of the coarctation and the presence or absence of associated anomalies affect the clinical presentation. Associated anomalies include PDA, VSD, and bicuspid aortic valve

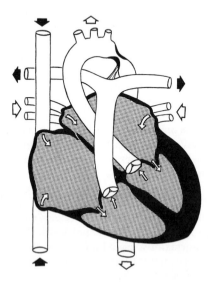

Figure 23-3 Coarctation of aorta. (Courtesy Ross Laboratories, Columbus, Ohio.)

(50%). Coarctation is frequently observed in infants with Turner's syndrome.

Data Collection

Physical Findings.   Newborns with critical coarctation of the aorta usually have signs and symptoms of congestive heart failure and low cardiac output. Coarctation of the aorta is a medical and surgical emergency.

Cyanosis.   Generally, cyanosis in the newborn is not present in the isolated coarctation of the aorta.

Heart Sounds.   Cardiac murmurs are generally not found in an isolated, severe coarctation of the aorta. If other associated cardiac defects are present, however, a murmur may be heard. A soft, grade I to II/VI systolic murmur may be present at the left sternal border, radiating to the left axilla and to the back. A gallop rhythm is usually present. The murmurs of associated anomalies, however, are usually dominant.

Pulses and Blood Pressure.   The blood pressure proximal to the area of obstruction is higher than the blood pressure distal to the area of obstruction.

The most consistent physical finding in infants with critical coarctation of the aorta is a higher systolic blood pressure (>15 mm Hg) in the upper extremities than in the lower extremities. This blood pressure must be measured with the appropriate-size cuff. In addition, pulses are easily palpable in one or both upper extremities but are difficult to palpate or are absent in the lower extremities. Pulses should be carefully evaluated in all extremities and blood pressures obtained in *both arms* and either leg. The coarctation may occur between the subclavian arteries, or the right or left subclavian artery may arise aberrantly distal to the coarctation, resulting in a differential pulse and blood pressure between the right and left arms.

Congestive Heart Failure.   Congestive heart failure is a common finding in infants with severe coarctation as a result of a pressure overload on the left ventricle (see section on congestive heart failure).

Laboratory Data

Arterial Blood Gases.   Arterial blood gases are normal.

Chest X-ray Examination.   Cardiomegaly may be seen on the x-ray film. Pulmonary vascularity is normal unless associated anomalies are present.

Electrocardiogram.   Right ventricular hypertrophy is frequently present. Left ventricular hypertrophy or combined ventricular hypertrophy is rarely seen in the newborn period. The ECG may be normal.

Echocardiogram.   The area of coarctation can often be visualized using two-dimensional techniques and color flow mapping. Abnormal Doppler blood flow is diagnostic. However, cautious interpretation of the findings is suggested.

Cardiac Catheterization.   Cardiac catheterization is diagnostic and is commonly performed before any surgical procedure is undertaken to evaluate other associated anomalies.

Treatment

Medical Management.   Congestive heart failure should be treated aggressively. Intractable congestive heart failure, acidosis, oliguria, and hypertension are indications for corrective surgery as soon as possible. (See section on general treatment strategy of congenital heart disease.) Balloon dilation of the coarcted site has been performed in the catheterization laboratory at some institutions with variable success. A significant incidence of aortic wall aneurysm formation has been identified 6 to 12 months later.

Surgical Treatment.   The two most common surgical procedures are resection of the coarctation with end-to-end anastomosis or the subclavian flap aortoplasty. With the former, the coarcted segment is resected and the ends of the aorta reanastomosed together. With the latter, a longitudinal incision is made in the aorta across the coarctated site and continued to the end of the distally divided left subclavian artery. The left subclavian artery is used as a patch or flap to increase the diameter of the aorta. Both procedures are performed through a lateral thoracotomy incision and have been highly successful in relieving coarctation and providing for future growth of the aorta. Absorbable suture material is often used with the intention of decreasing the incidence of recoarctation from rigid suture lines.

Complications and Residual Effects

Complications and residual effects include (1) diminished or absent pulses in the left arm, (2) persistent hypertension, (3) Horner's syndrome, (4) paraplegia (<0.5 %), (5) mesenteric vasculitis, and (6) residual coarctation.

The overall operative mortality is 38% in infancy. However, the high mortality is usually related to preoperative status and associated lesions. Early detection and referral in addition to the use of prostaglandin E_1 may dramatically reduce this mortality in the future.

Prognosis and Follow-Up

Infants with mild coarctation require minimal care until later in life. If these patients are medically managed, close follow-up is mandatory, with cardiac catheterization and surgery expected at a later date.

Infants with severe coarctation require prompt medical and surgical treatment. If this therapy is instituted early, the prognosis is generally favorable. Untreated infants with severe coarctation often have a rapidly deteriorating clinical course with left ventricular failure, severe hypertension, or intractable congestive heart failure, and the prognosis is guarded. After surgical repair, frequent follow-up is required to ensure adequate coarctation repair. Cardiac catheterization may be required several months to years after the surgical procedure is completed.

Critical Aortic Stenosis

Physiology

Obstruction of the left ventricular outlet may occur below the aortic valve, at the aortic valve, or above the aortic valve (subvalvular, valvular, or supravalvular aortic stenosis) (Fig. 23-4). Valvular aortic stenosis is the most common type and is discussed here. A pressure gradient (the pressure difference from the left ventricle to the ascending aorta) of 50 mm Hg or more is indicative of significant aortic stenosis in the newborn.

Data Collection

Physical Findings.   Although most infants with aortic stenosis are asymptomatic in the neonatal period, an infant who is symptomatic from critical or severe aortic stenosis needs medical and surgical emergency treatment. The infant with critical aortic stenosis will have pale, gray, cool skin with decreased perfusion and peripheral pulses.

Cyanosis.   Cyanosis is generally not present in isolated valvular aortic stenosis.

Heart Sounds.   A grade II to IV/VI harsh systolic murmur is typically heard in the upper right sternal border, radiating to the upper left sternal border and faintly to the neck. The intensity of the murmur is unrelated to the severity of the obstruction. An ejection click may be heard at the apex, radiating to the lower left sternal border. A suprasternal notch thrill is often palpable.

Congestive Heart Failure.   Infants with critical aortic stenosis have congestive heart failure caused by a pressure overload of the left ventricle (see section on congestive heart failure).

Laboratory Data

Arterial Blood Gases.   Arterial blood gases are generally normal.

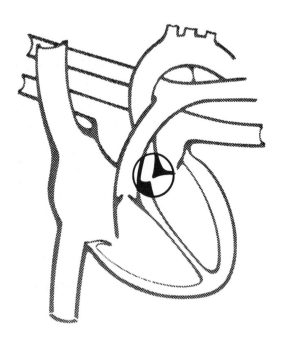

Figure 23-4   Aortic stenosis. (Courtesy Ross Laboratories, Columbus, Ohio.)

Chest X-ray Examination.   A chest x-ray examination shows cardiomegaly with normal pulmonary vascularity.

Electrocardiogram.   The ECG may be normal or demonstrate left ventricular hypertrophy. It is important to remember that there is poor correlation between an electrocardiographic abnormality and the degree of aortic stenosis present.

Echocardiogram.   The aortic valve is usually thickened and appears to close abnormally on an echocardiogram. Doppler interrogation can accurately estimate the systolic pressure gradient from the left ventricle to the ascending aorta and identify the level or levels of obstruction.

Cardiac Catheterization.   Cardiac catheterization is diagnostic and may or may not be performed in cases of critical aortic stenosis. Some centers are performing balloon dilation of the aortic valve during the cardiac catheterization.

Treatment

Medical Management.   Medical management is usually unsatisfactory, and surgical intervention is necessary for critical aortic stenosis in the newborn (see section on general treatment strategies). However, balloon dilatation of aortic valve stenosis in the cardiac catheterization laboratory has been a successful alternative to surgical intervention in selected newborns.

Surgical Treatment.   Aortic valvulotomy through a median sternotomy incision is the surgical procedure for correcting critical aortic stenosis in infants. This procedure can usually be accomplished in the newborn with inflow occlusion and circulatory arrest for 1 to 2 minutes. In older infants, cardiopulmonary bypass should be performed. The fused commissures of the valve are incised, permitting the leaflets to open freely during systole.

Complications and Residual Effects

Complications and residual effects include aortic insufficiency and residual aortic stenosis. The mortality in infancy ranges from 5% to 50%, with the highest risk involving the newborn with critical obstruction. It is hoped that avoidance of a cardio-pulmonary bypass operation will reduce the mortality in this group.

Prognosis and Follow-Up

Surgery for critical aortic stenosis in the neonatal period is considered a palliative measure for relief of the obstruction. Repeated catheterization and further surgical repair of the valve should be expected in the next several months to years.

Critical Pulmonary Stenosis with Intact Ventricular Septum

Physiology

In critical pulmonary stenosis with intact ventricular septum, the flow to the pulmonary artery from the right ventricle is obstructed. The obstruction may occur below the valve in the infundibular area, above the valve, or at the valve (subvalvular, supravalvular, or valvular). In valvular stenosis the orifice of the pulmonary valve is markedly narrowed, and the valvular tissue may assume the shape of a cone (Fig. 23-5). The pulmonary artery

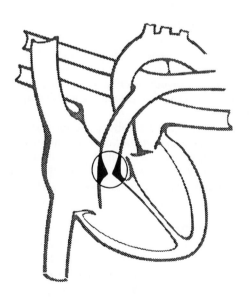

Figure 23-5 Pulmonary stenosis. (Courtesy Ross Laboratories, Columbus, Ohio.)

distal to this area of stenosis may be dilated. Because the ventricular septum is intact, the right ventricle is subjected to a marked increase in pressure and becomes hypertrophied. A pressure gradient from the right ventricle to the pulmonary artery of 50 mm Hg or more is indicative of significant pulmonary stenosis in the newborn.

Data Collection

Physical Findings

Cyanosis.   Cyanosis is generally not present in an isolated lesion but may occur in the presence of a right-to-left atrial shunt.

Heart Sounds.   A harsh, grade II to III/VI systolic murmur is heard in the upper left sternal border, radiating to both axillae and faintly to the back. Diastole is quiet. A murmur of tricuspid insufficiency (Grade I/VI, soft, systolic murmur at the lower left sternal border) may be heard. An ejection click may also be heard at the left sternal border.

Congestive Heart Failure.   The infant with critical pulmonary stenosis typically has signs and symptoms of right-sided congestive heart failure resulting from excessive pressure overload (see section on congestive heart failure).

Laboratory Data

Arterial Blood Gases.   Arterial blood gases are generally normal.

Chest X-ray Examination.   The chest x-ray examination may be normal but usually demonstrates cardiomegaly with normal or decreased pulmonary vascularity.

Electrocardiogram.   The ECG may be normal or demonstrate right ventricular hypertrophy.

Echocardiogram.   An abnormal pulmonary valve pattern on a two-dimensional echocardiogram is diagnostic. Doppler interrogation and color flow mapping can accurately estimate the systolic pressure gradient from the right ventricle to the pulmonary artery and identify the level or levels of obstruction.

Cardiac Catheterization.   Infants suspected of having critical pulmonary stenosis with an intact ventricular septum usually undergo cardiac catheterization as soon as possible. Balloon dilation of the pulmonic valve during catheterization has been successfully performed in many institutions.

Treatment

Medical Management. Prostaglandin E₁ has been used successfully to maintain the patency of the ductus arteriosus, thereby allowing adequate pulmonary blood flow until surgery or balloon dilation is performed. If balloon dilation has been successful, surgical intervention may be postponed or may not be necessary at all.

Surgical Treatment. The degree of pulmonary stenosis and the size of the pulmonary arteries determine surgical approach. If the right ventricle and pulmonary arteries are of adequate size, then pulmonary valvulotomy through a median sternotomy incision is the preferable procedure. This involves incising the pulmonary valve commissures, allowing the leaflets to open freely during systole. Like aortic valvulotomy, this procedure can often be performed under inflow occlusion.

Complications and Residual Effects

Complications and residual effects include pulmonary insufficiency and residual pulmonary stenosis. The mortality of pulmonary valvulotomy is 17% in newborns.

If the right ventricle and pulmonary arteries are too small to allow antegrade flow, then a palliative procedure such as the Blalock-Taussig operation is performed. This procedure consists of bringing down the subclavian artery opposite the aortic arch and anastomosing it to the ipsilateral pulmonary artery or placing a Gore-tex or Dacron tube graft (conduit) between the subclavian artery and the pulmonary artery.

Complications and residual side effects of Blalock-Taussig shunts include (1) diminished or absent pulses in the affected arm, (2) congestive heart failure from an overlarge shunt, and (3) inadequacy of the shunt. The mortality in this group is higher than in infants with adequately sized right ventricles and pulmonary arteries.

Prognosis and Follow-Up

If a palliative shunt has been used, follow-up catheterization and surgical procedures should be anticipated either when the shunt becomes nonfunctional or when total repair is expected. If the lesion has been primarily corrected surgically in the neonatal period, repeated catheterization is routinely performed several months later to evaluate the residual obstruction. However, evaluation by echocardiogram may be sufficient without catheterization.

Atrioventricular Septal Defect, Endocardial Cushion Defect (AV Canal)

Physiology

The complete type of endocardial cushion defect is characterized by a large central hole in the endocardial cushion of the heart with free communication among all four chambers. The anterior leaflet of the mitral valve and the septal leaflet of the tricuspid valve both have clefts and are continuous with each other through the defect. Thus the atrioventricular (AV) valves are represented by a valve common to both sides of the heart.

These infants usually have a left-to-right shunt at both the atrial and ventricular levels. If the cleft in the mitral valve is substantial, mitral insufficiency may also be present. The symptomatology depends on the degree of shunting at the atrial and ventricular levels and the amount of mitral insufficiency present. There is an association between endocardial cushion defects and Down syndrome.

Data Collection

Physical Findings
Cyanosis. Generally, cyanosis is not present with an isolated endocardial cushion defect.

Heart Sounds. If mitral insufficiency is present, a blowing, systolic, apical murmur with radiation to the left axilla and/or a VSD murmur is heard.

Congestive Heart Failure. Congestive heart failure may be present because of volume overload of the ventricles as a result of mitral insufficiency and left-to-right shunting at either the atrial or ventricular level (see section on congestive heart failure).

Laboratory Data
Arterial Blood Gases. The Paco₂ may be elevated if there is severe mitral insufficiency and pulmonary edema. The pH is usually normal. The Pao₂ is also usually normal.

Chest X-ray Examination. The heart size may be normal or increased. The pulmonary vascularity is generally increased.

Electrocardiogram. An ECG with a left axis deviation, counterclockwise loop in the frontal plane, and superior axis suggests AV septal defect.

Echocardiogram. A two-dimensional echocardiogram with doppler and color flow mapping demonstrates the atrial septal defect (ASD), VSD, and common AV valves, and the degree of AV valve insufficiency. This technique is diagnostic.

Cardiac Catheterization. Cardiac catheterization is diagnostic but generally not performed in the neonatal period in a typical AV septal defect. An echocardiographic diagnosis may be sufficient without cardiac catheterization.

Treatment

Medical Management. See general section on medical therapy.

Surgical Treatment. If the infant does not respond to medical treatment and exhibits congestive heart failure, severe mitral regurgitation, or pulmonary hypertension, surgical repair is necessary. The surgical procedure through a median sternotomy incision involves closing the ASD and VSD, separating the common leaflets of the mitral and tricuspid valves, and reconstructing the mitral valve.

Complications and Residual Effects

Complications and residual effects include (1) persistent shunt (residual ASD or VSD); (2) conduction abnormalities (dysrhythmias and third-degree heart block), (3) mitral regurgitation, and (4) tricuspid regurgitation. The mortality in infancy is 10% to 25%.

The alternative to total repair is pulmonary artery banding. This is, however, contraindicated when mitral regurgitation or atrial shunting is severe. The risk of banding plus later debanding and repair approaches the risk of primary total repair.

Prognosis and Follow-Up

In the complete AV septal defect, congestive heart failure is a frequent problem and early surgical intervention is generally required. The prognosis of surgical repair in the neonatal period is guarded, with a generally favorable outcome if the surgery can be postponed until the infant is older than 6 months of age. The prognosis is guarded if pulmonary hypertension develops before surgical intervention.

Ebstein's Anomaly

Physiology

Ebstein's anomaly consists of an abnormally low insertion of the tricuspid valve, incorporating a portion of the right ventricle into the right atrium. The resultant right ventricular cavity is small, and because the elevated pulmonary artery pressure is normally present in the newborn period, the cardiac output from the right ventricle to the pulmonary artery is decreased. This cardiac output generally increases as the pulmonary artery pressure decreases after birth. Tricuspid insufficiency is present in varying degrees in the infant.

Data Collection

Physical Findings

Cyanosis. Varying degrees of cyanosis are present and depend on (1) the amount of right-to-left shunting at the foramen ovale and (2) the amount of blood that enters the pulmonary circulation by the right ventricle. In severe cases, the amount of pulmonary blood flow is markedly decreased, and these infants may be deeply cyanotic.

Heart Sounds. The second heart sound, S_2, is normal in the mildly affected infant, but the pulmonary component of S_2 may be diminished or inaudible in severely affected patients. A nonspecific systolic murmur is usually present and varies from a grade I/VI to a grade V/VI, representing tricuspid insufficiency. Diastolic murmurs, ejection clicks, and triple or quadruple rhythms are frequently heard.

Congestive Heart Failure. Newborns who are symptomatic usually have congestive heart failure resulting from volume overload of the left ventricle (see section on congestive heart failure).

Laboratory Data

Arterial Blood Gases. The Pa_{O_2} may be normal to very low, depending on the amount of ante-grade blood flow through the pulmonary valve. Pa_{O_2} in the low 20s is not uncommon.

Chest X-ray Examination. The chest x-ray examination shows cardiomegaly with decreased pulmonary vascularity. Massive cardiomegaly generally indicates severe tricuspid insufficiency.

Electrocardiogram. An ECG shows abnormal P waves and various degrees of heart block. The QRS generally demonstrates a right bundle-branch block pattern. Wolff-Parkinson-White (preexcitation) syndrome is frequently present, and dysrhythmias are common.

Echocardiogram. An echocardiogram with abnormal tricuspid valve patterns on an M mode suggests Ebstein's anomaly. A two-dimensional echocardiogram is diagnostic. Doppler interrogation and color flow mapping are very useful in evaluating the amount of antegrade blood flow through the pulmonary valve and the degree of tricuspid insufficiency present.

Cardiac Catheterization. There is an increased risk of dysrhythmias during catheterization. This procedure is not generally performed in the neonatal period unless a question regarding the differential diagnosis exists (to rule out pulmonary atresia).

Treatment

Medical Management. Dysrhythmias, especially supraventricular tachycardia, should be anticipated and appropriately managed (see section on general treatment strategies).

Surgical Treatment. Surgical treatment for Ebstein's anomaly is rarely indicated in infancy. The procedure through a median sternotomy incision involves repositioning the tricuspid valve and an anuloplasty to improve the competency of the valve. In addition, plication of the atrialized ventricle is performed. Replacing the tricuspid valve may be required.

Complications and Residual Effects

Complications and residual effects include tricuspid insufficiency and dysrhythmias. The mortality in infancy is unknown because of insufficient data.

Prognosis and Follow-Up

The prognosis of mild Ebstein's anomaly is generally favorable. Infants with severe Ebstein's anomaly generally improve as the right ventricular output increases. Although surgery has been used successfully in the more severe forms of Ebstein's anomaly, the prognosis is less favorable in patients requiring surgical intervention.

Persistent Pulmonary Hypertension in the Newborn

Physiology

Infants with abnormally elevated pulmonary vascular resistance have persistent fetal circulation or PPHN. These infants are generally hypoxic and acidotic but usually do not have severe pulmonary parenchymal disease or underlying cardiac disease. These infants have a right-to-left shunt at the ductal or atrial level.

Data Collection

History. PPHN is usually associated with severe antepartum or peripartum conditions that involve hypoxia reflected by low Apgar scores. These infants are generally term or near term and are symptomatic within the first hours after birth. Associated findings include hyperviscosity, hypoglycemia, or a congenital diaphragmatic hernia.

Physical Findings
  Cyanosis. The milder cases of PPHN have minimal transient tachypnea and cyanosis associated with stress (crying or feeding). Severe cases have marked cyanosis, tachypnea, acidosis, and decreased peripheral perfusion.
  Heart Sounds. A loud pulmonary component of S_2 and occasionally a nonspecific systolic ejection murmur are heard.
  Congestive Heart Failure. Infants with PPHN usually have congestive heart failure because of pressure overload of the right ventricle (see section on congestive heart failure).

Laboratory Data
  Arterial Blood Gases. Arterial blood gases demonstrate acidosis, hypoxia, and increased $Paco_2$. If a blood gas is obtained simultaneously in the right radial artery (preductal) and in the descending aorta with a UAC (postductal), the right-

to-left shunt at the ductal level can be documented. If blood gases are repeated after intubation and pharmacologic intervention (see section on treatment), the amount of hypoxia is often reduced. Simultaneous preductal and postductal transcutaneous oxygen measurement may also be used.

Chest X-ray Examination. The chest x-ray examination demonstrates mild to moderate cardiomegaly with normal pulmonary vascular markings. The lung fields may be clear.

Electrocardiogram. The ECG frequently is normal but may demonstrate right ventricular hypertrophy and signs of myocardial ischemia.

Echocardiogram. An echocardiogram helps to evaluate cardiac structures and rule out cyanotic lesions. Evaluating the right ventricular and pulmonary artery pressures by Doppler and the degree of right-to-left shunting at the atrial and ductal levels is helpful.

Cardiac Catheterization. Cardiac catheterization is usually not performed.

Treatment

Medical Management. (See Chapter 22).

Complete ᴅ-Transposition of the Great Arteries

Physiology

Complete ᴅ-transposition of the great arteries (Fig. 23-6) is one of the most common forms of serious heart disease. The aorta arises from the right ventricle, receives unoxygenated systemic venous blood, and returns this blood to the systemic arterial circulation. The pulmonary artery arises from the left ventricle, receives oxygenated pulmonary venous blood, and returns this blood to the pulmonary circulation. ᴅ-transposition can occur by itself or can be associated with other defects (PDA, ASD, VSD, or pulmonary stenosis).

Data Collection

History. Transposition of the great arteries is more prevalent in males and is typically found in infants who are full term.

Physical Findings. The major physiologic abnormalities in ᴅ-transposition of the great arteries are

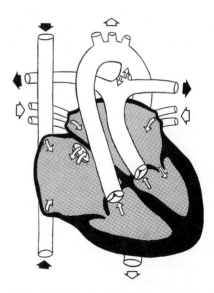

Figure 23-6 Complete transposition of the great arteries. (Courtesy Ross Laboratories, Columbus, Ohio.)

an oxygen deficiency in the tissues and excessive work load of the right and left ventricles. The only mixing of oxygenated and unoxygenated blood occurs in the presence of associated lesions (patent foramen ovale, ASD, VSD, PDA, or collateral circulation). The extent of the mixing depends on the number, size, and position of the anatomic communications, the pressure differential between the two systems, and changes in the systemic and pulmonary vascular resistance.

Cyanosis. Cyanosis is present in varying degrees, depending on the amount of intercirculatory mixing present. Cyanosis may be mild if the mixing occurs through a significant VSD or PDA. Cyanosis is profound with intact ventricular septum or a closing PDA. Oxygen therapy will be of limited benefit. Only a certain amount of oxygenated blood is able to reach the systemic circulation, and administration of additional oxygen does not improve this situation. Enlargement of the interatrial communication by balloon septostomy (Rashkind procedure) during cardiac catheterization is commonly performed to establish adequate intercirculatory mixing for these infants. Additional management may include surgical removal of the atrial septum (Blalock-Hanlon operation).

After these palliative procedures, the infant will continue to be cyanotic, especially in times of stress (crying, feeding, or exposure to cold temperatures). If the Pao_2 at rest in room air is not greater than 35 mm torr or if persistent metabolic acidosis is present, inadequate intercardiac mixing should be suspected.

Heart Sounds.   The aorta arises from the anterior (right) ventricle, and the closure of the aortic valve is easily heard. The S_2 is single with an increased intensity. Murmurs if present are usually those of associated lesions (see section on individual lesions).

Congestive Heart Failure.   As a result of the volume and pressure overload experienced by both ventricles, the infant may show signs of congestive heart failure. This is especially true if there is a large VSD or PDA present (see section on congestive heart failure). Digoxin should be used with caution if subvalvular pulmonary stenosis is present.

Laboratory Data

Arterial Blood Gases.   The pH and $Paco_2$ are normal. The Pao_2 is typically low (20 to 40 torr), but if a large VSD or PDA is present, the Pao_2 may approach normal levels.

Chest X-ray Examination.   The chest x-ray examination may be normal or demonstrate either decreased or increased pulmonary vascularity. The cardiac silhouette may assume the shape of an egg lying on a string. However, this finding is not diagnostic.

Electrocardiogram.   The ECG may be normal or demonstrate right ventricular hypertrophy. Left ventricular hypertrophy and combined ventricular hypertrophy are uncommon.

Echocardiogram.   The echocardiogram is extremely useful in establishing the diagnosis and evaluating associated lesions in infants with transposition of the great arteries.

Cardiac Catheterization.   Cardiac catheterization is diagnostic. A balloon septostomy is commonly performed to improve interatrial mixing.

Treatment

Medical Management.   Serial venous and arterial pH measurements should be obtained to rule out the presence of a persistent metabolic acidosis that would suggest inadequate intercardiac mixing.

In addition, congestive heart failure should be continually anticipated and treated appropriately if it occurs (see section on general treatment strategies).

Surgical Treatment.   The arterial switch procedure in most centers is the treatment of choice for D-transposition of the great arteries. This procedure through a median sternotomy incision involves amputation of the main pulmonary artery and the aorta above the respective valves. The pulmonary artery is anastomosed to the right ventricle, and the aorta is anastomosed to the left ventricle (the aortic valve becomes a functional pulmonary valve, and the pulmonary valve becomes a functional aortic valve). The coronary arteries are resected with a button of surrounding tissue and reanastomosed to the supravalvular area of the ascending aorta.

It is essential in performing this procedure that the left ventricular pressure is systemic. In infants with a VSD, the pressure tends to remain elevated; therefore this procedure may be postponed for several days or even months. However, once the left ventricular pressure decreases below that of the right ventricle, the morbidity and mortality increase dramatically. Therefore infants with an intact ventricular septum require surgery within the first few days of life.

If the arterial switch procedure is not performed and the infant becomes refractory to medical management and exhibits congestive heart failure, failure to thrive, pulmonary hypertension, or severe hypoxia, an alternative surgical procedure is necessary. The most common procedures other than the arterial switch for repair of D-transposition with an intact ventricular septum are the Mustard and the Senning procedures. Both of these procedures performed through a median sternotomy incision involve intraatrial redirection of blood flow. The oxygenated blood returning from the lungs through the pulmonary veins is redirected to the tricuspid valve and right ventricle, while the systemic venous return from inferior and superior venae cavae is redirected to the mitral valve and left ventricle.

Complications and Residual Effects

Complications and residual effects of the arterial switch procedure include (1) dysrhythmias,

(2) myocardial ischemia and infarction, and (3) aortic and/or pulmonary supravalvular stenosis.

Complications and residual effects of the Mustard and Senning procedures include (1) dysrhythmias, (2) superior vena cava or inferior vena cava obstruction, (3) tricuspid regurgitation, and (4) pulmonary venous obstruction. The latter is a severe complication warranting early detection and immediate correction. The mortality to infants is 8% and is even higher in the neonatal period.

Prognosis and Follow-Up

Without treatment, 30% of these infants die within the first week of life, 50% die within the first month, 70% die within the first 6 months, and 90% die within the first year. With treatment, the mortality is reduced to approximately 20%.

Tetralogy of Fallot

Physiology

Tetralogy of Fallot is the most common form of cyanotic congenital heart disease. The four components of tetralogy of Fallot are (1) VSD, (2) overriding of the ascending aorta, (3) obstruction to the right ventricular outflow tract, and (4) right ventricular hypertrophy (Fig. 23-7).

Data Collection

Physical Findings. The degree of symptomatology in these infants depends on the degree of right ventricular outflow tract obstruction. Newborns who are symptomatic usually have severe right ventricular outflow tract obstruction.

Cyanosis. The predominant intercardiac shunt is right to left; therefore most infants with tetralogy of Fallot are cyanotic. However, if the right ventricular outflow obstruction is only mild or moderate, the intercardiac shunt is left to right and the infant initially will be acyanotic.

Infants with tetralogy of Fallot occasionally have a "TET," or hypercyanotic spell. These spells consist of cyanosis, irritability, pallor, tachypnea, flaccidity, and possible loss of consciousness. TETs may be the result of a transient increase in the obstruction of the right ventricular outflow tract (usually the muscular infundibular area) and usually respond to knee-chest positioning, oxygen, propranolol, or morphine.

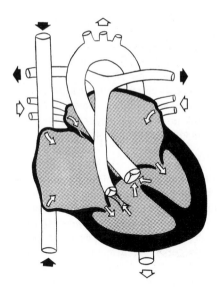

Figure 23-7 Tetralogy of Fallot. (Courtesy Ross Laboratories, Columbus, Ohio.)

Heart Sounds. A grade II to IV/VI harsh systolic murmur at the mid to upper left sternal border is usually present but is diminished or absent during a TET. The S_2 is usually loud and single (representing aortic closure).

Congestive Heart Failure. Congestive heart failure is uncommon in tetralogy of Fallot.

Laboratory Data

Arterial Blood Gases. The $Paco_2$ and pH are normal. The Pao_2 is normal if the pulmonary stenosis is mild and there is little right-to-left shunting at the ventricular level. If the pulmonary stenosis, however, is more severe, the amount of right-to-left shunting increases and the Pao_2 falls.

Chest X-ray Examination. The classic chest x-ray examination of tetralogy of Fallot resembles the shape of a boot with a normal-sized heart. However, the classic chest x-ray pattern described is not common in the newborn. Pulmonary vascularity is either normal or decreased.

Electrocardiogram. The ECG demonstrates right ventricular hypertrophy.

Echocardiogram. The echocardiogram is suggestive when the overriding aorta can be demonstrated. Echocardiograms help identify the pulmonary valve to rule out pulmonary atresia. Doppler interrogation helps to define the degree and level of pulmonary stenosis. Color flow mapping identifies the VSD as well as the direction of blood flow across the VSD.

 Cardiac Catheterization.   Cardiac catheterization is diagnostic and performed in the newborn when there is a question regarding the differential diagnosis (pulmonary atresia).

Treatment

Medical Management.   Digoxin is not routinely used because it may increase the amount of infundibular obstruction present. Propranolol is the preferable drug for treating hypercyanotic infants, although morphine has been used successfully (see section on general treatment strategies).

Surgical Treatment.   Total repair of tetralogy of Fallot involves patch closure of the large VSD and relief of the right ventricular outflow obstruction performed through a median sternotomy incision. Often a pericardial patch across the pulmonary valve annulus is required. The use of homograft conduits for relief of right-sided obstruction is also common. Contraindications include small size of the child, anomalous left anterior descending coronary artery, and hypoplastic pulmonary arteries.

 Total surgical repair of tetralogy of Fallot is not usually recommended in the neonatal period. If surgical intervention is warranted (i.e., the infant is severely hypoxic because of inadequate pulmonary blood flow), a systemic-to-pulmonary shunt is performed. The Blalock-Taussig operation is usually preferred (see previous description of the Blalock-Taussig operation).

Complications and Residual Effects

Complications and residual effects include (1) diminished or absent pulses in the affected arm, (2) congestive heart failure from an overlarge shunt, and (3) inadequate shunt. Mortality in infancy is 10%.

Prognosis And Follow-Up

Early cardiac catheterization with subsequent surgery is recommended if the child is symptomatic or refractory to medical care. Tetralogy of Fallot without surgery has a grave prognosis.

Parent Teaching

Parents should be instructed to place the infant in a knee-chest position during a TET spell and to notify the physician immediately.

Pulmonary Atresia with Intact Ventricular Septum

Physiology

Pulmonary atresia is characterized by complete agenesis of the pulmonary valve. This lesion produces severe signs or symptoms soon after birth and is not compatible with life unless there is an associated interatrial communication and an additional pathway of entry for blood into the pulmonary circulation (through a PDA and/or collateral blood flow). Because flow to the lungs may depend on a PDA, death may occur when this structure closes. The right ventricle is usually hypoplastic but may be normal or dilated, depending on the degree of tricuspid insufficiency present.

Data Collection

Physical Findings

 Cyanosis.   Cyanosis is always present in varying degrees, depending on the amount of pulmonary blood flow from the PDA and/or collateral blood flow.

 Heart Sounds.   The S_2 is single, and a soft systolic murmur is heard as a result of either the PDA or tricuspid insufficiency in about one half of the infants with pulmonary atresia.

 Congestive Heart Failure.   Congestive heart failure is usually present with moderate to severe tricuspid insufficiency (see section on congestive heart failure).

Laboratory Data

 Arterial Blood Gases.   The pH and Pa_{CO_2} are usually within normal range. The Pa_{O_2}, however, is usually very low (20 to 30 torr), unless there is a large shunt at the ductal or bronchial collateral level. In some cases the amount of pulmonary blood flow is insufficient, and the pH may be low, reflecting metabolic acidosis.

 Chest X-ray Examination.   The heart appears enlarged on x-ray examination if tricuspid insufficiency is present. Pulmonary vascularity is either decreased or normal, depending on the amount of shunting through the PDA and/or collateral blood flow.

Electrocardiogram. The ECG is usually normal but may demonstrate left ventricular hypertrophy. It is important to differentiate this lesion from tricuspid atresia that shows a counterclockwise loop in the frontal planes with a superior axis.

Echocardiogram. The two-dimensional echocardiogram with Doppler and color flow mapping can identify absence of blood flow across the pulmonary valve and is diagnostic.

Cardiac Catheterization. Cardiac catheterization is diagnostic and may be performed if the diagnosis is suspected. A balloon atrial septostomy may be performed at the time of catheterization.

Treatment

Medical Management Prostaglandin E_1 is used to maintain patency of the ductus arteriosus until surgical intervention (see section on general treatment strategy).

Surgical Treatment. In most medical centers a systemic-to-pulmonary shunt such as the Blalock-Taussig operation is performed through a lateral thoracotomy incision. However, some institutions are performing a pulmonary valvulotomy or a pulmonary outflow patch procedure in addition to a shunt. This establishes an open pathway through the atretic valve area between the pulmonary artery and the right ventricle. Antegrade blood flow through the right ventricle and pulmonary artery will then promote growth of these areas. The pulmonary valvotomy and pulmonary outflow patch procedures are performed through a median sternotomy incision.

Complications and Residual Effects

Complications and residual effects of the Blalock-Taussig operation include (1) diminished or absent pulses in the affected arm, (2) congestive heart failure from an overlarge shunt, and (3) inadequate shunt. The mortality in infants is 25% or higher.

Prognosis and Follow-Up

Pulmonary atresia is fatal without surgical intervention. If a palliative shunt is performed, catheterization and further surgical procedures should be anticipated when the shunt becomes nonfunctional. If primary surgical correction is undertaken in the newborn period, catheterization should be anticipated to evaluate residual obstruction. Despite the development of newer surgical techniques, the prognosis in these infants is guarded.

Total Anomalous Pulmonary Venous Return

Physiology

Total anomalous pulmonary venous return (TAPVR) is characterized by all the pulmonary veins returning directly or indirectly into the right atrium rather than the left atrium. The presence of an ASD is necessary to sustain life (Fig. 23-8). The four main varieties of TAPVR are (1) supracardiac (most common), in which the drainage is to the superior vena cava through the innominate vein; (2) cardiac, in which the pulmonary veins drain into the coronary, sinus or directly into the right atrium; (3) infracardiac, in which the four veins join behind the heart, flow through the diaphragm, and connect to the portal venous system; and (4) mixed. Each of the various types of anomalous drainage can occur with or without obstruction along the pulmonary venous pathway. The presence or absence of obstruction profoundly affects the clinical course.

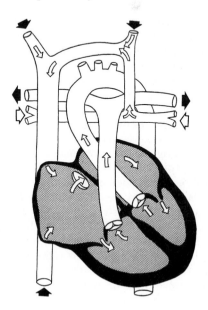

Figure 23-8 Anomalous venous return. (Courtesy Ross Laboratories, Columbus, Ohio.)

Data Collection

Physical Findings

Cyanosis.   Infants with obstructed or unobstructed TAPVR are typically cyanotic. Because all pulmonary venous return (oxygenated blood) ultimately enters the right atrium (as opposed to the left atrium), a right-to-left shunt at the atrial level is required to sustain life.

Heart Sounds.   Murmurs are rarely heard in infants with TAPVR and when present are nonspecific.

Congestive Heart Failure.   Infants with unobstructed TAPVR usually show signs of congestive heart failure resulting from volume overload of the right ventricle. Infants with obstructed TAPVR generally do not demonstrate evidence of congestive heart failure but typically demonstrate pulmonary venous congestion (see section on congestive heart failure).

Laboratory Data

Arterial Blood Gases.   The pH and Pa_{CO_2} are usually normal. The Pa_{O_2} may be within the normal range if there is a large amount of pulmonary blood flow (always associated with severe congestive heart failure). If the pulmonary blood flow is limited, secondary to obstruction of blood flow, the Pa_{O_2} may be low.

Chest X-ray Examination.   If the TAPVR is obstructed, the chest x-ray examination will demonstrate pulmonary venous congestion without cardiomegaly. If the TAPVR is unobstructed, the chest x-ray examination will demonstrate a marked increase in pulmonary vascularity and cardiomegaly.

Electrocardiogram.   An ECG may demonstrate right axis deviation, right ventricular hypertrophy, and right atrial enlargement.

Echocardiogram.   An echocardiogram is diagnostic; however, it is sometimes difficult to visualize the pulmonary veins by this method. The diagnosis of TAPVR is strongly suggested when an extra cavity is seen behind the small left atrium. With color flow mapping, the right-to-left shunting across the atrial septum, as well as the anomalous venous return as it enters through the atrium, superior vena cava, or coronary sinus can be visualized.

Cardiac Catheterization.   Infants suspected of having TAPVR may undergo cardiac catheterization to define the type of TAPVR and presence or absence of obstruction. A Rashkind balloon septostomy may be performed at that time to improve intraatrial mixing.

Treatment

Medical Management.   Obstructed TAPVR is a surgical emergency. Nonobstructed TAPVR may be medically treated temporarily, although early surgery is generally recommended (see section on general treatment strategy).

Surgical Treatment.   Surgical correction of TAPVR depends on the variety. Supracardiac and infracardiac varieties require surgical reimplantation of the common vein into the left atrium. Intracardiac TAPVR can usually be surgically repaired by realigning the atrial septum during closure of the ASD and directing the anomalous veins to the left atrial side. All repairs are performed through a median sternotomy incision.

Complications and Residual Effects

Complications and residual effects include pulmonary venous obstruction and dysrhythmias. The mortality varies from 5% to 25% in infancy, depending on the anatomic type.

Prognosis and Follow-Up

Infants with nonobstructed TAPVR generally do well if the lesion is recognized early and early corrective surgery is performed. The prognosis for obstructed TAPVR is less favorable despite early surgical intervention.

Tricuspid Atresia

Physiology

In tricuspid atresia there is complete agenesis of the tricuspid valve with no direct communication between the right atrium and right ventricle. Systemic venous blood entering the right atrium is shunted through a patent foramen ovale or ASD into the left atrium. A VSD may be present, and the right ventricle and pulmonary arteries may be normal in size. If the ventricular septum is intact but a large PDA is present, the right ventricular cavity may be hypoplastic and the pulmonary arteries are usually slightly decreased or normal in size (Fig.

23-9). About 30% of these infants will have transposition of the great arteries.

Data Collection

Physical Findings

Cyanosis.   The degree of cyanosis present varies. Newborns will have marked cyanosis if the pulmonary blood flow is compromised.

Heart Sounds.   A single S_2 is present in infants with tricuspid atresia. Murmurs of associated shunts (VSD and PDA) are typically present.

Congestive Heart Failure.   Congestive heart failure may be present with a large shunt (PDA or VSD) (see section on congestive heart failure).

Laboratory Data

Arterial Blood Gases.   The pH and Pa_{CO_2} are usually normal. The Pa_{O_2} may vary from near normal if there is a large VSD or PDA to extremely low if there is limited shunting into the pulmonary system.

Chest X-ray Examination.   A chest x-ray examination is nondiagnostic and may show a normal heart size or cardiomegaly. Pulmonary vascularity may be normal, decreased, or increased, depending on the degree of pulmonary blood flow.

Electrocardiogram.   An ECG is highly suggestive and usually demonstrates left axis deviation with a counterclockwise loop, a superior axis in the frontal plane, and left ventricular hypertrophy.

Echocardiogram.   Absence of the tricuspid valve and presence of a small hypoplastic right ventricle echocardiographically is highly suggestive of tricuspid atresia. Color flow mapping can identify the right-to-left shunt at the atrial level and the presence of a VSD and/or PDA.

Cardiac Catheterization.   An infant suspected of having tricuspid atresia usually undergoes cardiac catheterization and a balloon septostomy. A balloon septostomy is performed to improve intraatrial mixing.

Treatment

Medical Management.   See section on general treatment strategy.

Surgical Treatment.   When surgery is indicated, the preferred procedure in the neonatal period is a systemic-to-pulmonary shunt such as the Blalock-Taussig operation performed through a lateral thoracotomy incision.

Definitive repair of tricuspid atresia (Fontan procedure) involves the creation of a communication between the right atrium and pulmonary artery or right ventricular outflow chamber by direct anastomosis or conduit. Closure of the ASD and any VSDs present is also performed. Definitive repair is performed through a median sternotomy incision.

Complications and Residual Effects

Complications and residual effects include (1) heart failure, (2) pleural effusions, (3) renal or liver failure, (4) persistent shunts, (5) conduit obstruction, and (6) dysrhythmia. The mortality in infancy is unknown, but in older children it is approximately 10% to 25%.

Prognosis and Follow-Up

The prognosis of tricuspid atresia is guarded. The Fontan procedure may improve this prognosis.

Truncus Arteriosus

Physiology

Truncus arteriosus is characterized by one great artery arising from the left and right ventricles,

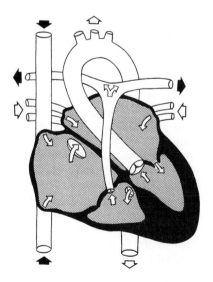

Figure 23-9   Tricuspid atresia. (Courtesy Ross Laboratories, Columbus, Ohio.)

overriding a VSD. This common artery has one valve and gives rise to the pulmonary, coronary, and systemic arteries (Fig. 23-10). Truncus arteriosus is classified into three types depending on the origin of the pulmonary arteries.

- Type I—A short, main pulmonary artery arises from the common trunk that bifurcates into the right and left pulmonary arteries.
- Type II—The right and left pulmonary arteries arise directly from the posterior surface of the common trunk.
- Type III—The right and left pulmonary arteries arise directly from the lateral walls of the common trunk.

The ductus arteriosus is absent in approximately 50% of infants with truncus arteriosus. Between 30% and 35% have a right aortic arch.

Data Collection

Physical Findings.   In truncus arteriosus the common trunk receives a mixture of unoxygenated blood from the right ventricle and oxygenated blood from the left ventricle. Blood flow to the

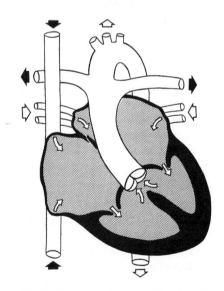

Figure 23-10   Truncus arteriosus. (Courtesy Ross Laboratories, Columbus, Ohio.)

lungs varies with the type of truncus but is usually increased and at systemic level pressure.

Cyanosis.   Cyanosis is present at birth but varies in intensity according to the amount of pulmonary blood flow. Minimal cyanosis indicates adequate pulmonary blood flow.

Heart Sounds.   The first heart sound, S_1, will be normal, but the S_2 will be single and loud because of the single valve of the common trunk. A loud systolic ejection click is frequently heard. A loud pansystolic murmur maximal at the lower left sternal border that radiates to the entire precordium is commonly heard. A middiastolic rumble may be present. If the truncal valve is insufficient, a blowing diastolic murmur may be heard. A wide pulse pressure may also be present.

Congestive Heart Failure.   Congestive heart failure may be present shortly after birth or appear between 2 and 3 weeks of age. The presence of congestive heart failure depends on the amount of pulmonary blood flow. Persistent high pulmonary arteriolar resistance in the first few weeks of life will decrease pulmonary blood flow, and congestive heart failure may not be present. However, if the truncal valve is severely damaged, congestive heart failure will be present shortly after birth (see section on congestive heart failure).

Laboratory Data

Arterial Blood Gases.   The pH and Pa_{CO_2} are usually normal. If there is no obstruction to pulmonary blood flow, the Pa_{O_2} may be near normal (usually associated with severe congestive heart failure). If the pulmonary blood flow is restricted, the Pa_{O_2} may be extremely low.

Chest X-ray Examination.   Cardiomegaly, displayed pulmonary arteries, and increased vascular markings are typical findings on the chest x-ray examination.

Electrocardiogram.   Combined ventricular hypertrophy is most often seen in an ECG. Left atrial enlargement is also commonly found.

Echocardiogram.   A two-dimensional echocardiogram is helpful in establishing the diagnosis and in differentiating tetralogy of Fallot from truncus arteriosus. In addition, the echocardiogram is used to identify the number of truncal valve leaflets, the presence of truncal valve insufficiency, and the presence of pulmonary stenosis.

Cardiac Catheterization.   A cardiac catheterization is diagnostic and is usually performed on an infant suspected of having truncus arteriosus.

Treatment

Medical Management.   Medical management of these infants consists of stabilizing and treating congestive heart failure when present. Calcium should be closely monitored because of the possibility of DiGeorge syndrome.

Surgical Treatment.   Totally repairing truncus arteriosus is rare in the newborn period. It consists of separating the pulmonary artery from the common trunk, closing the VSD with a patch, and inserting a right ventricular-to-pulmonary artery valved conduit. The use of homograft conduits for repair of truncus arteriosus has become more common. Total repair of truncus arteriosus is performed through a median sternotomy incision.

Complications and Residual Effects

Complications and side effects include (1) pulmonary vascular disease, (2) residual shunts, (3) truncal valve incompetence, and (4) conduit obstruction. The mortality is 40% to 50% in infancy.

   Prognosis and Follow-Up.   The natural history depends on the amount of pulmonary blood flow and the competency of the truncal valve. Without treatment, more than half of these infants die before 3 months of age. Survival past 1 year of age ranges from 15% to 30%. Truncus arteriosus is often associated with DiGeorge syndrome, which has a guarded prognosis.

Hypoplastic Left Heart Syndrome

Physiology

Hypoplastic left heart syndrome represents a clinical spectrum that includes severe coarctation of the aorta, severe aortic valve stenosis or atresia, and severe mitral valve stenosis or atresia. The left ventricle and ascending aorta are hypoplastic. Coronary blood flow occurs in a retrograde fashion into the small ascending aorta through the PDA. The resultant poor myocardial perfusion leads to rapid decompensation.

Data Collection
Physical Findings
   Cyanosis.   These infants are usually not truly cyanotic but rather have severe pallor and a grayish skin color as a result of marked vasoconstriction and congestive heart failure.
   Heart Sounds.   A nonspecific systolic murmur is heard in approximately two thirds of infants with hypoplastic left heart syndrome.
   Congestive Heart Failure.   Congestive heart failure is present in all cases as a result of right ventricular volume and pressure overload (see section on congestive heart failure).

Laboratory Data
   Arterial Blood Gases.   The arterial blood gases are typically normal until the infant begins to deteriorate, at which time the baby will become acidotic.
   Chest X-ray Examination.   Cardiomegaly with increased pulmonary vascularity and pulmonary edema is seen on the x-ray examination.
   Electrocardiogram.   An ECG frequently demonstrates right axis deviation and right ventricular hypertrophy. However, the electrocardiogram may be normal.
   Echocardiogram.   An echocardiogram is usually diagnostic with a small left ventricular cavity and ascending aorta with an abnormal aortic valve pattern.
   Cardiac Catheterization.   Cardiac catheterization is diagnostic. In some cases only an aortic root contrast study using a UAC is required to demonstrate the typical small ascending aorta. If there is a question regarding the differential diagnosis, a heart catheterization is indicated.

Treatment

Medical Management.   Hypoplastic left heart syndrome is a lethal lesion, and currently no medical therapy is effective. Surgical intervention offers the only chance of survival. Patency of the ductus arteriosus is maintained with infusion of prostaglandin E_1 (PGE) until surgical intervention. (see Table 23-4). (See section on general treatment strategy.)

Surgical Treatment.   Recent advances in surgical treatment have made it possible to treat this lesion with a multistaged approach. The Norwood procedure is performed initially, consisting of enlargement of the atrial septal defect, ligation of the PDA, anastomosis of the pulmonary artery to the ascending aorta and the aortic arch, and creation of an aortopulmonary shunt (Blalock-Taussig shunt) to maintain pulmonary blood flow. In the second stage the aortopulmonary shunt is removed and an anastomosis is made between the superior vena cava and the pulmonary artery, which is called the bidirectional Glenn shunt and is performed at 6 to 12 months of age. The final stage is the Fontan procedure connecting the inferior vena cava to the pulmonary artery at 18 to 36 months of age. The mortality is high, but surgery offers a chance for survival. Cardiac transplantation is an alternative surgical option. In some centers the Norwood procedure is performed as a bridge to transplant, allowing the infant to survive until a donor heart is available.

Heart Transplantation in Infants Approximately 10% of infants born with congenital heart disease have severe, complex lesions that preclude corrective surgery. For some of these infants, heart transplantation may offer a chance of long-term survival. Hypoplastic left heart syndrome is the most common of these defects and is the most common indication for heart transplantation in early infancy. Cardiomyopathies are another indication.

Heart transplantation in infancy is severely limited by donor availability. There is a scarcity of donor hearts in this age and size group, and 31% of infants less than 6 months of age on transplant lists die waiting for donors.

Contraindications for donor hearts are cardiac dysfunction and congenital heart disease (screened by echocardiogram), infection, systemic illness, and prolonged cardiac arrest. Acceptable hearts are matched with recipients by ABO blood group and approximate body weight and heart size. Specific human leukocyte antigen (HLA) matching is not done. Contraindications for recipients include major CNS abnormalities, irreversible failure of other organ systems, uncontrolled infections, and severe dysmorphism. Relative contraindications include marked prematurity (less than 36 weeks' gestational age), low birth weight (less than 2000 grams),

positive drug screen, and a family structure that is unable to support the long-term medical needs of the patient.[4] Abnormal structural relationships (i.e., situs inversus, dextrocardia, and abnormalities of systemic and pulmonary veins) are not contraindications to heart transplantation.[4]

Pretransplant care involves the support of the infant to maintain systemic perfusion, adequate oxygenation, and control of congestive heart failure. Great caution is used to avoid infection and maintain optimal nutritional status. If blood transfusions are necessary, washed, leukocyte-filtered red blood cells and blood products negative for CMV are used.

In performing the transplant, the donor heart atria are anastomosed to the posterior walls of the recipient atria, thus leaving the infant with two sinoatrial (SA) nodes, the native recipient SA node and the donor SA node. This will give a characteristic ECG postoperatively, with both the recipient and donor P waves present. The donor SA node controls the rhythm of the transplanted heart; therefore donor P waves will be related to the QRS complex.

Postoperative management of these infants involves isolation for prevention of infection, inotropic support as needed, immunosuppression, and surveillance for rejection. Rejection is closely monitored by clinical examination, ECG, echocardiogram, and myocardial biopsy. Rejections are treated with pulsed corticosteroids and other agents.

Immunosuppression is achieved through the administration of a variety of drugs, including cyclosporine, OKT3, FK-506, azathioprine, and corticosteroids. Each institution performing transplants uses some variation of combination of the above drugs for both immediate and long-term immunosuppression. The highest incidence of rejection occurs in the first 6 months posttransplant. Death in the perioperative period can be from graft failure, rejection, or infection.

Long-term complications include rejection, infection, impairment of renal function, hypertension, growth restriction, neurologic sequelae, lymphoproliferative disease, and graft atherosclerosis. Most of these complications are secondary to chronic immunosuppression.

Prognosis and Follow-Up

The prognosis is grim. Without surgical intervention, all infants die within several days or months of birth. Even with surgical intervention, the mortality is still high.

Dysrhythmias

Physiology

The development of the cardiac conduction system continues after birth with a steady increase in the sympathetic innervation of the heart. This accounts for the observed heart rate variability and the high frequency of benign dysrhythmias in the newborn. Premature ventricular beats (Fig. 23-11), brief episodes of ectopic atrial rhythms, wandering atrial pacemakers (Fig. 23-12), and even brief episodes of sinus arrest are all frequently seen in the newborn

period. The majority of these dysrhythmias do not require immediate treatment; however, if they persist, the presence of congenital heart disease, sepsis, drug toxicity, persistent hypoxia, adrenal insufficiency, disorders of electrolyte and acid-base balance, hypoglycemia, and hypocalcemia should be considered.

All cardiac tissue is capable of generating a spontaneous depolarization. However, the SA node, AV node, and His-Purkinje system consist of specialized conductive tissue with rapid spontaneous depolarization. The SA node is the normal pacemaker of the heart because it has the fastest rate of spontaneous depolarization. If, however, the spontaneous depolarization of the SA node is delayed or slower than normal, an escape rhythm (Fig. 23-12) is generated by either the AV node or His-Purkinje system (these rhythms are called nodal escape or ventricular escape, respectively).

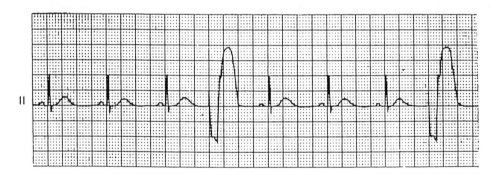

Figure 23-11   Premature ventricular beats.

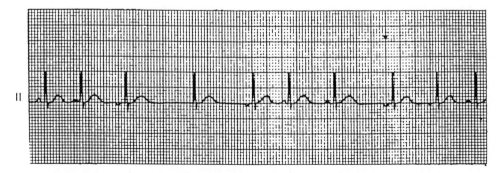

Figure 23-12   Wandering atrial pacemaker with junctional escape (fourth complex).

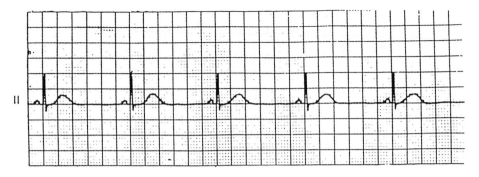

Figure 23-13   Sinus bradycardia.

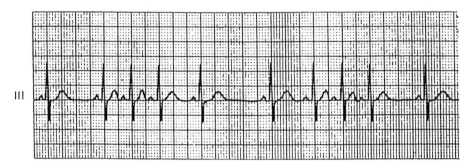

Figure 23-14   Sinus dysrhythmia.

Dysrhythmias can also originate from an automatic "ectopic" pacemaker located anywhere in the heart. These ectopic pacemakers become more active in the presence of hypoxia, acidosis, digoxin toxicity, abnormal sympathetic nervous system stimulation, increased wall tension (congestive heart failure), or altered electrolyte balance. Drug therapy for dysrhythmias is based on the ability of certain medications to alter the electrophysiologic properties of cardiac tissue. One class of antidysrhythmic drugs directly increases the automaticity of certain cardiac fibers. Examples of such drugs include quinidine, procainamide, lidocaine, and phenytoin (see Table 23-4). Other drugs directly or indirectly affect the autonomic nervous system activity. Propranolol is a beta-adrenergic blocker and works in this fashion. Digoxin exerts its chronotropic activity by altering the sympathetic and parasympathetic nervous system response within the heart.

Benign Dysrhythmias: Sinus Bradycardia, Sinus Tachycardia, and Sinus Dysrhythmia

Of normal premature infants, 35% to 40% have brief episodes of sinus bradycardia (Fig. 23-13), sinus tachycardia, or sinus dysrhythmia (Fig. 23-14) that are benign and require no treatment. Healthy premature and term infants may have heart rates that range from 90 to 200 beats/min. Sustained heart rates (greater than 15 seconds) above or below this range should be evaluated with a 12-lead electrocardiogram and rhythm strip. These are important, because artifact created by the bedside monitors often makes accurate interpretations of dysrhythmias impossible.

Supraventricular Tachycardia

Supraventricular tachycardia (SVT) (Fig. 23-15) is the most common tachydysrhythmia in the newborn period. It is the result of dual AV nodal pathways, rapid conduction through an accessory

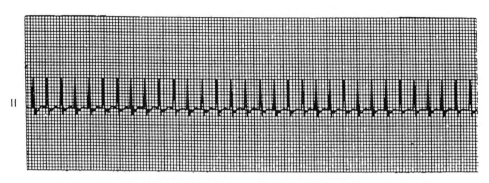

Figure 23-15   Supraventricular tachycardia.

bundle (Wolff-Parkinson-White syndrome), or the existence of an ectopic atrial pacemaker. SVT is commonly associated with Ebstein's anomaly of the tricuspid valve, L-transposition of the great vessels, cardiomyopathy, or myocarditis. These lesions are present in 10% to 25% of infants with SVT and should be excluded with the appropriate evaluation. Newborns with SVT will have a history of gradually developing congestive heart failure with findings of anxiousness, restlessness, tachypnea, and poor feeding. These symptoms develop after 12 to 24 hours of SVT. SVT often starts and ceases abruptly.

Criteria for SVT include (1) persistent ventricular rate over 200 beats/min, (2) a fixed and regular R-R interval, and (3) little change in heart rate with various activities (crying, feeding, or apnea).

Treatment.   Various maneuvers may be used to attempt to convert the infant to normal sinus rhythm (NSR). Vagal maneuvers (unilateral carotid pressure, gagging, rectal stimulation) may be attempted but rarely work. Ocular compression should never be used. Stimulation of the diving reflex using an ice bag applied to the infant's face may be attempted. (Caution must be used in this procedure to ensure adequate ventilation for the infant.) Adenosine, a purinergic agonist, is an especially effective antidysrhythmic drug for treatment of SVT. Adenosine slows the sinus rate and produces transient AV block, interrupting the SVT. Overdrive atrial pacing has been successful in converting SVT to NSR. However, direct-current

(DC) cardioversion (1 to 2 watt seconds/kg) is the most effective mode of treatment. The defibrillator must always be in the synchronous mode. If cardioversion is successful, maintenance drug therapy should be initiated. Other antidysrhythmic drugs such as digoxin have been used to treat this disorder. Recently, however, it has been suggested that digoxin not be used in Wolff-Parkinson-White syndrome and that this disorder be ruled out before digoxin is used. If not contraindicated, digoxin should be administered using standard doses (see Box 23-2).

Propranolol administered IV may be used if the patient is not in congestive heart failure. Beta-blocking agents may inhibit circulating catecholamines, which are needed for the maintenance of adequate cardiac output in the face of congestive heart failure.

Verapamil is a calcium channel blocker and when first introduced was thought to be the drug of choice in SVT. However, this drug should not be used in children under 1 year of age and should never be used in a patient in congestive heart failure.

If the SVT fails to convert using the methods outlined above, other drugs such as amiodarone flecanide procainamide may be required. After conversion to NSR, maintenance drug therapy should be continued for 12 months or longer. Relapses during the first 48 hours are common (70%) and should be anticipated.

Fetal SVT is uncommon, but when present can be associated with severe congestive heart failure and hydrops fetalis. Fetal SVT requires aggressive management, including conversion with maternally administered propranolol and digoxin.

Atrial Flutter and Fibrillation

The presence of atrial flutter (Fig. 23-16) usually indicates severe organic heart disease (endocardial fibroelastosis, Ebstein's anomaly of the tricuspid valve, or complex heart defects). Atrial flutter is diagnosed when (1) the atrial rate is greater than 220 beats/min; (2) the P waves are very regular; and (3) there is a characteristic sawtooth pattern, indicating a flutter wave. The ventricular rate will vary depending on the degree of AV block present. Atrial fibrillation is extremely rare and almost always indicates a serious organic heart disease.

Treatment.   The treatment of atrial flutter or fibrillation is DC cardioversion or overdrive atrial pacing followed by maintenance therapy with digoxin.

Ventricular Tachycardia

Ventricular tachycardia is frequently associated with severe organic heart disease.

Treatment.   Ventricular tachycardia is best treated with immediate DC cardioversion. Lidocaine may be used as a bolus (1 to 2 mg/kg IV) or as a continuous IV infusion of 20 to 30 µg/min. After conversion, maintenance therapy should be initiated using phenytoin, Inderal, lidocaine, procainamide, or amiodarone.

Complete Atrioventricular Block

In complete heart block, the ventricular rate is slower than the atrial rate and there is no associa- tion between the ventricular and atrial rates. Complete heart block can be seen in infants with myocarditis or endocardial fibroelastosis. There is a strong association between congenital heart block and maternal collagen diseases such as SLE. Often these mothers have no signs or symptoms of lupus, but laboratory confirmation is often possible.

Treatment.   No treatment is required unless the ventricular rate falls below 55 beats/min or the infant becomes symptomatic, in which case a pacemaker is required. Isoproterenol may increase the ventricular rate until a pacemaker is placed.

Parent Teaching[1,5,8,12]

The diagnosis of congenital heart disease in their child is a frightening experience for parents. Depending on the family background, educational level, and emotional state, parents may think their infant will die regardless of the severity of the heart defect. In addition, parents may have an overwhelming sense of guilt at having borne a child with a heart defect. Frequently they ask, "What did I do wrong to cause this?" Therefore comprehensive teaching, reassurance, and support are essential for the well-being of both the infant and the family. Understanding the heart defect aids in decreasing anxiety. Parents should also have a basic understanding of their child's heart defect to provide good care after discharge.

Explain the infant's heart defect to the parents. Draw or show a picture of the heart defect, explaining briefly and simply the normal circulation of the

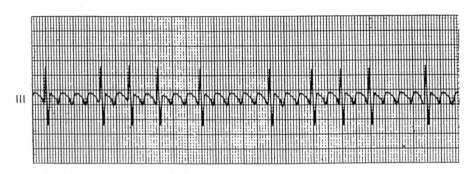

Figure 23-16   Atrial flutter.

heart and how the circulation of their child's heart differs from normal. This explanation should be repeated often for parental understanding and retention. Careful explanation of all tubes, monitors, equipment, and procedures in the nursery also helps decrease parental anxiety.

Heart defects are not visible lesions. Most of these infants will appear quite normal and healthy. It therefore may be difficult for some parents to accept that anything is wrong with their infant. In addition, parents are under great emotional and sometimes physical stress (from labor and delivery), which decreases their ability to hear and retain explanations about the defect. Repetition of explanations is important.

Medical and nursing personnel should facilitate bonding and decrease the parents' fear of holding or caring for their infant by encouraging interaction with the infant and enabling parents to participate in their infant's care. The parents' confidence in caring for their infant at home is established in the nursery. Parents must feel comfortable caring for their infant and have the opportunity to demonstrate their ability to do so before discharge from the hospital.

Teaching home care of the infant before discharge should be detailed and include medications, signs and symptoms to observe, and guidelines for care. Ideally these should be written instructions. The parents should telephone the physician if the infant demonstrates (1) poor feeding for 1 to 2 days or sweating with feeds, (2) vomiting most of feedings for a 12- to 24-hour period, (3) fast or labored breathing for several hours, (4) decreased activity level, (5) weight loss or failure to gain weight, and (6) frequent respiratory illnesses.

All medications should be explained in detail, including their purpose, action, and administration. Parents should be made aware of the potential adverse effects (side effects) of all of their infant's medications. Parents should be observed giving medications in the nursery before the infant is discharged.

Cyanotic heart disease is particularly disturbing to parents because their infant's skin color is "blue." Parents should be cautioned that their infant will appear blue, especially around the mouth, mucous membranes, hands, and feet, and the blueness will increase with activity such as crying, feeding, and bowel movements. Parents should notify the physician about any of the previously listed symptoms in addition to (1) greatly increased cyanosis, especially if associated with fast or labored breathing, (2) decreased movement in any or all of the extremities, (3) decreased responsiveness or eyes deviating to one side, and (4) seizure activity such as jerking motions or stiffness followed by the infant becoming floppy or limp.

It is important to emphasize to parents that their infant should be treated as normally as possible. There is no activity restriction for infants with heart disease because infants will "self-limit" themselves according to their capacities. It is difficult for parents with a firstborn child with heart disease to differentiate "normal baby problems" from cardiac-related problems. For these parents, as well as other parents of children with cardiac defects, it is particularly important to have open communication between the family, the primary care provider, and the cardiologist. Parents should be encouraged to call these medical personnel as needed for support, answers to questions, and reassurance. Support groups of parents whose children have heart defects provide information, empathy, and practical tips to parents dealing with medical and/or surgical interventions for their child's heart defect.

Acknowledgment

We would like to thank David Clark, M.D., F.A.C.S., F.A.C.C. for his contribution to the sections on surgical management.

References

1. American Heart Association: *If your child has a congenital heart disease: a guide for parents* (free on request), Dallas, American Heart Association.

2. Baum MF et al: Physiologic and psychological growth and development in pediatric heart transplant recipients, *J Heart Lung Transplant* 10:848, 1991.

3. Benson LN, Freedom RM: The clinical diagnostic approach in congenital heart disease. In Freedom RM, Benson LN, Smallhorn JF, editors: *Neonatal heart disease,* London, 1992, Springer-Verlag.

4. Clark EB: Epidemiology of congenital cardiovascular malformation. In Emmanouilides GC et al, editors: *Moss and Adams heart disease in infants, children and adolescents,* Baltimore, 1995, Williams & Wilkins.

5. Freedom RM, Benson LN, Smallhorn JF, editors: *Neonatal heart disease,* London, 1992, Springer-Verlag.

6. Fyler DC: Report of the New England Regional Infant Cardiac Program, *Pediatrics* 65(suppl):375, 1980.

7. Garson A et al: Parental reactions to children with congenital heart disease, *Child Psych Hum Dev* 9:86, 1978.

8. Garson A, Bricker JT, McNamara DG: *The science and practice of pediatric cardiology,* Philadelphia, 1990, Lea & Febiger.

9. Gillette PC, Garson A: *Pediatric arrhythmias: electrophysiology and pacing,* Philadelphia, 1990, WB Saunders.

10. Gottesfeld IB: The family of the child with congenital heart disease, *ECN* 4:101, 1979.

11. Moller JH, Neal WA: *Fetal, neonatal, and infant cardiac disease,* Norwalk, Conn, 1990, Appleton & Lange.

12. Perry LW et al: Infants with congenital heart disease: the case. In Fernandez C et al, editors: *Epidemiology of congenital heart disease: the Baltimore-Washington infant heart study 1981-1989,* Mount Kisco, NY, 1993, Futura.

13. Rose V, Clark E: Etiology of congenital heart disease. In Freedom RM, Benson LN, Smallhorn JF, editors: *Neonatal heart disease,* London, 1992, Springer-Verlag.

14. Rudolph A: *Congenital diseases of the heart; clinical-physiologic considerations of the heart,* Chicago, 1974, Year Book Medical Publishers.

15. Wolterman M, Miller M: Caring for parents in crises, *Nurs Forum* 22:34, 1985.

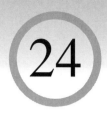

24 Neonatal Nephrology

Melvin Bonilla-Felix, Patricia Brannan, Ronald J. Portman

In utero the placenta is the organ responsible for toxin removal and fluid and electrolyte homeostasis. The fetal kidney is not required for this role in utero, but it plays an essential role in the development of the fetus by the generation of amniotic fluid. Postnatally the kidney assumes its role as the regulator of fluid and electrolyte homeostasis as the body adapts to the external milieu. There is a rapid change in renal function that is clinically difficult to assess. This task is even more difficult in the premature infant whose kidneys must perform a role for which they are not ready. In fact, nephrogenesis continues to progress until 36 weeks' postconceptional age whether the infant is in utero or ex utero. The genitourinary system has the highest percentage of anomalies, congenital or genetic, of all of the organ systems (10%).

In some series the genitourinary system represents 22% to 50% of all abnormalities found on in utero ultrasound examinations.[34] They frequently present during the neonatal period, but some cases are diagnosed later in childhood. The variability in renal function and maturation combined with the high frequency of anomalies makes a prediction of the neonatal kidneys' response to an insult very complicated. Our knowledge of these changes is very limited but growing.

This chapter discusses the anatomic and physiologic development of the kidney and its clinical assessment. Prenatal and postnatal indicators of renal disease are presented, followed by a discussion of the most common and important clinical conditions involving the genitourinary system in the neonatal period.

General Physiology

Normal Development of the Kidney*

The two primitive kidneys, the pronephros and the mesonephros, regress in the human but induce the definitive kidney, the metanephros (Fig. 24-1). The pronephros, a solid mass of cells along the nephrogenic cord, is located at the cervical level at approximately 3 weeks' gestation. Degeneration of the pronephros begins soon after its formation, and no excretory function occurs. Infection or other insults at this stage in development may result in agenesis or abnormal development of the kidney. The ureter of the pronephros forms the Wolffian, or mesonephric, duct, which induces the formation of the second kidney, the mesonephros. It is speculated that retention of abnormal pronephric tissue may be one cause of mediastinal cysts.

The mesonephros originates at approximately 31 days' gestation more caudally. It evolves from the nephrogenic cord and forms 40 pairs of thin-walled tubules and glomeruli with excretory function. At the end of the fourth month, these degenerate as the metanephric kidney develops. Portions of the mesonephric duct system retained in males have been shown to form the ducts of the epididymis, the ductus deferens, and the ejaculatory duct. In the female, near-complete degeneration occurs.

The metanephros appears at 31 to 34 days' gestation. The uretic bud or duct grows from the posteromedial wall of the mesonephric duct near its junction with the cloaca. This bud migrates to the most caudal end of the nephrogenic cord and finally

---

* References 39, 64.

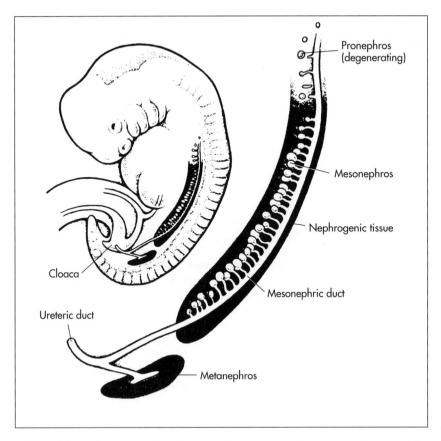

Figure 24-1 Schematic representation of overlapping stages in embryogenesis of human kidney. See text for detailed description. (From Holliday MA: *Hosp Pract* 13:101, 1978.)

to the lumbar region and rotates medially along the longitudinal axis. Cephalic migration of the kidney to its normal position is due to straightening of the fetus from the curled position. Abnormalities in the ascent or rotation can lead to pelvic kidneys, horseshoe kidneys, or crossed fused ectopia.

The ureteric bud grows into the metanephric blastema (metanephros), then repeatedly branches dichotomously, determining the number and location of the renal pelvis, calyces, and collecting ducts. The cells of the metanephric blastema clump around the ureteric bud and stimulate the formation of the glomerulus, proximal tubule, loop of Henle, and distal tubule, which then empty into the collecting duct.

Nephrogenesis begins in the renal cortex closest

to the medulla (juxtamedullary nephrons). The process continues in a centrifugal pattern with the outermost (superficial cortical) nephrons forming last. The process of forming the lifelong complement of 1 million nephrons in each kidney is complete by 34 to 36 weeks' post-conceptional age (i.e., from the time of conception). The kidneys will continue their development at approximately the same rate whether in utero or ex utero. For example, a 28-week-gestation premature infant will not complete nephrogenesis for 6 to 8 more weeks (Fig. 24-2). How insults such as hypoxia, asphyxia, and various toxins affect this development is not yet clear. The newborn kidney may be relatively protected from these insults, because the superficial cortical nephrons are not fully developed and the juxtamedullary nephrons are more resistant to hypoxic damage.

Physiologic Development and Clinical Assessment

Glomerular Filtration Rate*

In utero the placenta serves as the major organ for maintenance of body fluid, electrolyte composition, and clearance of metabolic wastes. It is not surprising that the percentage of cardiac output to the kidneys is low (2.2% to 3.7%) compared with the 25% observed in the adult. Renal blood flow is similarly depressed and distributed mainly to the more mature juxtamedullary nephrons. A high renal vascular resistance is a primary determinant of this reduced flow. The GFR is also quite low and increases proportional to changes in body mass and gestational age. Postnatally there is a dramatic increase in GFR as the kidney assumes its functional role. The GFR doubles in the first weeks of life to 30 to 40 ml/min/1.73 m² (see Figs. 24-2 and 24-3) and then further increases to the adult normal of 100 to 120 ml/min/1.73 m² by between 1 and 2 years of life. During this period the GFR is increasing at a rate greater than the growth in body mass. Factors responsible for the rise in GFR are an expansion in filtration surface area caused by a greater perfusion of the superficial cortical nephrons and a decrease in renal vascular resistance. Premature infants of less than 34 weeks' postconceptional age have a rather stable and low GFR until nephrogenesis is completed. At this point, a threefold to fivefold rise in GFR can be observed (see Fig. 24-2). Factors contributing to this phenomenon are not yet determined.

The clinical assessment of GFR is very difficult in a newborn for several reasons. Although inulin and iothalamate clearances in the infant are accurate, they are not a practical clinical tool. New developments in this area, such as iohexol clearances, are needed. The usual endogenous marker of GFR is the serum creatinine level. At birth, the serum creatinine reflects maternal values as creatinine freely crosses the placenta. As the GFR increases, the creatinine level decreases by 50% to a

* References 6, 7, 21, 33, 78, 79, 83.

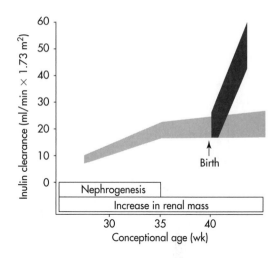

Figure 24-2 Correlation of glomular filtration rate (GFR) as measured by insulin clearance and postconceptional age. Note marked increase in GFR postnatally. However, this increase in GFR does not occur after 40 weeks unless birth occurs. If birth occurs before nephrogenesis is complete (usually at 35 weeks), this increase will not occur until 34 to 36 weeks' post-conceptional age. (From Guignard JP: Neonatal nephrology. In Holliday MA, Barratt TM, Vernier RL, editors: *Pediatric nephrology,* ed 2, Baltimore, 1987, Williams & Wilkins.)

level of approximately 0.4 mg/dl in the term infant over the first week of life (see Fig. 21-3). The rate of this decrease can be quite variable depending on the infant's hydration and clinical status. This lack of steady state makes accurate creatinine clearance measurement troublesome. Also, the laboratory measurement of creatinine has a very low sensitivity for any changes in GFR. A true increase in creatinine from 0.4 to 0.5 mg/dl could reflect a decrease in GFR of as much as 25%. However, a rising serum creatinine is never normal.

In an effort to enhance the sensitivity of the serum creatinine, Schwartz[78] developed a formula correlating creatinine clearance to body length and plasma creatinine values:

$$\text{GFR (ml/min/1.73 m}^2) = \frac{k}{\text{Length (cm)} \times \text{Plasma creatinine (mg/dl)}}$$

The proportionality constant, *k,* is a function of urine creatinine excretion per unit of body size.

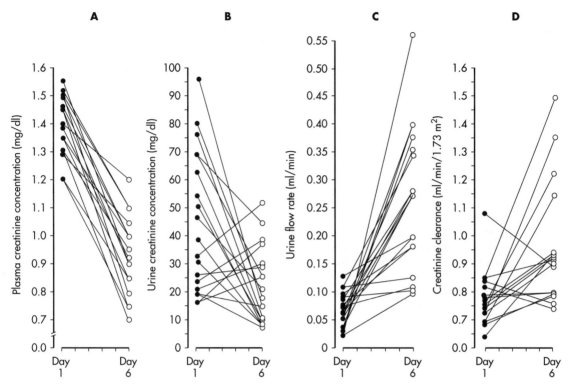

Figure 24-3   **A,** Change in plasma creatinine concentrations on day 1 *(solid circle)* and day 6 *(open circle)* of life. *Solid line* connects values of individual infant. **B,** Urinary creatinine concentrations. **C,** Urinary flow rate. **D,** GFR as measured by creatinine clearance. Note that increase in GFR is accompanied by decrease in creatinine concentrations as infant excretes maternal creatinine and by increase in urine flow rate. (From Sertel H, Scops J: *Arch Dis Child* 48:717, 1973.)

For the infant less than 2500 g at birth, the mean value of k is 0.33 throughout the first year of life. For the full-term infant during the same period, k is 0.45. Other k values are available for older children.

The determination of GFR in the preterm infant is much more complicated. The GFR generally does not increase until nephrogenesis is complete. Until this time the infant's creatinine reflects maternal creatinine or creatinine in transfused blood. The only reasonable assessment of renal function in the premature infant is a relative change in creatinine on serial determinations. Values in excess of maternal creatinine or greater than 1.5 mg/dl may be considered abnormal.

If measurement of creatinine clearance is de-sired, it is best performed by serial-timed voids. When the infant voids, Credé's maneuver is per-formed on the bladder, a timer is set, and a urine bag is applied. At the next void the timer is stopped, Credé's maneuver is performed, and the volume is noted. This can be done two or three times, and an average value can be used for the clearance result. The clearance formula is:

$$\text{Clearance (ml/min/1.73 m}^2) = \frac{UV}{P} \times \frac{1.73}{BSA}$$

where U is the urine creatinine concentration (milligrams per deciliter), P is the plasma concen-tration, V is the volume of urine divided by the time of collection in minutes, and BSA is the body surface area in square meters. However, such maneuvers are rarely indicated, because a precise determination of GFR during the newborn period is usually not necessary.

Urine Flow Rate[6,7,21,79,83]

Urine flow in utero is important for its contribution to amniotic fluid and for the development of the urinary tract. Sufficient amniotic fluid volume is critical for fetal development, because compression of the fetus by the uterus can lead to fetal akinesia syndrome.

The fetal kidney excretes a hypotonic urine (10 ml/kg/hr) with a large sodium content. After birth, the urine flow rate increases in the first week of life (see Fig. 24-3). Quite often, infants will void unnoticed in the delivery room. Fifty percent of infants void in the first 12 hours, 92% in the first 24 hours, and 99% in the first 48 hours of life. Causes for failure to void by this time must be carefully evaluated, including abnormalities in volume status or renal function, or anatomic abnormalities such as obstruction. A diuresis occurs in the first 5 days of life as the expanded extracellular fluid volume of the neonate is excreted. A 10% loss of body weight can be normally seen in those first few days of life. Stimuli for this diuresis are unknown but may be related to the rise in renal blood flow and GFR, and possibly to atrial natriuretic factor release.

Oliguria is generally defined as urine output of less than 1 ml/kg/hr. This definition should not be used for the first 48 hours of life, however, because the infant who typically has a poor oral intake may be conserving fluid appropriately. One must not necessarily equate oliguria with an abnormality in renal function. Further assessment of function must be undertaken as previously discussed.

Urine flow depends on fluid intake and solute load, as noted in Chapter 13. The neonatal kidney can dilute urine to the same degree as an adult kidney (i.e., 50 mOsm/L); however, the neonate can have difficulty excreting a water load, because it cannot raise the GFR quickly enough to excrete it. This ability to dilute appears to be well developed, because the neonate receives its nutrition in a calorically diluted solution (breast milk) and thus needs to be able to excrete water freely. The term neonatal kidney cannot concentrate well (maximum concentration 700 mOsm/L) for several

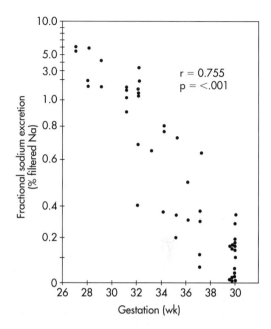

Figure 24-4   Decrease in fractional excretion of sodium occurs with increasing postconceptional age. (From Siegel S, Oh W: *Acta Paediatr Scand* 65:481, 1976.)

reasons. A low medullary urea content, low peritubular capillary oncotic pressure, resistance to antidiuretic hormone, decreased expression of water channels, and a short loop of Henle are all postulated mechanisms. The kidneys of most infants can fully concentrate by 1 year of age.

Sodium[7,21,33,80,84]

The fractional excretion of sodium (FENa) is high (15%) in utero and in premature infants but decreases with increasing gestational age (Fig. 24-4). FENa is defined as the clearance of sodium factored by the GFR:

$$\frac{\dfrac{U_{Na}V}{P_{Na}}}{\dfrac{U_{cre}V}{P_{cre}}} \xrightarrow[\substack{volume\\cancels}]{\text{On the same}\\ \text{sample}} \frac{\dfrac{U_{Na}}{P_{Na}}}{\dfrac{U_{cre}}{P_{cre}}} \times 100 = FENa(\%)$$

The FENa is 5% to 6% in a 28-week-gestation premature infant, 3% to 5% in a 33-week-gestation

infant, and 1% to 3% in a term infant. The extra-cellular fluid volume is expanded in the newborn, and the aforementioned diuresis is accompanied by a natriuresis. The ability of the neonatal kidney to handle rapid challenges in sodium balance is relatively fixed. The immature proximal tubule cannot reabsorb adequate amounts of sodium, and thus the distal nephron must compensate with an increase in sodium reabsorption. This is mediated by the increase in the renin, angiotensin, and aldosterone (RAA) levels seen in the newborn.[84] This mechanism cannot completely compensate for the increased distal sodium delivery; thus the "salt wasting" of the newborn is observed. Conversely, the neonatal kidney cannot increase the FENa rapidly and thus cannot handle a large sodium load. Such a load would lead to edema and volume overload. Urinary prostaglandin levels are also quite high and may also account for the increase in RAA levels. With tubular maturity and increased proximal sodium reabsorption, the RAA and prostaglandin levels gradually fall. Abnormalities in sodium concentration are discussed in Chapter 13 and are primarily problems with water balance. Sodium losses are also increased in the stressed, hypoxic infant as the major oxygen consumption of the kidney is used for sodium reabsorption.

Proximal Tubular Function[7,21,83,89]

The proximal tubule appears to be less well developed anatomically than the glomerulus at birth. Additionally, the neonatal increase in urinary glucose and amino acid excretion have led to the consideration of a possible imbalance of function between the glomeruli and tubules. In fact, there is a balance in each individual nephron for glomerular and tubular function. The tremendous heterogenicity in nephron development can lead to an enhanced delivery of these substrates to certain nephrons. The transport systems are overwhelmed by this filtered load, and thus glucose and amino acids are spilled into the urine. This is termed an increase in "splay." The neonatal expansion of extracellular fluid volume may also lead to a decrease in proximal tubular absorption of these compounds in the first days of life.

Low-molecular-weight proteins such as beta-2-microglobulin (β_2M) are also absorbed exclusively in the proximal tubule. β_2M is the small subunit of the HLA class I antigen. As cells die, β_2M is released into the circulation and is excreted solely by the kidney. After being freely filtered by the glomerulus, β_2M is 99.9% reabsorbed by the proximal tubule and metabolized to amino acids. Any increase in urinary β_2M levels is suggestive of proximal tubular dysfunction. Whether an increased excretion in more premature infants is a marker of tubular immaturity is a matter of some debate. β_2M is, however, a very sensitive marker of damage to the proximal tubule by hypoxia or toxins and has been used clinically for this purpose.[89]

Potassium[7,77,83]

Potassium levels in the newborn are quite frequently higher than later in childhood, (e.g., 5.5 to 6.0 mEq/L). This level is rarely of pathologic significance. The renal clearance of potassium in the neonate is lower (9%) than observed later in life (15%), even after correcting for GFR. This is most likely the result of resistance of the immature cortical collecting duct to aldosterone.

Acid-Base Balance[7,14,21,33,83]

Serum bicarbonate levels are lower in the newborn (19 to 21 mEq/L). This is a result of increased endogenous acid production, decreased bicarbonate reabsorption in the proximal tubule, and decreased proton secretion in the collecting duct. Another contributing factor is the neonate's expanded extracellular fluid volume, which leads to a reduction in sodium and bicarbonate reabsorption in the proximal tubule. Carbonic anhydrase activity is decreased bicarbonate in the newborn. The tubular maximum gradually increases to near-adult levels by the first year of life (21 to 24 mEq/L). Urine pH in the newborn is frequently greater than 6, but the appropriateness of urinary pH can only be gauged by comparison with systemic acid-base studies. Renal failure, shock, and many inborn errors of metabolism may lead to an increased anion gap metabolic acidosis. Renal tubular acidosis (RTA) may account for a metabolic acidosis with a normal anion gap.[14]

RTA can be seen transiently as the neonatal tubule recovers from acute renal failure or renal vein thrombosis. Diarrhea is another cause of normal anion gap acidosis. In older children and adults, an increased urinary anion gap signifies

RTA, whereas a normal gap signifies gastrointestinal bicarbonate loss.[9] However, the urinary anion gap is not a valuable index of urinary ammonium excretion in the newborn.[88] Rapid expansion of extracellular fluid, addition of acid (most commonly seen with parenteral nutrition), and urinary diversions into an ileal segment are other major causes of normal anion gap acidosis in the newborn.

Uric Acid[33,85]

Serum uric acid levels are elevated in the newborn because of an increase in production. Infants who are stressed have particularly high levels from nucleotide breakdown. There is also a fivefold to sevenfold increase in uric acid excretion in the newborn later in life. The fractional excretion of uric acid is 30% at 30 weeks' gestation and 18% at 40 weeks' gestation as opposed to 5% noted in the adult. Infarcts in the kidney have been noted distal to an obstruction from uric acid. The newborn is relatively protected from this excessive uric acid excretion by the normal alkalinity of the urine improving the solubility of uric acid. Uric acid crystals can appear reddish in the diaper and have been mistaken for blood.

General Etiology and Prevention

Prenatal*

Most congenital abnormalities of the urinary tract are presumed to be sporadic, genetic (either alone or as a part of a syndrome), or to result from environmental factors (e.g., cocaine, alcohol, organic solvents, and maternal fever [>101° F]).[14,24,51,91] Exposure to environmental agents must occur early in pregnancy during morphogenesis. Recently, significant fetal and neonatal damage has been reported with maternal administration of angiotensin converting enzyme (ACE) inhibitors (i.e., ACE fetopathy).[35] These agents easily cross the placenta and affect fetal RAA levels, resulting in oligohydramnios, fetal hypotension, renal tubular maldevelopment, renal failure, and death. The use of maternal nephrotoxic agents (i.e., ACE inhibitors) should be avoided when possible.

Prenatal care enables patients at risk for these conditions to be monitored closely. When hydronephrosis is present, serial ultrasound should be done to determine amniotic fluid changes that may warrant early intervention. **Early diagnosis and treatment of these anomalies may improve the long-term prognosis for renal function.[69]** Educating professionals and the public about the medications, drugs, and toxins that cause renal damage in utero and furthering such research are critically important preventive measures.

Neonatal

Renal involvement in the neonate should be considered with the use of three categories of drugs: diuretics, aminoglycosides, and indomethacin.† The neonatal kidney's immature GFR must be considered when administering certain drugs. Complicating the issue of dosage is the rapid maturation of the neonate's GFR.

Furosemide may have significant side effects when used in the newborn. It is filtered by the glomerulus but primarily secreted in the proximal tubule. An increased dose is required in the newborn because of the low GFR. The loss of potassium through the kidney is well documented and must be treated with potassium supplementation. With furosemide, increased excretion of calcium in urine is associated with renal calcifications, including renal stones and interstitial calcifications (in neonates receiving more than a week of furosemide therapy).[40] Although nephrocalcinosis occurs in prematures without the use of furosemide, it is the single major risk factor in this form of renal damage.[41] This type of calcification may be reversed by the addition of a thiazide diuretic that promotes the reabsorption of calcium.

Furosemide is freely used in infants with RDS and BPD (with little evidence of its effectiveness in improving lung compliance). **Because of the aforementioned complications and a controlled trial showing benefit in BPD,[47] thiazides should be used as the drug of choice. If needed, furosemide can then be added to the regimen. Thiazides should**

---

* References 11, 52.

† References 5, 22, 31, 34, 40, 41, 47.

always be used with chronic furosemide administration to prevent hypercalciuria. The possibility also exists that the incidence of PDA is increased with the use of furosemide from an increased prostaglandin synthesis.[31] The potential for furosemide ototoxicity is also a significant complication, especially when used in combination with aminoglycosides.

Aminoglycosides are also excreted by glomerular filtration. Drug levels need to be assessed frequently because of the uncertainty of the rate of renal excretion. The neonatal kidney may be at less risk for nephrotoxicity from aminoglycosides than is the mature kidney. However, gentamicin-induced renal toxicity was recently confirmed in the neonatal kidney without any relationship to peak and trough serum levels.[5] In fact, the long-term effects of neonatal aminoglycoside exposure on renal development have yet to be adequately evaluated.

Renal failure may be induced or exacerbated by the use of indomethacin for the closure of PDA. Prostaglandin synthesis inhibitors may decrease renal blood flow and affect water excretion by removal of the inhibition by prostaglandins of the vasopressin effect. Transient side effects include hyponatremia, decreased urine flow rate, decreased GFR, and abnormal electrolyte excretion. Normal renal function often returns a few days after discontinuation of the drug. If renal compromise is already present, surgical management for the PDA should be considered.

Simultaneous administration of these potentially nephrotoxic agents should be done when absolutely required. Aggressive management of patients with asphyxia, sepsis, hypotension, and dehydration is important to prevent renal damage.

General Data Collection*

History

Obviously critical in the prenatal assessment is a family history of renal diseases or syndromes involving the kidneys. A history of prenatal maternal infections, drugs, toxin, or medication intake is important data because these may be risk factors

---

* References 11, 33, 52, 68.

for the development of fetal nephropathy. Paternal smoking and advanced age may be associated with an increased risk of urinary tract anomalies.

The quantity of aminiotic fluid is the only reliable indicator of renal function in the fetus. A clinical change in volume and its subsequent correlation to impaired renal function may be assessed in utero in selected abnormalities. Fetal swallowing, breathing, and urination are thought to regulate amniotic fluid volume beginning in the second trimester. Abnormalities in these regulatory mechanisms result in alteration of amniotic fluid volume. Normally, amniotic fluid volume increases during gestation, peaking at 34 weeks' gestation. Decreased volume, or oligohydramnios, is caused by fetal genitourinary abnormalities (Table 24-1). Polyhydramnios, or excessive amniotic fluid, occurs in varying degrees with moderate (2000 ml) to extreme (15,000 ml) increases in fluid volume. A correlation between perinatal outcome and the degree of hydramnios has been reported. Gastrointestinal abnormalities that inhibit fetal swallowing are implicated as a major etiological factor in polyhydramnios. Conditions characterized by a severe urinary concentrating defect such as diabetes insipidus and Bartter's syndrome, have been associated with polyhydramnios.

A perinatal asphyxia scoring system that utilizes fetal heart rate monitoring, Apgar scores, and metabolic acidosis has been developed. A high score is an excellent predictor of renal damage.[63]

Signs and Symptoms

Physical findings that are indicators of genitourinary tract abnormalities are outlined in Table 24-1. The table points out the importance of a careful physical examination as a first step in a nephrologic evaluation.

Laboratory Data

Ultrasound

Ultrasound and amniocentesis are technologies used to assess fetal and amniotic fluid status. Noninvasive in nature, ultrasound creates an image by bouncing sound waves off a selected target tissue and projecting the image on a screen.

Table 24-1
Perinatal Indicators of Abnormalities of the Genitourinary Tract

Finding	Suspected Abnormality
Oligohydramnios	Bilateral renal agenesis, PKD, or dysplasia
	Amnion nodosum
Polyhydramnios	Nephrogenic diabetes insipidus, trisomy 18 or 21, anencephaly, esophageal or duodenal obstruction, Klippel-Feil syndrome, Bartter's syndrome
Enlarged placenta (>25% of infant birth weight)	Congenital nephrotic syndrome
Velamentous insertion of umbilical cord	Increased congenital anomalies
Asphyxia neonatorum	Renal failure
Physical Examination	
Hypertension	See text
Skin	
Hemangioma	Hemangioma of kidney or bladder
Edema	Congenital nephrotic syndrome, hydrops fetalis
Adenoma sebaceum	Tuberous sclerosis—cystic kidneys
Head	
Encephalocele	Meckel's or Meckel-Gruber syndrome—polycystic kidney disease
Cleft lip and palate	Urinary tract anomalies
Macroglossia	Beckwith-Wiedemann syndrome—renal dysplasia
	Johanson-Blizzard syndrome—hydronephrosis, oro-facial-digital syndrome—renal microcystic disease
Eyes	
Phakoma (tubular sclerosis)	Angiomyolipoma of the kidney
Retinitis pigmentosa	Medullary cystic disease of the kidney
Cataracts	Cystic diseases, Lowe's syndrome, Wilms' tumor, congenital rubella
Aniridia	Wilms' tumor
Ears	
Low set or malformed	Increased risk of renal abnormalities, Potter's syndrome
Ear tags	Brancho-oto-renal (BOR) syndrome
Preauricular pits	
Skeleton	
Hemihypertrophy	Wilms' tumor
Spina bifida	Neurogenic bladder
Arthrogryposis	Oligohydramnios, Potter's syndrome
Dyplastic nails	Nail patella syndrome
Vertebral anomalies	VATER syndrome—renal dysplasia
Polydactyly	Meckel's or Meckel-Gruber syndrome—polycystic kidneys
Abdomen	
Absence of abdominal musculature	Prune-belly syndrome
Single umbilical artery	Increased congenital anomalies of the urinary tract

Modified from Retek AB: *Hosp Pract* 11:133, 1976.   *Continued*

Table 24-1
Perinatal Indicators of Abnormalities of the Genitourinary Tract—cont'd

Finding	Suspected Abnormality
Abdomen—cont'd	
Umbilical discharge	Patent urachus
Abdominal mass	See Table 24-6
Hepatomegaly	Storage diseases—renal tubular dysfunction, Beckwith-Wiedemann syndrome, Zellweger's syndrome
Pulmonary	
Spontaneous pneumothorax	Increase in renal abnormalities
Pulmonary hypoplasia	Oligohydramnios
Genitourinary—Male	
Undescended testes	Prune-belly syndrome, Noonan's syndrome, Lawrence-Moon-Biedel sydnrome
Congenital absence of vas deferens	Renal agenesis or ectopia
Hypospadias	Increase in renal abnormalities
Abnormal urinary stream	Bladder dysfunction or urethral outlet obstruction
Genitourinary—Female	
Enlarged clitoris	Adrenogenital syndrome
Cystic mass in urethral region	Ectopic ureterocele, paraurethral cyst
	Sarcoma botryoides
Bulging in vagina	Hydrometrocolpos
Abnormal urinary stream or dribbling	Bladder dysfunction, urethral obstruction
Common cloaca	Urinary tract abnormalities
Rectal	
Deficient anal sphincter tone	Neurogenic bladder dysfunction
Dilated prostatic urethra	Posterior urethral valves, prune-belly syndrome
Masses	Tumor
Anal atresia	VATER syndrome—renal dysplasia
Urinalysis	See text

Modified from Retek AB: *Hosp Pract* 11:133, 1976.

Ultrasound identifies urinary tract dilation between the seventeenth and twenty-fourth weeks of gestation. Fetal ultrasound for the assessment of renal function provides information about (1) amniotic fluid volume, (2) appearance and echogenicity of kidneys on ultrasound, and (3) degree of upper urinary tract dilatation, and (4) provides guidance for amniocentesis to analyze fetal urine electrolytes. Ultrasonographic diagnosis of oligohydramnios involves measuring the largest pocket of fluid in two perpendicular planes. Measurements of fluid pockets less than 1 cm are associated with perinatal morbidity.[52] Up to 20% to 50% of all abnormal in utero ultrasound examinations represent urinary tract abnormalities.[36] The term *dilatation* does not always imply urinary tract obstruction and must be used in conjunction with the amount of amniotic fluid in determining kidney function. Antenatal diagnosis of renal abnormalities has a sensitivity of 85% and a specificity of 99%. A definitive renal anomaly postnatally is found in 86% of the cases.[72] Dysplastic kidneys, which may be caused by early obstruction in utero, often have cortical cysts on ultrasound and an increased echogenicity.

Amniocentesis

Amniocentesis, performed during the second trimester, involves the aspiration of amniotic fluid with a needle transabdominally under ultrasound guidance for safety of the fetus and to increase the likelihood of a successful tap.[11,52] **Amniocentesis reveals information on fetal lung maturity, presence of fetal chromosomal abnormalities, Rh isoimmunization, and prenatal diagnosis of many inherited disorders.** The determination of alpha fetoprotein (AFP), the major serum protein present in early gestation, yields important data from amniocentesis. Produced initially by the yolk sac, levels of AFP peak between 14 and 18 weeks' gestation. High concentrations of AFP are associated with open neural tube defects and other conditions such as congenital nephrosis, hydrocele, esophageal atresia, and Meckel's syndrome. Cystinosis can be diagnosed by measuring the cystine content of cells obtained by amniocentesis. Fetal urinary electrolytes as determined by amniocentesis have recently been studied as biochemical indicators of fetal renal function, but many researchers argue against any relationship between urinary electrolytes and renal function. We would not recommend their use unless more convincing data become available.[94]

Urinalysis[88]

Urinalysis is a frequently overlooked but very important indicator of renal disease. After the perineum is cleansed with bactericidal solution and rinsed with water, a urine bag is applied to collect urine. Neonates requiring ongoing strict monitoring of urine output should have a fresh urine bag placed daily.

Specific Gravity

Specific gravity of the urine in the newborn reflects the ability to concentrate and dilute the urine. As the ability to dilute is fully developed, a specific gravity can be as low as 1.001 to 1.005. Concentration is limited in the term neonate, and the maximum specific gravity is usually 1.015 to 1.020. Other components of the urine, such as glucose, protein, and dyes, alter the specific gravity. Urine osmolality measurements should be obtained and correlated to serum osmolality if issues of concentration are being considered.

Glucosuria

Glucose may be found in trace quantities in a term infant's urine but more frequently is noted in the premature infant's urine. Even minor elevations of plasma glucose concentrations may cause significant glucosuria. Large glucose loads given during parenteral alimentation may lead to an osmotic diuresis.

Urinary pH

Urinary pH is relatively alkalotic at 6.0. Most neonates can acidify the urine to a pH of 5.0 if challenged.

Hematuria[48,83]

Hematuria (five or more red blood cells/high powered field [hpf]) is not normal in a neonate. A positive dipstick for heme occurs with hemoglobinuria, during hemolytic states, and with myoglobinuria from severe asphyxia. Inducing a rapid urine flow and alkalinizing the urine to a pH greater than 7 is important to prevent conversion to ferrihemate, the nephrotoxic breakdown product of these globin molecules. Hematuria may occur after the trauma of delivery, especially with an enlarged kidney (e.g., cystic disease or obstruction). Hematuria is most commonly seen in perinatal asphyxia. Other common conditions associated with hematuria include renal vein thrombosis, urinary tract infections, sepsis, embolization to the renal artery (especially from UACs), renal necrosis, hypercalciuria, coagulopathies and, rarely, congenital glomerulonephritis or nephrosis. Hematuria may also be observed from blood outside of the genitourinary tract that is mixed with urine. This includes blood from a circumcision, blood from perineal irritation, and uterine bleeding caused by withdrawal from the effects of maternal hormones. If the hematuria is persistent, it should be evaluated with urine culture, assessment of proteinuria and urine calcium excretion, measurement of GFR, and an anatomic evaluation of the kidneys, such as renal ultrasound.

Pyuria

Pyuria is frequently noted in the newborn, especially females. As many as 25 to 50 white blood cells/hpf may be observed in the first days of life. Pyuria may be a marker of infection, and urine

culture should be obtained where clinically indicated. However, pyuria may also be seen with stress, fever, sepsis, and other injuries to the kidney.

Proteinuria[43]

Proteinuria (greater than or equal to 1+) is frequently seen in the newborn and is related to gestational age. Protein excretion can range from 2.3 mg/m²/hr at 30 weeks' gestation to 1.29 mg/m²/hr at term. Proteinuria is highest in the first day of life but then rapidly decreases. $\beta_2\mu$ excretion is elevated between 3 and 5 days of life before decreasing. Proteinuria is seen in many renal parenchymal diseases and should be evaluated if it persists. Twenty-four hour urine collections for protein are difficult to perform in the newborn. Generally one would see less than 20 mg/m² of protein excretion in the neonate but would consider more than 400 mg/m²/day to be clearly abnormal. Spot urine protein/creatinine ratios are very effective in assessing proteinuria in most clinical situations.

Other Imaging Studies

The more invasive intravenous urographic studies should be done after the first week of life to allow the kidneys' concentrating ability to improve (so that the test will be more reliable). The resolution of neonatal nuclear scans may be inadequate for diagnosing all but the most glaring abnormalities (e.g., lack of renal perfusion). Voiding cystourethrogram is an invasive procedure used to evaluate the lower urinary tract. MRI studies of the kidney are difficult because of movement artifact.

Acute Renal Failure*

Pathophysiology†

Acute renal failure (ARF) is defined as the sudden deterioration of the kidneys' baseline function, resulting in an inability to maintain the body's fluid and electrolyte homeostasis. Even though this determination is particularly difficult in the newborn, the presence of a rising serum creatinine, when it

---

* References 23, 30, 33, 53, 63, 86.
† References 23, 86.

should be decreasing (see Figure 24-3), is one indicator. Some clinicians prefer to use an absolute creatinine value of greater than 1.5 mg/dl.

Etiology

Renal function is adversely affected by multiple insults. Perinatal asphyxia of mild to moderate severity, hypoxemia, hypotension, hypovolemia, acidosis, various medications, and positive pressure ventilation can cause abnormalities in GFR, urine flow rate, sodium and water excretion, and tubular protein handling (e.g., increased $\beta_2\mu$ excretion). These changes may be seen without actual failure of renal function. Acute renal failure has been reported to occur in up to 8% of neonates admitted to an NICU.[63,86] This is probably an underestimate because of the difficulty in making the diagnosis, especially in nonoliguric cases. A scoring system for diagnosing the severity of perinatal asphyxia suggests that up to 38% of patients with severe asphyxia may have acute renal failure.[63] In fact, asphyxia is the most common cause of acute tubular necrosis in the term neonate (65%); sepsis is the most common in the preterm infant (35%). Patients with congenital heart disease appear to be especially vulnerable to tubular necrosis after cardiac catheterization and cardiac surgery.

The etiology of ARF is divided into prerenal, renal parenchymal, and postrenal causes. Various urinary and blood indices have been used to separate these entities and are based on the appropriateness of the renal response to a challenge.[53] For example, an infant who is dehydrated with intact tubular function should be avidly conserving sodium and water, thus the FENa would be very low (less than 1%). If the infant had tubular damage, one would expect the FENa to be greater than 2.5% to 3%. Unfortunately there are some renal causes, such as glomerulonephritis, that can give prerenal values for these indices. When the tubules sense a decrease in filtration, they avidly reabsorb fluid but cannot differentiate between glomerular inflammation and dehydration. Thus we have categorized these groups into pretubular, tubular, and posttubular causes (Table 24-2). The use of these indices is effective in infants and older children, but the immaturity of the kidneys in premature infants leads to salt wasting (e.g., FENa

Table 24-2
Etiology of Acute Renal Failure in the Neonate

	Urinary Indexes of Acute Renal Failure				
	U_{Na} (mEq/L)	FENa (%)	RFI	U/P_{Cre}	U/P_{Osm}
Pretubular	31.4 ± 19.5	0.95 ± 0.55	1.29 ± 0.82	29.2 ± 15.6	>1.3
Renal parenchymal (tubular) obstruction	63.4 ± 34.7	4.25 ± 2.2	11.6 ± 9.6	9.6 ± 3.6	>1.0

Pretubular: hypotension-sepsis, shock, hypovolemia-dehydration, hemorrhage, hypoproteinemia, cardiac failure, renal artery stenosis, hypoxemia, asphyxia, glomerulonephritis, mechanical ventilation, pressor agents.
Renal parenchymal (tubular): acute tubular necrosis, corticomedullary necrosis, asphyxia neonatorum, pyelonephritis, interstitial nephritis, polycystic kidney disease, renal parenchymal/aplasia/hypoplasia, intrauterine infection, endogenous toxins (uric acid, hemoglobinuria, myoglobinuria), exogenous toxins (aminoglycosides, indomethacin, contrast media), renal vein thrombosis, disseminated intravascular coagulation, congenital nephrotic syndrome.
Obstruction: ureteral obstruction, urethral obstruction.
U, Urine concentration; *P,* plasma concentration; *FENa,* fractional excretion of sodium; *Cre,* creatinine (mg/dl); *Osm,* osmolarity (mOsm/L); *RFI,* renal failure index ($U_{Na} \times$ P/U creatinine).
Modified from Mathews OP et al: *Pediatrics* 65:57, 1980.

of as great as 5% to 7% and abnormalities in water handling that cause difficulty in interpretation). Also, the FENa and renal failure index (RFI) can be affected by salt loading and diuretic therapy. The U/P creatinine ratio is helpful and is not affected by diuretics.

Aside from the hypoxia and acidosis, other important contributing factors may be hemoglobinuria, myoglobinuria, and an increase in uric acid excretion. Inappropriate secretion of anti-diuretic hormone may also lead to oliguria; however, these patients have a normal serum creatinine, hyponatremia, a urine osmolarity that is inappropriately high for the serum osmolarity, and an increase in sodium excretion.

Prevention

Prevention of perinatal asphyxia, avoidance of maternal ACE-inhibitor use, aggressive management of hypoxemia, hypovolemia, hypotension, acidosis, and the early detection and treatment of infections decrease the risk of renal insults.

Data Collection

History

See preceding discussion of etiology of ARF.

Signs and Symptoms

Acute tubular necrosis (ATN) presents earlier in the term infant and is more likely to be oliguric, whereas the nonoliguric form predominates in the preterm infant, occurring in the second week of life. Oliguric renal failure includes a urine flow rate of less than 1 ml/kg/hr after the first 48 hours of life. Nonoliguric forms of ARF have a normal urine flow rate with an increase in creatinine.

Laboratory Data

A renal ultrasound should be performed in all neonates with suspected ARF to assess possible urinary tract obstruction, renal vein thrombosis, and congenital renal abnormalities such as dysplasia, polycystic disease, or aplasia.

Treatment*

Treatment involves removing the cause of the ARF. Prerenal causes require increasing perfusion of the kidney by fluid therapy and restoring cardiac output and blood pressure to normal. Any obstruction or thrombosis needs immediate attention.

A fluid challenge of 5 to 10 ml/kg of body weight of colloid should be attempted. These fluids may exacerbate lung disease or heart failure and

* References 23, 33, 86.

should be administered with caution. If heart failure is present, inotropic agents should be considered (see Chapter 23). Central venous pressure (CVP) is an important, underutilized parameter in measuring the appropriateness of fluid therapy. Use of CVP is especially important in infants with capillary leak syndrome or with third spacing of fluids postoperatively. These infants appear fluid overloaded but may be intravascularly depleted. Therapeutically, diuretic administration removes fluid, but it does not help diagnostically because an increase in urine output does not differentiate between renal involvement and prerenal causes. Diuretics may in fact cause dehydration. Mannitol should be avoided because of its hyperosmolarity and increased risk for IVH.

Conservative management must then be undertaken with careful attention to fluid and electrolyte balance, correction of acidosis, avoidance of nephrotoxins, aggressive nutritional therapy, diuretic therapy to maintain urine output, phosphate binders, and calcium supplements. Aggressive therapy

of any infections is also important, because sepsis can be fatal in the neonate with renal failure. As yet, there is no specific therapy for acute tubular necrosis. Many agents show promise in animal studies, including calcium channel blockers, adenosine triphosphate (ATP), magnesium chloride, and thyroxin, but no controlled trials in humans have as yet been performed.

Dialysis* should be used only when complications of ARF are no longer medically manageable. Indications include fluid overload, acidosis, hyperkalemia, symptomatic uremia, or prolonged malnutrition because of the inability to give enough fluid. Both continuous venovenous hemodialysis (CVVHD) and peritoneal dialysis (PD) are feasible for the neonate (Table 24-3).

Continuous Venovenous Hemodialysis (CVVHD)

The goal of CVVHD is to provide normal electrolyte balance and fluid removal while the kidneys

---

* References 16, 18, 19, 25, 32, 42, 44, 49, 50, 70, 71, 75.

Table 24-3
Comparison of the Types of Dialysis for the Neonate

Dialysis	Advantages	Complications/Disadvantages
Hemodialysis	Most effective form of dialysis	Requires large amount of blood extracorporeally Risk of exsanguination Risk of sepsis Marked fluid shifts and hypotension Difficulty maintaining vascular access
Peritoneal dialysis	No need for vascular access Adaptable for long-term and/or home care Effective in neonates because of larger peritoneal surface area relative to body weight Effective waste removal without massive fluid shifts	High risk of peritonitis High risk of leakage at catheter site Respiratory compromise caused by pressure on the diaphragm or hydrothorax Potential temperature irregularities Potential injury to internal organs during catheter insertion Hyperglycemia
CVVHD	Easy vascular access if umbilical vessels are available Effective removal of fluid in extremely fluid overloaded patients is possible	Risk of clotted filter membrane Risk of sepsis Risk of blood loss Risk of IVH and/or bleeding problems Only available for acute dialysis

CVVHD, Continuous venovenous hemodialysis; *IVH*, intraventricular hemorrhage.

recover from ARF or profound fluid overload. CVVHD is only feasible in the critical care setting and is not an alternative to chronic care. For the last few years, CVVHD has been our first choice for dialysis of small infants with ARF. The slow but continuous removal of fluid allows the clinician to remove massive amounts of fluid without adverse effects on the patient's hemodynamic status. We have been using the BM11 blood pump (Baxter) with the Renaflo II hemofilter (HF 400, Renal Systems), running at a blood flow of 30 ml/min (Fig. 24-5). Because the extracorporeal blood volume

will be in most cases more than 10% to 20% of the patient's blood volume, we routinely prime the lines with whole blood or packed red blood cells. In our experience, all the infants, including those below 1.5 kilograms, have tolerated the procedure well. The continuous dialysis maintains normal electrolyte balance. Hypophosphatemia is seen fairly frequently, requiring replacement with phosphate salts. Heparinization is often not necessary since most of these patients also have a coagulopathy. CVVHD offers a great alternative for acute dialysis, especially in the infant with labile hemodynamic status, in whom hemodialysis and peritoneal dialysis are not feasible.

Peritoneal Dialysis

PD is useful in acute and chronic care; therefore it is the intervention of choice for the neonate with end stage renal disease. The goal of chronic peritoneal dialysis treatment in pediatrics is to allow for normal growth and development. Peritoneal dialysis functions primarily through the principles of diffusion and ultrafiltration across the peritoneal membrane and begins with the insertion of the dialysis catheter.[32] (Fig. 24-6 and Table 24-4). Neonatal catheters are commercially available and are best inserted in the operating room. A full cycle of fill, dwell, and drain time usually lasts 1 hour. Dwell volume can be gradually increased from 20 to 50 ml/kg per exchange.[44,75] New cyclers are currently available that allow volume exchanges as low as 50 ml per exchange.

Before either type of intervention is chosen, several ethical concerns must be carefully addressed. Aggressive intervention with dialysis must be viewed as only one option that physicians and parents must consider during this decision-making process. Acute dialysis should be undertaken where reasonable expectations of the infant's recovery are foreseen. Leiberman has reported satisfactory continuous arteriovenous hemofiltration (CAVH) treatment on almost all the infants in his center.[49] Even though dialysis was effective, a mortality of almost 50% was reported as a result of the underlying disease.

Chronic dialysis is not considered the "standard of care" for the critically ill neonate.[16] Although peritoneal dialysis with aggressive dietary management[18] can provide some growth for the infant with

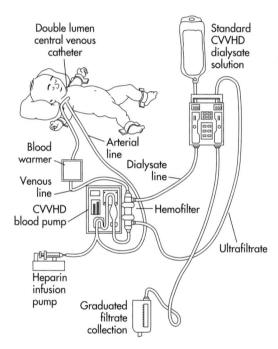

Figure 24-5 Continuous venovenous hemodialysis (CVVHD) in newborn. Blood access is provided by a central venous line. Blood is pumped through the system by a hemofiltration pump at a blood flow of 5 to 8 ml/kg/min (minimum 30 ml/min). A constant heparin infusion is maintained to keep an activated clotting time between 180 and 220 seconds. The amount of ultrafiltrate is regulated (according to the individualized needs) by using an infusion pump at filter outflow. A standard CVVHD dialysate solution is used unless severe metabolic acidosis develops. Before the blood is returned to the patient, it is passed through a blood warmer to prevent hypothermia.

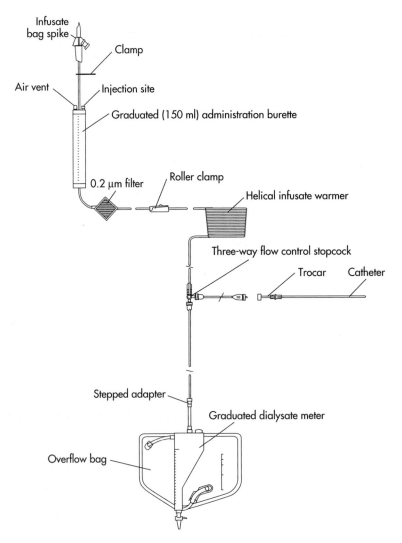

Figure 24-6 Example of a commercially available dialysis set for neonatal peritoneal dialysis. Graduated burette in this closed system allows for easily varying amount of dialysate delivered. Helical coils allow dialysate to be warmed in same manner as in exchange transfusion. Graduated meter allows for accurate measurement of outflow. (From Gesco International, San Antonio, Texas, 1987.)

end-stage renal disease (ESRD), chronic uremia still has well-documented effects on the neurologic development and growth of the infant.[73] Restoration of normal renal function via transplantation has provided better growth and normal development in many infants. Transplantation as an intervention in infants, however, carries its own risks, and there are as yet insufficient data to assess its effectiveness.

The decision to intervene with chronic dialysis should be made by physicians, parents, and possibly a medical ethics committee. Dialysis should not be started without the goal of ultimate transplantation. All persons involved in the decision making must be aware of the long-term nature of renal failure management, which may extend for months or years into the home and family setting. **If dialysis**

Table 24-4
Nursing Care Plan for Peritoneal Dialysis in the Neonate

Problems	Nursing Actions

Potential peritonitis	1. Sterile technique to be used at all tubing connections and bag spikes; all connections clamped and taped.
	2. Assess PD effluent with each drain for color, turbidity, and the presence of fibrin.
	3. Should turbidity exist:
	   a. Obtain cell count, differential, gram stain, and culture of PD fluid.
	   b. Administer antibiotics as ordered.
	4. Occlusive dressing at catheter site.

Potential fluid overload and/or dehydration	1. Measure and record the exact amount of inflow and outflow of dialysate with each exchange.
	2. Weigh neonate at regular intervals during drain to determine real weight of infant.
	3. Assess for fluid reabsorption:
	   a. Peripheral and dependent edema
	   b. Weight gain
	   c. Failure to drain out all of dwell volume
	4. Assess for dehydration:
	   a. Weight loss
	   b. Poor skin turgor and sunken eyes
	   c. Hypotension
	5. Notify physician of weight discrepancies or other symptoms.

Potential temperature maintenance problems	1. Warm all PD fluid to body temperature by blood warmer or heating pad immediately before inflow.
Inflow and/or outflow obstruction	1. Check for kinks in line. 2. Reposition patient, inflow and/or drain bags. 3. Plain radiograph of the abdomen to check position of catheter—should be toward pelvis. 4. Add heparin to dialysate if fibrin is present.
Potential respiratory compromise	1. Use smaller exchange volumes. 2. Position patient with elevated HOB to reduce pressure on the abdomen. 3. If distress exists after drain, obtain chest x-ray to rule out pneumonia or hydrothorax.

PD, Peritoneal dialysis.

is begun, all should realize that the decision is not irrevocable for either parents or physicians. The prognosis should be openly discussed with the parents, as well as the amount of suffering the infant may have to endure as a result of the many possible life-threatening complications. The best chance for success lies with an infant with all other organ systems intact and with a good family situation. Finally, the decision-makers, especially the parents, should understand that the choice not to intervene in some instances is a valid decision that may be in the infant's best interest. Having said this, we are still optimistic that dialysis and transplantation will become a very promising treatment modality. Infant transplantation should be performed at a center with experience in this area.

Complications*

The mortality of neonates with ARF ranges from 14% to 75%. Patients with the worst prognosis are those with congenital renal anomalies, those with

* Reference 86.

congenital heart disease, and those requiring dialysis. Patients with nonoliguric forms of ARF have the best prognosis. Recovery of function is unlikely if diffuse cortical necrosis or medullary necrosis has occurred. Reversal of the underlying condition is the most important factor for determining prognosis. The prognosis also appears to be better if renal perfusion is demonstrated on ^{99m}Tc glucoheptonate or I^{131} hippurate nuclear renal scan.[30]

For survivors, chronic renal failure has been seen in as many as 40% of the cases. Renal tubular abnormalities (i.e., RTA and concentrating defects) have been noted. Hypertension can also be seen. Renal growth can be affected, and a kidney can be noted years later to appear hypoplastic or dysplastic.

Hypertension*

In the past decade it has become apparent that hypertension is a significant clinical problem in the neonate cared for in a NICU setting. The incidence of hypertension in healthy term infants appears to be quite low, and the majority of hypertensive infants have a definable etiology. Nearly universal blood pressure monitoring in nurseries with established normal blood pressure ranges enables more frequent diagnosis. A hypertensive infant may be quite ill, with symptoms similar to those of an infant with sepsis or heart or lung disease. If the infant is properly diagnosed and treated, the outcome may be quite favorable.

Blood pressures (BPs) vary by gestational age, body weight, cuff size, and state of alertness. Normal values have been developed by body weight and by postnatal age, but no criteria combining these variables are available. BP begins low and postnatally increases by 1 to 2 mm Hg/day for the first 3 to 8 days and 1 mm Hg/week for 5 to 7 weeks, and reaches a steady value for the first year of life by 2 months of age.[20,90] Whether the percentile for an infant's BP will track into later childhood or adulthood is still controversial at this point. Normal values for BPs in infants are listed in Fig. 24-7.

Etiology†

The causes of hypertension can be seen in Box 24-1. Any infant with hypertension must be assumed to have a specific secondary etiology. The most common cause may be a complication of umbilical artery catheterization.

Prevention

Obtaining accurate, reliable measurements of BP is necessary to prevent falsely elevated (or depressed) values.[20,90] Under study conditions, the best determinator of BP is the direct arterial measurement, usually through a UAC. Older techniques such as auscultation, palpation, and flush blood pressure measurements have been replaced by Doppler measurements and oscillometry. These latter two techniques have correlated very well with direct arterial measurements for systolic BP but not as well with diastolic BP. Cuff selection is also important, because small cuffs give falsely high values. The cuff should completely encircle the extremity and be the largest cuff possible without impinging on the joints of the upper arm or leg. In this way, BP in the arms and legs should be equal. Frequently the same cuff is used for the arm and the leg, with the result that the leg pressures appear to be higher, because the cuff is too small. The size of the cuff and extremity used for measurement should be documented so that serial measurements will be consistent. The position for measuring BP is always supine. BPs taken on extremities elevated above the level of the heart may give erroneously low values; the converse is true of pressures taken on extremities lower than the level of the heart. BP can vary greatly with the state of alertness and with crying. Frequently a sick infant will have a BP measured directly through a UAC as well as by oscillometric techniques. Significant discrepancies between these measurements may be seen, and it is often difficult to discern which one is the "true" BP. Aside from equipment malfunction, discrepancies can be caused by a UAC with a caliber too small for the infant's size, a thrombus at the tip of the catheter, or poor peripheral perfusion.

---

* References 3, 4, 20, 26, 33.

† References 3, 26.

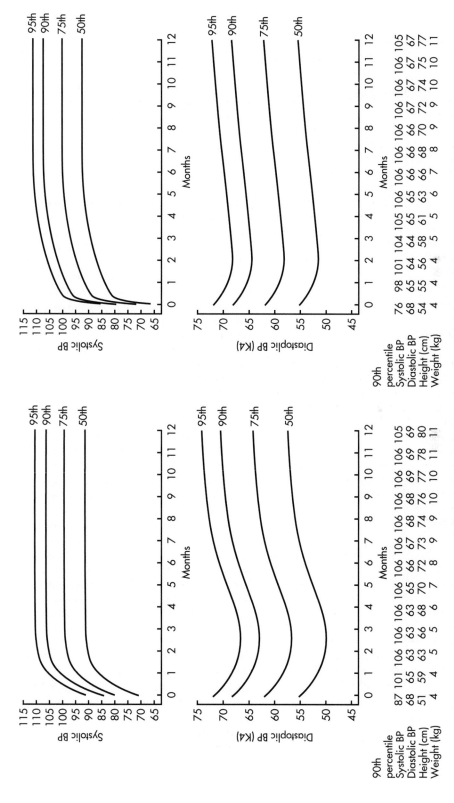

Figure 24-7 Age-specific percentiles of blood pressure measurements in males (*left*) and females (*right*). Korotkoff phase IV is used for diastolic blood pressure. Blood pressures exceeding 90th percentile are considered hypertensive unless infant's height and weight exceeds 90th percentile. Blood pressure exceeding 90th percentile are always considered hypertensive. (From Report on the Second Task Force on Blood Pressure Control in Children: *Pediatrics* 79:1, 1987.)

<table>
<tr><td>

Box 24-1

Etiology of Hypertension in the Neonate

Vascular
Renal artery stenosis
Renal artery thrombosis
Coarctation of the aorta
Hypoplastic abdominal aorta
Renal vein thrombosis
Idiopathic arterial calcification

Renal
Renal dysplasia and/or hypoplasia
Polycystic kidney disease (autosomal dominant or recessive)
Renal failure
Obstructive uropathy
Reflux nephropathy
Pyelonephritis
Glomerulonephritis
Tumors
   Wilms'
   Neuroblastoma

Endocrine
Adrenogenital syndrome
Cushing's disease
Hyperaldosteronism
Thyrotoxicosis

Other
Closure of abdominal wall defects
Fluid overload
Genitourinary surgery
Hypercalcemia
Increased intracranial pressure
Medications
   Phenylephrine
   Corticosteroids
   Theophylline
   Deoxycorticosterone
Seizures
Bronchopulmonary dysplasia

Modified from Adelman RD: Neonatal hypertension. In Loggie JMH et al, editors: *NHLBI workshop on juvenile hypertension,* New York, 1983, Biomedical Information; Gulgnard JP: Neonatal nephrology. In Holliday MA, Barratt TM, Vernier RL, editors: *Pediatric nephrology,* ed 2, Baltimore, 1987, Williams & Wilkins.

</td></tr>
</table>

Data Collection

History

Nearly all hypertensive infants (88%) have had a UAC. The incidence of renal artery thrombosis in neonates with indwelling UACs is 3% to 20%; however, only 13% of these infants were clinically diagnosed. Of patients with UACs, 3% develop hypertension.[3,26]

Signs and Symptoms [3,20,33]

Any infant exceeding the 95th percentile for BP is considered to be hypertensive. Thus 5% of the population on initial screening would be hypertensive. For the term infant, any BP exceeding 95 mm Hg systolic or 75 mm Hg diastolic is considered hypertensive. In prematures the definition is less clear but is considered to be 80 mm Hg systolic and 50 mm Hg diastolic.[2] Hypertension usually occurs during the first week of life in the full-term infant and in the second week in preterms. However, new data suggest that hypertension can occur much later in the course of a sick infant and even after discharge.

BP measurements should be taken in all extremities to seek evidence for coarctation of the aorta.

The symptoms of hypertension may be severe but very nonspecific. Hypertension presents with respiratory distress in 50% of infants; PDA in 50%; neurologic symptoms such as seizures, tremor, and abnormalities in tone in 30%; and congestive heart failure in 40%. Intracranial hemorrhage, hemiparesis, hepatosplenomegaly, and cyanosis may also occur. Approximately 50% of infants, however, are asymptomatic. Fundoscopic examination revealed typical changes of hypertensive retinopathy in 11 of 21 hypertensive infants studied. The true incidence of hypertension in the newborn has been reported to be 1.2% to 5% of NICU admissions.

Laboratory Data [3,26]

A hypertensive neonate demands a full evaluation seeking the etiology. In one study of 17 hypertensive infants, 5 had a definable cause, 2 had UACs, and 10 had no cause defined.[26] Evaluation should consist of a study of renal anatomy with an ultrasound. If this is unrevealing, a renal scan or

Table 24-5
Antihypertensive Medications for Use in the Neonatal Period*

Medications	Dose	Schedule	Route	Comments
Propranolol	1-4 mg/kg/dose	bid-tid	PO	Contraindicated in heart failure, possibly in BPD, sedation
Hydralazine	0.025-1 mg/kg/dose	bid	IV	
	0.25-1.5 mg/kg/dose (max 4.5 mg/kg/day)	bid-qid	PO	Tachycardia, sodium retention
	0.1-0.5 mg/kg/dose with beta blocker	q6h	IV	
	0.4-0.8 mg/kg/dose (sole agent)			
Captopril	0.1-2.0 mg/kg/dose	tid	PO	Leukopenia, rash, protein-uria, hyperkalemia, acute renal failure, seizures
Enalapril	0.1-0.3 mg/kg/dose	qd-q12h	PO	Hypotension
Enalaprilat	0.005-0.05 mg/kg/dose	qd-q12h	IV	Hypotension
Diazoxide	1-5 mg/kg/dose	q4-24h	IV	Hyperglycemia, fluid retention, hyperuricemia
Sodium nitroprusside	0.5-10 µg/kg/min	Continuous infusion	IV	Keep covered in foil, careful observation for infiltration of IV or varying rate of administration

BPD, Bronchopulmonary dysplasia.
*No reported experience in the newborn with nifedipine, Catapres, labetalol, or verapamil. Furosemide (Lasix) and thiazides are not antihypertensive mediations but are used for volume overload.

angiography should be performed. Serum creatinines are usually normal or slightly elevated. Urinalysis may be normal, but hematuria and proteinuria may also be noted (either as a sign of a cause of hypertension or as a result of the hypertension). Peripheral renin activities are generally elevated but must be compared with age-matched normal values.[84] Effects of hypertension should also be evaluated, including a fundoscopic examination by an ophthalmologist and cardiac evaluation for evidence of hypertensive damage.

Treatment*

Hypertension should be treated in the neonate, especially if it exceeds the definition of severe

hypertension (greater than 110 mm Hg systolic). However, normalization of BP should not be sought because an excessive lowering of BP may also be detrimental. A definable cause, such as a urinary tract obstruction, a tumor, or a coarctation, should be treated surgically. Rarely a nephrectomy of the involved kidney has been advocated in medically unmanageable, severe hypertension. Drugs and dosages commonly used in the neonate for controlling BP are found in Table 24-5. Captopril should be used with caution if there is possible bilateral renal artery stenosis because renal failure has been reported in this situation. For an acute hypertensive crisis, IV hydralazine, IV diazoxide, enalapril, or oral captopril are the drugs of choice.[57] Calcium channel blockers have great potential for the treatment of neonatal hypertension. They do not cause fluid retention nor reflex tachycardia and may even be mild bronchodilators.

* References 3, 26, 62, 93.

However, dosage forms small enough for study in neonates are not available. Some pharmacies are able to make a liquid preparation of nifedipine. Studies of these promising agents should be forthcoming.

Complications*

Prognosis for these patients is excellent if BP is well controlled medically or cured surgically. These infants have a normal somatic growth and development and most have their antihypertensive medications discontinued after several years of follow-up. Poor renal growth is noted on the side of the renal artery pathology, and renal scans tend to be persistently abnormal. Creatinine clearances appear to be normal in most infants.

Abdominal Mass†

Slightly more than half of abdominal masses present during the newborn period are of renal origin. The literature offers no consistent data on frequency of abdominal masses in infants, but there is general agreement regarding the urgent need to evaluate these patients quickly and thoroughly before planning intervention. The differential diagnosis in the infant with an abdominal mass is shown in Table 24-6.

Data Collection

Physical Examination

Visualization of the abdomen before manual exploration enables the examiner to note a mass that may be missed on a tense abdomen. Bimanual palpation using the flat surface of the fingers while supporting the infant's flank with the other hand allows for exploration of the abdomen during deep palpation. Renal masses are usually smooth to palpation and move with respirations. Size of the mass is not helpful in determining its etiology. Percussion may be used to outline the suspected area, and transillumination is sometimes helpful in

---

* References 3, 4, 26.
† References 33, 45, 46, 48, 55.

Table 24-6
Neonatal Abdominal Masses

Type of mass	Percent of total
Renal Masses	55
Hydronephrosis	
Multicystic dysplastic kidney	
Polycystic kidney disease	
Mesoblastic nephroma	
Renal ectopia	
Renal vein thrombosis	
Nephroblastomatosis	
Wilms' tumor	
Genital Masses	15
Hydrometrocolpos	
Ovarian cyst	
Gastrointestinal Masses	15
Duplication	
Volvulus	
Complicated meconium ileus	
Mesenteric-omental cyst	
"Pseudocyst" proximal to atresia	
Nonrenal Retroperitoneal Masses	10
Adrenal hemorrhage	
Neuroblastoma	
Teratoma	
Hepatosplenobiliar Masses	5
Hemangioendothelioma	
Hepatoblastoma	
Hepatic cyst	
Splenic hematoma	
Choledochal cyst	
Hydrops of gallbladder	

From Kirks DR et al: *Radiol Clin North Am* 19:527, 1981.

---

identifying hydronephrosis and multicystic kidneys, which are both positive when transilluminated. Some renal masses are quite soft, and excessive pressure during the examination will frequently cause the mass to be missed.

Laboratory Data

Ultrasonography is the most desirable diagnostic tool for initial evaluation of an abdominal mass in the newborn. The advantages of this technology include its noninvasive nature, accessibility for bedside studies, improved resolution, and relatively low cost.

Traditional studies such as IV pyelography are not done in the first weeks of life because of the neonatal kidney's inability to concentrate urine and decreased GFR. Ultrasound reveals a kidney with communicating cystic masses in hydronephrosis. Renal dysplasia most often is seen as non-communicating cyst formations on ultrasound. When this diagnostic tool is incapable of differentiating dysplasia and hydronephrosis, renal scintigraphy is indicated. With this modality, dysplasia is noted as having no functional activity on nuclear scan. A hydronephrotic kidney demonstrates "rim" activity with delayed accumulation of the radionuclide in the pelvis and calyces. Selected isotopes (glucoheptonate) used in renal scintigraphy will reveal fine anatomic detail, making this modality a useful tool in assessing renal function. Rarely, a percutaneous nephrostogram is performed to determine whether cysts are due to obstruction or dysplasia. A voiding cystourethrogram is the method of choice to diagnose vesicoureteral reflux. CT scans can be helpful, especially for differentiating renal masses.

Intrinsic Renal Parenchymal Abnormalities*

Renal abnormalities can be classified by the amount of tissue, the differentiation of tissue, and the position of the kidneys. A thorough summary of renal involvement with various syndromes is presented by Ronco et al.[70]

Amount of Tissue

Congenital absence or agenesis of renal tissue can occur unilaterally or bilaterally. Unilateral renal agenesis is seen more frequently (1:1000 live births) and may present as a solitary kidney on examination with enlargement caused by compensatory hypertrophy. Unilateral agenesis has been associated with Turner syndrome, Poland syn-

---

* References 46, 55, 64, 91.

drome, and VATER syndrome. Bilateral agenesis, also known as Potter's disease, is seen rarely, with an incidence of 1 per 4000 births.

Hypoplasia is a deficiency in the amount of renal tissue expressed as an abnormally small kidney. Morphologically, the kidney is normal, and renal function is unaffected in the neonatal period. Later in life patients can sometimes outgrow their renal function.

Signs and Symptoms

In unilateral agenesis, patients are often asymptomatic and are diagnosed inadvertently on ultrasound or based on the significant association with malformations of the lower genitourinary tract. There is no need for long-term follow-up in this group.

In bilateral agenesis the majority of affected infants are male and small for gestational age, with a history of maternal oligohydramnios. The characteristic facial features accompanying Potter's syndrome include wide-set eyes, parrot-beak nose, receding chin, and large, low-set ears with little cartilage. Other associated malformations include pulmonary hydroplasia, hydrocephalus, meningocele, multiple skeletal anomalies, and imperforate anus. Death usually occurs within hours to several days.

Differentiation of Tissue

Abnormalities in renal tissue differentiation are most commonly expressed as dysplastic kidneys. Renal dysplasia is a failure of the metanephrogenic tissue to mature appropriately, frequently because of obstruction of the urinary tract early in gestation. The result is a persistence of immature structures and very little normal functioning renal tissue.

Renal dysplasia may be seen in one or both kidneys, and involving the entire kidney, segments of the kidney, or microscopic areas (foci) of a kidney. Dysplasia is most commonly expressed as cyst formation. Bilateral multicystic dysplastic kidneys are nonfunctional and not compatible with life. Unilateral involvement is both the most common cystic lesion of the neonatal kidney and one of the most frequently palpated abdominal masses in the newborn. Unilateral dysplasia shows no predilection for males or females, nor for involvement of right or left kidney. **Usually the ureter is absent, atretic, or stenotic. No orifice is found in the bladder. Renal function and structure may be normal in the remaining kidney of infants with unilateral dysplasia; however, frequently vesicoureteral reflux or ureteropelvic (UPJ) obstruction is present in the contralateral kidney. Therefore a voiding cystourethrogram should be performed on every patient.**

Data Collection

Renal dysplasia is usually sporadic, but some familial cases have been reported.[60] A lack of blood flow on ^{99m}Tc DPTA nuclear renal scan confirms the diagnosis of dysplasia.

Treatment

Generally, these kidneys involute with time; therefore a conservative rather than surgical approach is recommended. The association between renal dysplasia and neoplasia has not been confirmed. However, removal of the kidney is sometimes indicated if its size prevents adequate nutrition.

Position

Abnormalities in position are described in the section on normal development. An ectopic kidney frequently located in the pelvis, crossed-fused ectopia, and a horseshoe kidney can present as an abdominal mass.

Polycystic Kidney Disease*

Pathophysiology

Polycystic kidney disease (PKD) may present as one of two types in the infant: (1) infantile type (ICPD), which is autosomal recessive, and (2) adult type, which is autosomal dominant. Traditionally, adult-type disease has not been associated with onset during the first year of life, but recent studies have confirmed both presentations in the infant. Thus an attempt should be made to discontinue use of the terms "infant" and "adult" forms.

---

* References 10, 17, 64.

Autosomal recessive PKD presents with varied severity, but it is always bilateral. The kidneys become enlarged with a proliferation of renal tubules and dilated collecting tubules. These are not true "cysts," and the kidney has a renoform shape. Autosomal dominant disease involves cyst formations in any portion of the nephron, Bowman's space, and liver. Rarely, cyst formation in the pancreas and spleen are present. There is a strong association with autosomal dominant PKD and cerebral artery aneurysms.

Data Collection

History

Criteria for making a definitive diagnosis for both diseases have been developed. Autosomal recessive disease includes infants with the following: (1) congenital hepatic fibrosis on liver biopsy or evidence of portal hypertension, (2) renal histologic studies consistent with collecting tubule ectasia or (3) a sibling with the disease. Infants diagnosed with adult (dominant) disease had the following: (1) positive parental history or (2) known liver cysts or Berry aneurysm.[17]

Signs and Symptoms

Both types of PKD can present initially with an abdominal mass. The infant may present with bilateral flank masses, hepatic enlargement, Potter's facies caused by oligohydramnios, oliguria, hypoplastic lungs, respiratory distress, and spontaneous pneumothorax. Hypertension is common in both types of the disease.

Laboratory Data

Differentiation of autosomal dominant versus recessive type is difficult because radiographic studies are not consistently accurate in discerning differences.

Treatment

Management consists of serial monitoring of blood pressure, renal function, and urine cultures. Neonates with either form of PKD need aggressive treatment of BP with captopril as the drug of

choice, treatment of any urinary tract infection, and aggressive nutritional management.

Hydronephrosis*

Physiology

The collecting system of the kidney is composed of the ureter, pelvis, and calyces, all of which function as a system for removing urine from the kidney. Hydronephrosis, one of the most common abdominal masses in the newborn, involves a dilation of the pelvis and calyces, most often as a result of congenital obstruction. The impaired movement of urine as a result of severe or chronic obstruction may lead to dysplastic and cystic changes that further impair kidney function if the obstruction occurs early in gestation.

The most common ureteral site of obstruction is the ureteropelvic junction. The infant presents with a ballooning of the renal pelvis. Obstruction at the ureterovesical junction, also known as congenital megaureter in its primary form, occurs more often in the male infant, and more frequently affects the left ureter. Posterior urethral valves (PUV) in males are the major cause of urethral obstruction. This distal obstruction may result in bladder hypertrophy, hydroureter, and hydronephrosis if severe. Dysplastic changes can be seen if the obstruction occurs early in gestation. The neonate with PUV is at risk for developing an ascending infection and subsequent renal damage. Prune-belly syndrome,[87] also known at Eagle-Barrett syndrome, is a less common cause of obstruction and dilation of the pelvis and calyces. There is a strong male predominance. This triad of anomalies includes (1) absence or hypoplasia of the abdominal wall muscles, (2) bilateral cryptorchidism, and (3) urinary tract abnormality. The loose, shriveled abdomen is responsible for the "prune belly" appearance, which diminishes with age and does not require surgical correction. Renal dysplasia is usually seen in prune-belly syndrome and may range from mild to severe involvement. The enlarged bladder may be seen in conjunction with a patent urachus draining urine. The prostatic urethra is usually hypoplastic.[11]

Etiology

The etiology of most types of hydronephrosis remains unclear. Primary prune-belly syndrome may be a result of a mesenchymal developmental arrest. A variant of the syndrome can also be seen as a sequela of an intrauterine distention of the abdomen by an obstructed urinary system. The existence of this secondary cause of prune-belly syndrome is controversial. Another cause of calyceal dilation not associated with obstruction is vesicoureteral reflux, as discussed further under urinary tract infections.

Data Collection

Infants may have few if any symptoms, and there are usually no physical findings unless a bladder or kidney is palpated on routine examination. These infants can present with a poor urinary stream and frequently with failure to thrive.

With the advent of frequent prenatal ultrasound examinations, the finding of a dilated collecting system is common.

Treatment†

Unilateral obstruction does not require immediate treatment. Close follow-up is indicated, because surgery may be a postnatal consideration. Bilateral dilation with *normal* amounts of amniotic fluid is treated with close observation. Treatment of bilateral dilation with *decreased* amniotic fluid depends on the gestational age of the fetus. In a previable fetus with bilateral obstruction and oligohydramnios, termination of the pregnancy should be considered. A viable fetus with bilateral obstruction and oligohydramnios is treated with steroids in an attempt to accelerate fetal lung maturity. The fetus is then delivered at 32 to 34 weeks of gestation and surgically corrected postnatally.

A viable fetus with dilated collecting systems,

---

* References 8, 54, 59, 61, 87.

† References 28, 29.

initial normal amount of amniotic fluid, and evidence of decreasing amniotic fluid should be delivered early. If the same fetus is previable, and termination of pregnancy is not a consideration, placement of in utero bladder-AF shunt is undertaken. Other conditions such as bilateral vesicoureteral reflux, prune-belly syndrome, and primary megaureter may present with dilated collecting systems and are not amenable to in utero surgery. Surgical intervention in utero is very controversial, and the morbidity of this therapy is very high.

Obstruction at the uteropelvic and/or uterovesical junctions is surgically corrected. For uterovesical obstructions, surgical correction involves excising the stenotic segment in the obstructed megaureter as well as ureteric reimplantation and is successful in the large majority of infants. Management of PUV depends on the age at presentation and infant's condition. After initial stabilization of the infant, relief of obstruction with a catheter provides quick decompression. Permanent repair consists of fulgarization of the valves. The use of a vesicostomy versus a higher diversion is controversial. Recent success in dialysis and renal transplantation is improving the outlook for infants with prune-belly syndrome and should be strongly considered as management for these infants if other organ systems are normal.

Complications

The mortality of these male infants has been very high, with 20% dying within 2 weeks and 50% dying within the first 2 years of life.

Renal Vein Thrombosis*

Renal vein thrombosis (RVT), an acute life-threatening condition, is seen most frequently in neonatal populations. Affecting males more frequently (1.9:1), RVT is associated with conditions that cause circulatory collapse and decreased oxygenation within the kidney.

---

* References 57, 65.

Etiology

Perinatal causes of neonatal RVT include maternal diabetes, toxemia, maternal thiazide therapy, polycythemia, placental insufficiency, birth asphyxia, prematurity, RDS, and sepsis. Angiography has also been associated with RVT. Thrombosis most often occurs in the smaller renal veins rather than the main renal vein.

Data Collection

Signs and Symptoms

The involved kidney engorges with blood because of obstruction to blood flow and forms a palpable flank mass. Other clinical symptoms may include hematuria (60% of cases), anemia, oliguria, and thrombocytopenia (less than 75,000 platelets).

Laboratory Data

Positive blood on dipstick, urine output of less than 1 ml/kg/hr, and a low platelet count may indicate RVT.

Treatment

Management includes treatment of the underlying illness, treatment of sepsis if suspected, fluid therapy, and possibly dialysis in select cases. Heparin therapy remains controversial for RVT. Surgical excision of the thrombus is not usually indicated during the acute phase but may be appropriate at a later time. Rarely, nephrectomy is required. Renal tubular dysfunction is often observed after recovery from RVT.

Miscellaneous Causes of Abdominal Mass

Wilms' tumor, also known as nephroblastoma, is the most common intraabdominal tumor seen in children and occurs at a rate of 8 to 9/100,000 per year in the United States. Two thirds of patients present in the first 3 to 6 months of life. The tumor is described as firm, smooth, and confluent with the kidney or attached to the organ. Both kidneys are involved in 10% of cases. This condition has an excellent prognosis with treatment. Surgical removal of the tumor is followed by irradiation for most patients and chemotherapy.

Neuroblastoma, on the other hand, is the most common malignant tumor in infancy. The primary site of the tumor may be any area of neural crest tissue, with the most common site identified in the adrenal gland. Presenting in the neonate as a palpable abdominal mass, this tumor may also cause urinary obstruction. Prognosis is related to the site of the primary tumor, histologic appearance of the tumor, staging of the disease, and age of the patient.

Renal Tubular Disorders

Although most of the renal tubular disorders are congenital, they rarely manifest clinically during the newborn period. However, in sick infants admitted to the intensive care unit, these tubular abnormalities can lead to severe, and frequently life-threatening, electrolyte disorders.

Etiology

With the advent of routine prenatal ultrasound, a number of newborns referred for evaluation of polyhydramnios and polyuria have been diagnosed with diabetes insipidus (central or nephrogenic) and Bartter's syndrome. In addition, obstruction of the urinary tract, which is frequently diagnosed prenatally, is commonly associated with RTA, particularly the hyperkalemic type (type IV).

Data Collection

History/Signs and Symptoms

Infants with Fanconi syndrome and distal RTA most commonly present after the neonatal period with the complaint of failure to thrive. Frequently a history of previous admissions to the hospital for evaluation of sepsis and/or dehydration is obtained.

Laboratory Data

The diagnosis of Fanconi syndrome is confirmed by demonstration of a generalized dysfunction in the proximal tubule, evidenced by the presence of glycosuria, proteinuria (low-molecular-weight proteins), bicarbonaturia, phosphaturia, and uricosuria. Distal RTA is diagnosed by demonstrating a decreased urinary excretion of ammonium. Since the measurement of urinary ammonium is cumbersome, calculation of the urine net charge by the formula

$$([Na^+] + [K^+]) - [Cl^-]$$

where $[NA^+]$, $[K^+]$, and $[Cl^-]$ represent the concentration of the respective electrolytes in a random urine sample (in mEq/L), has been proposed as a bedside tool for screening distal RTA. If the result of this calculation is a negative number (less than zero), then distal RTA is ruled out. A positive urine net charge (higher than zero) is consistent with RTA. However, because of the presence of other organic anions in the urine during the first 2 weeks of life, the validity of this test during the neonatal period has been questioned. Disorders of Vitamin D metabolism and/or phosphate reabsorption (rickets) usually present by the end of the first year of life, after the child starts walking. Infants with diabetes insipidus present during the first 2 months of life with dehydration and a sepsislike picture.

Complications

Thus, although most of the tubular disorders are not clinically evident at birth, it is important for the clinician to keep a high index of suspicion in those infants with prenatal diagnosis of urologic abnormalities or serious abnormalities in water and electrolyte metabolism. Early evaluation and treatment of renal tubular disorders may prevent catastrophic complications such as life-threatening episodes of dehydration and delayed growth and development.

Urinary Tract Infections*

Urinary tract infections (UTIs) affect approximately 1% of full-term infants and 3% of premature infants. Male infants are affected 5 times more frequently than females. Vesicoureteral reflux is a common radiographic finding in infants. Primary reflux is seen in abnormalities of the vesicoureteral

---

* References 2, 33, 38.

junction, ureteral duplication, and ureterocele. Secondary reflux is associated with infection, PUV, and neurogenic diseases.

Etiology

Abnormalities of the urinary tract are responsible for a large number of UTIs in the neonate. Whether the infection is ascending from the bladder or hemotogenously spread is a matter of debate. The high association of reflux with UTI makes determining the etiology of reflux a priority for planning appropriate treatment. Reflux is graded on a four-point scale, with grade IV denoting massive hydronephrosis and hydroureter.

Data Collection

Maternal urinary infections have also been associated with neonatal UTIs. **Symptomatic manifestations include abnormal weight loss during the first days of life, decreased feeding, dehydration, irritability, lethargy, cyanosis, jaundice, and septicemia. In some cases the affected kidneys are palpable. Infected infants may also be asymptomatic.**

Laboratory Data

Evaluation of a neonate with suspected UTI includes an immediate ultrasound to rule out upper tract abnormalities. Urine for culture, blood cultures, and a CBC should be obtained. The optimum method of obtaining urine for culture is a suprapubic aspiration of the bladder. Successful results depend on a full bladder. Catheterization may not be recommended in the neonate because of possible urethral stricture formation in the male and frequent culture contamination in the female. Urine obtained in a urine bag should not be used for cultures. Skin contamination frequently yields false positive cultures; conversely, one drop of betadine in a bag of urine can prevent in vitro bacterial growth. Grades of reflux are diagnosed by voiding cystourethrogram (VCUG). Sterile urine is necessary before a VCUG is undertaken.

Treatment

Pyuria (10 to 15 WBC/hpf) can be observed in the neonate normally. Treatment for UTI is indicated when an organism is cultured from the urine. Any

growth in a urine specimen obtained by suprapubic aspiration should be considered an infection if the procedure was cleanly done. Any aspiration of bowel contents must affect the interpretation of culture results. Traditional antibiotic coverage consists of both ampicillin and an aminoglycoside. The advent of third-generation cephalosporins has allowed for excellent gram-negative coverage without the nephrotoxicity of the aminoglycosides. *E. coli* is the organism most often implicated in neonatal UTIs, followed by *Klebsiella*. Sulfonamides are contraindicated in the neonate because of their potential to complicate hyperbilirubinemia.

Antibiotic therapy should continue for 14 days, with a follow-up urine culture 3 days after therapy is discontinued.

Complications

After urine is sterile, a VCUG is used to assess any lower urinary tract abnormalities, specifically reflux. A normal study indicates that antibiotic therapy may be discontinued. These patients should be followed with monthly urine cultures. Patients who demonstrate reflux should be maintained on suppressive antibiotic therapy. VCUG should be repeated in 12 months if reflux was initially present.

Neurogenic Bladder*

Neurogenic bladder is an anatomic interruption of the micturition reflex normally triggered by a full bladder. The bladder may be flaccid and unable to empty urine or spastic and hyperreflexive and unable to store urine. Infants with lumbosacral spinal malformations commonly have a urinary tract dysfunction known as neurogenic bladder. Lower motor neuron deficit causes bladder atony, and upper motor neuron deficit can cause spasticity.

Data Collection

Signs and Symptoms

Often there is a mixed presentation of symptoms. It is the flaccid bladder that requires aggressive

---

* References 1, 12, 74.

intervention in the neonate. Diagnosis begins immediately at the bedside when the newborn has no apparent voiding stream or the urine flow rate falls below expectations without other explanations. Further clarification of the diagnosis can be made by VCUG and by cystometric studies.

Treatment

Proper bladder management in the neonate is very important. If a VCUG shows no reflux and the urine appears to flow freely from the bladder with only a small amount of residual urine, no intervention is necessary. However, if the sphincter tone is such that urine is stagnant in the bladder, gentle Credé's maneuver at regular intervals can be initiated. Credé's maneuver should be performed only after a VCUG has documented the absence of reflux. Surgical intervention is indicated in the neonate with neurogenic bladder when there is severe reflux with renal damage present or recurrent UTI. The urologist creates a vesicostomy to allow the free flow of urine into diapers.

Complications

Early diagnosis and intervention for infants with neurogenic bladder can decrease the risks of the complications associated with this problem. Long-term complications of neurogenic bladder include UTI and vesicoureteral reflux leading to hydrone-phrosis, electrolyte imbalances, and permanent damage to the kidney.

Neonatal Chronobiology

The human time structure consists of a spectrum of rhythms of different frequencies, which are superimposed on trends such as development and aging. These rhythms are genetically determined and are adjusted in time (synchronized) by environmental factors, which adapt the organism to its periodic surroundings. The genetic environmental interactions in the establishment and maintenance of these rhythms begins in early intrauterine life and continues during infancy and childhood with the establishment of mature time structure similar to adults by 2 years of age. The rhythms reach their peak in amplitude in adolescence before stabiliza-

tion during adult life and return to a more infant-like pattern in old age. These rhythms are often defined as *circadian* (circa = about; dian = day) for 24 hour rhythms (e.g., heart rate and blood pressure), *ultradian* for rhythms of less than 24 hours (e.g., various cycles of sleep), and *infradian* for rhythms of greater than 24 hours (e.g., menstrual cycles). Hundreds of studies have defined the human time structure in health. Examples include body temperature, the circadian variations of gastrointestinal motility and blood flow, gastric acid secretion, hepatic enzyme activity, peripheral blood lymphocyte helper/suppressor ratios, adrenergic receptor activity, and many cardiovascular parameters.[82]

Disease states have very specific periodic rhythms as well. Examples include exacerbation of asthma at night, arthritis in the morning, and ulcer disease in the evening. The peak incidence of myocardial ischemia, migraine headache, angina pectoris, and thrombotic stroke occurs in the early morning hours when blood coagulation is at a peak and early morning rises in heart rate, blood pressure, sympathetic tone, and adrenergic receptor activity are observed. Diagnostic tests are also time-dependent with marked diurnal variations noted (e.g., in casual BP measurements, pulmonary function testing, glucose tolerance, and cutaneous antigen testing). Chronokinetics refers to rhythm effects on the rate and extent of drug absorption, distribution, and elimination. Circadian changes in gastric hydrogen ion excretion, gastric emptying, intestinal transit time, hepatic enzyme activity, and renal function lead to administration time differences in pharmacokinetic studies. The effects may also depend on the chemical nature of the medication or the attributes of new drug delivery systems. Chronokinetic data are known for many classes of medications, including β-adrenergic receptor agonists and antagonists, nonsteroidal antiinflammatory drugs, and antihypertensive medications. There also exists a rhythm dependency in the body's response to medications, termed *chronesthesy*. Chronesthesies may result from many factors, including rhythms in cell receptor number, rate limiting steps in metabolic pathways, and cell turnover. Variations in response to medications have been described for analgesics, IV heparin, β-adrenergic receptor antagonists, and cancer chemotherapy. The knowledge of these rhythms is important for the understanding of disease states and their development as well as administration of appropriate therapies. It is important to understand how these principles may be applied in neonatology.

The development of the time structure has two distinct phenomena: the spontaneous maturation within the framework of genetic make-up and the accumulation of experience by the child. It is now established that a biological clock, the suprachiasmatic nucleus, is oscillating in the mammalian fetus[67] and reflects the endocrine, metabolic, cardiovascular, and nutritional functions of the mother. The fetal clock is entrained by redundant circadian signals from the mother, which include feeding times, breathing movements, heart rate, and sleep-wake patterns.[66] While this maternal-fetal communication of circadian phase is apparent, the potential for direct perception of light by the fetus in utero also exists. An entrainable circadian clock during fetal life allows the developing mammal to prepare more readily for life outside the womb and confers a significant survival advantage for those species whose rhythms are fully developed at birth.

At the time of birth the transplacental maternal influences cease and direct environmental stimuli become operative. During the first week of life, some of the infant's rhythmicity may represent maternal influences. Ultradian rhythms predominate in the newborn at the time of birth and shortly thereafter. The development of recognizable circadian periodicity in the infant occurs gradually during the first month and may extend over the first 2 years of life by maturation of the infant and by environmental synchronization of the genetically determined circadian oscillators. After birth the child is exposed to new stimuli, which show marked circadian periodicity. These stimuli act as synchronizers of endogenous oscillators. The strongest of these stimuli are the alternation of light and dark, noise and silence, heat and cold, and hunger and satiety, and the relations of the neonate to its human environment. Circaseptan (weekly) rhythms based on the day of birth have also been found.[95] The effect of external stimuli for sick infants in an intensive care nursery on the development of rhythms is not well defined. During the first 2 years of life a variance transposition takes place with the circadian rhythms gaining in importance and de-

velopment of a time structure more and more similar to that seen in the adult.

The classic cross-sectional studies of circadian rhythms in infants of Hellbruegge[37] still provide the best information on the development of rhythms in human infants. Conclusions from this study of 297 children from the first week of life to 15 years of age include six important points: (1) physiologic functions develop circadian rhythms independently of each other; (2) rhythms develop at different times after birth; (3) increased range of oscillation occurs in all physiologic functions with age; (4) increase in oscillation can occur from increase of upper width of oscillation during light (activity) or increases in lower oscillation during dark hours (sleep); (5) in humans monophasic rhythms or circadian rhythms originate out of polyphasic or ultradian ones, and; (6) maturation of the infant at birth is essential to rhythm development. The details of the study can be seen in Figure 24-8.

More recent studies confirm Hellbruegge's findings. Mirmiran[56] found in a group of 12 premature infants 29 to 35 weeks of gestational age a circadian pattern of heart rate in about half of the subjects by 1 to 2 weeks of age. Gemelli[27] studied BP and heart rate patterns in 21 term newborns at 4 days of age. Single cosinor analysis reveals few significant rhythms. None of the subjects had rhythms of heart rate, but males had greater BP variability than did females. Sitka et al[81] examined circadian patterns in 17 infants on day 2 and at 4 weeks of age. Almost all subjects had rhythms in body temperature unrelated to activity, and greater than 50% had rhythms for systolic blood pressure. None demonstrated a circadian rhythm in diastolic blood pressure. In all of these studies, activity, environment, and feeding times played a significant role in pattern development. However, the infant rhythm was distinct and could be separated from maternal rhythms.

The suprachiasmatic nucleus is felt to be the master biological clock. The pineal gland is felt to be the effector of this clock through the production of the hormone melatonin. During intrauterine development, the fetus does not produce noteworthy amounts of melatonin.[13,92] However, because of melatonin's excellent placental permeability, maternal melatonin crosses the placenta freely in rhythmic fashion and thus the fetus is exposed to

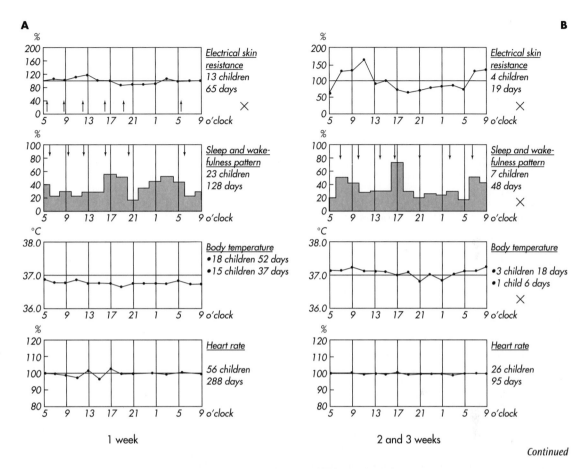

Figure 24-8 Development of circadian rhythms in children. Presented are six sets of graphs of 297 patients at different ages, with hours of the day along the x-axis. Arrows along this axis represent feeding times. The *X* at the right of each graph represents statistical significance of the circadian rhythm detected by cosinor analysis. During the first week of life, only electrical skin resistance demonstrates a circadian rhythm. Other variables such as sleep, body temperature, and heart rate (as well as urine output and sodium and potassium excretion, not shown) demonstrate no discernable circadian pattern. By 2 to 3 weeks of life, circadian patterns are demonstrated with skin resistance, sleep, and temperature. By 4 to 20 weeks of age, and certainly by 5 to 9 months, infants continue to have significant patterns for all variables with the same acrophase as earlier in life but with deeper amplitude. The MESOR (24-hour mean) increases with increasing age. The 1- to 7- and 7- to 15-year-old children continue to have significant rhythms now similar to an adult pattern.

the same environmental stimuli as the mother. Melatonin levels are slightly higher as pregnancy progresses. Labor and delivery do not alter the maternal circadian rhythm of melatonin. Shortly after birth, all maternal melatonin is cleared and there is a virtual lack of melatonin for a period of

2 to 3 months. Melatonin production then increases and becomes circadian with a steadily rising melatonin level and increased amplitude. The period of melatonin deficiency is longer for premature infants, suggesting the onset of melatonin production occurs approximately 10 to 12 months

C   **D**

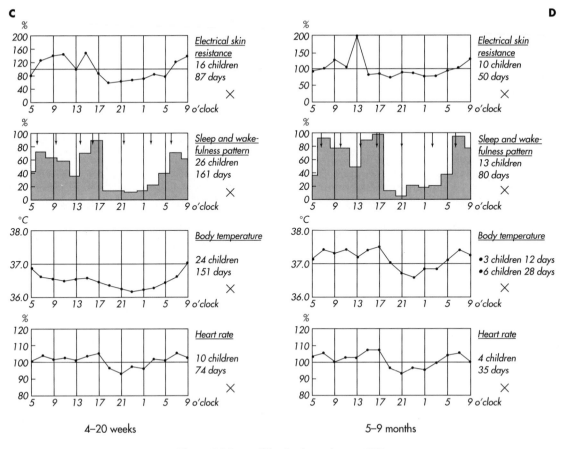

4–20 weeks   5–9 months

Figure 24-8, cont'd   For legend see p. 565.

after conception and may be the result of a genetically determined maturation process. Melatonin is stimulated by darkness but not by sleep. Peak lifetime levels occur in the first 3 to 7 years of life (250 pg/ml). There is a gradual decline in melatonin levels (120 pg/ml) until a marked decrease in melatonin levels occurs at the time of puberty (50 pg/ml). There is speculation that this marked melatonin decline not only marks the onset of puberty, but as in lower mammals may stimulate the onset of puberty. Delayed puberty has been noted with melatonin-producing tumors. Tumor removal normalizes melatonin levels and puberty then proceeds normally. The common calcification of the pineal gland has no known functional effect. During adult life, nocturnal

melatonin levels average 20 pg/ml and fall to much lower levels in the aged.

In adults, diurnal rhythms of hormones lead to as much as 70% variation in blood levels. In the newborn, many hormones do not have the same rhythms as later in life. It has been shown that a circadian rhythm in cortisol excretion is absent in the newborn. Variations do occur but are related more to stress than a specific circadian rhythm. Further, the rhythm of this vital hormone does not achieve a mature rhythm until 2 years of age. Growth hormone does not have a normal circadian pattern until approximately 10 weeks of age, but neonates have a very definable ultradian rhythm, and newborns, with their eyes covered for phototherapy, have a marked increase in growth

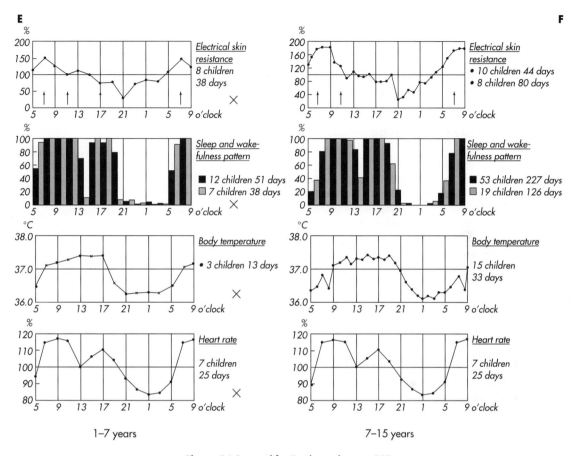

E

Electrical skin resistance
8 children
38 days

Sleep and wakefulness pattern
■ 12 children 51 days
▨ 7 children 38 days

Body temperature
• 3 children 13 days

Heart rate
7 children
25 days

1–7 years

F

Electrical skin resistance
• 10 children 44 days
• 8 children 80 days

Sleep and wakefulness pattern
■ 53 children 227 days
▨ 19 children 126 days

Body temperature
15 children
33 days

Heart rate
7 children
25 days

7–15 years

Figure 24-8, cont'd   For legend see p. 565.

hormone levels.[58] Certain enzymes such as glucose phosphate isomerase and hexosaminidase are circadian in the newborn at birth and synchronous with the mother. Sankaran et al showed in 17 infants with a mean gestational age of 32 weeks and birth weigh of 1790 ± 898 g at a mean of day 3 of life to have a marked circadian variation in plasma concentrations of β-endorphins.[76] Various other physiologic parameters rapidly become circadian, as noted in Hellbrugge's work, even in the absence of melatonin.

In summary, the fetal biological clock is entrained by the mother. The effects of maternal rhythms quickly abate after birth. Although infants of lower mammals have well defined and mature rhythms at birth, the human newborn's patterns are low in amplitude and ultradian in pattern with the virtual absence of melatonin. Statistically, significant circadian rhythms are often absent at birth, especially with increasing prematurity, and rhythms observed are most likely a reflection of activity. With age the rhythms become more organized, less ultradian and more circadian, less variable in acrophase and higher in amplitude. The circadian rhythms in children have the same pattern as seen in adults but with a lower 24-hour mean level and occasionally with the circadian peaks (acrophases) shifted because of earlier sleep or awake times. Since there are marked variations in body size, there are also marked individual variations in biological time structure. Whether these genetically based rhythms track throughout development is not established. The field of chronobiology itself is in its infancy and requires a great deal of investigation before neonatal rhythms are fully understood so that chronotherapeutics can be applied.

Parent Teaching

Because many renal problems are secondary to abnormalities, parents need the information that nothing they have done or did not do caused the anomaly. Grief work over the loss of the perfect infant is necessary before attachment and care giving is possible (see Chapters 28 and 29). Genetic counseling enables parents to make informed choices about subsequent pregnancies (see Chapter 26).

Most infants with renal problems require accurate intake and output measurement. The importance and necessity of measuring intake and not overfeeding must be stressed to parents, as well as the necessity of saving and weighing diapers. Infants who are fluid restricted may be "difficult" for care providers and parents because they are fussy and irritable. Holding, rocking, and using a pacifier for nonnutritive sucking is helpful in calming these infants. Adherence to the prescribed formula and/or breast milk is very important to regulate sodium intake and fluid retention.

Long-term complications that parents may have to recognize and/or manage must be explained and instructions given in writing. Because abnormalities in renal function and anatomy may be sequelae of renal diseases, follow-up by a pediatric nephrologist and/or urologist for urinalysis, cultures, and other diagnostic tests is important. General health maintenance is also important, because growth failure may be a manifestation of ongoing or recurring renal problems.

The importance of administering antihypertensive medications must be stressed to parents. Because hypertension is often a silent condition, the need for continuation of medications must be thoroughly explained. Side effects of hypertensive medications such as sedation, tachycardia, and excessive weight gain, as well as the necessity of medical follow-up, must also be emphasized.

References

1. Action Committee on Myelodysplasia: Current approaches to the evaluation and management of children with myelomeningocele, *Pediatrics* 63:663, 1979.
2. Adelman RD: Urinary tract infections in children. In Tune BM, Mendoza SH, editors: *Pediatric nephrology.* In Brenner BM, Stein JH, editors: *Contemporary issues in nephrology,* New York, 1984, Churchill-Livingstone.
3. Adelman RD: Neonatal hypertension. In Loggie JMH et al, editors: *NHLBI workshop on juvenile hypertension,* New York, 1983, Biomedical Information Corporation.
4. Adelman RD: Long-term followup of neonatal renovascular hypertension, *Pediatr Nephrol* 1:35, 1987.
5. Adelman RD, Wirth F, Rubio T: A controlled study of the nephrotoxicity of methicillin and gentimicin plus ampicillin in the neonate, *J Pediatr* 111 888, 1987.
6. Arant BS: Postnatal development of renal function during the first year of life, *Pediatr Nephrol* 1:308, 1987.
7. Arant BS: Renal disorders of the newborn infant. In Tune BM, Mendoza SH, editors: *Pediatric nephrology.* In Brenner BM, Stein JH, editors: *Contemporary issues in nephrology.* New York, 1984, Churchill-Livingstone.
8. Barrat TM, Manzoni GA: The dilated urinary tract. In Holliday MA, Vermier RL, editors: *Pediatric nephrology,* ed 2, Baltimore, 1987, Williams & Wilkins.
9. Battle DC et al: The use of the urinary anion gap in the diagnosis of hyperchloremic metabolic acidosis, *N Engl J Med* 318:594, 1988.
10. Blyth H, Ockenden BG: Polycystic disease of the kidneys and liver presenting in childhood, *J Med Genet* 8:257, 1971.
11. Boylan P, Parisi V: An overview of hydramnios, *Semin Perinatol* 10:136, 1986.
12. Borzyskowski M, Mundy AR: Management of the neuropathic bladder in childhood, *Pediatr Nephrol* 2:56, 1988.
13. Cavallo A: The pineal gland in human beings: relevance to pediatrics, *J Pediatr* 123:843, 1993.
14. Chan JCM: Renal tubular acidosis, *J Pediatr* 102:327, 1983.
15. Chavez GF, Mulinare J, Codero JF: Maternal cocaine use during early pregnancy as a risk factor for congenital urogenital anomalies, *JAMA* 262:795, 1989.
16. Cohen C: Ethical and legal considerations in the care of the infant with end stage renal disease whose parents elect conservative therapy, *Pediatr Nephrol* 1:166, 1987.
17. Cole BR, Conley SB, Stapleton SB, Southwest Pediatric Nephrology Study Group: Polycystic kidney disease presenting in the first year of life, *J Pediatr* 111:693, 1987.
18. Conley SB. Supplemental nasogastric feedings in infants undergoing continuous peritoneal dialysis. In Fine R, editor: *Chronic ambulatory peritoneal dialysis and chronic cycling peritoneal dialysis in children,* Boston, 1987, Martinus-Nyhoff.
19. Conley SB et al: Five years experience with cyclosporine in children, *Transplant Proc* 20(suppl 3):280, 1988.
20. DeSwiet M, Fayers P, Shinebourne EA: Systolic blood pressure in a population of infants in the first year of life: the Brompton study, *Pediatrics* 65:1028, 1980.
21. Edelmann CM Jr: Developmental renal physiology. In Gruskin AB, Norman ME, editors: *Pediatric nephrology,* Boston, 1980, Martinus-Nyhoff.

22. Elinder G et al: Development of glomerular filtration rate in excretion of beta 2 microglobulin in the neonate during gentamycin treatment, *Acta Paediatr Scand* 72:219, 1983.
23. Engle WD: Evaluation of renal function in acute renal failure in the neonate, *Pediatr Clin North Am* 33:129, 1986.
24. Ferris M et al: Is *in utero* cocaine exposure a risk factor for urinary tract anomalies? *J Am Soc Nephrol* 2:307A, 1991.
25. Fine RN, Gruskin AB, editors: *End stage renal diseases in children,* Philadelphia, 1984, WB Saunders.
26. Friedman AL, Hustead VA: Hypertension in babies following discharge from a neonatal intensive care unit, *Pediatr Nephrol* 1.30, 1987.
27. Gemelli M et al: Circadian blood pressure pattern in full-term newborn infants, *Biol Neonate* 56:315, 1989.
28. Glick PL et al: Management of the fetus with congenital hydronephrosis. II. Prognostic criteria and selection for treatment, *J Pediatr Surg* 20:376, 1985.
29. Golbus MS et al: Fetal urinary tract obstruction: management and selection for treatment, *Semin Perinatol* 9:91, 1985.
30. Gordon I, Barratt TM: Imaging the kidneys and urinary tract in the neonate with acute renal failure, *Pediatr Nephrol* 1:321, 1987.
31. Green TP et al: Furosemide promotes patent ductus arteriosus in premature infants with the respiratory distress syndrome, *N Engl J Med* 308:743, 1983.
32. Gruskin AB: Developmental aspects of peritoneal dialysis kinetics. In Fine R, editor: *Chronic ambulatory peritoneal dialysis and chronic cycling peritoneal dialysis in children,* Boston, 1987, Martinus-Nyhoff.
33. Guignard J-P: Neonatal nephrology. In Holliday MA, Barratt TM, Vernier RL, editors: *Pediatric nephrology,* ed 2, Baltimore, 1987, Williams & Wilkins.
34. Guignard J-P, Gouyan J-B: Adverse effects of drugs on the immature kidney, *Biol Neonate* 53:243, 1988.
35. Hanssens M et al: Fetal and neonatal effect of treatment with angiotensin converting enzyme inhibitors in pregnancy, *Obstet Gynecol* 78:128, 1991.
36. Helin I, Persson P-H: Prenatal diagnosis of urinary tract abnormalities by ultrasound, *Pediatrics* 78:879, 1986.
37. Helbrugge T et al: Circadian periodicity of physiological function in different stages of infancy and children, *N Y Acad Sci* 117:361, 1964.
38. Hellstrom M et al: Renal growth after neonatal urinary tract infection, *Pediatr Nephrol* 1:269, 1987.
39. Holliday MA: Developmental abnormalities of the kidney in children, *Hosp Pract* 13:101, 1978.
40. Hufnagle KG et al: Renal calcifications: a complication of long-term furosemide therapy in preterm infants, *Pediatrics* 70:360, 1982.
41. Jacinto JS et al: Renal calcification incidence in very low birth weight infants, *Pediatrics* 81:31, 1988.
42. Kalia A et al: Renal transplantation in the infant and young child, *Am J Dis Child* 143:47, 1988.
43. Karlsson FA, Hardell L-I, Hellsing K: A prospective study of urinary proteins in early infancy, *Acta Paediatr Scand* 68:663, 1979.
44. Kohaut EC, Alexander S: Ultrafiltration in the young patient on CAPD. In Moncrief J, Popovich R, editors: *CAPD update,* New York, 1981, Masson.

45. Kirks DR et al: Diagnostic imaging of pediatric abdominal masses: an overview, *Radiol Clin North Am* 19:527, 1981.
46. Kissane JM: Congenital malformations of the kidney. In Hamburger J, Crosnier T, Gruenfeld J-P, editors: *Nephrology,* 1979, Wiley-Flammarion.
47. Kao et al: Use of diuretics in bronchopulmonary dysplasia, *Pediatrics* 74:37, 1984.
48. Kleinman LI, Stewart CL, Kaskel FJ: Renal disease in the newborn. In Edelmann CM, editor: *Pediatric nephrology,* ed 2, Boston, 1992, Little, Brown.
49. Lieberman K et al: Treatment of acute renal failure in an infant using continuous arteriovenous hemofiltration, *J Pediatr* 106:646, 1985.
50. Lieberman K: Continuous arteriovenous hemofiltration in children, *Pediatr Nephrol* 1:330, 1987.
51. Lindemann R: Congenital renal tubular dysfunction associated with maternal sniffing of organic solvents, *Acta Paediatr Scand* 1991; 80:882-884.
52. Manning FA: Ultrasound in perinatal medicine. In Creasy RF, Resnik R, editors: *Maternal and fetal medicine principles and practice,* Philadelphia, 1984, WB Saunders.
53. Matthew OP et al: Neonatal renal failure: usefulness of diagnostic indices, *Pediatrics* 65:57, 1980.
54. McLean RH, Gearhart JP, Jeffs R: Neonatal obstructive uropathy, *Pediatr Nephrol* 2:48, 1988.
55. McVicar M, Margouleff D, Chandra M: Diagnosis and imaging of the fetal and neonatal abdominal mass: an integrated approach, *Adv Pediatr* 38:135, 1991.
56. Mirmiran M, Kok JHL: Circadian rhythms in early human development, *Early Hum Dev* 26:121, 1991.
57. Mocan H, Beattie TJ, Murphy AV: Renal vein thrombosis in infancy: long term follow-up, *Pediatr Nephrol* 5:45, 1991.
58. Muehlendahl KE, Ballowitz L: Growth hormone and cortisol in neonates during phototherapy, *Z Kinderheilk* 119:53, 1975.
59. Murphy JL et al: Prenatal diagnosis of severe urinary tract anomalies improves renal function and growth, *Child Nephrol Urol* 9:290, 1988.
60. Murugasu B et al: Familial renal adysplasia, *Am J Kid Dis* XVIII:490, 1991.
61. Parkhouse H, Barrett JM: Investigation of the dilated urinary tract, *Pediatr Nephrol* 2:43, 1988.
62. Perlman JM, Volpe JJ: Neurologic complications of captopril treatment of neonatal hypertension, *Pediatrics* 83:48, 1989.
63. Portman RJ et al: Predicting neonatal morbidity after perinatal asphyxia: a scoring system, *Am J Obstet Gynecol* 162:174, 1990.
64. Potter EL: *Normal and abnormal development of the kidney,* Chicago, 1972, Year Book Medical Publishers.
65. Rasoulpour M, McLean RH: Renal venous thrombosis in neonates, *Am J Dis Child* 134:276, 1980.
66. Reppert S, Weaver D: A biological clock is oscillating in the fetal suprchiasmatic nucleus. In Klein DC, Moore RY, Reppert SM, editors: *Suprachiasmatic nucleus: the mind's clock,* New York, 1991, Oxford University Press.
67. Reppert SM et al: Putative melatonin receptors in a human biological clock, *Science* 242:78, 1988.
68. Retik AB: Genitourinary problems in children, *Hosp Pract* 11:133, 1976.

69. Reznik VM et al: Follow-up of infants with bilateral renal disease detected in utero, *AJDC* 142:453, 1988.

70. Ronco C et al: Treatment of acute renal failure in newborns by continuous arteriovenous hemofiltration, *Kidney Int* 29:908, 1986.

71. Ronco C et al: Arteriovenous hemodiafiltration (CAVHD) combined with CAVH, *Trans Am Soc Prof Artif Organs* XXXI:349, 1985.

72. Rosendahl H: Ultrasound screening for fetal urinary tract malformations: a prospective study in general population, *Eur J Obstet Gynecol Reprod Biol* 36:27, 1990.

73. Rotundo A et al: Progressive encephalopathy in children with chronic renal insufficiency in infancy, *Kidney Int* 21.489, 1982.

74. Roussan MS: Neurogenic bladder dysfunction, *Med Times* 109:43, 1981.

75. Salusky IB et al: Experience with continuous cycling peritoneal dialysis during the first year of life, *Pediatr Nephrol* 1:172, 1987.

76. Sankaran K, Hindmarsh KW, Tan L: Diurnal rhythm of J-endorphin in neonates, *Dev Pharmacol Ther* 12:1, 1989.

77. Satlin LM: Maturation of renal potassium transport, *Pediatr Nephrol* 5:260, 1991.

78. Schwartz GJ, Brion LP, Spitzer A: The use of plasma creatinine concentration for estimating glomerular filtration rate in infants, children, and adolescents, *Pediatr Clin North Am* 34:571, 1987.

79. Sertel H, Scopes J: Rates of creatinine clearance in babies less than one week of age, *Arch Dis Child* 48:717, 1973.

80. Siegel S, Oh W: Renal function as a marker of human fetal maturation, *Acta Paediatr Scand* 65:481, 1976.

81. Sitka U et al: Investigation of the rhythmic function of heart rate, blood pressure, and temperature in neonates, *Eur J Pediatr* 153:117,

82. Smolensky MH, D'Alonzo GE: Medical chronobiology concepts and applications, *Am Rev Respir Dis* 147:S2, 1993.

83. Springate JE, Fildes RD, Feld LG: Assessment of renal function in newborn infants, *Pediatr Rev* 9:51, 1987.

84. Stalker HP et al: Plasma renin activity in healthy children, *J Pediatr* 89:256, 1976.

85. Stapleton FB: Renal uric acid clearance in human neonates, *J Pediatr* 103:290, 1983.

86. Stapleton FB, Jones DP, Green RS: Acute renal failure in neonates: incidence, etiology and outcome, *Pediatr Nephrol* 1:314, 1987.

87. Straub E, Spranger J: Etiology and pathogenesis of the prune belly syndrome, *Kidney Int* 20:695, 1981.

88. Sulyok E, Guigard J-P: Relationship of urinary anion gap to urinary ammonium excretion in the neonate, *Biol Neonate* 57:98, 1990.

89. Tack ED, Perlman JM, Robson AM: Renal injury in sick newborn infants: a prospective evaluation using urinary beta 2 microglobulin concentrations, *Pediatrics* 81.432, 1988.

90. Task Force on Blood Pressure Control in Children: Report of the Second Task Force on Blood Pressure Control in Children, 1987, *Pediatrics* 79:1, 1987.

91. Temple JK, Shapira E: Genetic determinants of renal disease in neonates, *Clin Perinatol* 8:361, 1981.

92. Walhauser F et al: Alterations in nocturnal serum melatonin levels in humans with growing and aging, *J Clin Endo Metab* 66:648, 1987.

93. Wells JG, Bunchman TE, Kearns GL: Treatment of neonatal hypertension with enalapril, *J Pediatr* 117:664, 1990.

94. Wilkins IA et al: The nonpredictive value of fetal urinary electrolyte: preliminary report of outcomes and correlates with pathologic diagnosis, *Am J Obstet Gynecol* 157:694, 1987.

95. Wu J et al: Circaseptan and circannual modulation of circadian rhythms in neonatal blood pressure and heart rate. In: Hayes D, Pauly J, Reiter R *Chronobiology: its role in clinical medicine, general biology and agriculture,* 1990, Wiley-Liss.

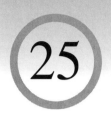

25 Neurologic Disorders

Paul Moe, Patti L. Paige

The developing nervous system provides an ongoing challenge for researchers and clinicians alike. Investigation continues in a wide variety of areas, yet basic mechanisms for a pathophysiologic understanding of common events such as neonatal seizures and IVHs remain unclear.

Improved neonatal care in recent years has not significantly reduced neurologic residua. How much of this is a reflection of sicker and more immature infants being salvaged is difficult to assess. Primary neurologic disease and secondary neurologic complications from such common conditions as cardiopulmonary disease, metabolic derangements, shock, infection, and coagulopathy still represent major problems encountered in every intensive care nursery. Serious anomalies still appear with regularity, albeit in small numbers.

This chapter deals with selected topics in neonatal neurology, including congenital malformations, trauma, seizures, hypoxic-ischemic encephalopathy, and IVH.

Congenital Malformations

Physiology, Etiology, and Clinical Features

Congenital malformations of the nervous system occur when the usual sequence of maturation and development is interrupted (Table 25-1).[53] By definition, the malformation is present at birth. Causes are multiple and largely unknown. Although strictly destructive lesions (such as hydranencephaly resulting from bilateral carotid artery occlusion) are separate from primary failures of morphogenesis, both may be included in the broad category of congenital malformations. The distinction between the two types lies in an understanding of the causes.

Understanding congenital malformations requires an appreciation of the normal embryologic sequence.[57] The clinical and pathologic identification of normal and abnormal structures allows for timing of the insult or development failure. Once timing is established, an appropriate search for the cause can be made.

Neural Tube Defects

At the end of the first embryonic week the *primitive streak* is present on the rostral surface of the embryo. A second streak, the *notochordal process,* develops alongside the primitive streak. The notochord is responsible for the induction of both the *neural plate* and the *neurenteric canal.* Cells proliferate along the lateral margin of the neural plate to form the *neural folds* around the central *neural groove.*

Cells at the apex of the neural folds make up the *neural crest.* Schwann cells, piarachnoid cells, sensory ganglia, melanocytes, and various secretory cells arise from the neural crest. The neural folds meet and fuse with the rostral (anterior) and caudal (posterior) ends (neuropore), closing approximately by the end of the fourth embryonic week.

Failure of development at this stage results in the defects of neurulation (or dorsal induction). The most severe of these defects is craniorrhachischisis, in which there is significant malformation of the brain (as in anencephaly), absence of the posterior skull, and an open spine the full length of the spinal cord.

Anencephaly is similar to craniorrhachischisis without the spinal defect. There is essentially no normal brain tissue above the brainstem and thalami, and parts of those structures are malformed.

Myeloschisis involves the failure of the posterior neural tube to close. No skull defect is present.

Encephaloceles are caused by a limited failure of closure at the rostral (head) end of the neural

Table 25-1
Central Nervous System Development and Related Defects

Maturational Process	Time	Associated Defects
Neural tube defects (dorsal induction, neurulation)	3-4 weeks	Craniorrhachischisis Anencephaly Myeloschisis Encephalocele Myelomeningocele Arnold-Chiari malformation
Prosencephalic development[13]	2-3 months	Cyclopia Holoprosencephaly Arhinencephaly Septooptic dysplasia Agenesis of corpus collosum Agenesis of septum pellucidum
Proliferation	2-4 months	Microcephaly Megalencephaly Neurocutaneous syndromes (?)
Migration	3-5+ months	Schizencephaly Lissencephaly Pachygyria (macrogyria) Microgyria (polymicrogyria) Neuronal heterotopias
Neuronal organization and functional organization	6 months	Down syndrome (?) Mental retardation (?) Genetic epilepsy (?)
Myelination	8 months	Anoxic/ischemic damage

tube. Extensions of meninges or brain tissue through the skull may occur on the ventral or rostral surface.

Myelomeningoceles (or even the more limited meningoceles) are a limited form of myeloschisis with failure of closure at the caudal (tail) end of the neural tube. The Arnold-Chiari deformities are usually included here. These malformations, often seen with myelomeningoceles, involve structures of the brainstem and cerebellum. Generally, the cerebellar tonsils are pulled down through the foramen magnum, and the brainstem is elongated in later life. Hydrocephalus is common. Symptoms of brainstem involvement may occur. Open myelomeningoceles and anencephaly (any defect in which the spinal or cranial contents are "open" to the outside) will cause an elevation of AFP in the amniotic fluid. This is important in prenatal diagnosis.

Segmentation Defects

After closure of the neural tube, suprasegmental structures are formed. The division of the brain into hemispheres, formation of the ventricular system, and formation of the major gyral patterns are all part of this period of development. Major areas of the brain, including the cerebellum, basal ganglia, brainstem nuclei, thalamus, and hypothalamus, form at this time. Defects of segmentation and cleavage occur during this phase of neural development. For unknown reasons, defects of segmentation and cleavage are far less common than defects of neurulation. Because these malformations involve abnormalities of ventral induction rather than dorsal induction (such as neurulation), the face, eyes, nose, mouth, and hair are also involved in the malformation. These features should always be investigated carefully for specific anomalies.

Holoprosencephaly is characterized by a single, midline, lateral ventricle; incomplete or absent interhemispheric fissure; absent olfactory system; midfacial clefts; and hypotelorism. The most severe form of holoprosencephaly is cyclopia, a single fused midline eye and supraorbital proboscis. An intermediate form is cebocephaly, which is phenotypically like trisomy D.

Archinencephaly involves aplasia of the olfactory bulbs and tracts.

When any of these malformations are suspected or when features suggestive of them are seen, careful examination of the hair, eyes, ears, mouth, and nose may reveal other related anomalies.

Septooptic dysplasia, with blindness and diabetes insipidus, may also be a malformation in this group.

Certain malformations of the base of the skull, cervical spine, and upper cervical cord are also grouped here, although there is less evidence that their embryogenic cause is the same. Malformations in this group include Klippel-Feil syndrome, platybasia, and Sprengel's deformity. These congenital malformations cause symptoms and signs related to the base of the skull and upper cervical spine. Short neck, restricted neck motion, and mirror movements of the upper extremities are commonly seen symptoms.

Migration and Cortical Organizational Defects

A critical aspect of brain development has yet to be described. The remaining development of the brain takes over twice as long as the previously described development and includes cellular proliferation, migration, organization, and myelination. The cells that later form the cerebral cortex begin in the germinal matrix (near the caudate nucleus around the lateral ventricles). These cells then migrate in a radial fashion to their final positions near the surface of the brain. Abnormalities of cellular migration result in collections of gray matter in unusual places (heterotopias), abnormal gyri and sulci, abnormal spaces in the brain, and frequent clinical signs of gray matter dysfunction. Frequently, these clinical problems are not apparent in the newborn period. The malformations in this grouping show no characteristic cranial or somatic features, because the timing of the malformations is

after the formation of large brain structures, divisions, and connections.[33]

Microcephaly means "small brain" and is manifested by a head circumference measuring greater than two standard deviations below average for infants at that gestational age. Microcephaly may be (1) genetic (dominant, recessive, sex-linked) or chromosomal (translocation [see Chapter 26]), (2) due to teratogens (radiation, cocaine, alcohol, phenylalanine), (3) due to infection (rubella, cytomegalovirus), or (4) of unknown cause. Occasionally, there is a paucity of germinal matrix cells or they fail to adequately migrate, resulting in a brain cortex with lessened neuronal cells.

Schizencephaly is a malformation in which atypical clefts, most often in the region of the sylvian fissue, are present within the brain substance. The clefts, covered only by meninges, may extend to the ventricles of the brain. Deep structures such as the thalamus and basal ganglia may be displaced.

In contrast to schizencephaly, porencephaly (not a malformation) is most often thought to be the result of destruction of previously normal tissue. Porencephaly is the occurrence of a cavity within the brain. This theory of porencephaly is confirmed by the identification of porencephalic cysts after strokes or meningitis.

The lissencephalic brain has a very smooth cortex with only a few small fissures and sulci. The brain is small, and the ventricles are enlarged. The organization of the cortex is abnormal with frequent heterotopias. Somatic anomalies (cardiac, renal, gastrointestinal, reproductive, and skeletal) may occasionally occur.

Macrogyria (pachygria) may be a localized hemispheric malformation or a diffuse malformation. The involved gyri show large, abnormal neurons and dense gliosis. Unusually wide gyri with compressed sulci can be seen.

Microgyria or polymicrogyria occurs as a response to an arrest in neuronal maturation before the fifth gestational month. CMV and maternal carbon monoxide poisoning (at 20 to 24 weeks' gestation) have been shown in some instances to produce this malformation, but most often the cause is unknown. Anatomically, areas of very small gyri are present in the involved area.

Agenesis of the corpus callosum most likely

represents a midline anomaly and is often seen as a part of a more extensive malformation such as Aicardi's syndrome, in which agenesis of the corpus callosum is accompanied by a chorioretinal lacuna and infantile spasms.

Schizencephaly and other malformations often have associated agenesis of the corpus calosum. In this malformation, there is a large subarachnoid space between the two hemispheres, and the lateral ventricles are displaced laterally (a commonly looked-for sign on a CT scan). The third ventricle is often dilated. An X-linked form has been reported, but most cases are sporadic. Clinically, the X-linked cases generally show multiple neurologic problems, whereas the isolated malformations of the corpus callosum have been found incidentally at autopsy in patients in whom it was not at all suspected.

Migrational anomalies easily lead to problems of gray matter dysfunction. These problems include seizures, mental retardation, motor dysfunction (cerebral palsy), and sensory dysfunction (blindness or deafness). Common manifestations in the newborn period are seizures, microcephaly, SGA, abnormal cry, and abnormal transillumination. Findings that are present later in life and probably not seen in neonates are mental retardation and spasticity.

Clinical features of schizencephaly include seizures, retardation, spastic quadriparesis, or minimal findings.

Clinical features of porencephaly include seizures, motor problems, increased intracranial pressure if the cyst is enlarging, and abnormal transillumination if the cyst is superficial. On occasion, no symptoms are perceptible.

Clinical features of lissencephaly include seizures, microcephaly, abnormal cry, SGA, polyhydramnios, micrognathia, downward-slanted palpebral fissures, anteverted nares, and prominent forehead and occiput. Later severe spasticity, hypsarrhythmia, and severe mental retardation may develop.

Clinical features of macrogyria include spastic hemiplegia or diplegia (depending on the site of involvement). If the area of involvement is very limited, there may be a paucity of findings. Clinical features of microgyria include absence of findings

in the newborn period. Later, spasticity and mental retardation are observable.

Signs and symptoms of absence of the corpus callosum are most often a result of associated malformations and anomalies. These include seizures, mental retardation, hydrocephalus, motor abnormalities, and asynchronous electroencephalogram.

Additional Defects

Cerebellar malformations are quite varied. Most often, at least a portion of the cerebellum is preserved, but total absence occurs. Hemispheric aplasia or vermal aplasia are seen, and familial forms have been reported. The Dandy-Walker cyst is another complex malformation involving the cerebellum. In it the fourth ventricle is dilated into a cystic structure. The foramina of Magendie and Lushka are atretic, and hydrocephalus results. The cerebellum is small and displaced upward. Associated anomalies include heterotopias, microgyria, agenesis of the corpus callosum, aqueductal stenosis, and syringomyelia. No specific causes are known. The differential diagnosis includes an arachnoid cyst of the posterior fossa. In the case of an arachnoid cyst, the fourth ventricle is not part of the malformation and is normal, although it may be displaced.

Clinical features of cerebellar malformations include absence of symptoms in the newborn period, cerebellar findings in family members, and the proband (hypotonia, incoordination, and nystagmus), especially in vermal aplasia, or total absence of symptoms throughout life.

Clinical features of the Dandy-Walker cyst include frequent progressive hydrocephalus, associated malformations that cause additional specific symptoms, possible absence of symptoms in the newborn period, enlargement of the occipital shelf and posterior part of the skull, positive transillumination in a triangular shape, nystagmus, lateral gaze palsy, abnormalities of respiratory control, and, later in life, ataxia.

Craniosynostosis is the abnormal fusion of the bones of the skull. The causes of this malformation are unknown. The premature closure of sutures may involve one or many sutures, with resulting deformity of the skull. Numerous terms are used to describe the shapes the skull assumes when craniosynostosis is present. Among these terms are plagiocephaly, scaphocephaly, dolichocephaly, keel-shaped deformity, and clover-leaf skull. Any of the atlases of human malformations give striking examples of these deformities.

Craniosynostosis should be suspected in the presence of microcephaly or a misshapen head. Appropriate evaluation requires x-ray films of the skull and a CT scan to define which if any of the sutures are stenosed and what problems might exist with brain structure (pressure or malformation).

Hydrocephalus may occur in many different situations from many separate causes. An inherited, X-linked form exists. Intrauterine infections are another cause. Hydrocephalus may be associated with many of the malformations listed above. Hydrocephalus results when the normal flow of ventriculospinal fluid is obstructed. This may be the result of an atretic portion of the ventricular system, blockage from the outside, inflammation within the ventricular system causing a permanent blockage, or (very rarely) overproduction of ventriculospinal fluid. Therefore if the cause is an inflammatory process that caused degeneration and destruction of part of the ventricular pathway, hydrocephalus may at times be more appropriately categorized with the destructive lesions. These infectious processes may also be responsible for some of the cases of congenital porencephaly. Vascular occlusion is the other cause thought to be responsible for some malformations in the "destructive lesion" category, including cases of porencephaly and hydranencephaly.

Data Collection

The diagnosis of malformations of the CNS may be quite obvious (as in anencephaly) or totally unrecognized during life (as in some cases of agenesis of the corpus callosum). Careful examination of all newborns will result in the identification of most malformations. At times the diagnosis will be suspected not on the basis of the examination but on the basis of an accompanying sign such as seizures.

When a congenital malformation is suspected, whether or not somatic signs are present, careful evaluation of the status of the CNS is in order. CT scanning is important for a better understanding of the intracranial structures, and electrophysiologic studies (EEG and evoked potentials) will help assess the functional aspects of the malformations. Clearly, there is no need for these studies in a seriously malformed infant who is not expected to survive.

Two very important tests have become available in recent years that allow for prenatal diagnosis of certain congenital malformations of the nervous system. Ultrasound examination (an abdominal ultrasound scan of the mother) provides an opportunity to identify certain malformations by viewing the fetus during development. Hydrocephalus, encephaloceles, myelomeningoceles, and anencephaly may be identified prenatally. Determination of AFP in the amniotic fluid allows for the identification of anencephaly and open myelomeningoceles. A nonenclosed nervous system will cause a significant rise in AFP in the amniotic fluid. Amniocentesis provides the amniotic fluid necessary for this determination. Testing of maternal serum for AFP is less specific and more controversial. At present, the combination of ultrasound examination and amniocentesis provides the most helpful information.

Clinical signs and symptoms have been described for each individual nervous system malformation presented earlier in this chapter.

Treatment

Very limited treatment is available for congenital malformations of the nervous system. A variety of strategies are available for making efforts at reducing secondary complications or providing earlier management to handle these complications more efficiently.

The greatest efforts and accomplishments have been made for those with congenital malformations who might be expected to live productive lives. When secondary complications are managed appropriately, children with myelomeningoceles often become well-adjusted, productive adults. This is not possible when the malformation causes severe retardation.

Some of the malformations are lethal in a short period of time (anencephaly and hydranencephaly) making intervention unnecessary and inappropriate. When intervention results only in increased time of survival without any improvement in profound physical and mental handicaps, the desirability of intervention should be questioned.

Treatment of many of the malformations of the brain is limited to the management of the manifestations of the malformation. These would include seizures, hearing impairment, spasticity, and secondary orthopedic problems. Because the primary defect cannot be changed, it is important to recognize that for many of the conditions, one cannot hope for substantial improvement.

In certain malformations, some specific treatment is indicated. If the encephalocele is small and a large amount of the brain is not contained in the sac, the defect should be closed. Associated neurologic problems such as seizures should be treated.

When treatment is thought to be appropriate, closure of the myelomeningocele should be performed as soon as possible. In this way the risk of meningitis and ventriculitis can be reduced. Untreated infants often die within the first year of life. Soon after closure of the primary defect, many infants develop hydrocephalus or experience a more severe case of antecedent hydrocephalus. Shunting then becomes necessary (Boxes 25-1 and 25-2 and Figs. 25-1 and 25-2).

The only situation in which microcephaly could be considered surgically treatable is total craniosynostosis. Generally, skull deformity is also present in these infants with craniosynostosis, but

---

Box 25-1

Post-OP Ventriculoperitoneal Shunt Care

I. Positioning
   A. Place on unaffected side (may position on shunt side with "donut" over operative site once incision has healed). Keep head of bed flat to 15 degrees to 30 degrees to prevent too-rapid fluid loss.
   B. Support head carefully when moving infant.
   C. Turn q2h from unaffected side of head to back.
II. Shunt site
   A. Use strict aseptic technique when changing dressing.
   B. Pump shunt if and only as directed by neurosurgeon.
   C. Observe for fluid leakage around pump.
III. Observe and document all intake and output. Watch for symptoms of excessive drainage of CSF:
   A. Sunken fontanel
   B. Increased urine output
   C. Increased sodium loss
IV. Observe, document, and report any seizure activity or paresis.
V. Observe for signs of ileus:
   A. Abdominal distention (serially measure abdominal girth)
   B. Absence of bowel sounds
   C. Loss of gastric content by emesis or through orogastric tube

VI. Perform range-of-motion exercises to all extremities.
VII. Observe and assess for symptoms of increased intracranial pressure (shunt failure):
   A. Increasing head circumference (measure head daily)
   B. Full and/or tense fontanel
   C. Sutures palpably more separated
   D. High-pitched, shrill cry
   E. Irritability and/or sleeplessness
   F. Vomiting
   G. Poor feeding
   H. Nystagmus
   I. Sunset sign of eyes
   J. Shiny scalp with distended vessels
   K. Hypotonia and/or hypertonia
VIII. Observe and assess for signs of infection:
   A. Redness or drainage at shunt site
   B. Hypothermia and/or hyperthermia
   C. Lethargy and/or irritability
   D. Poor feeding and/or weight gain
   E. Pallor
IX. Parent teaching (see Figure 25-1).
   A. Demonstrate and receive return demonstration of drug administration.
   B. Teach parents side effects of medications.
   C. Document on NICU's routine discharge teaching checklist with routine care.

it is always wise to consider the possibility of craniosynostosis in any infant with a small head. If present, total craniosynostosis should be treated surgically.

The management of congenital hydrocephalus consists primarily of early shunting as soon after birth as possible. Experimental procedures with fetal surgery in the early 1980s, including fetal ventriculostomy and multiple ventricular taps, held promise for earlier treatment of hydrocephalus.

Outcome was variable, and the procedures were not as reliable as hoped. It was not always possible to distinguish true hydrocephalus from ventriculomegaly without increased pressure. Shunting soon after birth often produces a far better outcome than would be assumed, with minimal motor deficit and only a mild to moderate deficit in intellect.

Monitoring of pregnancies with fetal ultrasound allows for the detection of congenital hydrocephalus. Induction of lung maturation with steroids has been suggested to allow a preterm delivery (with a smaller head) without excessive pulmonary complications. In this way, a permanent shunt can be placed sooner than with term delivery.[13]

Complications

Many of the expected complications are dealt with previously in the sections describing the malformations and their associated problems. It is difficult to separate true complications from problems occurring by nature of the malformation. For example, hydrocephalus after closure of a myelomeningocele is not truly a complication of the procedure or the disease but merely a condition brought out by the procedure.

Malformations carry with them disturbed anatomy and physiology that are reflected in abnormal function. General problems commonly encountered are seizures, retardation, sensorimotor abnormalities, disturbances in primary sensory function such as vision and hearing, orthopedic problems, and vegetative functions.

The problems encountered are ordinarily explainable on the basis of the malformation. Midline defects in the brain (particularly at the base of the brain) will often have clinical problems involving

the hypothalamus. Diabetes insipidis may be present. To some extent, the anatomy predicts the kinds of problems encountered. Involvement of the cortex causes seizures, retardation, and sensorimotor problems. White matter damage can cause spasticity. If the brainstem participates in the malformation, apnea, deafness, sleep disturbance, oculomotor disturbances, and problems with sucking and swallowing may be seen. Spinal cord lesions cause quadriplegia or paraplegia. Genitourinary problems, and to a lesser extent gastrointestinal problems, are also seen.

Apnea and other brainstem findings may occur when the malformation involves the brainstem, as in Arnold-Chiari deformities, Dandy-Walker cysts, occipital encephaloceles, and arachnoid cysts.

Pituitary-hypothalamic dysfunction may manifest itself in impaired temperature regulation, thyroid abnormalities, diabetes insipidus, and adrenal insufficiency.

Most of the complications occur after the newborn period, although the causes are already present at birth. These include seizures, retardation, spasticity, genitourinary problems, and orthopedic problems. In many of these circumstances the problem is already present, but the functional expression, such as impaired ambulation, retardation, and deafness, is lacking. In the infant's follow-up examinations, careful attention must be given to those problems likely to develop or intensify with age. When a specific malformation is identified, it is necessary to become familiar with the expected problems, not only to anticipate them as they appear, but also to lessen any secondary damage that might occur if they go unrecognized.

Parent Teaching

Parents of an infant born with congenital malformations are faced with a stressful event that may develop into a major life transition. Parents (especially mothers) report feelings of guilt and self-blame, although they may not initially share these feelings with hospital staff. After the birth of a malformed child, they go through stages of grief (see Chapters 28 and 29): shock and/or denial, anger, bargaining, depression, and acceptance. Some authors question whether full acceptance occurs for the family of the handicapped child

BAPTIST MEDICAL CENTER
WOLFSON CHILDREN'S HOSPITAL
JACKSONVILLE, FLORIDA

Wolfson
Children's
HOSPITAL
at Baptist Medical Center

VENTRICULOPERITONEAL (VP) SHUNT TEACHING CHECKLIST

GOAL/SKILL	NURSING (Date and Initials)	CARE GIVER #1	CARE GIVER #2	CARE GIVER #3
1. Verbalizes understanding of reason for VP shunt.	H - "An Introduction to Hydrocephalus" ☐			
2. Identifies the pathway of the VP shunt and the shunt's function.	H - "Ventriculo-Peritoneal Shunt" (Newborn) ☐ H - "Hydrocephalus and Shunts" (For infants with Cordis Shunts) ☐ H - "Your Valve System for Hydrocephalus" (For Cordis Valve System Shunts) ☐ H - "Just Like Any Other Little Beagle" ☐ V - "Just Like Any Other Little Beagle" ☐			
3. Lists signs and symptoms of shunt infection and emergent need to notify MD.				
4. Lists signs and symptoms of shunt failure and emergent need to notify MD.				
5. Discuss the reason and importance of prompt treatment of health problems.				
6. Verbalizes understanding of importance of close medical follow-up.				

SIGNATURE/INITIAL		TEACHING CODES	PARENT SIGNATURE(S)
		L - Lecture/Discussion	
		D - Demonstration (or return demo)	
		U - Verbalizes Understanding	
		R - Reinforced Teaching	PATIENT LABEL
		V - Video	
		H - Handout	
		E - Equipment	

20-207 Rev 5/96

Figure 25-1 Ventriculoperinatal (VP) shunt teaching checklist. (Courtesy of Wolfson Children's Hospital, Jacksonville, Fla, 1996.)

Box 25-2

Wolfson Children's Hospital Parent Handout
Newborn Ventriculoperitoneal (VP) Shunt
(For Use with VP Shunt Teaching Checklist)

Purpose of VP Shunt. Ventricles are compartment-like spaces that are located in the normal brain. Spinal fluid forms daily in these ventricles. This clear fluid flows out over the brain and down around the spinal cord. Spinal fluid helps cushion the brain from injury, keeps the brain moist, and carries away waste products.

Hydrocephalus is a condition when an abnormally large amount of spinal fluid builds up in your baby's ventricles and is usually caused by a blockage in the spinal fluid path. Because the ventricles continue to make spinal fluid daily, a build-up of fluid occurs when it can't escape. This excess fluid can cause pressure on the brain and result in permanent damage to the brain unless it is properly treated.

The purpose and function of your baby's VP shunt is to allow the excess spinal fluid to drain through a tube from the ventricle into the abdomen, where it is absorbed.

Pathway of the VP Shunt. A small incision is made on the scalp and the tube is passed through the skull and into the ventricle. Located under the skin, the tube passes behind the ear, down the side of the neck, and continues to the abdomen where a second incision is made to put the end of the tube into the abdominal cavity. A third incision is sometimes needed in the neck area with some babies.

The scalp incision will be hidden as your baby's hair grows. You'll see and feel the shunt tubing (like a large vein under the skin), but it is barely noticeable after the baby gains weight.

Signs and Symptoms of Shunt Infection. The shunt is at risk for infection because it is a foreign object located inside the body. You will need to watch for these signs of shunt infection and report them **immediately** to your doctor:

- Temperature of 101° F or higher
- Swelling, redness, and/or drainage along the pathway of the shunt tube
- Lethargy or irritability (change in behavior)
- Loss of appetite or poor feeding

Signs and Symptoms of Shunt Failure/Increased Intracranial Pressure (ICP). The spinal fluid contains proteins and chemicals that may build up and block off the shunt. It is also possible for tissue within the brain or abdomen to block the shunt or for the shunt device itself to fail. This shunt failure (malfunction) means that the spinal fluid will once again build up and result in pressure on the brain and possible irreversible damage. It is therefore very important for you to watch for the signs of increased pressure in the brain that occurs with shunt failure and report them immediately to your doctor.

- Lethargy or sleepiness
- Unusual irritability, fussiness, or excessive crying
- Repeated vomiting
- Poor feeding
- Bulging soft spot when baby is sitting up quietly
- Shrill, high-pitched cry
- Eyes that look downward
- Increase in spaces between the bones of the skull
- Seizures/posturing

Reason and Importance of Prompt Treatment of Health Problems. Prompt treatment of your baby's health problems (ear infections, skin infections, etc.) is important to prevent infections spreading to the shunt. It is also vital to seek medical care for signs of shunt infection or failure as noted above.

Importance of Close Medical Follow-up. Your baby will need to be followed up by a neurosurgeon and your pediatrician after being discharged. It is important for you to bring the baby to every follow-up appointment so that your baby's head can be measured and physical condition can be evaluated. Your baby will also go to the Developmental Evaluation Clinic where a specialist in baby development can examine him or her. If development problems occur, this will ensure early diagnosis and treatment.

Care of the Shunt: You can handle, cuddle, and play with your baby like any baby. Your baby can also sleep in any position after the initial postoperative period.

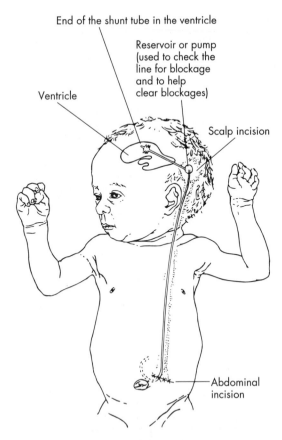

End of the shunt tube in the ventricle

Reservoir or pump (used to check the line for blockage and to help clear blockages)

Ventricle

Scalp incision

Abdominal incision

Figure 25-2   Ventricular peritoneal shunt. (Harrison H, Kositsky A: *The premature baby book,* New York, 1983, St Martin's Press.)

because of return of grief and sorrow each time a developmental milestone is missed or the child experiences illness.[26,36]

Social support received from hospital personnel, family, and friends can help parents feel less stressed and more able to cope with the illness of their infant. The ability of the staff to accurately anticipate and assess parental feelings and concerns can be invaluable when assisting families through this difficult time. Parents should be encouraged to verbalize their feelings and fears in a supportive environment. Reassurances, when appropriate, should be provided (e.g., parents were not responsible for the congenital malformation; it is normal for the mother to experience [or at least report] more fears than her husband, etc.) The ultimate goal of intervention is to reduce stress, assist families to confront fears, improve coping, and facilitate the bonding process.[17,36]

Infants with congenital malformations present such a complex variety of problems that parent teaching and emotional support needs to begin as early as possible. Often, parents will know from the time of birth or earlier that a major problem exists. In other circumstances the anomaly will be detected only after appropriate studies are performed.

When the infant is not viable, care should be directed to meeting the emotional needs of the family. Every effort should be made to give family members positive experiences and memories by encouraging early parental holding of the infant and participation whenever possible with care (see Chapter 29). Anticipatory counseling from social service and chaplain staff can help the family during grieving and with funeral arrangements. There will also be questions about etiology and genetics, which should be dealt with according to the family's wishes.

If serious handicaps are anticipated and the infant is expected to survive, the parents should be encouraged to participate in the care of the infant from the beginning. Not only will the adjustment occur more easily, but also the important aspects of care in special circumstances will be learned more effectively. A multidisciplinary team approach to parent education and support will allow hospital resources to be individualized to the specific needs of the patient and family. In addition to medical, nursing, social service, and chaplain involvement, team members can be drawn from psychologic, developmental, PT/OT, and other services based upon specific needs and circumstances. Parent teaching and support must be individualized according to the anomaly. When available, support groups and specialized clinics can help with postdischarge care and parent education.

Parent teaching for the mothers and fathers of infants with congenital anomalies should be started early, involve the parents in the care of the infant, use the resources of the hospital for specialized help, and continue after the infant has gone home from the hospital.

Birth Injuries

Physiology and Etiology

Birth injuries (birth trauma) are the direct result of difficulties encountered during the delivery process. They may be minor injuries without expected sequelae or may be the direct cause of death in the neonatal period. Classification of birth injuries is usually etiologic (predisposing factors or mechanisms of injury) or anatomic. An anatomic classification is used in this discussion to illustrate the commonly encountered problems (Table 25-2).

The timing of birth injuries can be used to describe causes. Etiologic classification of birth injuries includes uterine injury (antenatal), fetal monitoring procedures, abnormal or difficult presentations or methods of delivery, and multifactorial injuries. It should be recognized that the same injury might be caused in several ways. Thus a cephalhematoma could be the result of forceps delivery or vacuum extraction. A variety of specific predisposing factors increase the risk for birth injury:

- Macrosomia
- Cephalopelvic disproportion
- Dystocia
- Prematurity
- Prolonged or precipitous labor
- Breech presentation
- Forceps usage
- Rotation of fetus
- Version and extraction
- Handling after delivery

Multiple factors are often present. When multiple predisposing factors are present, they are often caused by a single underlying maternal disease. A common example would be a premature, macrosomic fetus with a diabetic mother in whom labor is not progressing properly.

The common factors that are present in deliveries complicated by birth injuries are as follows:

- **Unusual progress of labor**
- **Unusual size or shape to the fetus (large for gestational age and hydrocephalus)**
- **Problems encountered during delivery (dystocia and forceps application)**

Table 25-2	
Anatomic Classification of Birth Injuries	
Site of Injury	**Type of Injury**
Scalp	Caput succedaneum
	Subgaleal hemorrhage
	Cephalhematoma
Skull	Linear fracture
	Depressed fracture
	Occipital osteodiastasis
Intracranial	Epidural hematoma
	Subdural hematoma (laceration of falx, tentorium, or superficial veins)
	Subarachnoid hemorrhage
	Cerebral contusion
	Cerebellar contusion
	Intracerebellar hematoma
Spinal cord (cervical)	Vertebral artery injury
	Intraspinal hemorrhage
	Spinal cord transection or injury
Plexus injuries	Erb's palsy
	Klumpke's paralysis
	Total (mixed) brachial plexus injury
	Horner's syndrome
	Diaphragmatic paralysis
	Lumbosacral plexus injury
Cranial and peripheral nerve injuries	Radial nerve palsy
	Medial nerve palsy
	Sciatic nerve palsy
	Laryngeal nerve palsy
	Diaphragmatic paralysis
	Facial nerve palsy

- **Unusual or unexpected presentations (breech or unexpected twin)**

The maternal history must always be studied for the underlying disease process or conditions that might increase the risk for a birth injury.

Prevention

Most birth injuries may be preventable, at least in theory. Careful attention to risk factors and the appropriate planning of delivery should reduce the incidence of birth injuries to a minimum. Transabdominal ultrasonography allows for predelivery awareness of macrosomia, hydrocephalus, and unusual presentations. Particular pregnancies may then be delivered by controlled elective cesarean section to avoid significant birth injury. Care must be taken to avoid substituting a procedure of greater risk. Often, a small percentage of significant birth injuries cannot be anticipated until the specific circumstances are encountered during delivery. Emergency cesarean section may provide last-minute salvage, but in these circumstances the injury may truly be unavoidable.

Specific Birth Injuries

Injuries to the Scalp

The three commonly encountered forms of extra-cranial hemorrhage (caput succedaneum, subgaleal hemorrhage, and cephalhematoma) are distinguished not only in clinical manifestations, but also in pathophysiology. These three extracranial scalp injuries are included with neurologic birth injuries not because they have associated neurologic problems, but because the question of possible neurologic involvement is often raised by the family or health care providers.

Physiology and Etiology. The caput succedaneum is caused by trauma to the scalp, usually during a routine, vertex, vaginal delivery. The caput is the result of hemorrhagic edema superficial to the aponeurosis of the scalp. Spread of the edema is therefore not restricted to suture lines and is soft and pitting because of its superficial location.

Subgaleal hemorrhage is caused by forces that compress and then drag the head through the pelvic outlet. Significant acute blood loss can occur with shock as the presenting symptom. Bleeding may continue after birth with enlargement of the accumulated blood and dissection of the blood along tissue planes into the neck. Such a hemorrhage carries the greatest potential for complications, but fortunately it is the least common form of birth injury to the scalp.

Cephalhematoma is a subperiosteal collection of blood. The cause is uncertain, but its occurrence is more common in primiparous women and in forceps delivery. Males are generally more likely to be affected than females. The firm, tense collection of blood may increase in size after birth, but significant blood loss does not occur.

Data Collection. With caput succedaneum, physical examination reveals soft, pitting edema that is diffuse and crosses suture lines. There is no need for laboratory tests.

Because the subgaleal collection of blood is under the aponeurosis connecting the occipitofrontalis muscle and superficial to the periosteum, subgaleal hemorrhage crosses suture lines. It is firm but fluctuant to palpation. Vital signs should be carefully monitored for symptoms of shock. The hematocrit should be serially followed, and bilirubin levels should be determined during recovery.

Cephalhematoma may occur anywhere but is most commonly found in the parietal area on one side. Because the location of the blood is subperiosteal, it is confined by suture lines. Symptoms are normally absent. A skull fracture underlying the cephalhematoma is present in 10% to 25% of affected infants. X-ray examination of the skull defines the fracture. An occipital cephalhematoma may be mistaken for an occipital encephalocele. Lack of resolution and associated neurologic deficit aids in distinguishing the more severe pathologic process.

Treatment. No treatment is required for any of these three lesions. In subgaleal hemorrhage, treatment of blood loss and shock may be necessary. During resolution the breakdown of the blood may cause hyperbilirubinemia requiring treatment (see Chapter 20).

Parent Teaching. Careful preparation of the parents for the acute side effects of subgaleal hemorrhage is important. Parents should be warned of the possibility of swelling and discoloration of the face, head, and neck. Parents of an infant with a cephalhematoma can remain unconcerned unless localized changes occur, suggesting secondary infection (erythema, induration, or drainage). Cephalhematoma may be evident for 6 to 8 weeks. Outpatient biliruben levels may be required in some cases.

Skull Fractures

Three forms of skull fracture should be identified and differentiated: linear fractures, depressed fractures, and occipital osteodiastasis.

Physiology and Etiology.   Linear skull fracture is the most common type of skull fracture. The result of compression of the skull during delivery, a linear skull fracture most often has no associated injuries and causes no symptoms. Bleeding may be seen extracranially (common) or intracranially (rare). Intracranial bleeding causes symptoms referable to the bleeding rather than to the fracture itself.

The typical depressed skull fracture is of the "ping-pong" type, an indentation without loss of bony continuity. Forceps are usually the direct cause of injury, which most often is without complication or sequelae. When neurologic signs are present, direct cerebral injury, intracranial bleeding, or free bone fragments should be suspected.

Data Collection.   A linear skull fracture usually has no signs or symptoms unless intracranial bleeding has occurred. Skull x-ray films most frequently demonstrate a parietal fracture. A depressed skull fracture is usually a palpable "ping-pong" fracture in the parietal area. No other signs and symptoms are present unless they are caused by intracranial bleeding or focal irritation of the cortex. Evaluation with a skull x-ray examination or CT scan is necessary to delineate the fracture and to identify complications.

Treatment.   No treatment is necessary for a linear skull fracture. The controversy over treatment of a depressed skull fracture centers on the mode of treatment and the necessity for treatment. If free bone fragments are identified, neurosurgical intervention is required. More conservative approaches are indicated when no complications are present. Vacuum extractors and breast pumps have been used with variable success.

Complications.   With a linear skull fracture the single complication to be aware of is a "growing" skull fracture. A dural tear may allow leptomeninges to extrude into the fracture site, setting up the possibility of a leptomeningeal cyst. As the cyst enlarges, the edges of the fracture may fail to fuse and even spread apart, giving the appearance of a "growing" fracture. Palpation and x-ray examination demonstrate the lesion. Surgical correction may be required to ensure healing and prevent further complications. With a depressed skull fracture, intracranial bleeding and direct cerebral injury with seizures or residual neurologic deficit are rare.

Parent Teaching.   Parents should be instructed to have the fracture site checked for several months to ensure that reunion of the bone has taken place. Patients will have no other aftercare unless neurosurgical intervention was necessary or complications developed.

Intracranial Birth Injuries

Three major forms of bleeding occur intracranially: epidural hematoma, subdural hemorrhage, and subarachnoid hemorrhage. Added to these are cerebellar hemorrhages, cerebellar contusions, and cerebral contusions. Each has its own particular set of symptoms and signs, and complications and sequelae. IVH is usually not related to trauma and is covered separately in this chapter.

Physiology and Etiology.   Epidural hematoma is pathophysiologically difficult to form in newborns because of a relatively thick dura. When present, it is almost always accompanied by a linear skull fracture across the middle meningeal artery.

Subdural hemorrhage is more common in term infants than in preterm infants and occurs from trauma tearing veins and venous sinuses. Four major pathologic entities are defined: laceration of the tentorium, laceration of the falx, laceration of the superficial cerebral vein, and occipital osteodiastasis. Tentorial laceration causes a posterior fossa clot with compression of the brainstem. The straight sinus, Galen's vein, lateral sinus, and infratentorial veins may be involved. Laceration of the falx is caused by rupture of the inferior sagittal sinus. The laceration usually occurs at the junction of the tentorium and the falx, and the clot appears in the longitudinal cerebral fissure over the corpus callosum. Laceration of superficial cerebral veins causes subdural bleeding over the convexity of the brain. Subarachnoid bleeding or contusion of the brain may also be present.

Subarachnoid hemorrhage is the most common type of neonatal intracranial hemorrhage. In term infants, trauma is the most common cause, whereas in preterm infants hypoxia is more often the cause. Small hemorrhages are more common than massive ones and usually result from venous bleeding. Underlying contusion may occur.

Cerebral contusion is uncommon as an isolated event. Focal blunt trauma is necessary to produce a contusion. Pathologically, focal areas of hemorrhage and necrosis are seen. Shearing forces may cause slitlike tears in the white matter.

Cerebellar contusion and intracerebellar hemorrhage are uncommon events usually seen in association with occipital osteodiastasis and infratentorial subdural hemorrhage. These are catastrophic events, as described previously, and most often result in the death of the patient.

Data Collection. For epidural hemorrhage the signs and symptoms may be diffuse (increased intracranial pressure with a bulging fontanel) or focal or lateralizing seizures, eye deviation, and hemisyndromes. Laboratory tests should include x-ray examination to look for fractures and CT scanning to identify bleeding.

Infants with subdural hemorrhage are neurologically abnormal at birth. Tentorial lacerations and laceration of the falx tend to produce signs by pressure on the brainstem. These signs include skew deviation of the eyes, apnea, coma, or unequal pupils. Nuchal rigidity and opisthotonos are signs of progressive herniation. Signs and symptoms of subdural hemorrhage from laceration of the superficial cerebral veins are variable. Small clots may produce no identifiable dysfunction. Typical symptoms are those of focal or lateralized cerebral dysfunction, although increased intracranial pressure may occur. CT scans including views of the posterior fossa should be obtained immediately when a subdural hemorrhage is suspected.

With subarachnoid hemorrhage, underlying contusions may cause focal neurologic signs. Often no significant increase in intracranial pressure is found acutely. Irritability and a depressed level of consciousness may persist. Seizures are frequent in term infants, whereas apnea is common in preterm infants. Useful laboratory data include lumbar puncture and CT scan results. Focal signs predominate in cerebral contusions.

Treatment. Surgical evacuation of epidural and subdural clots may be necessary as emergency procedures. Subdural taps may be useful in the symptomatic infant with subdural bleeding from laceration of superficial cerebral veins. Many infants with intracranial bleeding may require treatment of seizures.

Complications. The complications of epidural hemorrhage range from none to permanent neurologic deficits with or without seizure. Sequelae of subdural hemorrhage occur in 20% to 25% of affected infants. The most common sequelae are focal neurologic signs. Seizures and hydrocephalus are seen less often. Hydrocephalus is the major potential complication of subarachnoid hemorrhage and directly alters outcome. If hydrocephalus is not present, as many as 90% of affected infants are normal at follow-up. Only 35% to 50% of those in whom hydrocephalus develops will be normal.

Parent Teaching. Because the long-term outcome is variable and may be abnormal even in infants normal at the time they leave the nursery, parent teaching must be individualized. The need for appropriate follow-up and intervention must be emphasized. Referral to available support groups is usually beneficial.

Spinal Cord Injuries

Physiology and Etiology. Injuries to the spinal cord (usually the cervical portion) are most often seen in complicated breech deliveries. Before cesarean sections were performed routinely for breech delivery, fatal attempts to deliver vaginally were often associated with interspinal hemorrhage. The breech presentation in conjunction with a hyperextended head is the most dangerous situation and is worsened by a depressed fetus. Traction, rotation, and torsion cause mechanical strain on the vertebral column. Cephalic deliveries are not entirely safe, because of the difference in mechanical forces; a different clinical picture is seen with a higher lesion.

Data Collection. Clinical manifestations depend on the severity and location of the injury. Clinical syndromes include stillbirth or rapid neonatal death, respiratory failure, and spinal shock syndrome. High cervical cord injuries are more likely to cause stillbirths or rapid death of the neonate. Lower lesions cause an acute cord syndrome. Common signs of spinal shock include flaccid extremities (may just involve the lower extremities if the cervical cord is spared), a sensory level, diaphragmatic breathing, paralyzed abdominal movements, atonic anal sphincter, and distended bladder. Useful laboratory tests include myelography, an MRI or CT scan of the spine, and somatosensory-evoked potentials to help determine the extent and site of the lesion. The differential diagnosis includes dysraphism, neuromuscular disease, and cord tumors.

Complications. After the acute phase, chronic lesions include cysts, vascular occlusions, adhesions, and necrosis of the spinal cord. Flaccid or spastic quadriplegia is expected. Some infants with spinal cord injuries will be respirator-dependent. Bowel and bladder problems will continue.

Parent Teaching. Parents need to understand fully the implications of severe injury to the spinal cord. Recovery is frequently minimal to nonexistent. Continued specialized care may be required, including ventilator therapy. The overwhelming implications for the family cannot be emphasized strongly enough.

An individualized multidisciplinary team approach to discharge planning is vital to parental confidence and a timely discharge. The problems of both patient and family are complex and not limited to medical concerns. A successful discharge is unlikely unless family emotional, financial, and educational concerns are addressed early in the planning process. The timely assessment of needs and involvement of supportive agencies will allow resolution of problems well before the projected discharge date. Such assistance should include early family referral to available federal programs for financial aid (SSI, etc.) and assistance with patient transportation to their multiple outpatient follow-up appointments. Early assessment of equipment needs and home nursing requirements is also of primary importance and should include a determination of the availability of these resources in the community, parent acceptance of their use, and whether the home can accommodate them (adequate electrical system, space, etc.).

Plexus Injuries

Physiology and Etiology. Plexus injuries occur much more commonly than cord injuries and result from lateral traction on the shoulder (vertex deliveries) or the head (breech deliveries).[40,50] Most often a depressed fetus or dystocia from a large infant is a contributing factor. Inappropriate augmentation of labor is another possible additive cause. Estimates of the incidence of brachial plexus injuries range from 0.5 to 1.9 per 1000 live births. Extremely mild cases may have undetectable findings and may remain unidentified.

Pathologic changes range from edema and hemorrhage of the nerve sheath to actual avulsion of the nerve root from the spinal cord. Of the reported cases of plexus injuries, 90% involve the C5-7 nerve roots and are classified as Erb's palsy. In a small minority of cases, the C4 nerve root is also affected, causing diaphragmatic problems. The site of injury in Erb's palsy is Erb's point where C5 and C6 nerve roots join to form the upper trunk. Total brachial plexus palsy occurs in 8% to 9% of the cases and has findings referable to C5 to T1 (and possibly C4). When T1 is involved, the sympathetic fibers become affected with an ipsilateral Horner's syndrome (ptosis, anhydrosis, and miosis) and possible delay in pigmentation of the iris. Less than 2% of the cases have Klumpke's paralysis involving only C8 to T1. In this form the site of pathologic conditions is the point at which C8 to T1 join to form the lower trunk.

Data Collection. Signs of brachial plexus palsies vary somewhat, most often because of overlap of the pure clinical syndromes. Shoulder and arm findings are characteristic of a true Erb's palsy. Involvement of the hand and fingers is seen in total forms or Klumpke's paralysis. Table 25-3 lists the specific cord levels involved in various functions that might be addressed.

Evaluation of diaphragmatic function by x-ray examination is at times necessary. Myelography or MRI may be required to identify nerve root avulsion, which generally should be suspected when recovery does not occur. Electromyography often shows abnormalities early in the course of the injury, suggesting that the process may actually have begun in the last weeks of pregnancy rather than at the time of delivery.

Clinical syndromes of plexus injuries include

Table 25-3
Brachial Plexus Examination:
Distinguishing Features

Part Examined	Spinal Level
Diaphragm movement (downward)	C4 (C3-5)
Deltoid muscle	C5
Spinatus muscle	C5
Biceps muscle	C5-6
Brachioradialis muscle	C5-6
Supinator of arm	C5-6
Biceps tendon reflex	C5-6
Wrist extensors	C6-7
Long extensor of the digits	C6-7
Triceps tendon reflex	C6-7
Wrist flexors	C7-8, T1
Finger flexors	C7-8, T1
Dilator of iris	T1
Eyelid elevator (full elevation)	T1
Moro reflex (shoulder abduction)	C5
Moro reflex (hand motion)	C8-T1
Palmar grasp	C8-T1

Erb's palsy, total palsy, and Klumpke's paralysis. Erb's palsy accounts for about 90% of plexus injuries. It involves the upper part of the plexus, C5-7 and occasionally C4. The shoulder and upper arm are involved, and the biceps reflex is decreased. When C4 is involved, diaphragmatic dysfunction is present.

Total palsy occurs in 8% to 9% of the cases. Plexus involvement is diffuse (C5 to T1 and occasionally C4). The upper and lower arm and hand are involved. Horner's syndrome (ptosis, anhydrosis, and miosis) exists when T1 is involved. The diaphragm is affected when C4 is involved. Biceps and triceps reflexes are decreased.

Klumpke's paralysis is seen in less than 2% of cases. The lower part of the plexus, C8 to T1, is involved. The lower arm and hand are involved. T1 involvement is associated with Horner's syndrome. Triceps reflex is decreased.

Treatment. Treatment may include immobilization for 1 to 5 days. Finger and wrist splints may be necessary. Passive range-of-motion exercises follow, and then gradual increase of activity to the affected limb is permitted.

Complications. Associated trauma may occur and should be carefully investigated. Common associated injuries include clavicular fracture, shoulder dislocation, cord injury, facial nerve injury, and humeral fracture. Full recovery of plexus function is seen in 88% to 92% of cases in the first year of life.[56]

Parent Teaching. Parents should be taught passive range-of-motion exercises to encourage mobility and prevent contractures. Instructions should begin before discharge from the hospital. Most often the instructions are given by a neonatal nurse or an occupational or physical therapist.

Parents may equate the presence of a brachial plexus injury with poor obstetric care. Most often this will not be the case. The awareness of early changes on electromyography should be used to help families understand that the factors causing injury to the plexus may begin long before the onset of labor.

Cranial and Peripheral Nerve Injuries

Median and sciatic nerve injuries are usually postnatal and result from brachial and radial artery punctures (median nerve) and inferior gluteal artery spasm (umbilical artery line drug instillation). Recovery is variable.

Median nerve palsy is manifested by decreased pincer grasp, decreased thumb strength, and the continuous flexed position of the fourth finger. Sciatic nerve palsy is manifested by decreased hip abduction and decreased distal joint movement. Hip adduction, flexion, and rotation are normal, because they are controlled by the femoral and obturator nerves.

Radial nerve damage is usually seen in conjunction with a humeral fracture. Prolonged labor is normally present. Congenital bands may also be causative. Recovery takes place in weeks to months.

Radial nerve palsy is manifested by wrist drop (decreased finger and wrist extension) and normal grasp.

Laryngeal nerve palsy may be seen in conjunction with facial or diaphragmatic paralysis. If the paralysis is unilateral, a hoarse cry may be heard. Bilateral involvement causes breathing to be difficult and the vocal cords to remain closed in the midline. It is important to rule out intrinsic brainstem disease. Often the presence of other brainstem findings such as oculomotor problems, apnea, or facial palsy will help clarify this. Evoked potentials, both brainstem auditory and somatosensory, may also help rule out brainstem involvement.

Laryngeal nerve palsy is manifested by difficulty in swallowing (superior branch), difficulty in breathing (bilateral), and difficulty in vocalizing (recurrent branch). Also, the head is held high and flexed laterally with slight rotation.

Diaphragmatic paralysis is most often seen in association with plexus injuries (80% to 90% have an associated plexus injury) and has the same cause. Some series involving unilateral paralysis have a mortality of 10% to 20%. Most patients recover fully in 6 to 12 months. Although less than 10% of patients have bilateral diaphragmatic paralysis, the mortality for these patients is higher (almost 50%). Treatment has consisted of using rocking beds, electric pacing of the diaphragm, CPAP, respirators, or plication. Because diaphragmatic paralysis may occur in other conditions such as a myotonic dystrophy, attention to the differential diagnosis is important, particularly when associated brachial plexus problem is not present.[56]

Diaphragmatic paralysis is demonstrated by respiratory difficulty in the first few hours of life. X-ray film shows elevation of the hemidiaphragm with paradoxic movement that may disappear on PEEP or CPAP.

Facial palsy may be part of intrinsic brainstem disease (see previous discussion of laryngeal nerve palsy) or other conditions such as Möbius syndrome, myotonic dystrophy, or facial muscle agenesis. When it is traumatic in origin, facial palsy is thought to be caused by the position of the face on the sacral promontory at the exit of the nerve from the stylomastoid foramen. It is debatable whether forceps delivery increases the incidence. Normally, both the upper (temporofacial) and lower (cervicofacial) branches are involved. Known complications (from lack of total resolution) include contractures and synkinesis. Cosmetic surgical procedures are occasionally necessary but are often delayed for years.

Facial palsy is seen on the left side in 75% of cases. Features include a widened palpebral fissure, flat nasolabial fold, and decreased facial expression. Most infants completely recover within 3 weeks, although some infants continue to have deficits months later.

Parent Teaching. Infants with facial palsy may require the use of artificial tears if unable to completely close the eye on the involved side. Occasionally, it may be necessary to tape the eye to prevent injury to the cornea. Parents should also be taught to expect some drooling of formula from the corner of the mouth during feedings.

Although most infants with laryngeal nerve palsy recover in the first 6 to 12 months of life, their symptoms will initially require supplemental parent education and support. Infant risk of aspiration necessitates careful feeding and appropriate response should choking occur. Additional education for gavage feedings, a tracheotomy, or an apnea monitor may be required for the parents of a few infants. The teaching requirements of the infant with diaphragmatic paralysis must also be tailored to meet the individual needs and circumstances of the child and family involved.

Neonatal Seizures

Physiology

Seizures are signs of malfunctioning neuronal systems. It is most useful to think of a localized or generalized loss of inhibitory control as the source of the seizure activity. This inhibitory loss may be the result of damage to the developing brain or transient effects such as disturbances in blood flow, glucose availability, or hypoxia. These disturbances may cause paroxysmal electrical activity recorded as seizures on the EEG. Ordinarily there are clinical signs that mimic what might, under other circumstances, be normal brain activity but, in the context of the seizure, cause stereotyped, repetitive, and inappropriate activity.

Seizures may be the only manifestation of brain dysfunction, but this is extremely uncommon in the neonate. Most often, seizures in the newborn period are the result of a very significant brain insult; the clinical signs of the insult are multiple.

Table 25-4
Common Causes of Neonatal Seizures

Classification	Causes
Acute metabolic conditions (Do blood gases, pH, HCO_3^-, Na, K, Ca, Mg, glucose, BUN)	Hypocalcemia Hypoglycemia; hyperglycemia Hypomagnesemia Pyridoxine dependency or deficiency Hyponatremia; hypernatremia
Inherited metabolic conditions (acidosis, common; do urine amino acids, organic acids, NH_3, galactose)	Maple syrup urine disease Nonketotic hyperglycemia Hyperprolinemia Galactosemia Urea cycle abnormalities Organic acidemias
Infections (12% of cases, assess CSF; cult blood; ?CSF, PCR of CSF; imaging)	Viral encephalitis, herpes, or enterovirus Congenital infections Bacterial meningitis Sepsis Brain abscess Septic venous thrombosis
Intracranial hemorrhage (15% of cases, imaging; ?CSF exam)	Subdural hematoma Cerebral contusion Subarachnoid hemorrhage Epidural hemorrhage Intraventricular hemorrhage (premature)
Hypoxic ischemic (0-3 day) most common (60%) Congenital malformations Neonatal drug withdrawal (see Chapter 8)(e.g., opiates) Local anesthetic intoxication Kernicterus Specific nongenetic syndromes Benign familial neonatal seizures Idiopathic (in only 10% no cause is found)	

Etiology and Data Collection

Neonatal seizures may be caused by a variety of acute and chronic stresses on the brain.[6,23,24,53] Table 25-4 lists the general groups of causes of neonatal seizures. The search for a cause proceeds in an orderly, methodic way. Most often the known history of perinatal problems will narrow the differential diagnosis to one or two likely causes. Acute metabolic changes that are likely to cause seizures should be rapidly investigated first.

Sepsis should never be overlooked as a potential cause. The infectious agent (meningitis, encephalitis, empyema, abscess, septic thrombosis, and ventriculitis) may directly affect the CNS. Systemic infection may cause seizures through the complication of shock, coagulopathy, impaired oxygenation, and multisystem organ failure. When the CSF is examined, not only will the changes associated with infection be identified, but evidence of bleeding (red blood cells) or cell destruction (protein) may also be found.

Structural studies are routinely performed as part of the evaluation. Presently, the most useful studies are CT scans and ultrasound examination.

The infant's history should be carefully reviewed to narrow the possible causes to the most likely ones. Physical examination may further narrow the differential diagnosis. Once these are quickly done, blood should be drawn for arterial blood gases, electrolytes, glucose, calcium, and magnesium.

Appropriate cultures must be obtained. Usual culture sites or specimens include blood, urine, spinal fluid, and pharyngeal or tracheal aspirate. The CSF should be examined for red blood cells and white blood cells, organisms (Gram's stain), protein, and sugar.

Ultrasound examinations are particularly useful for identifying and following intraventricular bleeding and hydrocephalus. The infant is exposed to no radiation, either immediately or long-term; no complications, either immediate or long-term, have been identified. The test may be repeated as often as needed and is usually performed at the bedside.

Although it provides better resolution for identifying subtle changes in brain structure, a CT scan exposes the developing brain to significant radiation. The larger the number of "cuts" made, the greater the exposure. The exact amount of

radiation varies with the type of machine and duration of the study. Short-term effects have not been detected, but the potential for long-term or cumulative effects of radiation exposure has not been determined. In addition, the use of contrast media is occasionally necessary for a complete study. This may be contraindicated in newborns with impaired renal function or in those with delicate fluid balance.

Although they provide interesting and helpful information in older patients with seizures, newer imaging techniques such as positron emission tomography have not been widely available and/or applied to newborns except as research. The potential hazards of isotopic scanning need further study before positron emission tomography can be put to general use in newborns.

MRI produces exceptional detail and is sensitive to changes in cellular composition. Presently the studies often require transport and up to an hour's time, limiting their practicality in the sick newborn.

Clinical Seizure Types

The application of technology used in the assessment of patients with epilepsy has finally been applied to neonates experiencing seizures. Simultaneous EEG and video recording allow for the accurate diagnosis of difficult-to-assess subtle behaviors, apneic and bradycardiac spells, and the jerks and twitches commonly seen in preterm newborns.[49] Many have been surprised to find no correlation between events thought to be seizures and changes on the EEG.[8]

It is now widely accepted that much of what had been called neonatal seizure activity represents nonseizure subcortical or brainstem activity that reflects poor brain functioning. Tonic episodes and so-called "subtle" seizures are frequently found to be in this category of "non-seizures."

Focal clonic, and multifocal clonic seizures are the most likely to have true cortical origins. Eye blinking (a clonic manifestation) may be seen, as may nystagmus. Focal clonic seizures have been seen as an important manifestation of stroke in the neonate.[10] Apnea has been seen as an ictal manifestation without any other evidence of seizure activity, although most apnea is not on this basis.

The lack of ongoing monitoring of brain activity in most neonatal units makes accurate iden-

tification of seizures extremely difficult. The best correlation can be made by obtaining an EEG during periods of presumed seizure activity. If the activity is confirmed as true seizures, then the same activity or closely related activity is also likely to be true seizure activity.

The traditional categorization of neonatal seizures is presented in Table 25-5. The classification does not have the same significance as the International Classification of Seizures in older individuals. Some general observations may pertain, even with the confusion surrounding the accurate diagnosis of neonatal seizures. Seizures, however, continue to be more difficult to recognize in the neonate. Compounding this difficulty is the confusion added in the presence of newborn jitteriness. Care must be taken to avoid mistaking this jitteriness for seizure activity[10,56] (Table 25-6).

Episodes characterized as tonic and subtle are most likely to be seen in premature infants. Tonic episodes are quite commonly associated with IVH. Clonic and multifocal clonic seizures are more common in term infants. Myoclonic seizures often include a metabolic etiology such as nonketotic hyperglycemia or urea cycle disorder.

Prevention

Many neonatal seizures can be successfully prevented through careful attention to possible metabolic changes expected on the basis of the infant's condition. Hypoglycemia, hypocalcemia, hypomagnesemia, and often hypoxia can be anticipated and controlled.

Seizures resulting from intracranial malformations, infections, or prenatal injury most often cannot be prevented. Inherited metabolic disorders may not be identified until after initial symptoms (often including seizures) appear.

Whether neonatal seizures can be prevented by pretreatment of the mother (in high-risk situations thought likely to result in neonatal seizures) has not been adequately investigated. As progress in antenatal treatment of the fetus continues, this may become an area for further investigation.[56]

Treatment

The rational treatment of neonatal seizures involves a vigorous attempt to achieve four specific

Table 25-5
Traditional Categorization of Neonatal Seizures

Classification/Types	Definition/Description	Clinical Manifestations
Clonic • Focal clonic • Multifocal clonic Tonic • Focal tonic • Generalized tonic	• Rhythmic jerks (1-3 per sec) • Rate slows during seizure • + EEG seizure activity • Characterized by posturing • Focal: + EEG seizure activity • Generalized: usually no EEG seizure activity seen	Focal: well-localized to a body part Multifocal: several body parts jerking simultaneously or in migrating order Focal: continued posturing of limb or a posturing (asymmetrical) of trunk or neck Generalized: extension of lower limbs with either upper limb extension (looks like decerebrate posturing) or with upper limb flexion (looks like decorticate posturing)
Myoclonic • Focal myoclonic • Generalized myoclonic Subtle (more common in the premature infant)	• Faster jerking than clonic seizures • Flexor muscles (limbs) involved • Focal: usually no EEG seizure activity • Generalized: + EEG seizure activity • Abnormal behavioral, autonomic, or motor activities that are not due to the other 3 seizure classifications • + EEG seizure activity only with some of the seizure activities	Focal: flexor jerking of upper limbs Generalized: bilateral jerking of upper extremities; sometimes lower limbs also are involved. **Ocular:** nystagmus, horizontal or vertical deviation of eyes, staring episodes, eyelid flutter or blinking **Facial:** repetitive sucking, mouth movements, tongue protrusion, chewing, drooling **Limb:** bicycling, swimming movements, "boxing" or "hooking" motions, stepping **Apnea:** only 2% due to seizures **Autonomic or vasomotor changes**

Table 25-6
Seizures vs Jitteriness

Clinical Observations	Seizure	Jitteriness
Ocular abnormalities (eye deviations or staring)	Yes	No
Gentle restraint of the involved body part halts the activity	No	Yes
Activity is easily elicited with stimulation (voice, motion, etc.)	No	Yes
Dominant movement is a rapid tremor where the amplitude and rate of the alternating movements is equal	No (Dominant movement is a slower clonic jerking having both a fast and slow element)	Yes
Autonomic changes are present: apnea, tachycardia, elevated BP, pupil changes, increased salivation, etc.	Yes	No

goals: acute treatment, correction, prevention, and minimization.

Acute Treatment

The first goal is acute treatment of prolonged or multiple seizures and status epilepticus. Prolonged seizures and frequent, multiple seizures may result in metabolic changes and cardiorespiratory difficulties. Whether seizures themselves may cause brain damage is an unanswered question. It seems appropriate to make vigorous efforts to control seizures completely, although this may not always

Box 25-3

Acute Management of Neonatal Seizures

Assess clinical situation—are the episodes seizures? (May need stat EEG if available.)

Draw blood for glucose, calcium, magnesium, blood gas analysis, and electrolytes.

Maintain adequate oxygenation and ventilation.

Remain prepared to intubate infant and provide respiratory support (especially after medications are given).

Perform Chemstrip/Dextrostix:

If value is <25-45, give 2 ml/kg of D_{10} W IV

If value is 45 or better, give 20 mg/kg phenobarbital IV (slowly over 10 to 15 min)

If seizures continue after 5-20 minutes, the following steps should be taken:

Give additional 5 mg/kg doses of phenobarbital IV over 10-15 min (max 20 mg/kg extra)
and/or

Give 20 mg/kg phenytoin (dilantin) IV slow push (no faster than 1 mg/kg/min);

*PRECIPITATES EASILY. Flush IV with normal saline before and after dose.

*Monitor ECG and BP during infusion.

If seizures continue or recur after the above steps,

Draw phenobarbital level (therapeutic serum level is 15 to 30 µg/ml).

Draw dilantin level (therapeutic serum level is 15 to 20 µg/ml).

Correct calcium or magnesium if low.

Give 100 mg pyridoxine (Vitamin B_6) IV push (protect from light)

If seizures continue with the above treatment:

Obtain imaging study to look for a major intracranial etiology (bleed, malformation, etc.)

Obtain metabolic studies (lactate, pyruvate, urine amino and organic acids, blood amino acids, and NH_4).

Give 0.05-0.1 mg/kg lorazepam (Ativan) IV slow push. May repeat dose if needed.

Give 0.3 mg/kg diazepam* (Valium) IV slow push. PRECIPITATES EASILY.

*CAUTION: There is a debate in literature about using diazepam for treatment of seizures in the neonatal population due to severe side effects (especially when phenobarbital is also in use). Volpe[56] does not use for multiple other reasons.

Once seizures are under control, maintain therapeutic serum phenobarbital level.

Cultures (blood and CSF) should be done as soon as possible. Treat with IV antibiotics (bacterial infection) and acyclovir (herpes) if pertinent.

---

be possible. When the administration of a single drug does not result in lasting control, a second or third should be tried. Box 25-3 outlines a plan for acute management.[19,23,34,47]

The most commonly used drugs for the control of acute seizures and status epilepticus in the newborn are phenobarbital and phenytoin (Box 25-3 and Table 25-7). Both are given in loading doses of 20 mg/kg. In most infants this load achieves a blood level within the therapeutic range. Because both drugs are always given intravenously (IV) for this indication, the blood level is promptly achieved.[4,56,64] **When these antiepileptic drugs are unsuccessful in bringing the seizure(s) under control, alternate drugs such as lorazepam or diazepam may be used.**[52]

Correction

The second goal is correction of underlying remediable causes. This goal is often more important than the first goal, because some seizures induced by metabolic abnormalities cannot be controlled with antiepileptic drugs until the metabolic derangement is corrected. It is especially inappropriate to treat a newborn with antiepileptic drugs before correctable causes have been excluded.

After the drawing of blood for glucose, calcium, magnesium, electrolytes, and blood gas determination, therapy may begin. It is always proper to administer glucose. Inspired oxygen concentration may be raised temporarily if hypoxia is suspected. The IV administration of 100 mg pyridoxine should ideally be done under electroenceph-

Table 25-7
Antiepileptic Drugs

Drug	Dose	Comments
Phenobarbital (drug of choice for neonatal seizures)	Loading: 20 mg/kg IV given slowly over 10-15 min; additional 5 mg/kg can be given to a maximum of 40 mg/kg total Maintenance: 5-7 mg/kg in 2 divided doses beginning 12 hr after last loading dose	Therapeutic level: 15-30 µg/ml (obtain levels any time 1 hr after dose); respiratory depressant; incompatible with other drugs in solution
Phenytoin (added if seizures not controlled by phenobarbital alone)	Loading: 10-20 mg/kg IV (no more rapidly than 1 mg/kg/min) Maintenance: 4-8 mg/kg in 1-2 doses/day beginning 12 hr after last loading dose	Therapeutic level: 15-20 µg/ml (obtain levels 1-10 hr after last loading or maintenance dose); incompatible with all other drugs, glucose, and pH <11.5; give slowly directly into vein; too-rapid administration causes dysrhythmias, bradycardia, hypotension, cardiovascular collapse, and/or respiratory distress
Pyridoxine (vitamin B_6)	100 mg IV bolus	Pyridoxine (vitamin B_6) deficiency or dependency as etiology of neonatal seizures is rare; seizures will cease and EEG normalize within 5 minutes after vitamin B_6 injection if deficient
Lorazepam (Ativan)	0.05-0.1 mg/kg/dose IV over 2-5 min	Use justified in severely ill newborns with seizures nonresponsive to other drugs
Primidone (Mysoline)	Loading: 15-20 mg PO Maintenance: 12-20 mg/kg/day	Use justified for refractory seizures; close monitoring of phenobarbital levels is necessary, because levels rise after primidone loading and fall precipitously with phenobarbital discontinuance
Valproic acid (Vepakene)	Initital dose: 15-30 mg/kg/day PO, PR Maintenance: 15-60 mg/kg/day PO q12h	Anticonvulsant for refractory neonatal seizures; complications include neutropenia, hepatic damage, hepatic failure, and hyperammonemia

alogram monitoring. In this way the true causes of pyridoxine dependency or deficiency can be detected.

Prevention

Prevention of further seizures is the third goal. Seizure prophylaxis is an admirable goal for patients of all ages, but it is often not easily achieved in newborns. Often, in spite of the appropriate and vigorous administration of several antiepileptic drugs, seizures persist for several days only to remit spontaneously and never return. Despite this rather frequent observation, attempts to provide adequate seizure prophylaxis seem justified.

Phenobarbital remains the most studied and most used drug for seizure control in the newborn.

Because the half-life of phenobarbital is long, it is not necessary to give routine maintenance doses on a fixed schedule.

Phenytoin is also used extensively. Although it may be very useful in acute treatment, phenytoin is often quite difficult to use as a maintenance drug. The most frequently encountered problem is the extremely variable half-life in newborns. It is not predictable, and frequent blood level determinations are necessary to estimate a useful half-life for the individual infant. Not uncommonly, repeated loading doses must be used several times a day to maintain an adequate blood level.[7] This pharmacokinetic problem is dramatically compounded by oral administration. It is reasonable to avoid the oral use of phenytoin in the newborn altogether.

A second problem is the variability in binding of phenytoin to albumin in blood. The binding is affected by the amount of albumin, concurrent drugs, and other poorly understood factors. Because changes in binding alter the amount of drug available to enter the brain, there is often little control over the true unbound "level." Whenever the unbound level of phenytoin (normal 1 to 3 mg/ml) can be measured, it is more useful than the total level. Using the unbound level does not make the calculation of an appropriate dosage any simpler, but it does give information that can help avoid needless toxicity.

Maintenance doses of phenobarbital (3 to 5 mg/kg) should be given after blood level determinations indicate that the level is dropping.[14,16] Phenytoin maintenance doses are difficult to predict. Frequent blood levels may be necessary to understand the way in which a given infant metabolizes phenytoin.

If unbound levels of phenytoin are available, these are often easier to use to ensure that a therapeutic range is maintained. Because the characteristic signs of phenytoin toxicity are cerebellar, they are ordinarily not recognized in the newborn. One must rely on the accurate determination of blood levels to safeguard against excessive administration. Maintenance doses for phenytoin range from 4 to 8 mg/kg IV every 24 hours for the neonate.[42,64]

Other antiepileptic agents such as primidone, carbomazepine, and valproic acid are used less frequently. Data about safety, effectiveness, and dosage are less available than for phenobarbital and phenytoin.

Minimization

The fourth goal is minimization of the side effects of antiepileptic drug therapy. In the attempt to control seizures, the potential of antiepileptic drugs to produce side effects must not be ignored. Drug-induced encephalopathy may mimic the clinical changes seen in hypoxic-ischemic encephalopathy (HIE) or numerous metabolic derangements. The possibility that the pharmaceutical agent may be causing some of the findings being attributed to the underlying disorder always exists. Likewise, improvement in the underlying disorder may be masked by changes induced by the drug.

More significant side effects such as respiratory or cardiovascular depression produced by large doses of any of the drugs, hepatotoxic changes induced by valproic acid, or hyperbilirubinemia intensified by diazepam are rare but worthy of recognition.

The issue of long-term side effects of the antiepileptic drugs is far from being settled. Virtually all of the drugs used have been shown in animal or tissue culture studies to have detrimental effects on the growth or development of the brain. The extent to which any of this information can be transferred to the human situation remains the subject of extensive investigation.

Complications and Outcome

The evidence for long-term clinical complications that can be directly related to the presence of neonatal seizures is limited and controversial.[62] This should not be surprising, because most neonatal seizures occur in the course of significant insults to the developing brain (hypoxia, ischemia, infection, and malformation).

Studies to date have been unable to separate satisfactorily the effect of the seizures from the effect of the cause of the seizures.[61] Hypoglycemia is a good example. Infants with significant hypoglycemia are likely to have identifiable problems, whether or not they actually had neonatal hypoglycemic seizures.

Another curious example is the syndrome of benign familial neonatal seizures. In this condition, even the day of life in which the seizures occur may be characteristic. No sequelae occur in this condition, which suggests that seizures alone can occur without resultant damage to the brain.

Early hypocalcemia (often seen in stressed newborns) is another example of a relatively benign cause of neonatal seizures. These infants have an excellent chance of recovery without complications. It is wise not to be overaggressive in the correction of low calcium levels.

Separate from any discussion of the direct effect of seizures on the developing brain is the question of whether seizures in the newborn period predispose to later seizures. Again, cause seems to be the most important factor. Those seizures caused by transient metabolic changes that do not cause other permanent neurologic dysfunction are themselves likely to be transient and not occur outside the neonatal period. Seizures caused by congenital anomalies or those accompanied by obvious permanent brain damage are likely to persist.

Persistent seizures with structural brain damage are among those seizures that even later in life are hardest to control. Children who develop infantile spasms or the Lennox-Gastaut syndrome frequently have significant problems, including seizures in the neonatal period.

Important prognostic findings and signs can be grouped to provide a general guide to assess newborns with seizures. Factors favoring a good prognosis include transient metabolic causes (hypocalcemia, hypomagnesemia), normal neurologic examination, normal EEG findings, and benign familial neonatal seizures.

Factors favoring a poorer prognosis include the presence of a congenital malformation, seizures persisting for more than several days, severe birth asphyxia as the cause, presence of a major IVH, severely abnormal EEG findings (burst suppression, extremely low voltage, or isoelectric), or major signs on neurologic examination (hemisyndrome, multiple brainstem signs, and severe hypotonia with unresponsiveness).

Factors not carrying any particular prognostic significance include duration of individual seizures (other than status epilepticus), total number of seizures in the first few days of life, initial response to antiepileptic drug therapy, and presence of epilepsy in the patient's family.

Parent Teaching

Lay terms such as "fit" or "spell" provide a hint of the fear that seizure activity can instill in parents. Parent teaching should focus not only on providing pertinent information but also on the correction of existing misinformation. Parents may initially have difficulty believing that an infant is seizing because neonatal seizure is difficult to recognize. It is also not unusual for parents to expect staff to insert items in the mouth, perform CPR, restrain or shake the infant, etc., once they understand that the infant is seizing.

Parents may express an urgent and under-standable need to know the cause and the long-term outcomes of the seizure activity. It is important to supply careful explanations of tests being performed and their purpose in identification of the cause of the seizure. The long-term impact on the infant can be harder to predict for the parents, although the presence of certain factors can result in a poorer or better prognosis (see Complications and Outcome). Close follow-up after discharge by both medical and developmental services is vital.

Once home with the infant, the ability of care givers to recognize seizures and appropriately intervene is crucial. Careful documentation of teaching and parent understanding will allow the nursing staff to build on previous knowledge and skills. Parent handouts should focus on the skills and goals listed on this teaching checklist (Fig. 25-3). Care should be taken to use short, easy-to-understand sentences and to explain all terminology that parents might find confusing (i.e., what EEG is, etc.). Without parent handouts, attempting to teach the volume of information required is more stressful on both the care giver and the family. Even more importantly, handouts improve the retention of what has been learned.

Providing parents with a form on which to document seizures is also helpful. It can guide the parents in the appropriate observations to make during seizure activity: date, time, duration, seizure activities observed, color changes, behavior after seizure, etc. Parents should practice using this form while the infant is in the hospital so that staff can assist them with their assessments and documentation until they gain confidence. Parents should also administer the medications whenever possible during the infant's hospitalization in order to establish skills and to reinforce their confidence.

With the transition to the use of neonatal nurse practitioners (NNP) and physician assistants (PA) in the NICU, collaboration has been identified as essential to the provision of effective health care.[29] Certainly this holds true for the provision of effective discharge teaching as well, because the involvement with the multidisciplinary team approach to discharge planning is crucial. This planning and parental education must be initiated early in the hospitalization for successful outcomes.

BAPTIST MEDICAL CENTER
WOLFSON CHILDREN'S HOSPITAL
JACKSONVILLE, FLORIDA

Wolfson
Children's
HOSPITAL
at Baptist Medical Center

SEIZURE DISORDER FAMILY TEACHING CHECKLIST

GOAL/SKILL	PRESENTATION/ NURSE DEMONSTRATION DATE AND INITIAL	CARE GIVER/ PATIENT DEMONSTRATION DATE AND INITIAL	CARE GIVER/ PATIENT DEMONSTRATION DATE AND INITIAL	COMMENTS/ HANDOUTS DATE AND INITIAL
1. Verbalizes understanding of seizure pathophysiology.				Handouts given:
2. Describes signs that indicate a seizure.				
3. Lists important observations to make during a seizure.				"Seizure Recognition"
4. Describes care of a child during a seizure.				
5. Identifies child's a. medication, dosage and schedule b. side effects of anticonvulsants c. consequences of non-compliance d. correct administration of medication				Medication _____ Dosage _____ Schedule _____ Medication handout given _____
6. Verbalizes how to seek emergency assistance from home.				
7. Identifies resources for families with a child with a seizure disorder.				
VIDEOS FOR PARENTS (Date that care giver/ patient views)	_____ "How Medications Work" _____ "Understanding Seizure Disorders"			

Figure 25-3   Seizure disorder Family Teaching checklist. (Courtesy of Wolfson Children's Hospital, Jacksonville, Fla, 1996.)

Hypoxic-Ischemic Encephalopathy

Physiology

A common identified cause of brain damage in newborns is HIE.[25,29,56,60] Hypoxemia refers to a diminished amount of oxygen in the blood, and ischemia refers to a diminished amount of blood perfused in the brain. Asphyxia refers to the impairment of the exchange of respiratory gases, implying low oxygen and high carbon dioxide in the blood.[35]

Etiology

The timing may be antepartum (i.e., before the onset of labor) with faulty placental gas exchange because of maladies such as diabetes or prediabetes in the mother or preeclampsia.[36] IUGR suggests a chronic antepartum circulatory insult.

The antepartum insult may be acute (e.g., acute hypotension in the mother or placental separation with uterine hemorrhage).

Intrapartum asphyxia may be due to cord strangulation or placental problems, such as abruptio, during labor. Difficult delivery with transverse arrest would be another example of intrapartum cause or contribution to asphyxia. More rare in the term infant are postnatal causes. In the premature infant, RDS, prolonged apnea, severe cyanotic congenital heart disease, or enlarged patent ductus might affect gas exchange enough to result in asphyxia. Many times, a combined insult (intrapartum and antepartum) may be causative.

About 1 to 2 per 1000 newborns experience HIE; 0.3 per 1000 have permanent sequelae.

Data Collection

Prevention

Prevention and management of this entity include optimizing prenatal, parturitional, and postnatal care.

History

Infants with intrapartum cause of HIE show symptoms as a newborn. These infants will have fetal distress in utero, will be depressed at birth, and will have prolonged low Apgar scores. Most have evidence of systemic organ damage: renal, cardiac, and sometimes pulmonary dysfunction will be readily apparent, accompanying the neurologic features of HIE. Diagnosis of HIE depends on careful prenatal and perinatal history and a thorough postnatal neurologic exam. Severe and persistent neurologic findings suggest an unfavorable prognosis.

Signs and Symptoms

Multiple diagnostic criteria have confused the recognition of intrapartum asphyxia in the term infant.[11] Diagnosis of acute perinatal asphyxia should meet one of the three sets of criteria in the Report of the Workshop on Acute Perinatal Asphyxia in Term Infants.[63] The basic requirement for making this diagnosis is a pH <7.0 with a five minute Apgar score of ≤3. The addition of abnormal fetal heart rate patterns to these two parameters has been used to develop a scoring system that improves the predictive value of these parameters.[47] The American Academy of Pediatrics/American College of Obstetricians and Gynecologists add multiple organ system failure and neurologic sequelae to their definition.[3]

The neurologic syndrome presents as stupor or coma, ventilatory problems (e.g., periodic breathing or apnea), hypotonia, and often, early onset seizures.[48] The seizures, often subtle, may be epileptic seizures (i.e., with brain electrical discharges), or the seizures may be nonepileptic release phenomenon such as decerebrate/decorticate posturing. There may be extraocular movement and pupillary irregularities (e.g., miosis or unequal pupils).

In the next few days, seizures, apnea, hypotonia, jitteriness, weakness, and even respiratory arrest may occur. In the premature infant, IVH may be catastrophic. Increased intracranial pressure with or without respiratory arrest may happen in the most severely involved infants. In those infants who survive, tube feedings, weak suck, and continued stupor may persist for days to weeks.

Laboratory Data

Metabolic or laboratory parameters will often be abnormal, and blood gases and pH should be assessed. Acidosis, hypoxemia, and hypercarbia are frequent findings. Other parameters possibly needing correction include a low blood sugar (hypoglycemia), hypocalcemia, hyponatremia, and more rarely, hyperammonemia. Creatine phosphokinase, especially the BB (brain fraction), correlates with parenchymal brain damage.

One should sample the spinal fluid to see if there is bleeding and to rule out infectious possibilities. The professional should also monitor the infant with an EEG for seizures. In a term infant, a severely abnormal pattern such as burst suppression, very low amplitude, or isoelectric EEG suggest an ominous prognosis.

Ultrasound done accurately may show periventricular increased echodensities, later to become lucencies, even large cysts or cystic encephalomalacia.

Early computerized axial tomography (CAT) scans may show cerebral edema, sometimes difficult to quantify and to differentiate from the normal brain in a newborn. Hemorrhagic lesions are clearly seen. The CAT scan has more utility in follow-up, showing location of white matter malacia, basal ganglia lesions, etc.

MRI may show cortical necrosis on a T1 weighted image and loss of the gray-white delineation on T2.

Treatment

Treatment includes the broad principles of adequate ventilation, gas exchange, and perfusion; maintenance of normal glucose and electrolyte levels; control of seizures; and prevention and control of brain swelling.

New therapies may include excitotoxic amino acid antagonists and free-radical scavengers.[31] These are the same new approaches taken for management of stroke and ischemic brain damage in adults.

Complications

A variety of sequelae may result from selective neuronal necrosis and periventricular leukomalacia.[18] The former often correlates with mental retardation, spastic quadriparesis, seizure disorder, ataxia, pseudo-bulbar palsy, and attention deficit hyperactivity disorder. Periventricular leukomala-

cia has been most commonly associated with spastic diplegia.

Prognosis, of course, depends on the severity of the insult, but in large studies, 50% of affected infants have normal outcome, 20% to 30% have abnormal sequelae, and 10% to 30% die with the more unfavorable statistics noted in prematures.[45,56]

Intraventricular Hemorrhage

Physiology

The problem of bleeding into and around the ventricular system has received more attention in the last decade than any other neurologic problem in the neonate. In large measure, this relates to the frequency with which the problem develops, generally estimated to be 20% to 30% in premature infants under 32 weeks' gestational age or less than 1500 g. The growth of routine cranial ultrasound examination in premature infants is directly due to this common problem. Recently, the incidence of these hemorrhages has appeared to be decreasing. With the advent of CT and ultrasound scanning, a large number of infants have been recognized who were not suspected of having an intraventricular bleed but who were diagnosed on scans.

Although the bleeding is regularly spoken of as intraventricular and intracranial hemorrhage, these terms do not accurately reflect its etiology. Highly vascularized areas, with relatively fragile and poorly supported blood vessels, are the source of bleeding.

In term infants the choroid plexus of the lateral ventricles is the most common site in which bleeding originates. In premature infants the germinal matrix, in the subependymal area adjacent to the caudate nucleus, is the primary site of bleeding. Both of these are areas of high arterial and capillary blood flow; in addition, they use an anatomically awkward venous drainage system, eventually draining into the internal cerebral vein (Fig. 25-4).

The extent of bleeding generally predicts the likelihood of complications and residua. Bleeding may be confined to the germinal matrix or the choroid plexus, or it may enter the ventricular system. When filled under pressure, the ventricular

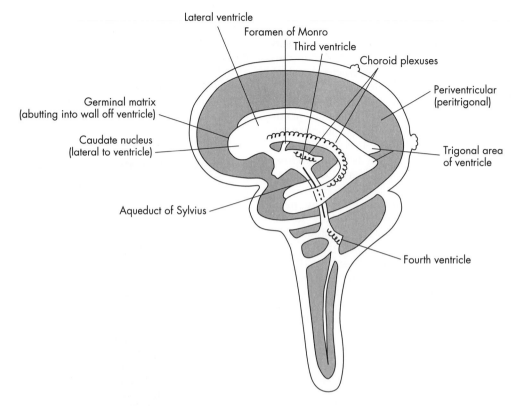

Lateral ventricle
Foramen of Monro
Third ventricle
Choroid plexuses
Periventricular
(peritrigonal)
Germinal matrix
(abutting into wall off ventricle)
Caudate nucleus
(lateral to ventricle)
Trigonal area
of ventricle
Aqueduct of Sylvius
Fourth ventricle

Figure 25-4   Central nervous system/ventricular system.

system may dilate. Blood may also extravasate out into the brain parenchyma (more likely with germinal matrix bleeding than with choroid plexus bleeding).

Several classification schemes have been used, each trying to assess the degree of bleeding or amount of blood present. Ideally, a classification should relate to pathophysiology, treatment, or outcome, but with present knowledge this is not possible.

A classification based on the extent of hemorrhage seen on the CT scan grades germinal matrix hemorrhages as follows (Fig. 25-5):

0—No bleeding
I—Germinal matrix only
II—Germinal matrix with blood in the ventricles

III—Germinal matrix with blood in the ventricles and hydrocephalus
IV—Intraventricular and parenchymal bleeding (other than germinal matrix)

Etiology

The factors identified in infants who have experienced IVH are multiple. These include asphyxia, severe respiratory distress, pneumothorax, hypoglycemia, shock, acidosis, blood transfusions, seizures, and rapid volume expansion. What appears to be the common factor underlying the pathology is a fluctuation in cerebral blood flow.[11,55,58,59]

At times, this may have a systemic counterpart, such as in shock. At other times, changes in brain perfusion occur without any reflection in systemic blood pressure, pulse, or respiration. The fragility

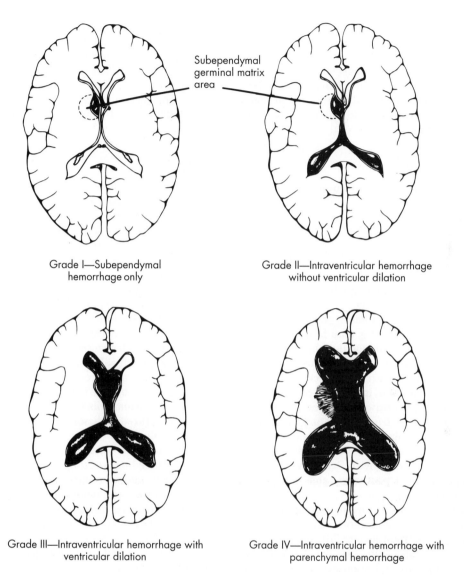

Subependymal
germinal matrix
area

Grade I—Subependymal
hemorrhage only

Grade II—Intraventricular hemorrhage
without ventricular dilation

Grade III—Intraventricular hemorrhage with
ventricular dilation

Grade IV—Intraventricular hemorrhage with
parenchymal hemorrhage

Figure 25-5 Periventricular-intraventricular hemorrhage, Grades I-IV. (Rozmus C: Periventricular-intraventricular hemorrhage in the newborn, *MCN* 17(2):79, 1992. Used with permission of Lippincott-Raven Publishers, Philadelphia, Pa.)

of the germinal matrix and choroid plexus seem to allow for the disruption of capillary or small blood vessel integrity with resultant bleeding.

Intraventricular bleeding tends to occur in the first few hours or days of life. The profound physiologic changes normally seen after birth are coupled with the multiple problems (primarily cardiorespiratory) typically experienced by the premature infant to make intraventricular bleeding common. The degree to which the aggressive management of premature newborns has a role in the development of bleeding cannot be accurately assessed. In general, although not exclusively, it is the sicker infants who both require more intervention and have a greater likelihood of bleeding. **The decreased incidence of intraventricular bleeding with antenatal (but not with neonatal) phenobarbital administration suggests a role for prenatal and intrapartum events in the etiology of intraventricular bleeding.**

Data Collection

As has been suggested previously, the historical information is somewhat varied. Some infants, generally those who are at term, will have IVH associated with severe asphyxia.

Premature infants often show one or more of the following: birth weight less than 1500 g, gestational age less than 34 weeks, shock, RDS, need for blood transfusions, coagulopathy, hyperviscosity, hypoxia, and birth asphyxia.

Because premature infants, particularly those weighing less than 1500 g, tend to have multiple problems, it is not surprising that the clinical presentation of germinal matrix hemorrhage may range from subtle (or even undetectable) to catastrophic. Deterioration in clinical condition followed by apnea, flaccid quadriparesis, unresponsiveness, and death from circulatory collapse is a recognizable syndrome. Common signs of germinal matrix hemorrhage include apnea, hypotension, drop in hematocrit, flaccidity, areflexia, full fontanel, tonic posturing, and oculomotor disturbances.

When intracranial bleeding is suspected, appropriate studies of intracranial structures should be performed as soon as possible. In the case of periventricular-intraventricular hemorrhage both ultrasonography and CT scanning are useful tools for defining the presence of bleeding and for following its evolution. Because sonography is the safer procedure and uses no radiation, it should be used for follow-up.

Treatment and Intervention

The primary treatment of IVH is confined to supportive care. Ventilatory support, maintenance of oxygenation, regulation of acid-base balance, suppression of seizures, and treatment of any attendant coagulopathy are all extremely important

in reducing mortality and morbidity. The role that successful management has in the amelioration or prevention of complications is unclear.

Many therapies have been proposed or used but remain unproved. These are listed here not to recommend them for general clinical use, but to suggest the ways in which the problem has been approached.

When the hemorrhage is confined to the germinal matrix, little can be done even from a theoretic standpoint.

The removal of blood from the ventricular system has been used for many years as a treatment for IVH. Many studies have shown it to have limited effectiveness. The rationale for removing blood is two-fold: (1) to remove an irritating substance from the ventricular system, at the same time reducing clot formation, and (2) to remove protein in the hope of preventing hydrocephalus. Yet, because of high spinal fluid protein levels and the potential for a block in the flow of fluid, there is a concern that repeated lumbar punctures may be ineffective in clearing blood from the ventricles.

Lumbar puncture has much less chance of morbidity and is the preferred procedure. Ventricular taps can be used but are rarely recommended.

Intraventricular fibrinolytics (streptokinase) have been utilized to dissolve the clot and prevent hydrocephalus.

Care must be given to reduce the risk for continued bleeding, working to maintain perfusion of the brain and to reduce wide fluctuations in blood pressure, oxygenation, and pH.

Another theoretical (and unproved) objection to these methods suggests that removing blood will allow for further bleeding by reducing the pressure in the ventricles and therefore upsetting the homeostatic balance.

Medications to reduce intracranial pressure and therefore treat secondary effects of the bleeding include furosemide, acetazolamide, and steroid agents. Mannitol and glycerol have also been used. The same unproved argument concerning upsetting the homeostatic balance may be applied here.

Helpful pharmacologic preventatives (glucocorticoids and possibly phenobarbital prenatally and indomethacin, vitamin E, and phenobarbital postnatally) have had some success.[28,35,43,46,54]

Apparently, the best recommendation for the treatment of IVH is to continue the management of

ensuing problems without undue attention to the intracranial bleeding.

Complications

The complications from IVH relate to the underlying causes and the extent of bleeding. Massive bleeding with dilation of the ventricular system is much more likely to cause an acute change in brain function, with increased intracranial pressure, brainstem findings, and apnea. Milder degrees of hemorrhage may be asymptomatic or associated with seizurelike events, changes in muscle tone, or apnea.

When bleeding extends into the parenchyma, porencephaly may result from liquefactive necrosis or ischemic-induced encephalomalacia. Follow-up structural brain studies may show hypodense areas where blood was present; later they may show areas of porencephaly.

The most common complication is posthemorrhagic hydrocephalus. The possibility of this developing is directly related to the severity of the hemorrhage, with up to 10% of survivors of mild IVH and 65% to 100% of survivors of severe IVH showing progressive ventricular dilation. Posthemorrhagic hydrocephalus should be sought in all survivors of germinal matrix hemorrhage. CT scanning or ultrasonography to assess ventricular size should be used. Clinical signs alone are not reliable.[30]

With the hope of avoiding a shunt, some attempts at control of the hydrocephalus have been attempted. Osmotic and diuretic agents, including furosemide, isosorbide, and acetazolamide, have been used to reduce the formation of CSF. Some clinicians have been enthusiastic about this approach, but it has not gained widespread acceptance. As mentioned previously, lumbar and intraventricular taps are sometimes used in an attempt to avoid shunting. This approach holds anecdotal promise but has not been adequately proved. In some small premature infants, ventricular drainage without a full shunt (to the peritoneal cavity) is used.

Outcome studies have been difficult to assess. Clearly, the sickest infants tend to do poorly. They also tend to have more complications, including CNS complications. There is a clear correlation between the grade of bleed and the likelihood of significant neurologic residua, but the correlation is far from perfect. The influence of other factors on neurologic outcome may be more significant than the actual bleed itself. Hypoxia, hypoperfusion, and other conditions known to damage the developing nervous system cannot easily be separated as individual factors in outcome.[51] Patients with grade 1 and 2 hemorrhages usually do as well as patients with no hemorrhage. Patients with grade 3 and 4 hemorrhages most often have long-term morbidity.

Parent Teaching

It is of particular importance to involve the parents of an infant with IVH with the care plan. The rationale for a minimal handling protocol needs to be explained. Encouraging parents to participate in setting "time out" and "touch me" times will facilitate their ability to visit and assist with care. During visits, they should be encouraged to recognize signs of overstimulation and appropriate interventions.[11,17,22]

The infant with IVH will have varying degrees of problems. Often the acute situation resolves without ongoing problems. In these cases, parents should understand the possible complications such as hydrocephalus that may occur in the short term. Teaching the parents to measure head circumference and alerting them to the signs of increased intracranial pressure such as poor feeding, posturing, eye movement difficulties, full fontanel, and lethargy will enable them to participate more fully in the medical follow-up (see Box 25-2).

Parents must understand the risk for long-term neurologic sequelae. Even though these sequelae are difficult to predict with any degree of certainty, parents should understand that mental and motor handicaps, delays in the acquisition of milestones, seizures, and problems associated with hydrocephalus and potential shunt placement may occur. Specific preparation for these potential problems should begin in the nursery but will be increased during follow-up visits if the possibility for such problems seems greater.

References

1. Aicardi J: Disorders of neuronal migration: a spectrum of cortical abnormalities, *Int Pediatr* 8:162, 1993.

2. Altman N et al: Advanced MRI of disorders of neuronal migration and sulcation, *Int Pediatr* 10 (Suppl 1):16, 1995.
3. American Academy of Pediatrics/American College of Obstetricians and Gynecologists: *Guidelines for perinatal care,* ed 3, Elk Grove Village, Ill, 1992, American Academy of Pediatrics.
4. Ballweg DD: Neonatal seizures: an overview, *Neonat Net* 10(1):15, 1991.
5. Barkovich AV et al: Normal maturation of neonatal and infant brain: MR imaging at 1.5 T., *Radiology* 166:173, 1988.
6. Bernes SM, Kaplan AM: Evolution of neonatal seizures, *Pediatr Clin North Am* 41:1069, 1994.
7. Bourgeois BFD, Dodson WE: Phenytoin elimination in newborns, *Neurology* 33:173, 1983.
8. Camfield PR, Camfield CS: Neonatal seizures: a commentary on selected aspects, *J Child Neurol* 2:244, 1987.
9. Carter BS, Haverkamp, AD, Merenstein GB: The definition of acute perinatal asphyxia, *Clin Perinatol* 20:287, 1993.
10. Clancy R et al: Focal motor seizures heralding stroke in full-term infants, *Am J Dis Child* 139:601, 1985.
11. Cordis Corporation: *Hydrocephalus and shunts; Your valve system for hydrocephalus; and Just like any other beagle,* parent handouts, 1989.
12. Dietch JS: Periventricular-intraventricular hemorrhage in the very low birth weight infant, *Neonat Net* 12(1):7, 1993.
13. Edwards MSB: Fetal hydrocephalus, *Int Pediatr* 2:89, 1987.
14. Fischer JH et al: Phenobarbital maintenance dose requirements in treating neonatal seizures, *Neurology* 31:1042, 1981.
15. Fujii et al: Corpus callosum in developmentally retarded infants, *Pediatr Neurol* 11:219, 1994.
16. Gal P et al: Efficacy of phenobarbital monotherapy in treatment of neonatal seizures: relationship to blood levels, *Neurology* 32:1401, 1982.
17. Gennaro S: Facilitating and parenting of the neonatal intensive care unit graduate, *J Perinat Neonat Nurs* 4(4):55, 1991.
18. Goetz MC et al: Incidence, timing, and follow-up of periventricular leukomalacia, *Am J Perinatol* 12:325, 1995.
19. Hahn JS: Controversies in treatment of neonatal seizures, *Pediatr Neurol* 9:330, 1993.
20. Hankins GDV, Clark SL: Brachial plexus palsy involving the posterior shoulder at spontaneous vaginal delivery, *Am J Periatol* 12:325, 1995.
21. Harrison H, Kositsky A: *The premature baby book,* New York, 1983, St Martin's Press.
22. Haskins R, Finkelstein NW, Stedman DJ: Infant stimulation programs and their effects, *Pediatr Ann* 7:123, 1978.
23. Halslam RAH: Section 543.5: neonatal seizures. In Behrman R, editor: *Nelson textbook of pediatrics,* ed 15, Philadelphia, 1996, WB Saunders.
24. Holmes GL: Neonatal seizures, *Acta Neuroped* 1:241, 1995.
25. Hull J, Dodd KL: Falling incidence of hypoxic-ischemic encephalopathy in term infants, *Br J Obstet Gynaecol* 99:386, 1992.
26. Hummel PA, Eastman DL: Do parents of preterm infants suffer chronic sorrow? *Neonat Net* 10(4):59, 1991.
27. Kaempf SW et al: Antenatal phenobarbital for the prevention of periventricular and intraventricular hemorrhage: a double-blind, randomized placebo controlled multihospital trial, *J Pediatr* 111:931, 1990.
28. Leviton A et al: Antenatal corticosteroids appear to reduce risk of postnatal germinal matrix hemorrhage in intubated low birth weight newborn, *Pediatrics* 81:1083, 1993.
29. Leviton A, Nelson KB: Problems with definitions and classifications of newborn ecephalopathy, *Pediatr Neurol* 8:85, 1992.
30. Lin JP et al: Neurological outcome following neonatal post-haemorrhagic hydrocephalus: the effects of maximum raised intracranial pressure and ventriculo-peritoneal shunting, *Child Nerv Syst* 8:190, 1992.
31. Little GA, Russ Frank ME: Transition from housestaff in neonatal intensive care unit, *Am J Perinatol* 13:127, 1996.
32. Lombroso C: Neonatal seizures: historic note and present controversies, *Epilepsia* 37(suppl 3):5, 1996.
33. Martin-Padilla M: Review of perinatal brain damage in premature born infant, *Int Pediatr* 10(suppl 1):26, 1995.
34. McLone D et al: *An introduction to hydrocephalus,* handout, Chicago, 1982, Children's Memorial Hospital.
35. Ment LR et al: Low-dose indomethacin and prevention of intraventricular hemorrhage: a multicenter randomized trial, *Pediatric* 93:543, 1994.
36. Miles MS et al: Sources of support reported by mothers and father of infants hospitalized in a neonatal intensive care unit, *Neonat Net* 15(3):45, 1996.
37. Nelson KB, Leviton A: Problems with definition and classification of newborn encephalopathy, *Pediatr Neurol* 8:85, 1992.
38. Nelson KB, Leviton A: How much of neonatal encephalopathy is due to birth asphyxia? *Am J Dis Child* 143:1325, 1991.
39. Painter MJ, Gaus LM: Neonatal seizures: diagnosis and treatment, *J Child Neurol* 6:101, 1991.
40. Painter MJ: Brachial plexus injuries in neonates, *Int Pediatr* 3:120, 1988.
41. Palmer C, Vannucci RC: Potential new therapies for perinatal cerebral hypoxia-ischemia, *Clin Perinatol* 20:411, 1953.
42. *Physician's Desk Reference (PDR),* ed 50, Montvale NJ, 1996, Medical Economics Data Production Company.
43. Poland SRL: Vitamin E for prevention of intracranial hemorrhage, *Pediatrics* 85:865, 1090.
44. Portman RJ et al: Predicting neonatal morbidity after perinatal asphyxia: a scoring system, *Am J Obstet Gynecol* 162:174, 1990.
45. Robertston CM, Finer NM: Long-term follow-up of term neonates with perinatal asphyxia, *Clin Perinatol* 20:483, 1993.
46. Rozmus C: Periventricular-intraventricular hemorrhage in the newborn, *Maternal Child Nurs* 17:74, 1992.
47. Rust RS, Volpe JJ: Neonatal seizures in pediatric epilepsy: diagnosis and therapy. In Dodson WE, Pellock JM, editors: Demos, NY, 1993, Demos.
48. Sarnat HB: Disturbances of late neuronal migrations in the perinatal period, *Am J Dis Child* 141:969, 1987.

49. Scher MS, Painter MJ et al: EEG diagnoses of neonatal seizures: clinical correlations and outcome, *Pediatr Neurol* 5:17, 1989.
50. Sellinger C: Brachial plexus injuries, *Pediatr Rev* 13:77, 1992.
51. Shinnar S et al: Intraventricular hemorrhage in the premature infant: a changing outlook, *N Engl J Med* 306:1464, 1982.
52. Smith BT, Masotti RE: Intravenous diazepam in the treatment of prolonged seizure activity in neonates and infants, *Dev Med Child Neurol* 13:630, 1971.
53. Stafstrom CE: Neonatal seizures, *Pediatr Rev* 16:248, 1995.
54. Thorp JA et al: Antepartum vitamin K and phenobarbital for preventing intraventricular hemorrhage in the premature newborn: a randomized, double-blind, placebo-controlled trial, *Obstet Gynecol* 83:70, 1994.
55. Volpe JJ: Neonatal intracranial hemorrhage: pathophysiology, neuropathology and clinical features, *Clin Perinatal* 4:77, 1977.
56. Volpe JJ: *Neurology of the newborn,* ed 3, Philadelphia, 1995, WB Saunders.
57. Volpe JJ: Normal and abnormal human brain development, *Clin Perinatol* 4:3, 1977.
58. Volpe JJ: Intraventricular hemorrhage and brain injury in the premature infant: neuropathology and pathogenesis, *Clin Perinatol* 16:361, 1989.
59. Volpe JJ: Intraventricular hemorrhage and brain injury in the premature infant: diagnosis, prognosis and prevention, *Clin Perinatol* 16:387, 1989.
60. Volpe JJ: Brain injury in the premature infant: current concepts, *Biol Neonat* 69:165, 1956.
61. Webb R, Bobele G: "Benign" familial neonatal convulsions, *J Child Neurol* 5:295, 1990.
62. Wiscal BS: Neonatal seizures and electrographic analysis: evaluation and outcomes, *Pediatr Neurol* 10:271, 1994.
63. Wright LL, Merenstein GB, Hirtz DG, editors: *Report of the workshop on acute perinatal asphyxia in term infants,* Bethesda, 1996, NIH.
64. Young TE, Mangum OB: *Neofax,* ed 9, Raleigh, NC, 1996, Acorn Publishing.

Selected Readings

Allan W, Volpe JJ: Periventricular-intraventricular hemorrhage, *Pediatr Clin North Am* 36:47, 1986.
Barkovich AJ: *Pediatric neuroimaging,* ed 2, New York, 1995, Raven Press.
Brazelton TB: *Neonatal behavioral assessment scale. Clinics in developmental medicine, No. 50,* Philadelphia, 1973, JB Lippincott.
Cunningham M: Intraventricular hemorrhage of the newborn, *Dimens Crit Care* 6:1, 1987.
Fenichel GM: *Neonatal neurology,* New York, 1980, Churchill-Livingstone.
Giles FH et al, editors: *The developing human brain,* Boston, 1983, John Wright/PSG.
Hellman J, Vannucci R: Intraventricular hemorrhage in premature infants, *Semin Perinatol* 6:42, 1982.
Korobkin R, Guilleminault C, editors: *Advances in perinatal neurology,* vol 1, New York, 1979, Spectrum Books.
Kuban K, Teale R: Rationale for grading intracranial hemorrhage in premature infants, *Pediatrics* 74:358, 1984.
Lemire RJ et al: *Normal and abnormal development of the nervous system,* New York, 1975, Harper & Row.
MacDonald M et al: Timing and antecedents of intracranial hemorrhage in the newborn, *Pediatrics* 74:32, 1984.
McLone DG et al: *An introduction to hydrocephalus,* Chicago, 1982, Children's Memorial Hospital.
Morselli PL et al, editors: *Antiepileptic drug therapy in pediatrics,* New York, 1983, Raven Press.
Painter MJ, Berman I, Crumrine P: Neonatal seizures, *Pediatr Clin North Am* 33:91, 1986.
Powell MJ, Painter MJ, Pippenger CE: Primidine therapy in refractory neonatal seizures, *J Pediatr* 15:651, 1984.
Shankaran S, Kottamasu S, Kuhns L: Perinatal asphyxia, *Clin Perinatol* 20:379, 1993.
Swaiman KF, Wright FS, editors: *The practice of pediatric neurology,* ed 2, St Louis, 1982, Mosby.

26 Genetic Disorders, Malformations, and Inborn Errors of Metabolism

Eva Sujansky, Anne L. Matthews

The neonate born with a malformation, genetic syndrome, or an acute metabolic disorder represents a management challenge for the staff of the NICU. If these conditions are not suspected and diagnosed in the critically ill neonate, an inappropriate course of action might be taken. Thus a specific diagnosis becomes imperative. An accurate diagnosis provides the staff with information regarding etiology, treatment, and prognosis necessary for initiation of the most appropriate care of the infant. Moreover, broader issues of providing supportive care and counseling for the affected infant's family can be addressed.

The genetic evaluation is a complex process that requires expertise in the ability to differentiate normal variations from abnormal and a knowledge of the principles of embryology and dysmorphology to provide an accurate diagnosis. Skills in obtaining detailed information of prenatal and family histories may be equally important.

The field of medical genetics has witnessed an explosion of new knowledge regarding the processes of heredity and its effect on human health. This chapter is a concise overview of the major categories of genetic disorders and the appropriate techniques to establish specific diagnoses. For an excellent review and detailed explanation of concepts, terminology, and specific genetic mechanisms refer to Thompson's text, *Genetics in Medicine,* fifth edition. See the Glossary for a comprehensive list of terms.

Genetic Principles

Gene

A **gene** is a segment of a DNA molecule coded for the synthesis of a single polypeptide and contains the hereditary information needed for development or function. DNA, which allows for the storing, duplicating, and processing of hereditary information, consists of two long strands twisted around each other to form a double helix. Each strand of DNA is composed of four nucleotides: guanine (G), adenine (A), thymine (T), and cytosine (C). The specific order of the nucleotides determines the precise information that will be coded at that site. Genes can regulate other genes by turning them on or off, specify the exact structure of proteins, which then control the activities of the cells, and specify RNA, which is required for protein synthesis.

Chromosomes

Genes are packed in linear order on chromosomes. **Chromosomes** are found in the nuclei of cells. In humans, normal somatic cells contain 46 chromosomes (**diploid** number), of which 44 are termed **autosomes** and 2 are **sex chromosomes.** Females have two X chromosomes (XX), and males have an X and a Y chromosome (XY). Gametes, eggs or sperm, contain 23 chromosomes (**haploid** number). In the zygote and somatic cells, chromosomes are paired (**homologs**). In each pair, one homolog is maternal and the other is paternal in origin. Each chromosomal pair has unique morphologic characteristics that allow it to be distinguished from other chromosomes, such as size, position of the centromere, and the unique banding pattern that is demonstrated by special staining techniques[3] (Fig. 26-1, *A* and *B*).

To pass on the genetic information to daughter cells, the chromosomes must replicate and then divide correctly. Somatic cells undergo **mitosis,** in which cells replicate and then divide chromosomal material into two genetically indentical daughter cells with 46 chromosomes each. In gametes, the

Glossary

Acrocentric chromosome Chromosomes with the centromere near the end of the chromosome.

Allele One of a series of alternate forms of a gene at the same locus.

Aneuploid Any chromosome number that is not an exact multiple of the haploid set.

Autosome A chromosome that is not a sex chromosome.

Centromere The primary constriction of a chromosome where the long and short arms meet.

Chromatid After replication of a chromosome, two subunits attached by the centromere can be seen; each is called a chromatid, and after separation each becomes a chromosome of a daughter cell.

Chromosome The microscopic structures in the cell nucleus composed of DNA and proteins that contain the genes.

Congenital Present at birth.

Dermatoglyphics The dermal ridge patterns on the digits, palms, and soles.

Diploid Two copies of all chromosomes; the number of chromosomes normally present in somatic cells. In humans, this is 46 and is sometimes symbolized as 2N.

Dominant A gene (allele) that is expressed clinically in the heterozygous state. In a dominant disorder the mutant allele overshadows the normal allele.

Dysmorphic Morphological abnormality, often a minor physical finding that may or may not have any cosmetic or functional significance and is present in less than 4% of the newborn population.

Fluorescent in situ hybridization (FISH) Molecular cytogenetic method for detection of microdeletions of chromosomes.

Gamete Mature reproductive cell, the egg or the sperm, containing the haploid number of chromosomes.

Gene The functional unit of heredity.

Genotype A person's genetic constitution.

Haploid One copy of all chromosomes; the number of chromosomes present in the gamete; in humans this is 23 and can be symbolized as N.

Hemizygous The condition in which only one copy of a gene is normally present, and so its effect is expressed because there is no counterpart gene present; e.g., the genes on the X or Y chromosome of the male.

Heterozygote An individual who has two different alleles at a given locus of two homologous chromosomes.

Homologous chromosomes Members of the same chromosome pair; normally they have the same number and arrangement of genes.

Homozygote An individual who has two identical alleles at a given locus of two homologous chromosomes.

Karyotype The standard pictorial arrangement of chromosome pairs, numbered according to centromere position and length.

Locus The position or place that a gene occupies on a chromosome.

Malformation A primary structural defect that results from a localized error of morphogenesis; abnormal development.

Metacentric chromosome Chromosomes with the centromere in the center of the chromosome.

Monosomy When one chromosome of one pair is missing.

Mosaicism Presence in the same individual of two or more different chromosomal constitutions.

Mutation A heritable alteration in the genetic material.

Nondisjunction Failure of two homologous chromosomes to separate equally during cell division into two daughter cells, resulting in abnormal chromosome numbers in gametes or somatic cells.

Phenotype The observable expression of traits either physically or biochemically.

Recessive A gene (allele) that is expressed clinically in the homozygous state. In a recessive disorder, both genes at a given locus must be abnormal to manifest the disorder.

Sex chromosomes The X and Y chromosomes.

Syndrome Recognizable pattern of multiple malformations that occur together and have the same etiology.

Transcription The process by which complementary messenger RNA is synthesized from a DNA template.

Translation The process whereby the amino acids in a given polypeptide are synthesized from the messenger RNA template.

Translocation Transfer of all or part of a chromosome to another location (i.e., on the same or another chromosome) after chromosome breakage.

Trisomy The presence of three homologous chromosomes rather than the normal two.

X-linked A gene located on an X chromosome.

Zygote A fertilized egg that develops into the embryo.

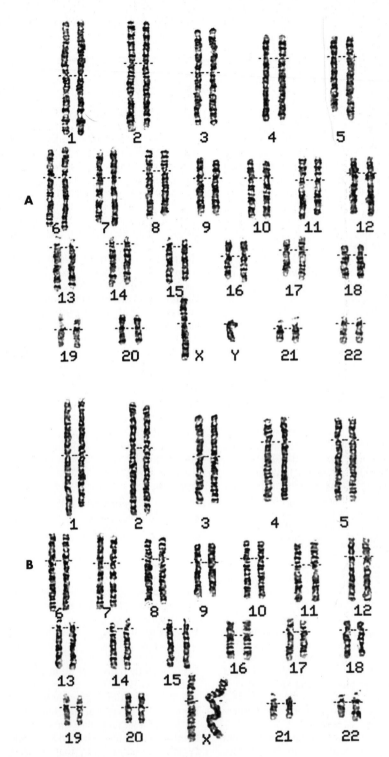

Figure 26-1 **A,** Normal male karyotype. **B,** Normal female karyotype. Each karyotype contains 46 chromosomes (44 autosomes and 2 sex chromosomes, *XY,* male; *XX,* female.) The autosomes are numbered from 1 to 22. Note banding pattern, unique for each chromosomal pair. (Courtesy Cytogenics, The Children's Hospital, Denver, Colorado.)

process is known as **meiosis,** which is different from mitotic division in that daughter cells contain the haploid number of chromosomes (23) and crossing over or recombination between two homologs occurs, thus facilitating genetic variation in offspring.[21]

An individual's chromosome constitution can be determined by examining dividing body cells under certain laboratory conditions from any accessible tissue such as blood lymphocytes or skin fibroblasts. The resulting **karyotype** (see Fig. 26-1, A and B) or pictorial arrangement demonstrates the number and structure of that individual's chromosomes.

Etiology

Malformations and genetic disorders caused wholly or partly by genetic factors can be categorized into four major areas: (1) chromosomal disorders caused by numeric or structural abnormalities of chromosomes; (2) single-gene or mendelian disorders, which are secondary to single-gene mutations; (3) multifactorial disorders resulting from interaction of multiple genes and environmental influences; and (4) abnormalities caused by environmental exposures of the fetus during development.

More recently, better understanding of molecular processes has allowed the identification of additional genetic mechanisms contributing to genetic disorders: gonadal mosaicism, genomic imprinting, and uniparental disomy.

Chromosomal Disorders

Chromosomal abnormalities are relatively common. Approximately 0.5% to 0.7% of all live newborns and 4% to 7% of perinatal deaths are the result of a chromosomal abnormality. Moreover, it is estimated that at least 50% of all recognized first-trimester miscarriages are due to a chromosomal aberration.[4] Newer cytogenetic techniques, such as high-resolution banding, have increased the detection rate of chromosomal aberrations. Minute deletions, duplications, or other abnormal rearrangements of chromosome material that may not have been identified a few years ago are now being detected in children with congenital malformations and/or mental retardation.

Chromosomal aberrations should be suspected in any of the following situations:

- **Small for gestational age for weight, length, and/or head circumference**
- **Presence of one or more congenital malformations**
- **Presence of dysmorphic features**
- **Neurologic/neuromuscular dysfunction**
- **Family history of multiple miscarriages or siblings with mental retardation or birth defects along with one of the above**

Chromosomal abnormalities can be classified into two major categories: abnormalities of chromosome number (**aneuploidy**), in which there is an extra or missing chromosome, and abnormalities of chromosome structure that result in the loss or duplication of part of the chromosomal material. Abnormalities of autosomes usually have more significant deleterious effects on the development of the infant than those seen with sex chromosome abnormalities.

Abnormalities of Chromosome Number

Numeric chromosomal abnormalities occur as a result of nondisjunction in which aberrant segregation leads to loss or gain of one or more chromosomes. Nondisjunction can occur during either meiosis or mitosis, resulting in an abnormal gamete (egg or sperm) or abnormal somatic cell, respectively (Fig. 26-2). Fertilization of an aneuploid gamete by a normal gamete produces a zygote with an extra chromosome (**trisomy**) or missing chromosome (**monosomy**). Aneuploidy in somatic cells results in chromosomal **mosaicism** (i.e., the presence of some cells with the normal number of chromosomes and other cells with an abnormal number of chromosomes) (Fig. 26-3). Although nondisjunction may affect any chromosomal pair, the most commonly recognized trisomies in liveborns are trisomy 21 (Down syndrome), trisomy 18 (Edward syndrome), and trisomy 13 (Patau syndrome). On the other hand, trisomy 16 has been found exclusively in spontaneous abortions.[4] The most common monosomy is 45,X,

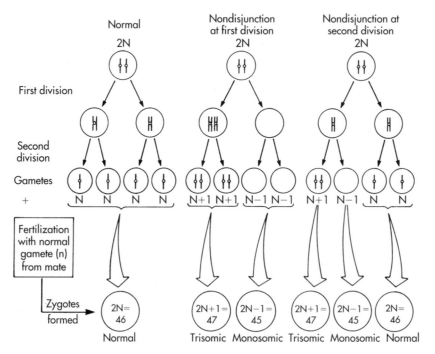

Figure 26-2   Nondisjunction. During formation of gametes, errors of nondisjunction can occur during either first or second meiotic division.

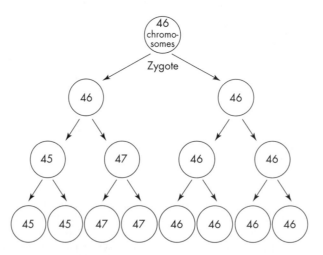

Figure 26-3   Mosaicism. Nondisjunction occurring after fertilization and zygote formation results in some cells containing the normal 46-chromosome complement and other cells having an abnormal number of chromosomes.

Turner syndrome. **As a rule, numeric chromosomal abnormalities are associated with IUGR, dysmorphic features, malformations, and mental retardation. Physical abnormalities may be milder or absent in the newborn with mosaicism.**

Abnormalities of Chromosome Structure

Structural abnormalities have been described in all chromosomes. These include deletions, translocations, duplications, and inversions (Fig. 26-4). A **deletion** is a loss of chromosome material and results in partial monosomy for the chromosome involved. Loss of material from the end of a chromosome is known as a **terminal deletion,** as seen in 5p −, cri du chat syndrome. An **interstitial deletion** involves a loss of chromosomal material that does not include the ends of the chromosome. A terminal deletion of both arms of a chromosome may result in reattachment of the remaining arms, leading to a formation of a **ring** chromosome. Presence of additional chromosome material results in **duplication** or partial trisomy of a chromosome. **Translocation** is the detachment of a chromosome segment from its normal location

and its attachment to another chromosome. The translocation is **balanced** if the cell contains two complete copies of all chromosomal material, although in different order. In an **unbalanced** translocation the rearrangement results in partial trisomy or monosomy.

Translocations can be reciprocal or Robertsonian. A reciprocal translocation involves exchange of segments between two chromosomes; (e.g., part of the short arm of the chromosome 4 trades a place with a part of chromosome 10). Robertsonian translocations involve two acrocentric chromosomes fused at their centromeres. The most frequent Robertsonian translocation is formed between chromosomes 14 and 21.[10]

Inversions are the result of a double break in a single chromosome and reinsertion of the chromosomal material that has been inverted. Inversions are either **pericentric** (including the centromere) or **paracentric** (without the centromere). The most common inversion is a small pericentric inversion of chromosome 9, which is considered to be a normal variant, found in approximately 1% of the general population.[21] All other inversions may

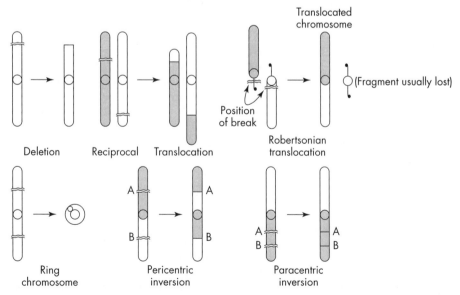

Figure 26-4 Schematic example of structural chromosomal abnormalities. (From Hathaway WE et al, editors: *Current pediatric diagnosis and treatment,* ed 10, Norwalk, Conn, 1991, Appleton & Lange.)

produce gametes that result in an individual with an unbalanced rearrangement (i.e., having both a duplication and a deletion of some chromosome material, such as that seen in recombinant 8 syndrome).

Microdeletions and Syndromes

At times, structural chromosomal abnormalities are submicroscopic and therefore cannot be detected by conventional cytogenic techniques. Fluorescent in situ hybridization (FISH) is a molecular-cytogenic method that facilitates the detection of microdeletions. FISH utilizes segments of fluorescently labeled DNA called probes, constructed so that each probe can attach only to a specific segment of a chromosome, which then will be fluorescent during a microscopic visualization. In the case of deletion of that chromosome segment, the probe cannot attach to the chromosome, thus the fluorescent segment is missing from the deleted chromosome.[22]

Microdeletions result in phenotypic abnormalities. Microdeletion syndromes that may be suspected in the NICU include Prader-Willi syndrome caused by interstitial deletion of chromosome 15 (q11q13), which may present in a newborn as severe hypotonia, feeding difficulties, and micropenis or hypoplastic labia[12]; and Shprintzen/DiGeorge spectrum caused by interstitial deletion of the long arm of chromosome 22 (22q11.21-22q11.23). The affected newborn may present with congenital heart defect in 85% (VSD 62%, right aortic arch 52%, tetralogy of Fallot 21%; and others), submucous or overt cleft palate, thymus hypoplasia, transient hypocalcemia in 20%, long slender digits, and dysmorphic facial features.[12]

Clinical Examples of Chromosomal Abnormalities

Down Syndrome. Down syndrome has an incidence of approximately 1 in 600 live births. Approximately 95% of cases are caused by nondisjunction involving chromosome 21, 5% are caused by a translocation, and 1% have a mosaicism. Down syndrome may present with marked hypotonia; a number of major malformations, most commonly congenital heart defects, duodenal atresia, and tracheoesophageal fistula; and a characteristic pattern of dysmorphic features. The classic phenotype seen in Down syndrome includes a flattened occiput, midfacial hypoplasia, depressed nasal bridge, upward slanting palpebral fissures (mongoloid slant), epicanthic folds, grayish speckling of the iris (Brushfield spots), micrognathia, excess nuchal skin, single palmar creases (simian creases), single flexion creases and incurving of the fifth fingers (clinodactyly), and increased distance between the first and second toes (Fig. 26-5, *A* and *B*).

In full-term infants with the classical phenotype of Down syndrome, the clinical diagnosis is not difficult. However, it is imperative that cytogenetic studies be done to confirm the diagnosis and to differentiate a nondisjunctional trisomy from a translocation. This distinction has important implications for recurrence risks (see discussion under Prevention). In premature infants the classical facial phenotype is frequently missing, making clinical diagnosis more difficult. The presence of an AV canal or duodenal atresia with minor malformations, such as abnormal dermatoglyphics, should alert the clinician to the possibility of Down syndrome.

Trisomy 18. Trisomy 18 has an incidence of 1 in 6000 live births. The major phenotypic features include prenatal growth restriction, complex cardiac malformations, abnormal muscle tone, microcephaly, prominent occiput, low-set and malformed ears, corneal opacities, micrognathia, peculiar hand posturing with the second and fifth digits overlapping the third and fourth, hypoplasia of fingernails, abnormal dermatoglyphics, prominent calcanei, and deep plantar furrows between the first and second toes (Fig. 26-6). The prognosis is poor, and the majority of infants with trisomy 18 will die within the first few months of life. Those infants who have survived into childhood are profoundly retarded.

Trisomy 13. Trisomy 13 is seen in approximately 1 in 15,000 live births. Phenotypic features include prenatal and postnatal growth restriction, microcephaly, sloping forehead, coloboma of the iris, microphthalmia or anophthalmia, low-set or malformed ears, cleft lip and palate, postaxial polydactyly, and abnormal palmar creases and dermatoglyphics (Fig. 26-7). Internal abnormalities may include a number of CNS malformations such as holoprosencephaly, cardiac malforma-

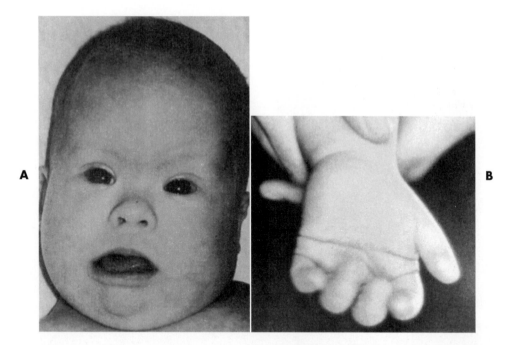

A   B

Figure 26-5   Infant with Down syndrome. **A,** Note midface hypoplasia, epicanthic folds, and depressed nasal bridge (From Gorlin RJ, Cohen MM, Levin LSW, editors: *Syndromes of the head and neck,* ed 3, New York, 1990, Oxford University Press). **B,** Single palmar crease (Courtesy Genetic Services, University of Colorado Health Sciences Center and The Children's Hospital, Denver, Colo).

tions, omphalocele, renal malformations, and urogenital abnormalities such as cryptorchidism in males and uterine malformations in females. The prognosis is extremely poor for these infants, with most dying within the first few months of life.

Turner Syndrome.   The only monosomy to be seen in live births is that of Turner syndrome— females with a 45,X, karyotype. Additionally, it is the only numeric abnormality of the sex chromosome that may be identifiable at birth. Turner syndrome has an incidence of 1 in 5000 female births.[18] Clinical features that may be evident in the newborn period are a short, webbed neck or redundant skin on the back of the neck and marked lymphedema of the dorsum of the hands and feet (Fig. 26-8, *A* and *B*). Congenital heart defects are seen in approximately half the patients, with 30% having a coarctation of the aorta. Renal anomalies may also be present.[12] Prognosis is usually excellent but depends on the presence and severity of

the congenital heart defect. Intelligence is normal; however, some females with Turner syndrome have been noted to have spatial perception or fine motor problems.[18]

Cri Du Chat.   Cri du chat, or cat cry syndrome, is the result of loss of the terminal end of the short arm of chromosome 5 (5p−). The name of the syndrome reflects the unusual cat-like weak cry these infants have in the neonatal period. These infants are usually small for gestational age, hypotonic, and microcephalic, and may have ocular hypertelorism, epicanthic folds, downward slant of the palpebral fissures, low-set ears, and micrognathia. They are significantly mentally retarded.

San Luis Valley Syndrome.   Recombinant 8, or the San Luis Valley syndrome, named for the area in which many of these individuals were first identified, is an example of an unbalanced pericentric inversion with both a duplication and a dele-

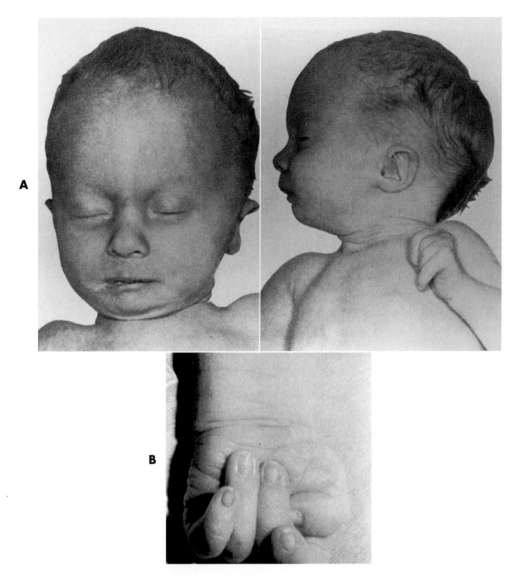

Figure 26-6   Infant with trisomy 18. **A,** Typical facies with small chin, abnormal pinna, and prominent occiput (From Gorlin RJ, Cohen MM, and Levin LSW, editors: *Syndromes of the head and neck,* ed 3, New York, 1990, Oxford University Press). **B,** Typical hand posturing with overlapping fingers (Courtesy Genetic Services, University of Colorado Health Sciences Center and The Children's Hospital, Denver, Colo).

tion of chromosome 8 material. The pericentric inversion of chromosome 8 found in a parent and other relatives of a child with recombinant 8 syndrome has no phenotypic consequence because it is a balanced rearrangement. However, a carrier is at risk for producing unbalanced gametes during meiosis. In recombinant 8 syndrome, there is a deletion of chromosomal material of the short arm of chromosome 8 and a duplication of chromosome material of the long arm of 8. The phenotype

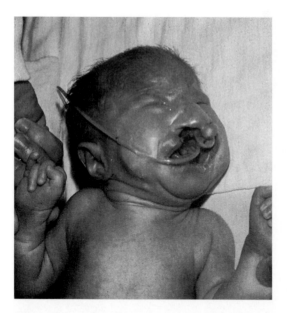

Figure 26-7 Infant with trisomy 13. Facial clefts and microcephaly; abnormal positioning of hands. (From Hathaway WE et al, editors: *Current pediatric diagnoses and treatment,* ed 10, Norwalk, Conn, 1991, Appleton & Lange.)

is characterized by unusual facial features, including a wide face, depressed nasal bridge, hypertelorism, antimongoloid slant of the palpebral fissures, upturned nose, long philtrum, low-set and malformed ears, cleft lip and/or cleft palate, congenital heart disease, and renal abnormalities.[20]

Prevention

The identification of chromosomal abnormalities in the newborn is important not only for management issues regarding the infant, but also because of the recurrence risks the abnormality carries for the family. In general, numerical chromosomal abnormalities carry low recurrence risks (approximately 1% to 2%).[4] In the presence of structural abnormalities, recurrence risks depend on whether one of the parents carries a balanced rearrangement. If parental chromosomes are normal, the recurrence risk is minimal. However, if a parent carries a balanced chromosomal rearrangement, the recurrence risk is significantly increased. The exact risk figure will vary with the nature of the specific chromosomal rearrangement and in some cases

the sex of the carrier parent. In either situation, for those parents and families concerned about recurrence risk, prenatal chromosomal analysis is available.

Single-Gene Disorders

McKusick's catalogue of mendelian inherited disorders currently lists more than 4000 single-gene disorders with known patterns of inheritance.[17] Many of these disorders are singularly rare; however, collectively, they affect about 1% of the population. Single-gene disorders are the result of either a single or double dose of an abnormal gene. Single-gene disorders are classified as autosomal dominant, autosomal recessive, X-linked dominant, and X-linked recessive. Humans have two copies of each gene located at identical places (gene **loci**) on homologous chromosomes. In a single-gene disorder, an abnormal or mutated **allele** (an alternate form of a gene) is found on one or both members of a pair of chromosomes.[21] Individuals with identical alleles at a particular locus are **homozygous** for the gene. Individuals with different alleles are **heterozygous** for the gene. Because males have only one X chromosome, and most genes located on the Y chromosome do not correspond to those located on the X, males are **hemizygous** for the genes on the X chromosome. Abnormal genes located on one of the 44 autosomes are the cause of **autosomal** disorders: abnormal genes located on the X chromosome are the cause of **X-linked** disorders. Disorders are **dominant** when the phenotype is expressed in the presence of only one copy of the abnormal gene. In **recessive** disorders the phenotype is expressed only when both the chromosomes carry the abnormal gene.

Autosomal Dominant Disorders

Autosomal dominant disorders are ones in which the disorder is expressed in the heterozygous state. Major characteristics include (1) multiple generations affected (i.e., an infant would have an affected parent), (2) both males and females are affected and both sexes can transmit the disorder to their offspring (i.e., male-to-male transmission can occur), (3) there is a 50% risk for each offspring to inherit the gene from an affected parent, and (4) individuals who do not have the gene cannot transmit the disorder to their offspring.

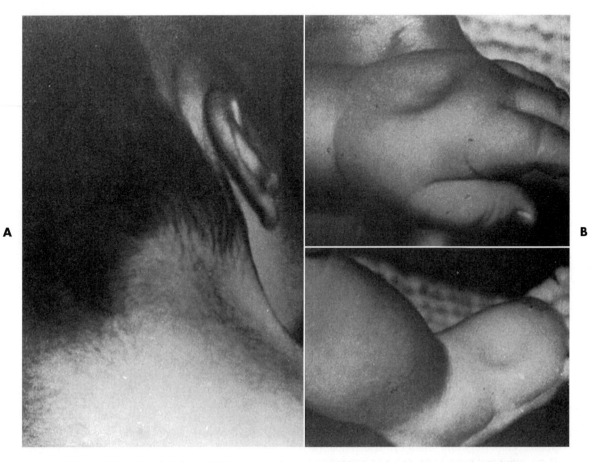

A

B

Figure 26-8 Female infant with Turner syndrome. **A,** Webbed neck with low posterior hairline. **B,** Lymphedema of dorsal surfaces of hands and feet. (From Knuppel R, Drukker JD, editors: *High risk pregnancy: a team approach,* Philadelphia, 1988, WB Saunders.)

A negative family history does not rule out the presence of an autosomal dominant disorder. Possible explanations for a negative family history are (1) the infant's disorder is a result of a new mutation, (2) a parent has a very mild expression of the disorder and may not have been previously diagnosed, (3) nonpaternity, (4) decreased penetrance (i.e., not all individuals with the gene have phenotypic abnormalities [skipped generation]), and (5) gonadal mosaicism for the mutation (see nontraditional inheritance).

Dominant disorders that may be seen in the NICU include skeletal dysplasias (such as achondroplasia), osteogenesis imperfecta, Apert syn-

drome, Crouzon syndrome, Treacher Collins syndrome, and ectrodactyly (Fig. 26-9).

Autosomal Recessive Disorders

Autosomal recessive disorders are expressed only in the homozygous state. Thus, to be affected, an individual usually inherits an abnormal gene from each parent. The parent who is heterozygous for an abnormal gene is usually phenotypically normal and is called a carrier. Major characteristics of autosomal recessive inheritance include (1) phenotypically normal parents, (2) affected siblings, (3) both males and females affected, (4) offspring of two carrier parents are at a 25% risk of being

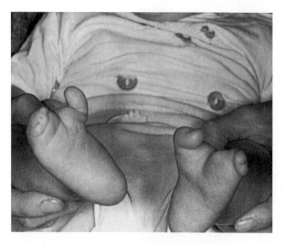

Figure 26-9 Ectrodactyly (lobster claw deformity) of the feet. (Courtesy Genetic Services, University of Colorado Health Sciences Center and The Children's Hospital, Denver, Colorado.)

affected, (5) unaffected siblings have a two-thirds chance of being carriers, and (6) there may be an increased incidence of consanguinity (mating between blood relatives). Autosomal recessive disorders that may be identified in the neonatal period include some of the metabolic disorders such as PKU, galactosemia, and isovaleric acidemia; as well as some of the multiple-malformation syndromes (such as Meckel-Gruber syndrome), cystic fibrosis presenting with meconium ileus, Zellweger (cerebral-hepato-renal) syndrome (Fig. 26-10), and skeletal dysplasias such as achondrogenesis.

X-Linked Disorders

X-linked disorders are caused by an abnormal gene(s) located on the X chromosome. Most X-linked disorders are recessive. The X-linked recessive disorders are phenotypically expressed in hemizygous males; heterozygous females are generally phenotypically normal and are referred to as carriers. Affected fathers do not have affected sons (no male-to-male transmission); however, all daughters of affected males are carriers. A carrier female has a 50% chance of having an affected male offspring.

Occasionally, there may be heterozygous females who are phenotypically affected, although usually less severely than males. If females are severely affected, other mechanisms, including homozygosity for the X-linked gene, may be responsible for the phenotype. X-linked recessive disorders that may be recognizable in the newborn period include factor VIII and IX deficiency (classical hemophilia A and B), X-linked hydrocephalus, and Opitz syndrome.

X-linked dominant disorders occur when the abnormal gene located on the X chromosome is expressed in both the hemizygous and heterozygous states. As in X-linked recessive conditions, there is no male-to-male transmission because the affected male passes his Y chromosome and not his X chromosome to his sons; however, all of the daughters of an affected male will inherit his X chromosome and thus be affected. Each son and daughter of an affected female has a 50% risk of being affected; males are usually more severely affected than females. There are only a few disorders that are known to be inherited as an X-linked dominant, such as incontinetia pigmenti, hypophosphatemia (vitamin D–resistant rickets), and ornithine transcarbamylase (OTC) deficiency. Early diagnosis of OTC is important because, if untreated, it leads to neonatal hyperammonemia and death in affected males. In affected females, the clinical picture can be variable, ranging from an asymptomatic infant to one who presents in the first week of life with lethargy, vomiting, and protein avoidance, ending in seizures and coma.

Multifactorial Disorders

Multifactorial disorders are caused by the interaction of multiple genes and environmental factors that are frequently unknown.[21] Most isolated single malformations, including congenital heart defects, neural tube defects, cleft lip and palate, pyloric stenosis, and club feet, are inherited in this manner. Additionally, the more common familial disorders, such as diabetes mellitus, coronary artery disease, affective disorders, and mild mental retardation, are the result of multifactorial inheritance. In contrast to single-gene inheritance, multifactorial disorders recur within families without a characteristic pedigree pattern, and recurrence risks are based on empiric data.[21] Multifactorial inheritance is explained as a liability model with a threshold effect.[21] The general population as a

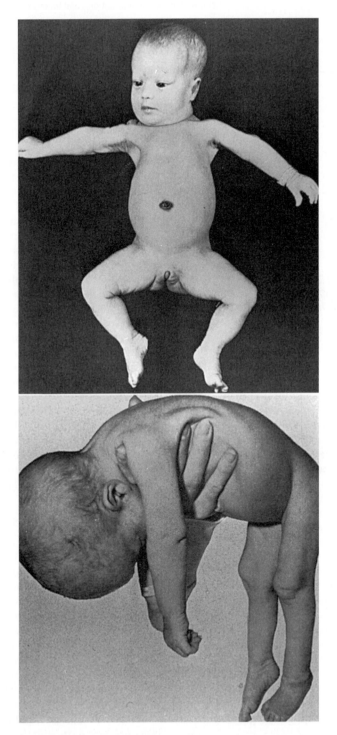

Figure 26-10 Infant with Zellweger syndrome, an autosomal recessive disorder. Note high forehead, narrow facies, and extreme hypotonia. (From Gorlin RJ, Cohen MM, Levin, LS, editors: *Syndromes of the head and neck,* ed 3, New York, 1990, Oxford University Press.)

whole has an underlying genetic predisposition for multifactorial traits and disorders that follow a normal distribution curve; only in those individuals in whom the genetic predisposition exceeds the threshold will the malformation actually be expressed (Fig. 26-11).

Major characteristics of multifactorial inheritance include (1) no consistent pedigree pattern between families (i.e., there may be only an isolated occurrence, or the disorder may be seen among siblings, in multiple generations, or scattered throughout the family); and (2) recurrence risks are not constant as in single-gene disorders but are influenced by a number of factors: (a) the number of family members affected (i.e., the more family members affected, the higher the recurrence risk becomes); (b) the degree of relatedness to those affected—first-degree relatives are at higher recurrence risk than second or third-degree relatives; (c) the severity of the defect—the more severely affected an individual is, the higher the recurrence risk; (d) the frequency of the disorder, which may vary with ethnic background (e.g., neural tube defects have a higher incidence among English and Irish populations); and (e) the sex of the individual (for disorders where one sex is more commonly affected than the other [e.g., pyloric stenosis is more common in males]; if the less commonly affected sex has the defect, then the recurrence risk is higher).

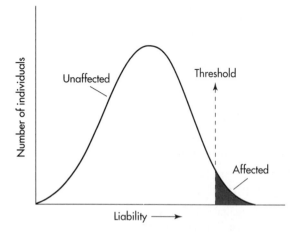

Figure 26-11 Multifactoral inheritance. Liability curve with a threshold beyond which the trait is expressed.

Nontraditional Inheritance

Gonadal Mosaicism

The spectacular growth in the field of molecular genetics and its technologies in only the past few years has enabled the clarification of the inheritance patterns of many genetic disorders and birth defects that were previously unknown or unclear. For example, the lethal form of osteogenesis imperfecta (OI) occurring in multiple offspring of unaffected parents was thought to be the result of autosomal recessive inheritance. However, improved molecular techniques have documented it to be the result of **gonadal mosaicism,** that is, the mutation occurs in the gonad of one of the parents, who then has some gametes with and others without the OI mutation. This distinction alters the recurrence risks and is very important for genetic counseling.[6]

Genomic Imprinting

In the past, little notice was given to whether the sex of the parent that transmitted an abnormal gene to offspring had any effect on the expression of genes. Now it is recognized that maternally and paternally derived genes may function differently, and this is called **genomic imprinting.**[7] For example, offspring who inherit the gene for Huntington's disease (autosomal dominant) from an affected father are more likely to have childhood onset of the disease than if they inherited the maternal gene.

Uniparental Disomy

Uniparental disomy is the result of inheriting both copies of a chromosome from one parent and none from the other.[7] It is assumed that for normal growth and development, a child must receive both maternal and paternal genes; if both copies of a gene originate only from one parent, the development is abnormal. This is based on finding uniparental disomy in cystic fibrosis with short stature, and in the Prader-Willi, Angelman, and Beckwith-Wiedemann syndromes. The parental origin of a child's chromosomes can be identified only by molecular analysis; chromosome analysis is usually not helpful.

The possibility of a nontraditional pattern of inheritance makes genetic counseling more complex than previously thought. Thus it is imperative that health care providers be aware of such complexities and refer families to a geneticist or genetic counselor for more detailed discussion.

Inborn Errors of Metabolism

Genetic disorders in which defects of single genes cause clinically significant blocks in metabolic pathways are known as inborn errors of metabolism. The recognition of disorders caused by inborn errors of metabolism has increased rapidly in recent years, and they are now recognized as important causes of disease in the newborn and pediatric age group.[5] Inborn errors of metabolism include defects of carbohydrate metabolism, amino acid metabolism, organic acid metabolism, and purine metabolism; disorders of fatty acid oxidation; lysosomal storage diseases; and disorders of peroxisomes. It is important to remember that inborn errors can present at any time and may affect almost any organ system. Specific disorders that need to be considered in symptomatic newborns include galactosemia, OTC, or carbamoyl-phosphate synthetase (CPS) deficiency, maple syrup urine disease, nonketotic hyperglycinemia, propionic and methylmalonic acidemias, isovaleric acidemia, and glutaric acidemia type II.[5] Although the majority of infants will not be found to have an inborn error of metabolism as the etiology of their illness, early recognition is imperative and may be considered a medical emergency if appropriate treatment is to be initiated. Many of these disorders can be effectively treated and if untreated are lethal in the newborn period. Moreover, without the appropriate diagnosis, parents would not be aware of recurrence risks in future offspring.

Inborn errors of metabolism should be included in the differential diagnosis of any critically ill newborn in the following instances: (1) suspicion of neonatal sepsis; (2) recurrent vomiting and/or altered consciousness; (3) clinical findings of hypoglycemia, seizures, parenchymal liver disease, unusual odor, hyperammonemia, or unexplained acidosis; and/or (4) a family history of a sibling affected with similar symptoms, mental retardation, or SIDS.[5]

In general, laboratory analysis will depend on the presenting symptoms seen in the newborn. Laboratory studies that should be obtained before any treatment is begun are electrolytes, ammonia, glucose, urine pH, urine-reducing substances, and urine ketones. Clues to suspecting an inborn error are (1) hypoglycemia and ketonuria in the newborn, (2) acidosis with recurrent vomiting and hyperammonemia, and (3) acidosis that is difficult to correct and is out of proportion to the clinical state. If other etiologies are not readily apparent, additional laboratory tests that may be appropriate are serum and urine amino acids and urine organic acids.[24]

Newborn Screening

Inborn errors of metabolism when unrecognized and untreated may lead to severe consequences, including mental retardation and death in some instances. Thus the goal is to identify, treat, and prevent major sequelae whenever possible. Newborn screening accomplishes this goal for a small number of disorders. Screening criteria that should be met are relatively high frequency of the disorder, severity of symptomatology in untreated individuals, availability of treatment, simplicity of obtaining tissue for testing, and availability of a simple screening test with high sensitivity and specificity and reasonable cost. Metabolic disorders that are currently screened for include PKU, homocystinuria, maple syrup urine disease, biotinidase deficiency, and galactosemia. Additionally, the newborn may be screened for hypothyroidism, hemoglobinopathies, and cystic fibrosis. Each state decides individually what will be included in the newborn screening program. Any screening test may give both false-positive and false-negative results. Thus a positive screen should be followed by a confirmatory diagnostic test. Moreover, if there is clinical suspicion of a particular disorder in spite of a negative screening result, further diagnostic testing is warranted. For an in-depth review of those disorders that may be part of the newborn screening program, refer to the American Academy of Pediatrics Newborn Screening Fact Sheets.[2]

Environmental Etiologies

Environmental exposures may have adverse effects on fetal development (teratogenic effect) resulting in malformations and functional, neurodevelopmental abnormalities in infants and children. There are four major prerequisites needed for teratogenic action[8]: (1) The agent must have the potential to be teratogenic. There are little conclusive data available regarding the teratogenicity of most chemicals and drugs in humans. Animal studies provide most of the data available regarding the teratogenicity of agents; however, not all are always applicable to human situations. To prove that an agent is teratogenic, a causal relationship between the exposure and presence of a malformation must be documented; just the history of an exposure to an agent is not sufficient. **Although very few agents have been documented to be teratogenic in humans, a few stand out, such as alcohol, cocaine, anticonvulsants, and isotretinoin (Accutane) (Fig. 26-12).** (2) The timing of the exposure during pregnancy is of major importance. For the agent to adversely affect the fetus, it must be present during organogenesis and/or histogenesis. Exposures occurring within the first 2 weeks postconception, before cell differentiation, will cause no damage or will result in fetal wastage; exposures occurring from 2 to 12 weeks of gestation (period of organogenesis) may result in major malformations; after completion of development of the major organ systems, harmful expo-

sures usually do not result in malformations but can be responsible for organ dysfunction. However, some agents may morphologically disrupt previously intact organs.[1] On the other hand, it has been shown that if the harmful exposure to an agent such as alcohol has been discontinued, the damage is less severe than if the exposure continues throughout the pregnancy. (3) Dosage of the teratogen is related to the severity of the teratogenic effect; the higher the dose, the more severe the effect and the higher the frequency of affected fetuses.[8] (4) Finally, genetic makeup or genetic susceptibility of the mother and fetus may affect the metabolism as well as tissue sensitivity to the teratogen.

Teratogenic agents may be divided into four categories: (1) infectious agents, (2) chemical agents (drugs and environmental agents), (3) radiation, and (4) maternal factors. Chapter 2 provides excellent overviews of most of these exposures.

Traditionally, only maternal exposures to teratogens have been implicated in malformations. There has been a concern that some paternal exposures also may be teratogenic. Theoretically, a teratogen excreted in the semen could be introduced into the fetal environment and could be potentially teratogenic to the developing fetus.[11]

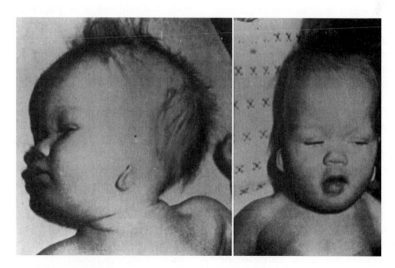

Figure 26-12   Infant exposed to Accutane in utero. Note dysmorphic face and auricles with atretic ear canal. (Courtesy Genetic Services, University of Colorado Health Sciences Center and The Children's Hospital, Denver, Colo.)

Teratogenic exposures should be considered in the differential diagnosis of congenital malformations and CNS dysfunction if one can document fetal exposure and the phenotype is compatible with the known effects of the suspected teratogen. The recognition of exposures is important for genetic counseling; if they can be avoided during subsequent pregnancies, recurrence risk is not increased. Frequently there is phenotypic overlap between the fetal abnormalities caused by specific teratogens and other syndromes. Referral to a genetics clinic should be made to rule out chromosomal, single-gene, and sporadic syndromes with overlapping phenotypes.

Data Collection

The genetic evaluation consists of the same components found in any medical evaluation; however, the emphasis may be different. Moreover, to make an accurate diagnosis and assessment, medical information regarding extended family members may need to be obtained.

History

Prenatal and perinatal histories, from a genetic standpoint, need to elicit information regarding potential teratogenic exposures including maternal disease and acute illness. Fetal growth and behavior (e.g., fetal movement and swallowing) provide important clues for the assessment of fetal neuromuscular function. Thus information regarding fetal position, movement, and amount of amniotic fluid should be obtained. Perinatal history should include the duration of gestation, anthropometric birth measurements, including head circumference, and information regarding perinatal adaptation. In a newborn with abnormal CNS functioning, it may be difficult to differentiate between primary maldevelopment and dysfunction caused by perinatal complications. An abnormal newborn with a genetic disorder may present with symptoms suggestive of birth asphyxia (i.e., hypoxia, acidosis, hypotonia, seizures). Moreover, because many a priori abnormal newborns have increased frequencies of perinatal complications, a documented birth injury does not rule out the presence of a genetic etiology.

Family history may be extremely helpful in clarifying the etiology and risk of recurrence. The information obtained from the parents may need to be complemented by physical examination of the parents and other family members and review of the medical records. This may be necessary because parents may not be aware that different defects in family members may be expression of the same disorder. For example, an autosomal dominant gene may cause mild hypoplasia of thumbs in one family member and complete absence of thumb and radii in another.

Physical Examination

The physical examination should detect major and minor malformations (dysmorphic features). Minor malformations are defined as structural variations found in less than 4% of the general population and having no significant medical or cosmetic effect.[1] This is in contrast to structural variations that are found in more than 4% of the newborn population and represent a normal variation, such as a mongolian spot and capillary hemangioma on the forehead. Minor malformations may provide important clues to the identification of a specific syndrome. None of the minor malformations as an isolated finding are clinically significant; however, a combination or pattern of minor malformations may indicate a specific disorder. For example, dysmorphic features such as up-slanted eyes, epicanthic folds, hypertelorism (Fig. 26-13),

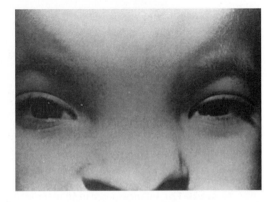

Figure 26-13   Dysmorphic feature of hypertelorism. Note wide-spaced eyes. (From Aase JM: *Diagnostic dysmorphology,* New York, 1991, Plenum Press.)

and abnormal dermatoglyphic pattern (Fig. 26-14, *A* and *B*) in an infant with a congenital heart defect, are suggestive of Down syndrome. Minor malformations may also alert the clinician to the presence of major malformations. For example, preauricular ear tags are associated with an increased frequency of inner ear malformations and hearing loss. Additionally, the greater the number of minor malformations an infant has, the higher the chance of finding one or more major malformations.[15]

If minor malformations are identified, the parents of the infant should be examined. Presence of the same minor malformation in one of the parents may indicate a benign familial feature. Alternatively, finding the same dysmorphic features in other family members may represent an inherited genetic disorder. A mild syndactyly between second and third toes is frequently an isolated, inherited finding without clinical significance. However, syndactyly associated with craniosynostosis may represent an autosomal dominant disorder with variable expression and significant clinical sequelae.

If an infant looks dysmorphic, documentation of specific features should be recorded. Actual measurements compared with age-related norms should be utilized to measure body proportions, length of extremities, and such facial features as distance between eyes, length of eye fissures, size of ears, and length of philtrum. Description of the other features, such as the shape of the neck (webbed) or the chest size (widely spaced nipples), or a specific description of any skin lesions as to size, shape, location, and color (hyperpigmented or hypopigmented), may provide important clues for a specific diagnosis. Dermatoglyphic analysis, the analysis of the dermal ridges on the digits, palms, and soles, may prove useful for the timing of a fetal insult.[25] Development of ridges begins during the thirteenth week of gestation and is complete by the nineteenth week. Thus many chromosomal and genetic disorders will have disruptions of the dermal ridge patterns. For example, an infant with Down syndrome may have a single palmar crease (simian crease), a single flexion crease of the fifth digit, and an open field pattern (arch tibial) on the hallucal area of the foot.[25] Moreover, specific descriptors, or even more useful, photographs, should be used to describe dysmorphic findings. Photographs are particularly important if the infant is critically ill and the constellation of findings

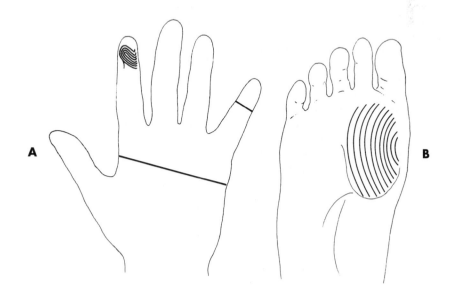

Figure 26-14 Dermatoglyphics commonly seen with infants with Down syndrome. **A,** Ulnar loop on second digit, single flexion crease on fifth digit, and single palmar crease (simian line). **B,** Arch tibial pattern in hallucal area of foot.

does not immediately suggest a specific syndrome. Thus the patient's findings may more accurately be shared with other clinicians in the future.

Smith's Recognizable Patterns of Human Malformations[12] and other texts contain a large number of syndromes, some of which are quite rare and may not be immediately recognized by neonatal staff. It may be helpful and important to consult a clinican who is familiar with dysmorphology and syndromology to help establish a diagnosis.

Laboratory Data

When suspecting a genetic disorder, a number of diagnostic studies may be useful in delineating a diagnosis, including chromosome analysis, biochemical studies to rule out inborn errors of metabolism, radiographs, organ imaging, and when appropriate, autopsy. Not all of these studies are routinely used in all patients but are based on clinical suspicion of a particular disorder.

Chromosome Analysis

Routinely, results of chromosome analysis may not be available for several weeks. However, if results of chromosome analysis are urgently needed for clinical management, chromosome analysis from bone marrow can be available within a few hours, and preliminary results from blood lymphocyte culture can be obtained in 48 hours. Indications for chromosome analysis have been listed previously. However, chromosome analysis should be obtained in all critically ill infants without a plausible explanation for their grave clinical course, before death occurs. Postmortem chromosomes may also be obtained from any tissue, in particular intracardiac blood, thymus, skin, and gonad. Under sterile conditions, these tissues should be obtained as soon as possible after the infant's demise. Tissue should be transported to the laboratory in tissue culture media or sterile saline and not in formalin.

Biochemical Studies

A critically ill neonate who has a condition suggestive of an inborn error of metabolism or who has no specific diagnosis should have blood and urine sent for appropriate biochemical studies (listed in the section on inborn errors of metabolism). If such studies have not been obtained, postmortem tissue such as liver should be obtained and frozen for later biochemical analysis. Care providers should request detailed instructions from a laboratory specializing in testing for inherited metabolic disorders regarding which tissue is appropriate and how it should be obtained, stored, and shipped to the laboratory.

Radiographs

X-ray examination should be obtained if a skeletal dysplasia or other skeletal abnormality is suspected or if the differential diagnosis includes a genetic syndrome that has skeletal defects as part of the phenotype. Moreover, if a localized skeletal defect is found, a skeletal survey should be obtained to identify other possible skeletal defects.

Organ Imaging

Organ imaging, ultrasound, MRI, and CT scan should be utilized to rule out structural abnormalities of major organs such as the brain, heart, and kidneys. Malformations may be suspected on the basis of clinical symptoms such as anuria or on the basis of known nonrandom associations of certain birth defects, such as the VATER association (vertebral, anal, T-E fistula, renal, and radial). In addition, some dysmorphic features are associated with major malformations, and one must rule out these features. For example, there is an increased incidence of underlying midline brain defects associated with some facial dysmorphic features.

Autopsy

In the event of a neonatal death, an autopsy may provide crucial information for the establishment of a correct diagnosis. As outlined previously, chromosome analysis, biochemical studies, X-ray examination, and photographs all should be included. In the absence of specific, confirmed diagnosis, the family should be strongly encouraged to consent to an autopsy and a tissue sample should be frozen for further testing. Without this valuable information, subsequent genetic counseling, including clarification of the etiology and recurrence risks, becomes impossible.

Treatment/Intervention

For most genetic disorders and malformations, there are no "cures," and only symptomatic treatment is available. That is, conventional medical and surgical interventions are instituted, although the basic genetic defect is not corrected. Surgical intervention for specific malformations will depend on the malformation, its etiology, and prognosis. For example, surgical repair of a cleft lip and palate usually has an excellent outcome, although the underlying genetic etiology has not been altered. In other instances, the diagnosis may provide direction and guidance to the health care professionals and family as to the appropriate course of action. An infant born with a hypoplastic left heart may be considered a candidate for a heart transplant. However, if the cardiac malformation is the result of a chromosomal abnormality with an extremely poor prognosis, such as trisomy 13, the management of that infant may be palliative as opposed to corrective. With the diagnosis of a metabolic disorder, treatment may be one of a nutritional or pharmacologic approach, such as the restriction of phenylalanine in an infant with PKU or the replacement of a deficient hormone, such as thyroid supplements in hypothyroidism. For some conditions, such as OI, the best approach may be educating the parents on specific techniques of holding and caring for an infant to prevent further fractures. In some disorders, organ or tissue transplantation may be appropriate. Bone marrow transplantation has been found to be effective in treating select genetic disorders, including lysosomal storage disorders[13] and beta thalassemia.[14] Because specific treatment leading to a cure is not available for most genetic disorders, the utilization of genetic counseling and available reproductive alternatives, such as prenatal diagnosis, in vitro fertilization, and artificial insemination by donor, are acceptable alternatives for some families.

With the numerous advances in molecular genetics leading to a better understanding of genetic disease, many genetic disorders and malformations may be amenable to treatment in utero or after birth. In utero correction of such birth defects as urinary tract malformations and diaphragmatic hernia have been attempted.[9] In 1990, the first human trial of gene therapy was undertaken at the National Institutes of Health. The treatment was somatic gene replacement in a 4-year-old with adenosine deaminase deficiency, a rare inherited disorder that destroys the immune system.[16] Since that time, a number of gene therapy trials for other genetic disorders have been done. Although the success of gene therapy has been thus far limited, the results have led to new areas of research and experimentations with new promising techniques.[19]

Parent Teaching

The birth of any infant with a malformation or genetic disorder is a devastating event for any family. The neonatal staff find themselves on the front lines helping families to deal with the infant's problems and provide the best environment for both the critically ill newborn and his or her family. In general, the most difficult factor for most parents and families to deal with is the unknown. Thus, once again, the need for an accurate diagnosis becomes paramount. Moreover, even when the diagnosis carries a very poor prognosis, parents would prefer having the information to realistically anticipate and prepare.[23] Currently, many parents obtain information about their infant's malformation or genetic disorder through prenatal diagnosis and have already begun the process of anticipatory grief by the time the infant is admitted to the NICU. Parental feelings of disbelief, shock, anger, or despair may have already been replaced with a "sense of relief" about confirmation of the abnormalities and a need to deal with the situation at hand.[23] Chapter 29 provides an excellent review of the grief and mourning process that parents will experience when their anticipated "perfect baby" is born with a malformation or genetic disorder.

From a genetic counseling standpoint, there are a number of principles that should be incorporated into the plan of care for the neonate and his or her family. First, and it cannot be overstated, an accurate diagnosis is essential if genetic counseling is to be provided. Even with what appears to be an isolated malformation, a genetics consultation may be appropriate to rule out other etiologies, such as single-gene disorders or chromosomal abnormalities. After establishing the diagnosis, one can realistically address the prognosis, treatment, and other management issues with the family. Finally, at the appropriate time for the family, recurrence risks and options for future pregnancies can be addressed. Certainly, the busy and stressful environment of the NICU is not the most conducive atmosphere to obtain and provide detailed information. However, it is very appropriate for the geneticist to make an initial contact with the family in the NICU, where basic information regarding pregnancy and perinatal and family histories can be obtained and aid in diagnosis and defining etiology. Diagnosis and management can then be addressed by the neonatal staff and geneticist. Later, at a time appropriate for the family, such issues as recurrence risks can be addressed. Eventually, the family should receive a written summary of all the issues discussed for their own documentation.

The genetic evaluation is a complex and multifaceted process that cannot be done in isolation; it requires a team approach. The geneticist can provide the neonatal intensive care staff with assistance in the diagnosis, etiology, management, prognosis, and future counseling of the families they serve. The neonatal staff should use the genetics team as a resource for consultation and assistance in providing infants and families with the most appropriate and complete health care available.

References

1. Clayton-Smith J, Donnai D: Human malformations. In Rimoin DL, Connor JM, Pyeritz RE, editors: *Emery and Rimoin's principles and practice of human genetics,* ed 3, New York, 1996, Churchill Livingstone.
2. Committee on genetics: Newborn screening fact sheets, *Pediatrics* 83(3): March, 1989.
3. DeGrouchy J, Turleau C: *Clinical atlas of human chromosomes,* ed 2, New York, 1984, John Wiley & Sons.
4. Gardner RJM, Sutherland GR: *Chromosome abnormalities and genetic counseling,* New York, 1989, Oxford University Press.
5. Goodman SI, Greene CL: Inborn errors as causes of acute disease in infancy, *Semin Perinatol* 15(suppl 1):31, 1991.
6. Hall JG: Somatic mosaicism observations related to human genetics, *Am J Hum Genet* 43:355, 1988.
7. Hall JG: Genetic imprinting: review and relevance to human disease, *Am J Hum Genet* 46:857, 1990.
8. Hanson JW: Human teratogens. In Rimoin DL, Connor JM, Pyeritz RE, editors: *Emery and Rimoin's principles and practice of human genetics,* ed 3, New York, 1996, Churchill Livingstone.
9. Harrison MR et al: Management of the fetus with a urinary tract malformation, *JAMA* 246:635, 1981.
10. Hay WW et al: *Current pediatric diagnosis and treatment,* ed 12, Norwalk, 1995, Appleton & Lange.
11. Joffe JM, Soyka LF: Paternal drug exposure: effects on reproduction and progeny, *Semin Perinatol* 6(2):116, 1982.
12. Jones KL, editor: *Smith's recognizable patterns of human malformation,* ed 4, Philadelphia, 1988, WB Saunders.
13. Krivit W, Whitley CB: Bone marrow transplantation for genetic diseases, *N Engl J Med* 3165:1085, 1987.
14. Lucarelli C et al: Marrow transplantation in patients with advanced thalassemia, *N Engl J Med* 316:1050, 1987.
15. Marden AM, Smith DW, McDonald MN: Congenital anomalies in the newborn infant, including minor variations, *J Pediatr* 64:357, 1964.
16. Marwick C: Two more cell infusions on schedule for gene replacement therapy patient, *JAMA* 265(18):2311, 1991.
17. McKusick VM: *Mendelian inheritance in man,* ed 9, Baltimore, 1990, The Johns Hopkins University Press.
18. Robinson A et al: Sex chromosome aneuploidy: the Denver prospective study, *BD OAS* 26:59, 1991.
19. Schuchman EH, Desnick RJ: Strategies for the treatment of genetic disease. In Rimoin DL, Connor JM, Pyeritz RE, editors: *Emery and Rimoin's principles and practice of human genetics,* ed 3, New York, 1996, Churchill Livingstone.
20. Sujansky E et al: Natural history of recombinant (8) syndrome, *Am J Med Genet* 47:512, 1993.
21. Thompson MW, McInnes RP, Willard HF: *Genetics in medicine,* ed 5, Philadelphia, 1991, WB Saunders.
22. Tcachuk DC et al: Clinical applications of fluorescence in situ hybridization, *Genet Anal Tech Appl* 7:49, 1991.
23. Walker AP: Genetic counseling. In Rimoin DL, Connor JM, Pyeritz RE, editors: *Emery and Rimoin's principles and practice of human genetics,* ed 3, New York, 1996, Churchill Livingstone.
24. Ward JC: Inborn errors of metabolism of acute onset in infancy, *Pediatr Rev* 11(7):205, 1990.
25. Wertelecy W: Dermatoglyphics. In Stevenson RE, Hall JG, Goodman RM, editors: *Human malformations and related anomalies,* ed 2, 1993, Oxford University Press.

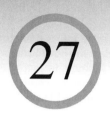

27

Neonatal Surgery

Randall M. Holland, Frances N. Price, Denis D. Bensard

Surgical problems in the neonate are often acute and potentially devastating. At no other time in life, however, is the human more hardy and resilient. Given early diagnosis and judicious surgical intervention, a high rate of success may be anticipated. This chapter briefly discusses clinical history, diagnostic evaluation, and therapeutic intervention of common neonatal surgical conditions.

Malrotation and Volvulus

Physiology and Etiology

The midgut normally herniates into the base of the umbilical cord at the beginning of the sixth week of development and returns to the abdominal cavity by the tenth or twelfth week. As it returns, the proximal midgut rotates posterior and counterclockwise to the superior mesenteric artery (SMA). Thus the duodenum comes to lie posterior to the SMA, forming the ligament of Treitz. Concomitantly, the colon and distal small bowel rotate anterior to the SMA until the cecum lies in the right lower quadrant.[2] Failure to undergo this rotation results in the clinical condition of "malrotation." Malrotation is seen in gastroschisis, omphalocele, and congenital diaphragmatic hernia because the bowel is malpositioned at the normal time of fixation. Malrotation can also occur in the absence of other anomalies.

The degree of malrotation covers a wide spectrum from complete nonrotation to partial malrotation or improper fixation of a segment of bowel.[26] There may also be a reversal of rotation such that the colon lies posterior to the SMA and the duodenum lies anterior. Nonrotation or total failure of rotation is the most common of these. In this situation the entire small bowel is on the right side of the abdomen and the colon is mainly on the left side.

Consequently, the root of the mesentery is not anchored, and the entire bowel is suspended by the superior mesenteric artery and vein. This long pedicle is prone to twisting (volvulus). Once volvulus occurs, the involved vessels occlude, leading to ischemia and infarction of the entire midgut.

The cause of malrotation and volvulus is unexplained in most cases. People may live their entire life with malrotation having no problems, but others may have severe symptoms in infancy.

Data Collection

History

Malrotation may present as a mechanical bowel obstruction caused by the abnormal attachments (Ladd's bands) or as a clinical emergency from a volvulus with impairment of the blood supply to a large segment of the bowel. In the former presentation, the first few days of life are normal, followed by the onset of abdominal distention and bilious vomiting. Presumably, dilation of the bowel by food and gas precipitates the obstructive process.

Signs and Symptoms

The symptoms of the infant with Ladd's bands are similar to those of an infant with duodenal stenosis or atresia, including bilious vomiting.

Midgut volvulus presents as the sudden onset of abdominal distention, lethargy, mottling, and hypovolemia. The infant may pass bloody, maroon stools indicating mucosal injury or necrosis. These neonates are gravely ill.

Laboratory Data

Plain films of the abdomen show a dilated stomach and proximal duodenum. An upper GI series will confirm the point of partial obstruction and an abnormal ligament of Treitz. A barium enema will

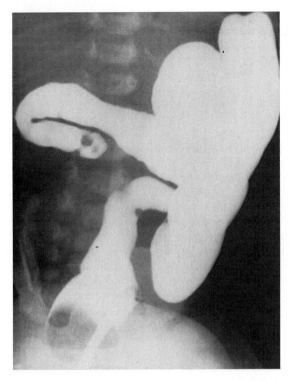

Figure 27-1 Midgut volulus in 2-day-old male infant who vomited bile-stained fluid for 12 to 24 hours before surgery. Barium enema shows high-lying cecum curved on itself in right upper quadrant.

also show an abnormal rotation. These infants should have an emergency barium enema (Fig. 27-1) that will show the colon's occlusion at the point it twists around the mesenteric vessels. Laboratory data may show severe acid-base derangement if there is significant bowel necrosis.

Treatment

Preoperative Care

Although distinguishing between volvulus in its early stages and malrotation with obstruction may be difficult, they are treated similarly. Gastric decompression, vigorous fluid hydration, correction of electrolyte and acid-base abnormalities, and parenteral antibiotics are instituted in the preoperative period.

Operative Intervention

Emergency abdominal exploration is necessary for the infant with volvulus because the bowel will be irreparably damaged within 4 hours. In fact, it is unwise to await total correction of metabolic abnormalities because it may be impossible until the bowel is revascularized.

Operative correction for malrotation includes division of Ladd's bands to relieve the duodenal obstruction and placement of the colon in the left side of the abdomen and the small bowel on the right. This will splay out the mesentery and prevent a subsequent twist. An appendectomy is performed because, in the future, abnormal location of the appendix makes the diagnosis of appendicitis difficult. If volvulus has occurred, it must be untwisted and frankly necrotic bowel resected. In some instances, marginal intestine is better left in place with plans to do a "second-look" abdominal exploration in 24 hours if necessary. This will allow marginally viable intestine time to recover or become frankly necrotic, thus short-gut syndrome may be prevented if the marginal bowel recovers.

Complications and Prognosis

Straightforward malrotation is cured by the Ladd procedure, and recurrence is very rare. If a major amount of bowel is resected because of volvulus and necrosis, short-gut syndrome may occur, requiring long-term TPN (see Chapter 16). At least 20 cm of small intestine is necessary for adequate bowel function.

Omphalocele and Gastroschisis

Physiology and Etiology

Omphalocele and gastroschisis are defects in the abdominal wall around the umbilicus. Omphaloceles are herniations through the base of the umbilical cord and are covered by a peritoneal sac (Fig. 27-2). The cause is not known but is likely to be abnormal abdominal wall development.[15] Omphalocele may be associated with trisomy and/or other midline congenital defects, including sternal and diaphragmatic defects and congenital heart lesions. Omphaloceles below the umbilicus are

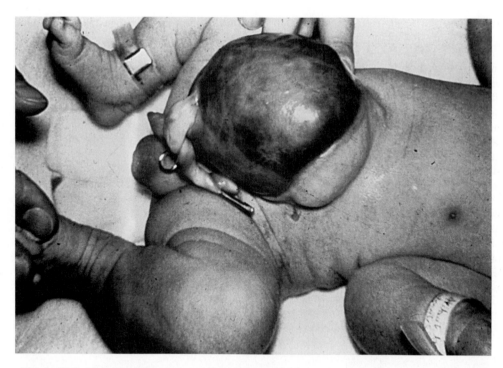

Figure 27-2   Omphalocele. Large umbilical defect with viscera protruding from abdominal cavity into transparent moist sac.

seen in conjunction with cloacal exstrophy, spinal abnormalities, and imperforate anus.

Gastroschisis is a defect just to the right of the umbilicus; in this disorder no sac covers the bowel (Fig. 27-3). Gastroschisis may be a herniation through a weak area of the umbilical cord caused by obliteration of the right umbilical vein. **Gastroschisis is not associated with other congenital anomalies or syndromes. A 5% to 10% incidence of bowel atresia may be due to mesenteric kinking and vascular compromise of the affected segment secondary to the small fascial defect.**

Malrotation of the intestine is found in both defects.

Data Collection

History

Many of these defects are diagnosed by antenatal ultrasound, which permits therapy to be planned. Normal vaginal delivery may be permit-ted since there is a low risk of bowel injury during delivery.

Preterm, prelabor Cesarean section may be elected to prevent severe bowel wall thickening or serositis. Severe serositis makes repair more difficult and delays the return of bowel function.

Signs and Symptoms

Both of these entities present as a mass of abdominal contents extruding through an anterior abdominal wall defect. Gastroschisis patients have only bowel eviscerated, whereas omphaloceles may contain liver as well. Gastroschisis is always to the right of the midline and will often have a skin bridge between the umbilicus and the defect.

Laboratory Data

If time permits, the neonate with omphalocele must be investigated for further defects. Echocardiography and plain x-ray examination of the chest and spine are done to rule out cardiac, chest wall, diaphragmatic, and spinal anomalies.

Treatment

Preoperative Care

Initial management includes preservation of body heat and fluid, gastric decompression, protection of the intestine, and prophylaxis against infection.

Heat and fluid loss are minimized by covering the exposed viscera. This may be accomplished by wrapping the intestines in warm, saline-soaked gauze and then covering in plastic wrap. Alternatively, the entire infant may be placed up to the axilla in an impermeable, clear plastic bowel bag. Both methods decrease evaporative losses; the bowel bag allows continuous visual monitoring as well. With either method, it is imperative that the bowel be positioned to prevent kinking at the fascial level.

Intravenous fluids and broad-spectrum antibiotics should be instituted early. To prevent bowel distention, an orogastric tube is placed on suction.

Operative Intervention

Rarely an infant with omphalocele may be too ill to undergo operation or may have other malformations inconsistent with long-term survival. Under these circumstances, daily application of 65% alcohol or silver sulfadine to the abdominal sac will cause eschar formation and subsequent epithelialization in 10 to 20 weeks. A large ventral hernia will remain and require later repair.

Primary surgical repair entails placing the abdominal contents into the abdominal cavity without increasing abdominal pressure to the point that ventilation, venous return, or intestinal blood supply are compromised. If the amount of eviscerated abdominal contents is small or moderate, primary repair is simple and safe.[8] Sometimes the fascial

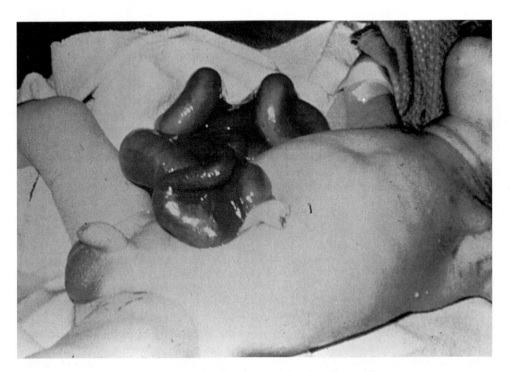

Figure 27-3   Gastroschisis. Abdominal wall defect to right of midline, without sac or sac remnant.

defect may have to be enlarged to allow replacement of the herniated organs into the abdomen. The abdominal wall is manually stretched to increase the capacity of the abdominal cavity to more easily allow reduction of the abdominal contents.

In large omphaloceles and some gastroschises, reduction is done over days. The herniated organs are placed into a silastic "silo" or pouch sewn to the fascia of the abdominal defect (Fig. 27-4). Daily, the silo is made smaller by a series of suture lines in the silo, which gradually forces the bowel into the abdomen. By this method, the abdomen is allowed time to accommodate the increased volume.

Complications and Prognosis

Bowel injury, respiratory compromise, and diminished venous return caused by increased abdominal pressure may complicate recovery. The silastic pouch may become infected, separate from the fascia, and make closure by this method impossible. **Bowel function is often delayed, especially in gastroschisis caused by exposure of the bowel to amniotic fluid. A central venous catheter may be needed for long-term TPN** (see Chapter 16). Incisional hernia and adhesive bowel obstruction are possible as short- and long-term complications. Otherwise, prognosis is good unless severe associated malformations are present.

Diaphragmatic Hernia

Physiology and Etiology

Diaphragmatic hernia occurs in 1 in 4000 live births. The defect is a result of failure of closure of the foramen of Bochdalek on the posterolateral portion of the diaphragm. This defect occurs early in gestation, allowing the bowel to migrate into the chest as it returns from the umbilical cord. Thus there is always a malrotation associated with a diaphragmatic hernia. From 85% to 90% of diaphragmatic hernias occur on the left side because the liver usually fills defects on the right side.[29]

As the bowel develops in utero it compresses the lung and leads to pulmonary hypoplasia, diminishing both the size of the lung and the number of

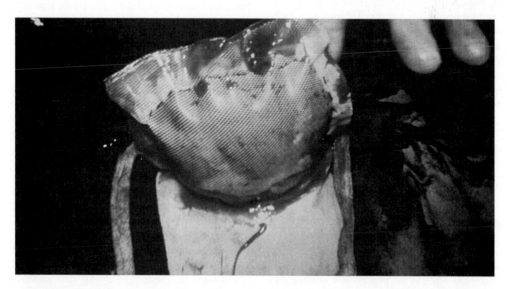

Figure 27-4 Silicone-coated mesh pouch containing abdominal contents that will be reduced daily into abdominal cavity as top is sewn down.

alveoli in the lung. Once the umbilical cord is clamped, the pulmonary hypoplasia becomes a serious problem as respiratory distress develops.

Data Collection

History

Ultrasound enables antenatal diagnosis of diaphragmatic hernias, which allows early planning or intervention. The mother may then deliver in a high-risk perinatal center with neonatal medical and surgical support on standby. Recently, in utero surgical repair has been attempted in several perinatal centers. This has not markedly altered outcome.

Signs and Symptoms

Respiratory distress commonly develops immediately after birth. Because most of the intestines are in the chest, the abdomen is scaphoid and the anteroposterior diameter of the chest may increase as the bowel distends with air. Breath sounds are diminished or absent on the affected side, and the mediastinum is displaced toward the contralateral side. Associated anomalies include hypoplasia of the lung, malrotation of the intestine, and DA. The ductus remains open in an attempt to maintain fetal circulation because of pulmonary hypertension caused by hypoplasia of the lung. There is also a slightly higher incidence of CNS malformations, genitourinary anomalies, esophageal atresia, omphalocele, cleft palate, and cardiovascular defects, which should be investigated.

Laboratory Data

A plain radiograph of the chest will confirm that the bowel is in the thoracic space and the heart is displaced (Fig. 27-5).

Treatment

Preoperative Care

As soon as diaphragmatic hernia is suspected, an orogastric tube should be placed for gastric decompression to prevent further distention of the bowel. The infant may require endotracheal intubation and positive pressure mechanical venti-

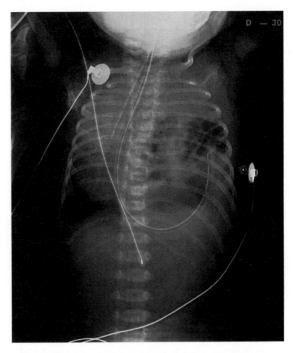

Figure 27-5 Diaphragmatic hernia in newborn female with respiratory distress. Note nasogastric tube that is below diaphragm, then curves upward into left hemithorax. Note loops of bowel in left chest. Endotracheal tube is in right mainstem bronchus, accounting for increased atelectasis of right upper lobe.

lation to maintain adequate respiratory status. The earlier the infant is symptomatic, the more severe the respiratory compromise and the poorer the prognosis. PPHN compromises the course (see Chapter 22).

Operative Intervention

Timing of surgical repair is not vital. The patient should be stable from a pulmonary standpoint. Early repair is not indicated if the patient has severe respiratory insufficiency. A period of stabilization with mechanical ventilation, high-frequency ventilation, pulmonary artery dilators, or ECMO is warranted. Surgical repair will not improve and may even worsen pulmonary function over the short-term.

Transabdominal operative repair is indicated.

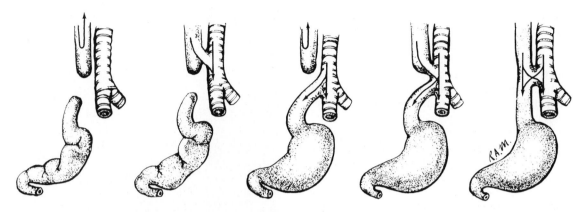

Figure 27-6   Most common types of esophageal atresia and tracheoesophageal fistula. (From Whaley LF, Wong DL: *Nursing care of infants and children,* ed 3, St Louis, 1987, Mosby.)

The abdominal contents are reduced from the chest and replaced into the abdominal cavity, and the diaphragmatic defect is closed. In rare instances it is necessary to use mesh or other prosthetic materials to close the defect because of an insufficient amount of diaphragm. Closure of the abdomen may be difficult because of an underdeveloped abdominal cavity. If closure is impossible, only the skin is closed over the top of the abdominal contents, leaving a large ventral hernia. A chest tube (to water seal rather than to suction) is placed on the affected side. Some surgeons advocate placement of a chest tube on the contralateral side to deal with possible pneumothorax and mediastinal shift.

Postoperative Care

The principal postoperative concern is ventilation. If conventional mechanical ventilators are insufficient, high-frequency ventilation may be instituted. If high-frequency ventilation is also unsuccessful, ECMO may be used (see Chapter 22). Inhaled nitric oxide is a new selective pulmonary vasodilator that shows promise in reversing pulmonary hypertension. Liquid ventilation is an even newer modality that is being investigated for respiratory failure in this and other situations. ECMO and nitric oxide have not greatly improved long-term survival in patients with diaphragmatic hernia, but trials continue in an effort to find optimal ventilator management.

Complications and Prognosis

The survival for infants who require mechanical ventilation in the first 18 to 24 hours of life is approximately 50%. If an infant with diaphragmatic hernia does not present with respiratory distress in the first 24 hours of life, survival approaches 100%. With improvements in ventilator management, there has been a gradual, albeit small, increase in survival. There are now investigations in repairing diaphragmatic hernias in utero with some success. Unfortunately, to prevent pulmonary hypoplasia, fetal repair must be done at a very early stage of development, when intrauterine operations are risky.[1]

Esophageal Atresia and Tracheoesophageal Fistula

Physiology and Etiology

Esophageal atresia (EA) occurs in 1 in 4500 live births. In 86% of patients, esophageal atresia is associated with a fistula between the distal esophagus and the trachea. Other combinations include esophageal atresia without a fistula (7.7%), "H" type tracheoesophageal fistula without esophageal atresia (4.2%), esophageal atresia with a proximal fistula (0.8%), and atresia with proximal and distal fistulae (0.7%) (Fig. 27-6).

The etiology of these defects is unknown, but the embryologic mechanism is well understood. At 34 to 36 days of gestation the esophagus separates completely from the trachea. Failure of separation leads to the tracheoesophageal fistula (TEF) defect. Other defects may occur in conjunction with TEF, including cardiac anomalies in 30% and anal anomalies in 12% of patients.

There is an increased incidence of TEF/EA in twins and in offspring of affected parents. The exact hereditary mechanism is unknown. The majority of cases, however, are sporadic.

Data Collection

History

Frequently there is a history of polyhydramnios because the fetus was unable to swallow amniotic fluid normally.

Signs and Symptoms

Most infants present soon after birth with copious secretions or inability to swallow feedings. After one or two sucks the child will begin coughing and then regurgitate unchanged formula. An orogastric tube should be passed and will meet an obstruction at 8 to 10 cm from the mouth if esophageal atresia is present. Patients with upper pouch fistulas will aspirate feedings. Infants with an "H" type fistula may have a more insidious onset of symptoms. They will cough and choke with feeding and may have intermittent abdominal distention or recurrent pneumonia over the first months of life.

Physical Examination

Once a TEF is diagnosed, the infant must be carefully examined to exclude the other anomalies of the VACTERL association, a combination of anomalies affecting the vertebrae, anus, heart (cardiac), trachea, esophagus, urinary tract (renal), and limbs. Further studies may be indicated to fully assess or rule out these defects.

Laboratory Data

A plain radiograph of the chest and abdomen should be obtained after orogastric (OG) tube placement. The OG tube will be visible at the second or third thoracic vertebra (Fig. 27-7). The stomach will contain air if there is a distal fistula. If there is

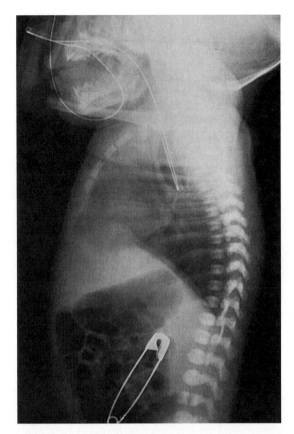

Figure 27-7 Esophageal atresia with tracheoesophageal fistula. Lateral x-ray film shows gastric tube in esophageal pouch and air in gastrointestinal tract.

not a distal fistula, the abdomen will be gasless (Fig. 27-8).

Treatment

Preoperative Care

Once the diagnosis is established, the catheter in the upper pouch should be placed on suction to prevent aspiration. While awaiting operation, the child should be kept in the head-up position to prevent gastroesophageal reflux, which will spill into the trachea through the fistula. If a proximal fistula is present, urgent operation is indicated because saliva will empty into the lungs despite the OG tube. While awaiting operation the child should

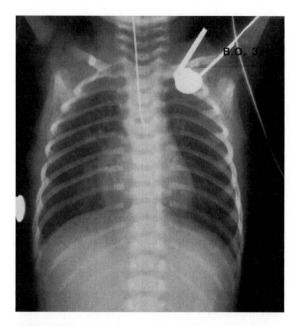

Figure 27-8 Esophageal atresia without tracheoesophageal fistula in a 3-hour-old, 36-week infant with feeding difficulty and inability to pass nasogastric tube. Note nasogastric tube in esophagus and gasless abdomen suggestive of absent distal fistula.

be kept in the head-down position to improve drainage of the upper esophagus.

Operative Intervention

The surgical repair of the standard esophageal atresia is not an emergency but should be carried out as soon as the patient is stable. If the infant is in otherwise good health and the gap between esophageal elements is not too large, primary anastomosis is indicated through a right retropleural approach.[9]

If the gap is too great or if the child is too ill, a delayed or staged repair is needed. This entails a gastrostomy for decompression and division of the fistula to prevent soilage of the tracheobronchial tree.[19] After a wait of several days to as long as 10 weeks to allow maximum growth of the distal esophagus, a second operation completes the repair.

Postoperative Care

Postoperative care includes pulmonary toilet, IV fluids, and antibiotics. Tracheal and esophageal suction catheters should not come in contact with the newly repaired esophagus since this may cause a leak or recurrent fistula. Antibiotics are continued for 3 to 5 days. A retropleural chest tube is placed on suction. Oral feedings may begin at 5 to 10 days after repair if an esophagram indicates no anastomotic leak. All of these infants have some degree of esophageal dysmotility and gastroesophageal reflux (GER). Elevating the head of the bed 35 to 45 degrees, employing the prone position, and feeding slowly helps control reflux symptoms.

If delayed or staged repair is planned, secretions must be controlled. Many infants are able to spit up their secretions, but others may require suction catheters in their pouch or pharynx.

Complications and Prognosis

Long-term problems include stricture, anastomotic leak, and esophageal dysmotility. Anastomotic leaks are approached conservatively with chest tube drainage, parenteral nutrition, antibiotics, and patience. The vast majority heal without operative intervention. Strictures are often associated with GER and are treated by repeated esophageal dilation. If GER is complicated by recurrent stricture, a fundoplication procedure may be necessary.

Symptomatic esophageal dysmotility is often self-limited. The child may adapt to a poorly functioning esophagus by altering his or her feeding habits. However, in infancy, gastrostomy feeding may be required to prevent vomiting and aspiration.

With modern surgical and medical techniques, long-term survival after repair of TEF/EA is very good. Prognosis depends on the presence of associated anomalies and their severity.

Bowel Atresia and Stenosis

Physiology and Etiology

Any segment of the bowel may be narrowed or discontinuous. Duodenal atresia is most common,[4,28] followed by ileum, jejunum, colon, and stomach atresia. The single most common site of atresia is at the papilla of Vater.

The cause of bowel atresia is either a vascular accident (e.g., intrauterine volvulus, vessel occlusion, or intussusception) during development or failure of vacuolization and recanalization. Atresias are classified as membranes, fibrous cords, gap defect including mesentery, and "apple-peel" atresia.[16] The apple-peel deformity is a proximal jejunal atresia with the distal small bowel corkscrewed around a single vessel filled retrograde by the ileocolic, right colic, or inferior mesenteric arteries. This distinct atresia appears to occur in a familial pattern while the others occur sporadically.[26]

Data Collection

History and Physical Examination

Typically, the neonate is small for gestational age and the mother has polyhydramnios. The more proximal the atresia, the more likely the polyhydramnios. The infant has bilious vomiting and abdominal distention. If the atresia occurs early in gestation, the infant will not pass meconium. Duodenal atresia is frequently associated with trisomy 21.

Laboratory Data

Plain abdominal films show dilated bowel proximal to the obstruction. A "double-bubble" is seen in patients with duodenal atresia.[28] The bubbles are air in the dilated stomach and duodenum (Fig. 27-9). Upper gastrointestinal series are not done unless the diagnosis is in doubt or the obstruction is only partial. Some surgeons advocate barium enema in all cases of neonatal bowel obstruction to distinguish small from large bowel obstruction, to determine whether microcolon is present, and to rule out malrotation.

Treatment

Preoperative Care

Preoperative care includes gastric decompression, intravenous hydration, and replacement of electrolytes. An orogastric tube empties the stomach to minimize vomiting and aspiration.

Operative Intervention

Duodenal atresia often requires repair through a side-to-side anastomosis to prevent injury to the bile and pancreatic ducts. Jejunoileal atresias may be repaired by a simple end-to-end anastomosis.

The size disparity between the dilated proximal loop and the decompressed distal loop may require that the proximal bowel be tapered and/or that the distal bowel be cut obliquely to allow anastomosis. If these methods are not possible, then both segments may be brought out as stomas. When they become more equal in size, anastomosis may be done.

Postoperative Care

Postoperatively the bowel is decompressed by an OG tube until bowel function begins. Stomas must be protected from desiccation by covering with saline-soaked gauze or petroleum jelly. When the stoma is functional, a stoma appliance should be applied. Proximal ostomies have high output because of a lack of absorptive capacity. When calculating fluid needs, ostomy output and sodium and bicarbonate losses should be measured and replaced appropriately. To avoid such losses the proximal output is often refed into the distal mucous fistula, although this can be technically difficult because of an inability to secure the infusion catheter.

Complications and Prognosis

Wound care and nutritional support minimize infectious problems. Prolapse of the proximal stoma may occur as it becomes smaller (allowing it to push through the large opening made for it in the abdominal wall) but rarely causes major problems. Short- or long-term bowel dysfunction can be devastating. The short-gut syndrome occurs if long segments of bowel are lost or if they function poorly, as is seen in "apple-peel" segments. Such infants may require long-term parenteral nutrition. The majority of patients have no long-term problems after postoperative recovery and return of bowel function.

Imperforate Anus

Physiology and Etiology

Imperforate anus occurs in 1 in 5000 live births; males are 57% of all cases. In a high imperforate anus, the rectum ends above the levator ani

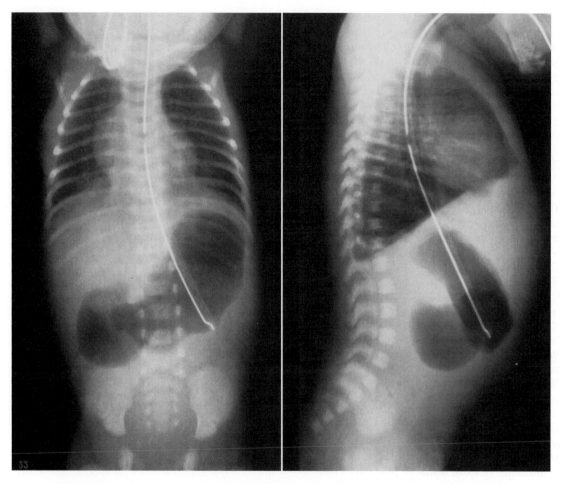

Figure 27-9   Duodenal atresia in 2-day-old, 36-week, SGA preterm infant who was unable to tolerate feedings. Classic double bubble sign of gastric and duodenal dilation secondary to duodenal atresia is noted on both x-ray films. Note airless abdomen; no bowel gas extends beyond duodenum.

muscles. If the rectum has descended below the levator mechanism, it is a low imperforate anus. High imperforate anus is twice as common in males; "low" lesions occur equally in males and females. Fistulae in high lesions most often enter the membranous urethra in the male and the vagina in the female.[18] Fistulae in the low lesion exit on the perineum or the posterior fourchette of the vagina. Imperforate anus may occur in conjunction with other congenital anomalies, such as the VACTERL association. If one of these lesions is found, the others must be sought by careful examination and further studies, including radiographs of the spine, echocardiography, passage of an orogastric tube, renal ultrasound, and limb examination.

Data Collection

Signs and Symptoms

Most of these anomalies are quite obvious but may be missed if a careful examination of the buttocks and anus is not done. This is particularly

true in the patient with a low imperforate anus. Once the diagnosis is made, a fistula should be sought. In low lesions there may be a thin membrane over the anal orifice, or there may be a fistula along the perineum and scrotal raphe. If meconium passes in the urine or from the vagina, a high lesion is present. If untreated, the subsequent intestinal obstruction will cause abdominal distention and vomiting.

Laboratory Data

A plain radiograph of the abdomen reveals bowel dilation without rectal gas, but it will not reliably show the distal extent of the rectum. Ultrasound may be used to establish the level of the obstruction and to outline the fistula.

Treatment

Preoperative Care

The infant should be kept NPO, and an orogastric tube should be placed. If a fistula is present on the perineum or fourchette, it should be dilated. If no fistula is visualized, a colostomy is necessary to decompress the colon.

Operative Intervention

After dilation in infants with a low imperforate anus, formal anoplasty is electively done. After colostomy in infants with a high imperforate anus, a formal repair is undertaken at 6 to 12 months of age. Approached via a posterior sacral incision, the blind-ending rectum is brought through the sphincter mechanism and anastomosed to the anal skin. The two forms of this procedure are the sacroperineal pull-through and the posterosagittal anorectoplasty.[20]

Postoperative Care

After anoplasty, simple skin care is all that is necessary. After a colostomy, stoma care is needed and should be taught to parents (Box 27-1).

Complications and Prognosis

Colostomy may be complicated by stenosis, urinary tract infections resulting from the fistulous opening into the urinary tract, and hyperchloremic acidosis caused by absorption of urine by the rectum.

After anoplasty for a low lesion, long-term obstipation may occur if the anoplasty is too tight. Anal dilation often makes this quite manageable; if not, the anoplasty should be redone or revised.

In high imperforate anus, continence will be of major concern. About 25% will have good continence, 50% will have fair continence, and 25% will have poor results. The amount of sphincter mechanism present and its innervation will give some clue as to the long-term outlook for continence. Those with poor outcomes may improve with further special procedures.

Hirschsprung's Disease

Physiology and Etiology

Hirschsprung's disease is a congenital, rarely hereditary, intestinal disorder caused by a lack of ganglion cells in the bowel wall, preventing effective peristalsis and resulting in an intestinal obstruction. It is seen four times more often in males than females, with an increased incidence reported in Down syndrome. The area of aganglionosis always originates at the rectum, extends a variable distance proximally, and may include the lower rectum, colon, small intestine, or rarely, entire gastrointestinal tract except for the stomach. A transition zone exists between abnormal and normal bowel with dilated, thickened, and hypertrophic intestine proximally and an aganglionic segment that is spastically contracted distally.[21] The most common transition zone is the sigmoid colon, seen in approximately 80% of cases.

Data Collection

Signs and Symptoms

Symptoms usually begin at birth with a failure to pass meconium during the first 48 hours of life, often accompanied by abdominal distention and vomiting. Evacuation of stool may be accomplished by rectal examination and, for a while, the infant appears to be in a normal state of health. However, episodes of obstipation, vomiting, and abdominal distention recur. Paradoxic diarrhea, watery stool escaping around obstipated stool, may also

---

Box 27-1

Instructions for Ostomy Care

Supplies

Skin-prep (United)*   Ostomy set-up (skin wafer and bag)
Stoma-adhesive paste (Convatec)*   Pattern for stoma

Application Instructions

1. Measure the diameter of the stoma, using the measuring guide circle enclosed in the wafer box.
2. Trace the appropriate circle onto the white paper backing of the wafer and cut out the hole. Gently bend and slightly stretch the opening with your finger. The goal is to have the hole 1/16 to 1/8 inch larger than the stoma. A snug but not constricting fit is needed to prevent stool from leaking onto the skin.
3. Clean and dry the skin around the stoma.
4. Apply a generous coat of Skin-prep (United) on the skin around the stoma.
5. Apply a thin border of Stoma-adhesive paste (Convatec) around the stoma.
6. Press wafer firmly to skin.
7. If using a two-piece appliance, snap on the bag and close the end of the bag with a clip or rubber band if it is open-ended. If using a one-piece appliance, the appliance may be applied directly to the skin or to a skin barrier such as Stoma-adhesive (Convatec).*

Helpful Hints

1. *Change the appliance as soon as there is any evidence of leaking!*
2. Rinsing the bags with some type of scented soap (peppermint or spice) will help cut down on the bag odor.
3. Pre-cut several wafers ahead of time.
4. When travelling, always have an extra set of clothes and a complete set of supplies as well as a new set-up with stoma holes already cut.

*Other products may be used in place of the brand names upon recommendation of your medical supplier, physician, or nurse. Provided by Kris Altzenbeck, R.N., The Children's Hospital, Denver, Colo.

---

occur. In milder cases of Hirschsprung's disease, chronic obstipation may be the only symptom. In the most severe cases, ischemic enterocolitis occurs and is manifested by acute abdominal distention, profuse vomiting, the passage of foul smelling gas, and large, loose, often bloody stools. The infant deteriorates rapidly with a potentially lethal outcome if a colostomy is not performed immediately. In most cases the infants are stable enough to allow for definitive diagnostic studies before surgical intervention.

Laboratory Data

The most useful diagnostic tests for Hirschsprung's disease are barium enema and rectal biopsy. Barium enema usually identifies the transition zone (Fig. 27-10). Rectal biopsy confirms the diagnosis. If ganglion cells are present on rectal biopsy a diagnosis of Hirschsprung's disease is eliminated.

Once the diagnosis of Hirschsprung's disease is confirmed, operative intervention is indicated.

Treatment

Preoperative Care

In infants with colitis, immediate resuscitation consists of passage of an orogastric tube, rapid vascular expansion, administration of antibiotics, and correction of acid-base deficits (see Chapters 4, 10, 13, and 21).

Operative Intervention

In the presence of ischemic enterocolitis, emergency colostomy is indicated. If the infant presents with milder symptoms, multiple biopsies are obtained at operation to determine the location of the transition zone, and a colostomy is performed just

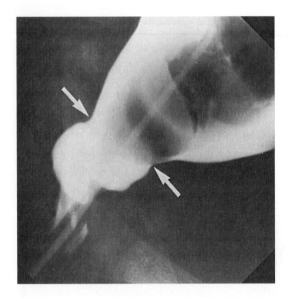

Figure 27-10   Lateral view of barium enema showing the transition zone *(arrows)* in child with Hirschsprung's disease.

proximal to the site. It is prudent to perform a biopsy on the colostomy to ensure that it does contain ganglion cells, because it will not function if aganglionosis exists at that site.

Postoperative Care

Postoperative care should include thorough parent education in ostomy care (see Box 27-1). The infant may be fed when gastrointestinal function returns. A definitive pull-through procedure is delayed until 6 months to 1 year of age, allowing the infant to reach an optimal nutritional state and the dilated bowel to return to normal size. The pull-through procedure entails resecting abnormal aganglionic bowel and bringing ganglionic bowel to the anus.[21,27] A protective colostomy is often made and subsequently closed after 4 to 6 weeks.

Complications and Prognosis

Complications of the pull-through operation include inadequate blood supply to the anastomoses, anastomotic dehiscence, or cuff abscess. The infant usually thrives postoperatively and grows normally.

It is not uncommon to have frequent stools during the immediate postoperative period.

Meconium Ileus

Physiology and Etiology

Meconium ileus is an intestinal obstruction caused by hyperviscous secretions from the intestinal glands coupled with a lack of the pancreatic enzymes that normally help break down intestinal secretions. This creates a sticky plug of meconium that cannot be propelled through the intestine.[16] Of patients with meconium ileus, 95% have cystic fibrosis. Meconium ileus occurs in 7% to 25% of patients with cystic fibrosis.

Uncomplicated meconium ileus manifests as a midileal obstruction with a small distal ileum that may contain the characteristic "gray pellets" of inspissated meconium. Meconium ileus is considered complicated when a volvulus, atresia, necrosis, or perforation occurs.

Data Collection

Signs and Symptoms

Symptoms of simple meconium ileus present as ileal obstruction 24 to 48 hours after birth and include increased abdominal girth, bilious vomiting, and the absence of stooling. The anus and rectum are small in caliber and contain a small amount of gray meconium. If the abdomen is not severely distended, the meconium may be palpated in dilated bowel loops as a doughy, rubbery mass on the right side of the abdomen. Complicated meconium ileus often presents more abruptly and progresses more quickly. Symptoms include abdominal distention within 24 hours of birth, respiratory distress (especially if a postnatal perforation has occurred), and prominent veins on an edematous, erythematous abdomen.

Laboratory Data

Abdominal x-ray examination demonstrates a "soap-bubble" appearance of the bowel caused by trapped gas within the meconium, and large dilated loops of bowel with air and/or fluid levels. Barium enema shows a microcolon and pellets of inspissated meconium distal to the obstruction.

Treatment

Preoperative Care

After gastric decompression, IV hydration, and electrolyte replacement, half-strength Gastrografin enema can be attempted. The hyperosmolarity of Gastrografin causes increased water return to the bowel lumen, which softens the meconium and facilitates passage. If unsuccessful, operative intervention is indicated.[17,24]

Operative Intervention

The goal of operation, to evacuate the small intestine of meconium, is rarely accomplished by enterotomies and manual extraction of the tenacious meconium. More often, resection of the obstructed segment, exteriorization of the affected segment, and postoperative irrigation are required.[17,24]

Postoperative Care

Postoperatively a nasogastric tube is connected to intermittent suction, and fluid maintenance offsets the fluid lost in the bowel. Feedings and pancreatic enzymes are begun when gastrointestinal function is established. To prevent pulmonary compromise caused by cystic fibrosis, pulmonary hygiene is begun. A sweat test, diagnostic for cystic fibrosis, can be performed when the patient is stable.

Complications and Prognosis

Postoperative complications include intestinal obstruction, anastomotic dehiscence, and volvulus if an enterostomy was done. Late complications are associated with cystic fibrosis.

Pyloric Stenosis

Physiology and Etiology

Pyloric stenosis, often called infantile congenital hypertrophic pyloric stenosis, is not exclusively congenital, although heredity is implicated. Approximately 7% of children with pyloric stenosis are born to affected parents, with affected mothers being four times more likely than fathers to pass it on to their offspring. Pyloric stenosis occurs four times more frequently in males than in females and is most often seen in the firstborn. The stenosis itself is due to the hypertrophic pyloric muscle, but the cause of the hypertrophy is unknown.[25]

Data Collection

History

Vomiting usually begins at approximately 3 weeks of age, increasing in frequency and force as the stenosis progresses until there is projectile vomiting. The vomiting may be less severe but of longer duration with associated failure to thrive, weight loss, dehydration, and alkalosis (caused by chloride losses).

Signs and Symptoms

In 70% to 90% of the patients a small, firm, olive-size mass can often be palpated under the liver. Gastric peristalsis may be seen as a wave progressing from the left upper quadrant to the right. Jaundice is associated in approximately 2% of these infants.

Laboratory Data

If the "olive" is not palpated, ultrasonography outlines the pyloric tumor in 95% of cases. Otherwise, an upper gastrointestinal series shows the markedly narrow pyloric channel and confirms the diagnosis.

Treatment

Preoperative Care

The goal is to restore fluid and electrolyte balance. D_5 half normal saline infused at a rate of 100 ml/kg/8 hr with KCl added to equal 40 mEq/L usually restores balance within 12 to 48 hours.

Operative Intervention and Postoperative Care

The Rammstedt pyloromyotomy is done through a right transverse incision.[7,22] The hypertrophic muscle is split longitudinally, leaving the mucosa and submucosa intact. **IV fluids are continued for**

6 to 12 hours postoperatively, and oral feeds are resumed. Most infants are ready for discharge on the second postoperative day.

Complications and Prognosis

Duodenal perforation, occurring in approximately 2% of operations, should be repaired, the myotomy closed, the pylorus rotated 90 to 180 degrees, and the myotomy repeated. Recurrent pyloric stenosis caused by incomplete myotomy is rare.

Gastroesophageal Reflux

Physiology and Etiology

Gastric contents are prevented from refluxing into the esophagus by (1) an area in the distal esophagus called the high pressure zone, (2) a sharp angle (of His) between the gastric fundus and the esophagus, and (3) a significant length of intraabdominal esophagus. At birth any or all of these components may be deficient, leading to free reflux into the esophagus. The antireflux mechanism may not be fully developed until 6 months of age. Minor problems with reflux before this time may be treated medically in hopes of spontaneous resolution.[6] Infants who are premature or have a TEF or a neurologic disorder are prone to GER.

Data Collection

Signs and Symptoms

Vomiting is the most obvious sign of reflux and may prohibit adequate nutritional intake.[5] The gastric contents may be aspirated, causing frequent, recurrent pneumonias. Apnea and bradycardia, a more severe manifestation of aspiration, are triggered by even small amounts of gastric juices in or around the larynx. Acidic fluid reflux into the esophagus may cause esophagitis, leading to anemia from bleeding, or may cause esophageal stricture formation.

Laboratory Data

Radiologic confirmation of suspected GER and anatomic abnormalities (e.g., hiatal hernia and stricture) is obtained by a barium esophagram. A pH probe placed in the distal esophagus for 8 to 24 hours is even more sensitive because it will show the frequency, severity, and duration of reflux episodes. Esophagospy and biopsy showing esophagitis may also be used to prove GER.

Treatment

Preoperative Care

A trial of nonoperative therapy is almost always indicated. Feedings are thickened with rice cereal and given more frequently and in smaller volumes. The child is placed in the prone position with the head elevated 30 to 45 degrees. An infant seat should not be used because it increases intraabdominal pressure, thereby increasing the amount of reflux. Ranitidine or omeprazole will decrease the volume and acidity of gastric juice. Metoclopramide and cisapride increase gastric emptying and improve lower esophageal sphincter function (Table 27-1).

Operative Intervention

Operation is indicated for failure to thrive, recurrent apneic spells, recurrent aspiration pneumonia, severe esophagitis, or stricture. Operations that are used in the treatment of reflux disease are the Nissen, Thal, and Toupet fundoplication procedures.[2,3,6] The common goal is to wrap the gastric fundus partially or completely around the gastroesophageal junction to prevent reflux. A gastrostomy is often added for feeding or for gastric decompression. A gastrojejunal feeding tube may be placed surgically rather than performing a fundoplication.

Postoperative Care

After an antireflux procedure, gastric decompression is continued for 1 to 2 days. Then the gastrostomy tube is elevated for a day to ensure that the infant tolerates his or her own secretions. Oral or tube feedings may be started and gradually advanced.

Proper care of a gastrostomy tube begins with securing it so that movement does not cause the wound to enlarge and leak. The tube should be secured protruding at a 90 degree angle from the

Table 27-1
Medications for Gastroesophageal Reflux

Drug	Dosage	Comments
Cisapride	0.2-0.3 mg/kg 20 min ac divided q8h	Increases gastric motility May cause QT prolongation
Metoclopramide	0.1 mg/kg divided q8h	GI smooth muscle stimulant May cause extrapyramidal symptoms (e.g., dystonic posturing)
Omperazole	Not currently recommended for neonates	Gastric acid pump inhibitor
Ranitidine	1-2 mg/kg divided q8h IV 3-4 mg/kg divided q8h PO	H₂ antagonist

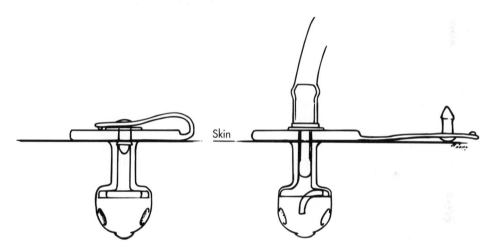

Figure 27-11   Gastrostomy button with one-way valve. Six weeks after gastrostomy, the initial tube can be replaced by a button. Having little external extension, the button is more comfortable and easier to care for.

abdomen. Cotton dental rolls are easily used to secure the tube by snugly "sandwiching" the tube between two dental rolls. This type of dressing serves two purposes. It secures the tube and absorbs drainage from around the tube. The dressing should be changed daily, and the area should be kept clean and dry. The tube is secured to the child's diaper or to a t-shirt with a safety pin. Taping the tube flat across the abdomen also prevents movement. If the tube is accidentally dislodged, it must be replaced quickly because the tract to the stomach shrinks in a few hours. Parents should be instructed to call the physician or take the infant to a facility where a physician can replace the tube. If the gastrostomy is more than 4 weeks old, the parents should be shown how to replace the tube with a Foley catheter.

Six weeks after the initial gastrostomy is done, a button gastrostomy can be placed. The gastrostomy button fits flush to the abdomen and has a one-way valve for feedings (Fig. 27-11). This allows for increased activity and easier care.

Complications and Prognosis

The Nissen fundoplication is probably the most effective in preventing reflux, but it has a higher incidence of postoperative gas-bloat syndrome.

Often the gastrostomy tube is left in place until burping occurs. The Thal and Toupet procedures have a lower incidence of distention and inability to vomit but have a slightly higher recurrence rate of GER. Recurrence may necessitate a second procedure, which is more difficult and will have a somewhat higher complication rate.

Biliary Atresia

Physiology and Etiology

Biliary atresia, once thought to be a congenital malformation, is now thought to be caused by a developmental insult of uncertain etiology. The extrahepatic bile ducts are grossly nonpatent. It is a dynamic disease process in which the disease progressively obliterates the ducts (Fig. 27-12), with complete obliteration occurring by 3 to 4 months of age. The disease process is panductal, affecting the intrahepatic (albeit not as severely), as well as the extrahepatic, biliary trees. The intrahepatic damage is often responsible for morbidity. Biliary atresia is the most common cause of obstructive jaundice in infants, affecting females slightly more often than males.[13]

Data Collection

History and Physical Examination

Because the gradual loss of patency of the bile ducts is not complete until around the time of birth, few newborns with biliary atresia are visibly jaundiced. They often eat and grow normally until about 1 month of age, when scleral icterus and clay-colored stools may first be noticed. Hepatomegaly is common, and splenomegaly also may be found.

Laboratory Data

Infantile jaundice may be due to obstructive or nonobstructive causes (infection, hematologic, metabolic). In the past, differentiation of these etiologies has been costly and time consuming. The best early diagnostic study that clearly differentiates obstructive and nonobstructive jaundice is the technetium 99m iminodiacetic acid, or IDA, scan. Uptake of the radioisotope by the liver is nor-

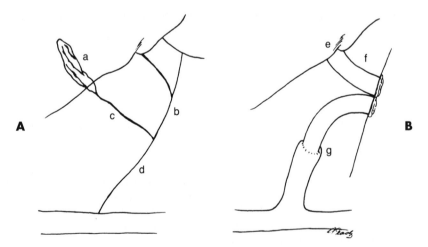

Figure 27-12 **A,** Extrahepatic biliary atresia is manifested as fibrosis of the gallbladder *(a)* and the hepatic *(b)*, cystic *(c)*, and common bile *(d)* ducts. **B,** After Kasai hepatic portoenterostomy, the jejunal limb is anastomosed to the portahepatis *(e)* and exteriorized *(f)* to allow daily bile measurement. The distal portion of the jejunal limb has an intussusception valve *(g)* to prevent reflux of bowel contents.

mal in early obstructive jaundice. In parenchymal disease, uptake is delayed.

Ultrasound may confirm the diagnosis of biliary atresia by showing a shrunken, empty gallbladder and increased echogenicity of hepatic parenchyma. Direct bilirubin and alkaline phosphatase are elevated. Diagnostic laboratory studies include liver function tests, total bilirubin, and alpha-I antitrypsin. A cholangiogram and liver biopsy are done intraoperatively for confirmation before correction is attempted.

Treatment

Operative Intervention

If the intraoperative cholangiogram shows patency of the gallbladder, cystic duct, and distal common duct (10% of cases), the gallbladder can be anastomosed to the transected proximal hepatic duct at the liver hilus. This is the optimal scenario because it virtually eliminates the chance for postoperative cholangitis.[12] In the usual case, however, the gallbladder is small and fibrotic, and a Kasai operation, or hepatic portoenterostomy, is indicated. This entails making a jejunal anastomosis (Roux-en-Y) to the transected hepatic duct at the hilus of the liver, which allows bile to flow from the liver directly to the gastrointestinal tract. The intestinal conduit is temporarily exteriorized to allow measurement of bile volume and bilirubin excretion (see Fig. 27-12).[11,12,14]

Kasai's operation provides adequate bile drainage in approximately 50% of infants under 4 months of age. An 80% success rate is reported in infants less than 10 weeks old. Early diagnosis and operative intervention are essential because the success rate is inversely proportional to the infant's age.

Postoperative Care

Postoperatively a nasogastric tube is required until bowel function returns. Bile flow from the intestinal conduit is measured and replaced unless it is replaced into the distal stoma. Failure to replace fluids may result in acute dehydration and electrolyte derangement. Bile drainage is expected to be sluggish for several weeks, and jaundice usually resolves in 2 to 3 months. Once steady bile flow has been established (usually in 6 weeks), the stomas are closed in the operating room.

Complications and Prognosis

Cholangitis is a frequent complication of Kasai's hepatic portoenterostomy operation caused by intrahepatic bile stasis and bacterial contamination of the intestinal conduit. Cholangitis, manifested by fever, leukocytosis, and decrease in quality and quantity of bile, is treated first with a 5- to 7-day course of antibiotics, followed by a short 3- to 5-day course of corticosteroids if it persists.[14] If adequate bile flow is achieved and the underlying hepatic parenchymal damage is minimal, good long-term result can be anticipated. If there is significant hepatic injury or poor bile flow, cirrhosis will occur. In this circumstance, patients often have portal hypertension with esophageal variceal bleeding. Fat-soluble-vitamin deficiency may also occur because of poor fat absorption. Children with poor results from Kasai's procedure become candidates for liver transplantation.

Necrotizing Enterocolitis

Physiology and Etiology

NEC is usually a disease of premature infants but is also seen in term infants. The pathogenesis of NEC remains unclear, but a common pathway appears to be mucosal injury. The cause of mucosal injury may be perinatal hypoxemia, polycythemia, hyperosmolar feedings, gastrointestinal infection (bacterial or viral), or severe cardiopulmonary disease. After mucosal injury has occurred, bacteria invade through the mucosa and cause gas formation in the submucosal plane.[13]

Prevention

Prevention appears to be better than the nonspecific treatment available for NEC. The best prevention is avoidance of the high-risk factors listed previously. If asphyxia, other perinatal stress, or trauma has occurred, delay in feedings may be beneficial. If polycythemia has occurred, especially in SGA infants, exchange transfusion may be beneficial. The incidence of NEC seems to be lower in breast-fed infants than in those on formula. The mechanism for this protective effect is unclear.[10]

Data Collection

History and Signs and Symptoms

Affected newborns are often the product of a complicated pregnancy and/or a premature birth. There is often a history of perinatal hypoxemia, respiratory distress, or other serious illness. Infants who had been feeding well may develop feeding intolerance with vomiting, distention, and/or increased gastric residuals. Nonspecific signs of apnea, bradycardia, temperature instability, and jaundice may be evident. Mucosal injury may manifest as bloody stools. There may be localized abdominal erythema with induration.

Laboratory Data

Laboratory findings include thrombocytopenia, leukocytosis, or leukopenia. Occult blood and reducing substances (i.e., positive occult blood or Clinitest) are often found in the stool. Blood cultures may be positive. Common x-ray findings include bowel distention with gas or a completely gasless abdomen. Pneumatosis intestinalis (intramural air) is pathognomonic. Air may extend into the portal venous system. Pneumoperitoneum is indicative of bowel perforation.

Treatment

Preoperative Care

Medical management is sufficient in many cases. Enteral feeding should be discontinued and gastric decompression instituted with an orogastric tube. Parenteral antibiotics covering gram-positive and gram-negative organisms should be instituted (see Chapter 21). Fluid volume and electrolytes should be restored and parenteral nutrition begun. Clinical examination and radiographic studies should be performed frequently for close follow-up.

Pneumoperitoneum is an obvious indication for operative intervention. Persistent acidemia is suggestive of bowel necrosis and may necessitate exploration. Surgical intervention must also be considered when there is persistence of abdominal wall erythema, a tender abdominal mass, or a persistent, dilated bowel loop.

Operative Intervention

At operation, frankly necrotic bowel requires resection with stoma formation or a primary anastomosis. Bowel of questionable viability is best left in place. Reexploration performed in 12 to 24 hours may be necessary to reassess bowel viability.[10] Every effort should be made to preserve bowel length. Proximal diversion by jejunostomy may diminish the insult in the distal bowel and allow recovery of questionable segments. Primary anastomoses or decompressive enterostomies are the options for dealing with the segments left in situ.[13]

Postoperative Care

General supportive care with antibiotics, parenteral nutrition, and cardiorespiratory support is the mainstay of postoperative treatment. After the infant has recovered, at about 10 days from the time of diagnosis, low-osmolar, elemental feedings can be introduced.

Complications and Prognosis

Early complications include abscess, fistula, or bowel obstruction. Stricture is a late finding in patients undergoing both surgical and medical management. If a large amount of bowel length is lost, the infant may have short-gut syndrome and require long-term parenteral nutrition. If adequate bowel length is maintained, and there are no other severe underlying illnesses, the long-term outlook for these infants is good.

Parent Teaching

Preoperative

Parents should be told before surgery about the anesthesia their infant will receive. The need for anesthesia and analgesia should be explained to parents, along with the physiologic and behavioral

benefits of pain relief. Care providers' sensitivity to the neonate's pain and advocating for pain relief are comforting for parents (see Chapter 11).[27]

The surgical procedure and what the infant will look like on return from surgery are explained. Providing written material with simple drawings of the operative procedure helps in retention of important facts. It is helpful for both nurse and physician to meet with the family to discuss the operation. This is especially important for the nurse, who must answer questions, interpret information, and reassure an anxious family when the physician leaves.

Because parental fears and fantasies about their infant's problem are frequently worse than reality, parents should see their infant before surgery (see Part VI). Infants who are extremely ill should have a picture taken before surgery. In the tragic situation of neonatal death during operation, these pictures may be very valuable to the family. It may also be helpful for parents to see an infant who has had a similar procedure and has the equipment that has been described (e.g., colostomy, orogastric tube, chest tube). If this is not possible, pictures or drawings are useful in preventing postoperative surprises.

Operative

Accompanying the infant to surgery and seeing the infant as soon as possible after surgery are comforting for the parents. Progress reports, if at all possible during surgery, are always appreciated by an anxious family. After the operation, the pediatric surgeon should immediately see the parents to explain the procedure and give a progress report on the infant.

Postoperative

After surgery, parents need to review the equipment and what it does to help their infant. It is important to help them focus their attention on their infant rather than merely on the machinery. Early involvement in care giving helps to personalize the newborn. Comfort measures are ideally provided by parents, who may then actively participate in their infant's pain relief.

If the infant will be discharged with an ostomy

or while receiving TPN, it is helpful to involve the parents in this care as early as possible. They may begin by cleansing the skin around the ostomy or helping to prepare the equipment. Gradually they are able to increase their responsibilities of care giving as their infant improves. Waiting to teach these special care needs until a few days before discharge does not give parents adequate time for practice and familiarity before being on their own.

The possibility of postoperative complications (such as leakage in a TEF at the anastomotic site) must always be discussed with parents. Although the development of complications is disappointing, they may be less difficult to handle when the parents are aware of their possibility. In preparation for discharge, parents should know what problems might develop and how to recognize them (e.g., late bowel obstruction). The ability to recognize excessive stooling and signs of dehydration should be taught to parents of any infant with an ostomy.

The importance of follow-up care must be stressed to parents. It may be helpful for parents to talk with a "graduate" parent who had an infant with similar problems. Parents should know what resource people, such as visiting nurses, graduate parents, and physicians, are available and how to contact them. It is important for the resource people in the community to know the infant's history and what information the parents have received. Ideally, a written discharge plan should be given to the parents and community resource people.

Acknowledgement

We would like to thank Carol Rumack, M.D., and the Department of Radiology, University of Colorado Health Sciences Center, for the use of material from their teaching files.

References

1. Adzick NS et al: Diaphragmatic hernia in the fetus: prenatal diagnosis and outcome in 94 cases, *J Pediatr Surg* 20(4):357, 1985.
2. Andrassy RJ, Mahour GH: Malrotation of the midgut in infants and children. A 25-year review, *Arch Surg* 116:158, 1981.
3. Ashcraft KW et al: The Thal fundoplication for gastroesophageal reflux, *J Pediatr Surg* 19(4):480, 1984.

4. Bailey PV et al: Congenital duodenal obstruction: a 32-year review, *J Pediatr Surg* 28(1):92, 1993.

5. Bartlett RH: Extracorporeal life support in neonatal respiratory failure, *Surgery Rounds* 41, August, 1989.

6. Bensauron AZ, Yaybeck S, Carceller-Blanchara A: Results and complications of Toupet partial posterior wrap: 10 year's experience, *J Pediatr Surg* 29:1215, 1991.

7. Dufour H, Fredet P: La stenose hypertrophique du pylore chez la nourisson et son traitement chirurgical, *Rev Chir* 37:208, 1908.

8. Filston HC: Gastroschisis—primary fascial closure, *Ann Surg* 197:260, 1983.

9. Holder TM, Manning PB: Esophageal atresia and tracheoesophageal fistula, *Surgical Rounds* 492, 1991.

10. Kosloske AM: Indications for operation in necrotizing enterocolitis revisited, *J Pediatr Surg* 29:663, 1994.

11. Kasai M: Treatment of biliary atresia with special reference to hepatic portoenterostomy and its modifications, *Prog Pediatr Surg* 6:5, 1974.

12. Kasai M et al: Surgical treatment of biliary atresia, *J Pediatr Surg* 3:665, 1968.

13. Kosloske AM, Musemeche CA: Necrotizing enterocolitis of the neonate, *Clin Perinatol* 16(1):97, 1989.

14. Lilly JR, Karrer FM: Contemporary surgery of biliary atresia, *Pediatr Clin North Am* 32(4):1233, 1985.

15. Mahour GH: Omphalocele, *Surg Gynecol Obstet* 143:821, 1976.

16. Martin LW, Zerella JT: Jejunoileal atresia: a proposed classification, *J Pediatr Surg* 11(3):399, 1976.

17. Mabogunje OA, Wang CI, Mahour H: Improved survival of neonates with meconium ileus, *Arch Surg* 117:37, 1982.

18. Nicolai I, Rehbein F: Management of imperforate anus with recto-urethral fistula, *Arch Dis Child* 38(198):167, 1963.

19. O'Neill JA Jr, Holcomb GW Jr, Neblett WW: Recent experience with esophageal atresia, *Ann Surg* 195:739, 1982.

20. Pena A, deVries PA: Posterior sagittal anorectoplasty: important technical considerations and new applications, *J Pediatr Surg* 17:796, 1982.

21. Raffensperger J: Hirschsprung's disease, *Surgical Rounds* 89, November, 1988.

22. Ramstedt C: Ziu operation der angetoreneu pylorusstenose, *Med Klin* 8.1702, 1912.

23. Randolph J: Experience with the Nissen fundoplication for correction of gastroesophageal reflux in infants, *Ann Surg* 198:579, 1983.

24. Rescorla FJ et al: Changing patterns of treatment and survival in neonates with meconium ileus, *Arch Surg* 124:837, 1989.

25. Robertson DE: Congenital pyloric stenosis, *Ann Surg* 112:687, 1940.

26. Seashore JH et al: Familial apple peel jejunal atresia: surgical, genetic, and radiographic aspects, *Pediatrics* 80:540, 1987.

27. Soave F: A new surgical technique for treatment of Hirschsprung's disease, *Surgery* 56(5):1007, 1964.

28. Wesley JR, Mahour GH: Congenital intrinsic duodenal obstruction: a twenty-five year review, *Surgery* 82:716, 1977.

29. Woolley MM: Congenital posterolateral diaphragmatic hernia, *Surg Clinic North Am* 565:317, 1976.

Resources for Parents

American Association of Critical Care Nurses. It's critical that you know . . . what you should do when your baby is in the NICU, *AACN,* California, 1987.

Butler NC: Questions parents and concerned professionals might ask of their local health care institutions, *Birth* 15:40, 1988.

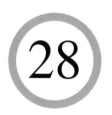

28 Families in Crisis: Theoretical and Practical Considerations

Roberta Siegel, Sandra L. Gardner, Gerald B. Merenstein

The technical advances that have characterized newborn care in the last 40 years have resulted in marked improvement in the mortality and morbidity of the high-risk infant. These developments have been accompanied by a heightened appreciation of the psychologic strain and emotional stresses encountered by the family of the sick neonate.[33] Realization of the need for a family-centered approach to perinatal care has emerged out of an enhanced understanding of individual and family functioning and their adaptation to stress.[41,85] It has become essential for perinatal health care teams to address the psychologic needs of families who are experiencing the painful crisis of the birth of a sick newborn. The purpose of this chapter is to discuss the complex psychosocial needs of families during this stressful period and to offer concrete suggestions for intervention.

Normal Attachment

Emotional investment in the child begins not at birth, but during the pregnancy. The terms *attachment* and *bonding*[49] are used to describe this process of relating between parents and their infant. Attachment behavior is characterized by the same qualities used to describe love: care, responsibility, and knowledge.[27]

The infant's need for the parent is absolute, but the parent's need for the infant is only relative. The neonate is totally dependent, both physically and emotionally, on the care givers. Recognition of this unique relationship is evidenced cross-culturally by immediate and prolonged contact with no evidence of separation.[44,61] In most animal species the mother engages in species-specific behaviors[49] that enable her to become acquainted with and claim the newborn. Interference during this critical period results in rejection by the animal mother and death of the young. Parental attachment and care giving behaviors are crucial for the infant's physical, psychologic, and emotional health and survival.[43,79] Ultimately, this influence will affect the child's well-being as an adult and a potential parent for a subsequent generation.

Critical and Sensitive Period

In the period immediately after birth, both mother and infant are physiologically and psychologically ready for reciprocal interaction.[49] Physiologically, even though labor and birth are tiring, most mothers feel "high" and have an incredible surge of energy after birth. Psychologically, the family is ready to meet and interact with the long-awaited newcomer. Physiologically, the first hour of life is a time of alertness for the newborn. Before the sleep phase the newborn is alert, makes eye-to-eye contact, fixes and follows, begins to search, unassisted, for the maternal nipple, and begins to feed.[91] At birth, all five senses are operational, and the infant is ready to cue and shape the environment (see Chapter 12).

This period of mutual readiness has been compared with the critical period in animals. This human "maternal sensitive period"[49] is the time immediately after birth in which the attachment process is initiated. Called the optimal, but not the sole, period for attachment to develop, the human critical period represents a reciprocal readiness for acquaintance. Positive effects of early and extended contact, rather than initial separation, have shown significant differences in care giving behaviors that persist over time.

Sustained and early contact between parents and infant completes the process of labor and birth and gives the family the opportunity for interaction. The presence of the infant enables the parents to begin knowing the reality and individuality of their infant. Early parent-infant contact facilitates parent-infant attachment and contributes to the regulation of the newborn's physiology and behavior.[18,43,78] Unnecessary "routines" and procedures that interfere with initial contact should be deferred until the initial acquaintance process is completed.[8,43,91]

Failure to establish immediate contact because of medically indicated interventions necessary to sustain life does not promote attachment, but it also does not undermine the entire process of attachment. Unlike animals, human mothers do not automatically reject their infant if they are unable to interact immediately. Interference or failure to interact during the critical period does not condemn the resilient and adaptable human parent to rejection of or maladaptation to the infant.

Crisis Event: Pregnancy and Parenthood

Pregnancy, birth, and parenthood are almost universally defined as a life crisis.[44,53] Parenting is a major adjustment of the prepregnancy roles, lifestyle, and relationships. Because previous ideas and coping styles may not be helpful, life crisis situations challenge the individual with the potential for growth as new responses and solutions are used for problem solving. Periods of upheaval, change, and vulnerability provide a time of openness, receptiveness, and readiness for help from significant others (including professionals).

Influences on Parenting

Opportunities to experience parenting and to observe others parent within a social setting are essential learning experiences for the development of parenting behaviors. The ability to parent is influenced by a multitude of factors that occur before, during, and after the birth of the infant. Previous life events, including genetic endowment,[49] cultural practices,[44,61] being parented,[36] previous pregnancies,[45] and interpersonal relationships,[36] affect the experience of pregnancy and parenthood. The events of the current pregnancy,[49,88] their significance to the parent, and the availability of support and assistance influence parenting ability. After birth, infant characteristics, behavior of health professionals,[23,28,38,49] separation from the infant,[10,52,78] and hospital practices[23,28,50,90] may positively or negatively influence parents. Not only the occurrence of these events, but also their meaning to the individual and the type of assistance received, influence parenting abilities.

Steps of Attachment

Klaus and Kennell[49] have proposed nine steps in the process of attachment.

Step 1. Planning the Pregnancy

This is the initial step of investment in the life-altering prospect of parenthood. Pregnancies are planned in one of two ways: consciously or unconsciously. Who planned the pregnancy and why this particular time has been chosen are important indicators of the investment of each individual in the decision and in the pregnancy.

Carrying a pregnancy is not assurance that the baby is wanted. Although it may be a legal option, abortion may not be a cultural, moral, financial, or ethical option for the individual woman. Attachment of the mother (or father) to the infant is not assured merely by the mother's remaining pregnant, giving birth, and keeping the infant.

Step 2. Confirming the Pregnancy

This occurs after the first and often subtle signs of pregnancy appear. Pregnancy confirmation begins the psychologic acceptance of the pregnancy. Delaying confirmation enables the fact of pregnancy to be denied and prevents progression to the acceptance stage.

Step 3. Accepting the Pregnancy

This usually begins early in the pregnancy and is characterized by the emotional changes of primary narcissism, introversion, and passivity. Being less interested in the outside world and more interested in her own inner world, the mother is able to become attuned to her own needs. Although she was previously engaged in active, extroverted behaviors, she may, during the pregnancy, contentedly participate in quieter, more introspective activities.

At this early stage of pregnancy the fetus is not perceived by the woman as separate from herself but as an extension of her body. The psychologic changes of pregnancy have survival significance in that caring for herself assures caring for the fetus as an integral part of herself.[12]

During the early months of pregnancy, the man and woman realize that parenting will require a major adjustment of prepregnancy roles, lifestyle, and relationships. The adaptation of parenthood is characterized by upheaval and change, losses and gains. Bombarded with phenomenal lifelong changes, the future parents experience the normal feeling of ambivalence.

Step 4. Fetal Movement

Fetal movement, felt by the mother between 16 and 32 weeks of gestation, is the beginning of the acceptance of the fetus as an individual. Fetal movement is the first concrete evidence to the mother of the existence of another person within her. Hearing the baby's heartbeat, seeing the ultrasound readings, or experiencing an amniocentesis also confirms the reality of the fetus.[42] Fetal movement is such a significant event that often a pregnancy that began as unplanned and unwanted becomes wanted.

Perception of the first fetal movement is a happy event. When asked, "How did you feel when the baby first moved?" most women respond in a happy tone and with a smile. A negative tone or negative words used to describe fetal movement is a concern because the individual (fetus) may already be perceived as an intruder.

Step 5. Accepting the Fetus

Accepting the fetus as an individual begins with fetal movement. The fetus asserts individuality in controlling the movement; the mother can neither start nor stop these movements. With the realization

of the concrete evidence of the presence of another person, parents begin the psychologic acceptance and personification of the fetus as a separate individual. Love for the fetus as a separate individual occurs through the parents' investing a personality in the fetus and establishing a relationship with that personality. Fantasies about how the baby looks, the sex, and the wish for a perfect, healthy infant are common.

Outwardly, preparations are made for the acceptance of an infant into the home; baby clothes and furniture are purchased, and a room is prepared. The fetus may be referred to by a nickname or a term of endearment. The baby's name may be chosen. Choosing a name is a highly personal and significant event. The meaning of the name and who chooses it illustrate the power holder and decision-maker within the family. Prenatal questions such as "Do you have a nickname for the baby?" "Do you have a name picked out for the baby?" and "Who picked it out?" may be asked after the birth to elicit information.

Whether the newborn meets parental expectations for "the right sex" may be crucially important in the parent's ability to attach to the infant. "Do you have a sex preference for the baby?" may be asked before or after the birth to elicit this information. Often parents with a strong sex preference have chosen no names for a baby of the "wrong" sex.

"It doesn't matter as long as it's healthy," is often heard and may indicate no conscious sex preference. However, unconsciously the parents may have a strong sex preference as evidenced by a predominance of dreams about one sex. If dreams are equally divided between male and female children, there may indeed be no sex preference at the unconscious level.

Most parents are fearful of producing a defective child. This fear is experienced as dreams about dead, deformed, or damaged fetuses and babies, or dreams with a central theme of destruction. These unconscious contents are often experienced as frightening nightmares that may often be imbued with magical ideas such as, "If I think (or talk about) it, it will come true." Both before and after birth, it is reassuring for parents to know that this is a common and scary phenomenon, that they aren't "crazy," and that the fears are not magical.

Parental expectations of the newborn are established before birth in the personification and relationship with the unseen, unheard fetus. After birth the developmental task of parenthood is a working out of the discrepancy between the wished for and the actual infant.[87] Before attachment to the actual infant is able to proceed, the fantasized child must be mourned.

Step 6. Labor and Birth

Labor is a physiologic, maturational, and psychologic crisis for the family. Birth is the culmination of pregnancy and the reward for the work of labor. Parents' attitudes about the labor and birth experiences affect their reactions to the infant. Newton and Newton[67] found mothers more likely to be pleased with their infant at first sight if the mothers were relaxed, calm, and cooperative; had rapport with the attendants; and received personalized, solicitous care.

Paternal participation in labor and birth is an important issue. In the past, health care professionals saw no benefit to the presence of the father and even wished to exclude him because of imagined "horribles" such as increased infection rate, malpractice suits, and disruption of routines.

Birth is a powerfully emotional experience, so that those who attend birth are more attached to the infant than those who do not attend.[49] Benefits attributed to a father's participation at labor and birth include use of less analgesia, a more supportive environment, and deepened relationship[8] between parents and between parents and their infant.[75] Inclusion of the father in perinatal events may "hook" him for inclusion in parenting activities. Rather than just a financial provider, fathering may be perceived as a psychologic necessity for both fathers and children.

Parental behaviors at birth indicate involvement and investment in the infant*:

- "How does the mother or father *look?*" At the sound of the infant's cry, parents smile and breathe a sigh of relief at this first breath of life. Support, joy, and happiness are positive feelings shared by couples at birth.
- "What does the mother or father *say?*" By

speaking in a positive tone with words of affection and endearment, the parents relate to each other and to the new infant.
- "What does the mother or father *do?*" When offered the infant, both parents will reach out to take the infant. Spontaneously, parents engage in eye-to-eye contact and touch and explore the infant. Affectionate behaviors such as kissing, fondling, cuddling, and claiming characterize positive parental reactions.

A positive, self-affirming birth experience for the mother enhances her feelings of self-esteem, thus her self-concept as a woman and mother.[28] A birth experience that does not meet parental expectations may have a negative effect on the self-concept of the mother, her perception of her ability to parent, and her relationship with the infant.[23,28] In fact, "so intricately are mother and infant entwined in a symbiotic relationship, that what is psychically positive for the mother is positive for the infant. What is psychically negative for the mother will affect the infant."[27] Labor and delivery that have been difficult or prolonged may influence parental overprotection, resentment, or antagonism toward the infant.[2,23]

So powerful is the labor and birth experience that women are unable to proceed with parenting until psychic closure of the experience has been obtained. Even women who experience a normal labor and birth process need to recount the experience to others. Maternal perception of the events is obvious in tone and content of the recounting. *Missing pieces*[2] is the term used to describe the aspects of labor and birth that are forgotten or unavailable to recall. Long labor, short labor, or medicated labor can cause missing pieces in the mother's memory of the birth. Labor that did not meet expectations because of difficulty, cesarean section, use of forceps, or episiotomy could also affect the mother.[2] To proceed with parenting, these women need to fill in their knowledge gaps by asking questions or looking at pictures or films of the birth to reconstruct the situation.

Step 7. Seeing

Seeing and touching, are the species-specific ways in which humans attach to their young.[49]

Eye contact between parents and their infant in

---

* From Helfer B, Kempe CH, editors: *Child abuse and neglect: the family and the community,* 1976, Ballinger Publishing Company.

the initial period after birth may be a positive release of parental feelings of warmth, closeness, and caring. As parents see and inspect the newborn, they begin claiming their infant: "He has my eyes; she has your nose" and begin "letting go" of the prenatally fantasized child. Characteristics of each parent and the family are identified in the infant, and the newborn is claimed as a member of the family.

The term *en face position* is used to describe the mother's (father's) eyes and the infant's eyes positioned in the same vertical plane.[49] This positioning enables the parent and infant to look directly into each other's eyes, to focus, and to regard each other (Fig. 28-1).

The newborn infant is an active participant in the acquaintance process, as he or she cues the mother with eye-to-eye contact. Even minutes old[25] newborns see and show a preference for the human face (within 7 to 12 inches from their face). The newborn is able to visually follow the parent's face and voice and to signal the parent with facial expressions, movement, and vocalization, includ-

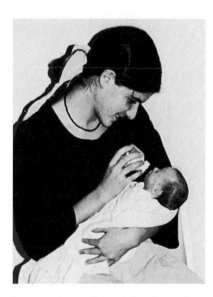

Figure 28-1 En face position: infant is held in close contact (mother's body touching infant's); mother is looking at infant en face; bottle is perpendicular to mouth; milk is in tip of nipple. (From Klaus MH, Kennel JH: *Parent-infant bonding,* ed 2, St Louis, 1982, Mosby.)

ing a distress cry when separated from body contact with mother.[18]

Deterrents to the infant's full participation include removal to the nursery, medication (from analgesia), and eye prophylaxis. Unless medically indicated (necessary for physical survival), newborns should remain with their parents after birth.[78,90] Because eye prophylaxis irritates and interferes with vision, the "routine" instillation immediately after birth (in the delivery room) can be delayed until after the initial acquaintance process is completed.

Step 8. Touching

This behavior is important to the adult as a means of tactile and sensory knowledge of the infant. To the neonate the "stimulus hunger"[77] is satisfied by parental touch and ministrations.

In exploring the infant, parents systematically use fingertip contact with the infant's extremities. Gradually, there is progression to palm contact with the infant's trunk (Fig. 28-2). With the healthy term infant, this progression occurs within minutes of the first contact. After gaining confidence and preliminary knowledge, the parent will enfold the infant close to the ventrum of the adult (a cuddling position).

With the preterm infant, this characteristic progression may take hours, days, or several visits (see Fig. 28-2). Fear of harming the small, fragile preterm infant prevents parents from feeling at ease in touching their infant. Until the parents feel confident that their actions will not harm the infant, they may be reticent to use palm contact with the trunk (vital organs).

Holding and cuddling the infant are significantly different from touching and exploring. Mothers who have only seen and touched their infant still experience "empty arms." The species-specific behavior of touch is not completely satisfied until the parent is able "to hold" the infant.

Step 9. Care Giving

The final step of attachment, care giving is important for psychic closure of the task of bonding. The relationship between the primary care giver and the infant is a reciprocal relationship. In the care giving relationship both care provider and infant give to and receive from each other.[18,38,43] The physical

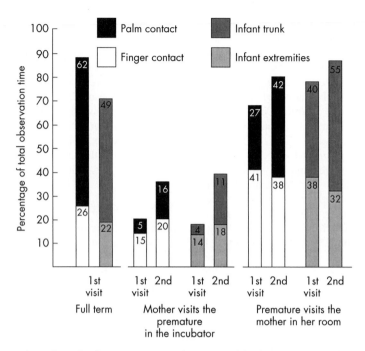

Figure 28-2   Fingertip and palm contact on trunk or extremities in three groups of mothers: (1) 12 mothers of term infants at their first visit, (2) 9 mothers who visited their premature infants in incubators in NICU, and (3) 14 mothers whose premature infants were brought to their maternity rooms and placed in their beds. (From Klaus MH, Kennell JH: *Parent-infant bonding,* ed 2, St Louis, 1982, Mosby.)

and emotional needs of the helpless infant are satisfied by parental care giving behaviors such as feeding, soothing, grooming, and playing. Based on the infant's ability to perceive and receive these ministrations, the infant responds to the care provider. Parental expectations of newborn responses include quieting, sucking, clinging and cuddling, looking, smiling, and vocalizing. Parental capability to soothe and satisfy the infant provides emotional satisfaction and positive feedback about the parent's competency.

Personal needs for comfort, maintenance of homeostasis, and relief from painful experiences are infant expectations of the relationship with the care provider. Care-eliciting behaviors (crying, visual following, and smiling) are neonatal cues used to signal the care provider that attention is needed. Relief from discomfort enables the infant to respond positively to the care provider. The

infant experiences the world through the care giver and quickly learns that the environment is either nurturing and loving or hostile and nonresponsive. Consistent, predictable nurturing and care giving enable the infant to develop a sense of trust in the care giver, the world, and self (see Chapter 12).

Care by parents is the ideal neonatal care situation, because the infant learns and reacts to one set of cues or care giving behaviors. Cared for by one or two people, the infant is able to regulate his physiologic behavioral processes (i.e., autonomic, neuroendocrine, behavioral, and electrophysiologic) and develop synchrony with the parents.[43] Single care giving improves the establishment of biorhythms of the neonate[23,43] for sleep-wake cycles, feeding, and visual attentiveness. Multiple care giving confuses the infant, increases distress with feeding, causes irritability, and upsets visual attention. Care by parents provides for mutual cuing and acquaintance and a natural setting for observation of parent-infant interaction.[90]

Psychologic Adjustments to a Sick Newborn

The birth of a sick newborn with its consequent family disruption represents to the perinatal health care team a unique crisis, a dangerous opportunity[6] within which to practice preventive health care.[65] For the involved individual and family this stressful event results in a period of psychologic disorganization during which their usual problem-solving mechanisms may not be adequate to cope with the events presented to them.[16] In addition to confronting this situational crisis, the individual or family must master the normal developmental process of parenthood.

Parental behavior and responses are determined not only by preexisting personality factors, social and cultural variables, and interactions with significant others[16,48] but also by the immediate situation in which the parents are placed.[79] Situational factors can have an important bearing on the family's ability to cope with the crisis and thus affect the overall outcome (Box 28-1).

Families are psychologically vulnerable after the birth of a sick infant. During this period of temporary disorganization, there is a heightened receptivity to accepting help and being responsive to change, because the family is struggling for a way to cope with the crisis. Significant potentialities exist for individual and family emotional growth and development.[15,16] The perinatal health team has an opportunity to influence how the individual and family adapt to the crisis. By providing appropriate supportive interventions coupled with enlightened policies and attitudes that reflect family-centered principles (Box 28-2), the team can positively influence the family's coping, thus enhancing the likelihood for a successful resolution of the crisis and ultimately a healthy parent-child relationship.[22,80,83,85]

As discussed earlier, attachment is a complex developmental process. There are many interrelated factors that influence parental behavior and attachment toward the infant.[14,40] These include the in-

---

Box 28-1

Situational Factors Affecting Parental Coping[13,29,38,83,85]

1. The behaviors and attitudes of the hospital staff (physicians, nurses, and allied health professionals)
2. The sensitivity used in the process of separation and transfer of the infant to the intensive care unit or in some cases the referral hospital
3. The flexibility of hospital policy concerning parental and sibling involvement and visitation in the nursery
4. The instruction of parents in their infant's individual behaviors and characteristics (thus facilitating appropriate parent-child interaction and reciprocity) (see Chapter 12)
5. The staff's comprehension and appreciation of the psychosocial functioning of families and the family's responses and adaptation to stress and crisis
6. The employment of emotionally supportive intervention programs for parents within the nursery setting
7. The development of appropriate discharge planning to provide adequate follow-up care to the infant and family

---

fant, sex of the infant, social class, birth order, parental attitudes and expectations, events of the newborn period and postdischarge period, and level of family functioning.[50,56,76,85] Very important in any neonatal illness and subsequent hospitalization is the disruption and stress that is frequently created in the nuclear family system. It has been demonstrated that the family's functioning and its adaptation to stress have important effects on the family's relationship with the infant and the infant's later development. A crucial task of the perinatal health care team is to intervene in such a way as to assist families in using the unfortunate event of the birth of their sick infant to maximize their growth, adaptation, and reorganization during this period.[22,43,61]

To assist parents through the difficult experience of having a sick infant, it is helpful to identify the psychologic tasks and emotional reactions they experience. This section describes the six psycho-

---

Box 28-2

The Principles for Family-Centered Neonatal Care

1. Family-centered neonatal care should be based on open and honest communication between parents and professionals on medical and ethical issues.
2. To work with professionals in making informed treatment choices, parents must have available to them the same facts and interpretation of those facts as the professionals, including medical information presented in meaningful formats, information about uncertainties surrounding treatments, information from parents whose children have been in similar medical situations, and access to the chart and rounds discussions.
3. In medical situations involving very high mortality and morbidity, great suffering, and/or significant medical controversy, fully informed parents should have the right to make decisions regarding aggressive treatment for their infants.
4. Expectant parents should be offered information about adverse pregnancy outcomes and be given the opportunity to state in advance their treatment preferences if their infant is born extremely prematurely and/or critically ill.
5. Parents and professionals must work together to acknowledge and alleviate the pain of infants in the NICU.
6. Parents and professionals must work together to ensure an appropriate environment for infants in the NICU.
7. Parents and professionals must work together to ensure the safety and efficacy of neonatal treatments.
8. Parents and professionals should work together to develop nursery policies and programs that promote parenting skills and encourage maximum involvement of families with their hospitalized infant.
9. Parents and professionals must work together to promote meaningful long-term follow-up for all high-risk NICU survivors.
10. Parents and professionals must acknowledge that critically-ill newborns can be harmed by overtreatment as well as by undertreatment, and we must insist that our laws and treatment policies be based on compassion. We must work together to promote awareness of the needs of NICU survivors with disabilities to ensure adequate support for them and their families. We must work together to decrease disability through universal prenatal care.

Adapted from Harrison H: The principles for family-centered neonatal care, *Pediatrics* 82(5):643, 1993.

---

logic issues facing families; it discusses the clinical and behavioral indicators that parents are struggling with and then suggests interventions that the perinatal health care team can employ to help families. It is extremely important to remember that these are generalizations and that each family or person must be approached individually. Additionally, in assessing families' reactions, it is critical to look at how they cope over a period of time. Initially there may be a tremendous amount of upset, disruption, and upheaval within the individual or family system that eventually may lead to improved functioning and a sense of growth and mastery. The key is how the individuals or families reorganize, how able they are to return to a state of equilibrium, the coping strategies they are able to develop, and whether they are adaptive or maladaptive. Attachment and parenthood are complex, interactional developmental processes that must evolve and unfold over time.

Kaplan and Mason[45] describe four psychologic tasks that parents of premature infants must deal with:

- Anticipatory grieving and withdrawal from the relationship established during pregnancy
- Parental acknowledgment of feelings of guilt and failure
- Resumption of the relationship with the infant that had been previously disrupted

- Preparation to take the infant home

Two additional tasks are significant:

- Crisis events related to labor and delivery
- Adaptation to the intensive care environment[35,73]

In general, these six psychologic tasks can be applied to any parent's reaction to a sick infant, with additional specific issues arising depending on whether the infant was premature or born with a congenital anomaly.

Labor and Delivery

The first psychologic task involves working through the crisis events surrounding the labor and delivery. Medical problems occurring at any point during the pregnancy or delivery that threaten the health or survival of the fetus or the mother can result in the parents' delaying their planning and making an emotional investment in the fetus or infant. Parents may psychologically withdraw from the pregnancy as a way of protecting themselves. The parents of an infant born prematurely often do not have the necessary psychologic and physical time to prepare. This deprivation of time may interfere with the parents' ability to complete the final steps of attachment described earlier.[34] Parents who have been concentrating on themselves in a healthy, narcissistic way may not yet be ready to transfer their investment to the infant because they have been prematurely thrust into the role of parents. There is an overwhelming sense of losing control of the events of the labor and delivery and their timing. Parental wishes to retain the pregnancy can influence their attitude about the delivery and the infant.[89] On the other hand, some parents react oppositely; they may wish to be rid of the pregnancy as a way of dealing with their ambivalent feelings about the infant or their fear of the unknown and the uncertainty facing them. Many mothers of premature infants feel alien to their infants. They do not feel that the infants are really theirs, making it easier to have feelings of rejection toward the infant. In addition to feeling insufficient and inadequate about the ability to deliver an infant

at term, they feel empty inside, as if something is missing. This seems to occur because the mother who has been predominantly concerned about herself, her body, and the fetus growing inside is not ready to transfer that emotional investment outside of herself. With a premature birth there is usually a heightened sense of emergency and concern about the health and survival of the infant and at times the mother, who herself may have suffered complications.

In the case of a full-term infant born with a problem despite a problem-free pregnancy, there is a sense of overwhelming shock and disappointment. Parents immediately sense the problem; as their apprehension mounts, they frequently imagine and fantasize the worst. Parents of a newborn with a malformation normally experience lowered self-esteem and view this event as an affront to their reproductive capabilities. The mother specifically views it as a failure of her feminine role. Parents often feel that they have failed and that the infant symbolically represents their own defectiveness. Parents not only fear for the infant, they fear for themselves and what this child may mean to their future. The reaction of the parents is based on the specific psychologic, social, and cultural meaning of the defect to the parents and the manner in which the problem is discussed and handled with the parents by the health care team.[49]

The emotional reactions and feelings that parents have at and after the delivery of a sick infant range from shock, fright, and panic to anxiety and helplessness.[70] Parents may be so overwhelmed by the events that initially they may block any observable emotional response or affect. Staff interventions at this time are extremely important because they lay the foundations for subsequent interactions between parents and health professionals. Early comments and influential statements during this critical time can have lasting impressions in the minds of parents. This is also an emotionally difficult time for physicians and nurses, because they too are struggling with their own feelings of inadequacy, failure, and helplessness. Unconsciously, in an attempt to deal with their own feelings, staff may withdraw from parents and not be emotionally available to help. This is a normal response, but one that needs to be guarded against because it only perpetuates a breakdown in relationships and communication with parents that are so greatly needed at this time. Many helpful interventions can be employed that are sensitive and supportive, and that facilitate the emerging relationship between the parents and their infant.

Early Communication

In the labor and delivery phase, early communication with both parents is essential. Parents normally are apprehensive and extremely sensitive to explicit or implicit cues such as actual statements by the staff, the atmosphere, looks, or a tone of voice that may indicate how things are progressing. Because of the emphasis on prepared childbirth, parents are extremely sophisticated in their knowledge of labor and delivery practices and immediately sense some deviation from what they expected. Prompt, direct explanations presented in a calm manner are important and reassuring to parents. This explanation of the process of what is or will be happening can be effective because it helps to organize the parents at a time when they are extremely vulnerable and feeling out of control. Although it is normal for the staff to be guarded, members of the health care team should tell the parents the known facts and what actually is being done for their infant without giving any diagnosis, prognosis, or forecast for the future course of the infant. Avoiding or not talking to parents only accelerates parental anxiety and adds to their growing fantasies or distortions. It has been well established and documented that parents' fantasies about their infant's problems are usually worse than the reality.[49] Parents often report that when they actually saw their infant, they were relieved because they had imagined the infant to appear worse.

Support of Staff

It is also important that one of the staff stay with the parents through labor, delivery, and recovery to offer continual support and to reassure parents that communication will continue as soon as more information is known. This is, again, an uncomfortable time for the staff because they may feel helpless and useless and as a result may avoid parents or revert to performing more technical activities. Some parents may need someone to be with them, not only to talk to them, but, more importantly, to listen; on the other hand, some parents may not be able to talk or verbalize their concerns or fears. Others may wish to be alone with each other or any other significant person in their life. Because of the varying responses and needs of people, it is extremely important to be sensitive to individual differences in approaching parents.

As much as possible, talking to both parents at the same time is helpful when discussing the infant's condition. This decreases their distortions and misconceptions, increases the communication and support between parents, and prevents either parent from feeling excluded. The assumption is commonly made that the father is in a better emotional state to hear about the infant; this misconception leads health professionals to mistakenly exclude or "spare" the mother, which only postpones her ability to begin to cope with the reality of her infant's condition. Sparing the mother may cause the parents to be in different stages of their understanding of the infant's medical condition and in their emotional state. Because emotional support between parents is so critical, the staff should avoid sparing, because it can add to the parents' difficulty in being attuned to each other's needs and creates more opportunities for the parents to be out of synchrony with each other. Both mothers and fathers of critically ill newborns generally find each other to be the greatest source of support in the first 2 weeks of NICU hospitalization.[62]

Seeing the Infant

The question usually arises about the value of the parents seeing their infant, especially if the infant is very small, is not likely to survive, or is profoundly malformed. Generally, it is assumed that it is psychologically better for parents to have had the opportunity to see their infant, but this must be individualized for each family and newborn. Seeing the infant helps to facilitate attachment, decrease exaggerated fantasies, decrease withdrawal from the infant, and enhance the parents' ability to grasp the reality of the situation. Because of the need to respect individual differences in people, the best approach is to give parents the opportunity to decide whether they together or individually want to see the infant.

This decision should be ultimately made by the parents with the support of the health care team. It is not uncommon to find a well-meaning family member, physician, nurse, or social worker advising the parents or making the decision himself or herself and concluding it would be in the parents' best interests not to see the infant. The argument is given that, "It's better not to get attached," or "It would make them cry or upset them to see the anomaly," or "They could not handle it," or "They would lose control." This decision is for the parents, not the professional, to make.

Some parents may know unequivocally what they want to do; others may be ambivalent, unsure, and indecisive. It is the role of the professional to give the parents assistance (information and support) in making the decision. The parents may need time to think about it or may need to discuss their fear and ambivalence first, before being able to decide. They may need some factual information and preparation from the professional, such as the appearance of the infant and a description of the equipment. They may need assurance that someone will stay with them. Although time often is a factor and a decision must be made quickly, it is important to move at the parents' pace. The professional should still follow as much as possible the principle of allowing the parents the option of seeing the infant. If for medical reasons of the mother this is not possible, a self-developing picture can be taken.[64] If it is medically possible for the parents to touch or hold the infant, the parents should be offered the opportunity. Touching or holding not only facilitates attachment but can provide parents with an emotional experience that is very sustaining and reassuring, helping them proceed through a very critical time of separation.

The parents are very sensitive to the staff's attitude toward the infant as reflected by their comments and the manner in which the staff handle the infant. If the infant is regarded with respect and treated as important, the parent is given the feeling that the infant is seen as valued and worthwhile. This is especially important for parents of an infant with a congenital anomaly; the parents could wonder if their infant is viewed as "damaged goods" by society. In describing the infant to the parent, it is important to present a balanced picture of both the normal and abnormal aspects of the infant. In discussing the infant with the parents, reference to the infant by name, if they have named the infant, helps personalize the infant and establish the infant's unique identity.

Care Giving

To reinforce the care giving needs of parents, it is important to discuss with them their plans to feed their infant. Support and encouragement should be given whether the parents have decided on breast-feeding or bottle-feeding. In many situations, breastfeeding a sick infant may be possible. Many mothers are able to pump their breasts for milk that eventually will be given to the infant. There are many psychologic and physiologic reasons why breastfeeding or pumping may be beneficial for mothers and infants alike (see Chapter 18). The breastfeeding or pumping experience helps the mother to feel close to her infant and that she has some control over what is happening to her infant; she can uniquely contribute to her infant's care in a way no one else can. Fathers, too, can participate in this activity by their support and interest in the actual breastfeeding or the pumping and milk collection activities. Many mothers are able to successfully pump and eventually put the infant to breast, but others are not, because of emotional stresses, the condition of the infant, the length of time until the infant can feed, and the waning interest of the mother. Regardless of eventual success, the mother should be encouraged to try if she has an interest; then she can feel that she made an attempt to relate to her infant in this way. If a mother does not plan to breastfeed or pump, or if she tries but does not continue, she should not be made to feel guilty or that she failed in her role. She is already vulnerable to these feelings, having had an infant born with problems.

After the delivery when the mother returns to her room without a healthy infant, she usually experiences a void; an amputation has occurred.[49] She and those around her are beginning to grieve. The interventions of the staff should be flexible and sensitive to the individual needs of the family. Empathy, responsiveness, and an ability to listen to the parents are important at this time.

Encouraging parents to verbalize and express their feelings and concerns (at their own pace), although difficult to do at times, is useful to the parents. Avoiding their grief gives the mother and father the impression that they are "bad parents" for having feelings of sadness, anger, guilt, or loss; this only increases their level of guilt and isolation. Prescribing tranquilizers also gives the message that is it not permissible to talk about what has happened to them and their infant. Tranquilizers only increase the feelings of unreality that normally are experienced. This stifles the parental coping mechanisms at a time when the parents need to begin to come to terms with what has happened.

Room assignments are a very personal matter and one that the mother should decide. Some mothers want to return to the regular maternity ward; for others it is too painful, and they want to be in a separate area. Flexible visiting regulations for the father and other significant persons are necessary to facilitate support to one another through a very difficult, uncertain period.

In talking to parents, it is important to bear in mind that the parents do not remember much of what has been said; it is very difficult for them to assimilate both cognitively and emotionally all that has happened. It is important for the staff to move at the parents' own pace. If the infant has been transferred or the chances for survival are limited, the mother should be discharged or given a pass to visit the infant as soon as possible. It is also important to acknowledge to the mother (and father) that they are parents and that they did give birth to a baby. They need the congratulatory cards, gifts, and attention that they would have normally received.

Anticipatory Grieving

After labor and delivery, parents are struggling with the second psychologic task of anticipatory grieving and withdrawal from the relationship established during pregnancy. This task requires that parents acknowledge that their infant's life is endangered or that the newborn might die. Events surrounding the labor, delivery, and postpartum period may have indicated to the parents that their infant's chances for survival are diminished. If this has occurred, parents can then become involved in anticipatory grieving and withdrawal from the relationship established during pregnancy. Studies have shown that the decision to transfer an infant to an NICU alone is likely to initiate an anticipatory grief reaction.[11]

Parents may also be experiencing feelings of grief and sadness over the loss of the expected, idealized child that they had wished for during the pregnancy. For some parents, attaching to a critically ill or malformed infant may be too overwhelming; parents may withdraw from the infant in an attempt to protect themselves from their feelings of hurt, disappointment, and guilt.[35,65] Some parents may feel ambivalent about the infant; they may feel they could not love or cope with an infant who might die or who would have significant physical or mental problems. Feeling uncertain about whether they want the infant to survive can cause feelings of guilt that may cause the parents to withdraw from the infant as a way of avoiding confronting these difficult, painful feelings.

During this period, parents may find themselves in a very stressful position; they are faced with the task of balancing the painful realities of confronting a possible loss against their hopes of the intact survival of their infant. The emotional withdrawal and grieving that parents experience is normal during the critical time that the infant's life is endangered or when parents are faced with the possibility that their infant may have a life-long problem. This withdrawal becomes pathologic only if it continues beyond the time the infant demonstrates definite signs (to the parents) of improvement and survival. In the case of a permanently handicapped newborn, parents unable to grieve their idealized infant may maintain this withdrawal, which might lead to attachment difficulties.[87]

Parental Responses

Parents exhibit many emotional responses and behaviors that indicate they are struggling with the anticipatory grieving and withdrawal. Some parents are very sad, depressed, and teary, and others may be highly anxious, at times bordering on panic states; others react by having a flat affect, being withdrawn, and appearing apathetic. Some parents may exhibit very angry, hostile, confrontational behavior as a way of dealing with their distress, others may deny the situation by optimistically feeling that "everything will be OK."

Parents who typically are verbal may ask questions reflecting their concerns about their infant's survival; this is especially true after the child has received medical attention and decisions are being made about treatment for the infant, including transfer to an NICU. The questions they ask physicians and nurses are "Is he going to make it?" "What do you think his chances are?" "He'll be OK, won't he?" "Have you seen other babies with this problem?" "Do other babies make it?" "How long will he be in the hospital?" Parents struggling with their fears may resist seeing, touching, or visiting the infant. If they do visit the infant in the NICU, they may remain distant by having little or no eye contact with the infant, refusing to touch, standing far from the warmer or incubator, and asking few or no questions of the staff. The parents may be reluctant to name the infant; when they do refer to the infant, they say "it," "she," "he," or "the baby." If the infant has been given a special or treasured family name, they may be reluctant to use it.

A very common phenomenon occurs when parents, being protective of each other, discourage each other's involvement with the infant. This is especially true at the time of transport when the transport nurse may suggest to the father or family members that the infant be shown to the mother before leaving. Many fathers are afraid this will increase the emotional attachment to the infant and thus the feelings of disappointment and loss if the infant should die. The father is usually very apprehensive about how to handle the mother's feelings of grief in addition to his own. This type of behavior also is true with regard to medical information; it is not uncommon for one parent to request that all communication go through that parent. The response is that "my spouse is too upset or anxious and couldn't handle hearing any bad news." Many times it is actually the parent making the request who is most anxious and who is dealing with this anxiety by projecting it onto the other partner. Work and child care responsibilities, transportation difficulties, and financial limitations are all legitimate reasons why parents may be unable to have frequent contact with their infant. However, these factors may also serve as unconscious ways to maintain distance from the infant.

It is important to keep in mind that this withdrawal and grieving is a necessary and natural process. For parents to develop an attachment to and accept the reality of their infant's condition, they must experience their feelings of grief, sadness, anger, guilt, and disappointment over the loss of the expected child.[87] This grieving serves to free the parents' emotional energy so that they can interact with and become attuned to their infant. Grieving enhances the parents' availability to the infant. This availability aids in their feeling competent to handle their infant.[89] The goal, then, of the perinatal health care team's interventions is to help the family realize that their feelings are natural and normal and will be accepted. Parents need permission to have their feelings. It is essential to acknowledge to parents that it is normal to be afraid of attaching to an infant who might die or have a handicap. Giving permission diminishes the guilt that the parents may feel about their behavior being abnormal or about being bad parents because they are afraid. Simple statements such as, "Many parents tell us they are afraid of getting close to their baby," or "It's scary to attach when you think the baby may die," are helpful.

It is sometimes useful for parents to verbalize what their fears actually are. They may fear their infant's dying, being retarded, or being paralyzed. Once their fears are clarified in the minds of the parents and either confirmed or refuted by the medical staff, it is usually easier for parents to begin to accept their infant's diagnosis and prognosis and begin relating to the infant. Social workers can provide valuable emotional support to families in helping them deal with their realistic and unrealistic concerns.[68]

Communicating Medical Information

The role of the physician in communicating medical information is extremely important. There are many schools of thought about how to approach parents, ranging from being extremely cautious and pessimistic ("paint the bleakest picture") to being encouraging and optimistic ("give parents hope"). Although the approach should be individualized for each family, a balanced approach is the most beneficial. Parents need a realistic assessment of the situation that is honest and direct. It is important to acknowledge the infant's condition and possible problems, but not to inundate parents with every potential problem that can arise. Parents who hear "brain damage," "retarded," or "the baby will die" are not likely to forget these statements. These statements can linger in the minds of parents and adversely influence how the parents relate to their newborn. They may believe that some day "brain damage will show up" or that the infant is susceptible and frail and needs to be treated cautiously for fear of a life-threatening condition. These children may become victims of the vulnerable child syndrome,[37,74] a condition in which a child is overprotected by his or her parents and treated as if he or she had a medical problem or is in danger of death when neither is any longer the case. Parents who are told their newborn may die may have trouble attaching or becoming emotionally invested. When talking to parents, physicians and nurses should be very judicious and careful in making dramatic statements of a sensitive nature. Definitive statements should be used only when appropriate and necessary. The long-term emotional implications of such statements need to be weighed.

There are several other rules or guidelines in communicating medical information to parents.[89] As mentioned earlier, parents' perceptions of their infant's condition are extremely important, remain in parents' minds, and can affect their relationship with the infant. Parents easily misperceive information given to them. They may believe that a PDA indicates open-heart surgery and therefore worry that their infant has a heart condition. Or perhaps they think a bilirubin problem means their infant has liver disease. Therefore, in beginning any discussion with parents, it is essential to determine and address their perceptions. A staff member might say, "Could you tell me what you understand about your baby's condition?" This will give the physician or nurse the opportunity to correct any misinformation or misconceptions and to hear about the parents' concerns. Parents' perceptions of the severity of their infant's illness are complex, change over time, and are affected by (1) parental anxiety, (2) infant size, (3) amount and type of equipment and treatments, and (4) amount and type of information received from health care providers.[17,39] A team member might specifically ask about the parents' concerns or worries: "Could you tell me what concerns you have about your baby?" Asking this can make communication between the perinatal health care team and the parents more meaningful and helpful; unless the team deals with the parents' anxiety, discussions become one-sided lectures and

only benefit the professional. Discussions need to be a dialogue between parent and professional.

During the course of a discussion and again at the end, it is useful to determine parents' interpretations of what has been said and to modify and clarify as needed. The staff needs to avoid overloading a parent with lengthy explanations that are too technical. It is more productive to move at a pace so that the parent can assimilate the information presented; it is not necessary to describe the entire course of RDS or BPD. It is always preferable to use simple language that is understandable to a lay person and to avoid the use of statistics and vivid modifiers. Statistics are confusing because they do not apply to the individual case and can easily be misinterpreted. When asked about the frequency of brain damage with a grade III IVH, a team member might say, "A majority of these babies have some neurologic problem, but there are some who do not." Vivid modifiers such as "This is the worst case of sepsis we have ever had" or "Your baby is the sickest baby in the nursery" are of no real benefit to the parents and only accelerate their fantasies and anxieties. Finally, if a referring physician and the nursery team are both communicating with the parents, it is essential to coordinate the particular approach. It is very confusing to parents and decreases their trust level for one to be pessimistic and the other optimistic.

Acknowledgment of Guilt Feelings

The third psychologic task parents are dealing with simultaneously with anticipatory grieving and withdrawal is confronting and recognizing their feelings of failure and guilt in not delivering a healthy infant. Most parents struggling with feelings of inadequacy and guilt are likely to search for answers to the causes of their infant's situation. The mother may focus on concrete things such as not eating well, the flu, intercourse, birth control pills, or an unwanted pregnancy. The father may also be concerned about his role in not helping his wife enough, placing too many demands on her, an argument he provoked that precipitated labor, or another family member with the same chromosomal abnormality. Parents search for reasons because they need to find a cause for such an event happening to them. It is harder for them to feel out of control and helpless than to feel guilty. Some parents place responsibility on themselves, but others shift the blame to others in their external world, such as their spouse, extended family, doctor, nurses, or God. Often both parents are concerned with the disappointment that they have caused the other. They may withdraw from each other at a time when they both need acceptance and support. Realistic answers from the medical team are helpful for some parents in diminishing guilt feelings; in other parents the guilt may be so deeply integrated in the parents' thinking that it is less easily overcome. For example, some parents may focus on irrational, unrealistic factors such as, "This is my punishment for not being a good wife or daughter" or "This is my punishment for running away from home when I was 15." It seems that the more irrational the parental thinking, the harder it is to assuage and resolve the guilt. Many feelings of guilt and failure are normal and expected; the feelings are a problem when the parent does not respond to the infant's progress because the infant may continue to represent the parent's failure.

Parental Responses

Parents demonstrate many behaviors that indicate they are struggling with guilt and failure. Some parents directly verbalize these feelings and attempt to obtain helpful answers from the staff. Less obvious are the parents who are markedly depressed and remain so despite any improvement in the infant. These parents demonstrate the classic signs of depression such as apathy, loss of interest in appearance and self, withdrawal, and loss of self-esteem. They exhibit an overwhelming sense of helplessness because they feel responsible for causing their infant's problem and are helpless to remedy the situation. Their guilt feelings cause them to be very self-deprecating and angry themselves, a state that often results in depression. Other parents struggling with guilt are highly anxious about their ability to handle their infant; they feel they have harmed their infant and cannot tolerate facing that infant. Another manifestation of guilt is hostility and anger that is usually directed toward others, such as the spouse, the staff, or God. Instead of focusing their

anger on themselves like a depressed parent, they direct it outward to rid themselves of their feelings of responsibility, projecting the guilt feelings onto others in their life. They may be angry at the physicians, nurses, or social workers for not making their infant healthy (if the child is premature) or perfect (if the child has a congenital defect). They may be hostile toward the social worker for not being able to help them with their financial problems. Unconsciously, they are trying to make the staff feel as guilty, helpless, and responsible as they do.

Facilitating Adaptation

To intervene with parents, it is useful to help the parents become aware of and acknowledge their feelings of failure and guilt.[35] By verbalizing their feelings, they can begin to identify the source of the guilt feelings, which may not always be clear to them. The staff can then intervene with appropriate information to modify and clarify the perceptions that may be the source of some of the parents' guilt feelings. Many parents directly ask about the causes of their infant's problem, and the medical team should provide them with appropriate information. Other parents are not as direct and verbal; they need to have the subject introduced. "Have you wondered why this has happened?" or "Many parents find themselves feeling responsible for their baby's problem, as if they failed. Have you had these feelings?" As parents begin to talk about their feelings, they themselves are often able to test reality and discover the irrationality in their thinking. Some parents, however, continue to feel guilty even though they have been told they are not to blame. Guilt feelings are very complex and may take a long time to resolve; for some they may never be completely resolved, but at least the intensity of the feelings may diminish. If a child recovers from the illness, guilt can be more easily relinquished. If the child has a chronic problem, the parent is daily confronted with feelings of responsibility. The more irrational the source of the guilt, the harder it will be to dispel. Because this persistent guilt can cause problems in the parental relationship to the child, a referral to a perinatal social worker or other mental health professional may be indicated.

To facilitate support between parents, it is useful to ask whether they have shared their feelings of guilt and failure with each other. Often a spouse may assume that one is angry at or disappointed with the other. Discussing this may bring a tremendous sense of relief and reassurance. However, if the parents are blaming each other and relationship problems develop, a referral to a perinatal social worker or counselor is appropriate.[69]

In some cases there may be realistic reasons (either intentional or unintentional) why the parent may feel guilty about the infant's problem. Parental drug or alcohol abuse, an accident, or an inherited genetic problem may be real reasons. In these cases the staff must acknowledge to the parent that there is a causal relationship and then give the parents support by allowing them to talk about their feelings. If causes were not intentional, it is helpful to acknowledge that fact: if they were, it is important to be nonjudgmental. A judging attitude only reinforces the feelings parents are already experiencing and further alienates them from the child and the staff. The parents need help with the problem that initially led to the impairment of the fetus. When this type of psychosocial problem arises, the involvement of a perinatal social worker or counselor is essential.

Adaptation to the Intensive Care Environment

The fourth psychologic task involves adaptation to the intensive care environment.[85] All of the reactions of guilt, anxiety, fear, anger, and disappointment become heightened when parents attempt to adapt to this unfamiliar environment. They must learn a new language, establish trust in new relationships, and adapt to their role in this setting. The intense and sometimes chaotic appearance of a high-risk nursery makes it a frightening experience that serves to increase parental feelings of helplessness and anxiety. Parents need to gain a sense of security in this environment before initiating a care-giving role with their infant. There may be cultural adaptations and geographic obstacles for families who live in small, rural communities and must travel to large, unfamiliar cities and become adapted to a large hospital. Locating the hospital and finding accommodations and meals can become overwhelming to parents who have under-

gone much emotional turmoil. Meeting the infant's care provider, the competent physician and nurse, can sometimes evoke a mixture of positive and negative feelings. Parents may experience reassurance and gratitude for care being given, yet at the same time a reinforcement of their feelings of uselessness, helplessness, and inadequacy can ensue. The sophistication of the highly technical care and heroic measures provided to attain survival may be met with both awe and uncertainty. Family disruption is exaggerated by distance, especially if the infant was transported and the father must decide whether he is most needed with the infant, the infant's mother, or perhaps other children at home. Decisions must be made about work responsibilities as well as child care. The financial concerns related to providing intensive care become an added stress on families and are often compounded by the travel expenditures necessary to visit the infant.

Parental Responses

There are a number of nonverbal and verbal signs that indicate parents are struggling to gain a sense of security in the NICU. Some parents appear frightened, overwhelmed, nervous, and withdrawn, asking few questions or being reluctant to call or visit. Others may be highly anxious and unable to focus on their infant and may instead concentrate on other activities or infants in the nursery. Some parents may ask many questions and become very interested in the technical aspects of their infant's treatment, such as respirator settings and laboratory values. Some parents, uneasy with entrusting their child to strangers, may initially feel a need to remain at their infant's side, maintaining a vigil. Some may request to read the infant's chart or attempt to read material on their infant's particular condition. Others may become angry or upset at minor differences in the infant's care or the nursery policies, such as a respiratory setting being off a point or the need to limit visitation of friends and relatives.

Facilitating Adaptation

There are many interventions that can be employed to familiarize and orient families.[85] First, the obstetrician, transport team, or any other professional who has initial contact with parents can give them preparatory information and a description of intensive care. A booklet or video that includes basic information and illustrative pictures is extremely useful and should include a discussion of the type of care being provided, normal feelings and reactions parents experience, financial information, a glossary of terms, breastfeeding information, available accommodations and meals, calling and visitation policies, the discharge policy, and a city map. Both at the time of transfer and later in the nursery, a self-developing picture can be taken of the infant for the parents. If the infant is being transported, information should be given as to the approximate length of time of transport and by whom and when the parents will be contacted after the infant has been admitted and evaluated. A personal phone call from the staff with an introduction, information about the infant and unit, and an inquiry regarding parental visitation plans are useful. Parents feel less anxious when they have an orientation and a name to relate to. The staff can then be prepared to be available when the parents arrive.

Certainly, the first visit to the NICU is stressful, and members of the team should welcome the parents and stay with them to explain the equipment and procedures, answer questions, review the infant's course, give emotional support, and in general, orient the parents to this new experience. It is important to be attentive to the mother's physical need; comfortable chairs or perhaps a wheelchair if the mother has had a cesarean section are helpful. The message needs to be conveyed that parents are welcome and that their visits do make a difference in that they have a useful role to play with their infant. Because many parents are uncertain about what questions to ask, it may be necessary at times to help parents construct questions ("Do you understand why we start IVs in the head?" or "Do you know what blood gases, hood oxygen, and CPAP are?") and to repeat explanations using simple, nontechnical language. Relating to the parent's affect or emotional state seems to establish a rapport with the family and helps them feel that the staff is empathetic and understanding. If parents sense the staff's genuine concern and interest in them and their infant, it is easier for them to leave their infant in the staff's care. A team member might say, "You look frightened or scared," or "This can be an overwhelming situation," or "You look like you want to cry." Facilitating the parents' relationship with the infant is essential and can be done by offering the parents the opportunity to touch or stroke their infant, hold the infant if possible, or at least remove eye patches. Pointing out some of the unique personal characteristics of the infant is helpful. A staff member might say, "Your baby is very active," or "He responds well to touch," or "She seems to prefer lying on her side."

Families coming from out of town should be provided with a list of inexpensive housing and restaurants located near the hospital. In many cities, national and local businesses have established nearby homes run by local volunteer organizations for housing parents on a temporary basis. The homes have several sleeping rooms in addition to kitchen and laundry facilities and provide parents with a comfortable, homelike atmosphere at a nominal charge. A natural support system generally emerges among the parents using the home. A list of apartments, hotels and boarding rooms reasonably priced and rented by the day or week can also be made available.

Parents are usually concerned with the cost of their infant's hospitalization. Some parents feel that if they are unable to pay, their child will receive less attention. Parents should be reassured that their infant's care will not depend on their ability to pay. They should, however, be referred to the appropriate funding agencies, such as the Handicapped or Crippled Children's Program, Social Security Disability, and Medicaid, that provide financial assistance.

Because communication is so critical, regular conferences between the family and staff (physician, nurses, and social workers) should be instituted to give consistent medical information and emotional support; this is especially helpful with both extremely critical and long-term infants. Parents should be given the names of the physicians and nurses taking care of their infant and the personnel's specific role in providing both care to the infant and communication to the family. If the physicians and nurses have a rotation system, this also should be explained from the beginning. At the end of a rotation the transition can be facilitated by the on-coming physician's participation in even a brief conference with the out-going physician, primary nurse, and parents. Primary nursing, especially for long-term infants, can be very helpful in providing for continuity of care. The primary nurse has been identified by parents as the primary source and facilitator of information to parents and between parents and other health care providers and as the link between parents and infant.

For out-of-town families the telephone plays a major role in staff-to-parent communication. The establishment of a telephone calling schedule with families and the use of a toll-free number, if available, can be useful. If the family is out of town and unable to visit frequently, the local or referring physician can supplement the communication. That physician often knows the family and can talk with them in person. The physician should, of course, communicate regularly with the nursery team to obtain the current medical information and present a consistent approach to the family.

Resumption of the Relationship with the Infant

The fifth psychologic task entails the parents' reestablishment of a relationship with their infant and initiating their care-giving role, a process that usually begins when the child's improvement revives previous hopes after a disappointing experience. Certain medical events may signal to the parents that it is safe to risk a relationship with the infant. These events may be a regular weight gain, changes in feeding patterns or methods, elimination of life support equipment, the infant crying for the first time or becoming more active and responsive, or the infant's transfer from the NICU to a level II nursery. The parents may begin to read baby books or pamphlets about their infant's condition, buy clothes, set up the baby's room, send out birth announcements, or name the baby. If the infant has a congenital defect, the parents may become involved with genetic counseling and other parents whose infants have similar deficits.

Parents must begin to shift their level of involvement and activity from that of a passive participant to that of an active primary care giver.[47] The shift includes the parents gaining confi-

dence in their ability to care for their infant. The family that has been disrupted must reestablish itself and recover from the crisis in an environment that is sensitive and supportive to this essential task.[3,29,38] The transfer of care from staff to parent is influenced by (1) the stability or lability of the infant's condition, (2) physical health of the mother, (3) level of parental support, and (4) staff expectations.[81]

Involvement in care giving lessens the parents' feelings of helplessness and frustration and facilitates their identification with their role as parents.[83] When parents visit, they can help by providing skin care for their infant, learning to read and respond to infant cues, helping turn the infant even if a respirator is attached, diapering the infant, and feeding the infant if this is possible. If the parents are separated by distance, they can send family pictures that can be posted at the infant's bed; periodic pictures of the infant taken by the staff can be sent back to the family. Parents can send clothing, mobiles, simple toys, and even cassette tapes so that the infant can hear the parents' voices. Some mothers who are pumping send frozen breast milk. All of these reminders help the nursery staff be aware of the real family that is genuinely interested. These personal attempts made by parents that help them feel they are important to their infants' development should be encouraged. Sometimes foster grandparents or volunteers can hold, feed, and talk to infants whose parents cannot visit frequently.

Kangaroo care, skin-to-skin contact between mother and infant by placing the infant in a vertical position between the mother's breasts, has positive maternal as well as neonatal responses. Use of kangaroo care activates the maternal processes of a search for meaning and mastery of the experience of preterm birth and a recovery of self-esteem and enhancement in the parenting of a high-risk neonate.[3,5] Successive sessions of kangaroo care ease the pain and emotional suffering as mothers deal with loss and letting go and develop competence and confidence.

The use of "graduate parents," parents who have had an infant in the NICU and who have successfully dealt with and resolved the crisis of the birth of their infant, can be extremely valuable.[54,57,72] They provide support to parents by sharing common feelings, reactions, and experiences about having a hospitalized infant. Graduate parents also visit selected infants whose parents are unable to visit. They can establish written correspondence with the parents and perhaps include a picture of the infant. Graduate parents can provide support and practical assistance for mothers interested in breastfeeding, parents who take their infant home on oxygen, or parents whose infant requires special medical care such as a shunt, tracheostomy, colostomy care, or gavage feedings. Organized graduate parent groups in large tertiary settings have become a very popular means of providing support, but locating one parent or couple to talk with parents in a small community can be just as helpful.[63]

Parent classes can also be offered on a variety of topics such as breastfeeding, infant development, premature infant development, sibling and family reactions, discharge, CPR, coping with the hospitalization, and special medical needs. These classes provide specific, didactic information combined with group discussions that are mutually supportive in nature. Social workers, nurses, and other related health care professionals (respiratory, occupational, and physical therapists) facilitate the group; graduate parents also participate as a resource group.

A third type of support group is counseling sessions.[58] The purpose of these sessions is to discuss and deal with common issues among parents arising from the hospitalization of their infant and the effects on their marriage and family life. This type of group has also been helpful for parents whose infant has died. The group is usually short term and is conducted by the perinatal social worker and another staff member such as a physician, nurse, or chaplain. The focus of the group is not to give specific medical information, but rather to provide parents with an opportunity to verbalize their feelings about their infant's hospitalization and to receive emotional support.

In 1982 the national organization Parent Care, Inc.* was established and dedicated to parents and professionals concerned with infants requiring special care after birth. Parent Care's mission is "to

---

* Parent Care, Inc., 9041 Colgate Street, Indianapolis, IN 46268. (317) 872-9913.

improve neonatal intensive care experiences and futures of babies, families, and care givers"[72] by promoting activities that support family-centered services in the NICU and after discharge.

Sibling Relationships

The inclusion of other children in the events surrounding the birth of a sick newborn is important.[66] From a sibling's viewpoint the anticipated birth of a new infant is a stressful time of noticeable physical and psychologic changes within the family. In preparation for the impending birth, the child is told that the mother will be going to the hospital for a few days and will return with a baby brother or sister. With the birth of a premature or ill infant the mother may go to the hospital unexpectedly, stay a long time, and not return home with the anticipated playmate. Instead of a celebration of the expected happy event, parents are grieving the loss of the normal newborn and the current crisis of their sick infant.

Parents are often unsure what to tell the other children and whether or not the children should see the infant. The siblings themselves may feel left out, rejected, or worried that they, too, may get sick. They may feel they are to blame and that their jealous feelings about their new rival may have caused this tragedy. Confused by their parents' distress, the other children may speculate that it is related to them and their "bad" behaviors. They may be disappointed and angry that they did not get the "playmate" they had wanted. Because parents are unsure and confused about how to manage these issues, it is often helpful for the staff to introduce the topic.

Because children will make up an explanation for the infant's illness, it is better to have it based on accurate information. Before explaining the infant's condition to siblings, elicit their ideas and perceptions about "what is the matter." Any fears, fantasies, misconceptions, or proper information is thus used to begin the explanation of "where the baby is." Explanations must be tailored to the individual child's cognitive and developmental level. The child should be told that the infant is sick but in a way that is different from his or her illnesses; the infant's illness is not "catching," and it is not like any of the illnesses that child has experienced. To allay the siblings' fears about medical personnel, they should also be told that the nurses and physicians are trying to help the infant "get better." Because children between 2 and 6 years are involved in magical thinking, they should be told they are not to blame and that they did not cause the infant's problem. If the infant is premature, a team member might say to the child, "The baby came out too early or too soon; he needed more time to grow inside." If the infant has spina bifida a staff member might say, "The baby's spine did not grow right, so he may have trouble lifting his legs or walking."

A child of 3 years or younger usually does not understand much about the coming infant. More important to this age group is the separation from parents who are frequently at the hospital. To ameliorate the separation, child-care arrangements should be structured so that the child is cared for by familiar people in a familiar environment. The best care arrangement would be with a familiar person in the child's own home; second best would be a familiar person in the care giver's home; and third best, an unfamiliar person in the child's own home. Least favorable, of course, would be an unfamiliar person in an unfamiliar setting. Many hospitals have a child-care facility run by volunteers that allows the child the opportunity to go to the hospital to "see where Mommy and Daddy are going" yet allows the parents the chance to see their infant without having to care for their older child(ren). Parents may also choose to include the young child in all or selected visits.

Children ages 3 and older have more interest in babies and a better grasp about the physical meaning of life. Sometimes a picture of the baby or a look into the nursery through the windows is helpful to the other children. Many children benefit from visits to the nursery to see their brother or sister. The natural curiosity of the child about "what is going on" in the family is answered when the child actually sees the baby. Behavior problems such as bed-wetting, sleeping and eating difficulties, and difficult separations from parents may be prevented or reduced by the reassurance of a visit that decreases the sibling's worry about the baby.[5] Sibling visitation must be individualized for every family.

Sibling Visits

The decision to include siblings in the NICU depends to a great extent on the views, beliefs, and attitudes of the hospital staff.[24,66] Generally, the staff's concerns about and resistance to sibling visitation focus on a fear of an increase in nosocomial infection, disruption of unit routine and order, and potential harm to young children from exposure to the NICU environment. Infection control is the responsibility of parents and professionals. Parents must be educated about the dangers of infection and instructed on how to screen their children for symptoms such as fever, cough, or diarrhea. Professional staff must inquire about the health of visiting siblings, including their exposure to communicable diseases. Both parents and children must wash their hands and may don cover gowns. Pediatric patient gowns and small stools to help children reach the sink are used. With vigilance, no increased bacterial colonization and no increased incidence of infection occur with sibling visits.[8,86]

Because sibling visitation may be beneficial, each NICU must evaluate the center's situation and consider instituting a sibling visitation policy.[66,82] The following general principles may be used in developing this policy:

- Communication and coordination between staff and family are necessary to promote successful sibling visitation.
- Children must be prepared, according to their age and development, for what they will see, hear, and feel in the NICU.[24] Language should be simple and honest; pictures of the infant or other infants can be helpful.
- Parents and staff screen the visiting sibling for signs of illness that would exclude the child from visiting.
- Parents and child must scrub and may gown.
- The initial visit should be held at a relatively quiet time in the nursery when a care provider is able to stay with the family. If the infant can be moved to a private room or family room area, this is preferable.

At the bedside the child is introduced to the infant and seated on a chair or stool at eye level with the infant. The care provider then again explains the equipment the child sees and any of the infant's "interesting" behaviors such as crying because of hunger, sucking on a pacifier, or eyes open "looking at you." Children may even be included in age-appropriate caregiving tasks. Choosing clothes, handling diapers and blankets, holding the bottle, or touching and talking to the infant are all ways "to help." The child may bring a present to the infant such as a simple toy, music box, or handmade picture or photograph of the family. After a visit, both parents and staff should be available to talk about the visit or answer any questions. Some children, however, will not discuss the visit or ask questions until some later time. A method for enabling children to express their feelings in a nonverbal way is through play or books. A child who receives a book about physicians and hospitals or a "doctor" or "nurse" doll, may "play out" feelings about the brother or sister and the hospital experience.

Creating a comfortable environment in which children feel free to ask questions is essential when siblings visit.[55] Every question deserves an answer, even "I don't know," when appropriate. Children are often quite unrestrained in their remarks and questions. Comments such as, "He's sure ugly!" or "Is he going to die?" or "Why is she tied up (restrained)?" are common. These may be embarrassing to parents who hesitate to make the same remarks or ask the same questions.

If the infant is hospitalized for a long time, the other children may lose interest or even wish it were all over. This response may upset parents who themselves may be struggling with the same feelings. The longer the infant is hospitalized, the greater the pressure on time and financial resources. Family routines are disrupted by continuing hospitalization, and the disruption may strain family relationships.

Staff and parent response to sibling visitation has been positive in hospitals where the policy has been implemented. Such a policy may facilitate family integrity and promotes mutual support during the stressful time of hospitalization.[8] Another advantage of visitation is that the older siblings do not endure repeated separations caused by parental visits to the hospital but are included as important and special family members. The presence of siblings in a nursery can be a rewarding experience for family and staff alike and perhaps is the ideal example of providing safe yet comprehensive family-centered care.

Although a flexible sibling visitation policy is viewed as the best possible situation, some alternatives such as coloring books and children's books should be considered (see Resource Materials for Parents). Staff should be sensitive to the needs of the siblings and understand that the parents must deal with both time and financial constraints.

Psychosocial Conferences

Psychosocial conferences for staff members to discuss the dynamics of family functioning and the effect of a seriously ill newborn on the family can be quite useful. These conferences, usually led by perinatal social workers, can give staff the opportunity to discuss and better understand their own feelings and reactions to families, infants, and the many stresses related to working in an NICU. In addition, weekly rounds with the entire multidisciplinary team (physicians, nurses, home health nurse coordinator, social workers, and financial counselors) are an effective vehicle to discuss and develop medical discharge and psychosocial care plans about each infant and family. The involvement of perinatal social workers to assess and evaluate the psychosocial functioning of families, to provide support and counseling services, and to coordinate the discharge planning and follow-up care for the infant and family is essential. Social workers need to evaluate all high-risk cases in addition to providing support in complicated medical conditions, including death of the infant (Box 28-3).

Transfer Back to Referring Hospital

Transfer of the infant from a tertiary center back to the referral or local community center for convalescent care and discharge is a frequent occurrence. This can be helpful in facilitating the relationship between the infant and parents, because the infant will be more accessible. Parents generally view the transfer as positive if the hospital is closer to home and if they feel comfortable with the level of care provided. Transfer is stressful, and there is always an adjustment period any time a transfer occurs.[26,51] Parents must adapt to different personalities of medical personnel and different procedures

---

Box 28-3

High-Risk Factors Needing Social Work Intervention

1. Teenage pregnancy (ages 11 to 18)
2. Single parent
3. Substance abuse
4. Psychiatric history of present problem that interferes with appropriate functioning, especially as related to parenting abilities
5. Mother or father with a history of being abused or early deprivation by own family, or history of having abused or neglected own children
6. Battered women/domestic violence
7. Mental retardation, borderline intelligence, or significant physical handicaps
8. History of loss with previous pregnancy or child because of stillbirth, birth defect, prematurity, abortion, custody case, or death
9. Rejection or ambivalence of current pregnancy as manifested by requests for termination of pregnancy, attempted abortion, or relinquishment
10. No prenatal care with previous or current pregnancies
11. Pregnancy exacerbating extreme depression, anxiety, or suicidal thoughts
12. Stressful home or personal situation because of marital or financial problems or lack of support systems
13. Long-term hospitalization during pregnancy requiring intervention in helping family adjust by arranging for younger children at home or for financial assistance
14. Other children with physical or mental handicaps
15. Attachment difficulties with the infant
16. Prior history with social services

---

and visiting policies. Preparing the parents for the transfer, orienting them to the new hospital, and talking to the staff of the referral hospital about the infant and the parents is important to help ease the transition.[4,26,51,71,83]

Preparation to Take the Infant Home

The sixth psychologic task for parents concerns preparations for taking the infant home. Parents must understand their infant's individual needs and personality characteristics in addition to feeling a sense of competency in relating to their infant. Discharge is an anxiety-provoking event and ushers in the "crisis" of homecoming, which parents must face and master. The unsuccessful resolution of the previously discussed five psychologic tasks can contribute to maladaptive parenting and a poor outcome for the infant, including the possibilities of attachment difficulties, overprotectiveness, failure to thrive, vulnerable child syndrome, emotional deprivation, and battering.[49,84] To achieve a positive parent-child relationship after the hospitalization and through the transitional period that ensues,

provision of appropriate follow-up support through the home adjustment period is crucial.[30,49,59]

Several behaviors demonstrate that parents are trying to understand the infant's care in preparation for discharge. First, parents may ask questions verbalizing a variety of concerns. For a premature infant, they might ask, "Do I need an apnea monitor at home?" or "Can the baby have visitors?" or "Do I need to wash my hands when handling the baby?" For a child with a congenital defect such as spina bifida, the parents might ask, "Can I lay the baby on his back?" or "Can I bathe him?" or "Do I need to pump the shunt?" For a child with a heart defect the staff might be asked, "Do I need oxygen?" or "Do I need to handle him differently?" or "What about going to higher altitudes?" All of these questions on the part of parents are typical and normal and represent the parents' working through their fears and anxieties.

On the other hand, parents who are highly anxious, extremely overprotective, or very indifferent should be a concern to the health care personnel. The inability to deal with the task of taking the infant home may indicate some unresolved feelings related to the previous psychologic tasks. Although most parents whose infants have been in an NICU do admit to initially treating their infant differently until they "got to know their child," a group of parents who are excessively overprotective does exist. This type of behavior often stems from parents who are struggling with intense feelings of guilt and failure. These parents either protect their child from everything because they feel so responsible for having caused the infant's initial problem or they demonstrate an indifference or lack of concern for the infant and the infant's welfare. Such parents may have an ambivalent attachment to their infant, who may continue to represent the threat of death or the parents' personal failure. This group of parents should be considered high risk for potential parent-child relationship difficulties and should be evaluated to determine an appropriate intervention.

At discharge, there are infants whose medical conditions are still fragile, a substantial indication that these infants may not be normal and have long-term problems. These infants may be temperamentally difficult to manage, and parents understandably treat them differently.[9] Both parents and infants need additional support and appropriate intervention.[21,59]

There are many interventions that the perinatal health care team can employ to assist parents with discharge and through the transitional period that follows. In the hospital, adequate teaching of care-giving skills that allow the parent to develop a sense of mastery and competence is of paramount importance. Maternal concerns about neonatal care center on elimination, feeding, and the infant's health.[47] If parents do not feel comfortable with their infant, their anxiety can cause adverse interactions with the infant. The parent needs to know the infant's mannerisms and behaviors; otherwise the parent may feel exhausted and resentful and then guilty. Teaching care-giving skills can often be facilitated in an environment that is less intense and crisis oriented than the NICU. Whenever possible, an infant should be transferred to a setting that is more conducive to the parents' initiation of the primary care-giving role; a more conducive setting might be a special care or transitional nursery,[7,31] a level II unit, or a general pediatric ward.

Adequate discharge planning and follow-up arrangements should include general pediatric care, home health care, lay home visitors, and parenting classes, especially for young or psychosocially high-risk parents.[20,60] Referrals to county social service departments should be made for single mothers who are eligible for Aid to Families of Dependent Children and Medicaid. For infants with special problems (spina bifida, cerebral palsy, or Down syndrome), referrals should be made for special programs that provide services for the infants and support groups of parents. Parents whose infants have special medical needs (gavage feedings, tracheostomy or colostomy care, oxygen or ventilators) should be evaluated by the medical and nursing personnel to determine helpful community resources (equipment, supplies, respite or emergency care) and to make appropriate referrals. Home nursing care and homemaker services are sometimes covered by medical insurance and may be necessary to provide actual nursing activities and to relieve parents from the emotional burden inherent in caring for an infant with medical problems.[19] For infants who are developmentally disabled, developmental intervention programs and follow-up programs provided by many hospitals that have NICUs are extremely valuable. These infants are eligible for Part H of the Individuals with Disabilities Education Act (IDEA). Locating babysitters who will care for a child with special problems can be an overwhelming task for parents; cultivating a resource list for parents and suggesting that parents exchange services with each other can also be helpful. Graduate parents, neonatal nurses, or respite care organizations can provide a useful service to parents in this situation. Lastly, parents should be referred to appropriate funding agencies (Handicapped or Crippled Children's Program, Medicaid, or Social Security Disability) that provide financial assistance.

References

1. Able-Boon H, Dokecki P, Smith M: Parents and health care providers communication and decision making in the intensive care nursery, *Child Health Care* 18:133, 1989.
2. Affonso D: Missing pieces: a study of post-partum feelings, *Birth Fam J* 4:159, 1977.

3. Affonso D et al: Exploration of mother's reactions to the kangaroo method of prematurity care, *Neonat Net* 7:43, 1989.

4. Affonso D et al: Stressors reported by mothers of hospitalized premature infants, *Neonat Net* 11:63, 1992.

5. Affonso D et al: Reconciliation and healing for mothers through skin-to-skin contact provided in an American tertiary level intensive care nursery, *Neonat Net* 12:25, 1993.

6. Aguilera D, Messick J. *Crisis intervention theory and methodology*, ed 3, St Louis, 1978, Mosby.

7. Bachrach S et al: A model transitional-care program for premature infants, *Perinat Neonat* 9:31, 1985.

8. Ballard J et al: Sibling visits to a newborn intensive care unit: implications for siblings, parents and infants, *Child Psychiatry Hum Dev* 14.203, 1984.

9. Barnard K, Kelly J: Assessment of parent-child interaction. In Meisels S, Shankoff J, editors: *Handbook of early childhood intervention*, Cambridge, Mass, 1990, Cambridge University Press.

10. Barnett C et al: Neonatal separation: the maternal side of interactional deprivation, *Pediatrics* 54:197, 1970.

11. Benfield DG et al: Grief response to parents after referral of the critically ill newborn to a regional center, *N Engl J Med* 294:975, 1976.

12. Bibring G et al: A study of the psychological processes in pregnancy and of the earliest mother-child relationship: some propositions and comments, *Psychoanal Study Child* 16:9, 1961.

13. Browne J, Smith-Sharpe S: The Colorado consortium of intensive care nurseries: spinning webs of support for Colorado infants and families, *Zero to Three,* June/July 1995.

14. Campbell S, Taylor P. Bonding and attachment: theoretical issues, *Semin Perinatol* 3:3, 1979.

15. Caplan G: Patterns of parental response to the crisis of premature birth, *Psychiatry* 23:365, 1960.

16. Caplan G et al: Four studies of crisis in parents of prematures, *Community Ment Health J* 1:149, 1965.

17. Catletta A, Miles M, Holditch-Davis D: Matenal perceptions of illness severity in premature infants, *Neonat Net* 13:45, 1994.

18. Christensson K et al: Separation distress call in the human neonate in the absence of maternal body contact, *Acta Paediatr Scand* 84:468, 1994.

19. Colt D, Beyers J: Baby Saige goes home, *Continuing Care* 12:25, 1993.

20. Community Caring Project, C. Henry Kempe, National Center for the Prevention and Treatment of Child Abuse and Neglect, Denver, Colo, 1990.

21. Cronin C et al: The impact of very low-birth-weight infants on the family is long lasting, *Arch Pediatr Adoles Med* 149:151, 1995.

22. Davis JA et al: *Parent-baby attachments in premature infants,* New York, 1983, St Martin's Press.

23. DeChateau P: The importance of the neonatal period for the development of synchrony in the maternal-fetal dyad: a review, *Birth Fam J* 4:10, 1977.

24. Doll Speck L, Miller B, Rohrs K: Sibling education: implementing a program for the NICU, *Neonat Net* 12:49, 1993.

25. Fantz RL et al: Early visual selectivity as a function of pattern variables, previous exposure, age from birth and conception and expected cognitive deficit. In Cohen L, Salapatic P, editors: *Infant perception,* vol 1, New York, 1975, Academic Press.

26. Flanagan V et al: Mothers' perception of the quality of their infant's back transfer: pilot study results, *Neonat Net* 15:27, 1996.

27. Fromm E: *The art of loving,* New York, 1965, Harper & Row.

28. Gardner SL: Mothering: the unconscious conflict between nurses and new mothers, *Keep Abreast J* 3:192, 1978.

29. Gennaro S: Facilitating parenting of the neonatal intensive care unit graduate. *J Perinat Neonatol Nurs* 4(4):55, 1991.

30. Goldberg S: Prematurity: effects on parent-infant interaction, *J Pediatr Psychol* 3:137, 1978.

31. Goldson E: The family care center: a model for the transitional care of the sick infant and his family, *Child Today* 10:51, 1981.

32. Goldson E: The neonatal intensive care unit: premature infants and parents. *Infants Young Child* 4:31, 1992.

33. Gottfried AW, Gaiter JL: *Infant stress under intensive care,* Baltimore, 1985, University Park Press.

34. Grace J: Development of maternal-fetal attachment during pregnancy, *Nurs Res* 38:228, 1989.

35. Grant P, Siegel R: Families in crisis: birth of a sick infant. Presented at the Perinatal Section Meeting of the American Academy of Pediatrics, District VIII, Scottsdale, Ariz, April, 1978.

36. Gray J et al: Perinatal assessment of mother-baby interaction. In Helfer B, Kempe CH, editors: *Child abuse and neglect: the family and the community,* Cambridge, Mass, 1976, Ballinger Publishing.

37. Green M, Solnit A: Reactions to the threatened loss of a child: a vulnerable child syndrome, *Pediatrics* 34:58, 1964.

38. Griffin T: Nurse barriers to parenting in the special care nursery, *J Perinat Neonatal Nurs* 4(2):56, 1990.

39. Haines C, Perger C, Nagy S: A comparison of the stressors experienced by parents of intubated and extubated children, *J Adv Nurs* 21:350, 1995.

40. Harmon RJ: The perinatal period: infants and parents. In Spittell JA, Brody E, editors: *Clinical medicine, vol 12, Psychiatry,* Hagerstown, Md, 1981, Harper & Row.

41. Harrison H: The principles of family-centered neonatal care, *Pediatrics* 92:643, 1993.

42. Heidrich S, Cranley M: Effect of fetal movement, ultrasound scans, and amniocentesis on maternal-infant attachment, *Nurs Res* 38:81, 1989.

43. Hofer M: Early relationships as regulators of infant physiology and behavior, *Acta Paediatr Scand* 397 (Suppl):9, 1994.

44. Jordan B: *Birth in four cultures,* St Albans, Vt, 1978, Eden Press.

45. Kaplan DM, Mason EA: Maternal reactions to premature birth viewed as an emotional disorder, *Am J Orthopsychiatry* 30:539, 1960.

46. Kennell JH et al: Maternal behavior one year after early and extended post-partum contact. *Dev Med Child Neurol* 16:172, 1974.

47. Kenner C, Lott JW: Parent transition after discharge from the NICU, *Neonatal Network* 9:31, 1990.

48. Klaus MH, Kennell JH: Mothers separated from their newborn infants, *Pediatr Clin North Am* 17:1015, 1970.

49. Klaus MH, Kennell JH: *Parent-infant bonding,* ed 2, St Louis, 1982, Mosby.

50. Klaus MH et al: Maternal attachment: importance of the first post-partum days, *N Engl J Med* 286:460, 1972.

51. Kuhnly J, Freston M: Back transport: exploration of parents feelings regarding the transition, *Neonat Net* 14:69, 1995.

52. Leifer A et al: Effects of mother-infant separation on maternal attachment behavior, *Child Dev* 43:1203, 1972.

53. LeMasters EE: Parenthood as cirsis, *Marriage and Family Living* 19:352, 1957.

54. Levick J, Lindsay J: Parent-to-parent support: enriching traditional prenatal and NICU care, *National Association of Perinatal Workers Forum* 12:9, 1992.

55. Levick J, Munch S: "I'm special too." Psychosocial aspects of sibling adjustment in the NICU, *National Association of Perinatal Social Workers Forum* 13:1, 1993.

56. Liederman PH, Seashore MJ: Mother-infant neonatal separation: some delayed consequences. Parent-infant interaction, Ciba Foundation Symposium 33, Amsterdam, 1975, Elsevier.

57. Lindsay J et al: Creative caring in the NICU: parent-to-parent support, *Neonat Net* 12:37, 1993.

58. Macnab A et al: Group support for parents of high-risk neonates: an interdisciplinary approach. *Soc Work Health Care* 10:63, 1985.

59. Marony D: Realities of a premature infant's first year: helping parents cope, *J Perinatol* 15:418, 1995.

60. McKim E: The difficult first week at home with a premature infant, *Neonat Net* 12:72, 1993.

61. Mead M, Newton N: Cultural patterning of perinatal behaviors. In Richardson S, Guttmacher A, editors: *Childbearing: its social and psychological aspects,* Baltimore, 1957, Williams & Wilkins.

62. Miles M, Carlson J, Fink S: Sources of support reported by mothers and fathers in infants hospitalized in an NICU, *Neonat Net* 15:45, 1996.

63. Minde K: The impact of prematurity on the later behavior of children and their families, *Clin Perinatal,* 11:227, 1984.

64. Minton C: Uses of photographs in perinatal social work, *Health Soc Work* 8:121, 1983.

65. Murphy K: Threatened perinatal loss: defining and managing strategies used by parents of critically ill infants, Doctoral dissertation, University of Illinois, Chicago, 1989.

66. Newman CB, McSweeney M: A descriptive study of sibling visitation in the NICU, *Neonat Net* 9:27, 1990.

67. Newton N, Newton M: Mothers' reaction to their newborn babies. *JAMA* 181:206, 1962.

68. Noble DN, Hamilton AK: Families under stress: perinatal social work, *Health Soc Work* 6:28, 1981.

69. O'Brien M, Solidy E, McClusky-Fawcett K: Prematurity and the neonatal intensive care unit. In Roberts M, editor: *Handbook of pediatric psychology,* ed 2, New York, 1995, Guilford Press.

70. Oehler J, Hannan T, Catlett S: Maternal views of preterm infants' responsiveness to social interaction, *Neonat Net* 12:67, 1993.

71. Page J, Lunyk-Child O: Parental perceptions of infant transfer from an NICU to a community nursery: implication for research and practice, *Neonat Net* 14:69, 1995.

72. Parent Care, Inc.: *Developing support programs, a how-to guide,* Indianapolis, 1995, Parent Care, Inc.

73. Perehudoff B: Parent's perceptions on environment stressors in the special care nursery, *Neonatal Network* 9:39, 1990.

74. Perrin EC et al: Is my child normal yet? Correlates of vulnerability, *Pediatrics* 83:355, 1989.

75. Phillips C, Anzalone J: *Fathering: participation in labor and birth,* ed 2, St Louis, 1982, Mosby.

76. Plunkett JW et al: Patterns of attachment among preterm infants of varying biological risk, *J Am Acad Child Psychiatry* 25:794, 1986.

77. Rice RD: Maternal-infant bonding: the profound long-term benefits of immediate continuous skin and eye contact at birth. In Stewart D, Stewart L, editors: *21st century OB: now,* Marble Hill, Mo, 1977, NAPSAC.

78. Rosenblatt J: Psychobiology of maternal behavior: contribution to the clinical understanding of maternal behavior among humans, *Acta Paediatr Scand Suppl* 3978:3, 1994.

79. Rosenblum L, Andrews M: Influences of environmental demand on maternal behavior and infant development, *Acta Paediatr Scand Suppl* 397:57, 1994.

80. Rostow P: The family's perspective. In Jones MJ et al, editors: *Hospital care of the recovering NICU infant,* Baltimore, 1991, Williams & Wilkins.

81. Scharer K, Brooks G: Mothers of chronically ill neonates and primary care in the NICU: transfer of care, *Neonat Net* 13:37, 1994.

82. Shea-McAleavey C, Janusz H: Sibling visiting—a plan for change, *Dimens Crit Care Nurs,* 10:218, 1991.

83. Shellbarger S, Thompson T: The critical times: meeting parental communication needs throughout the NICU experience, *Neonat Net* 12:39, 1993.

84. Siefert K et al: Perinatal stress: a study of factors linked to the risk of parenting problems, *Health Soc Work* 8:107, 1983.

85. Siegel R. A family-centered program of neonatal intensive care, *Health Soc Work* 7:50, 1982

86. Solheim K. Spellacy C: Sibling visitation: effects on newborn infection rates, *J Obstet Gynecol Neonat Nurs* 17:43, 1988.

87. Solnit AJ, Stark MH: Mourning and the birth of a defective child, *Psychoanal Study Child* 16:523, 1961.

88. Stainton M: Parents' awareness of their unborn infant in third trimester, *Birth* 17:92, 1990.

89. Taylor PM, Hall BL: Parent-infant bonding: problems and opportunities in a perinatal center, *Semin Perinatol* 3:73, 1979.
90. Thomson M, Westreich R: Restriction of mother-infant contact in the immediate postnatal period. In Chalmers I, Enkin M, Keirse M, editors: *Effective care in pregnancy and childbirth,* Oxford, 1989, Oxford University Press.
91. Widstrom A et al: Gastric suction in newborn infants: effects on circulation and developing feeding behaviors, *Acta Paediatr Scand* 76:566, 1987.

Resource Materials for Parents

Brazelton TB: *On becoming a family: the growth of attachment,* New York, 1981, Delacorte Press.
Harrison H, Kositsky A: *The premature baby book: a parent's guide to coping and caring in the first years,* New York, 1990, St Martin's Press.
Hatcher D, Lehman K: *Baby talk for parents who are getting to know their special care baby,* Omaha, 1985, Centering, Corp.

Hawkins-Walsh E, Borum S: *Kate's premature brother,* Omaha, 1985, Centering Corp.
Johnson B: Institute for Family-Centered Care, 7900 Wisconsin Avenue, Suite 405, Bethesda, Md, 20814.
Johnson J, Johnson M, Hatcher D: *Special beginnings,* Omaha, 1994, Centering Corp.
O'Brien M et al: *An introduction to the NICU and caring for your NICU baby* (videotapes), Baltimore, Md, 1994, Brookes.
Oehler J: *The frogs have a baby, a very small baby (a coloring book for children),* Durham, NC, 1979, Duke University Medical Center.
Sammons WAH, Lewis J: *Premature babies: a different beginning,* St Louis, 1985, Mosby.
Special care for your baby, Columbus, Ohio, 1982, Ross Laboratories.
The intensive care infant communicator: a different start, Philadelphia, Penn, 1988 and 1989. Wyeth-Ayerst Laboratories.
Your special newborn, Evansville, Ind, 1982, Mead Johnson Nutritional Division.

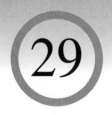

29 Grief and Perinatal Loss

Sandra L. Gardner, Gerald B. Merenstein, Audrey J. Costello

As a life passage, pregnancy and birth are associated with hopes and expectations, and joy and happiness for the future. Even though pregnancy and birth constitute a developmental crisis and major life change, expectant parents believe the gains of a healthy, happy child and family life offset any losses. Unfortunately, not all perinatal events have a happy ending. When pregnancy fails to produce a normal, healthy infant, it is a tragedy for the parents whose expectations of childbearing have not been fulfilled. Perinatal loss also affects their friends, family, and professional care providers.

Perinatal loss may be the first time the young adult has had the experience of coping with the illness or death of a loved one. Perinatal loss is especially significant because (1) it is sudden and unexpected, the most difficult loss to resolve[9]; (2) it interrupts the significant developmental stage of pregnancy, and the situational crisis of pregnancy[9]; (3) it is the loss of a child who did not have the opportunity to live a full life[17,59] and (4) it prevents progression into the next developmental stage of parenting that has been anticipated and rehearsed (at least in fantasy) during the pregnancy. Additionally, perinatal loss often means interpersonal exclusion from the activities of childbearing friends and siblings.[38]

Unfortunately, loss and grief are often only thought of in relation to death. However, as final and irreversible as death is, it is just one form of separation and loss. Although less obvious, other loss situations may have an equally crucial effect. Loss comes in many forms and during the perinatal period may occur without necessarily resulting in death. Circumstances of perinatal loss are at the same time parallel and different, because they all entail grief and mourning, and yet each has unique dimensions and characteristics.

The process of grief, its stages, and its symptoms are reviewed as a framework for understanding one's own feelings and those of others experiencing a loss. A desire to help and an idea of what is helpful and what is not helpful are presented as a basis for effective intervention by professionals.

The Grief Process

Grief, the characteristic response to the loss of a valued object, is not an intellectual and rational response.[18] Rather, it is personally experienced as the deep emotion of profound sadness and sorrow. To the individual, grief feels overwhelming, irrational, out of control, "crazy," and all-consuming. Mourning occurs in phases over time. After acknowledging that the loved object no longer exists, gradual withdrawal of emotion and feeling occurs, so that eventual psychologic investment in a new relationship is possible.

For grief to occur, the object must have been valued by the individual, so that its loss is perceived as significant and meaningful.[2] Because prenatally there is an investment of love in the fetus or newborn, the neonate is a valued object. To the extent the prenatal attachment has occurred, grief should be expected and felt at the loss of the fetus or newborn. Therefore loss at birth is a significant loss of a valued (although as yet only fantasized) person.

Loss, whether real or imagined, or actual or possible, is traumatic. The individual is no longer self-confident or confident about the surroundings, because both have been altered. Mourning and grief are forms of separation reactions. Fears of separation and abandonment are the universal fears of childhood regardless of age or developmental stage.

Perhaps loss of a significant other awakens these childhood fears and reminds us of the basic "insecurity of all our attachments."[43]

Life changes are stressful to the individual because they threaten to disrupt continuity and a state of equilibrium.[54] Marked changes in the family configuration, such as accession of a new member, are normally a stressful occasion for family members. Perinatal complication or loss is even more of a stressful event, for which the family has little or no preparation. The results of a crisis may be personal growth, maintaining the status quo, regression, or mental illness.[9,55] Often outcome depends on the type of help received during the crisis.

Decreasing the element of surprise through preparation for the situation to be encountered may modulate the effect of the event. Anticipatory grief[42,48,60] functions both to prepare and to protect the individual from the pain of impending loss. Prenatal diagnostic procedures, such as ultrasonography, amniocentesis, and fetoscopy, can now detect a variety of severe or lethal birth defects. When there is forewarning that the pregnancy or newborn is not healthy, the parents may begin a process of anticipatory grief and psychologically prepare for the loss of their child while simultaneously hoping for the neonate's survival.[1]

Parental withdrawal from the relationship established during pregnancy accompanies the intense emotions of anticipatory grief. Detachment protects and defends the parent from further painful feelings associated with the investment of self in a doomed relationship. If anticipatory grief proceeds, the parent may detach to the point of being unable to reattach to the infant should he or she survive. In this situation, the infant survives but the relationship with the parents may be significantly impaired. Maintaining even a remote hope that the fetus or newborn will survive protects the parents from the full experience of grief and total detachment from the child.

The degree of parental anticipatory grief is correlated with positive feelings about the pregnancy and the mode of delivery but not with the severity of the infant's illness. The more the parental investment and the higher the expectations for the pregnancy, the more anticipatory grief is associated with the development of a perinatal complication. The relative severity of the medical problem is not associated with the degree of anticipatory grief.

Perinatal Situations in Which Grief is Expected

Loss is a fact of life, and not just of death. Every stage of development requires a loss of the privileges of the preceding stage and movement into the unknown of the next stage. Any life event involving change or loss is accompanied by grief work, including moving, divorce, separation, death of a spouse or family member, injury or illness, retirement, job change, menopause, and even success.[10,54] The concept of loss is even applicable to the physiologic and psychologic events of normal pregnancy and birth. Certainly, when pregnancy fails to produce a live, healthy infant, a perinatal loss situation exists (Box 29-1). These perinatal losses, including stillbirth, loss of the perfect child,

---

Box 29-1

Perinatal Situations in Which Grief Reaction is Expected

I. Pregnancy
II. Birth
  A. Normal
  B. Cesarean section
  C. Forceps
  D. Episiotomy
  E. Medicated
  F. Prolonged or short labor
  G. Place of birth
III. Postpartum
  A. "Postpartum blues"
  B. Depression
  C. Psychosis
IV. Abortion
  A. Spontaneous
  B. Therapeutic
    1. Elective
    2. Selective
V. Stillbirth
VI. Loss of the perfect child
  A. Premature
  B. Deformed or anomalied baby
  C. Sick newborn
  D. "Wrong" sex
VII. Neonatal death
VIII. Relinquishment

and neonatal death, are discussed in detail in this chapter.

Stillbirth

Stillbirth is the demise of a viable fetus that occurs after fetal movement when the infant is invested by the parents with a personality and individuality. Because stillbirth occurs later in pregnancy than most abortions, there are increased parental expectations about the baby and the birth process. Selective abortions for genetic indications often occur in the second trimester of pregnancy and involve the death of a wanted child. Even though parents understand the validity of the reason for terminating the pregnancy, sadness, guilt, and self-doubt often accompany the decision to abort. The anxieties related to termination procedures that include labor and birth, and the feelings of helplessness, isolation, and depression should be acknowledged and handled as in a stillbirth.

Fetal demise in utero happens either prenatally or in the intrapartum period. For 50% of stillbirths, death was sudden, without warning, and from unexplainable causes.[15] The majority of women whose fetus has died in utero spontaneously begin labor within 2 weeks of fetal demise.[15] Carrying the dead fetus and waiting for spontaneous labor or induction is sad and difficult for the woman and her entire family. Feelings such as helplessness, disbelief, and powerlessness characterize this period.[29] There is often an uncontrollable urge to flee and escape the unpleasant situation.[11,29]

For the family who experiences an intrapartum demise, the joyous expectations of labor and birth suddenly change to fear, anxiety, and dread that the "worst" could have possibly happened to them. The suddenness of fetal demise in labor and birth affects both parents and professionals with feelings of shock, denial, and anxiety. Whether the loss is an early or late fetal loss, the woman and her family maintain hope by believing that the professional has made a mistake and that the infant is still alive.[58] The onset (or continuation) of labor is approached with both hope and dread—hope that the infant may be born alive and dread that the infant's death will soon be a stark reality.

The discomfort of labor and birth is particularly difficult for the woman whose infant has died, because her work will not be rewarded with a healthy infant.[61] Oversolicitous use of drugs at birth is not recommended, because they relegate the experience to unreality and give it a dreamlike quality.[75] Keeping parents together through this crisis is important for mutual support and sharing of the birth.[61,73] The deadening (and deafening) silence of a stillbirth forces the reality of the infant's death on both the parents and the professionals present at birth.[61]

In the past at the birth of a stillborn, the mother was heavily sedated or anesthetized and the infant was hidden and whisked away immediately. These women were often left with fears and fantasies: "Was the baby normal?" "What was the sex?" "What did the baby look like?" Seeing, touching, and holding the infant promote completion of the attachment cycle, confirm the reality of the stillbirth for both parents, and allow grief to begin.[5,58,75] Because it is easier to grieve the reality of a situation than a mystical and dreamlike fantasy, contact with the stillborn enables parents to grieve the infant's reality rather than their most frightening fantasies about the infant.[35,40,41,73]

After confirming the reality of the infant's death, a search for the cause, characterized by the universal question, "Why did the baby die?" begins. Either or both parents may blame themselves or feel guilty about real or imagined acts of omission or commission. An autopsy may determine the cause of death, but most often the cause is unknown, even after an autopsy; however, an autopsy may be useful in reducing parental guilt and uncertainty about future pregnancies, as well as in aiding the recovery from the loss.[29,75] The "empty tragedy"[41] of stillbirth forces the mother to deal with both the inner loss of the fetus and the outer loss of the expected newborn.

Loss of the Perfect Child

Even though pregnancy ends in the birth of a live child, the pregnancy outcome may not be what the parents had anticipated. Birth of an infant who does not meet parental expectations represents the realization of the parents' worst fears: a damaged child. Newborns who are preterm, anomalied, sick, or the "wrong" sex, or who ultimately die represent the loss of the fantasized perfect child.

After the birth of such a child, parental reactions include grief and mourning for the loss of the loved object (the perfect child) while simultaneously adapting to the reality and investing love in the defective child.[65,69] This reaction is analogous to parental mourning at the death of a child.[65] However, unlike the finality of death, birth of a living, defective child entails a persistent, constant reminder of the feelings of loss and grief because of parental investment of time, attention, and care for either a short time (preterm or sick newborn) or a lifetime (physically or mentally afflicted child).[65]

The psychic work involved in coping with the reality of the imperfect child and the inner feelings of loss is slow and emotionally painful.[69] The process is gradual and proceeds at an individual pace that cannot be hurried but can be facilitated and supported. Detachment from and mourning the loss of their fantasized child is necessary before parents are able to attach to the actual child.

Birth of an imperfect child represents multiple losses for parents. A primary narcissistic injury, a threat to the female's self-concept as a woman and mother and the male's self-concept as a man and a father, occurs when a less-than-perfect child is born.[13,14,32,37,38,69] Because the child is an extension of both parents, a less-than-perfect (i.e., deformed) child is equated with the perceived less-than-perfect part of the parental self.[69] In the mind of the parent, the imagined inadequate self has failed and caused the birth of the damaged child.[32]

Prematurity

Every woman expects to deliver a normal, healthy infant at term. Therefore the onset of premature labor is both physiologically and psychologically unexpected. Premature birth is a crisis and an emergency situation characterized by an increased concern for the survival of the infant and often the mother. Premature labor and birth are accompanied by feelings of helplessness, isolation, failure, emptiness, and no control.[32,65] The negative and dangerous atmosphere surrounding the premature birth experience may influence the relationship with the premature infant, who may also be perceived as dangerous and negative.

Normal adaptations to pregnancy are abruptly terminated by the birth of a premature infant.[32] Prenatal fantasies about the infant and the new roles of mother and father are interrupted by a premature birth. This forces parents who are "not ready to not be pregnant" to grieve the loss of a term infant and imposes premature parenting on individuals not yet ready for the experience.

As discussed in Chapter 28, anticipatory grief is one of the normal psychologic tasks accompanying premature birth. Anticipatory grief may be decreased by early contact between parents and infant and conversely increased by separation of parents from preterm infants.[32] Prolonging anticipatory grief with failure to progress through the other tasks results in altered relationships with the parents if the preterm infant survives.

Deformed or Anomalied Infants

In approximately 2 of every 100 births,[32] an infant is born with a birth defect. Because society values physical beauty, intelligence, and success, the birth of a physically or mentally defective child is seen as a catastrophe in our culture.[69,74]

Recent medical advances now make it possible to identify potential fetal problems in utero. As parents receive the information antenatally, they begin the process of anticipatory grief. They experience feelings of shock, anger, guilt, and hope. At the birth of their infant, there usually is the confirmation of the anomaly, and parents must deal with the reality of the situation. Whether anticipated or not, however, the birth of a child with a congenital defect is accompanied by ambivalent feelings for all concerned (parents, relatives, friends, and professionals). The first reactions to the reality of the situation are feelings of disbelief and shock. Feelings of shame, revulsion, and embarrassment at creating a damaged and devalued child are common.[61] Guilt, self-blame, and a search for a cause or reason for the tragedy are intermixed with feelings of anger.

The severity of loss and feelings of disappointment heavily burden the parents, a burden they feel no one else has experienced.[32] Their loneliness and isolation may be intensified by their self-imposed withdrawal from others. Unlike the birth of a healthy infant, the birth of an anomalied or sick child is not celebrated by society with announcements, visits, and gifts from friends and family. The negative responses of society's representatives (family, friends, acquaintances, and professionals) may increase the parents' negative feelings for a defective child.[74]

The extent of the infant's anomaly cannot be used as a criterion for the degree of parental grief reaction,[37] although a gross, visible anomaly may elicit more emotional reaction than a hidden or more minor one.[32] A seemingly "minor" anomaly as defined by the professional may represent a severe impairment to individual parents. The professional, who has had more contact with infants with a wide range of anomalies, views the individual infant's anomaly in a different context than the parents, who may have limited or no experience with a deformed child or adult. The professional also views the infant's defect from a less personal, more objective, and less narcissistic position than the new parents.

When the newborn is sick, the degree of mourning and parental feelings of grief and loss are not equated with the severity of the neonate's illness.[1] Even seemingly "minor" illnesses such as jaundice or respiratory difficulty requiring phototherapy or minimal oxygen supplementation are associated with parental concern for survival and feelings of grief and loss. These feelings are often not acknowledged by the parents or professional care providers because of the nonserious medical nature of the condition. In the mind of the care provider, self-limiting and treatable conditions are compared with more serious and often fatal neonatal illnesses. The care provider feels relieved about the "minor" nature of the neonate's condition and conveys this to the parents. "This is an easy condition to remedy. You don't have anything to worry about. The baby will go home in a few days."

Thus only the medical aspects of the newborn's illness are dealt with, whereas parental feelings remain unspoken and unresolved. In an altruistic attempt to reassure and comfort the family about the newborn's complete recovery, the professional unwittingly may discount the parents' real feelings. If the care provider is not concerned, parents may feel that they, too, should not be concerned and thus distrust and discount their own feelings.

Neonatal Deaths

The reactions accompanying neonatal illnesses are similar to the grief reactions experienced by parents whose infant dies.[1] Failure to acknowledge (even minor) neonatal illness as a loss situation and to work through the associated grief prevents parents from detaching from the image of the perfect child and taking on the sick newborn as a person to love. This may result in an aberrant parent-infant attachment. The liveborn infant who is critically ill or has a severe anomaly represents a "painful time of waiting"[5] for the family. They must deal with the uncertainty of whether their child will live and be healthy, live and continue to need extensive medical or special care, or die.

More deaths occur in the first 24 hours of life than in any other period of life. Yet death of a newborn is not the expected outcome of pregnancy. The majority of neonatal losses are caused by prematurity (80% to 90%) and congenital anomalies that are incompatible with life (15% to 20%). Regardless of the cause of death, even infants who live only a short time are mourned by their parents.[31] Prenatal attachment and investment of love in the newborn result in a classic grief reaction at the newborn's death.[33]

Even a short period of life between birth and death gives parents an opportunity to know their child. Completion of the attachment process enables parents to psychically begin the next process of detachment. Attachment to the child's reality encourages detachment from that reality, rather than from the parents' most dreaded fears and fantasies about their infant. Parental contact with the child before death enables them to share life for a brief time.

In the case of multiple births when one (or more) child dies and the other(s) lives, parents simultaneously grieve the loss of the dead infant(s) while attaching to the survivor(s). In many situations of multiple birth, the surviving infant(s) is in an intensive care nursery. The diametrically opposite feelings of love and attachment and grief and detachment, as well as the anxiety associated with the care and well-being of the surviving infant(s) are emotionally draining for new parents. The process of grief may slow the parents' ability to become intimately involved with their surviving infant(s).[71] They may have ambivalent feelings toward the infant(s) who survives or toward the infant(s) who dies. With the loss of one of a multiple birth there is less support for the grieving parents, as the frequent response by everyone is that they should be thankful for the survival of one (or more) of their infants.

Generally, death of the newborn occurs despite everything done to prevent it. This provides parents with some measure of comfort in knowing "that we did everything that could have been done." Yet when the neonate is so severely ill or deformed that a decision about initiating or continuing life support is necessary, the parents have an extra burden. The situation may involve conflicts between physicians, nurses, and family wishes, causing significant personal anguish. As part of the Federal Baby Doe regulations, most hospitals now have ethics committees that address the medical, legal, and ethical controversies (see Chapter 30). Regardless of who makes this decision, it is first and foremost the parents who will live with the ramifications of that decision. When parents are involved in the decision-making process, they wonder if theirs was the right decision regardless of what the decision is. If the child lives or dies, they wonder how a different decision would have changed their lives.

Stages of Grief

The experience of grief is a staged process that occurs over time. To detach both externally and internally from the lost loved object, emotional investment is withdrawn so that it may be invested in new love relationships.[42] Each stage of grief represents a psychologic defense mechanism used to help the individual to adapt slowly to the crisis. This slow adaptation is purposeful, because it prevents the individual psyche from being overwhelmed by the pain and anguish of loss.[44,50]

Although the stage of grief is recognizable, the process of grief is dynamic and fluid rather than static and rigid. Parents, families, and professionals progress cyclically through the stages of grief rather than in an orderly progression from beginning to end. However, each person experiences the process of grief uniquely and at an individual rate. Knowledge of each stage is necessary to assess where an individual family member, the family as a unit, and the staff are in their grief process. This information is then used to support individuals when they are in their particular stage of grief (rather than attempting to maneuver them from stage to stage), contributing to the defense, or stripping the individuals of their

defenses. Regardless of the type of perinatal loss, the experience of that loss through staged grief work closely parallels the grief stages of Elisabeth Kübler-Ross.[36]

The feelings of *disbelief and rejection* of the news are reflected in the responses "No! This couldn't happen to me!" "It isn't true! They've made a mistake!" This immediate response protects the individual from the shocking reality of loss by postponing the full effect of reality until the psyche is able to handle it.[58] By holding on to the fantasy of a positive outcome (e.g., the loss of the heartbeat is only temporary or the dead infant belongs to someone else), facing the awful truth and the grief associated with it is delayed at least temporarily.[44,58,61]

The initial stage of grief is characterized by overwhelming feelings of being stunned and surprised—often seen as emotional numbness, flat affect, or immobility.[74] Emotional detachment is often expressed as an inability to cope or respond with activities of daily living, an inability to remember what others have said, and a tendency to repeat the same question.[18,32,36,44,74] For the tragedy to be handled in manageable pieces without overwhelming the individual, the mind may acknowledge the event only intellectually, and there is a corresponding lack of emotional reaction,[44,74] or the event may be compartmentalized so that only a part of the situation rather than the whole becomes the focal point of attention.

Anger is the result of a gradually developing awareness of the situation's reality. As the significance of their perinatal loss begins to dawn on them, parents (and significant others) experience the diffuse emotions of anxiety and anger.[32] With the full effect of their loss comes more focused feelings of bitterness, resentment, blame, rage, and envy of those with normal pregnancy outcomes.[36]

Social prohibitions against the expression of anger, especially for women, encourage this powerful emotion to be turned inward toward the self. Anger directed inward results in depression and a deepening sense of guilt. "Why?" "What did I do wrong or not do right to have caused this to happen?" are the hallmarks of the self-examination and self-blame that accompany perinatal loss.[32,44,74] Answers are often irrational and have no cause-and-effect relationship with the reality of the circumstances. Irrational, feared causes include sexual intercourse (common worry of both men and women), career (of the mother) outside the home, superstitions, dietary habits, or lifting of heavy objects.[75] Ideas of punishment (for past wrongs, for negative or ambivalent feelings, or for an unwanted pregnancy)[3,69] are often thought to be the reason for the failed outcome. The search for a reason to answer the question "Why me?" requires correct information to dispel unrealistic fantasies of causation. However, the question does not require a literal answer (often no concrete answer exists) but is merely a wish for a change in the situation.[3]

Anger directed outward is usually expressed as overt hostility to those in the immediate environment (family, children, care providers, and infant)[39,44,74] or toward God.[39,50] Fathers exhibit more anger than mothers.[23] Blame and anger may be a destructive force in the relationships among family members and prevent these relationships from being a source of comfort and support.[44] Ventilation of angry feelings toward professional care providers protects these family relationships for more positive interactions. Anger moves the grieving process along, but persistence of anger may prevent grief work from progressing to subsequent stages.

Bargaining may occur concomitantly with denial and shock as an attempt to prevent or at least delay the loss.[49,70] Bargaining usually occurs with whomever the parents (family or staff) believe the supreme being to be. The "Yes, but" of this stage is a form of "conditional acceptance," while still attempting to make the reality other than what it is.[3,36] With the defective child, bargaining may take the form of shopping for a physician or searching for the magic cure.[74]

The onset of *depression and withdrawal* marks the stage of a greater level of acceptance of the tragedy. With the true realization of the effect of the loss, the individual acknowledges that indeed there is a reason to be sad. The predominant feelings of this stage are overwhelming sorrow and sadness[44] evidenced by tearfulness, crying, and weeping.[58,61] Feelings of helplessness, worthlessness, and powerlessness contribute to the sense that life is empty and futile. Withdrawal may be evidenced by requests to be left alone, by decreased or complete cessation of visits to the infant, and by silence.[36,49] The degree of withdrawal may be indicative of the depth of depression and the extent to which there is guilt and self-blame.[58]

Acceptance is the resolution stage of the grief process that is heralded by resumption of usual daily activities and a noticeable decrease in preoccupation with the image of the lost infant.[42] This stage most often is not witnessed by the perinatal professionals. The acceptance stage is characterized by emotional detachment of life's meaning from the lost relationship and reestablishing it independent of the lost object.[36,43] The lost relationship is seen in a new light—as giving meaning to the present.[43] The aggrieved person relinquishes that part of himself or herself that was defined in the lost relationship and establishes a new identity that is emotionally free to attach in another relationship.

For the family of a deformed child, acceptance is not an all-or-nothing proposition, but rather a daily adaptation and coping with the child and the defect.[62] For the family, periods of frustration and sorrow alternate with periods of delight and enjoyment of the child.[39] Because of the chronic sorrow experienced throughout the life of a defective child, the final stage of resolution of the family's grief is only possible after the child's death.[48,74]

The acceptance stage represents the ability to remember both the joys and sorrows of the lost relationship without undue discomfort.[18] With gradual integration of the loss, there are progressively fewer attacks of acute, all-consuming pain.[43] When recalling the lost infant, there are fewer feelings of devastation and more a feeling of sadness. The ability to "celebrate the loss" also identifies grief resolution. Celebration of the loss does not mean recall without sadness and sorrow but with an ability to find some meaning, some good, and some positive aspects in the situation (e.g., "At least we had our child for a time, even though it was a short time.").

Symptoms of Grief

Although each person copes with grief in individual ways, there are expected reactions to loss situations. Knowledge of the differences and commonalities of the grief experience enables care providers to understand their own reactions as well as to share their thoughts and feelings with the grieving family. The professional care provider must learn to "hear" what the family says about how and where each member is in the process of grief resolution. Often the "message" is not a direct reference to the loss or one's feelings, but rather nonverbal communication. The professional must learn to recognize that individuals often communicate more by what they do and what they omit than by what they say.

The signs and symptoms of acute grief have been well described and include both somatic and behavioral manifestations of the emotional experience of the loss (Box 29-2). The behavior of the bereaved is characterized as ambivalent.[43] In perinatal situations, parents simultaneously hope that the infant will live and wish for the infant to die; they want to love and care for the child while at the same time wish to reject the child.[32,39] These feelings are frightening and socially unacceptable, and therefore often remain unspoken.

Often the intensity of grief is greater when the relationship and feelings of the lost person are ambivalent.[43] Even with the most positive of pregnancy outcomes, taking a new infant into the family results in ambivalent feelings for all family members. The degree of disruption that a perinatal loss brings to the family is equated with the severity of grief, especially because reproduction and a healthy perinatal outcome are highly valued in our society.[43]

Box 29-2
Signs and Symptoms of Grief

I. Somatic (physiologic)
 A. Gastrointestinal system
  1. Anorexia and weight loss
  2. Overeating
  3. Nausea or vomiting
  4. Abdominal pains or feelings of emptiness
  5. Diarrhea or constipation
 B. Respiratory system
  1. Sighing respiration
  2. Choking or coughing
  3. Shortness of breath
  4. Hyperventilation
 C. Cardiovascular system
  1. Cardiac palpitations or "fluttering" in chest
  2. "Heavy" feeling in chest
 D. Neuromuscular system
  1. Headaches
  2. Vertigo
  3. Syncope
  4. Brisaud's disease (tics)
  5. Muscular weakness or loss of strength
II. Behavioral (psychologic)
 A. Feelings of
  1. Guilt
  2. Sadness
  3. Anger and hostility

  4. Emptiness and apathy
  5. Helplessness
  6. Pain, desperation, and pessimism
  7. Shame
  8. Loneliness
 B. Preoccupation with image of the lost infant
  1. Daydreams and fantasies
  2. Nightmares
  3. Longing
 C. Disturbed interpersonal relationships
  1. Increased irritability and restlessness
  2. Decreased sexual interest and drive
  3. Withdrawal
 D. Crying
 E. Inability to return to normal activities
  1. Fatigue and exhaustion or aimless overactivity
  2. Insomnia or oversleeping
  3. Short attention span
  4. Slow speech, movement, and thought process
  5. Loss of concentration and motivation

Modified from Lindemann E: *Am J Psychiatry* 101:144, 1944; Marris P: *Loss and change,* New York, 1974, Pantheon Books; and Colgrove M: *How to survive the loss of a love,* New York, 1976, Lion Publishing.

Male-Female Differences

Although members of both sexes have the same grief reactions, women express more symptoms (crying, sadness, anger, guilt, and use of medications)[13,14,45] than men. This difference in symptomatology does not represent a different experience of grief, but merely a different expression of it. Understanding these differences and the reasons for them are crucial for care providers working with parents at the time of perinatal loss.

The father's degree of investment in the pregnancy, impending parenthood, and the circumstances of birth all affect his feelings of loss. Because the father's body does not directly experience the changes of pregnancy, the pregnancy may initially be less of a reality to him than to the pregnant woman. This lag in the physiologic reality contributes to a lag in the psychologic investment of the father in the child. Fathers often comment that the infant became real when he felt the fetus move in the mother or at first sight of the new infant. Fathers who form an early attachment to the child feel sadness, disappointment, and often anger at being denied the expected son or daughter.[23,61] Conversely, fathers who have been normally ambivalent or overtly negative about the pregnancy may feel guilt and responsibility for the failed outcome.[61]

Participation of the father in the events of labor and birth also influences his attachment and ultimately his feelings of loss. Exclusion decreases his involvement in these life-crisis events, whereas inclusion has many advantages for the mother, infant, and self (see Chapter 28). If the infant is ill, the father may initially have more and closer contact than the mother.[1,49] In the birth place, the father may see, touch, or hold the infant before the mother. The father observes the initial resuscitation and stabilization and may accompany the infant to the nursery and on transport to a regional center. Often the father receives the first information and support[47] about the infant's condition and returns to the hospitalized mother with the news. This early, prolonged contact coupled with the father's increased responsibility often contributes to the development of a closer and earlier bond between father and child than between mother and child. The initial lag in prenatal investment may be offset after birth by concentrated contact between the father and child, so that a loss is highly significant to the father.

Societal expectations about masculinity and femininity markedly influence the expression of grief. Society's message to men starts early in life: "Big boys don't cry." "Don't cry, you'll be a sissy" (i.e., girl). The preferred male image in our society is the autonomous, independent achiever who is always strong and in control, even in the face of disaster.[24] In keeping with this image, the father may feel that he must make all the decisions and have all information filtered through him to protect the mother. However, this altruistic gesture prevents full disclosure and involvement of the mother. Assuming the role of strong protector also involves a heavy price for the father in suppression of his own feelings and delay of his own grief work. The role of "tower of strength" often engenders feelings of resentment from the mother. While he attempts to live up to his (and society's) expectations of himself, the woman views his lack of feelings and emotions, especially crying, as "He doesn't care."

Many men have difficulty dealing with irrational behaviors as well as with the normal ambiguity and conflict of life.[24] This difficulty makes the emotional response of grief and its accompanying ambivalent feelings and conflicts produce discomfort and anxiety in many men. The expression of appropriate human emotions becomes threatening and makes them feel vulnerable.[24] To decrease the anxiety associated with grief and its expression, men often deal with feelings by denying them, increasing their work load, or withdrawing from the situation and refusing to discuss it.[32,42]

The father's attitude and ability to communicate about the loss may help or impede the mother's grief work.[58] Lack of communication between a couple may contribute to intense mourning, psychiatric disturbances, and severe family disruption.[12,31] Synchrony of grieving between the mother and father is important in an ultimate healthy resolution for the family.[11] If the father denies and suppresses his own feelings of loss and grief, he may react to the normal signs and symptoms of grief in his partner as if they were abnormal. Often the father is able to resolve his grief faster than the mother, and he may become impatient with her continual "dwelling" on the loss.[45] Sometimes fearing the woman's prolonged grief, the man decides to "spare her" from his feelings and does not discuss them with her. Instead of being comforting as intended, failure to share grief leads to isolation and alienation within the relationship.[32]

In some situations the man may experience intense emotions, not unlike those his partner experienced at the time of the crisis, several months after the death. Because these intense emotions occur so long after the crisis, he may not even associate them with the death.[32]

Timing of Grief Resolution

Parents

Emotional recovery from the pain of perinatal loss occurs with time. There is no complete agreement on the length of time necessary for the individual to resolve grief. Indeed, a specific timetable for mourning may be impossible to establish.[3,12] However, some general time frames are available for the duration of a normal grief reaction.

Acute grief reactions are the most intense during the first 4 to 6 weeks after the loss,[42,43,50] with some improvement noted 6 to 10 weeks later. Normal grief reactions may be expected to last from 6 months to 1 year[18,32,50] or 2 years.[43] Indeed, significant losses of a spouse or child may never be completely resolved.[44] "I'll never get over it."

One parameter for differentiating normal from pathologic grief has been the length of time for grief to be resolved. Grief work may still be categorized as normal even if it lasts longer than 1 year, especially if the person is working through unresolved grief from the past. Grief work is normally energy draining. Dealing with more than one grief or loss situation compounds the intensity of mourning and may prolong the grief reaction. Because perinatal loss represents more than the loss of the child (loss of the perfect child, loss of plans for the future, and loss of self-esteem)[38] feelings of sadness and depression may still be evident for a year or longer.[32,75]

Sorrow and grief may even last a lifetime. For families of defective children, "chronic sorrow"[48,65] is experienced as long as the child lives. These parents live with the constant reminder of what is not and what the child will never be and can never do. The grief of death is final—parents do the work and go on; chronic sorrow is grieving on a daily basis. Expecting the parents to "adjust to" or "accept" their child's defect without any elements of lingering sadness is unrealistic. Chronic sorrow is a justifiable reaction to the daily stresses and coping necessary when a child is defective. The final stage of grief resolution is only possible with the finality of the death of the child.

Even when grief has been resolved, anniversary grief reactions are normal. Renewal of sadness, crying, and normal grieving behaviors may be reactivated at certain times. These anniversary reactions may not be limited to the infant's date of death but may also be felt on the expected date of delivery, on the actual birthday, or when seeing an infant of the same age and sex as the lost child. Holidays may also reactivate grieving behaviors, especially those that bring together family and friends and recall memories of joy and happiness.

Staff

Those sharing a crisis (complication, illness, or death) often become closely attached, so that the loss is felt not only by the family but also by the professional care providers.[16,21] Repeatedly dealing with death and deformity increases the professional's exposure to personal feelings of grief and loss. This may be perceived either as a threat or a personal opportunity for growth.

The critical variable in the ability to face or assist others in handling loss is the manner in which the care providers have been able to resolve their own personal losses.[72,73] Unless the care providers are able to cope with personal feelings of loss and grief, they may not be able to give of the "self" to others. Care given without genuine involvement and responsiveness to the family's feelings does not facilitate and may actually impede the mourning process. Professionals who are able to deal honestly with their own feelings will be able to help others cope with theirs.

Helping parents deal with their grief may be difficult for professionals because of their attitudes and feelings about perinatal loss. For professionals trained to preserve life, loss of the best pregnancy outcome or death itself represents both a personal and professional failure.[32] When success is equated with life, the failure of death (or loss) is associated with feelings of guilt, anger, depression, and hostility.[44,66,75] Just when professionals are expected to be supportive and therapeutic, they may be overwhelmed with their own feelings. Professionally, the care providers may feel helpless when all efforts inevitably result in no change in the outcome.

The feelings and stages of grief experienced by the family are the same ones felt by the staff who are attached to the parents and their newborn. Many professionals working in perinatal care are of childbearing age, so that identifying with the parents and their plight is relatively easy. Because the sick, deformed, or dead infant could easily be that of the staff, they share with the parents the special stress of the loss of a child. The care provider often experiences the same fantasies of blame as the parents. "What did I do (or not do) to cause this?"

Repetitive contact with loss situations and death exposes the staff to recurring feelings of frustration, guilt, self-doubt, depression, anger, classic grief reactions, helplessness, sadness, hopelessness, loneliness, and relief.[16] Such uncomfortable feelings often lead to behaviors of avoidance and withdrawal as a means of self-protection.[12,21,22] Adequate medical care may be given, but psychologic care of the family may be neglected. The involved primary care providers may decrease their attachment to both parents and infant when an unfavorable outcome is inevitable. Withdrawing emotional support and involvement may spare the professional but only adds to parental feelings of isolation, inadequacy, and worthlessness. Professionals who have risked family attachment and shared grief work may be more cautious in future involvements to protect themselves from the pain of loss.

Asynchrony and individual differences in handling grief reactions may also cause problems among the professional staff. Constant exposure to perinatal loss may desensitize some individuals until they are blasé or even callous about the crisis, whereas others have grief reactions that parallel the family's reaction. Some staff members may have

reached the stage of acceptance, while others who are unable to let the infant go persist in the idea of a magical cure,[12] a characteristic of denial. The rationale of prolonging the child's life may in reality be prolonging death, and inevitably one needs to accept death's finality.

The staff cannot offer support to families experiencing loss unless they receive support in dealing with their own grief reactions. Those who receive support learn about their feelings and how to handle them, and so have no need to displace their pain to others. The three most effective ways that NICU nurses have identified to manage their stress after neonatal death are (1) discussion with coworkers, (2) supporting and comforting the grieving family, and (3) talking with their own families.[16] Various formats are available for meeting staff needs, such as mutual support of colleagues or group sessions involving peer counseling on a long-term or short-term basis.[16,32,46,72] Group meetings provide a vehicle for support and for sharing information and feelings among staff members.[16,21,32,72] Facilitated by an objective person with expertise in group process and the concepts of grief, the goal is to help the staff deal with their reactions so they will be better equipped to help the parents. Group sessions also serve to decrease stress, increase job satisfaction, and ultimately help prevent burnout. Staff members are encouraged to retain their humanity when an environment is created in which emotions are valued and their healthy expression facilitated, both at the time of loss and in its resolution.[30]

Sharing grief work with a family gives the care provider a chance for personal growth, to review past personal losses, and to evaluate the adequacy of their resolution. Helping others with loss or grief provides the professional with the opportunity to contemplate present and future losses, including one's own mortality. By working with those who have suffered a significant loss or death, a health care provider may gain a deeper perspective about life.

Interventions

Those in a crisis feel an openness to help and assistance from others, so that those in the crisis emerge either stronger or weaker, depending on the help they receive.[6,55] This increased openness also makes those in a crisis more vulnerable to the reactions of others—to their facial expression, tone of voice, and choice of words. Helpful professional interventions provide psychologic assistance during a highly vulnerable period of personal development. The goal of intervention is to maintain the precrisis level of functioning and improve coping and problem-solving skills beyond the precrisis level (i.e., to facilitate personal growth). Effective intervention is characterized by helping grief work get started, by supporting those who are grieving adaptively, and by intervening with individuals who display maladaptive reactions.[11]

Nonhelpful Interventions

Caring for pregnant women and their infants is supposed to be a "happy" job. Birthing and caring for infants are supposed to be times of joy and celebration. Because no one expects death or loss to occur in maternity or nursery areas, when it does, both staff and families are shocked. To protect themselves from the reality of the situation or to "spare" the family, professionals may engage in interventions that do not help themselves or their patients.[26] Such interventions may be meant altruistically, but do not have the characteristics of effective intervention.

Maintaining the state of denial arrests grief work by preventing or delaying the acceptance of the reality of the loss situation. Progress toward resolution is not begun until the stage of disbelief is relinquished. Using drugs, not talking or crying about the loss, and using distraction all contribute to maladaptive reactions by maintaining the state of denial. The use of tranquilizers, sedatives, and other drugs does not help the recipient, but rather the giver. Excessive use of these medications prolongs the denial stage by making the feelings and emotions foggy and dreamlike.[22,31,37] The energy needed to begin the grief work is dissipated by the effect of the medications. Avoiding the reality of the situation becomes easier when mind-altering drugs makes the tragedy even more unbelievable.

Not talking about the loss is a powerful way of denying that it ever existed. The inability of

professionals to acknowledge that the loss has occurred and that the family is in pain maintains denial and repression.[35,44,73] Not discussing the loss prevents parents from learning the facts and facing its reality. Because a fantasy will be created to substitute for the unknown, the fantasy of what happened and why will be worse than the reality. By receiving truthful, honest communication, parents are not left to spend energy dealing with frightening fantasies.

Professional avoidance and unwillingness to talk with parents after a loss communicates other powerful messages that impede grief work. If the loss is not important enough to discuss, then perhaps it is not important at all. Not talking about the loss serves to reduce it and communicates to the parents, "I don't care; therefore neither should you." Avoidance of the topic or a hurried, businesslike or social communication that skirts the issue tells the parent that grief work is dangerous, that grief emotions are dangerous, and that others are afraid of grief and those experiencing it. In essence, not discussing the loss gives a loud and clear nonverbal message to not grieve.

An inability to cry in response to a significant loss is not helpful and impedes grief work. The prohibition against crying may have been learned early in life or may be the result of unresolved grief work. Parents may feel the need to be strong for each other, their family, or the staff and thus do not cry. Sometimes role reversal occurs, so that the grieving person feels the need to support others rather than be the recipient of support. Often the significance of parental loss is neither recognized nor acknowledged by the professional for fear that "she or he will cry." Rather than talking about the loss as a technique to facilitate tears, no one says anything so no one will cry, and no one's grief progresses through the grief stages.

Distraction is another way of denying the loss or its significance. Professionals, a spouse, or other family members try to distract parents from the feelings and emotions of acute grief by engaging in light, social conversation or by keeping them busy with work or recreation. Dealing only with the physical care and not the need for psychologic care after birth is a form of distraction used by care providers.[26] Parents are preoccupied with their shattered expectations of the past and the stark reality of the present, and they are not interested in distractions.

After an unfavorable perinatal outcome, there is often confusion by the couple about their status: "Am I a mother or father . . . or not?" Failure to acknowledge the newly acquired role of mother or father (even if the fetus or newborn dies) discounts their psychologic investment in the pregnancy, fetus, and newborn. Quickly removing the infant from the maternity or nursery areas or removing all the baby items from the home negates the infant's existence.[32] This is not helpful for grief resolution and prevents parents from making choices and decisions and thus maintaining control over the reality of the situation.[28]

Isolation of the grieving family prevents the development of dependent relationships with others who might potentially provide support and comfort. Without others, parents are unable to share their grief and may thus increase their feelings of guilt, anger, blame, and lack of self-worth at their failed pregnancy. Those directly experiencing a perinatal loss may be isolated from the rest of society, including their families, who do not view loss of a pregnancy or neonate as significant.[5,32] Empathy with the parents' definition of the loss as important is necessary for society to be supportive. The goal of recent research, professional literature, and education has been to sensitize the care provider to the effect of perinatal loss. Only recently have books specifically about perinatal loss become available to give information and assistance to parents.

To decrease contact with the grieving mother, the staff may neglect her or perform cursory physical care, or there may be overconcern for providing physical care.[44] Assigning a room at the end of the hall, not going into the room, delay in answering requests, or placing the mother on another floor are ways of avoiding families. Use of private rooms and room assignments off the maternity floor may be helpful but may be used by staff to remove the unpleasant and uncomfortable situation. Early discharge to a supportive environment may be helpful, but without plans for follow-up may merely be a way to remove the constant, painful reminder.

Keeping the childbearing couple together throughout the perinatal events facilitates a shared experience of the reality of the situation.[35,73] Separation of the mother and father or of the couple from friends, family, and other children is not helpful. Exclusion of family members from the experience also excludes them from providing support for the mother and the couple. Relaxed visiting policies and as much contact as possible between the hospitalized mother and father (and other family members) are important.[73]

Prohibiting contact between the parents and the infant allows for fearful fantasies of the truth that are always more frightening than the reality of the situation. Delayed contact prolongs the state of disbelief and denial.[11] Restrictive visiting policies in the nursery, institutionalizing an infant without looking at all alternatives, or any other policy that separates parents from their infant, does not facilitate grief. Especially in the case of a deformed, stillborn, or dead infant, the message of delayed or no contact is that the infant is too horrible and too unacceptable to be seen or touched. Because parental egos are so symbiotically attached to their offspring, an unacceptable child is equated with an unacceptable and unworthy self. The fantasy that the damaged or dead child is representative of the damaged and defective self is borne out in the behavior and separation policies of the care providers.

In an attempt to offer the grieving family comfort, friends, relatives, and even professionals often make comments that are nonsupportive and nonhelpful.[29,32,66]

- "Well, you're young. You can have more babies."
- "Just have another baby right away."
- "Well, at least you have others at home."
- "It's better to lose her now when she's a baby than when she's 4 years old."
- "He never would have been totally normal anyway."
- "He was born dead. You didn't get a chance to know or get attached to him anyway."
- "It's God's will."

Cliches and platitudes such as these do not help because of the message they give about the parents and the infant.[46,58] These comments at best reduce and at worst negate the effect of prenatal attachment to the fetus. The importance of pyschologic investment and attachment by the parents to this fetus or newborn is said to be basically unimportant and essentially nonexistent.[32] Because infants are viewed as an extension of the parents' self, "by a not very subtle process of identification, the parents see a part of themselves in the baby, and nobody likes to be told that part of them is better off dead."[58] Also, comforting parents whose infant has died with the information that the child was not perfect and never would have been normal and healthy reinforces their belief that they are as defective and unsatisfactory as their dead child.[32]

Such comments also convey a message about the importance of an individual life.[35] Essentially, they say that one fetus or newborn is fairly interchangeable with another. They negate the importance of and indeed the existence of the infant for the parents, siblings, family, and society. The life of the individual is devalued, because he or she is easily replaced by "another baby." Comparing one infant's illness or deformity with another's is not helpful for parents whose own infant's deformity is certainly more important than any other infant's problem.[46]

The power of words to help during grief is outweighed only by their power to not help. Because parents are increasingly open during a perinatal crisis, they are sensitive not only to what is said and how it is said but also to the nonverbal message. Giving premature or false reassurance may be more for relief of the professionals than for the parents[6,29,46] Comments such as "It's okay" and "Everything's going to be all right" must be genuine and timed appropriately for the parent. Telling parents that they have a child with Down syndrome and then saying, "But everything will be all right" is hardly helpful. Giving reassurance that subsequent pregnancies and infants will be all right or unaffected is not helpful before the parents are ready to think about and project into the future.

The basic terminology accompanying perinatal grief situations may be upsetting to parents. Instead of "dead," professionals substitute less frightening and less final words. The use of "loss" when "death" is appropriate may be misinterpreted (especially by children). The terms "lose, loss, and lost" connote misplacing, so that comments such as "I'm sorry you lost your baby" may be responded to by "I didn't lose (misplace) my baby. My child died." Medical professionals skirt the use of the words "dead, died, and die." Care providers are taught as students to use the word "expired" when referring to a patient who has died. Meant to soften the effect of "dead," the word "expired" may have its own effect, as a mother whose infant son died wrote in a poem: "The baby expired they said, as if you were a credit card."[67]

Other situations that do not facilitate grief work include dealing with multiple losses or stresses and ambivalence or mental illness.[75] The reaction to the loss of a significant relationship is intensified in the context of multiple losses, stresses, and problems.[2,75] Because perinatal losses represent not only a loss of the wished-for perfect child, but a threat to the parental self, self-concept, and self-worth, they represent situations of multiple loss.

Helpful Interventions

Professionals have an opportunity to make a significant difference in the outcome after the crisis of perinatal loss for the individual, the couple, and the family. A care provider who is knowledgeable about the grief process and comfortable in sharing another's grief is equipped to assist the family and its members toward a long-term healthy adjustment rather than a dysfunctional and pathologic one. Interventions that are helpful for family members also assist staff members in their own grief work.

Factors that influence an individual's personal experience of grief (and ultimately appropriate interventions) are outlined in Box 29-3. Care for the grieving is individualized through assessing these factors, planning, and continually evaluating the individual. Eliciting such personal information may not be as difficult as it first seems. Those in crisis often spontaneously share crucial data with little prompting. The importance of active listening to questions and comments or a more formalized therapeutic interview process may provide the needed encouragement and permission to begin communication.

A history of previous losses and their type and timing in the life cycle are important data for the

---

Box 29-3

Factors to Evaluate in Individualizing Grief Interventions

I. Previous losses
  A. Type
    1. Separation
    2. Divorce
    3. Death
    4. Spontaneous abortion (miscarriage)
    5. Elective or selective abortion
    6. Period of infertility
    7. Relinquishment of child
    8. Perinatal loss
  B. Timing in the life cycle
    1. Distant
    2. Recent
  C. Coping styles (of each individual and the family as a unit)
  D. Grief work
    1. Resolved
    2. Unresolved
II. Prenatal attachment
  A. Degree of psychologic investment in relationship with fetus or newborn
  B. Decision making about pregnancy and infant
    1. Planned or unplanned
    2. Wanted or unwanted
  C. Meaning of pregnancy and infant to individual and family
  D. Parental expectation about child-bearing
III. Nature of the current loss
  A. Timing
    1. Sudden and expected
    2. Anticipatory grief
  B. Definition and meaning of the event (death, deformity) to individual members of the family
  C. Multiple losses
    1. Self
    2. Perfect child
  D. Nature and severity
    1. Of loss
    2. Of defect
IV. Cultural influences
  A. On experience and the expression of grief
  B. Societal expectations dictate acceptable and unacceptable behaviors of mourning
V. Strengths (individual and family)
  A. Support system (family, friends, religious, community, or social agencies) mobilized when necessary
  B. Stable relationships—couple supportive of each other
  C. Financial stability
  D. Coping abilities—can evaluate, plan, and adjust to novel situations
  E. Good health
  F. Receptive and intelligent
  G. Realistic expectations about child-bearing and child rearing

---

care provider dealing with the current loss. Past experiences with a crisis or loss influence an individual's behavioral and coping style with current problems. Dealing with problems alone, with help and support from others, or withdrawing altogether are possible ways of coping with the loss.

The degree of attachment and the meaning of the pregnancy and impending parenthood to the family define expectations and influence reactions if an optimal outcome does not occur. The experience of grief depends on whether the loss situation was sudden and unexpected or if there was forewarning about a problem or complication. The definition and meaning of the crisis (i.e., the nature and severity of a deformity, the finality of death, or the chronic sorrow of a defective infant) reflect the individual's and family's value system and previous crisis experience. The process of grief is affected by the event itself, the previous and current coping mechanisms, and the family's definition of the event.[27] Consideration of all these factors is crucial in instituting appropriate intervention.

The national association SHARE: Pregnancy and Infant Loss Support has revised the Rights of Parents When a Baby Dies and Rights of the Baby (Box 29-4). These documents serve as (1) guide-

---

Box 29-4

Rights of Parents and Infant when an Infant Dies

Rights of Parents

1. To be given the opportunity to see, hold, and touch their baby at any time before and/or after death, within reason
2. To have photographs of their baby taken and made available to the parents or held in security until the parents want to see them
3. To be given as many mementos as possible (i.e., crib card, baby beads or bracelet, ultrasound and/or other photographs, lock of hair, feet and hand prints, and record of weight and length)
4. To name their child and bond with him or her
5. To observe cultural and religious practices
6. To be cared for by an empathetic staff who will respect their feelings, thoughts, beliefs, and individual requests
7. To be with each other throughout hospitalization as much as possible
8. To be given time alone with their baby, allowing for individual needs
9. To be informed about the grieving process

10. To request an autopsy; in the case of a miscarriage, to request to have or *not* have an autopsy or pathology exam as determined by applicable law
11. To plan a farewell ritual, burial, or cremation in compliance with local and state regulations and according to their personal beliefs, religion, or cultural tradition
12. To be provided information on support resources that assist in the healing process (i.e., support groups, counseling, reading material, and perinatal loss newsletters)

Rights of the Infant

1. To be recognized as a person who was born and died
2. To be named
3. To be seen, touched, and held by the family
4. To have life-ending acknowledged
5. To be put to rest with dignity

From SHARE: Pregnancy and infant loss support, 1995.

---

lines for creation of protocols, checklists, and bereavement programs;[57] (2) affirmation and empowering tools for bereaved parents, and (3) communication points for parents and care providers initiating the grief process.[53]

Environment

The first step in facilitating grief work is to create an environment that is supportive, permissive, and conducive to the expression of feelings. This type of environment does not depend on physical surroundings but rather is created and maintained by a warm, receptive, accepting, and caring staff. Such an environment centers its concern more on the people giving and receiving care than on the tasks of care.[32] This type of environment is nonjudgmental and is characterized by an attitude of openness and freedom.[58] People feel safe enough to ventilate a full range of feelings—sadness, anger, despair, and even humor—without the fear of

condemnation or rejection. The staff become role models of open communication, facing grief and feeling comfortable in an uncomfortable situation. The safety of such an environment generates feelings of acceptance and understanding so that grieving and healing may proceed.

Professional presence and support is essential to families in crisis because of the increased dependency needs that accompany grief and loss. Yet certain aspects of a conducive environment such as privacy, quiet, and comfort may be difficult to obtain in a noisy and busy perinatal setting. The recommendation to never leave the family alone must be balanced with their need for privacy and personal time alone with their infant (stillborn, ill, or dying).[73] Simply saying, "I will stay with you unless you ask me to leave so that you can have some private time alone with your child" or "Would you like me to leave for a while so that you can be alone with your baby?" offers both support and privacy. Many parents later regret not having time alone and not thinking to ask to be alone with their infant.

A quiet place away from the hustle and bustle of the routine may facilitate both attachment and detachment. The mother of a stillborn child who is quickly shown her infant in the delivery room as her episiotomy is being repaired is not in an optimal physical (or psychologic) environment. Attaching to and saying good-bye to her infant is better accomplished in a quieter and more private setting with significant others present. Active participation of parents at the death of their newborn may not optimally occur in a busy intensive care unit. Rather, adaptation of hospice concepts to neonatal care provides a private, homelike room and more palliative care than cure to the dying newborn and the family.[70]

Supportive, Trusting Relationships

A relationship with a caring individual who offers consistency and support is the foundation of a therapeutic environment. During periods of crisis, when there is a temporary increase in dependency needs and feelings of loneliness, it is an adaptive behavior to seek emotional support from family, friends, and professionals.[43,44,47] Even the crisis of normal childbearing prompts many cultures to provide a "doula"[56] to teach the new mother and give her emotional support. For the mourning family, the relationships established with helpful professionals are more important than the physical care given.[21]

Support, "sharing one's ego strength with another in a time of need,"[25] is particularly helpful in perinatal loss because of the threat to self-concept and self-esteem suffered by parents. Support may be as simple as remaining with the parents. "Being there" indicates not merely physical presence, but an emotional availability and willingness to share their experience of loss. Often professionals, family, and friends are hampered by "not knowing what to say." Usually words are initially unnecessary or do not adequately describe the moment, and silent presence may better convey the message. Often it is not what is said but the mere presence of loving others that conveys empathy and support to parents and colleagues. Yet presence is not enough; meaningful interaction between parents and professionals is also necessary for a trusting relationship to develop.

The initial meeting with the professionals, including verbal and nonverbal cues, leaves a lasting impression on the family. Addressing family members by name personalizes the encounter, and a brief touch or handshake represents an extension of self, a gesture of warmth, concern, and acceptance from professional to parents. An introduction that includes a brief explanation of the professional's role in relation to them and their infant helps to orient them: "Good morning, Mr. and Mrs. Black. I'm Sue, your baby's primary nurse. That means that I will be caring for Jason while he is here and working with you." Orientation to the physical surroundings and technical equipment eases the transition to an unfamiliar and often intimidating hospital environment. Providing physical comfort such as rocking chairs, privacy for interaction, and sleeping facilities for parents demonstrates the philosophy of the parents' worth and importance to their infant.

Empathy, an emotional understanding and identification with the plight of another, characterizes a helping relationship. In such a relationship, "How are you?" is asked with the emphasis on *you* and a genuine interest in the answer, unlike a social inquiry in which an automatic "Fine" is expected. Recognition of verbal and nonverbal cues of parental feelings (e.g., "You look tired" and "I hear that you are frustrated") communicates that these emotions are legitimate, understood, and accepted. A willingness to help, listen, console, and give encouragement and positive feedback establishes the professional as a sensitive, responsive person whom parents will trust. Supporting any and all parental involvement, supporting damaged parental egos, and helping parents to succeed in the tasks of attachment and detachment are goals of effective intervention.

The tone of in-hospital perinatal settings is often determined by the nursing staff. Generally, residents, interns, and specialists remain for short periods, and the private physician or permanent medical staff are not available on a minute-to-minute basis. Development of a safe, trusting environment depends on viewing parents as essential and not as visitors or "disruptors" of the ward routine.[26] Pleasant and relaxed surroundings convey the message of hospitality and "You are welcome here."

Both professional and nonprofessional support systems are available in the crisis of perinatal loss. Yet relating to many people during crisis is difficult for parents. Primary care (both medical and nursing) provides the same care provider for both the physiologic and psychologic care of the infant and the family. Thus the family is able to relate to as few professionals as possible. This special caring reassures parents that a few special people love, know, and are invested in their infant. Primary care providers share with the parents the joys of even small gains and the sorrows and tears of complications or death. Professionals and parents benefit from primary care systems in the emotional and psychologic satisfaction of such involvement. Yet this involvement is not without a price of vulnerability to an individual's feelings of loss and grief. Peer support on an individual basis or in a group setting is essential in dealing with the stress of continual attachment and loss.[16]

Normal grief reactions may be facilitated by nursing and medical professionals using others (social workers or counselors) when necessary.[1] Collaboration and consultation with these professionals help the staff gain insight into parental and personal behaviors and appropriate intervention strategies. The staff may also benefit from the expertise of a trained counselor in dealing with their own feelings of loss and grief.[46]

Maladaptive responses (see following list) to perinatal loss are indications for referral for specialized care.[74]

Pathologic Grief[42]

- Overactivity without a sense of loss
- Acquisition of symptoms belonging to the last illness of the deceased
- Psychosomatic conditions
- Altered relationships to friends and relatives
- Furious hostility against specific others
- Formal manner resembling schizophrenia
- Lasting loss of social interaction patterns
- Assuming activities detrimental to social and economic existence
- Agitated depression

Involvement of clergy and religious organizations is often comforting and supportive to the family. Religious rituals (i.e., baptism, prayer service, or anointing) may be advocated by certain denominations and provide a measure of comfort and hope. Often parents in crisis do not think to request infant baptism or calling their priest, minister, or rabbi. Offering to call a clergy member of their choice or the hospital chaplain may be helpful.[8] Primary care providers who have shared intimately with the parents the experience of their child's life and death may be invited to attend the funeral or memorial service. For both care providers and parents, this may represent the final act of caring for the infant.[16]

Nonprofessional support systems such as the couple, family, friends, and parent groups are often forgotten as sources of potential help to grieving parents. In our society of isolated, mobile, nuclear families, it may be erroneous to assume that a support system exists. On the other hand, it may be unrecognized because it does not fall into a traditional definition (the next-door neighbor or other friend who may be more supportive [and available] than the grandparents). Biologic kinship is not the only valid criterion for a support system; an emotional kinship is the most important factor.

Because professional availability and involvement with the parents is not lasting, the professional has a responsibility to identify, foster, and facilitate a nonprofessional (social) support system. Simply identifying supportive others and expecting them to automatically help in a perinatal loss situation may not be realistic. Unless those who constitute the support system are as well informed and instructed as the parents about the situation, they will not be able to offer emotional comfort. For example, if the parents wish to talk about their loss but the support system empathically wishes to spare them by not discussing it, no help will be given or received.

Open communication between the parents is essential in preserving and fostering a close relationship by the giving and receiving of mutual support. Sharing the experience presents the couple with the opportunity for personal growth and growth as a couple. Yet the individual experience of grief within the context of a couple is all too often fertile ground for misunderstanding and resentment.

Parental support groups offer their members an opportunity to discuss their feelings with others who have been through similar traumas. Knowing how others who have experienced perinatal loss have felt and dealt with similar situations is emotionally comforting and stabilizing to parents experiencing their own loss. Parents provide each other with validation for their feelings and a sense that they are not alone in their pain.

Each individual has different needs, different ways of adapting to crisis, and different ways of giving and receiving support. It is essential that the professional use those techniques that are real and spontaneous and not adopt words or actions that are foreign to one's own self. Interventions must also be gauged to the parents' needs and pace.

Information

Information aids in intellectually understanding the crisis, thus facilitating a sense of control over it. Actively seeking and using information enables confrontation and mastery of the crisis. Knowledge about a situation strengthens the ego, because it enables "worry work" and psychologic preparation for expected events. Because "the void of the unknown is more frightening than the known; facts are more reassuring than awesome speculations,"[6] a major role of the professional is to provide and clarify facts and information relevant to the perinatal loss situation. In the search for meaning that always accompanies loss, medical facts may help alleviate some parental guilt about causing the tragedy. Repeating to the parents that "Nothing you did or did not do could have caused this problem" is reassuring. Sketchy or no information only serves to contribute to parental denial of the reality or to their fantasies of causation.[46,58] Confronting the crisis and realizing its real element of danger and trouble starts the process of grief by giving permission for the expression of feelings of fear, sadness, and loss.

Because the family as a unit, composed of each individual member, must deal with perinatal loss, it is important to encourage and support open, interfamily communications. Keeping secrets, especially between the parents, should be discouraged because this eventually undermines trust and promotes asynchronous grief work. When parents are given the same information and talk with each other

about their loss and their feelings, more synchronous grief reactions develop.[32,46] Telling parents together with the infant present prevents misunderstanding, misinterpretations, and "shading" of information to one parent.[32] Informed parents are better able to share their experience with each other and to participate in joint decision making with the professional.

The question often arises, "When to tell?" and "How much to tell?" the parents. Parents should be told as soon as possible about perinatal complications or problems.[32,46] Receiving this information at the earliest possible time helps parents establish trust in the care provider, appreciate the reality of the situation, begin the grief process, and mobilize both internal and external support. Information must be given in its entirety, because attempts "to spare" parents by staging the truth only serve to undermine their trust in professional credibility. The couple's relationship may also suffer if one parent colludes with the professional in a conspiracy of silence. This is best illustrated by the following incident.

> To spare a diabetic mother from the truth about her infant's congenitally absent limbs, the physician and father decided to tell her about his missing legs, but not the missing arm. On arriving to transport the baby, the nurse asked if the mother had been told. "Yes" was the response, so she took the infant to the mother's room before transport. As she uncovered the infant, the mother gasped and looked at the physician and father and said, "You lied to me. You didn't tell me about his arm, too."

When given the unedited truth, parents are able to face reality and begin the grief process without fear that "something else is the matter that they aren't telling me about."

The individual's stage of grief influences not when or what will be said, but how the information will be given and received. During the initial stage of shock, information—if processed—is processed slowly.[32] Often events take on a foggy, dreamlike quality so that sensory information remembered is not believed. Yet to give no information only perpetuates this frightening feeling. Communication to those in shock and denial must proceed simply, slowly, and with much repetition and reinforcement. Giving information once does not ensure it will be either retained or understood. Repetition by the professionals is necessary for gradual acceptance of the reality of the situation. This may be a nuisance for the professional who "has already told her that. Why can't she remember it?" Parents are so shocked they do not hear what is said and information must be patiently repeated.

Even though an early contact with parents almost ensures they will be in a state of shock, the tone and content of the first meeting is not forgotten.[32] Initial information about the infant and his or her condition may have long-term effects on the parents' ability to attach or detach. In the past, parents were given a pessimistic outlook with the belief that "It will be easier for them. They won't get so involved." Negative descriptions and initial pessimism only increase the amount of grief and detachment while effectively blocking attachment behaviors. Should the sick or defective infant survive, the parents may have detached to the point of at least emotionally burying the infant. Knowledge of better survival rates and the quality of survival enables a truthfully optimistic outcome for many sick neonates. Therefore information must be given clearly (not medical jargon) with a minimum focus on possible complications and medical odds.[32,74]

Volunteering information to parents is essential, but encouraging their questions is equally important. As the normal mechanism for adapting to crisis and gaining mastery over a situation, questions help the professional "to start where the parents are" and to begin communication with their concerns. Questions and comments unrelated to the discussion may indicate either failure to comprehend or failure to send the information clearly.[74] Direct questions deserve direct answers, because they indicate a readiness and desire for information. Indirect questions or comments by the parents may indicate concern about their own infant that cannot be directly expressed. "Baby Stevie (who died yesterday) had severe respiratory distress syndrome, didn't he?" The parents want to be reassured that their infant is not going to die, too.

During the crisis of perinatal loss, interpersonal communication is difficult. Therefore it is important that as few professionals as possible relay information to the parents. Primary care providers (nurse and physician) should coordinate and provide continuity in giving information to parents because individual care providers will supply information about the same topic in different ways. The use of varied terms, inflections, and attitudes by a multitude of professionals becomes a monumental source of confusion and anxiety for parents. A trusted relationship with a primary nurse and physician through whom all communication flows minimizes unnecessary anxiety and concern for parents.

It is absolutely essential that the nurse (or primary nurse) be present and assist the physician in communication with the parents. Any anxiety-producing information (poor prognosis, complication, or impending death) may not be heard or understood initially by the parents. The nurse must know exactly what information was given and how parents were given this information. After the physician departs, the nurse must be able to offer clarification, explanation, and support to distraught parents. Nothing is more distressing than finding a crying, upset mother who is unable to relate what the physician said, why she is upset, or even if she understood what was said.

No family or parent should have to wonder and worry about a dreaded or feared outcome without being given the proper information. If the primary care physician is unavailable to speak with the family, then someone from the health care team must assume this responsibility. No mother whose infant is ill, deformed, or dead should awaken from an anesthetized birth to find her physician absent and the nurses unable to answer "How's my baby?" A plan of action for telling individual parents must be decided and agreed on by all care providers.

Parents are interested in the daily (or hourly) progress of their infant, including both positive and negative developments. A crisis or negative development in an infant's condition is important for parents to know about as soon as possible. They are then able to participate and care for their infant through the difficulty and to trust professional communication. Parents should have unlimited access to phone and/or personal contact with the staff in the perinatal care setting. Phone calls into the hospital from concerned parents should be possible any time of the day or night. The knowledge that information about their infant and a caring professional are available at any hour often is enough to comfort parents of a critically ill infant.

Encouraging Expression of Emotions

Because grief is an emotional reaction to loss, expression of these emotions is necessary for grief work to begin and proceed. Verbalizing thoughts and feelings provides an outlet for the intense emotions accompanying grief and signifies to others that emotional support is needed.[44] For some the open expression of emotions may be difficult because of influence from culture, sex roles, and social status. Yet the containment of intense feelings uses a great deal of emotional and physical energy that could be more productively used in "moving on" with the grief work. Those who are stoic and noncommunicative have symptoms of grief for a longer period of time than those who freely express their feelings and emotions.[4]

Talking about the loss helps parents to validate and assimilate the experience. Timing and events are clarified, including forgotten details, by discussion with each other and with their care providers. Confronting the reality enables them to work through the shock and disbelief, verbalize their fears and disappointments, and begin to cry and grieve. Expression of feelings gradually permits a clarification of the meaning of the loss to the parents.[73] Talking lightens the burden of loss because every time the experience is shared with another, half of the experience and the accompanying emotions are given away. Telling, retelling, reviewing, and reliving the experience are all necessary ways to understand and gain mastery over a frightening and most often unexpected situation.[39,49,61,66]

Verbal and nonverbal cues tell professionals "where the parents are" in their grief process. To elicit feelings, the professional may verbalize his or her own perceptions and observations:

- "Mrs. Green, you sound tense (upset, tired) today."
- "Mr. Brown, you look worried today."
- "I'm sorry that your baby died."

These statements indicate the listening ear and observing eye of one who cares. They set the stage for communication: "It's okay to talk with me about how you are feeling because I acknowledge your pain."

Feeling scared, alone, and out of control, parents often deny their feelings under direct questioning. Thus "Do you think you did or didn't do something to cause your baby's problem?" may be answered negatively, even though parents are consumed with guilt. Direct questioning places parents in an awkward and vulnerable position of revealing their most personal doubts and fears. Direct questions may be reworded with safer and more indirect statements:

- "Most parents feel overwhelmed and sad when their baby is sick."
- "Many parents wonder if the cause of their baby's death is something they did or didn't do."
- "It is helpful to many parents to talk about their doubts and fears. These feelings are common and normal in such a difficult situation."

The professional gives parents information about the feelings and emotions commonly felt in similar situations. Because there is safety in numbers, if "most" or "many" parents feel this way and it is expected, then it might be safe to share their feelings. Validating parental reactions as appropriate reassures them that they are not crazy. With this type of invitation, the feelings may be free to come spilling forth or the parents may need time to establish a relationship with this professional before they are ready to talk about such personal emotions.

Empathetic actions and comments may open communication pathways with parents. A professional presence that is warm and caring may facilitate more communication than any words. Touching or holding grieving parents may help feelings be expressed. Nonverbal cues such as nodding, direct eye contact, uninterrupted attention, and the physical closeness of pulling up a chair and sitting down gives positive feedback to verbal communication and indicates active listening by the professional.

Crying is the expression of feelings of sadness, sorrow, and intense longing that accompany the pain of loss.[42,75] A healthy catharsis, crying should be expected and encouraged in any loss situation. Yet the cultural, sexual, and professional taboo against crying has defined it as an unacceptable and inappropriate response, and one that should be suppressed. Because tears are healing and therapeutic, professionals must learn to be comfortable with the crying of others. "Don't cry" is often heard from those attempting to comfort grieving parents (or colleagues). This is an admonition against the behavior rather than an empathetic comment. "It's okay to cry" or "Go ahead and cry—let it out" gives permission and acceptance to the behavior and the need for it.

By expecting tears, providing a safe environment for their expression, and encouraging the behavior by words and actions, the professional may facilitate crying in both mothers and fathers. All too often, tears are blocked in a relationship in which one partner (usually the man) is expected to be stoic and in control, while the other's (usually the woman's) tears are defined as too upsetting or difficult. Because the ability to cry is a healthy response, the couple must be encouraged to use this outlet together.

In the past, crying in the presence of patients and their families was defined as "unprofessional." Yet the cool, controlled exterior defined as "professional" was seen by others as noncaring and nonfeeling. When the professional cries with the parents, it is an acceptable expression of genuine emotion, a demonstration of empathy, and a role model of the appropriateness of tears given the situation. Parents do not define the tears of care providers as weak or unprofessional. Rather, they feel a special bond of love and care with professionals who have been free enough to share their grief. Instead of relearning that crying is acceptable, many parents and care providers must learn for the first time.

Talking and crying about the loss are easier to facilitate than the expression of anger. Because of the social expectations of dependency of the patient role and real or imagined consequences of retaliation (against the infant or against job status), perinatal care settings are not safe environments for the expression of anger. Parents (and colleagues) will only be able to vent anger in an environment free of punishment or retaliation for their behaviors.

It is the responsibility of the professionals to create an environment that allows open expression of negative criticism and anger.

Seeing and Touching

Seeing and touching are as important to the parents of a sick, deformed, or dead infant as they are to the parents of a normal, healthy one. In the past, fear that seeing a deformed or dead infant would intensify grief and be overly upsetting resulted in no contact between parents and their newborn. Despite the fact that many mothers wished to see their infants, the prevailing practice was to discourage and prevent it. Often no information, including sex or physical characteristics, was given to grieving parents who were left to fantasize about their newborn's problems or cause of death. More recently, research and practice indicate that parental contact with the infant does not cause "unduly upsetting immediate reactions or appear to result in pathologic mourning."[31]

The decision to see and touch their infant is ultimately a parental one.[35,75] Making decisions for clients is not the professional's role; making decisions *with* clients is the professional's role. Each parent must make the decision for himself or herself; neither may decide for the other. Altruistic others such as professionals, spouse, or other family members must not usurp the right to individual decision making. Often in an attempt to protect the mother, the father or professional decides that she should not have contact with her infant. They either actually discourage it or do nothing to facilitate it. Mothers who have not seen their infants always know who prohibited it. The couple's relationship may suffer irreparable damage if one decides for the other, even if the motive is altruistic. The professional's role is to facilitate a healthy decision by each parent so that their individual needs to see or not to see the infant are met.

Parents may not realize that seeing and touching their infant is an option.[73] Or they may just be too overwhelmed or afraid to ask if it is possible. Instead of waiting for parents to ask, the professional care provider takes a more active role by offering the possibility to the parents: "Would you like to hold your baby?"

Time is often required to make the decision because initially parents are ambivalent about seeing and holding a deformed or dead infant. Most mothers and fathers want to see their child but fear what they might see and how they may feel.[61] The care provider may alleviate parental ambivalence by acknowledging that being with the infant will be difficult but that the professional will remain with them unless asked to leave. The emotional support of the physical presence of an empathetic professional may allay the fear of becoming out of control. The professional can reassure the family by explaining what they will see before they hold their infant. Making such a crucial decision in the initial stages of loss is difficult. Giving parents information about the positive aspects of seeing and holding the infant in facilitating their grief process helps make their decision an informed one.[8,75]

Seeing the infant brings the dreaded impossibility of perinatal loss into stark reality.[46,75] Parents confirm with their own eyes that the infant is alive or dead, or normal or abnormal. Contact enables claiming behaviors and identification of the infant as their own. While holding their infant, parents examine it and begin to recognize familiar family characteristics: "She has my long fingers and her father's red hair." Even small, severely deformed, or macerated infants are able to be recognized and claimed by the parents as part of their family.[35] The normal, endearing characteristics that identify the child as "mine" are remembered.

Parental contact confirms the infant's own reality and eliminates the prenatal fantasy of the expected child. For the parents of an anomalied infant, grief work about the fantasized perfect child may begin, so that the actual child may become the object of love. Early and frequent contact between the parents and the infant encourages a realistic perspective of the infant's problems. The stillborn or aborted fetus may be physically normal rather than the deformed infant imagined by the parents. Seeing the infant allays doubts and fears about the infant's normal state and about the parents' ability to subsequently have a normal child.[40,41,58] Seeing and touching enables parents to grieve the infant's reality rather than a feared and dreaded, thus more frightening, fantasy. It is easier to grieve a real infant than a mystical dreamlike fantasy of the infant.[32,35,40,41]

Whether the ultimate decision is to see or not see the infant, the professional must honor and respect that choice.[75] Cultural taboos against viewing dead bodies may preclude some parents from seeing and touching their infant. Yet many such cultures support their members by formalizing the grief process in sanctioned ritual and ceremony. For those parents who decide not to see and touch, it is important for the professional to reassure them of their infant's normal condition (e.g., "He had ten fingers and toes"). Describe the infant in as much detail as necessary to give parents a mental picture. Include sex, size, hair color, skin, weight, and distinguishing characteristics. A simple, realistic description of any anomaly is also helpful, because the fantasy of the defect is worse than its reality.

Adequate preparation for the first encounter with their infant includes a description of everything parents will see, hear, and feel.[35,75] Verbal preparation for viewing an infant with a congenital anomaly includes not only a simple description of the abnormality, but also the infant's normal characteristics. Seeing a picture of the abnormality first may help parents prepare for seeing their infant. Remaining with the parents at the initial visit, the professional describes the anomaly and points out normal findings. Focusing by parents on the normal familial characteristics helps in attaching to the less-than-perfect child. Although parents of a dead, deformed child view the abnormality, they often focus on the normal traits and remember the infant not as "monstrous" but as beautiful.

For those who have never seen a dead body, the mind may invent frightening images and sensations. Certainly, "dead" is associated with the temperature sensation of cold. However, a newborn who has been placed under a radiant warmer or in an incubator may feel warm rather than cold shortly after death. Hence, the statement by a mother, "You couldn't be dead. You feel so warm." The professional must touch the infant and prepare the parents for the tactile sensation of warm or cold: "The baby will feel warm to you because she (or he) has been under the radiant warmer."

To prepare parents for seeing their infant, the professional must observe the child. Color, skin condition, and size must all be described: maceration, "peeling of the skin," peripheral shutdown, "the blue-white discoloration," and the small size, "as long as the length of my hand" are not shocking with adequate preparation. Any equipment that must remain on the body should be described and explained before viewing. Even an umbilical cord clamp may cause concern in a parent who has never seen one. The reason for not removing equipment must also be explained. Respectful care of the infant's body after death shows respect for the person of the infant and for the grieving parents. Attention to details such as wrapping the infant in a blanket rather than a surgical drape or towel, cleaning the infant, and holding the infant in a cuddling position indicate care and concern.

Parents whose infant has died, is deformed, or is ill proceed with attachment behaviors of seeing and touching in the same manner as parents of normal, healthy infants.[32,35] Touching is important, but the distinction must be made between touching and holding. Cradling one's infant is quite different from merely touching with a hand. Holding the infant, whether healthy, sick, or dead, for the first time is a momentous event. Touching the infant who has died is not sufficient; parents must be given the opportunity to hold and cuddle the child before, during, and after death. Other parenting behaviors such as bathing and dressing their infant should also be offered to parents.[8]

Parents of a dead infant may need more than one chance to see and touch the infant. The first time, they attach to the reality of their infant. Subsequent encounters allow a final chance to see and hold their child. Parents have described the initial encounter as saying "Hello" and the subsequent one as saying "Good-bye." Some parents may be able to accomplish closure with one visit, whereas others who might benefit from a final visit may not ask or think to ask. Offering another contact with their infant leaves the decision with the parents.

The emotional effect of seeing the infant requires support, time, and permission to cry. Attaching is a process that occurs over time. Providing parents sufficient time with their infant takes precedence over paperwork, ward routine, or taking the infant to the morgue. Parents have indicated a need to hold their infant for a "longer" time and not feel pushed by care providers.[8] Even infants who have been removed to the morgue may be returned if parents need more time and contact for detachment.

When an infant dies, there are limited opportunities for memories. Professionals have the responsibility of helping parents make memories in order to have a tangible person to mourn. Encouraging parents to name their infant gives the child a separate identity, which helps facilitate the grieving process. Tangible mementos may include photographs, handprints and footprints, a lock of hair, measurements of the infant, identification bands, the blanket the infant was wrapped in, a blessing or baptismal certificate, and birth and death certificates. Parents find most beneficial interventions that acknowledged the infant (e.g., photographs, holding the infant, and receiving personal mementos).[8,28,52,63] Even when parents say they do not want mementos, they should be kept in hospital files and parents made aware that they will be available to them in the future if they want them. Taking a picture(s) of the infant, obtaining other mementos, and telling the parents that they will be available to them on request respects their immediate decision not to see or have information on the infant, but also provides a mechanism for them to "know" their infant at a later date if they wish to do so.

Before an infant is transported to a newborn special care unit, a photograph(s) should be taken and given to the parents to promote bonding. If the infant remains hospitalized for a long time or requires surgery, pictures taken at weekly intervals or before and after surgery can help confirm the reality of the child's condition and progress and assist with bonding as well as the grief process. Despite the outcome, parents will appreciate some lasting record of their child's life.

The staff who provides emotional support for parents must also receive support from each other.[16] Expecting the staff to immediately return to work is unrealistic. Such an emotional experience takes time and space for decompression, which is facilitated by the use of exercise, crying, and being alone for quiet time.[16]

Open Visiting and Caretaking Policies

Perinatal care settings with open visiting and care giving policies foster a shared family experience and support from others. Regardless of the type of perinatal loss, no mother should experience it alone—a spouse, friend, family member, or identified supportive other should remain with her.[8,35] Members of the mother's support system will also need an outlet for the expression of their grief.

Women suffering the grief of perinatal loss

should be given a choice about their room assignment. Arbitrary removal from the obstetric unit may deny the mother's maternity: "Am I a mother or not?" It may also escalate her feelings of failure, guilt, and worthlessness as a woman and a mother. Because she did not produce a normal, healthy infant, she may feel punished and banished from the maternity area by isolation on another floor. Her care may be entrusted to those without expertise in the physiologic and psychologic care of the normal postpartum period, much less a postpartum complicated by loss. Placement at the end of the hall far from the nurse's station, with the door closed and no company from staff and family, only increases her feelings of loneliness and isolation. Yet being on a happy maternity floor with normal, healthy infants and their mothers may be an exceedingly difficult and constant reminder of her loss and even complicate her recovery.[31,73] Information about the advantages and disadvantages of staying or leaving the maternity ward should be given by the professional. The mother, knowing what will be helpful, makes the decision.[75]

The alternative to maternal hospitalization is early discharge as soon as medically possible so the mother may join her infant when the infant has been transported to another hospital. Early discharge also facilitates an easier mobilization of supportive others in the familiar surroundings of home. Removal from the constant reminder of one's failure (i.e., other healthy infants) may let the grief work begin.[75] Early discharge is not therapeutic when the professional assumes there is a support system to provide care and no one is available. Without a plan for follow-up care and contact, early discharge merely relocates the problem.

Care giving is as important for the parents of a sick deformed, or dead infant as it is for the parents of a normal infant. Open visiting and care giving policies increase interaction between the parents and their infant by actively involving them in the reality of their child's illness, deformity, or impending death. Even if the child lives only a short time, parental access and taking care of the infant complete the attachment process and enable them to begin the detachment of grief work. Even minimal care giving helps parents overcome their sense of helplessness and be comforted by "We did all that we could have done. We cared, we made a

difference to our baby." Active parental involvement decreases poor outcomes such as aberrant parenting styles, attachment problems, and unresolved grief.[32]

The loneliness and isolation of death is decreased for both parents and infant when they are together at the time of death. Parents are often comforted and relieved that their fantasy of the agony of the death scene is not borne out in the quiet, peaceful reality of death.[32,72] Having experienced the beginning of life together, experiencing the ending of life as a family symbolizes closure and completion. Parents who are able to share even a brief life with their child and the moment of death are able to face death's finality knowing they did not abandon their child but provided the infant with love and care. Parents who are not present at death may take care of the infant afterward by seeing and holding their infant.

Parents need to be given the opportunity to make final plans for their deceased infant. The planning will help them face the death and facilitate the grief process. For many parents, this is their first experience with death and making final arrangements, and they are not aware of the options. Provision to the family of detailed, specific verbal and written information about cremation, burial, funeral, or hospital disposal is helpful.[8,28]

A funeral may be chosen for religious reasons or as a declaration of the fetus or newborn as a person befitting burial rather than disposal. Burial leaves a specific place of remembrance that this infant lived. Care for the infant after death may include funeral arrangements such as choosing the clothes, bathing, and even dressing the infant.[8,72] If parents choose not to have a funeral, they may wish to have a memorial service or do something special, such as plant a rosebush or tree, in memory of their infant. Regardless of their decision, the birth and death of their infant is a life event for the family, and it is important to recognize it.

Autopsy

For parents who experience a stillbirth, spontaneous abortion, or neonatal death, knowing why the infant was deformed or died eases their recovery from grief.[32] In the search for a cause, many parents blame themselves for doing too much or too little to favorably influence the outcome. Knowing why the infant died or the converse, that not even the "experts" know why the infant died, may help assuage their personal feelings of guilt and failure.

Approaching the family for permission for an autopsy must be done by the primary care providers (physician and nurse) with the utmost of tact and respect for the family's feelings.[72] Too often the permission for autopsy is denied because of the way the subject is broached by professionals. Telling the family about their infant's death in one breath and asking for an autopsy with the next breath is not appropriate. Parents need time to deal with the reality of the death, including seeing and holding their infant and being with each other and supportive others before they are even ready to think about an autopsy. Consideration of the family's feelings and stage of grief greatly enhances communication with the professional.[72] Reasons for the autopsy, including a possible answer to the question of "Why?" their infant died or was deformed, are important to discuss in a relaxed and unhurried manner. Parents may feel rushed to make a decision without clearly understanding the advantages and disadvantages and resist the emotional topic of a postmortem examination. Time for discussion with an empathetic professional as well as between themselves facilitates an informed parental decision.

The professional who receives permission for an autopsy is then obliged to discuss with the parents all findings.[22,31] This may entail more than one meeting with the parents, because they should be informed of the findings as soon as they are available. Therefore the professional may meet with them within 24 hours of completing the autopsy to discuss gross and preliminary findings and again 6 to 8 weeks later to discuss microscopic results.[32,72] Autopsy data may indicate either a condition that has implications for subsequent pregnancies or one that has little chance of recurrence. The need for genetic counseling for future pregnancies may be evident from autopsy results. Discussing the results with the report in hand and offering parents a copy for future reference is also important.

Anticipatory Guidance

Encounters with parents after the death of their infant give professionals the opportunity for *antici-*

patory guidance—information about what to expect from themselves and from others. Reactions to perinatal loss differ markedly, so that family, friends, and acquaintances may not act as parents might expect. Some will be supportive and emotionally empathetic, especially if they have suffered a perinatal loss. Others will be uncomfortable and, not knowing what to say or do, may choose to avoid the couple and never mention the loss, even in future conversations. Those who are unaware of the loss may question the newly nonpregnant parents about the new infant. These inquiries are both awkward and painful.

Knowledge of the universal feelings and behaviors associated with grief gives comfort and relief to parents. Knowing what to expect from grief (i.e., how it progresses and how long it takes) is valuable to those who are or will be experiencing it.[32,63,75] Knowing the stages of grief and that the accompanying behaviors and emotions are normal decreases the feeling of "going crazy." Recovery from the loss takes time and cannot be hurried or ignored. The most difficult time is immediately after birth and the first few months after the loss (2 to 4 months).[64] The emotions of grief begin to lessen toward the end of the first year.

Parents should be encouraged to support and care for each other in their time of loss. Professionals should advocate mutual support by a free expression of feelings and emotions between the parents. Although parents need each other during grief, they also need an identified support system with whom to talk and cry. The ability to reach outside of the nuclear family to friends, extended family, and professionals should be encouraged. Professionals have a responsibility to ask whom parents turn to for help and support in a crisis. If there are no identified supportive others, parents must know whom to call for help in the initial bereavement period.

Anticipatory guidance is also essential at the discharge of an anomalied, preterm, or previously ill newborn.[32] Knowing what to expect when going home with an infant with a defect or an infant who has been hospitalized for months makes the transition from hospital to society easier for parents. Evaluation of the grief process and the attachment level of the parents to a less-than-perfect infant is vital.

Long-Term Follow-Up Care

Follow-up care and contact with professionals are needed by grieving parents.[21,28] Follow-up meetings function as a catharsis for parents, as well as an opportunity for assessment, counseling, and possibly referral. Primary care providers (physicians, nurses, and social workers) from the perinatal care setting may provide follow-up. For the family, relating to providers with whom a relationship has been established may be easier than establishing a new relationship with a stranger.[28] However, being with those who are associated with the loss event may be uncomfortable for the parents at the height of their grief. For the professional, the ability to continue to be a source of help and comfort to families with whom one has established a relationship may help complete their grief reactions. Maintaining contact with the family may be painful as the professional relives the feelings of grief and loss associated with sharing their tragedy. Although painful, this reexperience of intense feelings gives both parents and professionals another opportunity to work toward grief resolution.

When and where to provide continuing care for families are crucial questions. Contact in the perinatal care setting both at the time of death and daily until discharge provides immediate care. However, when discharged, all too often the family returns home alone to face weeks and months of unsupported and lonely grief. Without feedback about their normal reaction and society's expectation that they will shortly be "back to normal," they are abandoned to their emotions. They suffer in silence and often drift apart in their misery. With their support system withdrawn but still feeling overwhelmed with grief, parents describe the period between 2 and 4 months after the loss as the most difficult time.[31,64,72] At 2 months after perinatal loss, parents show increased symptoms of anxiety and depression that are reduced by 8 months but still higher than in parents not experiencing perinatal loss.[68] Follow-up care from professionals is most meaningful and needed by parents during this period when they feel deserted by previously supportive others. Parents experience a need for spiritual support weeks and months after the loss. Meeting with families sooner (within weeks of their loss) may alleviate the effect of decreasing support as the months go by.[72] The

professional who acknowledges the withdrawal of others but can be relied on to be available provides the parents with the emotional anchor of long-term care and support.

Breaking appointments or continually not being available may be resistance to follow-up contact with the professionals but also represents a reluctance to return to the perinatal care setting with its painful memories. A visit from the professional in the home provides a non-threatening, familiar environment for follow-up care. The more comfortable home environment enables assessment of family interactions and facilitates communication at the "feeling" level.

Each family member and the family as a unit must be assessed for their place in the grief process:

- In what stage of grief is each family member?
- Is anyone "stuck" in a stage of grief?
- Are behaviors appropriate for normal grief reactions, or do altered behaviors represent pathologic grief reactions?
- Do altered behaviors warrant referral for further treatment and evaluation?
- Do the care giving and attachment behaviors of the parents reflect resolution of grief over loss of the perfect child and adoption of the less-than-perfect child as the love object?

Just because everything was progressing normally at previous encounters does not mean that it should be assumed to still be so. As the flood of initial grief subsides, problems and questions that were not considered suddenly become of great concern. For the first time in months, the regressive behavior of siblings may not only be noticed but may be extremely annoying to parents. The beginning of grief resolution may allow future projections such as "When can I have another baby?" or the dread of the painful anniversary of the loss.[72]

Referral to public health nurses or visiting nursing services in the community for follow-up care is appropriate. However, a written referral alone is not enough. Involving them in the hospital care and discharge planning is essential for a smooth transition to home care. Having the new professional meet the family in the hospital with the primary care providers facilitates trust transference from the familiar to the unfamiliar. Traditionally, home care providers have been involved in care of normal mothers and infants in the community. Involvement in perinatal loss situations requires knowledge about the process of grief and willingness to share the grief of the parents. Because these may be new skills for many, continuing education programs that teach the theory and skills of effective intervention help the professional be more comfortable with a perinatal loss situation.

Additional expertise may be warranted when the professional recognizes signs and symptoms of pathologic grief, delayed or absent grief, or concurrent multiple stresses or losses. Parents may not be ready for genetic counseling, infant stimulation programs, or financial programs until months later. Between 3 and 6 months after their loss, parents may be ready to reach outside of the nuclear and extended family for help and support for the first time. Suggesting a local hospital support group or the local chapter of a national support organization may at first be met with resistance. Leaving the names and phone numbers of such organizations ensures that the parents have the information at their disposal when they are ready to use it. Until their own support system has withdrawn, parents may not be ready for a support group of other parents.

Throughout this section, examples of "what to say" and "how to say it" have been used to illustrate helpful interventions for grieving families. It is essential to state that "there are no scripts." Parents do not say one thing and the professionals answer with a parroted response. Each encounter is a unique situation consisting of distinct parental and professional personalities. Each situation must be evaluated separately and individual interventions instituted.[28] It is recommended that the professional learn by observing an experienced colleague with grieving families and that the professional "practice" with role playing and situation solving before actually attempting to intervene with the parents.

Children and Grief

Explaining and helping a surviving child to understand the loss of an infant is an enormous task for parents. Facilitating the child's normal feelings of sadness, worry, and anger after a loss may be difficult for parents who fear being flooded with their own emotions. Unresolved grief from the parents' own childhood may prevent the expression of grief by their children.

To maintain the myth of childhood (innocent happiness), children are often shielded from any knowledge about death, even when it is an inevitable event in their lives. Thus children are prevented from full realization, validation, and expression of their feelings and emotions. They are not able to formalize and express their grief over the loss of a significant person.

Even though adults are encouraged to cry, talk, and gradually understand and integrate their feelings of grief, no one helps the child deal with the same frightening feelings. No one discusses the loss with the child, because "He might cry" and because of the adult's inadequacy and lack of understanding of how and what to say. No amount of secrecy or denial of the situation will hide the fact that the child is being excluded from an important family event.

Attempts to protect children from feelings of grief and mourning because of death or other important losses isolate the child. Age and developmentally appropriate explanations include the child in the family's experience, rather than separating and excluding him from "what is going on." Shielding children from the knowledge of death denies them the reality of life and the opportunity for personal growth and mastery of the experience. Like the subject of sex, death is taboo for children.

A child's grief and mourning in response to perinatal loss depend on his cognitive and developmental level, the extent of prenatal attachment and expectation about the infant, the degree of ambivalent feelings, and the response of his or her parents to the death. Because the child's understanding of death differs from that of adults, knowledge of the stages of growing awareness is essential for both parents and professionals working with children experiencing grief[33,34] (Table 29-1). Regardless of age or developmental stage, the universal fear of childhood is the fear of separation and abandonment. For the young child (under age 5), the loss of the infant is experienced indirectly through parental grief. The young child reacts to the emotional withdrawal of grieving parents and fears loss of them (and their love).

Table 29-1
A Child's Developing Concept of Death

Age	Cognitive Understanding	How Experienced
Infant (to 12 mo)	None	Indirectly through parental grief expressed in: Emotional withdrawal Inability to provide concern and continuity in caregiving behaviors Overconcern because of fear of recurrent loss
Toddler (1-3 yr)	Little understanding of cause and effect Death may be confused with sleeping or being away	Reacts to changes in behavior of grieving parents and reflects their feelings and anxiety
Preschooler (3-6 yr)	View death as a temporary state and not an inevitable occurrence Believe that they are the center of the universe and can do anything, and that thinking is doing (thoughts have the power of actions)	Expect the dead to return—ask questions about "when?" Fear (and feel guilty) that negative thoughts or actual death wishes caused the death
School age (6-12 yr)	Understand that death is inevitable and irreversible 6-9 year olds: personify death as a separate person (skeleton, boogey man) About 8 years old: "death phobia," a normal developmental stage characterized by preoccupation with thoughts of own death or that of a loved one	Realize death occurs in adults like parents and even in children; realize death is permanent, not temporary, state May show interest in biological aspects of death and details of funeral
Adolescents (12 yr)	Able to think abstractly about death like the adult	Similar to adult

Modified from Gardner SL, Merenstein GB: *Neonat Net* 5:17, 1986.

Although children at different developmental stages have their own conceptions of death, adults must provide them with the facts about the situation in language that they are able to understand. They may benefit from guidance by the nurse, social worker, or other health professional regarding beneficial approaches to facilitate the child's grief work. The professional serves as a resource, role model, and support system to parents caring for their surviving children. Printed materials are also available to assist parents in helping their other children understand death (see resource materials for parents at the end of this chapter). Age-appropriate story books concerning death can facilitate grief discussion and elicit questions and feelings from children.

Just as grieving adults need repetition, children need repeated explanations and discussions about the loss. Constantly in a state of developmental flux, the child attempts to view the loss in new ways as a result of increasing maturation. Asking questions (usually at inopportune times) and making comments about the infant are ways the child continues to process the experience, often long after the parents have completed it. These questions and comments may seem endless and resurrect the parent's own grief. The child's inquiries must be encouraged and supported so that he or she knows that talking about the loss or death is acceptable. Exploring the child's feelings for fears of causation, guilt, or the wonder if "death is catching" enables them to be dealt with appropriately. Truthful discussion with the child dispels the worst fears and fantasies and replaces them with reality that is "not too horrible to discuss" with parents. If the cause of the infant's death is known, it is explained to the child in simple, direct terms: "Baby Bobby couldn't breathe by himself because his lungs were sick. His sick lungs only happen to little babies."

A subsequent illness may precipitate worry by the child that he or she, too, will die. Often this fear is not verbalized but acted out by significant behavioral changes such as withdrawal, clinging and whining, or overactivity that are uncharacteristic for the child. Verbal reassurance that the child is not going to die and a reminder that "the baby died of a sickness that only little babies get; big boys and girls can't get it" are helpful.

The normal feelings that accompany grief should be acknowledged and explained to the child. "Mommy and Daddy feel sad that Baby Jean died. Sometimes we will cry because we feel sad. It's okay to cry when you feel sad." Permission for the expression of the child's feelings should also be given verbally: "You might feel sad, too. It's okay for you to cry when you're sad. Then we will talk about how you are feeling." Encouraging children to draw or write their feelings is another way of giving them permission to express their grief.

Using words such as "went away," "expired," "lost," or "went to sleep" is dangerous in describing death to children. Because young children are concrete and literal, they think they might die if they "go to sleep," or that anyone who leaves them is in danger of dying. Children also relate current experiences to past ones and interpret "lost" quite literally. In the mind of the child, if the parent only searched well enough, the misplaced (i.e., "lost") child would be found.

Including children at funeral or memorial services facilitates their grief and prevents exclusion from a significant family event. Consideration of the family value system, age of the child, and religious custom must enter into the decision to include the child. Adequate preparation includes a discussion of everything the child will see, hear, and feel, including the normal adult emotions of crying and sadness. An adult besides the grieving parents should accompany the child to reiterate what is happening and to meet the child's physical and psychologic needs. Adult support is necessary so that the child is able to express and deal with his or her feelings.

Helping children with their grief is also thera-peutic for parents. Assisting children to master the crisis of loss ultimately augments the parents' self-esteem and restores confidence in their parenting skills.[32] Parents are able to deal in a healthy way with their own grief when they are able to facilitate the grief of their other children.

Pathologic Grief

The absence of grief when it would be expected is not a healthy sign but rather a cause for concern. The emotions of grief and their expression are healing. Early and full expression of grief is associated with an optimal outcome.[32] However, many people in grief-producing situations attempt to avoid the pain of grief and the expression of emotions, the result of which prolongs mourning, delays a return to the previous lifestyle, prevents the creation of new attachments and relationships, and ultimately results in pathologic grief (see list on p. 690).[12,32,42]

Not grieving precludes opportunities for growth and change. No new coping styles will be attempted. No novel alternatives to problem solving and adapting to a crisis will be added to the repertoire of behavior for future use. In other words, those who choose not to do grief work say "no" to their own potential and remain frozen in development.[30] Under the stress of not resolving their grief, some may even regress in their development.

Reproductive loss is a blow to self-concept and self-esteem, as well as loss of the infant. Blocking appropriate feelings of loss, grief, and anger results in a significant decrease in one's sense of self-esteem.[14] After death of their neonates, 33% of mothers suffered severe and tragic outcomes (including psychoses, phobias, anxiety attacks, and deep depression).[12,32,75] Those who are unable to effectively resolve their grief may suffer lifelong emotional damage.[43]

Not working through grief associated with repetitive contact with perinatal loss also affects the staff. To cope with feelings, they may hide behind a "professional" demeanor characterized by decreased spontaneity and withdrawal. Such a provider defends against the repeated pain of loss by emotional dissociation from the situation; the real self does not respond, but the role of the omnipotent, unemotional physician or nurse responds. The result, self-alienation, eventually desensitizes the professional to the experience and ultimately prevents any empathy with the experience of others.[30] Emotions that are unable to be acknowledged or expressed healthily are vented in ways that may be destructive to relationships in personal and professional life.

Unresolved grief does not disappear and is not dissipated. The emotions accompanying grief may never be expressed but are not forgotten by the unconscious mind. Containment of these emotions through repression or suppression takes psychic energy. A conscious, intentional decision to postpone or dismiss grief to meet others' needs or to meet immediate demands of the loss situation (e.g., funeral arrangements) is called delayed grief.[42,43] For a period of time (days, weeks, or longer), there is little or no grief response when such a reaction would be expected and appropriate. Delayed grief may also be the result of repression, the unconscious contents that seem to have a life and energy of their own that become the sources of later emotional conflict.

Grief that is inhibited and never resolved is called abortive.[43] Those who have aborted their grief work often live bereft of "joie de vivre" with no interest, concern, or enthusiasm for life. Chronic grief is characterized by an indefinite prolonging of the acute stage of depression.[43] Indeed, chronic depression may be traceable to unresolved grief from the past.

Grief that is not resolved remains buried in the psyche, waiting for an opportunity to "rear its ugly head." A current loss may remind the psyche of the unmourned grief from a previous loss or losses.[17,44] As the two (or more) losses become intertwined and are experienced as one and the same, repressed emotions of unresolved grief pour forth.[44,66] Grieving more than one loss or a lifetime of losses is more difficult and emotionally draining than grieving one event at a time.[17] Cumulative grief work may also be occurring when a current loss of seemingly little importance overwhelms the person with intense emotions.[17,43] This flood of emotions seems disproportionate to the current loss and is only peripherally related to it. The unconscious, unre-

solved grief is finally uncovered when the individual is flooded with emotions. Thus the emotional components of any grief reaction may be influenced by aspects of unresolved grief from the past.[44]

Grief and loss events of the perinatal period have only been equated for a relatively short time (approximately 25 years). Because loss during the perinatal period is a common experience, many childbearing and older women (and men) have never grieved over their spontaneous abortion, stillbirth, or neonatal death, even 10 to 20 years after its occurrence. Parents in a current perinatal loss may also be dealing with unresolved grief from a previous perinatal loss. Unresolved grief (whether from perinatal or other loss events of life) may become available for resolution in subsequent crisis events. A mother who delivers a normal healthy newborn, yet is depressed postpartally, may not have postpartum depression. Instead she may be grieving the unresolved loss of a spontaneous abortion, therapeutic abortion, or other perinatal loss.[61,66] Her depressed mood could also be resulting from unresolved grief from the loss of a parent, spouse, or child. Depressed menopausal women may be experiencing the cumulative effects of a lifetime of unresolved grief. The symptomatology of unresolved grief is as follows[66]:

- Vivid memory for the details of the perinatal loss event
- Flashback to the event
- Anniversary grief (date of birth or expected date of delivery)
- Emotions of grief (sadness, anger, or crying) when talking about loss
- Intense emotions with subsequent loss or crisis

Recognizing unresolved grief has implications for facilitating grief work in a current loss, episodic care, and health maintenance. The energy to keep unresolved emotions restrained could better be used in personal growth and development, grieving, and maintaining and establishing relationships.[19] The lifelong stress of unresolved grief contributes to both psychologic and physical illness, including increased death rates and an earlier death.[54,72]

Not grieving a perinatal loss affects the individual involved and the relationships with significant others, including present and future children. Asynchronous grief and the absence of grief in one or more family members weaken and strain family relationships.[32] The irritability and preoccupation of normal grief may overly disrupt the family. Differences may be magnified to the extent that major rifts and disruptions in the relationship occur, resulting in increased incidence of separation and divorce.[32]

Exclusive dedication to the care of a deformed or ill child to the detriment of other family relationships is symptomatic of a pathologic grief reaction.[32,65,74] The parent who neglects other children, the couple's relationship, and social outlets is so overwhelmed with guilt about having caused the child's defect that nothing else in life matters. This guilty attachment and exclusive dedication are ways of avoiding grief work.[65] Other forms of pathologic reactions include parental rejection and intolerance of the deformed or ill child.[32]

The parent who is emotionally withdrawn and unavailable to the family because of chronic grief and depression is not able to attach and care for present or subsequent children. Aberrant parenting styles (resulting in a vulnerable, battered, or failure-to-thrive child) may be the result of prolonged separation, unresolved grief, or grief that has progressed beyond the anticipatory phase, so that emotional ties with the infant have been severed.[32] These difficulties with caring and parenting may affect the deformed or ill child and all the children in the family. In turn, these children may grow up unable to parent subsequent generations because of the type of ineffectual parenting they received. Parents who grieve inappropriately may leave their children a legacy of psychosocial problems such as difficulty with separation, independence, and control (e.g., school phobia and toilet training); a failure to thrive; and sleep disturbances.

Because detachment is necessary before a healthy attachment may again occur, unresolved grief affects future children. It is necessary to first complete the grief work over the loss of one child to be optimally ready to emotionally invest in a new infant.[32] The replacement child, a well-documented psychiatric syndrome, is associated with unresolved parental grief after the death (or loss) of a child.[17,51] Without withdrawing their emotional attachment to the lost child, parents plan, conceive, and bear another to replace their loss and alleviate their grief. Parental hopes, desires, and fantasies invested in the lost child are not relinquished but merely transferred to the replacement child. Planning for a new pregnancy and another child should begin only after the grief process for the lost child is completed.[32,66] Generally, 6 months to 1 year is the earliest that grief will be resolved so that the ego is free to invest in a relationship with another fetus and newborn.

References

1. Benfield D et al: Grief response of parents after referral of the critically ill newborn to a regional center, *N Engl J Med* 294:975, 1976.
2. Benoliel JQ: Assessment of loss and grief, *J Thanatology* 1:182, 1971.
3. Berezin N: *After a loss in pregnancy, help for families affected by a miscarriage, a stillbirth, or the loss of a newborn,* New York, 1982, Fireside Books.
4. Bibring GL: The death of an infant: a psychological study, *N Engl J Med* 283:370, 1970.
5. Borg S, Lasker J: *When pregnancy fails: families coping with miscarriage, stillbirth, and infant death,* Boston, 1981, Beacon Press.
6. Cadden V: Crisis in the family. In Caplan G, editor: *Principles of preventive psychiatry,* New York, 1964, Basic Books.
7. Cain A, Cain B: On replacing a child, *J Am Acad Child Psychiatry* 3:443, 1964.
8. Calhoun L: Parent perceptions of nursing support following perinatal loss, *J Perinat Neonat Nurs* 8:57, 1994.
9. Caplan G. *Principles of preventive psychiatry,* New York, 1964, Basic Books.
10. Colgrove M et al: *How to survive the loss of a love,* New York, 1976, Lion Books.
11. Costello AC, Gardner SL, Merenstein GB: Perinatal grief and loss, *J Perinatol* 8:41, 1988.
12. Cullberg J: Mental reactions of women to perinatal death. In Morris N, editor: *Psychosomatic medicine in obstetrics and gynecology,* New York, 1972, S Karger.
13. Cummings ST: The impact of the child's defect on the father, *Am J Orthopsychiatry* 46:246, 1976.
14. Cummings ST St et al: Effects of the child's deficiency on the mother: a study of mothers of mentally retarded, chronically ill, and neurotic children, *Am J Orthopsychiatry* 36:595, 1966.
15. Danforth DN: *Obstetrics and gynecology,* Philadelphia, 1990, JB Lippincott.
16. Downey V et al: Dying babies and associated stress in NICU nurses, *Neonat Net* 14:41, 1995.

17. Eason WM: *The dying child,* Springfield, Ill, 1970, Charles C Thomas, Publisher.
18. Engel GL: Grief and grieving, *Am J Nurs* 64:93 1964.
19. Garland KG: Unresolved grief, *Neonat Net* 5:29, 1986.
20. Gardner SL, Merenstein GB: Helping families deal with perinatal loss, *Neonat Net* 5:17, 1986.
21. Geis DP: Mothers' perceptions of care given their dying child, *Am J Nurs* 65:103, 1965.
22. Giles PFH: Reactions of women to perinatal death, *Aust NZ J Obstet Gynaecol* 10:207, 1970.
23. Goldbach K et al: The effects of gestational age and gender on grief after pregnancy loss, *Am J Orthopsych* 61:461, 1991.
24. Goldberg H: *The hazards of being male,* New York, 1976, Sanford J Greenberger, Assoc.
25. Gonzalez MT: Nursing support of the family with an abnormal infant, *Hosp Top* 15:68, 1971.
26. Griffin T: Nurse barriers to parenting in the special care nursery, *J Perinat Neonat Nurs* 4(2):56, 1990.
27. Hill R: Generic features of families under stress. In Parad H, editor: *Crisis intervention,* New York, 1965, Family Service Association of America.
28. Jack A: Current Canadian neonatal research: memories of a gentle presence, *Neonat Net* 14:49, 1995.
29. Johnson JM: Stillbirth: a personal experience, *Am J Nurs* 72:1595, 1972.
30. Jourard S: *The transparent self,* rev ed, New York, 1971, Van Nostrand Reinhold.
31. Kennell J et al: Mourning response of parents to death of a newborn infant, *N Engl J Med* 283:344, 1970.
32. Klaus M, Kennell J: *Parent-infant bonding,* ed 2, St Louis, 1982, Mosby
33. Koocher GP: Children, death, and cognitive development, *Dev Psychobiol* 9:369, 1973.
34. Koocher GP: Talking to children about death, *Am J Orthopsychiatry* 44:404, 1974.
35. Kowalski K, Osborn M: Helping mothers of stillborn infants to grieve, *Matern Child Nurs J* 2:29, 1977.
36. Kübler-Ross E: *On death and dying,* New York, 1969, Macmillan Publishing.
37. Lax RF: Some aspects of the interaction between mother and impaired child: mother's narcissistic trauma, *Int J Psychoanal* 53:339, 1972.
38. Leon I: The psychoanalytic conceptualization of perinatal loss: a multidimensional model, *Am J Psych* 149:1464, 1992.
39. Lepler M: Having a handicapped child, *Matern Child Nurs J* 3:32, 1978.
40. Lewis E: The management of stillbirth: coping with an unreality, *Lancet* 18:619, 1976.
41. Lewis E, Page A: Failure to mourn a stillbirth: an overlooked catastrophe, *Br J Med Psychol* 51:237, 1978.
42. Lindemann E: Symptomatology and management of acute grief, *Am J Psychiatry* 101:141, 1994.
43. Marris P: *Loss and change,* New York, 1974, Pantheon Books.
44. McCollum A, Schwartz H: Social work and the mourning parent, *Social Work* 17:25, 1972.
45. Menke J, McClead R: Perinatal grief and mourning, *Adv Pediatr* 37:261, 1990.
46. Mercer R: Crisis: a baby born with a defect, *Nursing '77* 7:45, 1977.
47. Miles M, Carlson J, Fink S: Sources of support reported by mothers and fathers of infants hospitalized in NICU, *Neonat Net* 15:45, 1996.
48. Ohlshansky S: Chronic sorrow: a response to having a mentally defective child, *Social Casework* 43:190, 1962.
49. Opirhory GJ: Counseling the parents of a critically ill newborn, *J Obstet Gynecol Neonatal Nurs* 8:179, 1979.
50. Parkes CM: *Bereavement: studies of grief in adult life,* New York, 1972, International Universities Press.
51. Pozanski E: The replacement child: a saga of unresolved parental grief, *J Pediatr* 81:1190, 1972.
52. Primeau M, Recht C: Professional bereavement photos: one aspect of a perinatal bereavement program, *J Obstet Gynecol Neonatal Nurs* 23:22, 1994.
53. Primeau M, Lamb J: When a baby dies: rights of the baby and parents, *J Obstet Gynecol Neonatal Nurs* 24:206, 1995.
54. Rahe R et al: Social stress and illness onset, *J Psychosom Res* 8:35, 1964.
55. Rapaport L: The state of crisis: some theoretical considerations. In Parad H: *Crisis intervention,* New York, 1965, Family Service Association of America.
56. Raphael D: *The tender gift: breastfeeding,* New York, 1973, Schoken Books.
57. Ryan P, Cote-Arsenault D, Sugarman L: Facilitating care after perinatal loss: a comprehensive checklist, *J Obstet Gynecol Neonatal Nurs* 20:385, 1991.
58. Saylor D: Nursing response to mothers of stillborn infants, *J Obstet Gynecol Neonatal Nurs* 8:39, 1977.
59. Schoenberg BA et al: *Loss and grief: psychological management in medical practice,* New York, 1970, Columbia University Press.
60. Schoenberg BA et al: *Anticipatory grief,* New York, 1974, Columbia University Press.
61. Seitz P, Warrick L: Perinatal death: the grieving mother, *Am J Nurs* 74:2028, 1974.
62. Seidman R, Kleine P: A theory of transformed parenting: parenting a child with developmental delay/mental retardation, *Nurs Res* 44:38, 1995.
63. Sexton P, Stephens S: Postpartum mother's perceptions of nursing interventions for perinatal grief, *Neonat Net* 9:47, 1991.
64. Siegel R et al: The impact of neonatal loss, *Pediatr Res* 16:93A, 1982.
65. Solnit A, Stark M: Mourning and the birth of a defective child, *Psychoanal Study Child* 16:523, 1961.
66. Stack J: Spontaneous abortion and grieving, *Am Fam Pract* 21:99, 1980
67. Traxler P: *Poem for my son, Blood calendar,* New York, 1975, William Morrow.
68. Vance J et al: Psychological changes in parents 8 months after the loss of an infant from stillbirth, neonatal death, or SIDS—a longitudinal study, *Pediatrics* 96:933, 1995.
69. Waechter E: The birth of an exceptional child, *Nurs Forum* 9:202, 1970.

70. Whitfield J et al: The application of hospice concepts to neonatal care, *Am J Dis Child* 136:521, 1982.
71. Wilson AL et al: The death of a newborn twin: an analysis of parental bereavement, *Pediatrics* 70:587, 1982.
72. Wooten B: Death of an infant, *Matern Child Nurs J* 6:257, 1981.
73. Yates SA: Stillbirth: what staff can do, *Am J Nurs* 72:1592, 1972.
74. Young RK: Chronic sorrow, parent's response to the birth of a child with a defect, *Matern Child Nurs J* 2.38, 1977.
75. Zahourek R, Jensen J: Grieving and the loss of the newborn, *Am J Nurs* 73:836, 1973.

Resource Materials for Parents

Balter L: *A funeral for Whiskers,* New York, 1991, Barron's Educational Services.

Buscaglia L: *The fall of Freddie the leaf,* New Jersey, 1982, Leo Buscaglia, Slack.

Bell J, Esterling LS: *What will I tell the children?* Omaha, Neb, 1986, American Cancer Society.

Eddy ML, Raydo L: *Making loving memories, a gentle guide to what you can do when your baby dies,* Omaha, Neb, 1990, Centering Corp.

Leon IC: *When a baby dies: psychotherapy for pregnancy and newborn loss,* New Haven. Conn, 1990, Yale University Press.

Mellonie B, Ingpen R: *Lifetimes,* New York, 1983, Bantam Books.

National Center for Education in Maternal and Child Health: *A guide to resources in perinatal bereavement,* Washington, DC, 1988, National Maternal and Child Health Clearing House, 38th & R Streets NW, Washington, DC 20057.

Simon N: *The saddest time,* Chicago, 1986, Whitman and Co.

Wass H, Coor C: *Helping children cope with death: guidelines and resources,* Washington, DC, 1984. Hemisphere.

Woods JR, Esposito JL, editors: *Pregnancy loss: medical therapeutics and practical considerations,* Baltimore, 1987, Williams & Wilkins.

Viorst J: *The tenth good thing about Barney,* New York, 1971, MacMillan Publishing Co.

Videos

"What do I tell my children?" Newton, Mass, 1990, Life-cycle Productions.

When a baby dies, LaCrosse, Wisc, 1991, Resolve through Sharing, LaCrosse Lutheran Hospital.

National Organizations

Bereavement Services/RTS, 1910 South Avenue, La Crosse, WI 54601, (608) 791-4747. E-mail: berservs@1:hl.gundluth.org.

Centering Corporation, Box 3367, Omaha, NE, 68103-0367, (402) 553-1200.

Climb, Inc., Center for Losing Multiple Births, P.O. Box 1064, Palmer, AK, 99645, (907) 746-6123.

On-line bereavement resource webpage: http://sids-network.org.

Parents of Stillborn, 5570 South Langston Road, Seattle, WA, 98718, (206) 772-5338.

SHARE Pregnancy and Infant Loss, St. Joseph's Health Center, 300 First Capitol Drive, St. Charles, Mo 63301, (314) 947-6164.

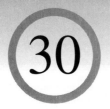

30 Ethics in Neonatal Intensive Care

Julie Sandling Swaney, Brian Carter, Claudia A. Moore, John W. Sparks

Clinical decision making is influenced by the values of the individuals involved. In the NICU, these values include preserving life, decreasing morbidity, and relieving pain and suffering. Sound clinical skills and judgment, combined with societal and personal values, result in the art of clinical practice.

Recent technologic advances in medicine have benefited many patients. We are better able to prolong life; at the same time, we are more often in a position to make deliberate decisions about when and how death will occur. Concomitantly, it has become necessary for society to reassess whether the value of prolonging life conflicts with other values, such as relieving pain and suffering, and reducing morbidity. In such cases, values of society, the family, and the health care professional necessarily enter into and influence the decision-making process.

Ethical reasoning insists that we understand the role of values as well as medical data in making decisions.

Treatment and Nontreatment

Numerous ethical issues arise in the context of all treatment decisions. Certainly, infants should be treated humanely and with respect in an environment that is conducive to maximum comfort and healing. For parents to be involved in determining overall treatment goals and in the decision-making process, they must be fully informed to consent to or reject treatment for their child. Humane judgments should be made in determining how infants can most benefit from treatment in any given situation. As noted in a previous chapter, sufficient analgesia should be administered to infants having surgery because they can, indeed, experience physical and psychologic pain. Staff and parents should maximize the development of premature infants and offer every possible benefit to them.

Other perplexing ethical questions arise when the benefit of treatment is unclear. Even the most perfunctory of decisions should be based on the patient's best interests, yet "best interests" are often difficult to determine. Should a child born with anencephaly be resuscitated or receive life-sustaining interventions solely for the purpose of organ transplantation? Should an ELBW infant be aggressively ventilated? Medical and ethical decisions involve not only the question of what kind of treatment serves the patient's best interest but also of the appropriateness of treatment at all. Limited or non-treatment decisions are agonizing and regularly result in ethical discussions. The more difficult or conflicting the decision to be made, the more ethical questions are raised. Therefore this chapter discusses both treatment and nontreatment decisions.

History

Historically, ethical concerns in neonatal care focused on the risks and benefits of available technology (Table 30-1). An example is oxygen therapy with the offsetting dilemma that treatment could cause degrees of blindness and/or residual lung damage, whereas nontreatment might result in death or brain damage (1960s). Treatment of premature infants and those with birth defects became technically possible in the 1950s with development of infant ventilators and refined surgical techniques. Because these new technologies not only failed to eliminate all bad outcomes and added new problems, controversies developed over when and how much to use them. Care of newborns with spinal cord defects is illustrative.

Table 30-1
Selected Issues in Perinatal/Neonatal History of Ethical Import

Time	Fetal Diagnosis	Fetal Therapy	Neonatal therapy
1900s (early)			Temperature regulation, nutrition; limited survival in LBW and anomalied infants Recognition of congenital rubella syndrome Cardiovascular surgery in the newborn period Modern incubator developed Oxygen therapy for respiratory distress
1950s		Tocolysis (ETOH)	EBF (Rh) incompatibility recognized Oxygen toxicity recognized: RLF/blindness in treated infants; CP and mortality in those untreated Other iatrogenic diseases Antibiotic usage broadens
1960s	Placentocentesis Early ultrasound FHR monitoring Fetal scalp pH assessment Amniocentesis Chromosomal analysis	Intraperitoneal blood transfusion for EBF	Birth of "modern" NICUs Field of teratology develops after thalidomide diaster Improved outcome for infants <2500 g Surgical management of meningomyelocele becomes an issue
1970s	Fetoscopy Real-time ultrasound Improved structural, chromosomal, and metabolic diagnostics	Intravascular blood transfusion for EBF Beta-adrenergic agonists for tocolysis Corticosteroids for lung maturation Legalization of abortion	CPAP, modern neonatal ventilator Improved outcome for infants <1500 g BPD recognized Problems of the VLBW infant: IVH, BPD, NEC TPN/HAL becomes available Improved pediatric surgery Newborn metabolic screening
1980s	Chorionic villous sampling Cordocentesis Doppler flow studies of placenta and umbilical vessels New reproductive technology AFP monitoring	Fetal surgery Prophylactic penicillin for group B streptococcus infection Treatment of fetal dysrhythmias via maternal medications	High-frequency ventilation Surfactant replacement therapy Improved survival in infants <1000 g ECMO IV immunoglobulin
1990s	Fetal cell isolation in maternal blood PCR (polymerase chain reaction) and genetic amplification		Liquid ventilation Recombinant erythropoietin Nitric oxide therapy

Zachary[64] and Shurtleff[54] advocated aggressive management, which increased survival rates but offered questionable quality of life for those more severely affected. Lorber[36,37] was less optimistic about the effects of aggressive management of infants with meningomyelocele and is recognized for his selective nontreatment of some of these infants.

Discussion of treatment of seriously ill newborns was stimulated by the 1973 publication of

Duff and Campbell.[19] Their seminal article described the selective nontreatment or withdrawal of treatment for 43 seriously ill newborns at Yale-New Haven Hospital (between 1970 and 1972) whose "prognosis for meaningful life was extremely poor or hopeless." According to Duff and Campbell[19]:

> Both treatment and nontreatment constitute unsatisfactory dilemmas for everyone. . . . When maximum treatment was viewed as unacceptable by families and physicians in our unit, there was a growing tendency to seek early death as a management option, to avoid that cruel choice of gradual, often slow, but progressive deterioration of the child.

They recognized that most survivors of NICUs are healthy; they also recognized that some infants remain severely disabled by congenital malformations that, until recently, would have resulted in premature death. They were legitimately concerned about the quality of life for these infants and their families.

The majority of newborns treated in NICUs do grow up to lead active, productive lives, but not all fare well with even the most aggressive of treatments.[37] Consequently, there is increasing concern over what is "appropriate" treatment of newborns, particularly seriously ill or disabled ones. Recognizing the risks and benefits of technology, Eisenberg[20] stated, "At long last, we are beginning to ask, not *can* it be done, but *should* it be done."

Baby Doe (1982) and Baby Jane Doe (1983) became the focus of controversy over the issue of withholding treatment and nutrition from handicapped infants.[10,17,45,59] One infant was born with Down syndrome and intestinal atresia, the other with meningomyelocele. Both were denied relatively uncomplicated surgery and died. In the Bloomington Baby Doe case the court upheld the parents' decision to deny treatment. The federal government later responded to this case with regulations monitoring and intervening in the medical care of handicapped newborns (Baby Doe I Rule, March, 1983).

Throughout this short but focused "history" of ethical issues in neonatal care, it has become increasingly apparent that there are significant issues regarding appropriate treatment and the limits of treatment. Not only numerous issues, but numerous individuals are involved in the decision-making process regarding treatment and nontreatment options. More people become involved as technologic advances increase treatment options. Parents have always been presumed to be the best decision makers on their child's behalf. Health care providers have also been committed to providing what is in the best interests of their patients. Historically, decisions were made privately between parents and their physician. In the modern NICU, treatment goals and decisions are made in the context of a health care team composed of professionals from various moral communities who offer specialized input into the care of the neonate and the family. Parents must be included in the team because their values are of paramount importance in establishing goals and making decisions about their infant's care. Societal concerns have generally focused on protecting infants against decisions that are detrimental to their best interests by statutes on child abuse and neglect. Professional groups such as the American Academy of Pediatrics (AAP),[3,4] American College of Obstetrics and Gynecology (ACOG),[6] and the Canadian Pediatric Society (CPS)[16] have now addressed these concerns in published guidelines for care of critically-ill infants. Community groups[18] are addressing limitations of care for high-risk newborns as well. Clinical decision making is impacted by parents, the health care team, professional groups, and society. Respect for clinical decision making, preferably made by parents and clinicians together, the appropriateness of care, and the protection of children against harm are constantly being balanced.

Definition of Bioethics

Ethics is the study of rational processes for determining the most morally desirable course of action in view of conflicting value choices. Ethics is a branch of philosophy that considers competing values in order to obtain the best possible outcome to a given situation. When values conflict and each value is morally justifiable, an ethical dilemma exists. For an ethical dilemma to exist, a real choice between possible courses of action must exist.

Bioethics seeks to determine the most morally desirable course of action in health care given the conflicting values inherent in varying treatment options.[7] Most often, when a conflict of values does not exist, moral conflict does not exist. That is, when the health care providers and parents all agree that it is most beneficial to an infant not to treat the infant aggressively and to allow the infant to die, no dilemma or conflict between them exists. Of course, that they agree does not mean that conflict does not exist with moral views of outside parties or principles. Regardless, the goal is to determine the most morally desirable course of action under a given set of circumstances.

Theories of Ethics

An ethical theory provides a basis for making morally appropriate decisions. There are many theories or approaches to ethics to consider. *Principle-based* ethics indentifies fundamental principles that form the foundation of ethical deliberation. This approach emphasizes the centrality of principles and rules to determine moral duty. *Virtue* ethics is character-based and as such identifies the virtues of the moral agents involved, rather than the applied principles, as essential to ethical outcome. Various views of the moral life emphasize different virtues as more primary than others. In modern bioethics, primary virtues include respect, fidelity, honesty, and benevolence. *Casuistry* is case-based ethics in which the claims, grounds, and warrants of a particular case are compared with similar cases. The basic question for moral casuistry is how a general moral precept is to be understood in similar sets of circumstances. *Narrative* ethics is story-based in which the narrative itself is a method of ethical reasoning. Every case has different "narratives" to consider, such as medical knowledge, personal identity, patient experience, and the doctor-patient relationship. Although the medical model may focus on disease, psychopathology, objectivity, and diagnosis, the narrative model may focus correspondingly on illness, "the person," subjective experience, and caring. *Feminist* ethics is relationship-based and considers primarily the ethics of care. Table 30-2 identifies these and other moral theories worthy of consideration.

All of these approaches are important to consider. Since theories are based on some foundational principles, principle-based ethics will be dis-

Table 30-2 Moral Theory	
Types	**Focus**
Utilitarian	Consequence based
Kantian	Obligation based
Liberal individualism	Rights based
Common morality	Principle based
Communitarian	Community based
Feminist/ethics of care	Relationship based
Casuistry	Case based
Virtue	Character based
Narrative	Story based

cussed in more detail. Again, principle-based ethics is only one of the many approaches to ethics reasoning, but the principles themselves are useful in any ethics consideration. Deciding which moral theory is operative is important to proceeding.

Principles of Ethics

Bioethical principles are at the heart of principle-based decision making in the NICU. These principles aid individual decision makers in determining what their moral obligations and duties are in times of moral dilemma.

The major principles are autonomy, beneficence and nonmaleficence, and justice. Although each principle can be theoretically defined, in the clinical setting they have a multitude of interpretations and applications. Each principle carries with it a significant interrelationship with the others. Often health care professionals and parents find themselves in situations where following one principle violates another. Deciding which principles and consequences should prevail is at the center of principle-based bioethics. Remember that each decision maker brings with him or her a personal, and perhaps an ethical, theory. It is *how* individuals apply these theories and principles that creates the basis for decision making in the NICU.

Principle of Autonomy

The principle of autonomy is based on the right to self-determination. This principle cannot be applied directly to the neonate, because he or she is not competent and never has been. The neonate has no known values, morals, or beliefs to bring to the decision-making process. Decisions must always be made for this patient by other parties. These other parties extend from the parents to the health care team, ethics committees, and possibly to the court system. Each member of the decision-making process brings with him or her an idea of what type of care is best for the patient. Each consideration carries with it personal values and morals demanding that certain duties and obligations be met. And each consideration must be based on adequate information being understood and applied to the particular situation.

In the NICU, autonomy applies to the right of the parents or designated guardian to make a decision about their infant's care. They are considered to be proxy, or surrogate, decision makers because their infant is, by nature, incompetent.

One standard of proxy action seeks to determine the patient's "best interest." This standard asks "What is in the best interest of this child?" and "requires a surrogate to do what, from an objective standpoint, appears to promote a patient's good, without reference to the patient's actual or supposed preferences." Another standard of proxy action is "substituted judgment." This standard asks "What would this child want if he or she could speak for him or herself?" The responsibility of the proxy is to make the decision the incompetent person would have made if competent. This grants the incompetent patient respect as a moral agent deserving autonomy, but because newborns are incompetent and have no expressed wishes, this standard is difficult, if not impossible, to invoke, thus the "best interest" standard is preferred.

In today's NICU, it is preferable to have informed parents involved in goal setting and decision making. When parents are well informed and involved, they can then best express the autonomy of their child. Some people believe, however, that the autonomy of the parents is conditional and that it must be so because the stress inherent in having a sick or dying newborn. Others believe to the contrary; they trust that parents can and should make these difficult decisions because they will eventually live with the results. Still others believe that parents can never understand the problems in-

volved in the decision-making process and that difficult decisions should therefore be made by the physician and the health care team.

When conflict arises, whose values take precedence? Shelp[53] suggests that parents' views of best interest should take precedence, within reason. He established a "standard of reasonableness" to guide the discretion of parents toward "reasonable" treatment or refusal of treatment. Harrison[30] and Raines[47] emphasize that parents should be informed and involved in goal setting and decision making. The AAP[3] supports individualized decision making, jointly deliberated by physicians and parents, within the bounds of legal and public policy guidelines for child protection and resource allocation.

Paternalism

Paternalism views the best-interest standard from the perspective that one individual, historically the physician, knows best. The Hippocratic image of physicians and their authority over patients was not only accepted, but expected, by society over the last 2500 years. Only recently has our society's increasing emphasis on self-knowledge and self-determinism led us to a position where the traditional physician is no longer considered purely autonomous in patient care discussions.

Paternalism is formally defined as "(1) the intentional limitation of the autonomy of one person by another, (2) where the person who limits autonomy appeals exclusively to grounds of beneficence for the person whose autonomy is limited. . . . The essence of paternalism, then, is an overriding of the principle of respect for autonomy on grounds of the principle of beneficence."[14]

Paternalistic interventions restrict the patient's autonomy and freedom. Engelhardt[23] upholds the need for some paternalism. However, he, like others, acknowledges the inherent and continuing problem with deciding whose paternalistic judgment should prevail. Whose substituted judgment brings the best outcome for the patient? Although the physician's knowledge and authority is still of utmost importance in decision making, it is now being considered with much more care and discretion by the family members, the health care team, and society as a whole.[43]

Sometimes situations exist where paternalism is

justified in the NICU. For example, if a family is obviously too stressed to give an informed consent in an emergency situation, the health care team must do what is in the best interest of the patient first. Often emergency care is required for a period of time before long-term treatment plans can be made. Time is frequently a critical factor with sick neonates, requiring instantaneous decisions by the health care team. Without such paternalistic interventions the neonate may die. The best-interest standard in the NICU continues to side with life until there is information available to the contrary.

In the past the physician usually belonged to the same moral community as the patient and his or her family. Values were generally similar and options generally limited. Today's high-tech NICUs and mobile society inhibit the simple best-interest standards of the past. Consequently, it is imperative to construct avenues for consideration of the varied and divergent moral communities present today. However, resolving the dilemma of who should decide does not solve the problem of what ought to be done. The principle of beneficence works to answer this question.

Principles of Beneficence and Nonmaleficence

Beneficence is broadly defined as "active goodness, kindness, charity."[13] Yet what is "good" for one may not be "good" for another. So, for example, preserving life may be a general "good," but in some instances allowing someone to die may be the greater "good." The variety of personal interpretations of "good" necessitates careful and deliberate communication among the parties involved.

So beneficence involves defining the "good." Further, the Hippocratic Oath expresses a duty of beneficence: "I will use treatment to help the sick according to my ability and judgment, but I will never use it to injure or wrong them." While one's duty is to do "good" (i.e., help the sick—beneficence), it is also expected that one will do no "harm" (i.e., never injure or wrong them—nonmaleficence).

Nonmaleficence is primarily associated with the maxim "primum non nocere—above all, or first, do no harm." Although the exact origin of this maxim is unknown, its importance is not questioned. Often in conflict situations, we can expect nonmaleficence to be overriding the principle of beneficence.[13] Although the principle of beneficence requires positive acts such as preventing or removing evil and doing or promoting good, the principle of nonmaleficence requires avoidance of certain acts that inflict harm or injury to the patient. Beauchamp and Childress[13] have constructed a model that shows today's clinical interpretation of the "goods" and "harms":

Goods	Harms
Health	Illness
Prevention, elimination, or control of disease and injury	Disease (morbidity and injury)
Relief from unnecessary pain and suffering	Unnecessary pain and suffering
Amelioration of handicapping conditions	Handicapping conditions
Prolonged life	Premature death

Where withdrawing or withholding treatment from a very anomalous infant would be viewed as inflicting harm and morally wrong by some, it could also be viewed by others as harmful *not* to withdraw or withhold treatment so as not to prolong pain and suffering or continue a life too tragic to exist. Finding an answer frequently entails weighing the "goods" against the "harms." Often there is a very fine line between doing "good" for the patient and doing "harm."

The principles of beneficence and nonmaleficence and the moral rules and obligations they require are not absolute. They are at best prima facie principles. For example, it is acceptable to inflict some pain and suffering in order to achieve a cure or to prevent a worse harm (i.e., death). However, any time harm is inflicted, there is a need for moral justification.[13]

Engelhardt[24] and Shelp[53] agree that the difficulty with the principle of beneficence lies in the fact that it is not able to reach across varied communities. Shelp[53] considers this possible scenario in the NICU:

> The parents may be Southern Baptist, the nurse a Reform Jew, the neonatologist an atheist, and

the social worker a Roman Catholic. It is possible, even probable, that each party could reach a different reasonable decision, given their individual moral commitments, about what interventions ought to occur.

When confronted with such a diversity of perspectives and values, one no doubt wonders how to proceed. Some ethicists believe that the parents as decision makers are motivated by beneficence and can best determine what is the "greatest good" for their child. But because no one can know what the patient would consider "good," surrogates must effect beneficence and nonmaleficence in deciding what is reasonable treatment in each situation.

Beauchamp and Childress[13] state that the duty of nonmaleficence includes not only actual harms, but also risks of harm. The greater the risk of harm, the greater the need for solid moral reasoning as justification. This is a standard of care maintained by all health care professionals. It reduces the probability of errors in diagnosis and treatment by requiring that moral agents act thoughtfully, carefully, and reasonably. Harms are not always intentional; in fact, it is possible to violate the principle of nonmaleficence by accident. Concern for the patient's "greatest good" inherently examines what risks or actual harms could be involved in treatment or nontreatment—too little technologic support or too much. Because uncertainty is common in the NICU, each team member should consider the balance between these two principles on a daily basis. The decision-making dilemma can be best approached with mutual respect for varied moral viewpoints, recognizing that there are no moral absolutes of right and wrong and that no moral agent need violate his or her own moral stance.

Principle of Justice

The concept of justice dates back to the Greek philosophers. Aristotle has been credited with one of the most basic premises of justice: equals ought to be treated equally and unequals may be treated unequally. This principle of formal justice does not give specific prescriptions for interpreting equals or unequals. In the NICU, each neonate is potentially equal to all other humans. His or her potential, however, is not only immeasurable at the time of treatment, it is also one with varied interpretations (i.e., potential for what?). For example, can we compare the potential life of a 480-gram 24-week infant with a teenage suicidal mother with that of a term infant with Down syndrome who has two loving parents? Some would say yes, and some would say emphatically no. Controversy over what is "due" each neonate often hinges on one's interpretation of "personhood" and consequent rights.

The concept of justice entails "giving to each his right or due."[13] Although our society generally believes all individuals are of equal worth, disparities of allocation still exist. The material principles of justice help to identify alternative bases on which to balance the distribution or allocation of benefits and burdens.[13]

- To each person an equal share
- To each person according to individual need
- To each person according to individual effort
- To each person according to societal contribution
- To each person according to merit

It is likely that when one basis for justice is used, an alternative basis for justice is negated or at least neglected. These material principles specify only prima facie duties. They must be weighed with other bioethical principles in particular situations. The acceptability of each material principle of justice rests on its moral justification. For example, critically ill neonates use health care dollars at an unequal rate compared with those newborns who do not need extraordinary high-tech help. Is it morally "just" to use $175,000 to produce one 700 g survivor when the money could be used to feed, counsel, and educate dozens of socially deprived children instead? Because resources are limited, trying to do everything for everyone leaves fewer resources to meet the needs of those who are unserved or underserved.[38]

How might we properly allocate our health care dollars? How can we help families to make the best decision for their neonate considering their own personal resources? Some advise that a basic health care minimum be provided for all individuals. Others suggest that health care dollars would be better spent on preventive care for many rather than intensive care for a few. Many infants and their families could avoid the trauma of a premature birth if research and education were given higher priority in resource allocation.

Just distribution of resources to meet an acceptable standard of health care is particularly problematic as resources become increasingly scarce. On a societal or macroeconomic scale, we question how best to distribute our scarce resources. These are issues of distributive justice. On an individual or microeconomic scale, we consider the competing claims for resources between affected individuals. It can be considerably problematic to balance macroeconomic theories with microeconomic claims. For example, if a hospital's ability to stay open depends on the majority of the patients paying their bills, then one must consider the consequences of frequently giving free care. On a microlevel, it is morally wrong to allow finances to enter into the allocation of health care. However, on a macrolevel, finances can determine whether a hospital stays open. Do we provide health care to all no matter what the consequences? Do we provide all that is available to each individual, or do we allocate our scarce resources by setting standards and limits to care? Macroallocation and microallocation policies are not mutually exclusive. They influence each other in the determination of goods and services available.

The fundamental needs of individuals are met because our society feels a moral obligation to us— rich or poor. Some consider equal access to a respectable minimum of health care to be the right of all members of society, whereas others consider health care to be a superogatory (not obligatory) duty of society. The problem with supplying all of society with minimum health care comes both in setting limits so that there is enough to go around and in specifying standards so that all get equal treatment. Inherent in this problem is who should set these limits and standards. Should it be the government? Society? Hospitals? Ethics Committees? Clinicians? These are moral questions underlying the principle of distributive justice.

Medical technology is moving ahead faster than morals. Specifically with neonatal care, there has been a revolution in technologic advances over the past 30 years. "The cost of intensive care for tiny babies of less than 800 grams birth weight is of the same order as that of heart transplants, liver transplants and bone-marrow transplants."[44] Consequently, the resources needed to maintain this population constitute a significant part of our limited health care resources. Priority setting becomes increasingly necessary as technology expands treatment options. New technologies do not promise certain cures; however, they do promise new controversies over resource allocation. A technologic imperative does not necessarily optimize health care. Health care can evolve and improve on a balanced scale with our available resources if we set humane and compassionate goals.

Ethical Issues of Particular Importance in the NICU

Personhood

Decision making in the NICU often revolves around the concept of "personhood." Determining what this means depends on which moral community is consulted. Designation of personhood is morally significant because it determines whether and what duties and obligations are owed to a particular newborn.

Some communities believe personhood is present at the moment of conception; they equate "human" with "person." Shelp[53] refers to this as the "genetic theory of personhood." Others believe personhood depends on the presence or absence of certain basic human qualities. Shelp calls this moral theory "property based." Although with the latter theory there is agreement that the concept of personhood is nongenetic, there are differences regarding which qualities qualify for "person" status.

Fletcher[27] and Engelhardt[22] support the "property-based" stance. They believe that there are human lives that are "subpersonal." They say that "it is not what is natural but what is personal which has the first-order value in ethics."[27] They believe that neocortical function is required for personhood. Engelhardt[22] relates qualities such as self-consciousness, rationality, and self-determination to personhood. He distinguishes between persons in a moral sense and persons in a social sense. Infants are deemed persons only in a social sense, not a strict sense where societal rights are obligatory. The rights of the infant, according to Engelhardt, are held in trust by his or her parents; therefore "decision(s) about treatment . . . belong properly to the parents because the child belongs to them in a sense that it does not belong to anyone else, even to itself."[22] In this sense, then, infanticide does carry moral significance. All such decisions must be properly justified. Engelhardt does consider that financial, emotional, and spiritual costs can be morally valid reasons to justify infanticide.

Tooley[57] suggests "that the ability to see oneself as existing over time is a necessary condition for the possession of a right to life."[33] If Tooley's reasoning is correct, then no infant has a right to life, at least not for some time. Although the "pro life" moral community assigns person status to all with potential life, Tooley denies that potential has anything to do with a right to life. Advocates of quality-of-life standards for personhood give a qualified endorsement to infanticide. When a life is full of intractable pain and suffering, death is seen as a morally acceptable option. In fact, it is sometimes considered a relatively better outcome than continuing life.

Ramsey,[49] Robertson,[51] and the Catholic church hold a contrasting view. For them, death is never better than life; quality-of-life assessments are not part of their moral reasoning. Life is considered sacred—an absolute good. Both the fetus and newborn are considered a person with a right to live. Therefore "death must always be imposed nonhumanly by God or nature or some other cosmic arbiter."[27] This "pro life" position supports the moral right of deformed fetuses and deformed newborns to whatever care would be given a normal infant, implying that abortion and infanticide are morally reprehensible. If antibiotics would be given to a normal infant, then they must also be administered to a newborn infant with trisomy 18.

If one is deemed a "person," then society owes one certain obligations and expects certain duties. If one is not deemed a "person," then it is morally reasonable for societal benefits to be withheld or withdrawn. Whatever justification is needed for a particular moral dilemma in the NICU extends from this beginning. There is no final answer, no final definition of personhood, and there likely never will be one.

Patienthood

A primary problem confronting the perinatal clinician is the fundamental question: Who is the patient? The adult patient is generally competent and worthy of respect as a moral agent. However, in the case of a newborn, the newborn, the family, and, in some circumstances, society have been variously considered the "patient." The accordance of rights to the newborn as an independent agent is a relatively recent occurrence. Neonatal cases are inextricably bound in the context of complicated family and societal situations. Nonetheless, decisions need to be made in perinatal cases, often in the face of societal disagreement and indecision, perhaps unduly posing special burdens on perinatal clinicians. The fundamental question remains: To whom is the moral duty owed?

Professional-Patient Relationship

The importance of the professional-patient relationship cannot be underestimated, because this is the human context in which decision making occurs. With neonates, this includes a relationship between parents as surrogates and the health care team.

When the four major principles—autonomy, beneficence, nonmaleficence, and justice—are applied to health care relationships, several moral rules can be derived. These moral rules include fidelity, truth telling, and confidentiality. The professional-patient relationship is considerably affected by the meaning and extent of these rules.

Fidelity, or promise keeping, may be derived from the principle of autonomy. The duty to keep promises may promote the greatest good (utilitarian) or be seen as an obligation (formalist). Many relationships between professionals and patients (or surrogates) involve promises or contracts, whether implicitly or explicitly made. For example, once professionals have established a relationship with a patient, their duty of fidelity includes not abandoning or neglecting that patient. An obvious problem in dealing with surrogates may be conflicting duties to the parents and the patient. Promises made by professionals are binding except when they are superseded by stronger obligations.

Truth telling, like fidelity, can be derived from the principle of autonomy or respect for persons. It implies an implicit contract between parties that the truth will be told. At the heart of truth telling is trust, which gives professional-patient relationships their integrity. Lying violates implicit contracts, respect for persons, and trust. It also impedes informed consent.

Utilitarians and formalists may agree on the duty to tell the truth, though they may disagree on the duty not to deceive. Cases have been made for "benevolent deception," when intentional deception is morally justifiable if its primary intent is for the benefit of the patient. In such cases telling the truth may be a violation of beneficence and nonmaleficence. Others argue that deception, benevolent or not, is morally wrong because it violates respect for persons and trust. Ultimately, the professional-patient relationship erodes. Respect for persons involves acknowledging patient autonomy to know, or not to know, the truth of his or her particular situation.

It is generally agreed that confidentiality should prevail in professional-patient relationships. With minors, confidentiality extends to the parents or legal guardians. Part of the implied contract is that information gained by both parties will be kept confidential. From the earliest days of medicine, protecting the patient's privacy has been a fundamental tenet of clinical practice. There are, of course, instances where confidentiality is justifiably breached. It is at this point that many ethical dilemmas arise.

Breach of confidentiality may be morally and legally justified to protect the life of a patient or the lives of others who may be endangered. The value of human life overrides the relationship, but the professional should be able to demonstrate clear danger before violating a patient's privacy. This may also be seen as a violation of autonomy. "The health care professional's breach of confidentiality thus cannot be justified unless it is necessary to meet a strong conflicting duty."[13]

Obviously, health care professionals can be torn between conflicting moral obligations, such as between the patient and society. Such instances where a breach may be justified include child abuse and neglect, and certain communicable diseases. But there is strong justification among both utilitarians and formalists for maintaining the privacy and confidentiality of patient information. Most important, the genuine integrity of the professional-patient relationship will be enhanced and preserved when confidentiality, like fidelity and truth telling, is respected and upheld. This integrity of relationship then becomes the basis of the decision-making process.

Nursing Ethics

Nurses are on the front line of neonatal care. Nurses care for the patient for 8- to 12-hour stretches, and they closely monitor the subtle changes, the rapid changes, and the intricate responses inherent in neonatal care. Nurses form close relationships with the families, coordinate the support services needed by the patient and/or family, and provide the continuity of care required by families in stressful situations. Parents vent frustrations to nurses; they ask questions, they seek certainty, reassurance, and compassion. They want their fears allayed, their anxieties lessened, and their problems solved.

At the same time, nurses are expected to maintain their expertise with rapidly changing technology. This is crucial not only for patient care, but for informed communication with parents. Nurses play an important role in communicating medical data and valuable information between the health care team and the parents. Of course, there will be times when nurses are caught between conflicting viewpoints. Sometimes this will be conflict between physician and parents; sometimes this will be conflict between nurse and physician. In the latter, not only are nurses dealing with helpless, incompetent patients whose potentials are uncertain, but they "must implement interventions resulting from decisions made about treatment options for each newborn—even when they have no input into the decision-making process."[21]

In any constellation of conflict, nurses are aware of their competing obligations, the first being to carry out the physician's orders and the other to ensure that the patient's best interest comes first. It is always the nurse's obligation to make sure the patient's best interest is being met. Mappes and Kroeger[39] suggest that such situations are not really moral dilemmas but instead manifest "a tension between doing what is morally right and what is least difficult practically . . . the problem is not that the nurse's obligation is unclear, but that in actual situations fulfilling this moral obligation is extremely difficult."

Nurses should have the relationships and technical skills to advocate for their patient's best interest. When parents consent to treatment without being informed, the nurse should speak up. When treatment goals are not clearly articulated by physicians or parents, the nurse should speak up. When the nurse perceives the burden of any action to be greater than the benefit—even if everyone is in agreement—he or she should speak up for the patient. When the nurse perceives the patient to be experiencing pain, he or she should speak up. In brief, nurses can utilize their hourly familiarity with their patient, as well as their technical knowledge, to contribute significantly to the discussion of what is in that neonate's best interest.

At least two things should inform, perhaps caution, a nurse's judgment about "best interest." First, a recent study of neonatal nurses' definitions of best interest "reflected the infant's characteristics, the nurse's value system, and the nurse's clinical knowledge, with little attention to the participation of the family."[48] Second, Guillemin and Holmstrom[29] found that health care professionals and parents have very different perceptions of an infant's condition and progress. Professionals may focus on the incremental changes in vital organ functioning while the parents are focusing on whether or not the infant responds to them. Physiologic improvement (or deterioration) may not mean subjective improvement (or deterioration) to parents.

An important consideration for nurses in their critical role as communicators for and with patient and/or families and the NICU team is that of neonatal pain and suffering. The neonatal patient both experiences and reacts to numerous noxious stimuli throughout his or her stay in the NICU.[9] The NICU staff, and perhaps nurses in particular, are called upon to recognize the sometimes subtle physiologic and behavioral cues for neonatal pain and discomfort (see Box 11-1). To be aware of a neonatal patient's pain, but not advocate for the patient by bringing it to the attention of the neonatal management team, is to fail to live up to the professional obligation to avoid harm (nonmaleficence) and to relieve suffering. To disregard the positive duties to relieve suffering is to ignore the generally beneficent obligations of the professional. Both are deleterious to patients in that they result in physiologic harm and suboptimal outcomes, break down the confidence that team members have in one another, and undermine the trusting relationships that (should) exist in families. Given the current understanding of the physiology of pain, the value of its prevention, and the benefit of its treatment, such omissions of responsible action clearly do not support the best interest of the vulnerable neonatal patient (see Chapter 11).

Informed Consent

The issue of valid informed consent is repeatedly raised in the environment of the NICU. Information given to parents may be poorly understood for many reasons, including the complex nature of the information; the emotional or physical state of the parents after the birth of a sick, premature, or anomalous infant; physical separation of the parents from their newborn; or feelings of bewilderment and intimidation leading to uncontested paternalism. Indeed, there are indications that valid informed consent is an ideal toward which we work but one that, within the realities of practice, may rarely be obtained. Consent should be sought, however, and open lines of communication and parental education established to facilitate some level of understanding and enable more than token participation in decision making by the parents.

One standard that has been put forth in an effort to accomplish informed consent is the "reasonable person standard," which consists of the following considerations:

- All relevant material information for a decision must be given.
- All known risks of significant bodily harm or death must be given.
- The "reasonable person" reflects an ideal composite of what a reasonable person in society is—the individual person in the case at hand is not in question unless he or she is extraordinary in some aspect (e.g., family values, etc.).
- The standards of disclosure in medicine are the same as in other professions in which relationships are built on trust.

There are several ways in which the reasonable

person standard might be enacted in the NICU, thus ensuring that more valid informed consent is obtained. First, early contact should be made with the parents or family regarding the expected course of problems and special management needs of the newborn. This consultation may even be initiated before delivery. Second, information should be provided by the clinical staff in a factual, compassionate manner. Parents may need continued orientation or reorientation to the NICU environment. This may be especially necessary for parents who are geographically separated from their child. Third, phone calls and photographs are important means for parents to maintain emotional involvement with their child. Fourth, social workers, clergy, or other support resources should be contacted and utilized early to manage emotional distress and to facilitate communication. Fifth, regular patient care conferences with the parents should be scheduled. This will keep parents apprised of the newborn's status and will keep the staff informed about the parents' level of understanding, perspectives, and values. Additional efforts to communicate must be made at the time of special procedures, tests, or therapies to enhance everybody's understanding and the informed consent process.

An integral part of the informed consent process and one that directly affects decision making is the principle of fidelity, commonly referred to as truth telling. Issues of what to tell, how and when to tell, and whom to tell become a daily part of the staff's interaction with each other and the families of affected newborns. A high level of respect for patient and family confidentiality needs to be maintained, and members of the staff need to be cautious about discussing cases and exchanging information given in confidence. Once again, however, open lines of communication and exchange of relevant information regularly will facilitate smooth operation in the NICU.

In practice, the issue of truth telling is considered an essential component of the physician-family relationship, thus allowing for ethical decision making and generally not conflicting with other competing values such as nonmaleficence, beneficence, autonomy, or justice. Information should be shared among staff members and presented to the family truthfully, compassionately, and without bias.

Double Effect

The principle of "double effect" asserts that an action may be considered good if the intent of the action is a positive value, even if the secondary effects of the action might be considered harmful if undertaken as the primary goal; further, the good effect should be commensurate with the harm. Double effect is used frequently in the NICU. An example is the use of narcotics in a dying newborn: the positive goal is reduction of suffering, even at the expense of shortening life.

Decision Making in the NICU

In the NICU, decisions of serious proportion are encountered regularly, based on medical facts and nonmedical values. From the moment of birth, and in some cases even earlier, a foremost issue is that of determining the appropriate level of treatment (or nontreatment) of sick or anomalous newborns. Entire texts have been devoted to this issue[33,61]; some of the primary concerns are outlined here regarding decisions of when to treat, when to limit treatment or not treat at all, and who should be involved in the decision-making process.

A frequently encountered treatment problem requiring attention, other than the much publicized anomalous infant, is the extremely premature or VLBW infant whose course is marked by slow or absent progress despite appropriate and seemingly heroic intervention. The development of complications from disease is of further concern. In concert, these may portend a guarded or very poor prognosis.

Recognizing this, the CPS and the Society of Obstetricians and Gynecologists of Canada have published guidelines for the care of women at 22 to 25 weeks' gestation.[16]

These cases may prompt "quality of life" and "ordinary versus extraordinary treatment" discussions. The President's Commission[46] noted that "there is no basis for holding that whether a treatment is common or unusual, or whether it is simple or complex, is in itself significant to a moral analysis of whether treatment is warranted or obligatory"—a view that had been previously voiced by moral philosophers. The AAP recently published a strategy for the initiation and withdrawal of treatment for high-risk newborns.[5] General recommendations include the importance of ongoing evaluation, parental participation, establishing the goals of humane care, and upholding the best interests standard seeking to benefit the infant. "It is inappropriate for life-prolonging treatment to be continued when the condition is incompatible with life or when the treatment is judged to be futile.[5] The AAP Committee on Bioethics further "supports individualized decision making about life-sustaining medical treatment for all children, regardless of age. These decisions should be jointly made by physicians and parents. . ."[5] If we are honest about our professions, we must realize that "quality of life" is what we are all about. Health care professionals are entrusted by society to advance the health and well being of the mind and body of all persons, such that they can lead their lives and function as part of the human family, individually or collectively. No individual is capable of establishing what is an acceptable "quality of life" for all persons in all circumstances. Each case requires our collective efforts to facilitate the best decision for that particular patient.

Steps in Ethical Decision Making

The approach should follow a method that clearly demonstrates the practice of applied clinical ethics. As stated by Pellegrino,[42] the goal of applied ethics is making right and good moral decisions for and with a particular patient. Such a decision requires first, however, that the decision maker, whether that be a parent, health care provider, or other, understand his or her own (1) philosophy of relationship to the patient (or family), (2) interpretation of ethical principles and values, (3) theoretical basis of ethics used (utilitarian, deontologic, etc.), and (4) source from which morality is derived. An ethical "workup" is then undertaken in which substantive issues are identified and worked through, resulting in a decision.[56] Implementing decisions requires determining who shall decide, by

what criteria they shall be allowed to do so, and subsequently how the decisions or actions are to be implemented in an acceptable fashion that does not override the values of others.

Box 30-1 presents the essential steps to decision making in neonatal cases where a dilemma exists. Consider all possible solutions to the problem, realizing that alternative solutions may uphold different principles and result in different (positive or negative) consequences. Options that may appear acceptable to the family may be unacceptable to the health care team, or vice versa. There may be societal (legal) constraints on certain actions. In some instances, only one option will be consistent with the rules and principles to which the decision maker subscribes. Other options may present apparent conflicts between competing values or result in unacceptable consequences. In a decision, there will more than likely be some give and take. Some priority must be assigned to a certain set of values, rules, principles, or resultant effects of any action or inaction. A decision should be made in light of these issues. This process need not always

---

Box 30-1

Approach to Ethical Dilemmas in Neonatal Care[15,28]

1. Consider who is involved in making and implementing the decision (family, guardians, clinicians, society).
2. Decide who will make the final decision. Is referral to an ethics committee indicated?
3. Clarify all of the medical facts within the case; consider indications, alternatives, and consequences of each action or inaction.
4. Understand significant human factors and values (for patient, family, and health care team).
5. Identify the ethical dilemma or conflict.
6. Make a decision.
   a. List options as solutions to the problem.
   b. Weigh and prioritize values.
   c. Make a decision.
7. Check for moral and rational defensibility.

be invoked in full. Often, when the case is carefully dissected and medical facts, treatment alternatives, and expected prognoses are revealed, issues that at first seemed in question are clarified, and it becomes apparent that no real dilemma exists.

Good ethics, then, start with good facts and effective communication. Clinicians should be aware of all relevant facts, be they medical, social, human value, or legal in nature. Decisions should not be based on personal opinion or insufficient data. The value placed on one's medical well-being may differ between the health care team and the patient and/or family, and discrepancy may lead to a perceived problem. This serves to remind us of the need for a formal approach to problem solving in hard cases.

A viable patient-professional relationship that facilitates the clarification of facts, human values and feelings, and the interests of all relevant parties is essential to ethical decision making. Decisions made should ideally reflect a moral choice that is good for the patient involved and is morally and rationally defensible. We should all work toward achieving a position that is both morally congruent with the values deemed of greatest worth in an individual case and applicable within the moral community as a whole. In the NICU the values most often dealt with are expressed in the principles described earlier.

Certain problems may arise. Often there is inadequate information or time, but decisions must be made, even at odd hours and with limited reflection on process. Limited foresight is available in prognosticating, especially in the individual case, and often very difficult value-laden predictors are required. Some have gone so far as to say that imagination is at least as important as facts in making decisions. But this is not unique to ethical decision making. As Brody[15] states, "We must always take action on the basis of some degree of uncertainty. The goal is to reduce that uncertainty to manageable proportions, and to insure that we have at least considered all the major consequences that we are able to predict with our current level of understanding of the world."

Although it may be arguable whether the patient is the neonate, the nuclear family, the extended family, or another societal group, it would appear prudent to develop a consensus wherever possible and thus minimize conflict among the interested parties. Early involvement of the parents in the care of their child, along with sensitive and thorough presentation of clinical information to the parents, helps minimize the stresses on the parents and prepares them to participate in decision making regarding the care of their child. With careful attention to the needs of patients, families, and staff, many conflicts can be resolved at an early stage before positions are hardened and emotional investment is high, resulting in a development of consensus and minimization of conflict.

In a minority of cases, conflict is unavoidable. In some cases, medical care raises issues that are highly controversial either within the group of clinicians providing care or in the broader context of societal problems. In many cases the family is far from homogeneous in its expression of wishes. Many parents are young and in the process of achieving independent adulthood with well-developed values. Single-parent families are not uncommon. The birth of a critically ill infant may serve as a focus to crystallize disagreements between spouses or may aggravate conflicts between the parent(s) and the extended family. In such cases a more formal process, such as a formal conference between clinicians and the family, appeal to an ethics committee, or even involvement of the legal system, may help to resolve or minimize conflicts of values.

Problems of Uncertainty

A major difficulty in ethical considerations is the medical uncertainty on which they are based. It is difficult to determine what may be in the best interest of the child when the prognosis remains unclear. And even when the prognosis seems clear, there are always those children who confound science, whose outcomes are far from expected.

Some of the most frequent problems in working with perinatal cases arise as a result of this uncertainty. Parents always ask, "Will my baby be okay when he (or she) grows up?" Answers are often unsatisfying or incomprehensible. In most cases with premature infants, "truth telling" may compel an answer that when reduced to its simplest form says, "I don't know." A statistical approach to answer the question may be: "Most babies like yours grow up to be normal." Or, "Some babies like yours have serious problems." These answers are often followed by a litany of statistical probabilities of each morbidity. Neither approach answers the mother's question of what *her particular* baby will be like. Such approaches serve to complicate the clinician's relationship with parents over issues such as expertise, veracity, and disclosure. The statistical approach may answer the NICU's question of quality of care, but few parents understand such statistics or are willing to apply them to a loved one. Nonetheless, uncertainty is a way of life in many perinatal cases, and this observation significantly compromises the resolution of ethical problems in the NICU.

In considering medical uncertainty, however, it is important to recognize two general classes of perinatal cases. NICU patients can be generally classified as either (1) premature infants without known anomalies or (2) near-term infants with major anomalies, either syndromic or nonsyndromic. For infants with known syndromes or major anomalies, prognoses from the literature are describable with reasonable accuracy. Thus the prognosis for an infant with trisomy 18 can be given with a fairly high degree of accuracy, permitting reasonable application of these processes.

A detailed review of neonatal outcome is beyond the scope of this chapter, but several conclusions appear justified. First, infant mortality has declined rapidly since the establishment of NICUs, and the major mortality groups are in lower weight and younger gestational age groups.[31,41] Second, coincident with the decline in mortality have come major improvements in neonatal morbidity from nearly 50% in the pre-NICU era to current figures in the range of 15% from many institutions.[41] Third, the absolute number of normal premature survivors has increased dramatically, and the absolute number of moderately and severely affected survivors appears to have increased as well.[41]

"Extreme prematurity, on the other hand, is characterized by an enormous uncertainty . . . In these cases predictions of outcome at birth are probablistic at best."[50] Recognizing this, attempts have been made to establish guidelines for treatment of ELBW infants.[6,16,18] The morbidities in premature survivors are variable in nature, but CNS morbidities generally include visual impairment and blindness, speech and hearing impairment, neuromuscular impairment, and serious retardation. Few premature survivors require long-term institutional care.[41] The combined risk for one or more of these handicaps is in the range of 15% to 20%. Most would agree that these are indeed serious handicaps, with major effect on the patient and family. However, do they justify withholding or withdrawing care and under what circumstances?

For perinatal clinicians who consider quality of life a major consideration, it remains an exceedingly difficult practical problem to predict which particular child will be significantly handicapped. The predictive value of nursery evaluations in estimating long-term handicap is low.

The intent of raising these questions is to underscore the complexity of ethical discussions as particularly applied to problems in the modern NICU. This in no way reduces the enormity of such problems for the patient, the family, health care providers, or society. Technologic advances may resolve old uncertainties but often seem to carry new uncertainties that are equally perplexing.

Strategies for Dealing with Factual Uncertainty in Ethical Discussions

Rhoden[50] has summarized several strategies for dealing with uncertainty in perinatal cases: (1) the "wait until certainty" approach, (2) the statistical prognosis approach, and (3) the individualized prognostic strategy.

In the first approach, aggressive care is continued until the clinical situation becomes more medically certain. Then ethical principles may be applied to evaluate the clinical situation. Such an approach "errs on the side of life." It supports the value of preserving life and may have other positive values for the patient, clinician, and society, while at the same time it has the major potential drawbacks of interfering with the autonomy of the patient (best interest) or parents (substituted judgment), increasing suffering (nonmaleficence), and perhaps increasing morbidity.

In the second approach, statistical prognosis is accepted as the basis for withholding or withdrawing care, with the positive goal of minimizing the number of infants who suffer long drawn-out deaths or who live with serious handicaps. According to Rhoden[50]:

> Since statistical data about categories of infants are seldom as good as information about a particular infant gained during a trial period of treatment, the statistical approach undoubtedly loses more salvageable survivors than is necessary or justifiable. . . . A pure statistical strategy brings with it the dual dangers of rigidity and minimization of the ethical component.

The individualized prognostic strategy involves starting treatment and then reevaluating it based on response. Thus initial treatment is a diagnostic as well as therapeutic trial, and the initial decision to treat is not irrevocable. Ethically speaking, there is no difference between withholding and withdrawing treatment. Psychological or emotional differences are recognized and may be experienced by any of the staff, as well as family members. However, the advantages of an individualized approach are that it provides the opportunity for preserving the chance of life in borderline cases, while at the same time it permits withdrawal of support based on individualized information. This strategy permits a wide variation in care within a statistical group and leads to potential confusion and errors in execution. It also supports the role of parents and other surrogate agents in ethical decision making. "When medical uncertainty leads to moral uncertainty, it seems preferable, albeit harder, to confront these dual ambiguities than to bury them under statistical criteria or unrelenting moral certitude."[50] Clearly, such an approach leads to practical difficulties. As noted above, the process of prognostication is usually far from precise, and judgments may frequently be made that later prove to be incorrect at the time when the withdrawal or withholding of support may no longer be an issue.

Setting Goals

Treatment goals need to be established in order to make incremental decisions. Preferably, goals should be established by the parents based on their values for their child. Parents need to be involved, not just informed, in determining the overall goals of treatment; then decisions toward that end can be made. Goals may be living a "normal" life, living with a debilitating outcome but without excruciating pain or suffering, existence without any notable "quality of life," and so on. All too frequently, decisions are made before the treatment goal is established. The physician, health care team, and parents all need to be guided by established goals in order to offer beneficial treatment. Importantly, while the role of parents in goal setting and decision making must be respected, "physicians should not be forced to undertreat or overtreat an infant if, in their best medical knowledge, the treatment is not in compliance with the standard of care for that infant."[3]

Proxy Decision Makers

In dealing with newborns who are, by their very nature, incompetent and cannot make decisions for themselves, value conflicts must be resolved with the input of a proxy or surrogate decision maker acting on the infant's behalf. This may be the parents, a family member, friend, guardian ad litem, or the physician. To be considered a valid surrogate, the person should be competent, knowledgeable of integral values of the patient or family, free from conflicting interests, and without serious emotional conflicts in dealing with the case.

Society has for many reasons allocated to the parents the primary authoritative role in collaboration with health care providers in making decisions about their newborn's care. In most instances the parents are best suited for such matters and have the infant's best interests in mind. They are usually present when possible, are concerned for their infant's well-being, and are willing to hear the facts of their infant's condition, as well as learn of needed therapies. Of all people, they also know best the values of the family culture or environment in which the infant will be raised.

Yet parents may be less than dispassionate decision makers. They are understandably overwhelmed at times, both physically and emotionally exhausted, and baffled or intimidated by the hi-tech environment of the NICU and the complexities of their infant's care. Amidst feelings of grief, fear, anxiety, and wonderment over their premature or anomalous infant, they may be uncertain of their proper role and responsibilities as parents. Health care providers need to give daily updates on the infant's condition and anticipated course. Parents' needs for emotional support and avenues to both vent their frustrations and explore their concerns over economic, marital, family and/or sibling, and career effects of their predicament make resources such as nurses, social workers, and chaplains essential in providing assistance to allow them to participate in goal setting and difficult decision making. Occasionally it will be necessary to assess the level of parental competency in assuming the role of surrogate, recognizing when additional help or support for them is needed to fulfill this role.

Physicians as decision makers, an oft-cited traditional paternalistic role, are yet another option. They know and understand the complexities of the medical condition and treatment more than do parents, and should promote the patient's best interests in advocating treatment. They may be more objective about individual cases and are not emotionally overwhelmed, as the parents might be. Also, based on experience, they offer a perspective of effectiveness of treatments and can be consistent in treating similar cases.

However, physicians may also encounter problems when they act as the principal decision makers. Although their knowledge of medical facts is the most complete of all persons, it is at the same time, unfortunately, incomplete. Accurate diagnoses and certainty in prognoses are at times elusive. Medical knowledge does have limits. Statistics are helpful for groups of similarly affected patients, but individual outcomes are difficult to predict. Further, while having the degree of specialized information and knowledge they do, physicians do not necessarily possess any more moral expertise than do parents or others.

Treatment versus nontreatment decisions are ultimately moral, not simply medical, decisions. These decisions are weightier than most clinical decisions that physicians make. There is more involved than a rote, rational process employed in isolation from the family or health care team. The physician must contend with his or her own values and emotions, as well as the medical facts, in each

individual case. He or she must facilitate parental and health care team communication and interaction and ultimately order the provision or withdrawal of care.

Fortunately, physicians do not work in isolation from the health care team when making decisions about patients. Nurses, social workers, and chaplains are vital members of the decision-making team. A potential problem with each of these clinicians as surrogates is that there may be a conflict of interest between them and the patients for whom they are deciding. Members of the health care team may be biased toward the prolongation of life, have preconceived and strong biases about euthanasia, or be influenced by issues unrelated to the patient, including advancement of care, financial issues, or societal issues. Hence they may not fully take into account the best interests of the patient or the values of the involved family. In contrast to parents, they do not live with the results of their decisions and actions. There may also be a lack of consistency in their application of principles to similar cases, and they may give in to strong pressures (real or perceived) exerted by the law or very assertive parents.

Various factors should contribute to minimizing the potential problems in parents and health care professionals reaching morally defensible decisions in the best interest of the premature or anomalous infant. The professionalism of health care team members who are committed to serving the health and interests of their patients is a foremost consideration that serves this purpose. A sense of duty leads these professionals to assist families in achieving their life goals through facilitating open communication and discussion of their varied concerns. A great sense of personal and professional satisfaction may be derived by helping families accept and deal with their emotions, questions, and concerns for their infant and their own circumstances. Professionals may benefit from the support afforded by each other and certainly will avoid problems if efforts are made to communicate well with each other.

In recent years, hospital ethics committees have been given an increasing role in facilitating ethical decision making for sick neonates and have, in rare instances, actually functioned as proxy decision makers. As more institutions are establishing committees, their roles are more focused on education, policy interpretation, and advisory functions than on decision making. Decision making by committees might be problematic in that it may threaten the traditional physician-patient and/or family relationship and usurp both the physician's authority and the parents' autonomy. Siegler[55] noted a number of ways in which a committee "can constrain and modify physician-patient decisions," including the imposition of administrative and regulatory burdens. The mechanics of the committee process, time, and distant relationship to the family and case have also been raised as problems in utilizing committees.

Weir[61] notes that a committee, especially an infant bioethics committee, may have the potential of meeting all of the criteria for a proxy decision maker. Ethics committees are multidisciplinary in composition and have the goals of emotional stability, objectivity, impartiality, and consistency. Ideally they may facilitate the resolution of conflicts between parents and physicians in matters of treatment and be more capable of both addressing and working through the ethical or moral aspects of cases than parents, health care professionals, or other individuals. In reality, their most useful role seems to be one of improving effective communication between staff and families. Finally, they may prove to be a safeguard for infants where parents and professionals are working toward an end that may be perceived as contrary to the infant's best interests.

Surely, much reflective thinking should be invested in our decisions, as individuals, parents, or members of a committee. However, a small number of cases will proceed beyond institutional review to a court. Courts may present many of the criteria for being good proxies—they are disinterested parties, free of emotional involvement, and mostly consistent in reasoning from case to case. They can ensure that all relevant facts are presented and considered, and judges are capable of exercising unmatched control of data collection, investigation, questioning of experts, and seeking of alternative solutions. A judge can also appoint a guardian ad litem to be the patient's advocate when necessary.

Yet, there are at least a few weaknesses in courts as proxies. They are removed from the NICU and have no contact with the case, patient, staff, or family whose problem they are deciding—as such they are more remote than other possible proxy decision makers. Time may be consumed in working through cases, which may result in additional problems, changes in pertinent facts, or prolongation of suffering. Decisions rendered by judges may also reflect some bias based on personal considerations of the judge rather than consistent judicial decisions across lines of legal jurisdiction. Also, some would argue that courts are by design adversarial, using force to resolve conflict rather than promoting cooperation.

Standard of Best Interest

The best-interest standard has been advocated by the President's Commission and others seeking to accomplish valid moral decision making in difficult neonatal cases.[46,60,61] We are obliged "to try to evaluate benefits and burdens from the infant's own perspective."[46] This standard is accepted in the case of newborns over the autonomy-promoting "substituted judgment," because substituted judgment can only be applied hypothetically to a never-competent newborn. This standard is accepted as the best method available to "reasonable" adults who have to make decisions for neonates.

The potential for self-seeking by the decision maker is easy to understand and has been recognized. The interests of parents, siblings, physicians, hospital staff or administration, and society may all seem to compete with those of the newborn. But the interests of others—be they emotional, economic, or otherwise problematic—cannot justifiably override those of the patient[11] based on the actual or potential personhood of the critically ill neonate. Individual or societal problems or perceived burdens are generally not viewed on the same moral plane as a person's claim to life.

Certainly there will be cases that stretch the best-interest standard to its limits. Cases of protracted treatment with uncertain prognoses beg the question of quality of existence (in which nonmaleficence is the principle of concern) and will require consideration of more than mere suffering and pain. Indeed, in the words of Arras,[11] "sometimes circumstances may be so extreme and the consequences so dreadful that the priority of justice can no longer be maintained." In this sense, we need to find the best balance of beneficence, nonmaleficence, and justice.

We must also consider other morally relevant concerns of neonates who may be doomed to brief lives with less than recognizably "human" existence. Human capacities (ability to think, be aware of self, and relate to other people) may be different from biologic human life. The preservation of biologic human life bereft of the benefit of distinctly human capacities is controversial and has been challenged in quality-of-life decisions.[11,19,33,36,61] Arras[11] suggests the "relational potential standard" (Does this child have the ability, or potential, to relate to physical space and time and to communicate to others?) as a means to address these concerns more aptly than the "misapplied best interest standard," calling on society itself to give inquiry "into the conditions of valuable human life."

Priority should be given to attempts at effecting a cure in these ill infants; when a cure cannot be achieved, patient comfort should be sought. Some maintain that life itself may not always be an absolute good; thus it may be morally justifiable to withhold or withdraw futile treatment associated with inhumane risks or harms that would prolong dying. Mitchell,[40] a member of the American Nurses Association Committee on Ethics, has stated:

> Some infants are so premature and underweight, so profoundly impaired, so hopelessly diseased, or so severely asphyxiated that their foreshortened lives are full of misery for them and those around them. For infants who are so impaired that medical therapies are futile or . . . would only prolong suffering, invasive medical procedures and surgery are morally as well as medically inappropriate.

She calls on nurses to shift their focus in such cases to "seek primarily to provide comfort, relieve suffering and help a grieving family."

Killing versus Letting Die

A controversial area in treatment and nontreatment decisions is that of the moral decision of killing versus letting die. One model of reasoning is to deny or to promote the distinction between active (killing) and passive (letting die) euthanasia. Many believe that philosophically and morally there is no difference between these two actions (i.e., allowing someone to die is the same as killing that person). Ramsey[49] argues that in the context of neonatal medicine, "letting die" actually connotes "benign neglect." No moral distinction can be made between this neglect—presumably taken as an act of beneficence—and euthanasia. He states that the "benign neglect of defective infants—who are not dying, who cannot themselves refuse treatment, who are most in need of human help—is the same as directly dispatching them: involuntary euthanasia," a course he clearly rejects.

Yet, when the neonate is determined to be dying and decisions to withhold further treatment have been made, taking the step of active euthanasia (i.e., actively doing something to effect the neonate's death) is considered by some to be more beneficent and nonmaleficent than purporting to enact passive euthanasia, or letting the neonate die. Such advocates claim that by "letting nature take its course" one simply avoids the difficult decision-making process of convenience, yet does not ensure imminent death—and may even prolong suffering.[33,61]

Another model of reasoning is to make the distinction between absolute and conditional treatment. The former emphasizes the technical and moral imperative to intervene within the NICU. Some individuals, as well as certain religious groups, believe that it is imperative to implement any means to treat patients. They call on technical, religious, and ethical arguments to support the prolongation of life.

In contrast, many individuals favor the rejection of the technical or moral imperative to preserve life at all costs. Vaux[58] reflects this view by calling for the withdrawal of our dependence on perceived technical, legal, and economic necessities and accepting an ethic that "honors the intrinsic value of newborns, the crucial capacities and needs of the family and community, and the finality of God."

Either of these models may lead one to consider the distinctions between what is termed the "sanctity of life" (holding life and its preservation in all circumstances as the preeminent condition or rule), and the "quality of life" (realizing or assigning value to life based on the conditions in which it will exist or by its possessing certain, characteristically human, attributes). Either line of reasoning can lead to acceptance or rejection of the idea of withholding or withdrawing treatment or life support, and either will conclude that society can or cannot apply certain standards that would justify actively seeking or bringing about a dying newborn's death.

Some would advocate selective euthanasia for suffering neonates in whom treatment has been withheld or withdrawn, although this is certainly not the normal process in this country. It is also entangled with legal considerations, uncertain consequences, and slippery moral slopes. Similar discussion arises in the debate about the use of anencephalic neonates as organ donors. A notable position of the Council on Ethical and Judicial Affairs of the AMA[8] is that it is ethically permissible to transplant organs of anencephalic donors while they are still alive if the diagnosis of anencephaly is certain, if the parents initiate discussion and desire donation, and if there is compliance with transplantation guidelines. "The use of the anencephalic neonate as a live donor is a limited exception to the general standard ("dead donor rule") because of the fact that the infant has never experienced, and will never experience, consciousness."[8]

Futility

The notion of futility of medical treatment may be as perplexing as the notion of benefit. It does, however, deserve attention because there are increasing circumstances where treatment may be considered to be futile and thus withheld or withdrawn. There is no ethical obligation to offer futile treatment, yet there is no one definition of futility.

Most often, futility is based on medical or physiologic data. It may be medically futile to resuscitate an infant under certain conditions because the treatment cannot alter the course of the illness or problem, yet there are psychologic, social, and religious reasons why such treatment might be offered. If, because of the treatment, the family has time to hold the infant and say goodbye, the resuscitation may not be considered by them to have been futile. Of course the opposite is also true. That is, what may not be physiologically futile may be considered to be futile by the family and/or

surrogates based on religious or other reasons. Again, there is no ethical obligation to offer futile treatment. It is possible to get a medical effect but not a medical benefit.[52] The distinction can be significant. Determination of futility should be based on medical benefit as determined by family goals for the patient, which include physiologic, psychologic, social, and religious data.[34] By attending to all of these aspects of care, which include staff and family input alike, a determination of what is futile therapy, and thus what is beneficial therapy, can be made.

Ethics Committees and Infant Bioethics Committees

It is preferable to keep the decision-making responsibility within the professional-patient relationship. In the vast majority of cases, members of the health care team and the parents do have the infant's best interests in mind. Yet, in view of the vast dimensions and difficulties of some of these decisions, many people may consult with an Infant Bioethics Committee (IBC). Where there is agreement about a treatment plan, the committee might be consulted for confirmation of that plan; where there is a dispute about a proposed course of treatment, the committee might be consulted for clarification of ethical principles, values, and various treatment options that would be consistent with ethical and legal standards.

The stimulus to the establishment of IBCs in the United States was the controversy over and death of Baby Doe in Bloomington, Indiana, when society (and government) became acutely aware of the moral issues surrounding what many perceived to be wrongful nontreatment. This incident provided strong moral justification for committee review of infant cases, particularly when treatment is being withheld or withdrawn to effect the termination of life. The government, in response, proposed a series of regulations to monitor the medical treatment of handicapped newborns.* The most recent regulation is the Child Abuse Prevention and Treatment

---

* The original statute stated that no handicapped individual could be discriminated against solely on the basis of handicap.[1] See also articles by Angell[10] and Victoroff.[59]

Act amendment[1] to protect disabled infants with life-threatening conditions from medical neglect. These guidelines, along with the recommendations of the AAP, encourage hospitals to create IBCs or to have access to one for consultation. "The Academy believes the creation of infant bioethical review committees constitutes a direct, effective, and appropriate means of addressing the existing education and information gaps."[2] Members are necessarily from various disciplines and areas of expertise: physicians, nurses, lawyers, clergy, social workers, ethicists, administrators, and community representatives. It is intended that such an interdisciplinary group will represent both the practical knowledge that is crucial to total case management and the various values that enter into treatment decisions. Their purpose is to promote quality decisions regarding treatment of ill newborns.

IBCs are a resource for consultation and advice. They are not a decision-making body, although some groups are moving toward a consensus model. Different committees have different procedures.[25,35] Committee functions and responsibilities may include (1) offering counsel and ethical review in cases involving disabled infants, (2) educating hospital personnel and families of disabled infants with life-threatening conditions, (3) reviewing prospectively the components of federal and state guidelines regarding care and management of such infants, (4) reviewing retrospectively case management and any deviations from federal and state guidelines as they exist, and (5) developing any policy statements for the institution as they are appropriate or necessary. Typically, anyone involved in a particular case may request a consultation from the IBC. The legal responsibility of all participants in case management and decision-making, including ethics committee members, is consistent with that of any surrogate.

"Baby Doe" Regulations

The 1985 amendments to the Child Abuse Prevention and Treatment Act of 1978 (which had been amended in 1984), more commonly known as the "Baby Doe" guidelines,[1] consider medical neglect a form of child abuse. To invoke these regulations may mean to bring allegations of child abuse or neglect against the parents (or health care team)

who would, purportedly, be denying appropriate care for an infant.

The guidelines state that "it is ethically and legally justified to withhold medical or surgical procedures which are clearly futile and will only prolong the act of dying.[1] They also require that everything reasonable be done to protect the disabled infant's life. There are three exceptions to the requirement that treatment, other than "appropriate nutrition, hydration and medication,"[1] must be provided to disabled infants. Exceptions, as determined by medical judgment, are as follows[1]:

- The infant is irreversibly comatose.
- The provision of such treatment would merely prolong dying and would be futile in terms of the infant's survival.
- The provision of such treatment would be virtually futile in terms of the infant's survival, and the treatment itself would be inhumane.

Federal guidelines deliberately specify that "quality of life" may not be considered in determining an exception.

In modern practice, until an accurate diagnosis and prognosis are determined, liveborn infants who might survive are resuscitated. In most instances it is deemed better to "err on the side of life" until appropriate evaluation is completed. If the infant can be stabilized, further decisions based on "reasonable medical judgment" are made. Ethically, legally, and practically speaking, treatment begun can be withdrawn.

Treatment should be attempted if it is clearly beneficial, possibly beneficial with minimal burden to the infant, or remotely beneficial but prognosis is fatal without it and it is in accordance with the parents' wishes. Treatment may be foregone if the infant is permanently comatose, treatment is clearly futile, or treatment is virtually futile and is unacceptably burdensome for the infant.

Perhaps most important, these guidelines advise hospitals to establish IBCs to offer counsel in those cases involving disabled infants with life-threatening conditions. In hospitals with NICUs or annual births of 1500 or more, over 50% have IBCs.[26] If, after consultation with an IBC, treatment dispute persists, the state child protection professionals may need to be consulted. They may, if necessary, obtain temporary guardianship to seek court-ordered treatment of a disabled infant to ensure that the infant receives what the court determines to be humane and ethical treatment of that child.

These guidelines have been in effect since 1985, but they have not been unanimously well received. Their intent is to protect handicapped newborns from medical neglect; their frequent effect is overtreatment of critically ill newborns. Kopelman[25] reports that many physicians changed their management of critically ill newborns (even against their own judgment) because they believed the regulations compelled them to do so. A fair number of other physicians were not sure what was required by the law. And, perhaps most significant, 56% of physicians agreed with the statement, "Most critically ill infants are overtreated when the chances for their survival are very poor."[32] Barnett[12] notes that the government really cannot dictate clinical decisions. We certainly share the belief that "ethically and medically, decisions to provide or withhold treatment are better made by loving parents based on physician advice from case-specific facts than by politicians and bureaucrats based on ideology and generalities."[12]

Social Ethics

Moral judgments made in the hospital setting do not occur in isolation from the larger social context of which institutions and individuals are a part. Such judgments can be considerably affected by prevailing social values and perspectives. Further, while decisions in the nursery generally are interpersonal in nature, they may also have a significant effect on the larger community. Technologic advancements have enabled some severely disabled infants to survive and grow, albeit with mental and physical handicaps. Indeed, these are not the majority of newborns, but they often require numerous hospitalizations and costly rehabilitation. Society frequently bears the financial, physical, and social costs of these individuals.

Social ethics reflects on the sociocultural aspects of human life. It considers how individuals as moral agents are accountable for their behavior in social structures and public policy issues. It can also refer to shared patterns of moral judgment. Moreover, it focuses on how social contexts influence individual moral behavior and the range of moral responsibility.

In a pluralistic society such as ours, there is no one social ethic. Some believe in rugged individualism, others in equality of opportunity, worth, and treatment; others believe that we bear mutual responsibility for one another. An underlying concern of most socioethical systems is concern for both the individual and the common good.

In NICUs, bioethics and social ethics converge. Treatment decisions have social implications; societal values influence treatment decisions. As described, government regulations highlight the paradox of societal values regarding the treatment of disabled infants. These federal guidelines advocate the use of "reasonable medical judgment" in treating disabled infants, yet their effect has been to increase the obligation to treat to the point of "unreasonable." Through government, society expresses the determination to treat; yet, societal commitment to long-term care of these patients and families is wholly insufficient. Public funds for such care have been reduced, while urgency for treatment of these infants has increased. The values inherent in our public policy decisions regarding initial and long-term treatment are curiously disparate.

After comparing the health care and social policies of the United States with the seemingly more equitable policies of Great Britain and Sweden, Young[63] concludes, "We need to strive for a better balance between aggressive treatment in the neonatal intensive care units initially, and the resources currently allocated for the long-term care of the disabled." Such a balance might include being more selective about aggressive treatment, as well as learning more about prematurity and trying to prevent it. "To the extent that society fails to ensure that seriously ill newborns have the opportunity for an adequate level of continuing care, its moral authority, to intervene on behalf of a newborn whose life is in jeopardy, is compromised."[63]

Recognizing this disparity, various community groups (such as the Colorado Collective for Medical Decision Making)[18] are establishing guidelines for standards of care that are fiscally, morally, and medically responsible in order to guide parents and clinicians in goal setting and decision making. They recognize the high cost, in every respect, of neonatal and pediatric intensive care. Their impetus has largely been to determine community "agreed upon" values for treatment and nontreatment of disabled infants in order to effect a standard of care for the extreme premature, severely disabled, and critically ill infant. Managed care organizations are also assessing the ethics of reasonable care and the limits of care to be offered. These community and professional groups offer an important social voice to the complexity of neonatal care.

Psychologic Effect of Ethical Decision Making

The psychologic effect of ethical decision making must not be neglected or negated, because in any given clinical situation human life is at stake. Philosophical constructs, when applied, must take into consideration human realities and capacities to tolerate and integrate the awesome responsibilities concerning life and death issues. What parents would not be distraught over the premature birth of their infant? Overwhelmed by their severely disabled infant? The prospect of lifetime rehabilitation? The reality or prospect of suffering? The prospect of death of their newborn?

Parents play a vital role in the decision-making process because they, along with the infant, are the most affected. No matter what their religious or sociocultural background, almost all parents experience shock and grief over their child's need for intensive care. They deal with this in better and worse ways. For many parents the ability to participate in ethical decision making is impaired while they are in such an acute stage of shock. Usually, prenatal diagnosis of anomalies gives parents time to adjust to their child's condition before birth and/or before decisions have to be made. This adjustment time can be most valuable. To participate in ethical decision making, particularly decisions about withholding or withdrawing treatment, parents must have achieved some degree of emotional reorganization and acceptance. Staff assistance in helping them move from emotional disorganization to reorganization is crucial to

further decisions that need to be made. At this point, parents may be better able to absorb medical data, ethical values, and principles. While there may not be a theoretical difference between withholding and withdrawing treatment, there is a large emotional difference. The sound clinician, as well as the ethicist, must be sensitive to both.

The stage of the parents in their grief and adaptation will affect their decision-making capacities. For instance, a mother's desire to treat even the most severely disabled child may evidence her denial (or misunderstanding) of her child's condition rather than a sanctity-of-life ethic. The already grief-stricken parents are faced with an overlay of agonizing decisions about letting their child die.

Choices about treatment and nontreatment do affect the grieving process. Questions such as "Am I just prolonging suffering by keeping her alive?" are countered by, "Am I not giving her a chance and playing God by allowing her to die?" Duff and Campbell[9] report families experiencing "a normal mourning for their losses" after allowing their seriously ill infants to die. What remains for many parents are doubts that their choice was correct. For some, decisions based on certain religious principles or other value criteria offer moral justification of behavior that assists in the mourning process. For others, the justification may be logically, but not emotionally, clear. In these instances, grieving can become more complex and difficult.

A valuable role of an IBC may be to offer input into, if not confirmation of, the parents' decision in a way that helps to allay guilt that can interrupt normal grieving. Ethics, while at once highly theoretical and intellectual, must consider that the situations with which it most intimately deals are highly emotional. For parents the psychologic trauma will affect their ethical considerations, and ethical decisions will have further psychologic effect.

A real value of an interdisciplinary health care team is the particular attention paid to the many complex aspects of a patient's living and dying. When parents are facing the death of their child, the entire team may be involved in assisting them. Nurses and physicians, social workers, clergy, and psychologists may all be intimately involved with monitoring the patient's comfort level and deteriorating course and with comforting grieving parents.

Baptisms (when appropriate) and, especially, funerals are important ritualistic ways of organizing the meaning of the traumatic event. The entire staff should encourage parents to offer all that they can to their dying child. They should provide maximum comfort for the patient and maximum support to the family. Helping patients and families cope with death is a privilege. It can be personally and professionally satisfying, and ultimately immeasurably helpful to everyone involved, to enter emotionally into this process. Often, care of the living means care of the dying.

Psychologic trauma and effect should also be recognized among the health care team, because their concern and involvement with the infant are usually significant. Helping someone through the dying process can be a traumatic, though rewarding, experience. In such instances professionals may agree with the decision (preferably the parents') to withhold or withdraw treatment. Professionals may also disagree with the decision but may place a higher value on the parents' autonomy to decide than on the decision itself. Respecting this,

they may abide by the parents' wishes for their child. No one should be forced to compromise personal or professional integrity, however, and in such cases where one's ethical integrity is being violated, the case may be transferred. Preferably, professionals can learn about the range of ethically defensible options and can support the parents in choices different from their own.

Effect of New Technologies

There are a number of technologies and ideologies in reproductive medicine, perinatology, and neonatology that are currently in use, under study, or being developed that may pose questions of ethical import. The issues in Box 30-2 are offered in an effort to raise the level of awareness among health care providers and to stimulate inquiry into the moral and ethical appropriateness of these advances and their consequences for individuals and our society. Should parents be told of these advances? Should parents be offered these advances regard-

---

Box 30-2
Ethical Implications of New Technologies

Liquid Ventilation
Which infants should receive liquid ventilation?
Which institutions should provide these experimental therapies?

Anencephalic Infants as Transplantation Donors
Are such infants brain dead? Born dying?
Should the definition of brain death be changed for these infants?
Are such infants "persons?" If personhood is denied, what does this say about the value of the pregnancy (or subsequent pregnancies)?
Does such an infant have any "rights" to health care for its brief life?
Is prolonging such an infant's life or arranging for transplantation simply "using" the infant, leading us to do what ordinarily would not be done in order to attain a "justifiable" end?
What abusive potentials exist for such a practice?

Managed Care
How should the patients best interest be balanced with that of the managed care organization?
Who manages technology/dependent children?
Who determines the overall goals for care of the neonate?

less of their experimental nature? Because we have these new technologies and methodologies, are we obligated to use them?

We can attempt to answer these and countless other questions by understanding what ethical issues they raise and by looking at what individual as well as social values are at stake. In doing so, we can apply the ethical workup in an effort to come up with rationally defensible solutions to these continually vexing issues.

The history of neonatal care has been, and continues to be, one of rapid technologic development, imposing new confrontations in values. We believe that professional development of ethical as well as clinical skills will help to meet these ongoing challenges.

Glossary

Best Interest A standard used to determine the validity of proxy consent in decision making. Treatment decisions are based on what most "reasonable persons" would assess as the burdens and benefits that would likely accompany the child's life. This standard leads clinicians to seek treatment resulting in a "net benefit" to the child.

Deontology (formalism) A theory of ethics that holds that the moral rightness of an act must be decided totally independent of the consequences of that act. Duty is independent of consequential good, and certain moral commands (rules) operative under fundamental principles must be obeyed under all circumstances.

Dilemma A situation that exists when more than one possible course of action exists and differing values are held of each possible course of action by the parties involved. Moral dilemmas arise when an appeal to moral considerations can be made for opposing courses of action; when it is apparent that an act can be considered both morally right *and* morally wrong, and that on moral grounds there is a sense of "ought" *and* "ought not" to perform the act.

Double Effect A principle, often viewed within the larger context of nonmaleficence, that claims that an act having a harmful effect is not always morally prohibited. Any harmful effect of an act is viewed as indirect, unintended, or simply a foreseen effect but not as the direct and intended effect (e.g., if an act, as in treatment, brings about death, it is not always to be prohibited). Four

conditions are often given to clarify this principle for specific acts:
- The action itself must be "good" or at least morally indifferent.
- The agent must intend only the good effect and not the evil effect.
- The evil effect cannot be a means to the good effect.
- There should be a favorable balance between the good and evil effects of the action.

Ethics The study of moral conduct, systems, and ideas.

Futility The notion that the efficacy of treatment is very low. There is no ethical obligation to offer futile treatment. Futility may best be judged by the overall medical benefit, not just effect, that a given treatment has on a patient. Treatment is futile if it is useless. Physiologic, psychologic, religious, and social data should be considered in making a determination of futility. Determination of futility should be based on medical benefit in consort with family goals for the patient.

Moral Rules Rules that are founded or justified by principles and state that actions of a certain kind ought (or ought not) to be done because they are right (or wrong).

Morals The conduct and codes of conduct of individuals and groups. Three popular uses exist: (1) in contrast to immoral (right versus wrong), (2) in contrast to nonmoral (actions that have no bearing or question of right and wrong), and (3) "morals" (the behavior pattern of an individual or group).

Continued

Glossary—cont'd

Morals The conduct and codes of conduct of individuals and groups. Three popular uses exist: (1) in contrast to immoral (right versus wrong), (2) in contrast to nonmoral (actions that have no bearing or question of right and wrong), and (3) "morals" (the behavior pattern of an individual or group).

Paternalism The principle and practice of ruling like a "father." This typically presupposes benevolence and making decisions for others—overriding of a person's wishes or actions (autonomy) for beneficent reasons.

Personhood A characteristic that may be used in decision making that is based on the idea that possession of certain capabilities (typically higher brain functions such as consciousness, rationality, perception of space and time, and the ability to communicate) constitute personhood; and that only "persons" have any moral claim to life, treatment, etc.

Prima Facie A term that qualifies a "right," "wrong," "duty," or "obligation," indicating a first appearance or self-evident/apparent condition of facts. Prima facie duties, for example, are those that are binding in all circumstances except when they are in conflict with equal or stronger duties.

"Proxy" Decision Maker (surrogate) A designated person who will act on behalf of an individual who is incapable of making decisions.

Reasonable Person Standard A standard by which the validity of informed consent is measured. Information to be disclosed is determined by referring to a hypothetical "reasonable person" and determining whether such a person would see any significance in the information in assessing risk and deciding whether to submit to a treatment or procedure.

Rights Those things to which people have a just claim; a claim to a condition to which the individual is entitled.

Substituted Judgment A standard used to determine the validity of proxy consent in decision making. Treatment decisions are based on what has been determined to be that choice an incompetent person would make in a given situation if that person were actually competent. This standard attempts to uphold patient autonomy even in the incompetent.

Utilitarianism (consequentialism) A theory in ethics that holds that an act is right when it brings about a good outcome for the greatest number of people, upholds the greatest balance of "good" over "evil," and seeks to effect "utility" or the most useful outcome. "The end justifies the means." This may be developed into rules that are adhered to in order to maximize benefits and minimize harms (rule utilitarian) or simply appealed to in individual actions (act utilitarian).

Values Those things that have worth or are desirable to an individual or group.

Virtues A habit, disposition, or trait that a person may possess or aspire to possess; specifically, a moral virtue upholds what is morally right or praiseworthy.

Wrongful Birth A legal action (a tort suit) sought by the parents of a handicapped child in which the claim is made that such handicaps are the result of the defendant's negligence.

Wrongful Life A legal action (typically a tort suit) sought by a handicapped child in which the claim is made that birth (and the ensuing life) resulted from the defendant's negligence.

References

1. Amendments to the Child Abuse Prevention and Treatment Act, 98 Stat 1749, 1984, 45 CFR PART 1340, April 15, 1985.
2. American Academy of Pediatrics: Components of the American Academy of Pediatrics on proposed rule regarding nondiscrimination on the basis of handicap relating to health care for handicapped infants. Undated manuscript.
3. AAP Committee of Fetus and Newborn: The initiation or withdrawal of treatment for high-risk newborns, *Pediatrics* 96:362, 1995.
4. AAP Committee on Fetus and Newborn: Perinatal care at the threshold of viability, *Pediatrics* 96:974, 1995.
5. AAP Committee on Bioethics: Ethics and the care of critically ill infants and children, *Pediatrics* 98:149, 1995.
6. American College of Obstetricians and Gynecologists Committee on ethics: Patient choice: maternal-fetal conflict, ACOG committee opinion 55, 1987.
7. American Hospital Association: *Report of the Special Committee on Biomedical Ethics: values in conflict: resolving ethical issues in hospital care,* Chicago, 1985, American Hospital Publishing.

8. AMA Council on Ethical and Judicial Affairs: The use of anencephalic neonates as organ donors, *JAMA* 273:1614, 1995.

9. Anand KJS, Hickey PR: Pain and its effects in the human neonate and fetus, *N Engl J Med* 317:1321, 1987.

10. Angell M: The Baby Doe rules, *N Engl J Med* 314:642, 1986 (editorial).

11. Arras JD: Toward an ethic of ambiguity, *Hastings Cent Rep* 14:25, 1984.

12. Barnett TJ, Baby Doe: nothing to fear but fear itself, *J Perinatol* 10:307, 1990.

13. Beauchamp T, Childress J: *Principles of biomedical ethics,* ed 2, New York, 1983, Oxford University Press.

14. Beauchamp T. McCulloch L. *Medical ethics: the moral responsibility of physicians,* Englewood Cliffs, NJ, 1984, Prentice-Hall.

15. Brody H: *Ethical decisions in medicine,* Boston, 1981, Little, Brown.

16. Canadian Pediatric Society and Society of Obstetricians and Gynecologists of Canada: Management of the woman with threatened birth of an infant with extremely low gestational age, *Can Med Assoc J* 155:547, 1994.

17. Caplan AL, Murray TH, editors: *Which babies shall live? Humanistic dimensions of the care of imperiled newborns,* Clifton, NJ, 1985, Humana Press.

18. Colorado Collective for Medical Decision Making (CCMD) in Denver, Colorado.

19. Duff R, Campbell AGM: Moral and ethical dilemmas in the special care nursery, *N Engl J Med* 289:890, 1973.

20. Eisenberg L: The human nature of human nature, *Science* 176:123, 1972.

21. Elisando A: Nurse participation in ethical decision making in the neonatal intensive care unit, *Neonat Net* 10:55, 1991.

22. Engelhardt HT Jr: Viability and use of the fetus. In Bondeson WB et al, editors. *Abortion and the status of the fetus,* Dordrecht, Netherlands, 1983, D Reidel Publishing.

23. Engelhardt HT Jr: Ethical issues in aiding the death of young children. In Mappes TA, Zembaty JS, editors: *Biomedical ethics,* ed 2, New York, 1986, McGraw-Hill.

24. Engelhardt HT Jr: *The foundations of bioethics,* New York, 1986, Oxford University Press.

25. Fleischman A, Murray T: Ethics committees for infants Doe? *Hastings Cent Rep* 13:5, 1983.

26. Fleming GV et al: Infant care review committees: the response to federal guidelines, *Am J Dis Child* 144:778, 1990.

27. Fletcher J: *Humanhood: essays in biomedical ethics,* Buffalo, New York, 1979, Prometheus Books.

28. Francoeur RT: From then to now. In Harris CC, Snowden F, editors: *Bioethical frontiers in perinatal intensive care,* Natchitoches, La, 1985, Northwestern State University Press.

29. Guillemin J, Holstrom L: Legal cases, government regulations and clinical realities in newborn intensive care, *Am J Perinatol* 1 (1):89, 1983.

30. Harrison H: The principles for family-centered neonatal care, *Pediatrics* 92:643, 1993.

31. Koops BL, Morgan LJ, Battaglia FC: Neonatal mortality risk in relation to birth weight and gestational age: update, *J Pediatr* 101:969, 1982.

32. Kopelman LM, Irons TG, Kopelman AE: Neonatologists judge the Baby Doe regulations, *N Engl J Med* 318:677, 1988.

33. Kuhse H, Singer P: *Should the baby live?* New York, 1985, Oxford University Press.

34. Lantos J et al: The illusion of futility in clinical practice, *Am J Med* 87:81, 1989.

35. Leiken S: Children's hospital ethics committees, *Am J Dis Child* 141:954, 1987.

36. Lorber J: Results of treatment of myelomeningocele, *Dev Med Child Neurol* 13:279, 1971.

37. Lorber J: Early results of selective treatment of spina bifida cystica, *Br Med J* 4:201, 1973.

38. Lyon J: *Playing god in the nursery,* New York, 1985, WW Norton.

39. Mappes E, Kroeger J: Ethical dilemmas for nurses: physician's orders versus patient's rights. In Mappes TA, Zembaty JS, editors: *Biomedical ethics,* ed 2, New York, 1986, McGraw-Hill.

40. Mitchell C: Care of severely impaired infant raises ethical issues, *Am Nurse* 16:9, 1984.

41. *Neonatal intensive care for low birth weight infants: costs and effectiveness,* December 1987, Health Technology Case Study 38, Congress of the United States, Office of Technology Assessment, Washington, DC, US Government Printing Office.

42. Pellegrino ED: The anatomy of clinical ethical judgments in perinatology, *Semin Perinatol* 11:202, 1987.

43. Pellegrino ED, Thomasma DC: *A philosophical basis of medical practice: toward a philosophical ethic of healing professions,* New York, 1981, Oxford University Press.

44. Pemberton PJ: The tiniest babies—can we afford them? *Med J Aust* 146:63, 1987.

45. Pless JE: The story of Baby Doe, *N Engl J Med* 309:663, 1983.

46. President's Commission for the Study of Ethical Problems in Medicine and Biomedical and Behavioral Research: *Deciding to forego life-sustaining treatment,* Washington, DC, 1983.

47. Raines D: Parents' values: a missing link in the neonatal intensive care equation, *Neonat Net* 15 (3):12, 1996.

48. Raines D: Deciding what to do when the patient can't speak, *Neonat Net* 12 (6):43, 1993.

49. Ramsey P: *Ethics at the edges of life,* New Haven, Conn, 1978, Yale University Press.

50. Rhoden NK: Treating Baby Doe: the ethics of uncertainty, *Hastings Cent Rep* 16:34, 1986

51. Robertson JA: Involuntary euthanasia of defective newborns. In Mappes TA, Zembaty JS, editors: *Biomedical ethics,* ed 2, New York, 1986, McGraw-Hill.

52. Schneiderman LJ, Jecker NS, Jonsen AR: Medical futility: its meaning and ethical implications, *Ann Intern Med* 112:949, 1990.

53. Shelp EE: *Born to die? Deciding the fate of critically ill newborns,* New York, 1986, The Free Press.

54. Shurtleff D: Care of the myelodysplastic patient. In Green M, Haggerty R, editors: *Ambulatory pediatrics,* Philadelphia, 1986, WB Saunders.

55. Siegler M: Ethics committees: decisions by bureaucracy, *Hastings Cent Rep* 16:22, 1986.

56. Thomasma DC: Training in medical ethics: an ethical workup, *Forum Med* 33, 1978.

57. Tooley M: *Abortion and infanticide,* New York, 1983, Oxford University Press.

58. Vaux KL: Ethical issues in caring for tiny infants, *Clin Perinatol* 13:477, 1986.

59. Victoroff M: The ballad of Baby Doe: parental discretion or medical neglect? *Prim Care* 13:271, 1986.

60. Weil WB: Issues associated with treatment and non-treatment decisions, *Am J Dis Child* 138:519, 1984.

61. Weir RF: *Selective nontreatment of handicapped newborns,* New York, 1984, Oxford University Press.

62. Wolf S: Ethics committees in the courts, *Hastings Cent Rep* 16:9, 1986.

63. Young EWD: Caring for disabled infants, *Hastings Cent Rep* 13:15, 1983.

64. Zachary R. Ethical and social aspects of treatment of spina bifida, *Lancet* 2.274, 1968.

Index